Acute Care Surgery

Acute Care Surgery

Principles and Practice

Editor-in-Chief

L.D. Britt, MD, MPH
Brickhouse Professor of Surgery and Chairman
Department of Surgery
Eastern Virginia Medical School
Norfolk, Virginia

Editors

Donald D. Trunkey, MD
Professor
Department of Surgery
Oregon Health Sciences University
Portland, Oregon

David V. Feliciano, MD
Professor of Surgery, Emory University School of Medicine
Chief of Surgery, Grady Memorial Hospital
Atlanta, Georgia

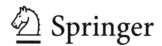 Springer

Editor-in-Chief:
L.D. Britt, MD, MPH
Brickhouse Professor of Surgery and Chairman
Department of Surgery
Eastern Virginia Medical School
Norfolk, VA, USA

Editors:
Donald D. Trunkey, MD
Professor
Department of Surgery
Oregon Health Sciences University
Portland, OR, USA

David V. Feliciano, MD
Professor of Surgery
Emory University School of Medicine
Chief of Surgery
Grady Memorial Hospital
Atlanta, GA, USA

Library of Congress Control Number: 2006925630

ISBN: 10: 0-387-34470-5   e-ISBN-10: 0-387-69012-3
ISBN: 13: 978-0-387-34470-6   e-ISBN-13: 978-0-387-69012-4

Printed on acid-free paper.

9 8 7 6 5 4 3 2 1

springer.com

Preface

The genesis of this project is a direct result of the fact that there is no substantive textbook that addresses the full-spectrum of surgical emergencies. Even in a field in which there is a plethora of excellent textbooks on a variety of surgical topics (including trauma), there is no one reference book with a dedicated emphasis on both traumatic and nontraumatic conditions potentially necessitating surgical intervention in the acute setting. This project became even more unique when its stepwise development paralleled the evolution of a new specialty–acute care surgery. This was far from a serendipitous link. On the contrary, my editorial colleagues and I, along with many of the contributors, have recently been part of a major effort to build the foundation for this new specialty. As with any proposed new specialty, there have been a few rough interfaces with some of the other surgical specialties regarding the scope of practice of the acute care surgeon. Fortunately, the key to this conflict resolution will revolve around what is best for the patient. However, irrespective of these dynamics, there is a worsening crisis in acute care in this nation.

The anatomy of the textbook has five parts: Each chapter in the first two parts is preceded by a case scenario and multiple choice questions. At the end of each chapter in Part I (General Principles) and Part II (Principles and Practice of Acute Care Surgery: Organ-Based Approach), there is a critique for the case scenario and the associated answer. This format is designed to have the reader focus on a specific clinical management or system-based problem prior to reading the chapter. An entire section (Part III) is dedicated to administration, ethics, and law as it relates to issues and situations in the acute surgical setting. Another important feature of the book is the emphasis on system development (Part IV). Similar to the current trauma systems throughout the nation, there should be a more comprehensive network to facilitate optimal management of all surgical emergencies. These issues are addressed. Also, in the same section, there is a proposed training curriculum for Acute Care Surgery along with a model of an existing emergency surgical service that could serve as a foundation for the development of a more broad-based specialty. How our international colleagues are addressing emergency surgical needs is highlighted in the final section (Part V). Experts from three different continents provide focused insight into the intricacies of their respective systems with respect to acute care surgery.

In summary, this inaugural edition of this textbook is designed to be a comprehensive and definitive reference of the full spectrum of Acute Care Surgery. With contributions from the top experts throughout the world, I do feel this goal has been accomplished.

L.D. Britt, MD, MPH
Editor-in-Chief

A Tribute

This textbook is dedicated to one of the true giants in American surgery. He was a contributor to and a major inspiration for this project. If Dr. Claude Organ were to be described in one statement, it would be the following: "He was a monument to excellence." With talents that transcended medicine, he was often highlighted as a legitimate renaissance man. Whatever he engaged in, Dr. Organ made better. It could be argued that the popular label "Midas touch" is more applicable to the life and times of Dr. Organ, for he was highly successful in all the arenas he entered. He consistently downplayed the litany of awards and accolades he accumulated

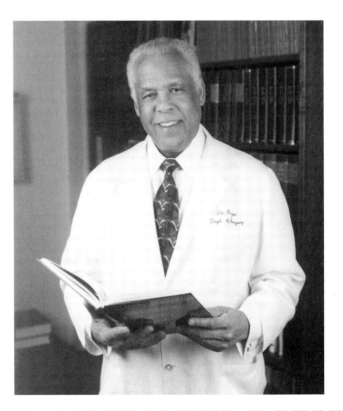

Claude H. Organ, Jr., MD, MS (Surg), FACS, FRCSSA, FRACS, FRCS, FRCSEd
Professor Emeritus, Department of Surgery
University of California San Francisco-East Bay
Oakland, California
(Deceased)

throughout his illustrious career, including being elected Chairman of the American Board of Surgery, President of the American College of Surgeons, and Editor-in-Chief of the Archives of Surgery. He was the recipient of the highest award given by the American College of Surgeons: The Distinguished Service Award. Dr. Organ, the author of more than 250 scientific journal articles and book chapters, was an invited lecturer and visiting professor at many of the great institutions throughout the world.

This tribute provides only a glimpse of the impact that Dr. Organ had over his 78 year lifespan. Merely highlighting his professional career inadequately covers the full spectrum of his legacy, for the "big picture" view of Dr. Organ also includes that man who portrayed the consummate husband, father, grandfather, friend, colleague, and mentor. Perhaps his crowning achievement is his tremendously accomplished family. Even with this recognition, Dr. Organ would be quick to give the credit for the success of his seven children to his equally talented wife, Elizabeth (Betty). He stated on numerous occasions that his wife was the chief architect of the social and professional development of their children. Each child has become a prominent professional in various fields, including medicine, banking, art, and education. An argument could be made that this is one of the most successful American families – essentially, a guarantee that the Organ legacy will continue.

I am one of the many who was mentored by Dr. Organ and who profited from his endless wisdom and guidance. In fact, his last advice to me just prior to his untimely death was a firm charge to me to find a way to accelerate the completion and production of this textbook so that it would match the timing of the unveiling of the new specialty – Acute Care Surgery. With Dr. Organ being such a driving force in the first phase of the development of this project, my editorial colleagues and I can think of no one more deserving of this tribute.

L.D. Britt, MD, MPH
Editor-in-Chief

Contents

Part I   General Principles

Contributors

Herand Abcarian, MD
Department of Surgery, University of Illinois at Chicago, University of Illinois at Chicago Medial Center, Chicago, IL, USA

Michel B. Aboutanos, MD, MPH
Division of Trauma, Critical Care, and Emergency Surgery, Virginia Commonwealth University Medical Center, Medical College of Virginia Hospitals and Physicians, Richmond, VA, USA

Jeffrey E. Abrams, MD
Department of Surgery, University of North Carolina, Chapel Hill, NC, USA

Murat Akyol, MD
University Department of Surgery and The Transplant Unit, The Royal Infirmary of Edinburgh, Edinburgh, Scotland, UK

Louis H. Alarcon, MD
Departments of Critical Care Medicine and Surgery, University of Pittsburgh School of Medicine, Pittsburgh, PA, USA

Nejd F. Alsikafi, MD
Department of Urology, University of Chicago, Mount Sinai Hospital, Chicago, IL, USA

Juan A. Asensio, MD
Department of Surgery/Division of Trauma, University of Medicine and Dentistry of New Jersey at Newark, Newark, NJ, USA

Christopher Aylwin, BSc, MBBS, MRCS
Department of General Surgery, Trauma Service, Royal London Hospital, London, England, UK

Philip S. Barie, MD, MBA
Departments of Surgery and Public Health, Weill Medical College of Cornell University, New York, NY, USA

Michael J. Bosse, MD
Department of Orthopaedic Surgery, Carolinas Medical Center, Charlotte, NC, USA

Thomas L. Bosshardt, MD
Department of Surgery, Marian Medical Center, Santa Maria, CA, USA

L.D. Britt, MD, MPH
Department of Surgery, Eastern Virginia Medical School, Norfolk, VA, USA

Bruce D. Browner, MD
Department of Orthopaedic Surgery, University of Connecticut Health Sciences Center, Farmington CT, USA; Department of Orthopaedics, Hartford Hospital, Hartford, CT, USA

Timothy G. Buchman, PhD, MD
Departments of Surgery, Anesthesiology, and Medicine, Washington University School of Medicine, St. Louis, MO, USA

Karyl J. Burns, RN, PhD
Department of Traumatology, Hartford Hospital/University of Connecticut, Hartford, CT, USA

David J. Ciesla, MD
Departments of Surgery and Trauma, University of Colorado Health Sciences Center, Denver Health Medical Center, Denver, CO, USA

Jeffrey A. Claridge, MD
Department of Surgery, MetroHealth Medical Center, Case Western Reserve University School of Medicine, Cleveland, OH, USA

Frederic J. Cole, Jr., MD
Department of Surgery, Eastern Virginia Medical School, Sentara Norfolk General Hospital, Norfolk, VA, USA

Jay N. Collins, MD
Department of Surgery, Eastern Virginia Medical School, Sentara Norfolk General Hospital, Norfolk, VA, USA

Craig M. Coopersmith, MD
Departments of Surgery and Anesthesiology, Washington University School of Medicine, St. Louis, MO, USA

Edward E. Cornwell III, MD
Department of Surgery, Johns Hopkins School of Medicine, Johns Hopkins Hospital, Baltimore, MD, USA

Martin A. Croce, MD
Department of Surgery, Regional Medical Center at Memphis, University of Tennessee, Presley Memorial Trauma Center, Memphis, TN, USA

Peter F. Crookes, MD
Department of Surgery, University of Southern California, Los Angeles, CA, USA

Edwin A. Deitch, MD
Department of Surgery, University of Medicine and Dentistry of New Jersey—New Jersey Medical School, University of Medicine and Dentistry of New Jersey—University Hospital, Newark, NJ, USA

Demetrios Demetriades, MD, PhD
Department of Surgery, Division of Trauma and Surgical Critical Care, University of Southern California, Los Angeles, CA, USA

José J. Diaz, Jr., MD, CNS
Department of Surgery, Division of Trauma and Surgical Critical Care, Vanderbilt University Medical Center, Vanderbilt University Hospital, Nashville, TN, USA

Philip E. Donahue, MD
Department of Surgery, University of Illinois at Chicago, John H. Stroger Hospital of Cook County, Chicago, IL, USA

Thérèse M. Duane, MD
Division of Trauma, Critical Care, and Emergency Surgery, Virginia Commonwealth University Medical Center, Medical College of Virginia Hospitals and Physicians, Richmond, VA, USA

Richard P. Dutton, MD, MBA
Division of Trauma Anesthesiology, R. Adams Cowley Shock Trauma Center, University of Maryland Medical System, Baltimore, MD, USA

Soumitra R. Eachempati, MD
Department of Surgery, Weill Medical College of Cornell University/New York Presbyterian Hospital, New York, NY, USA

A. Brent Eastman, MD
Department of Trauma, Scripps Memorial Hospital La Jolla, La Jolla, CA, USA

Sean P. Elliott, MD
Department of Urology, University of California San Francisco, San Francisco General Hospital, San Francisco, CA, USA

Peter I. Ellman, MD
Department of General Surgery, University of Virginia, University of Virginia Health Sciences Center, Charlottesville, VA, USA

Hosam F. El Sayed, MD, PhD
Department of Surgery, Division of Vascular Surgery, Eastern Virginia Medical School, Norfolk, VA, USA

Thomas J. Esposito, MD, MPH
Department of Surgery, Section of Trauma, Injury Analysis, and Prevention Programs, Loyola University Medical Center, Foster G. McGaw Hospital, Maywood, IL, USA

David V. Feliciano, MD
Department of Surgery, Emory University School of Medicine, Grady Memorial Hospital, Atlanta, GA, USA

Ilan S. Freedman, MBBS
Department of Orthopaedic Surgery, The Alfred Hospital, Melbourne, Victoria, Australia

Daniel M. Freeman, AB, JD
Einstein Institute for Science, Health, and the Courts, Chevy Chase, MD, USA

Eric R. Frykberg, MD
Department of Surgery, University of Florida College of Medicine, Shands Jacksonville Medical Center, Jacksonville, FL, USA

Richard L. Gamelli, MD
Department of Surgery, Loyola University Medical Center, Maywood, IL, USA

Maurice M. Garcia, MD
Department of Urology, University of California San Francisco, San Francisco, CA, USA

Idris Gharbaoui, MD
Department of Orthopaedics, University of Texas Health Science Center at Houston, Houston, TX, USA

Oscar D. Guillamondegui, MD
Department of Surgery, Division of Trauma and Surgical Critical Care, Vanderbilt University, Vanderbilt University Medical Center, Nashville, TN, USA

Nahid Hamoui, MD
Department of General Surgery, University of Southern California, Los Angeles, CA, USA

Gerald B. Healy, MD
Department of Otolaryngology, Harvard University, Children's Hospital, Boston, MA, USA

Spiros P. Hiotis, MD, PhD
Department of Surgery, New York University School of Medicine, New York, NY, USA

David B. Hoyt, MD
Department of Surgery, University of California San Diego Medical Center, San Diego, CA, USA

John G. Hunter, MD
Department of Surgery, Oregon Health and Science University, Portland, OR, USA

Rao R. Ivatury, MD, MS
Department of Surgery, Virginia Commonwealth University, Virginia Commonwealth University Medical Center, Richmond, VA, USA

Jondavid H. Jabush, MD
Department of Surgery, University of Medicine and Dentistry of New Jersey—New Jersey Medical School, University of Medicine and Dentistry of New Jersey—University Hospital, Newark, NJ, USA

David G. Jacobs, MD
Department of Surgery, Carolinas Medical Center, Charlotte, NC, USA

Lenworth M. Jacobs, MD, MPH
Department of Traumatology, Hartford Hospital/University of Connecticut, Hartford, CT, USA

Preeti R. John, MD, MPH
Department of Surgery, Johns Hopkins University, The Johns Hopkins Hospital, Baltimore, MD, USA

Riyad Karmy-Jones, MD
Department of Cardiothoracic Surgery, Harborview Medical Center, Seattle, WA, USA

Donald R. Kauder, MD
Department of Surgery, Division of Traumatology and Surgical Critical Care, University of Pennsylvania School of Medicine, Hospital of the University of Pennsylvania, Philadelphia, PA, USA

Patrick K. Kim, MD
Department of Surgery, Division of Traumatology and Surgical Critical Care, University of Pennsylvania School of Medicine, Hospital of the University of Pennsylvania, Philadelphia, PA, USA

M. Margaret Knudson, MD
Department of Surgery, University of California San Francisco, San Francisco General Hospital, San Francisco, CA, USA

Ira J. Kodner, MD
Department of Colon and Rectal Surgery, Washington University in St. Louis, Barnes-Jewish Hospital, St. Louis, MO, USA

Thomas Kossmann, MD
Department of Trauma Surgery, The Alfred Hospital, Melbourne, Victoria, Australia

Irving L. Kron, MD
Departments of Surgery and Thoracic and Cardiovascular Surgery, University of Virginia, University of Virginia Health Sciences Center, Charlottesville, VA, USA

Linda S. Laibstain, JD
Williams Mullen Hofheimer Nusbaum, Norfolk, VA, USA

Juliet Lee, MD
Department of Surgery, George Washington University, Washington, DC, USA

Raphael C. Lee, MD, ScD, DSc (Hon)
Departments of Surgery (Plastic), Medicine (Dermatology), Organismal Biology (Biomechanics), and Molecular Medicine, University of Chicago, Chicago, IL, USA

Peter B. Letarte, MD
Department of Neurosurgery, Hines Veterans Hospital, La Grange Park, IL, USA

Fred A. Luchette, MD
Department of Surgery, Division of Trauma, Surgical Critical Care, and Burns, Loyola University Medical Center, Foster G. McGaw Hospital, Maywood, IL, USA

Dana Christian Lynge, MD, CM
Department of Surgery, University of Washington, Seattle Veterans Affairs Medical Center, Seattle, WA, USA

Ajai K. Malhotra, MD
Division of Trauma, Critical Care, and Emergency Surgery, Virginia Commonwealth University Medical Center, Medical College of Virginia Hospitals and Physicians, Richmond, VA, USA

Kenneth L. Mattox, MD
Department of Surgery, Baylor College of Medicine, Ben Taub General Hospital, Houston, TX, USA

Tina A. Maxian, MD, PhD
Department of Orthopaedic Surgery, State University of New York Upstate Medical University, Syracuse, NY, USA

John C. Mayberry, MD
Department of Surgery, Oregon Health and Science University, Portland, OR, USA

Jack W. McAninch, MD
Department of Urology, University of California San Francisco, San Francisco, CA, USA

Norman E. McSwain, Jr., MD
Department of Surgery, Tulane University School of Medicine, Charity Hospital Trauma Center, New Orleans, LA

George H. Meier III, MD
Department of Vascular Surgery, Eastern Virginia Medical School, Norfolk, VA, USA

J. Wayne Meredith, MD
Department of Surgery, Wake Forest University School of Medicine, Winston-Salem, NC, USA

Anthony A. Meyer, MD, PhD
Department of Surgery, University of North Carolina, Chapel Hill, NC, USA

Omid Moayed, MD
Division of Trauma Anesthesiology, R. Adams Cowley Shock Trauma Center, University of Maryland Medical System, Baltimore, MD, USA

Ernest E. Moore, MD
Departments of Surgery and Trauma, University of Colorado Health Sciences Center, Denver Health Medical Center, Denver, CO, USA

John A. Morris, Jr., MD
Section of Surgical Sciences, Division of Trauma, Vanderbilt University School of Medicine, Vanderbilt University Medical Center, Nashville, TN, USA

Nicholas W. Morris, MD
Department of General Surgery, Powell Valley Health Care and Hospital, Powell, WY, USA

Ernest M. Myers, MD
Department of Surgery, Division of Otolaryngology, Head and Neck Surgery, Howard University Hospital, Washington, DC, USA

David T. Netscher, MD
Department of Surgery, Division of Plastic Surgery, Baylor College of Medicine, Veterans Affairs Medical Center, Houston, TX, USA

Robert C. Nusbaum, LLB, JD (Hon)
Williams Mullen Hofheimer Nusbaum, Norfolk, VA, USA

Claude H. Organ, Jr., MD, MS (Surg)
Deceased, Department of Surgery, University of California San Francisco-East Bay, Oakland, CA, USA

Hersh L. Pachter, MD
Department of Surgery, New York University School of Medicine, New York, NY, USA

Simon Paterson-Brown, MBBS, MPh
Department of Surgery, The Royal Infirmary Edinburgh, Edinburgh, Scotland, UK

Andrew B. Peitzman, MD
Department of Surgery, University of Pittsburgh, Pittsburgh, PA, USA

Patrizio Petrone, MD
Department of Surgery, Division of Trauma Surgery and Surgical Critical Care, Los Angeles County and The University of Southern California Medical Center, Los Angeles, CA, USA

Jeffrey L. Ponsky, MD
Department of Surgery, University Hospitals and Case Western Reserve University, Cleveland, OH, USA

Todd Ponsky, MD
Department of Pediatric Surgery, Children's National Medical Center, Washington, DC, USA

Stathis J. Poulakidas, MD
Department of Surgery, Loyola University Medical Center, Foster G. McGaw Hospital, Maywood, IL, USA

Basil A. Pruitt, Jr., MD
Department of Surgery, University of Texas Health Science Center at San Antonio, San Antonio, TX, USA

Reza Rahbar, DMD, MD
Department of Otolaryngology, Harvard Medical School, Boston Children's Hospital, Boston, MA, USA

Bernard F. Ribeiro, MB, BS
Department of Surgery, Basildon University Hospital, Basildon, England, UK

Craig M. Rodner, MD
Department of Orthopaedic Surgery, University of Connecticut Health System, Farmington, CT, USA

Michael F. Rotondo, MD
Department of Surgery, The Brody School of Medicine, East Carolina University, Greenville, NC, USA

Bobby Rupani, MD
Department of Surgery, University of Medicine and Dentistry of New Jersey—New Jersey Medical School, University of Medicine and Dentistry of New Jersey—University Hospital, Newark, NJ, USA

Thomas R. Russell, MD
American College of Surgeons, Chicago, IL, USA

Douglas J.E. Schuerer, MD
Department of Surgery, Washington University in St. Louis, St. Louis, MO, USA

C. William Schwab, MD
Department of Surgery, Division of Traumatology and Surgical Critical Care, University of Pennsylvania Medical Center, Philadelphia, PA, USA

Maheswari Senthil, MD
Department of Surgery, University of Medicine and Dentistry of New Jersey—New Jersey Medical School, University of Medicine and Dentistry of New Jersey—University Hospital, Newark, NJ, USA

Jian Shou, MD
Department of Surgery, Weill Medical College of Cornell University, New York, NY, USA

Andrew Sim, MBBS, MS
Department of Surgery and Remote and Rural Medicine, University of Highlands and Islands, Western Isles Hospital, Stornoway, Scotland, UK

Matthew S. Slater, MD
Department of Cardiothoracic Surgery, Oregon Health and Science University, Portland, OR, USA

Larisa S. Speetzen, BA
San Francisco Injury Center, University of California San Francisco, San Francisco, CA, USA

Kyoichi Takaori, MD, PhD
Department of General and Gastroenterological Surgery, Osaka Medical College, Takatsuki, Osaka, Japan

Nobuhiko Tanigawa, MD, PhD
Department of General and Gastroenterological Surgery, Osaka Medical College, Takatsuki, Osaka, Japan

Donald D. Trunkey, MD
Department of Surgery, Oregon Health and Sciences University, Portland, OR, USA

George C. Velmahos, MD, PhD, MSEd
Department of Surgery, Harvard Medical School/Massachusetts General Hospital, Boston, MA, USA

Michael Walsh, BSc, MS
Department of Vascular and Trauma Surgery, The Royal London Hospital, London, England, UK

Leonard J. Weireter, Jr., MD
Department of Surgery, Eastern Virginia Medical School, Sentara Norfolk General Hospital, Norfolk, VA, USA

Robb R. Whinney, DO
Department of Surgery, Washington University in St. Louis, St. Louis, MO, USA

Part I
General Principles

1
Initial Assessment and Early Resuscitation

Louis H. Alarcon and Andrew B. Peitzman

Case Scenario

During the initial assessment and early resuscitation phase, a multiple trauma patient (25-year-old man) is determined to be in hemorrhagic shock and has the following findings:

- Multiple abrasions (head, torso, and extremities)
- Dilated right pupil
- Precordial bruises (chest x-ray demonstrates fully expanded bilateral lungs with an endotracheal tube above the carina; a widened mediastinum; obliterated pulmonary-aortic window and aortic knob)
- Soft abdomen
- Unstable pelvic fracture (pneumatic garment is now inflated)

With a worsening hemodynamic status systolic blood pressure at 70 mm Hg and pulse, what is the top management priority for this patient (who required translaryngeal endotracheal intubation in the field because of his comatose state after an initial lucid period)?

(A) Immediate craniotomy
(B) Placement of an external pelvic fixator
(C) Repair of traumatic aortic rupture
(D) Further evaluation by computed tomography
(E) Abdominal ultrasonography

The purpose of this chapter is to describe the assessment and resuscitation of both acute care surgery and trauma patients. Although differences exist in the initial evaluation and management of these categories of patients, certain principles can be applied to all critically ill and injured patients. Both the similarities and the differences are addressed. The specifics of the subsequent management of these patients are discussed in other chapters.

During the initial encounter with a patient, determination of severity of illness, identification of life-threatening conditions, and resuscitation must occur. The Latin word *resuscitare* is the origin of the term *resuscitation* and means to reanimate or revive. Resuscitation implies restoring adequate tissue perfusion with oxygenated and nutrient-rich blood. As this chapter emphasizes, it is within the first minutes and hours of patient–physician interaction that subsequent organ dysfunction can be either aborted or allowed to progress. An essential tenet in the early management of the critically ill acute care surgery or trauma patient is immediate initiation of therapy to correct abnormal physiology, as evaluation and diagnosis proceed.

The classic approach taught to medical students in the evaluation of a new patient is to complete a detailed history and physical examination and then formulate a differential diagnosis. However, when dealing with the severely ill or injured patient, this approach is not appropriate. Recognition and treatment of life-threatening conditions may be necessary before a definitive diagnosis can be determined. This is the approach adopted by the American College of Surgeons in the Advanced Trauma Life Support (ATLS) course.[1] This organized and prioritized philosophy can be applied not only to trauma patients but also to any critically ill surgical or nonsurgical patient.

Triage

The word *triage* is derived from the French word meaning "to sort." In the context of medicine, it implies the sorting and classification of injured or ill patients according to the severity of illness and prioritization of care according to available resources. Historically, war has provided the impetus to develop and refine triage systems. The lessons learned from the triage and care of casualties of war were eventually adapted to civilian medicine.

Unique Aspects of the Trauma and Acute Care Surgical Patient

Trauma and acute care surgical patients present with acute anatomic and physiologic derangements that can be life or limb threatening. These problems often require immediate identification and treatment, making these patients very different from the patient who presents in a nonacute care setting. The early recognition that a patient is "sick" requires an astute clinician and can sometimes be made by quick examination of the patient. Aggressive and timely resuscitation efforts must be promptly initiated. It must be recognized that the patient has severe physiologic disturbances, and these need to be addressed before a definitive diagnosis can be entertained. This modus operandi, which places emphasis on physiologic stabilization rather than on exhaustive diagnostic maneuvers, is in contradistinction of the classic approach, which is to diagnose first and treat the definitive diagnosis. Thus, critical diagnostic and therapeutic decisions are made based on incomplete information.

Another aspect that makes these patients unique is that the acute nature of their illness allows little or no preoperative evaluation. Complete evaluation and optimization of cardiovascular and pulmonary status is not feasible. In addition, these patients often present with full stomachs and/or substance intoxication, which can complicate airway and anesthetic management. The patients may also have injuries that complicate airway management, such as head, cervical spine, maxillofacial, or tracheobronchial trauma. Perhaps contrary to Occam's razor,[2] trauma patients often have multiple injuries. However, these are not random and often do present in predictable constellations based on mechanism of injury.

Today, it is clear that the primary goal in the stabilization of trauma and critically ill surgical patients is correction of *physiologic* derangements. The sequential approach to patients condoned by the ATLS course can be applied to all cases of critically ill patients, acute care surgery, and trauma (Table 1.1).[1] The goals of the primary survey are to identify immediate threats to life and to stabilize the patient. These may require laparotomy or thoracotomy, control of hemorrhage or gastrointestinal contamination, and transfer to the intensive care unit for further optimization of hemodynamics and tissue perfusion. Definitive correction of *anatomic* disturbances may often need to be postponed until physiologic stabilization has occurred (e.g., the damage-control laparotomy).[3]

Systematic Evaluation and Treatment

The initial priorities in the management of all critically ill or injured patients are the same: verify the patency of the airway, ensure adequacy of breathing and ventilation, and restore circulation to vital organs. Airway, breathing, and circulation (commonly referred to as the *ABCs*) remain the basic tenets of life support. During the primary survey of the patient, life-threatening conditions are identified and treated immediately in this orderly fashion. This is an essential principle of the ATLS algorithm.[1] In the first few seconds of the patient encounter, the gravity of the patient's condition can be quickly ascertained; this brief assessment will dictate the tempo and aggressiveness of the resuscitation efforts. Patients should be categorized according to hemodynamic status: *agonal*, *unstable*, or *hemodynamically normal*. Terms such as *hemodynamic stability* should be avoided. While this phrase attempts to convey hemodynamic normalcy over time, it is more appropriate to accurately describe the patient's condition and its variability over the period of observation.

The patient who is *unstable hemodynamically* is hypotensive, tachycardic, or both. This represents physiologic decompensation and should be recognized as such and corrected expeditiously. The agonal patient is clearly profoundly ill with obvious clinical signs of shock. Such patients will not tolerate inadequate treatment. Time wasted on simply diagnostic procedures will increase the likelihood of a poor outcome for such patients. All maneuvers must be potentially therapeutic. For example, if the agonal patient may have a pneumothorax or hemothorax, this should be diagnosed by chest tube rather than chest radiograph, providing both diagnosis and therapy.

TABLE 1.1. Initial evaluation and management of critically ill or injured patients.

Primary survey
Airway
Breathing
Circulation
Disability
Expose the patient
Resuscitation
Secondary survey
Definitive care

Source: Data from American College of Surgeons Committee.[1]

Airway and Breathing

The airway is assessed first to ascertain patency. If the patient is able to speak clearly, the airway is not likely to be in immediate threat. However, repeated reassessment is essential. Continuous determination of arterial oxygen hemoglobin saturation via pulse oximetry serves as an adjunct to airway monitoring. However, changes in pulse oximetry temporally lag behind significant alterations in alveolar oxygenation and ventilation[4,5] and cannot be solely relied on to make this detection in a timely fashion. Supplemental oxygen should be provided via a mask.

The basic airway management strategy is to relieve the airway of obstruction. In unconscious patients, the most common cause of airway obstruction is the tongue, which moves posteriorly against the pharyngeal wall. A Glasgow Coma Scale (GCS) of 8 or less strongly suggests the need for a definitive airway immediately. Other causes of glottic obstruction are secretions, blood, vomitus, teeth, and or foreign materials. Edema of laryngeal structures may also lead to airway obstruction, as is seen with anaphylaxis, thermal injury, smoke inhalation, or epiglottitis. Facial, mandibular, or tracheolaryngeal fractures may also compromise the airway and complicate the ability to establish a definitive airway. Partial airway obstruction is evidenced by gurgling, stridor, hoarseness, or choking. The use of accessory respiratory muscles, paradoxical respiratory effort, or gasping signifies respiratory distress due to impending airway obstruction. These patients should have definitive airway control with the placement of an endotracheal tube.

For many patients with airway obstruction, simple maneuvers may open the airway and improve the ability of the patient to ventilate. These maneuvers are designed to displace the mandible anteriorly, thus moving the tongue forward and alleviating the obstruction. The head tilt–chin thrust maneuvers may be used initially for nontrauma patients. The head tilt is performed by placing the palm of the hand on the patient's forehead and the other hand behind the neck. The head is tilted posteriorly. The chin lift is done by hooking the second and third fingers beneath the chin, and pulling the chin upward, bringing the teeth to near occlusion. These maneuvers provide significant anterior displacement of the mandible and significantly open the glottis. To reemphasize, these maneuvers are contraindicated for patients who may have blunt cervical spine injury.

The jaw thrust is another maneuver that may relieve airway obstruction, and, if performed correctly, it can be done while maintaining cervical spine immobilization. By grasping the angles of the mandible and lifting anteriorly, the mandible can be displaced anteriorly without movement of the spine. For unconscious patients, these maneuvers in combination with an oropharyngeal airway can facilitate adequate ventilation with a bag-valve-mask device until definitive airway can be established. Appropriate head positioning and a tight seal of the mask on the face are critical for the success of this procedure.

Application of cricoid pressure, the Sellick maneuver, reduces but does not eliminate the risk of gastric insufflation, with subsequent vomiting and aspiration. Definitive airway management is best accomplished with tracheal intubation. The decision to intubate is made for patients who show signs of inadequate respiration despite the basic airway maneuvers described previously or for whom these interventions alone are unlikely to sustain

TABLE 1.2. Indications for endotracheal intubation.

Absolute indications
  Airway obstruction or near obstruction (e.g., stridor)
  Apnea or near apnea
  Respiratory distress (dyspnea, tachypnea, cyanosis, hypoxemia, hypercarbia)
  Depressed level of consciousness (GCS ≤ 8)
Urgent indications
  Hypotension or cardiovascular instability
  Penetrating neck injury with airway compromise
  Chest wall injury or disturbance that impairs ventilation despite tube thoracostomy
  Risk of aspiration because of bleeding in the oropharynx or airway and vomiting
Relative indications
  Oromaxillofacial injuries
  Pulmonary contusion
  Need for diagnostic or therapeutic interventions in a patient who is at risk for deterioration
  Potential respiratory failure due to analgesic or sedative requirements

adequate respiration (Table 1.2). The most experienced operator should be designated to perform this task, as patients often will not tolerate prolonged attempts at intubation. Placement of an endotracheal tube is the best method to oxygenate and ventilate a patient, and, once secured, the tube reduces the risk of gross aspiration of gastric contents compared with bag-valve-mask ventilation.[6] The decision to secure the airway with a tracheal tube can be made by assessing a number of parameters: airway patency, adequacy of oxygenation, adequacy of ventilation, ability to protect the airway (level of consciousness), and overall severity of the patient's condition. The preferred route for definitive airway control for most patients is the orotracheal route. The nasal route should be avoided in patients with potential basilar skull or facial fractures. The surgical cricothyroidotomy is employed when the orotracheal route has failed or is deemed inappropriate because of significant midface or mandibular injuries or bleeding. Plans and preparations should always be made for this eventuality, because orotracheal intubation is not always successful.

The key to successful tracheal intubation is preparation of the patient and of the necessary equipment. Failure to position the patient appropriately or to test and prepare all necessary equipment is a frequent cause of unsuccessful intubation. For nontrauma patients, the head should be placed in the "sniffing position," which is facilitated by placing a small pillow or folded towels behind the head (not the back). This position is absolutely contraindicated for trauma patients, who must be presumed to have a cervical spine injury. The need for inline cervical stabilization for trauma patients increases the degree of difficulty in intubating these patients.

The use of pharmacologic agents during intubation of patients remains an area of debate. The risks of sedative or paralyzing agents are loss of the airway, loss of spontaneous respiratory effort, aspiration of gastric contents, and hypotension or cardiovascular collapse. For these reasons, the ATLS course does not encourage the use of these drugs. However, in skilled hands, rapid-sequence induction with a combination of an inducing agent and a short-acting paralytic agent, is a highly effective method for securing the airway.[7–9] The use of sedatives alone, without paralytic agents, may have a theoretical advantage, that is, the patient may continue to breathe spontaneously should the attempt at placing the airway prove unsuccessful. However, this theoretical advantage has not been proved. In fact, in acute care airway situations, complications were greater in number and severity for the nonparalyzed patients compared with standard rapid-sequence induction with a paralytic agent and included aspiration, airway trauma, and death.[10]

Intubation is carried out after preoxygenation and is performed under direct vision during direct laryngoscopy. Successful placement of the endotracheal tube is confirmed by visualization of the tube between the vocal cords as it is placed, detection of exhaled CO_2 using a disposable CO_2 detector, and auscultation over the epigastrium and chest.

A number of alternative techniques are available to establish a secure airway in patients who fail orotracheal intubation (such as nasotracheal intubation, laryngeal mask airway, combi-tube, bronchoscopic intubation, "blind" tactile intubation, the "lighted-stylet," needle cricothyroidotomy and jet ventilation, and retrograde airway placement). However, these methods are heavily dependent on highly trained individuals performing difficult airway techniques and may not be possible with significant blood or secretions in the airway (e.g., bronchoscopic intubation), and the instrumentation may not be available in the emergent situation. Therefore, the surgical cricothyroidotomy is the preferred backup method for acute care surgical airway treatment.[11] This is accomplished by stabilizing the thyroid cartilage with the nondominant hand while making a vertical or horizontal incision over the cricothyroid space, which is often easily palpable. If not palpable, a vertical incision in the approximate area is made and can be extended cephalad or caudally if needed. Palpation confirms the location of the cricothyroid membrane, and a transverse incision is made in this membrane. The back end of the scalpel or a hemostat clamp can be used to dilate the cricothyroidotomy, and an appropriately sized standard endotracheal tube (or tracheostomy tube if available) can be inserted and secured in place. Emergent tracheostomy is not favored because of the greater difficulty associated with this procedure when performed emergently outside of the operating room, requiring greater technical skills and therefore more prone to failure than cricothyroidotomy. However, tracheostomy may be necessary for patients

TABLE 1.3. The "deadly dozen" lethal and potentially lethal thoracic and airway injuries in trauma patients that should be detected and treated in the primary and secondary surveys.

"Lethal six"
Airway obstruction
Tension pneumothorax
Cardiac tamponade
Open pneumothorax
Massive hemothorax
Flail chest
"Hidden six"
Thoracic aorta disruption
Tracheobronchial injury
Blunt cardiac injury
Diaphragmatic injury
Esophageal injury
Pulmonary contusion

Source: Data from American College of Surgeons Committee.[1]

with tracheolaryngeal trauma, as this injury may preclude safe cricothyroidotomy.

In the primary survey, a number of life-threatening conditions should be sought and corrected immediately upon detection (Table 1.3).[1] Of these, tension pneumothorax, flail chest, massive hemothorax, and open pneumothorax are identified on physical examination, without the need or delay to obtain chest radiography, and should be treated immediately. The initial relief of a tension pneumothorax can be accomplished rapidly by inserting a 14- or 16-gauge needle into the second intercostal space in the midclavicular line. Insertion of a thoracostomy tube into the fourth or fifth intercostal space should then follow. A flail chest results from the fracture of three or more ribs in at least two places. This results in a segment of the chest wall that moves paradoxically with respirations. More important from a physiologic standpoint is the underlying pulmonary contusion,[12–15] which can lead to significant hypoxemic respiratory failure. The pulmonary contusion may require intubation and mechanical ventilation if severe or if the patient has labored respirations or respiratory compromise. Patient mortality more than doubles when pulmonary contusion and flail chest are combined compared with either injury alone.[13] However, more than half of these deaths are directly attributed to central nervous system injuries, with another third caused by massive hemorrhage, demonstrating that these patients often have significant associated injuries.

For patients with major chest wall injuries, adequate analgesia can often best be accomplished with the placement of a thoracic epidural catheter for the continuous infusion of opiates and/or regional anesthetics.[16–20] Thoracic epidural anesthesia has been shown to be superior to intravenous administration of opioids via patient-controlled analgesia devices.[21] Pain control is critical in the management of chest wall injuries. With inadequate pain control, hypoventilation and splinting may lead to atelectasis or pneumonia and worsen the alveolar hypoventilation and intrapulmonary shunt, resulting in hypoxia and hypercarbia. The use of continuous epidural analgesia is associated with significant improvement in vital capacity and maximum inspiratory pressure in these patients.[18]

Circulation

Assessment of circulation is done by palpation of pulses and checking skin color, temperature, capillary refill, and mentation. As a general guide, the rate and quality of the pulses can provide important information regarding the adequacy of peripheral circulation and volume status. A strong pulse is associated with adequate cardiac output, whereas a weak, thready pulse often indicates hypovolemia and inadequate cardiac output. Arterial blood pressure is measured. However, a significant drop in blood pressure is a late finding in hemorrhagic shock and may require a blood loss of >30% of total blood volume to manifest (Table 1.4). Thus, a patient with a normal blood pressure measurement may be hypovolemic with ongoing hypoperfusion. On the other hand, the hypotensive patient has decompensated physiologically. In trauma patients, a single systolic blood pressure less than 90 mm Hg has an associated mortality rate of 25%. Narrowing of the pulse pressure and mild tachycardia may be the first signs of hypovolemia and may require blood loss of 15% to 30% of total blood volume to become apparent. Normal mentation implies adequate cerebral perfusion, while diminished level of consciousness in the presence of tachycardia and/or hypotension may be associated with shock or hypoxia, irrespective of central nervous system injury. In patients with significant head injuries, secondary brain injury occurs with hypoxia and hypotension, and these two abnormalities need to be aggressively corrected. Morbidity and mortality rates are doubled for patients with traumatic brain injury who develop hypotension and nearly triple if the combination of hypotension and hypoxia occurs.[22]

Intravenous access should be established immediately in all patients in shock. This is most efficiently accomplished by the insertion of two large-bore (14 or 16 gauge) peripheral lines in the antecubital fossae. Occasionally, percutaneous central venous access or venous cut-downs at the saphenous vein at the ankle or groin will be necessary, although these procedures are more time consuming and require technical skill and therefore are not preferred when peripheral veins are accessible. The choice of intravenous catheter will determine the rapidity with which fluids or blood products can be administered to the patient. As determined by the law of Poiseuille, flow of a fluid through a catheter and intravenous tubing is proportional to the pressure gradient across the catheter, the fourth power of the catheter radius, and inversely proportional to the length of the catheter and the viscosity of the fluid. For this reason, wide catheters and tubing with short lengths will have the advantage of providing the best intravenous access and permit the most rapid delivery of fluids.[23]

If the trauma patient has signs of hypovolemia or shock, hemorrhage must be immediately identified and controlled. The possible sites of blood loss in the trauma patient include thorax, abdomen, pelvis, retroperitoneum, external hemorrhage, and long bone fractures. Physical examination, plain radiography, focused abdominal sonography for trauma (FAST), and diagnostic peritoneal lavage are the mainstay diagnostic maneuvers. Empiric placement of thoracostomy tubes is often the most efficient *diagnostic* and *therapeutic* maneuver for hypotensive patients with thoracic injuries. If this search for bleeding is unrevealing, other causes of shock to consider are tension pneumothorax, cardiac tamponade, high spinal cord injury (neurogenic shock), and severe blunt myocardial injury (rare).

TABLE 1.4. Estimated fluid and blood requirements for a 70-kg male patient with varying degrees of blood loss, based on initial presentation.

	Class I	Class II	Class III	Class IV
Blood loss (mL)	Up to 750	750–1,500	1,500–2,000	>2,000
Blood loss (% blood volume)	Up to 15%	15%–30%	30%–40%	>40%
Pulse rate	<100	>100	>120	>140
Blood pressure	Normal	Normal	Decreased	Decreased
Pulse pressure	Normal or increased	Decreased	Decreased	Decreased
Respiratory rate	14–20	20–30	30–40	>35
Urine output (mL/hr)	>30	20–30	5–15	Negligible
Mental status	Slightly anxious	Mildly anxious	Anxious and confused	Confused, lethargic
Fluid replacement	Crystalloid	Crystalloid	Crystalloid and blood	Crystalloid and blood

Source: Reproduced with permission from American College of Surgeons' Committee on Trauma, Advanced Trauma Life Support® for Doctors (ATLS®) Student Manual, 7th ed. Chicago: American College of Surgeons, 2004.

Fluid Resuscitation

Restoration of normal circulation implies prevention or reversal of shock. Shock is defined as the inadequate delivery of oxygen and other metabolic substrates necessary for normal function and survival of cells and tissues. It is important to realize that significant cellular hypoperfusion and death can occur despite normal arterial blood pressure. Equating shock with hypotension and cardiovascular collapse is a gross oversimplification that may result in undue patient morbidity. The optimal type, amount, and timing of fluid administration during the resuscitation of injured patients in hemorrhagic hypovolemic shock remain a subject of intense investigation and debate. Understand that the primary goal in management of active hemorrhage, whether trauma or nontrauma, is to stop the bleeding. With truncal hemorrhage that results in hypotension, these patients need rapid control of bleeding in the operating room: operating room resuscitation.

For patients with hemorrhagic shock in the prehospital setting, aggressive volume infusion in an attempt to normalize blood pressure may be harmful. Until surgical control of hemorrhage has been achieved, aggressive infusion of fluids may actually disrupt hemostatic clots and cause hemodilution and vasodilation, and it has been shown to worsen outcomes in animal models of hemorrhagic shock.[24-30] In a prospective randomized trial of patients with penetrating torso trauma, patients received either delayed fluid resuscitation upon arrival to the operating room or standard resuscitation by the paramedics. Although a number of technical limitations of this study exist, the trial demonstrated that delayed fluid administration was associated with lower patient mortality.[31] However, a review of the diverse literature on this topic was unable to demonstrate a survival advantage or disadvantage to early or larger volume of intravenous fluid resuscitation in uncontrolled hemorrhage.[32] The literature on this topic is difficult to analyze as a whole because of the inconsistent methodologies employed in the different studies.

Overly aggressive resuscitation may also have other deleterious effects. A study of supranormal resuscitation in severely injured trauma patients with >2 L blood loss targeted resuscitation to a supraphysiologic cardiac index (≥ 4.52 L/min/m^2) and oxygen delivery (≥ 670 mL/min/m^2).[33] In this small study, the ability to attain these supranormal hemodynamic values was associated with improved survival and decreased morbidity rates. However, this effect was more a reflection of the patients' abilities to achieve these parameters in this subset rather than benefits of therapy. Subsequent studies of supranormal resuscitation have not shown benefit.[34] In fact may demonstrate a detrimental effect of the supranormal resuscitation strategy. For trauma patients, resuscitation using oxygen delivery ≥ 500 mL/min/m^2 was indistinguishable from oxygen delivery at ≥ 600 mL/min/m^2. Less volume loading was required to attain and maintain oxygen delivery at ≥ 500 mL/min/m^2 than at 600 mL/min/m^2 using a computerized algorithm to standardize resuscitation during the first 24 hours.[34] Supranormal resuscitation, compared with standard resuscitation, is associated with more lactated Ringer's infusion, decreased intestinal perfusion, and increased incidence of abdominal compartment syndrome, multiple organ failure, and death in trauma patients.[35]

It is clear that both extremes—no fluid versus massive resuscitation—should be avoided as they are detrimental to patient outcome. What is also clear is that surgical control of hemorrhage should be considered part of the initial resuscitation of patients in hemorrhagic shock. Attempts at resuscitation in this situation will be futile and perhaps detrimental, as definitive control of bleeding will be delayed.

Much has been written with regard to the choice of fluid used for the resuscitation of patients in shock. Clearly, most critically ill patients will require volume expansion at some point with the goal of restoring intravascular volume and preserving tissue perfusion and oxygenation. Options include isotonic crystalloids, hypertonic fluids, natural and synthetic colloids, blood products, and other novel solutions. At present, the first-line fluid of choice for the resuscitation of patients in shock remains isotonic crystalloids, such as lactated Ringer's or normal saline solutions. These fluids have a long history of proven effectiveness and are inexpensive, readily available, and easy to preserve. The theoretical advantages of colloids such as albumin solutions include the possibility that they will provide more rapid restoration of intravascular volume with a smaller volume of infused fluid than crystalloids. Colloids may also be associated with less tissue and lung edema and may preserve plasma albumin levels. The potential disadvantages of colloids include their cost and the fact that, in the leaky capillary syndrome seen in many critically ill patients, albumin infusion may not preserve the intravascular oncotic pressure but rather leak into the extravascular space. Hypertonic saline solution combines some of the advantages of crystalloids and colloids. Hypertonic saline may cause less peripheral edema than isotonic fluids, as it draws intracellular fluid into the vascular space. It also may have fewer detrimental effects on immune function. Several studies have examined the role of hypertonic saline compared with isotonic saline in trauma patients, and no clear difference in outcomes could be shown.[36-38] However, some benefit may result from infusion of hypertonic saline in patients with penetrating injuries[39] or those with combined traumatic brain injury and shock.[40]

Several studies have attempted to answer the question as to the benefits of colloids and crystalloid solutions.

One large meta-analysis of the use of albumin versus crystalloids showed a trend toward an increased mortality rate for a variety of critically ill patients who received albumin.[41] However, in other large meta-analyses of the literature comparing albumin solutions with crystalloids for a wide variety of surgical and nonsurgical indications, no difference in mortality rate was detected based on the these choices of resuscitation fluid.[42,43] These meta-analyses include heterogeneous populations of patients and studies of differing designs, confounding the interpretation of the results. At this time, no strong recommendation can be made to support the use of colloids over crystalloids for patients in shock.

The availability of newer colloid solutions, such as hydroxyethyl starch (HES) have renewed this debate. Synthetic starch solutions HES have been used clinically to restore intravascular volume in patients with shock. Several HES solutions are available clinically that differ in the molecular mass fractions of HES and in the composition of the electrolyte solution. The studies that have analyzed the use of HES as a resuscitation fluid are encouraging. In a canine model of hemorrhagic shock, fluid resuscitation during uncontrolled bleeding resulted in higher oxygen delivery and lower systemic lactate concentrations when HES (6%) was used compared with lactated Ringer's solution during resuscitation to a target mean arterial blood pressure of 60 to 80 mm Hg.[44] Also, compared with administration of 0.9% saline, volume resuscitation with HES in balanced electrolyte solution (Hextend) is associated with less metabolic acidosis and longer survival in an experimental animal model of septic shock.[45]

There are concerns regarding the development of coagulopathy with the infusion of HES, because it is known to inhibit platelet function. However, fluid resuscitation with low-molecular-weight HES may reduce the risk of bleeding associated with HES of higher molecular weight and degree of substitution.[46] Also, a dilutional effect on coagulation function independent of the type of resuscitation fluid employed has been observed.[47] Furthermore, colloids with a more physiologically balanced electrolyte formulation may result in less metabolic acidosis and alteration of intestinal perfusion. In a prospective, randomized, blinded trial with elderly surgical patients, the use of balanced electrolyte HES helped prevent the development of hyperchloremic metabolic acidosis and provided better gastric mucosal perfusion than saline-based HES.[48] Clearly, not all resuscitation fluids are equivalent, and patient outcomes will depend on the timing and on the amount and type of fluid employed.

Alternative crystalloid resuscitation fluids are being evaluated. One promising option is Ringer's ethyl pyruvate solution (REPS), which has been assessed in a number of studies using animal models of mesenteric ischemia/reperfusion injury,[49] hemorrhagic shock,[50] and acute endotoxemia.[51,52] In these animal models, infusion of REPS, when compared with Ringer's lactate solution, was shown to improve survival and decrease expression of proinflammatory cytokines. Ringer's ethyl pyruvate solution merits further evaluation for the resuscitation of patients with hemorrhagic shock, sepsis, and trauma.[53]

There remains a need for well-designed clinical trials to determine whether colloids or crystalloids are better for the resuscitation of trauma patients. Because of many limitations, the existing meta-analyses must be interpreted with caution. However, with this in mind, a meta-analysis of this literature regarding humans suggests that trauma patients should continue to be initially resuscitated with crystalloids at this time.[54,55]

Transfusion

The use of blood products in the care of critically ill and injured patients has saved many lives. However, evidence-based practices are evolving regarding the use of blood products. A multicenter, randomized clinical trial has clearly shown that, for critically ill patients in the intensive care unit (predominantly nontrauma patients), a restrictive strategy that employs a hemoglobin transfusion trigger of 7 g/dL is as at least as effective and may be superior to a liberal transfusion threshold of 10 g/dL.[56] In fact, the 30-day mortality rate was lower for the subgroup of patients with an Acute Physiology and Chronic Health Evaluation (APACHE) II score of ≤20 who were randomized to the restrictive transfusion strategy. Patients who were deemed to have ongoing bleeding were excluded from this study. The same investigators published a subsequent study involving patients with known cardiovascular disease that showed similar 30- and 60-day survival rates for the restrictive and liberal transfusion strategies, with the exception of patients with acute myocardial infarction or unstable angina. For the patients with acute coronary syndromes (not simply a history of coronary artery disease), outcomes with a hemoglobin transfusion threshold of 10 g/dL were improved.[57] For the trauma population, red blood cell transfusion has been shown to be a predictor of mortality, independent of severity of shock as determined by arterial base deficit, serum lactate level, shock index, and degree of anemia.[58] In addition, there is a dose-dependent correlation between transfusions of packed red blood cells and the development of infection in trauma patients. Multivariate analyses show that transfusion of blood within 48 hours of hospital admission is an independent risk factor for the development of nosocomial infections.[59–61] For other critically ill patients, a similar association between blood transfusion dose and nosocomial infections has been demonstrated.[62] The administration of blood transfusions is also an independent risk factor for the development of multiorgan failure in trauma patients independent of other indices of shock.[63] On the other hand, empiric blood transfusions should be administered to trauma patients in shock who fail to respond to initial resuscitation with crystalloids. As mentioned earlier, this patient group often requires prompt operative control of hemorrhage.

Because of these and other known detrimental effects associated with blood transfusion, as well as the limitations related to cost and availability (e.g., in the battlefield or prehospital setting), hemoglobin-based oxygen carriers (HBOCs) are being evaluated as an alternative to blood transfusion. While several varieties of HBOCs have been developed, the polyhemoglobins are the most promising type at this time; these include human recombinant polymerized hemoglobin and bovine hemoglobin glutamer 250.[64] The HBOCs have been shown to be effective and safe for the resuscitation of shock in animal models and to improve survival rates better than resuscitation with crystalloids or HES solutions.[65–68] Small clinical studies show promise for the use of HBOCs for surgical and trauma patients.[69–71] There are currently phase III clinical trials in progress that will attempt to answer this question for human patients,[64,72,73] and the HBOCs may become important in the early resuscitation of patients with anemia and shock.

Other Resuscitation Efforts

Emergency department resuscitative thoracotomy, surgical exploration for control of active hemorrhage (e.g., repair of ruptured abdominal aortic aneurysm, splenectomy for active hemorrhage from splenic injury), stabilization of pelvic fractures, and control of external bleeding should all be considered part of the *stabilization of circulation* phase of the primary survey of hemodynamically abnormal and unstable patients. The best results for emergency department resuscitative thoracotomy are obtained for patients with penetrating injuries to the thorax, who had obtainable vital signs, and who suffer rapid deterioration in the emergency department, with up to 20% survivorship.[74] Patients with penetrating abdominal injuries had significantly lower survivorship (6.8%), and survivors with blunt thoracic trauma who required emergent thoracotomy were extremely rare (0.5%).[74,75] For patients with penetrating thoracic injuries who have vital signs at the scene or in the emergency department, survival is much higher than for those who did not have obtainable vital signs.[76,77] Meanwhile, trauma patients who are pulseless and whose electrical cardiac activity is asystolic or agonal (wide complex heart rate <40 beats/min) can be pronounced dead.[78] Thus, although all these data are understandably retrospective, significant judgment must be exercised in selecting patients for emergency department resuscitative thoracotomy.[79]

Assessment of Resuscitation

The ability to assess clinically relevant parameters of tissue and organ perfusion and to employ this knowledge to improve patient outcomes is the core of critical care medicine. Unfortunately, consensus is lacking regarding the most appropriate parameters to monitor to achieve this goal. Of the highest importance is the integration of physiologic data obtained from monitoring into a coherent treatment plan. Thus, endpoints of resuscitation must be defined.

Classic Physical Examination Findings and Vital Signs

Vital signs, namely, heart rate and blood pressure, can be monitored to formulate conclusions regarding volume status and adequacy of resuscitation. However, changes in blood pressure and heart rate are insensitive for the detection of early hypoperfusion.

Urine Output

Bladder catheterization with an indwelling catheter allows the monitoring of urine output, usually recorded hourly. Over a period of observation, urine output is a gross indicator of renal perfusion. The generally accepted normal urine output is 0.5 mL/g/hr for adults and 1–2 mL/kg/hr for neonates and infants. Oliguria may reflect inadequate renal artery perfusion caused by hypotension, hypovolemia, or low cardiac output state or may be associated with intrinsic renal pathology such as acute tubular necrosis. However, normal urine output does not exclude the possibility of hypoperfusion or impending renal failure. Therefore, the measurement of urinary electrolytes, calculation of the fractional excretion of sodium or urea, urinalysis with examination of sediment, and renal ultrasonography are often employed to elucidate the causes of rising blood urea nitrogen (BUN) and serum creatinine levels and the development of oliguria.

Bladder Pressure (Abdominal Compartment Syndrome)

The triad of oliguria, elevated peak airway pressures, and elevated intraabdominal pressure is termed the *abdominal compartment syndrome* (ACS). This syndrome was first described in patients after repair of ruptured abdominal aortic aneurysms,[80] and it is associated with interstitial edema of the abdominal organs, resulting in elevated intraabdominal pressure, which causes in decreased renal perfusion and oliguria as well as hypoperfusion to other intraabdominal viscera. Other common etiologies of ACS include blunt and penetrating abdominal trauma, often with liver, vascular, splenic injuries, or pelvic fractures, especially if abdominal packing is performed. Severe burns, massive resuscitation, or ischemia/reperfusion of the abdominal viscera may also produce intraabdominal hypertension.

Although the diagnosis of ACS is a clinical one, based on the presence of hypotension, oliguria, increased airway pressures, and abdominal distension, measuring intraabdominal pressure may assist in making the diagnosis. Ideally, a catheter inserted into the peritoneal cavity could measure intraabdominal pressure to substantiate the diagnosis. In practice, transurethral bladder pressure measurement reflects intraabdominal pressure and is most often used to confirm the presence of intraabdominal hypertension (IAH). After instilling 50 to 100 mL of sterile saline into the bladder via a Foley catheter, the tubing is connected to a transducing system to measure bladder pressure. A bladder pressure of 20 to 25 cm H_2O in the appropriate clinic setting suggests IAH.[81] Treatment consists primarily of abdominal decompression, most effectively accomplished by laparotomy, leaving the abdomen open. The mortality rate associated with ACS is high, reaching 60% to 70%, reflecting delayed diagnosis and the underlying pathophysiology in these critically ill patients.[82] Thus, prevention is critical. For patients with a high likelihood of development of abdominal compartment syndrome, a temporary abdominal closure with a plastic bag, vacuum pack, or sterile intravenous bag is prudent.

Ventricular Preload

Invasive measurements of ventricular preload such as right atrial and pulmonary artery occlusion pressures and their changes in response to volume loading are inadequate predictors of intravascular volume status and cardiac output.[83] Also, while cerebral and myocardial perfusion may be preserved in compensated shock, mesenteric perfusion may be seriously compromised.[84] Splanchnic hypoperfusion is associated with functional and structural changes in the intestinal mucosa, resulting in increased mucosal permeability and the translocation of bacteria and bacterial products.[85] Increased intestinal mucosal permeability has been associated with the development of multiorgan dysfunction in septic human patients.[86] The rapid detection and correction of tissue hypoperfusion may limit organ dysfunction, reduce complications, and improve patient outcome. It is intuitive that the earlier tissue hypoperfusion is detected and corrected the greater the likelihood that outcome may be improved.[87] This has now been shown by Rivers and colleagues,[88] who reported a 32% relative reduction in the 28-day mortality rate for patients with severe sepsis who received early aggressive volume resuscitation in the emergency department In this study, the central venous

oxygen saturation ($ScvO_2$) was used as the endpoint of resuscitation in the intervention group, whereas in the control group treatment was guided by standard clinical endpoints, including the central venous pressure.

Lactate Level

Hyperlactacidemia is thought to correlate with tissue hypoxia and anaerobic glycolysis, often in the setting of normal blood pressure and cardiac output. Lactate may be generated by well-oxygenated tissues. In injured patients, increased aerobic glycolysis in skeletal muscle secondary to epinephrine-stimulated Na^+,K^+-ATPase activity may increase blood lactate levels.[89] This may explain why hyperlactacidemia often does not correlate with traditional indicators of perfusion and fails to clear with increased oxygen delivery. Continued attempts at resuscitation based on elevated blood lactate level may lead to unnecessary use of blood transfusion and inotropic agents in an effort to increase oxygen delivery and lactate clearance.

Base Deficit

The base deficit (BD) is a commonly used endpoint of trauma resuscitation. The BD is of prognostic value and correlates with mortality rate and with the development of organ dysfunction in a number of retrospective studies.[90–96] In a retrospective review of nearly 3,000 patients admitted to a level I trauma center, an admission BD greater than 6 predicted likelihood for early transfusion, prolonged intensive care unit (ICU) and hospital length of stays, and increased risk for shock-related complications. The risks of developing adult respiratory distress syndrome, renal failure, coagulopathy, multiorgan failure, and death rose significantly with increasingly severe BD.[96] The use of an injury severity score (ISS) and the BD may identify patients who require more invasive monitoring and aggressive resuscitation.

In a large, prospective, multicenter, observational study of over 2,000 multitrauma patients, the arterial BD on hospital and intensive care unit (ICU) admission was an important predictor of hemodynamic instability, transfusion requirement, metabolic and coagulation abnormalities, and mortality.[97] In this study, mortality also increased significantly with a worsening of BD from hospital to ICU admission. Therefore, an elevated BD may help guide an early and aggressive resuscitation for the multitrauma patient. Trend and response to therapy with correction of the BD are more important than a single determination of BD.

The use of the BD is based on the principle that tissue hypoperfusion will result in the development of an "oxygen debt" and metabolic acidosis. However, tissue hypoperfusion may occur without a significant change in the BD. Furthermore, as it requires time for regeneration of bicarbonate by the liver and kidney,[98] a delay can be expected between the correction of tissue perfusion and normalization of the BD. This was demonstrated in a murine hemorrhagic shock model that showed that the BD responded slowly to changes in intravascular volume and that there was a significant increase in the BD only when the mean arterial blood pressure fell by greater than 50%.[99] In contrast, this study demonstrated that changes in the esophageal CO_2 gap correlated well with changes in intravascular volume status. Similar findings have been reported by other investigators. In patients with penetrating trauma, the sublingual CO_2 measurements correlate with the amount of blood loss.[100] Similarly, the gastric intramucosal pH has been reported to correlate with the severity of injury and hypoperfusion.[100–103] The BD may be a less sensitive indicator of the degree of intravascular volume deficit following hemorrhage, and it responds slowly to volume resuscitation.[99] Esophageal or sublingual capnometry, however, may provide real-time assessment of hypoperfusion and the adequacy of volume resuscitation.[104–107] This technology is simple, less invasive than pulmonary artery catheterization, and ideally suited for use in the trauma bay and ICU. Esophageal or sublingual capnography may prove to be a useful endpoint for the resuscitation of trauma patients in the future.

The Triad of Death: Hypothermia, Acidosis, and Coagulopathy

Postinjury life-threatening coagulopathy in the seriously injured person requiring massive transfusion is predicted by persistent hypothermia and progressive metabolic acidosis. The independent risk factors for the development of life-threatening coagulopathy in multitrauma patients receiving massive transfusion are acidosis (pH < 7.10), hypothermia (core temperature <34°C), ISS > 25, and systolic blood pressure <70mm Hg.[108] The most important and effective strategy is to prevent the development of this triad: active correction of hypothermia, hypovolemia, ongoing hemorrhage and acidosis. Admission hypothermia, defined as temperature <36°C, is present in as many as two-thirds of patients admitted to level I trauma centers[109] and therefore must be actively corrected.

Damage control procedures involve limited surgery for the immediate correction of ongoing hemorrhage and contamination, followed by resuscitation in the intensive care unit. During this ICU phase of resuscitation, physiologic abnormalities are corrected. Aggressive resuscitation of the patient occurs, with active rewarming of hypothermic patients, correction of acidosis and hypoperfusion with infusion of fluids and red blood cells, and correction of coagulopathy with rewarming and infusion of blood products. After correction of the physiologic abnormalities, subsequent reoperation can be performed for definitive correction of anatomic abnormalities.

In addition to the infusion of fresh-frozen plasma and platelets, other approaches available to correct coagulopathy include the infusion of specific coagulation factors. The most promising is recombinant activated factor VII (rFVIIa). Recombinant activated factor VII reduces blood loss in hypothermic and coagulopathic swine with severe hepatic injuries when used as an adjunct to packing.[110] Recombinant activated factor VII has been shown in small human series to be effective in treating bleeding associated with coagulopathy in obstetrical patients[111] and trauma patients with multifactorial coagulopathy.[112] This raises the possibility of therapeutic use of rFVIIa for patients with coagulopathy and ongoing blood loss.[113]

Damage control surgery has emerged as the preferred management strategy for trauma patients with abdominal injuries complicated by hypothermia, coagulopathy, and acidosis.[114–116] It appears that the concept of damage-control surgery and correction of hypothermia and coagulopathy have a positive impact on patient survival for those who have had massive blood transfusion[117] or who are in the early phases of the downward spiral of hypothermia, coagulopathy, and acidosis. This approach can be used for both critically ill trauma and nontrauma patients.

Shock

As stated earlier, shock is defined as inadequate delivery of oxygen and nutrients to cells and tissues.[118] It should be noted that significant tissue hypoperfusion can occur despite normal arterial blood pressure; the definition of shock is independent of this parameter. However, the presence of hypotension implies more severe physiologic insult and degree of decompensation. In 1934, Blalock[119] proposed four categories of shock: hypovolemic, vasogenic, cardiogenic, and neurologic. Two additional categories of shock have been described: obstructive and traumatic. From a clinical perspective, a simple differential diagnosis can often be formulated for hypotensive patients in shock based on the presence or absence of loss of vascular resistance, as evidenced by the pulse pressure (Table 1.5).

Hypovolemic and Hemorrhagic Shock

Hypovolemia in the presence of hemorrhage is the most common cause of shock in the trauma patient and results from the loss of circulating blood volume from either hemorrhage or loss of plasma fluid. Acute loss of circu-

TABLE 1.5. Differential diagnosis of hypotension based on the pulse pressure (systolic–diastolic blood pressure) as an indicator of systemic vascular resistance.

Hypotension with normal/wide pulse pressure
Septic shock, severe sepsis (define), adrenal insufficiency
High spinal cord injury
Liver failure
Anaphylaxis
Hypotension with narrow pulse pressure
Hemorrhage/hypovolemia
Blunt/penetrating trauma to vessels or solid organs
Ruptured abdominal aortic aneurysm, visceral aneurysm
Ectopic pregnancy
Gastrointestinal bleed
Peritonitis/pancreatitis
Spontaneous rupture of liver/spleen lesions
Cardiogenic shock (myocardial infarction, tamponade, arrhythmia)
Obstructive shock (PE, PTX)

lating blood volume results in compensatory mechanisms mediated by the cathecholamines, hypophyseal-pituitary-adrenal axis, and other mediators that result in peripheral vasoconstriction, tachycardia, and oliguria. The initial management of this type of shock has been addressed previously in this chapter.

Cardiogenic Shock

Cardiogenic shock refers to the inadequate tissue perfusion caused by cardiac dysfunction and is most often associated with acute coronary syndromes and myocardial infarction.[120] Other potential causes include dysrhythmias, acute valvular insufficiency, ventricular wall or septal rupture, and rarely blunt myocardial injury.[121] Cardiogenic shock is clinically defined when evidence of tissue hypoperfusion occurs in the setting of adequate intravascular volume. Hemodynamic criteria may be confirmatory, such as hypotension or reduced cardiac index ($<2.2\,L/min/m^2$) associated with normal or elevated pulmonary artery occlusion pressure ($>15\,mm\,Hg$).[120] The mortality associated with cardiogenic shock remains 50% to 80% in most series.[121] It is important to differentiate cardiogenic shock from other causes of shock in the patient who presents acutely to the emergency department, as the treatment is very different. The management of cardiogenic shock may involve the use of inotropic agents, intraaortic balloon counterpulsation, diuretics, thrombolytic therapy, and catheter-directed or surgical coronary reperfusion.[120] The data from the SHOCK trial strongly favor the use of mechanical revascularization strategies for patients with cardiogenic shock.[122]

Obstructive Shock

When cardiac output is decreased because of impaired venous return to the heart, the condition of obstructive shock occurs. The common causes of obstructive shock of concern to the surgeon are tension pneumothorax, cardiac tamponade, and massive pulmonary embolus. In the first two instances, reduced right ventricular preload occurs from either increased intrapleural pressure (tension pneumothorax) or increased pericardial pressure (tamponade). In the case of massive pulmonary embolism, reduced left ventricular filling and massive right ventricular dilatation and failure occur, resulting in low cardiac output and hypotension. The diagnosis of tension pneumothorax is clinical. In the presence of shock, diminished breath sounds on one side of the chest with hyperresonance to percussion, possibly accompanied by shift of the tracheal to the contralateral side, and jugular venous distension, the diagnosis is made and treatment should be carried out immediately. Decompression of the affected pleural space should be performed immediately by the most expeditious manner. If a thoracostomy tube is not immediately available, needle decompression can temporize until a chest tube is inserted.

Cardiac tamponade results when fluid or blood accumulates in the pericardial sac, compressing the cardiac chambers and impairing cardiac filling. The clinical diagnosis may be difficult, as the classic signs may be absent or difficult to detect. Bedside FAST is sensitive for the detection of fluid in the pericardium, but the results are operator dependent.[123–126] For the patient in extremis, emergency department left anterolateral thoracotomy and pericardial decompression should be performed immediately. In more stable patients, further evaluation may require subxiphoid pericardial window. Pericardiocentesis to detect and decompress pericardial tamponade, although advocated by ATLS,[1] may potentially produce cardiac injury, has a definite risk of false-negative results, and is often unable to evacuate clotted blood from the pericardium.

Traumatic Shock

Some authors consider traumatic shock a separate clinical entity.[127] This category is used to describe a series of insults after injury that produce profound hypoperfusion in combination. In addition to hemorrhage, ischemia, and reperfusion, traumatic shock involves the activation of proinflammatory cascades and can involve components of vasodilatory shock as well.[128] Examples of traumatic shock include hemorrhage plus soft tissue injury (such as crush injury) or any combination of other forms of shock that present simultaneously in the injured patient. Treatment of traumatic shock must be directed at correcting the underlying elements that contribute to its development and that promote the inflammatory cascade, such as ongoing hemorrhage, volume deficits, intestinal contamination, presence of nonviable or infected tissue, and unstable bony injuries.

Vasodilatory Shock

Vasodilatory shock occurs when there is a loss of vasoregulatory function, resulting in vasodilation of the capacitance vessels. This is most often seen in sepsis, but can also occur with high spinal cord injury (neurogenic shock), anaphylaxis, liver failure, and adrenal corticosteroid deficiency.[129]

From a clinical standpoint, the most frequent cause of vasodilatory shock is sepsis. A series of clinical definitions have been proposed by an American College of Chest Physicians and Society of Critical Care Medicine Consensus Conference.[130] The *systemic inflammatory response syndrome* (SIRS) is defined by the presence of two or more of the following: (1) temperature >38°C or <32°C; (2) heart rate >90 beats/min; (3) respiratory rate >20 breaths/min or $PaCO_2$ <32 mm Hg; (4) white blood cell count >12,000 μL^{-1} or <4,000 μL^{-1} or >10% immature forms.

Sepsis is defined when SIRS results from established or suspected infection (whether bacterial, fungal, viral, or parasitic). *Severe sepsis* is defined as sepsis associated with signs of at least one organ dysfunction or hypoperfusion, and septic shock is hypotension not reversed with fluid administration and associated with organ dysfunction or hypoperfusion. These definitions are widely used in clinical practice and serve as the basis for entry criteria in numerous clinical trials. However, some diagnostic ambiguity exists with these definitions, prompting the International Sepsis Definitions Conference to further refine them, as well as to introduce a staging system for sepsis in 2001.[131] Despite some evolution of their definitions, the mortality rate of severe sepsis and septic shock remain high.[132,133] Severe sepsis is now the most common cause of death in noncoronary critical care units in the United States.[133]

The initial resuscitation of patients in severe sepsis or septic shock should occur as soon as the syndrome is recognized and not be delayed for ICU admission.[134] Early goal-directed therapy improves survival for patients who present to the emergency department with septic shock. This was shown in a randomized, controlled trial of protocol-driven resuscitation within 6 hours of presentation to the emergency department.[88] The endpoints of resuscitation for the patients in the treatment arm were central venous pressure of 8 to 12 mm Hg, mean arterial pressure ≥65 mm Hg, urine output ≥0.5 mL/kg/hr, and central venous oxygen saturation ≥70%. The patients in the control arm received standard resuscitation guided by the first three endpoints only. Patients in the early-goal-directed arm also received red blood cell transfusion to maintain a hemoglobin level of 10 mg/dL and dobutamine infusion if central venous saturation was <70% despite these initial interventions. This study showed a significant reduction in 28-day mortality in the early-goal-

directed therapy group compared with the standard resuscitation group (33.3% vs. 49.2%, respectively). During the initial 6 hours of resuscitation, patients in the early-goal-directed group received significantly more fluid, red blood cell transfusion, and inotropic support than the patients in the standard group. Over the first 72 hours as a whole, both groups received similar amounts of fluids and use of inotropic support. This study clearly demonstrates that *early* resuscitation of patients with severe sepsis and septic shock improves survival. Prior studies of goal-directed therapy failed to show a benefit of this treatment modality. However, these studies enrolled patients after admission to the ICU,[135,136] which adds a significant delay in the initiation of resuscitation, and these studies targeted supranormal endpoints of resuscitation.

Intravenous antibiotics, directed at the most likely causative pathogens, should be given early (within 1 hour) of recognition of sepsis, after appropriate cultures have been obtained, if possible.[134] Initial empiric antimicrobial choices should include drug(s) that have activity against the suspected organisms, should be guided by the susceptibility patterns of bacteria isolated in the local community and hospital, and should not await results of the cultures obtained from the patient. If the initial antibiotic choice fails to adequately cover the susceptibility pattern of the responsible microorganisms in patients with bacteremia, increased patient morbidity and mortality will result.[137–139]

All patients who present with the sepsis syndrome should be evaluated for the presence of a source of infection that is amenable to drainage, surgical debridement, removal of an implanted device or catheter, or the definitive control of a source of ongoing bacterial contamination or release of bacterial products (such as colectomy for fulminant colitis associated with *Clostridium dificile*). Source control should be undertaken soon after the initial resuscitation of the patient has occurred and may often be performed using minimally invasive techniques, such as the percutaneous drainage of a diverticular abscess, thus minimizing patient morbidity associated with more invasive forms of source control. However, for cases of diffuse peritonitis from perforation of the gastrointestinal tract, exploratory surgery is necessary, whereas with necrotizing soft tissue infections, wide surgical debridement of nonviable and infected tissue is required.

When appropriate fluid administration fails to restore adequate arterial blood pressure and organ perfusion in sepsis, therapy using vasoactive agents should be instituted. It is important to note that the first line of resuscitation is the administration of fluids. In the septic patient, induction of the enzyme-inducible nitric oxide synthase (iNOS) occurs, resulting in the production of nitric oxide (NO) in the smooth muscle cells of blood vessels, further resulting in vasodilation.[140] Although there are insufficient experimental data to support the use of one vasopressor over another in sepsis, norepinephrine or dopamine infusions can be useful in the treatment of hypotension and vasodilation in sepsis and cause less tachycardia and reduction in mesenteric perfusion than epinephrine and less reduction in cardiac stroke volume than phenylephrine.[141–144] For patients with refractory septic shock, relative vasopressin deficiency has been identified.[145] Low-dose continuous infusion of vasopressin may be considered for patients who remain hypotensive despite fluids and vasopressors.[146,147] High doses of vasopressin may cause intestinal ischemia, reduced cardiac output, and cardiac arrest.[148]

For septic patients who have low cardiac output despite volume administration, inotropic support may be necessary. Dobutamine is the preferred agent for patients with low cardiac index and evidence of adequate cardiac preload. In the presence of arterial hypotension, it may be necessary to infuse a vasopressor simultaneously, as dobutamine may result in a further decrease in systemic vascular resistance. Although in the past some authorities have recommended increasing cardiac output and oxygen delivery to supranormal levels, two large prospective clinical trials of septic patients have shown no benefit to this strategy, and in fact it may be detrimental.[135,136]

Septic shock is often associated with a relative insufficiency of adrenal steroid hormone production[149,150] or glucocorticoid receptor resistance.[151] Steroid hormone supplementation therapy has been shown to improve survival in septic patients. In a large, multicenter, randomized clinical trial of patients with septic shock, a 7-day course of treatment with hydrocortisone and fludrocortisone significantly reduced mortality rate and the requirement for vasopressor therapy for patients with documented adrenal suppression and septic shock.[152] There are no studies supporting the use of steroid supplementation for septic patients who do not have shock. Thus, adrenal steroid supplementation should be given to patients with septic shock and laboratory evidence of adrenal suppression by a cosyntropin stimulation test.

The sepsis syndrome involves activation of the inflammatory cascade by a number of bacterial products such as endotoxin. A number of therapeutic strategies have been investigated in an attempt to modify this cytokine response, without demonstrable benefit to human patients,[153,154] with one recent exception. It is clear that the inflammatory and coagulation cascades are intimately intertwined. Activated protein C is an endogenous protein that stimulates fibrinolysis and inhibits thrombosis and inflammation. Therefore, it is an important modulator of the inflammatory and coagulation cascades. Patients with severe sepsis often have reduced levels of activated protein C, and this deficiency correlates with mortality.[155–157] Administration of recombinant human

activated protein C (rhAPC, drotrecogin alpha [activated]) has been evaluated in patients with severe sepsis in a large, multicenter, randomized trial.[158] This trial showed an statistically significant absolute reduction in the risk of death of 6.1% with treatment with rhAPC. However, a trend toward increased bleeding events was seen in the patients who received rhAPC, although this did not reach statistical significance. Recombinant human APC should be given early, as a continuous infusion, to patients with severe sepsis and a high risk of death (APACHE II score >25) and with no contraindication related to bleeding risk.[134]

Acute Abdominal Pain

Acute abdominal pain refers to pain of nontraumatic etiology of less than 6 hours duration (although some authors use a 1 week's duration). The evaluation of patients who present with acute abdominal pain comprises a large portion of referrals for general surgeons and emergency departments. From the preface of the first edition of *Cope's Early Diagnosis of the Acute Abdomen*[159]: "All who have had much experience of the group of cases known generally as the acute abdomen will probably agree that in that condition early diagnosis is exceptional." This statement remains as true today as it was in 1921. Although the differential diagnosis of abdominal pain is extensive, there are a number of causes of abdominal pain that are of concern to the surgeon because of their relative frequency or because they require immediate recognition and treatment. In a large survey of patients presenting with abdominal pain, the primary etiologies were documented (Table 1.6).[160] Other

TABLE 1.6. Etiologies of acute abdominal pain.*

Diagnosis	Relative frequency (% patients)
Nonspecific	34.0
Acute appendicitis	28.1
Acute cholecystitis	9.7
Small bowel obstruction	4.1
Acute gynecologic disorder	4.0
Acute pancreatitis	2.9
Renal colic	2.9
Perforated peptic ulcer	2.5
Cancer	1.5
Diverticular disease	1.5
Dyspepsia	1.4
Amebic hepatic abscess	1.2
Other	6

* Relative frequency of specific etiologies of acute abdominal pain (pain of less than 1 week's duration). Organisation Mondiale de Gastro-Entérologie (OMGE) survey of 10,320 patients from 26 medical centers in 17 countries from 1976 to 1986. Patients with obvious hernia or trauma were excluded. The ages of the patients were not provided.
Source: Reprinted with permission of Taylor and Francis from de Dombal.[160]

causes of acute abdominal pain merit special consideration and must be excluded in the initial evaluation of these patients. The pitfalls in their recognition and treatment may lead to undue morbidity and mortality, and timely diagnosis and treatment are critical. These include acute intestinal ischemia, ruptured abdominal aortic aneurysm or visceral aneurysm, ruptured ectopic pregnancy, acute myocardial infarction or *Clostridium difficile*–associated colitis.

Nongastrointestinal causes of abdominal pain must be considered as well. These include gynecologic etiologies such as pelvic inflammatory disease, ectopic pregnancy, ovarian torsion, and tubo-ovarian abscess. Urologic disorders are common causes of abdominal pain and include infections of the urinary tract, calculi, obstruction of the urinary tract, and acute testicular events. A number of nonsurgical causes of abdominal pain must be excluded, including pulmonary (lower lobe pneumonia, pulmonary embolism), cardiac (myocardial infarction), hematologic (sickle cell crisis), neurologic (tabes dorsalis, herpes zoster), metabolic (uremia, porphyria), and toxins (insect bites, venom, drugs, and lead poisoning). Abdominal wall hematomas, such as rectus muscle hematoma, may mimic a surgical abdomen in some patients.

A general working algorithm can be used to evaluate patients who present with acute abdominal pain (Figure 1.1). Thorough history and physical examination are crucial to the assessment of patients with acute abdominal pain. Information gained will guide the subsequent evaluation and management of these patients. Guided laboratory studies, not ordered in a shotgun approach, may be helpful. Among these, the white blood cell count, hemoglobin, pancreatic enzymes, liver function tests, urinalysis, and urine pregnancy test for women of childbearing age can be most useful. In general, tests should not be ordered unless their results are likely to alter the patient's management.

Directed radiographic studies may aid in establishing a diagnosis. Plain radiographs may be diagnostic of intestinal perforation (pneumoperitoneum) or obstruction or reveal other important information in some patients.[161] Abdominal computed tomography (CT) may be of value for patients who present to the emergency department with abdominal pain without peritoneal signs on physical examination.[162] In a prospective study of the use of CT scanning for the evaluation of nontraumatic abdominal pain, CT obviated the need for hospital admission in 17% of patients with abdominal pain who otherwise would have been admitted.[163] In addition, before CT, 13% of all patients in this study would have undergone immediate surgery; however, following CT, only 5% actually required immediate surgery. Thus, CT scanning has a large impact on the evaluation and management of patients with acute abdominal pain without peritonitis or hemodynamic instability.

In fact, most patients in need of emergent abdominal operations do not need advanced radiographic studies. The primary role of advanced radiographic studies for these patients is in the localization of a bleeding site in patients with gastrointestinal bleeding. With the exception of patients who present with hemorrhage, advanced radiologic tests often cause unnecessary delay in treatment.[164] For most patients with suspected gastrointestinal tract perforation or intestinal ischemia, the decision to operate can be made using clinical features and simple radiographic studies, avoiding delay and risk of unnecessary tests. Minimally invasive surgery is emerging as an option for the diagnosis and treatment of patients who present with acute abdominal pain and peritonitis.[165–170]

For patients who present with upper gastrointestinal bleeding, an aggressive diagnostic and therapeutic approach is recommended.[171] These patients should be admitted to a surgical service, generally with intensive care monitoring and endoscopy within 24 hours. Urgent

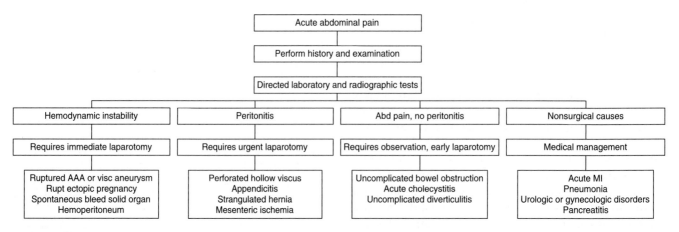

FIGURE 1.1. Initial management for patients who present with acute abdominal pain. AAA, abdominal aortic aneurysm; MI, myocardial infarction.

or acute care surgery is recommended for patients who present with shock, require greater than 4 units of blood transfusion, are elderly, or have a large ulcer (greater than 2 cm) or stigmata of recent hemorrhage.[171]

Patients who require acute care abdominal surgery, especially the elderly, often have postoperative morbidity and mortality rates that exceed those of patients who require elective surgery. These risks are further increased in patients who are inadequately volume resuscitated or have signs of SIRS,[172] and these patients must be adequately resuscitated before surgical exploration. Mortality correlates with advanced patient age, error in diagnosis,[173] delay in definitive therapy, high APACHE II score, low serum albumin level, and high New York Heart Association cardiac function status.[174]

Reevaluation and Definitive Care

Throughout the evaluation and treatment of acutely ill patients, simultaneous evaluation and treatment must occur. Constant reevaluation is mandatory, as these patients often suffer unexpected and sudden deterioration. Vigilance and constant reevaluation of the patient during the initial resuscitation are crucial. The patient's response to any intervention should be monitored to titrate ongoing resuscitation efforts. Stabilization of airway, breathing, and circulation must take precedence over definitive correction of most anatomic abnormalities. Failure to do so will seriously jeopardize the patient. Initial stabilization of the patient is followed by definitive management of the disease process. Note that, as described previously, initial stabilization may include operative intervention to correct ongoing hemorrhage or fecal contamination of the peritoneum. The outcome of critically ill patients will be most influenced by the adequacy and timeliness of the initial resuscitation.

Critique

With acute airway concerns already addressed, this patient, who is in hemorrhagic shock, needs expeditious determination and management of the source of bleeding. The three common cavities for such blood loss are the chest, abdomen, and pelvis. Chest radiography highlights a probable traumatic aortic rupture but no evidence of hemothorax. Therefore, the chest is not the site for this blood loss. The likely epidural hematoma also would not be the probable etiology for this shock state. With the pneumatic garments inflated, the pelvis could still be the source of original blood loss, particularly arterial bleeding. However, the intervention required in this situation would be arteriography and embolization. Although the patient has a soft abdomen, he could still have a substantial volume of blood in the abdominal cavity. Therefore, focused abdominal ultrasonography performed in the trauma bay, to determine if there is intraabdominal hemorrhage, is the next priority for this patient.

Answer (E)

References

1. American College of Surgeons Committee. Advanced Trauma Life Support Instructor Manual, 6th ed. Chicago: American College of Surgeons, 1997.
2. Lo RV, III, Bellini LM. William of Occam and Occam's razor. Ann Intern Med 2002; 136(8):634–635.
3. Nicholas JM, Rix EP, Easley KA, Feliciano DV, Cava RA, Ingram WL, et al. Changing patterns in the management of penetrating abdominal trauma: the more things change, the more they stay the same. J Trauma 2003; 55(6):1095–1108.
4. Miner JR, Heegaard W, Plummer D. End-tidal carbon dioxide monitoring during procedural sedation. Acad Emerg Med 2002; 9(4):275–280.
5. Baer GA, Paloheimo M, Rahnasto J, Pukander J. End-tidal oxygen concentration and pulse oximetry for monitoring oxygenation during intratracheal jet ventilation. J Clin Monit 1995; 11(6):373–380.
6. Rhee KJ, O'Malley RJ, Turner JE, Ward RE. Field airway management of the trauma patient: the efficacy of bag mask ventilation. Am J Emerg Med 1988; 6(4):333–336.
7. Mandavia DP, Qualls S, Rokos I. Emergency airway management in penetrating neck injury. Ann Emerg Med 2000; 35(3):221–225.
8. Sing RF, Rotondo MF, Zonies DH, Schwab CW, Kauder DR, Ross SE, et al. Rapid sequence induction for intubation by an aeromedical transport team: a critical analysis. Am J Emerg Med 1998; 16(6):598–602.
9. Wayne MA, Friedland E. Prehospital use of succinylcholine: a 20-year review. Prehosp Emerg Care 1999; 3(2):107–109.
10. Li J, Murphy-Lavoie H, Bugas C, Martinez J, Preston C. Complications of emergency intubation with and without paralysis. Am J Emerg Med 1999; 17(2):141–143.
11. Salvino CK, Dries D, Gamelli R, Murphy-Macabobby M, Marshall W. Emergency cricothyroidotomy in trauma victims. J Trauma 1993; 34(4):503–505.
12. Kishikawa M, Yoshioka T, Shimazu T, Sugimoto H, Yoshioka T, Sugimoto T. Pulmonary contusion causes long-term respiratory dysfunction with decreased functional residual capacity. J Trauma 1991; 31(9):1203–1208.
13. Clark GC, Schecter WP, Trunkey DD. Variables affecting outcome in blunt chest trauma: flail chest vs. pulmonary contusion. J Trauma 1988; 28(3):298–304.
14. Glinz W. Problems caused by the unstable thoracic wall and by cardiac injury due to blunt injury. Injury 1986; 17(5):322–326.

15. Johnson JA, Cogbill TH, Winga ER. Determinants of outcome after pulmonary contusion. J Trauma 1986; 26(8):695–697.

16. Abouhatem R, Hendrickx P, Titeca M, Guerisse P. Thoracic epidural analgesia in the treatment of rib fractures. Acta Anaesthesiol Belg 1984; 35(Suppl):271–275.

17. Luchette FA, Radafshar SM, Kaiser R, Flynn W, Hassett JM. Prospective evaluation of epidural versus intrapleural catheters for analgesia in chest wall trauma. J Trauma 1994; 36(6):865–869.

18. Mackersie RC, Shackford SR, Hoyt DB, Karagianes TG. Continuous epidural fentanyl analgesia: ventilatory function improvement with routine use in treatment of blunt chest injury. J Trauma 1987; 27(11):1207–1212.

19. Soliman IE, Safwat AM. Successful management of an elderly patient with multiple trauma. J Trauma 1985; 25(8):806–807.

20. Worthley LI. Thoracic epidural in the management of chest trauma. A study of 161 cases. Intensive Care Med 1985; 11(6):312–315.

21. Moon MR, Luchette FA, Gibson SW, Crews J, Sudarshan G, Hurst JM, et al. Prospective, randomized comparison of epidural versus parenteral opioid analgesia in thoracic trauma. Ann Surg 1999; 229(5):684–691.

22. Chesnut RM, Marshall LF, Klauber MR, Blunt BA, Baldwin N, Eisenberg HM, et al. The role of secondary brain injury in determining outcome from severe head injury. J Trauma 1993; 34(2):216–222.

23. Barcelona SL, Vilich F, Cote CJ. A comparison of flow rates and warming capabilities of the Level 1 and Rapid Infusion System with various-size intravenous catheters. Anesth Analg 2003; 97(2):358–363, table.

24. Burris D, Rhee P, Kaufmann C, Pikoulis E, Austin B, Eror A, et al. Controlled resuscitation for uncontrolled hemorrhagic shock. J Trauma 1999; 46(2):216–222.

25. Capone AC, Safar P, Stezoski W, Tisherman S, Peitzman AB. Improved outcome with fluid restriction in treatment of uncontrolled hemorrhagic-shock. J Am Coll Surgeons 1995; 180(1):49–56.

26. Kowalenko T, Stern S, Dronen S, Xu W. Improved outcome with hypotensive resuscitation of uncontrolled hemorrhagic-shock in a swine model. J Trauma 1992; 33(3):349–353.

27. Abu Hatoum O, Bashenko Y, Hirsh M, Krausz MM. Continuous fluid resuscitation and splenectomy for treatment of uncontrolled hemorrhagic shock after massive splenic injury. J Trauma 2002; 52(2):253–258.

28. Holmes JF, Sakles JC, Lewis G, Wisner DH. Effects of delaying fluid resuscitation on an injury to the systemic arterial vasculature. Acad Emerg Med 2002; 9(4):267–274.

29. Abu-Hatoum O, Bashenko Y, Hirsh M, Krausz MM. Continuous fluid resuscitation and splenectomy for treatment of uncontrolled hemorrhagic shock after massive splenic injury. J Trauma 2002; 52(2):253–258.

30. Krausz MM, Bashenko Y, Hirsh M. Crystalloid and colloid resuscitation of uncontrolled hemorrhagic shock following massive splenic injury. Shock 2001; 16(5):383–388.

31. Bickell WH, Wall MJ, Pepe PE, Martin RR, Ginger VF, Allen MK, et al. Immediate versus delayed fluid resusci-

tation for hypotensive patients with penetrating torso injuries. N Engl J Med 1994; 331(17):1105–1109.

32. Kwan I, Bunn F, Roberts I. Timing and volume of fluid administration for patients with bleeding. Cochrane Database Syst Rev 2003; (3):CD002245.

33. Fleming A, Bishop M, Shoemaker W, Appel P, Sufficool W, Kuvhenguwha A, et al. Prospective trial of supranormal values as goals of resuscitation in severe trauma. Arch Surg 1992; 127(10):1175–1179.

34. McKinley BA, Kozar RA, Cocanour CS, Valdivia A, Sailors RM, Ware DN, et al. Normal versus supranormal oxygen delivery goals in shock resuscitation: the response is the same. J Trauma 2002; 53(5):825–832.

35. Balogh Z, McKinley BA, Cocanour CS, Kozar RA, Valdivia A, Sailors RM, et al. Supranormal trauma resuscitation causes more cases of abdominal compartment syndrome. Arch Surg 2003; 138(6):637–642.

36. Younes RN, Aun F, Accioly CQ, Casale LP, Szajnbok I, Birolini D. Hypertonic solutions in the treatment of hypovolemic shock: a prospective, randomized study in patients admitted to the emergency room. Surgery 1992; 111(4):380–385.

37. Mattox KL, Maningas PA, Moore EE, Mateer JR, Marx JA, Aprahamian C, et al. Prehospital hypertonic saline/dextran infusion for post-traumatic hypotension. The U.S.A. Multicenter Trial. Ann Surg 1991; 213(5):482–491.

38. Wade CE, Kramer GC, Grady JJ, Fabian TC, Younes RN. Efficacy of hypertonic 7.5% saline and 6% dextran-70 in treating trauma: a meta-analysis of controlled clinical studies. Surgery 1997; 122(3):609–616.

39. Wade C, Grady J, Kramer G. Efficacy of hypertonic saline dextran (HSD) in patients with traumatic hypotension: meta-analysis of individual patient data. Acta Anaesthesiol Scand Suppl 1997; 110:77–79.

40. Wade CE, Grady JJ, Kramer GC, Younes RN, Gehlsen K, Holcroft JW. Individual patient cohort analysis of the efficacy of hypertonic saline/dextran in patients with traumatic brain injury and hypotension. J Trauma 1997; 42(5 Suppl):S61–S65.

41. Human albumin administration in critically ill patients: systematic review of randomised controlled trials. Cochrane Injuries Group Albumin Reviewers. BMJ 1998; 317(7153):235–240.

42. Wilkes MM, Navickis RJ. Patient survival after human albumin administration. A meta-analysis of randomized, controlled trials. Ann Intern Med 2001; 135(3):149–164.

43. Schierhout G, Roberts I. Fluid resuscitation with colloid or crystalloid solutions in critically ill patients: a systematic review of randomised trials. BMJ 1998; 316(7136):961–964.

44. Friedman Z, Berkenstadt H, Preisman S, Perel A. A comparison of lactated Ringer's solution to hydroxyethyl starch 6% in a model of severe hemorrhagic shock and continuous bleeding in dogs. Anesth Analg 2003; 96(1):39–45, table.

45. Kellum JA. Fluid resuscitation and hyperchloremic acidosis in experimental sepsis: improved short-term survival and acid–base balance with Hextend compared with saline. Crit Care Med 2002; 30(2):300–305.

46. Franz A, Braunlich P, Gamsjager T, Felfernig M, Gustorff B, Kozek-Langenecker SA. The effects of hydroxyethyl starches of varying molecular weights on platelet function. Anesth Analg 2001; 92(6):1402–1407.

47. Via D, Kaufmann C, Anderson D, Stanton K, Rhee P. Effect of hydroxyethyl starch on coagulopathy in a swine model of hemorrhagic shock resuscitation. J Trauma 2001; 50(6):1076–1082.

48. Wilkes NJ, Woolf R, Mutch M, Mallett SV, Peachey T, Stephens R, et al. The effects of balanced versus saline-based hetastarch and crystalloid solutions on acid–base and electrolyte status and gastric mucosal perfusion in elderly surgical patients. Anesth Analg 2001; 93(4):811–816.

49. Uchiyama T, Delude RL, Fink MP. Dose-dependent effects of ethyl pyruvate in mice subjected to mesenteric ischemia and reperfusion. Intensive Care Med 2003; 29(11):2050–2058.

50. Tawadrous ZS, Delude RL, Fink MP. Resuscitation from hemorrhagic shock with Ringer's ethyl pyruvate solution improves survival and ameliorates intestinal mucosal hyperpermeability in rats. Shock 2002; 17(6):473–477.

51. Ulloa L, Ochani M, Yang H, Tanovic M, Halperin D, Yang R, et al. Ethyl pyruvate prevents lethality in mice with established lethal sepsis and systemic inflammation. Proc Natl Acad Sci USA 2002; 99(19):12351–12356.

52. Venkataraman R, Kellum JA, Song M, Fink MP. Resuscitation with Ringer's ethyl pyruvate solution prolongs survival and modulates plasma cytokine and nitrite/nitrate concentrations in a rat model of lipopolysaccharide-induced shock. Shock 2002; 18(6):507–512.

53. Fink MP. Ringer's ethyl pyruvate solution: a novel resuscitation fluid for the treatment of hemorrhagic shock and sepsis. J Trauma 2003; 54(5 Suppl):S141–S143.

54. Rizoli SB. Crystalloids and colloids in trauma resuscitation: a brief overview of the current debate. J Trauma 2003; 54(5 Suppl):S82–S88.

55. Choi PT, Yip G, Quinonez LG, Cook DJ. Crystalloids vs. colloids in fluid resuscitation: a systematic review. Crit Care Med 1999; 27(1):200–210.

56. Hebert PC, Wells G, Blajchman MA, Marshall J, Martin C, Pagliarello G, et al. A multicenter, randomized, controlled clinical trial of transfusion requirements in critical care. Transfusion Requirements in Critical Care Investigators, Canadian Critical Care Trials Group. N Engl J Med 1999; 340(6):409–417.

57. Hebert PC, Yetisir E, Martin C, Blajchman MA, Wells G, Marshall J, et al. Is a low transfusion threshold safe in critically ill patients with cardiovascular diseases? Crit Care Med 2001; 29(2):227–234.

58. Malone DL, Dunne J, Tracy JK, Putnam AT, Scalea TM, Napolitano LM. Blood transfusion, independent of shock severity, is associated with worse outcome in trauma. J Trauma 2003; 54(5):898–905.

59. Claridge JA, Sawyer RG, Schulman AM, McLemore EC, Young JS. Blood transfusions correlate with infections in trauma patients in a dose-dependent manner. Am Surg 2002; 68(7):566–572.

60. Hill GE, Frawley WH, Griffith KE, Forestner JE, Minei JP. Allogeneic blood transfusion increases the risk of post-operative bacterial infection: a meta-analysis. J Trauma 2003; 54(5):908–914.

61. Offner PJ, Moore EE, Biffl WL, Johnson JL, Silliman CC. Increased rate of infection associated with transfusion of old blood after severe injury. Arch Surg 2002; 137(6):711–716.

62. Taylor RW, Manganaro L, O'Brien J, Trottier SJ, Parkar N, Veremakis C. Impact of allogenic packed red blood cell transfusion on nosocomial infection rates in the critically ill patient. Crit Care Med 2002; 30(10):2249–2254.

63. Moore FA, Moore EE, Sauaia A. Blood transfusion. An independent risk factor for postinjury multiple organ failure. Arch Surg 1997; 132(6):620–624.

64. Chang TM. A new red blood cell substitute. Crit Care Med 2004; 32(2):612–613.

65. Sampson JB, Davis MR, Mueller DL, Kashyap VS, Jenkins DH, Kerby JD. A comparison of the hemoglobin-based oxygen carrier HBOC-201 to other low-volume resuscitation fluids in a model of controlled hemorrhagic shock. J Trauma 2003; 55(4):747–754.

66. van Iterson M, Siegemund M, Burhop K, Ince C. Hemoglobin-based oxygen carrier provides heterogeneous microvascular oxygenation in heart and gut after hemorrhage in pigs. J Trauma 2003; 55(6):1111–1124.

67. Katz LM, Manning JE, McCurdy S, Pearce LB, Gawryl MS, Wang Y, et al. HBOC-201 improves survival in a swine model of hemorrhagic shock and liver injury. Resuscitation 2002; 54(1):77–87.

68. Manning JE, Katz LM, Brownstein MR, Pearce LB, Gawryl MS, Baker CC. Bovine hemoglobin-based oxygen carrier (HBOC-201) for resuscitation of uncontrolled, exsanguinating liver injury in swine. Carolina Resuscitation Research Group. Shock 2000; 13(2):152–159.

69. Gould SA, Moore EE, Hoyt DB, Burch JM, Haenel JB, Garcia J, et al. The first randomized trial of human polymerized hemoglobin as a blood substitute in acute trauma and emergent surgery. J Am Coll Surg 1998; 187(2):113–120.

70. Gould SA, Moore EE, Hoyt DB, Ness PM, Norris EJ, Carson JL, et al. The life-sustaining capacity of human polymerized hemoglobin when red cells might be unavailable. J Am Coll Surg 2002; 195(4):445–452.

71. Sprung J, Kindscher JD, Wahr JA, Levy JH, Monk TG, Moritz MW, et al. The use of bovine hemoglobin glutamer-250 (Hemopure) in surgical patients: results of a multicenter, randomized, single-blinded trial. Anesth Analg 2002; 94(4):799–808, table.

72. Creteur J, Vincent JL. Hemoglobin solutions. Crit Care Med 2003; 31(12 Suppl):S698–S707.

73. Arnoldo BD, Minei JP. Potential of hemoglobin-based oxygen carriers in trauma patients. Curr Opin Crit Care 2001; 7(6):431–436.

74. Velmahos GC, Degiannis E, Souter I, Allwood AC, Saadia R. Outcome of a strict policy on emergency department thoracotomies. Arch Surg 1995; 130(7):774–777.

75. Grove CA, Lemmon G, Anderson G, McCarthy M. Emergency thoracotomy: appropriate use in the resuscitation of trauma patients. Am Surg 2002; 68(4):313–316.

76. Aihara R, Millham FH, Blansfield J, Hirsch EF. Emergency room thoracotomy for penetrating chest injury: effect of

an institutional protocol. J Trauma 2001; 50(6):1027–1030.

77. Rhee PM, Acosta J, Bridgeman A, Wang D, Jordan M, Rich N. Survival after emergency department thoracotomy: review of published data from the past 25 years. J Am Coll Surg 2000; 190(3):288–298.

78. Battistella FD, Nugent W, Owings JT, Anderson JT. Field triage of the pulseless trauma patient. Arch Surg 1999; 134(7):742–745.

79. Working Group, Ad Hoc Subcommittee on Outcomes, American College of Surgeons-Committee on Trauma. Practice management guidelines for emergency department thoracotomy. J Am Coll Surg 2001; 193(3):303–309.

80. Kron IL, Harman PK, Nolan SP. The measurement of intra-abdominal pressure as a criterion for abdominal re-exploration. Ann Surg 1984; 199(1):28–30.

81. Ivatury RR, Porter JM, Simon RJ, Islam S, John R, Stahl WM. Intra-abdominal hypertension after life-threatening penetrating abdominal trauma: prophylaxis, incidence, and clinical relevance to gastric mucosal pH and abdominal compartment syndrome. J Trauma 1998; 44(6):1016–1021.

82. Tiwari A, Haq AI, Myint F, Hamilton G. Acute compartment syndromes. Br J Surg 2002; 89(4):397–412.

83. Michard F, Teboul JL. Predicting fluid responsiveness in ICU patients: a critical analysis of the evidence. Chest 2002; 121(6):2000–2008.

84. Ba ZF, Wang P, Koo DJ, Cioffi WG, Bland KI, Chaudry IH. Alterations in tissue oxygen consumption and extraction after trauma and hemorrhagic shock. Crit Care Med 2000; 28(8):2837–2842.

85. Pastores SM, Katz DP, Kvetan V. Splanchnic ischemia and gut mucosal injury in sepsis and the multiple organ dysfunction syndrome. Am J Gastroenterol 1996; 91(9):1697–1710.

86. Doig CJ, Sutherland LR, Sandham JD, Fick GH, Verhoef M, Meddings JB. Increased intestinal permeability is associated with the development of multiple organ dysfunction syndrome in critically ill ICU patients. Am J Respir Crit Care Med 1998; 158(2):444–451.

87. Third European Consensus Conference in Intensive Care Medicine. Tissue hypoxia: how to detect, how to correct, how to prevent. Societe de Reanimation de Langue Francaise. The American Thoracic Society. European Society of Intensive Care Medicine. Am J Respir Crit Care Med 1996; 154(5):1573–1578.

88. Rivers E, Nguyen B, Havstad S, Ressler J, Muzzin A, Knoblich B, et al. Early goal-directed therapy in the treatment of severe sepsis and septic shock. N Engl J Med 2001; 345(19):1368–1377.

89. James JH, Luchette FA, McCarter FD, Fischer JE. Lactate is an unreliable indicator of tissue hypoxia in injury or sepsis. Lancet 1999; 354(9177):505–508.

90. Ivatury RR, Sugerman H. In quest of optimal resuscitation: tissue specific, on to the microcirculation. Crit Care Med 2000; 28(8):3102–3103.

91. Kincaid EH, Chang MC, Letton RW, Chen JG, Meredith JW. Admission base deficit in pediatric trauma: a study using the National Trauma Data Bank. J Trauma 2001; 51(2):332–335.

92. Porter JM, Ivatury RR. In search of the optimal end points of resuscitation in trauma patients: a review. J Trauma 1998; 44(5):908–914.

93. Rixen D, Raum M, Bouillon B, Lefering R, Neugebauer E. Base deficit development and its prognostic significance in posttrauma critical illness: an analysis by the trauma registry of the Deutsche Gesellschaft fur Unfallchirurgie. Shock 2001; 15(2):83–89.

94. Rutherford EJ, Morris JA, Jr, Reed GW, Hall KS. Base deficit stratifies mortality and determines therapy. J Trauma 1992; 33(3):417–423.

95. Siegel JH, Rivkind AI, Dalal S, Goodarzi S. Early physiologic predictors of injury severity and death in blunt multiple trauma. Arch Surg 1990; 125(4):498–508.

96. Davis JW, Parks SN, Kaups KL, Gladen HE, O'Donnell-Nicol S. Admission base deficit predicts transfusion requirements and risk of complications. J Trauma 1996; 41(5):769–774.

97. Rixen D, Raum M, Bouillon B, Lefering R, Neugebauer E. Base deficit development and its prognostic significance in posttrauma critical illness: an analysis by the trauma registry of the Deutsche Gesellschaft fur Unfallchirurgie. Shock 2001; 15(2):83–89.

98. Stacpoole PW. Lactic acidosis. Endocrinol Metab Clin North Am 1993; 22(2):221–245.

99. Totapally BR, Fakioglu H, Torbati D, Wolfsdorf J. Esophageal capnometry during hemorrhagic shock and after resuscitation in rats. Crit Care 2003; 7(1):79–84.

100. Baron BJ, Inerrt R, Zehtabchi S, Stavile KL, Scalea TM. Diagnostic utility of sublingual PCO_2 for detecting hemorrhage in patients with penetrating trauma. Acad Emerg Med 2002; 9:492.

101. Barquist E, Kirton O, Windsor J, Hudson-Civetta J, Lynn M, Herman M, et al. The impact of antioxidant and splanchnic-directed therapy on persistent uncorrected gastric mucosal pH in the critically injured trauma patient. J Trauma 1998; 44(2):355–360.

102. Ivatury RR, Simon RJ, Havriliak D, Garcia C, Greenbarg J, Stahl WM. Gastric mucosal pH and oxygen delivery and oxygen consumption indices in the assessment of adequacy of resuscitation after trauma: a prospective, randomized study. J Trauma 1995; 39(1):128–134.

103. Ivatury RR, Simon RJ, Islam S, Fueg A, Rohman M, Stahl WM. A prospective randomized study of end points of resuscitation after major trauma: global oxygen transport indices versus organ-specific gastric mucosal pH. J Am Coll Surg 1996; 183(2):145–154.

104. Jin X, Weil MH, Sun S, Tang W, Bisera J, Mason EJ. Decreases in organ blood flows associated with increases in sublingual PCO_2 during hemorrhagic shock. J Appl Physiol 1998; 85(6):2360–2364.

105. Marik PE. Sublingual capnography: a clinical validation study. Chest 2001; 120(3):923–927.

106. Povoas HP, Weil MH, Tang W, Moran B, Kamohara T, Bisera J. Comparisons between sublingual and gastric tonometry during hemorrhagic shock. Chest 2000; 118(4): 1127–1132.

107. Weil MH, Nakagawa Y, Tang W, Sato Y, Ercoli F, Finegan R, et al. Sublingual capnometry: a new noninvasive meas-

urement for diagnosis and quantitation of severity of circulatory shock. Crit Care Med 1999; 27(7):1225–1229.

108. Cosgriff N, Moore EE, Sauaia A, Kenny-Moynihan M, Burch JM, Galloway B. Predicting life-threatening coagulopathy in the massively transfused trauma patient: hypothermia and acidoses revisited. J Trauma 1997; 42(5): 857–861.

109. Jurkovich GJ, Greiser WB, Luterman A, Curreri PW. Hypothermia in trauma victims: an ominous predictor of survival. J Trauma 1987; 27(9):1019–1024.

110. Schreiber MA, Holcomb JB, Hedner U, Brundage SI, Macaitis JM, Hoots K. The effect of recombinant factor VIIa on coagulopathic pigs with grade V liver injuries. J Trauma 2002; 53(2):252–257.

111. Segal S, Shemesh IY, Blumenthal R, Yoffe B, Laufer N, Ezra Y, et al. Treatment of obstetric hemorrhage with recombinant activated factor VII (rFVIIa). Arch Gynecol Obstet 2003; 268(4):266–267.

112. Martinowitz U, Kenet G, Lubetski A, Luboshitz J, Segal E. Possible role of recombinant activated factor VII (rFVIIa) in the control of hemorrhage associated with massive trauma. Can J Anaesth 2002; 49(10):S15–S20.

113. Hedner U, Erhardtsen E. Potential role for rFVIIa in transfusion medicine. Transfusion 2002; 42(1):114–124.

114. Asensio JA, McDuffie L, Petrone P, Roldan G, Forno W, Gambaro E, et al. Reliable variables in the exsanguinated patient which indicate damage control and predict outcome. Am J Surg 2001; 182(6):743–751.

115. Johnson JW, Gracias VH, Schwab CW, Reilly PM, Kauder DR, Shapiro MB, et al. Evolution in damage control for exsanguinating penetrating abdominal injury. J Trauma 2001; 51(2):261–269.

116. Rotondo MF, Schwab CW, McGonigal MD, Phillips GR, III, Fruchterman TM, Kauder DR, et al. "Damage control": an approach for improved survival in exsanguinating penetrating abdominal injury. J Trauma 1993; 35(3):375–382.

117. Cinat ME, Wallace WC, Nastanski F, West J, Sloan S, Ocariz J, et al. Improved survival following massive transfusion in patients who have undergone trauma. Arch Surg 1999; 134(9):964–968.

118. Harbrecht BG, Alarcon LH, Peitzman AP. Management of shock. In Moore EE, Feliciano DV, Mattox KL, eds. Trauma. New York: McGraw-Hill, 2004; 201–226.

119. Blalock A. Acute circulatory failure as exemplified by shock and haemorrhage. Surg Gynecol Obstet 1934; 58:551–566.

120. Hollenberg SM, Kavinsky CJ, Parrillo JE. Cardiogenic shock. Ann Intern Med 1999; 131(1):47–59.

121. Hochman JS, Boland J, Sleeper LA, Porway M, Brinker J, Col J, et al. Current spectrum of cardiogenic shock and effect of early revascularization on mortality. Results of an International Registry. SHOCK Registry Investigators. Circulation 1995; 91(3):873–881.

122. Hochman JS, Sleeper LA, Godfrey E, McKinlay SM, Sanborn T, Col J, et al. Should we emergently revascularize occluded coronaries for cardiogenic shock: an international randomized trial of emergency PTCA/CABG-trial design. The SHOCK Trial Study Group. Am Heart J 1999; 137(2):313–321.

123. Rozycki GS, Feliciano DV, Schmidt JA, Cushman JG, Sisley AC, Ingram W, et al. The role of surgeon-performed ultrasound in patients with possible cardiac wounds. Ann Surg 1996; 223(6):737–744.

124. Rozycki GS, Feliciano DV, Ochsner MG, Knudson MM, Hoyt DB, Davis F, et al. The role of ultrasound in patients with possible penetrating cardiac wounds: a prospective multicenter study. J Trauma 1999; 46(4):543–551.

125. Boulanger BR, Kearney PA, Tsuei B, Ochoa JB. The routine use of sonography in penetrating torso injury is beneficial. J Trauma 2001; 51(2):320–325.

126. Nagy KK, Lohmann C, Kim DO, Barrett J. Role of echocardiography in the diagnosis of occult penetrating cardiac injury. J Trauma 1995; 38(6):859–862.

127. Peitzman AB, Billiar TR, Harbrecht BG, Kelly E, Udekwu AO, Simmons RL. Hemorrhagic shock. Curr Probl Surg 1995; 32(11):925–1002.

128. Roumen RM, Hendriks T, van der Ven-Jongekrijg J, Nieuwenhuijzen GA, Sauerwein RW, van der Meer JW, et al. Cytokine patterns in patients after major vascular surgery, hemorrhagic shock, and severe blunt trauma. Relation with subsequent adult respiratory distress syndrome and multiple organ failure. Ann Surg 1993; 218(6):769–776.

129. Landry DW, Oliver JA. The pathogenesis of vasodilatory shock. N Engl J Med 2001; 345(8):588–595.

130. Bone RC, Balk RA, Cerra FB, Dellinger RP, Fein AM, Knaus WA, et al. Definitions for sepsis and organ failure and guidelines for the use of innovative therapies in sepsis. The ACCP/SCCM Consensus Conference Committee. American College of Chest Physicians/Society of Critical Care Medicine. Chest 1992; 101(6):1644–1655.

131. Levy MM, Fink MP, Marshall JC, Abraham E, Angus D, Cook D, et al. 2001 Sccm/Esicm/Accp/Ats/Sis International Sepsis Definitions Conference. Crit Care Med 2003; 31(4):1250–1256.

132. Friedman G, Silva E, Vincent JL. Has the mortality of septic shock changed with time? Crit Care Med 1998; 26(12):2078–2086.

133. Angus DC, Linde-Zwirble WT, Lidicker J, Clermont G, Carcillo J, Pinsky MR. Epidemiology of severe sepsis in the United States: analysis of incidence, outcome, and associated costs of care. Crit Care Med 2001; 29(7):1303–1310.

134. Dellinger RP, Carlet JM, Masur H, Gerlach H, Calandra T, Cohen J, et al. Surviving Sepsis Campaign guidelines for management of severe sepsis and septic shock. Crit Care Med 2004; 32(3):858–873.

135. Gattinoni L, Brazzi L, Pelosi P, Latini R, Tognoni G, Pesenti A, et al. A trial of goal-oriented hemodynamic therapy in critically ill patients. SvO_2 Collaborative Group. N Engl J Med 1995; 333(16):1025–1032.

136. Hayes MA, Timmins AC, Yau EH, Palazzo M, Hinds CJ, Watson D. Elevation of systemic oxygen delivery in the treatment of critically ill patients. N Engl J Med 1994; 330(24):1717–1722.

137. Kreger BE, Craven DE, McCabe WR. Gram-negative bacteremia. IV. Reevaluation of clinical features and treatment in 612 patients. Am J Med 1980; 68(3):344–355.

138. Leibovici L, Shraga I, Drucker M, Konigsberger H, Samra Z, Pitlik SD. The benefit of appropriate empirical

antibiotic treatment in patients with bloodstream infection. J Intern Med 1998; 244(5):379–386.

139. Ibrahim EH, Sherman G, Ward S, Fraser VJ, Kollef MH. The influence of inadequate antimicrobial treatment of bloodstream infections on patient outcomes in the ICU setting. Chest 2000; 118(1):146–155.

140. Vallance P, Moncada S. Role of endogenous nitric oxide in septic shock. New Horiz 1993; 1(1):77–86.

141. De Backer D, Creteur J, Silva E, Vincent JL. Effects of dopamine, norepinephrine, and epinephrine on the splanchnic circulation in septic shock: which is best? Crit Care Med 2003; 31(6):1659–1667.

142. Hollenberg SM, Ahrens TS, Astiz ME, Chalfin DB, Dasta JF, Heard SO, et al. Practice parameters for hemodynamic support of sepsis in adult patients in sepsis. Crit Care Med 1999; 27(3):639–660.

143. Martin C, Papazian L, Perrin G, Saux P, Gouin F. Norepinephrine or dopamine for the treatment of hyperdynamic septic shock? Chest 1993; 103(6):1826–1831.

144. Martin C, Viviand X, Leone M, Thirion X. Effect of norepinephrine on the outcome of septic shock. Crit Care Med 2000; 28(8):2758–2765.

145. Sharshar T, Blanchard A, Paillard M, Raphael JC, Gajdos P, Annane D. Circulating vasopressin levels in septic shock. Crit Care Med 2003; 31(6):1752–1758.

146. Holmes CL, Patel BM, Russell JA, Walley KR. Physiology of vasopressin relevant to management of septic shock. Chest 2001; 120(3):989–1002.

147. Malay MB, Ashton RC, Jr, Landry DW, Townsend RN. Low-dose vasopressin in the treatment of vasodilatory septic shock. J Trauma 1999; 47(4):699–703.

148. Holmes CL, Walley KR, Chittock DR, Lehman T, Russell JA. The effects of vasopressin on hemodynamics and renal function in severe septic shock: a case series. Intensive Care Med 2001; 27(8):1416–1421.

149. Annane D, Sebille V, Troche G, Raphael JC, Gajdos P, Bellissant E. A 3-level prognostic classification in septic shock based on cortisol levels and cortisol response to corticotropin. JAMA 2000; 283(8):1038–1045.

150. Rothwell PM, Udwadia ZF, Lawler PG. Cortisol response to corticotropin and survival in septic shock. Lancet 1991; 337(8741):582–583.

151. Molijn GJ, Spek JJ, van Uffelen JC, de Jong FH, Brinkmann AO, Bruining HA, et al. Differential adaptation of glucocorticoid sensitivity of peripheral blood mononuclear leukocytes in patients with sepsis or septic shock. J Clin Endocrinol Metab 1995; 80(6):1799–1803.

152. Annane D, Sebille V, Charpentier C, Bollaert PE, Francois B, Korach JM, et al. Effect of treatment with low doses of hydrocortisone and fludrocortisone on mortality in patients with septic shock. JAMA 2002; 288(7):862–871.

153. Zeni F, Freeman B, Natanson C. Anti-inflammatory therapies to treat sepsis and septic shock: a reassessment. Crit Care Med 1997; 25(7):1095–1100.

154. Wheeler AP, Bernard GR. Treating patients with severe sepsis. N Engl J Med 1999; 340(3):207–214.

155. Lorente JA, Garcia-Frade LJ, Landin L, De Pablo R, Torrado C, Renes E, et al. Time course of hemostatic abnormalities in sepsis and its relation to outcome. Chest 1993; 103(5):1536–1542.

156. Boldt J, Papsdorf M, Rothe A, Kumle B, Piper S. Changes of the hemostatic network in critically ill patients—is there a difference between sepsis, trauma, and neurosurgery patients? Crit Care Med 2000; 28(2):445–450.

157. Powars D, Larsen R, Johnson J, Hulbert T, Sun T, Patch MJ, et al. Epidemic meningococcemia and purpura fulminans with induced protein C deficiency. Clin Infect Dis 1993; 17(2):254–261.

158. Bernard GR, Vincent JL, Laterre PF, LaRosa SP, Dhainaut JF, Lopez-Rodriguez A, et al. Efficacy and safety of recombinant human activated protein C for severe sepsis. N Engl J Med 2001; 344(10):699–709.

159. Silen W. Cope's Early Diagnosis of the Acute Abdomen, 20th ed. New York: Oxford University Press, 2000.

160. de Dombal FT. The OMGE acute abdominal pain survey. Progress report, 1986. Scand J Gastroenterol Suppl 1988; 144:35–42.

161. Boleslawski E, Panis Y, Benoist S, Denet C, Mariani P, Valleur P. Plain abdominal radiography as a routine procedure for acute abdominal pain of the right lower quadrant: prospective evaluation. World J Surg 1999; 23(3):262–264.

162. Siewert B, Raptopoulos V, Mueller MF, Rosen MP, Steer M. Impact of CT on diagnosis and management of acute abdomen in patients initially treated without surgery. AJR Am J Roentgenol 1997; 168(1):173–178.

163. Rosen MP, Siewert B, Sands DZ, Bromberg R, Edlow J, Raptopoulos V. Value of abdominal CT in the emergency department for patients with abdominal pain. Eur Radiol 2003; 13(2):418–424.

164. Rozycki GS, Tremblay L, Feliciano DV, Joseph R, DeDelva P, Salomone JP, et al. Three hundred consecutive emergent celiotomies in general surgery patients: influence of advanced diagnostic imaging techniques and procedures on diagnosis. Ann Surg 2002; 235(5):681–688.

165. Ahmad TA, Shelbaya E, Razek SA, Mohamed RA, Tajima Y, Ali SM, et al. Experience of laparoscopic management in 100 patients with acute abdomen. Hepatogastroenterology 2001; 48(39):733–736.

166. Cohen SB, Weisz B, Seidman DS, Mashiach S, Lidor AL, Goldenberg M. Accuracy of the preoperative diagnosis in 100 emergency laparoscopies performed due to acute abdomen in nonpregnant women. J Am Assoc Gynecol Laparosc 2001; 8(1):92–94.

167. Ou CS, Rowbotham R. Laparoscopic diagnosis and treatment of nontraumatic acute abdominal pain in women. J Laparoendosc Adv Surg Tech A 2000; 10(1):41–45.

168. Memon MA, Fitzgibbons RJ, Jr. The role of minimal access surgery in the acute abdomen. Surg Clin North Am 1997; 77(6):1333–1353.

169. Geis WP, Kim HC. Use of laparoscopy in the diagnosis and treatment of patients with surgical abdominal sepsis. Surg Endosc 1995; 9(2):178–182.

170. Navez B, d'Udekem Y, Cambier E, Richir C, de Pierpont B, Guiot P. Laparoscopy for management of nontraumatic acute abdomen. World J Surg 1995; 19(3):382–386.

171. Bender JS, Bouwman DL, Weaver DW. Bleeding gastroduodenal ulcers: improved outcome from a unified surgical approach. Am Surg 1994; 60(5):313–315.

172. Nishida K, Okinaga K, Miyazawa Y, Suzuki K, Tanaka M, Hatano M, et al. Emergency abdominal surgery in patients aged 80 years and older. Surg Today 2000; 30(1): 22–27.

173. van Geloven AA, Biesheuvel TH, Luitse JS, Hoitsma HF, Obertop H. Hospital admissions of patients aged over 80 with acute abdominal complaints. Eur J Surg 2000; 166(11):866–871.

174. Christou NV, Barie PS, Dellinger EP, Waymack JP, Stone HH. Surgical Infection Society intra-abdominal infection study. Prospective evaluation of management techniques and outcome. Arch Surg 1993; 128(2):193–198.

2
The Operating Theater for Acute Care Surgery

Kenneth L. Mattox

Case Scenario

A patient requiring acute surgical intervention is taken from the field and brought directly to the operating room. Which of the following is an appropriate criterion for this type of triage?

(A) Better temperature control
(B) Cost effectiveness
(C) Radiographic capabilities
(D) Expedient management
(E) Enhanced monitoring

Acute care operative procedures in 2005 continue to occur in the ambulance, emergency center, operating room, interventional radiology suite, cardiac catheterization laboratory, intensive care unit, and outpatient clinics. The need to consolidate these locations as much as possible continues. This chapter focuses on a stylized concept of the operative venue that allows the surgeon to optimize the operative and interventional procedures needed for the injured patient. Emergency center and intensive care unit as operative sites are not addressed in this chapter.

Evolving since the early 1960s, a single site for evaluation, resuscitation, operation, and intensive care has been developed by one trauma center, Maryland Institute for Emergency Medical Services System (MIEMSS). This venue was built around an intensive care module, incorporating the needs for the other functions in this location. Patients in need of interventional radiology or cardiothoracic surgery requiring cardiopulmonary bypass were moved to secondary locations. This pioneering concept opened the door for modern innovations in the expanding need for repeated and diverse procedures in trauma patients.

For decades, several trauma centers in different countries have championed the concept and principle of using the operating theater as the site for resuscitation, evaluation, intervention, and packaging before going to the surgical intensive care unit.[1-3] The acute care surgery operating theater of the future should be a "one stop shopping" area for patients requiring procedures, intervention, operation, or whatever term is used for invasive procedures. Secondary movement of patients to two, three, and even four different sites for procedural intervention should be eliminated by the design of an operative suite that accommodates current and future concepts of the need for acute care surgery.[4-7] For this approach, the size of individual operating rooms will need to be 1.5 to 2.5 times larger than they currently are to accommodate required additional equipment. The types of patients requiring such acute care surgery are clearly defined in the various chapters of this book.

The "ideal" acute care operating suite has not yet been designed. Individual preferences, structure barriers, folklore, and tradition have kept most operating rooms locked in the past—serving as a site where only major operations are performed. Many of the known devices, imagers, computers, robots, and built-in accouterments of the future acute care operative suite are in existence, often scattered in other areas of the hospital, clinic, or office locations. The concepts, regulations, visions, and policies that should govern that location are discussed.

Location Within the Hospital

Positioning an essential service within the hospital is key to the success of the function and mission of that activity. Essential to acute care surgery is a site to accomplish the many potential interventions required for such patients. With proper planning, the strategic location of the operative suite will obviate the need for duplicative procedural locations.[8,9] Elimination of these often unnecessary and redundant locations can result in not only considerable capital cost savings but also marked overall

TABLE 2.1. Locations that can be consolidated in the acute care operative theater.

Surgical resuscitation area of the emergency center
Interventional radiology suite for acute care surgical patients
Routine imaging x-ray facilities
Cardiac evaluation laboratories
Emergency vascular laboratory

efficiency and improvement in patient care. Procedure consolidation is especially important for patients with severe and multisystem trauma and those with injury severity scores greater than 15 (Table 2.1). In older hospitals where the location of services and the operating room were established for agendas of former decades, deliberate planning to position the acute care operative theater strategically is essential, although often difficult.

Relationship to Ambulance Unloading Dock

The ambulance unloading location and any helicopter landing pad are often in juxtaposition to the acute care center or connected to the resuscitation area by elevator. The "new" acute care operating theater concept allows the patient with critical injuries or injury severity scores above 15 to go directly from the ambulance unloading area to the procedural/diagnostic intervention area. Acute care surgery patients can be from the ambulance to the operating theater in less than 60 seconds. This concept bypasses the emergency department and transports the defined patient directly to awaiting surgeons who perform evaluation, diagnosis, and therapy in one location.

Relationship to the Emergency Center

In the future, the emergency center will be a site only for patients with more minor problems, minimizing the need for a sophisticated resuscitation area in that location. Patients with low acuity injuries will be either treated by emergency physicians for minor conditions or triaged to receive specialty care. Screening imaging will be expeditiously performed, allowing rapid dismissal, transfer to an observation unit, or admission to specialized areas where care can be continued by hospital-based specialists, including acute care surgical hospitalists, whose functional base will be the acute care surgery operating theater and acute care surgery intensive care unit. As the emergency center is often in juxtaposition to imaging, operative, and critical care locations (although not necessarily so in the hospital of the future), a mechanism to rapidly transport the patient from the emergency center to the acute care operating theater is mandatory. Obviously, some patients who appear to have minor surgical problems deteriorate during evaluation, and immediate transport to the surgical evaluation area of the acute care surgery operating theater is required.

Relationship to the Intensive Care Unit

On admission, it is optimal to move the critical acute care surgery patient *only twice*: (1) from ambulance to acute care surgery evaluation and operating suite and (2) from operating suite to the intensive care unit. Secondary surgery performed hours, days, or weeks later may require that the patient be returned to the operating theater. Therefore, it is desirable to have the acute care surgery intensive care unit in immediate juxtaposition to the operating theater. This also offers the important advantage of sharing personnel, surgeons, and specialized equipment between the two units. The ideally architecturally designed operating rooms and surgical intensive care units of the future will have a common imaging suite, stat laboratory, and support equipment. The operating area and the surgical intensive care unit will be in the same location, as is the design at MIEMSS.

Life Science and Building Safety Considerations

A multitude of regulatory and engineering standards apply to the operating room environment, and most are beyond the knowledge base of surgeons. For future acute care operating theaters, surgeons will be better served to have at least a basic knowledge of these standards and, in some instances, insist that there be no conflict of frequencies, currents, computers, and imaging devices.

Air Exchanges

Infectious disease standards (supported by the Joint Council on Accreditation of Healthcare Organizations) require a minimum of 20 air exchanges per hour in any operating room environment. Air exchange below that level results in increased infection rates. For critical acute care surgery patients who often have multiple body cavities open simultaneously, monitoring of air exchange standards is especially important.

Victims of terrorist activities, including biologic, chemical, radiologic, and blast contamination, will be treated in the acute care/trauma operative theater. For this special group of patients, even more advanced isolation technology will have to be in place to monitor airflow direction and exchange.

Temperature and Humidity Control

Developed in the days of open drip ether anesthesia, regulator standards exist for temperature and humidity control in operating rooms. These initially were to minimize fire and explosive risks. Some of these standards have not kept pace with technology. The temperature in the operating room was often kept low for the comfort of the surgeons because of the heavy (and hot) operative gowns. For acute care surgery and trauma patients, surgeons often ask that the operating room temperature be elevated to reduce the incidence of hypothermia and its accompanying coagulopathy. While adhering to safe standards, temperature control in the operating rooms of the future will be amenable to immediate change, depending on the needs of the patient.

Lighting

Every surgeon recognizes that proper lighting is paramount to successful surgical intervention. Improvements in optics have allowed for many varied approaches to such visualization. The operating room of the future will have stationary direct overhead lighting as well as intracavitary lighting and image enhancement. As new operating rooms are developed, the ever-advancing technology relative to lighting must be taken into consideration and utilized.

Electrical Safe Current Leakage Standards

Both the Association for the Advancement of Medical Instrumentation (AAMI) and the American National Safety Institute (ANSI) have developed electrical safe current leakage standards for hospitals, especially operating rooms, intensive care units, and cardiac catheterization laboratories. The purpose of these standards is to prevent the many lines entering the patient's body from becoming conductors of electronic pulses, causing cardiac arrhythmias. Appropriate grounding circuits and built-in detectors exist relating to electrical safe current limits. When an alarm indicates unsafe grounding or leakage, the procedure is terminated, and all intravenous and monitoring lines that might contribute to intracavitary electrocution or electrical pulses must be investigated and/or removed. With the increase in lines, monitors, and varying new solutions, knowledge of electrical safe current leakage standards is needed. Machine monitors and alarms do exist for electrical safe current leakage, and biomedical engineering personnel are responsible for surveillance and maintenance of these alarms. It is presented here to make the surgeon aware of this potential current risk.

Competing Microwave Signals

In operating rooms and intensive care units, for the most part competing microwave signals have been eliminated. However, because microwaves are overwhelmingly endemic in our society (cell phones, telemetered medical information, wireless computer LAN networks, two-way beepers, wireless personal communicating devices, television waves, radio waves, commercial transmissions, garage door openers, burglar alarms), some hospitals continue to prohibit cell phones within the hospital. The acute care operating theater of the future will have numerous devices that use microwave wireless communication. Even some of the hard-wired devices send out radio waves that can create "static" in other devices. Many hospitals currently have installed repeater transmitters in the ceilings and halls of their operating rooms and critical care units for wireless transmission to physician laptop/beeper communication devices and for other hospital medical record and information technology transmission. Wireless nurse call systems and telemetered physiologic devices are in place in many operating rooms and intensive care units. Designers of future hospitals must address potential interference among the many microwave devices.

Medical Informatics Capabilities

Information technology is the key to current and future health care, and the future acute care operating suite epitomizes the area of greatest need for integration of medical information technology.[10,11] Interactive computer systems will allow instant review of past operations and known medical conditions, allow for timely entry of new data, including imaging, physical findings, and procedures performed, as well as review imaging from the current hospitalization and outside diagnostic tests. Patients might even have implantable or carried information chips. Integration and assimilation of this complex information will be part of a surgeon's challenge and opportunity.

Internet Access

The operating room of today (and tomorrow) must be computer compatible, complete with Internet, intranet, and web-based capabilities. The many stored and web-based images (PACS), past medical records, medication records, and physician visits and reports of consultants can be instantaneously available to the surgeon, anesthesiologists, and others in the acute care operating suite. Internet consultation from surgical colleagues worldwide should be available.[12] Such services and capabilities are available today and must be incorporated into the operating room of the future.

Interfacing with Real-Time Clinical Information

During the course of the procedure, operative team members generate new clinical information derived from the dissection, physiologic monitoring, and/or online imaging and may instantaneously enter data into the patient's electronic medical record. These findings, the interpretation, and details of the progress of interventions are recorded for review by other authorized practitioners and will include immediate transmission to health payers, such as insurance companies, for (hopefully) real-time prompt payment for services rendered. Such systems also will allow for real-time concurrent quality management review and comparison of quality indicators to established benchmarks.

Imaging Capability

Imaging has been integral to the workup and treatment of acute care surgery patients and has ranged from emergency center ultrasonography to routine x-ray and computed tomography (CT) scanning, as well as special imaging, such as arteriography, venography, insertion of inferior vena cava filters, and vascular Doppler evaluation.[13] With the miniaturization of equipment and digitizing of many of the "images," it is now possible to integrate and consolidate the imaging equipment into an acute care surgery utilitarian evaluation and treatment location. That location should be the acute care operating suite. The surgeon will direct the choice of imaging as well as interpret those images, dictating the report in real time and acting immediately on the information. The acute care surgery operative suite should have installed (not portable) imaging equipment capable of CT scanning, total body routine x-ray imaging, and catheter-based interventions, including arteriography, venography, insertion and removal of devices, placement of stents, and embolization of bleeding. The capability to perform these imaging diagnostics and interventions concurrently with open and minimally invasive surgical procedures, without moving the patient to multiple locations, is the goal.

In addition, the suite should have the capability to record specific interventions via light mounted and handheld cameras. Arteriography and Doppler evaluations should be available for intraprocedural and postprocedural evaluations. The surgeon is expected to be proficient in the performance and interpretation of imaging for the acute care surgery patient.

Equipment Considerations

The acute care surgery operating theater contains appropriate and immediately available equipment. Basic equipment such as anesthesia machines, power equipment for drills, saws, and so forth, suction equipment, monitoring devices and electrocoagulation devices are to be in every operating room. In addition, the acute care surgery operating theater must have additional available equipment, complete with trained personnel capable of operating these devices.

Cardiopulmonary bypass, rapid infusion, and auto-transfusion devices are often required during acute care surgery. Cardiopulmonary bypass is sometimes used for patients with thoracic aortic transaction and occasionally for rewarming. Recycling a patient's own shed blood should be part of every operating room's blood conservation protocols. The anesthesiologists usually operate rapid-infusing devices. Such devices can also be an aid to rewarming. They, however, do add to the possibility of fluid overload wherever they are used. Rewarming devices, such as the Bair Hugger, body-warming water circulating devices, and special veno/veno devices, are used for patients with severe hypothermia.

The acute care surgery operating theater should contain appropriate "point of service" laboratory equipment for tests needed in the evaluation of acute care surgery patients. Necessary equipment includes devices to measure arterial blood gasses, activated clotting time, selected electrolytes, and selected hematologic determinations, such as hematocrit. Interpretation of these tests will be accomplished and applied in real time by the operative team, with billing occurring from this initial point of service interpretation, negating the duplicative later interpretations made at a time and place that do not impact patient care decision making.[14]

Required "Zones" in the Operation Environment

The acute care surgery operating theater is a complex constellation of zones. Hospital architectural planners, working with the nursing, anesthesiology, administrative, and surgical personnel must ensure that these zones exist and are juxtaposed appropriately. Form must follow function.

Administrative Zone

The administrative zones of operating theaters have traditionally been standardized. Sufficient space should be available for support and management offices, surgeons' offices, anesthesiologists' offices, clothing change area, and lounge area and conference room, complete with library and computer access. For the acute care surgery operating theater, it is especially important that the surgeons' and anesthesiologists' offices as well as "on call sleep rooms" be immediately adjacent to the operating rooms.

The administrative zone also usually contains a *pathology zone* where frozen sections may be done and where blood and other needed pathology adjuncts are stored. This area should be in immediate juxtaposition to the operating theater but outside the area where scrub suits are required.

Operating Zone

The actual operating room is a symphony of professional coordination and cooperation. It involves a synergistic interaction of technical skills, communication, and technology. However, every member of this team has an assigned zone of function and must respect the other's work zone.

Anesthesia Zone

The anesthesia area is a like a sacred cockpit, full of instrumentation, devices, equipment, and drugs. The anesthesia record should be computerized and integrated with the electronic patient record. Communication between the anesthesiologist and surgeon is essential. Differences of opinion on patient management relating to blood, fluids, blood pressure, pressors, antibiotics, and other strategies and protocols should be discussed before the operation. In the future, decision algorithms and best-practice protocols will aid discussion and will often be implemented and integrated automatically.

Surgeon's Zone

The surgeon and surgical first assistant take strategic positions to maximize their operative intervention. This position should not compromise the anesthesia area and should allow the scrub nurse area to be in close proximity to the surgeon area. To shorten the distance between the dominant hands of the surgeon and the scrub nurse is undoubtedly one of the most important operational functions for the expeditious accomplishment of the procedure. Of all the positions, the surgeon first chooses and communicates his or her selected positional venue.

Scrub Nurse's Zone

For optimal success of the technical aspects of the operation, the proximity position and simultaneous interaction between the surgeon and the scrub nurse are essential.

Circulator's Zone

For the operating theater of the future, the circulating nurse's area(s) are extremely busy and even more important. It is this area where many of the supporting and ancillary equipment are positioned and function, and the circulating nurse will operate many of these specialized devices. Some of the technical record-keeping and real-time quality review occur in this area.

Imaging Zone

Although past operating rooms had a view box for static x-rays, operating theaters of the future will have multiple arrays of imaging capability and computer screen interaction. Some images will be a computer-type monitor with trend analysis and data integration. Entire walls will be taken up equipment projecting digital information. A new operating theater team member will be a biomedical technologist to ensure that this imaging area is functional and current.

Observer's Zone

For acute care surgery, there are always observers at various levels with varying objectives. These observers may be any member of the health team and/or trainees in any one of multiple heath interest areas. It is essential that the observers do not interfere with the conduct of the procedure or contribute to an increased infectious risk, which has always been the standard. In the larger operating room with more equipment and technology, some consideration will need to be given to the best way to position the observation area so that the educational experience is optimized.

Interactive/Internet/Robotic Zone

It is inevitable that the acute care/trauma operating room of the future will have active interaction with distant electronic health capabilities, including telemedicine, teleconsultation, and robotic surgery.[12,15–20] All hospital operating theaters will actively be senders and receivers of such electronic perioperative interaction.

Storage Zone

Ask any operating room director about storage space, and he or she will say there is not enough. Architects and operating room nursing supervisors develop operative space based on existing knowledge, technology, and devices. Inevitably, each year, newer, larger pieces of equipment are developed. The multifunction of operating theaters of the future will likewise require considerably more storage space. The exact location for this storage is a matter of logistics. In addition to equipment, space is needed for pharmacy supplies, backup supplies, and "surprise" supplies, and the needed space for the central processing, cleaning, and sterilization of instruments inevitably is larger each year. Many instruments and supplies are single use and disposable, and the storage zone must allocate space for these. While "trash" is not necessarily stored, it is imperative that the regulatory mandates relating to contaminated materials be taken into consideration when planning storage space.

Engineering Zone

An engineering zone is usually not considered an essential zone of the operating theater. Because of the complexity of the trauma/acute care operating theater, it is essential that space be dedicated to the biomedical engineering, Internet, repeater, electronic, and basic engineering functions of this complex and multiple function environment.

Policy Issues

Operating theaters have always had the most rigid functional policies in the hospital. Clean, sterile, and substerile areas are clearly defined. Regulatory agencies and professional organizations have developed increasingly complex and ever-evolving policies relating to operating room environment. For the acute care/trauma operating theater with its all-encompassing role and expanded range of technology and equipment, increasing vigilance with applicable new and innovative policies is imperative.

Critique

With the possible exception of life-threatening (mother and fetus) acute problems in the pregnant patient, emergency rooms (particularly trauma bays) at tertiary facilities can adequately accommodate the patient who requires an emergency admission. However, there are occasions when direct transport to the operating room is the best decision. Rhodes et al.[2] highlighted the need for direct transport of patients to the operating room for expedient management when acute care surgical intervention is likely and the patient is severely hemodynamically compromised. Enhanced monitoring, state of the art radiographic equipment, and heating devices are readily available in the emergency department at almost all comprehensive hospitals. Cost effectiveness should not be the sole criterion for this triage decision.

Answer (D)

References

1. Hoyt DB. The impact of in-house surgeons and operating room resuscitation on outcome of traumatic injuries. Arch Surg 1989; 124:906–910.
2. Rhodes M. Direct transport to the operating room for resuscitation of trauma patients. J Trauma 1989; 29:907–915.
3. Wooten C, Kessler D, Kracun M, et al. Choreographing trauma resuscitation in the OR of the future. J AORN 1996; 64(3):415–423.
4. Berci G, Phillips EH, Fujita F. The operating room of the future: what, when and why? Surg Endosc 2004; 118:1–5.
5. Bucholz R, Macneil W, Mcdurmont L. The operating room of the future. Clin Neurosurg 2004; 51:228–237.
6. Feussner H. The operating room of the future: a view from Europe. Semin Laparosc Surg 2003; 10:149–156.
7. Marshall N. Theatre of the future arrives. Health Estate 2004; 58:27–29.
8. Satava RM. The operating room of the future: observations and commentary. Semin Laparosc Surg 2003; 10:99–105.
9. Selvam A. Thinking ahead. Three hospitals demonstrate that you can plan for the future, even if you can't foresee it. Hosp Health Netw 2002; 76(1):52–53.
10. Macario A, Vasanawala M. Technology and computing in the surgical suite: key features of an OR management information system and opportunities for the future. Anesth Analg 2002; 95(4):1120–1121.
11. Moses GR, Farr JO. The operating room of the future; white paper summation. Stud Health Technol Inform 2003; 94:226–232.
12. Doarn CR. Telemedicine in tomorrow's operating room: a natural fit. Semin Laparosc Surg 2003; 10:121–126.
13. Kashyap VS, Ahn SS, Davis MR, Moore WS, Diethrich EB. Trends in endovascular surgery training. J Endovasc Ther 2002; 9(5):633–638.
14. Liu CY, Spicer M, Apuzzo ML. The genesis of neurosurgery and the evolution of the neurosurgical operative environment: part II—concepts for future development, 2003 and beyond. Neurosurgery 2003; 52(1):20–33.
15. Camarillo DB, Krummel TM, Salisbury JK, Jr. Robotic technology in surgery: past, present and future. Am J Surg 2004; 188(4A Suppl):2s–15s.
16. Federspil PA, Geisthoff UW, Henrich D, Plinkert PK. Development of the first force-controlled robot for otoneurosurgery. Laryngoscope 2003; 113(3):465–471.
17. Marohyn MR, Hanly EJ. Twenty-first century surgery using twenty-first century technology: surgical robotics. Curr Surg 2004; 61:466–473.
18. Marescaux J, Rubino F. The ZEUS robotic system; experimental and clinical applications. Surg Clin North Am 2003; 83(6):1305–1315.
19. Rattner DW, Park A. Advanced devices for the operating room of the future. Semin Laparosc Surg 2003; 10:85–89.
20. Ruurda JP, van Vroonhoven TJ, Broeders IA. Robot-assisted surgical systems: a new era in laparoscopic surgery. Ann R Coll Surg Engl 2002; 84(4):223–226.

3
Anesthesia and Acute Care Surgery

Omid Moayed and Richard P. Dutton

Case Scenario

A 22-year-old man, previously healthy with no comorbidities, is undergoing acute care surgery and suddenly becomes tachycardic with a documented increase in expired CO_2. The anesthesiologist notices rigidity of the masseter muscles. Which of the following is the most prudent management decision at this time?

(A) Immediate cessation of the operation
(B) Insertion of a pulmonary artery catheter
(C) Administration of benadryl
(D) Change from volatile anesthetic agents to a total intravenous technique
(E) Temperature control (warming maneuvers)

Good surgery deserves good anesthesia. Emergency surgery requires it.

—Anonymous

Surgeons and anesthesiologists must work together to bring their patients the best possible outcomes, and this is especially true in emergencies. A mutual understanding of the challenges posed by acute care surgery patients is the basis for communication, efficiency, and good clinical results. The goal of this chapter is to provide the surgeon with an understanding of the anesthetic challenges posed by emergency cases, as seen from the anesthesiologist's perspective.

Prioritizing

The anesthesiologist is frequently the "gatekeeper" of the operating room suite, with the authority to determine which case reaches which room at which time. In most large hospitals this role will be filled during busy daylight hours from a select group of anesthesiologists with both interest and experience in administrative juggling. These self-selected individuals will generally have a good idea of appropriate priorities for the common emergent, urgent, and elective cases seen in their practice. On nights and weekends, however, the anesthesiologist in charge may be less familiar with the surgeons and their cases, less experienced in assigning priorities, and less adept at communicating and implementing decisions. Multiple conflicting priorities confronting a single on-call provider may contribute to a lack of focus on individual cases, with potentially disastrous results.

The most important factor in determining surgical priority is the acuity of the patient, which should be directly assessed by the anesthesiologist whenever possible. Some cases are so urgent that no other factor matters: the operation must be done immediately to have any chance of success. Obtaining a definitive airway, relieving pericardial tamponade, and controlling exsanguinating hemorrhage are three examples. Secondary considerations come into play in inverse proportion to the acuity of the emergency case. Important secondary variables in assigning priority include the personal schedule of the surgeon, the desires of the patient or family, the availability of nurses and technicians, and hospital rules involving block room assignment. "Right now" is always the simplest time to do an emergency case, but reality dictates that some patients, surgeons, and medical systems will be best served by planning the case for a time in the near future, when the necessary resources can be brought to bear in the least disruptive fashion. Conflicts should be resolved by face-to-face discussion between the surgeon and the anesthesiologist, following assessment of the patient.

Figure 3.1 is a brief schematic for categorizing the urgency of acute care surgical cases, including both trauma and nontrauma. *Immediate* cases are those that should be taken at once to the first available operating room. These include any case in which the patient's airway is threatened and any patient with a progressive

FIGURE 3.1. Acute care surgical case priority.

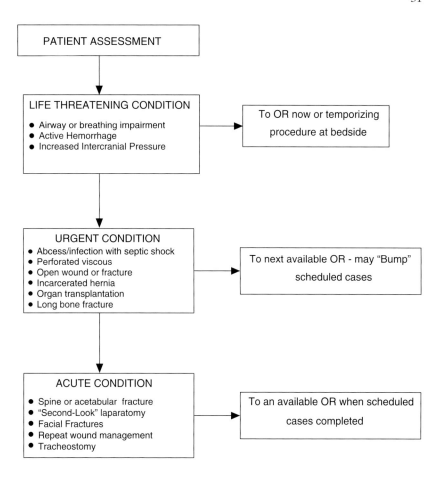

neurologic dysfunction, with cardiac tamponade, or with life-threatening hemorrhage. *Urgent* cases are those for which evidence suggests that the sooner they are completed, the better the patient's outcome will be. These include surgery for a perforated viscous, drainage of an abscess cavity, irrigation and debridement of open wounds, organ transplantation, relief of incarcerated hernias, and fixation of long-bone fractures. *Elective* emergency cases are not an oxymoronic concept but rather a large category of procedures that are not time sensitive except in the sense that the patient cannot leave the hospital until they are completed. These "add-on" cases are a challenge to the busy operating room because they must be fit into the operating room schedule as soon as possible, but without displacing previously scheduled patients. Examples include spinal and acetabular surgery, small bone and facial procedures, follow-on wound debridement and closure, tracheostomy, and feeding tube placement.

Preoperative Management

Preoperative assessment contributes strongly to good patient care. Preoperative assessment helps to avoid obvious pitfalls such as a critical medication allergy or a difficult airway. It also allows the formulation of an anesthetic plan to facilitate the proposed surgery. This can include elements as diverse as the choice of operating room to do the procedure in, the position of the operating room table, the amount of blood products ordered, or the specific medications administered. From the perspective of the patients and their families, a preoperative discussion with the anesthesiologist can reduce anxiety and facilitate postoperative analgesia.[1]

The preoperative assessment must be abridged in keeping with the urgency of the situation. For the patient presenting with severe respiratory, cardiovascular, or neurologic distress, there is little opportunity for discussion and no time for review of the medical records. The anesthesiologist must rely on the surgical team for a brief synopsis of the case, often at the same time as essential therapies are being provided (intubation, transport to the operating room, placement of arterial and venous access lines). Table 3.1 is a list of questions the anesthesiologist will consider when formulating an anesthetic plan, in approximate order of priority. Our usual policy is to begin asking these questions as soon as we encounter the patient and continue asking them while transporting to the operating room, attaching monitors, and making preparations for induction.

TABLE 3.1. Questions and considerations, in approximate order of relevance, for formulating an anesthetic plan.

- Chief complaint/indication for surgery
- Vital signs, including respiratory rate and volume
- Gross neurologic status: Glasgow Coma Score, cooperativity, movement of extremities
- Proposed surgery (patient position, likely blood loss)
- Major medical problems
- Medications
- Allergies to medication
- Personal or family history of anesthetic complications
- Recent consumption of alcohol or illegal drugs
- Examination of the airway: mouth opening, neck mobility, Mallampati class
- Further physical examination: heart sounds, breath sounds, open wounds, regional anesthesia site
- Results of diagnostic studies (arterial blood gas, complete blood count, coagulation factors, electrolytes, electrocardiogram, chest x-ray, assessments of cardiac risk, pregnancy test)
- Last meal (assume a full stomach in most cases)
- Detailed review of systems

The specific anesthetic plan will be determined by the nature of the surgical emergency. The anesthesiologist must consider what type of anesthesia to provide (regional vs. general), what drugs and techniques to use, what monitors and vascular access are indicated, what blood products to order, how to provide analgesia, and what postoperative care will be appropriate. Flexibility is required, as changing clinical circumstances frequently necessitate a change in anesthetic plans. To paraphrase von Clausewitz: No preoperative plan survives first contact with the actual patient.

Although regional anesthesia is safe and effective for most surgeries as compared with general anesthesia, the latter choice is almost always more appropriate in the emergency setting. Surgical extent and duration, blood loss, and patient condition are all unpredictable in emergency cases, making regional anesthesia problematic. The sudden fluid shifts produced by spinal or epidural anesthetics will complicate the management of shock, and any patient with a neurologic injury or intoxication will have difficulty cooperating with regional techniques. Furthermore, preemptive airway management allows for deeper levels of analgesia before, during, and after acute care surgery and frees the anesthesiologist for other tasks if a sudden deterioration occurs. Regional anesthetic techniques should be reserved for patients with the largest perceived benefit, motivation to cooperate with the procedure, and a surgical plan less likely to produce surprises. Regional analgesia *in combination* with general anesthesia is potentially more beneficial: adjuvant regional anesthesia will allow for lighter levels of sedation, more rapid emergence, and improved postoperative pain control, and it is a reasonable option in many emergency cases.[2] In some cases the regional anesthesia can

be performed before induction of general anesthesia; in other cases, pain with positioning, agitation, or patient preference necessitates placement following induction. The benefits of this approach must be carefully evaluated, because placement of an epidural catheter or regional block in an anesthetized patient is a controversial practice.[3] Improved analgesia must be weighed against the risk—slight but nonzero—of creating a new neurologic injury.

The American Society of Anesthesiology (ASA) has defined standard-of-care monitoring for any anesthetic (Table 3.2).[4] The anesthesiologist must consider the need for more advanced or invasive monitors based on the nature of the proposed surgery and on the patient's medical condition. Arterial access is indicated if frequent changes in blood pressure are likely or if there is a need for repeated laboratory assay. Central venous and pulmonary artery pressure monitoring is helpful for patients whose intravascular volume status and myocardial performance may be hard to determine. Transesophageal echocardiography (TEE) can be used in medical centers where this technology is readily available. Monitoring of intracranial pressure, somatosensory evoked responses, venous oxygen saturation, tissue oxygenation, or fetal heart rate may be indicated for specific emergency situations. In all cases, however, the anesthesiologist should not delay indicated surgery for the placement of monitors that can reasonably be placed once surgery is underway. The most important monitor during acute care surgery is the experienced anesthesiologist, who is able to integrate direct observation of surgical findings, including blood loss, with the patient's vital signs and response to anesthetic agents. From the surgical perspective, it is the presence and attention of an experienced anesthesia provider that should be insisted upon first in high-risk acute care surgeries or when a given case is going poorly.

TABLE 3.2. American Society of Anesthesiologists standard monitors for any anesthetic.

- A trained anesthesia provider continuously present during the procedure
- Oxygen content monitor and disconnect alarm for any mechanical ventilation system
- Exhaled oxygen and anesthetic gas analysis highly recommended for general anesthesia
- Continuous pulse oximetry
- Continuous electrocardiography
- Blood pressure monitoring: continuous or noninvasive at 5-minute (or less) intervals
- Continuous capnography
- Continuous temperature monitoring if appropriate

Source: Data from standards approved by the American Society of Anesthesiologists.[4]

Intraoperative Management

Intraoperative anesthetic care of the acute care surgery patient consists of the induction phase, in which the most likely cause of instability will be anesthesia related, and the maintenance phase, in which instability is more likely due to surgical manipulations and to the underlying pathophysiology of the patient. The choice of anesthetic agents and doses is important in preserving hemodynamic stability, interpreting changes in vital signs, and planning the postoperative course. Induction agents should be chosen based on the patient's fluid volume status and medical condition. Table 3.3 lists induction drugs and their most common side effects. It is important to recognize that even sympathomimetic agents such as ketamine may produce a profound decrease in blood pressure in the acute care surgery patient with a high circulating level of endogenous catecholamines.[5] This includes any patient who is hypovolemic from hemorrhage or sepsis, any patient with ongoing myocardial dysfunction, and any patient in significant pain. Medication-induced hypotension will be further exacerbated by the change from spontaneous ventilation to positive pressure mechanical ventilation following intubation. If uncertain regarding the patient's ability to tolerate a normal induction dose, the anesthesiologist should use smaller amounts in a titrated fashion. For the unstable patient, reduction of the induction dose may be more important than the choice of agent itself.

Most patients will receive a combination of intravenous narcotics and inhaled volatile gases for anesthetic maintenance. The ratio of one drug to the other has important implications. The more narcotic used, the less anesthetic-related vasodilation and negative inotropy will be present. This approach is appropriate for hemodynamically unstable patients who present to the operating room already in shock and for those patients with significant underlying myocardial dysfunction. Because narcotics have a much longer half-life than volatile gases, the patient maintained primarily on narcotics will emerge from anesthesia more slowly and will be more difficult to assess neurologically in the postoperative period. A volatile gas approach is more appropriate for the patient who is euvolemic and younger and for shorter procedures. Patients will emerge from anesthesia more rapidly if a larger proportion of their total anesthetic comes from volatile gases. The most common anesthetic pitfall, however, is failure to provide a sufficient anesthetic by either route, especially in the patient who is medically paralyzed to facilitate the surgical procedure. This can happen in the hypovolemic patient in whom hypotension leads to downward titration of anesthesia, using the patient's own sympathetic response to support the blood pressure. Because this is accomplished by way of significant vasoconstriction, the resulting hypoperfusion leads to an increased risk for organ system failure. A simple rule of thumb is that an otherwise healthy patient younger than 65 years of age should be able to tolerate the same quantity of anesthesia in either the elective or emergent situation. If the acute care surgery patient is not tolerating a normal dose of anesthesia, then hypovolemia or myocardial dysfunction should be suspected and must be definitively ruled out.

In addition to the patient's fluid volume status, there are other components of homeostasis that must be addressed during the maintenance phase of anesthesia. These include preservation of body temperature, continued administration of medically indicated drugs (beta-blockers, antibiotics), and attention to the prevention of positioning injuries. A fluid warmer should be used in any case requiring more than maintenance intravenous fluid therapy and in any case where packed red blood cells (PRBC) or plasma is administered. A forced hot air blanket should be used against the skin of any parts of the patient outside of the operative field, and the room temperature should be increased whenever the patient is significantly exposed. Active or passive humidification of the mechanical ventilation circuit will also reduce thermal loss. The anesthesiologist should be familiar with the patient's chronic medications and should continue to administer them as appropriate during the course of longer surgeries. Intravenous antibiotics are indicated for most acute care surgery patients; the choice of drug and the dosing interval should be discussed with the surgical team. Finally, the anesthesiologist should pay close attention to the patient's position throughout the intervention to avoid skin trauma and peripheral neurologic injury. Accessible portions of the body, such as the head and

TABLE 3.3. Induction drugs and common side effects.*

	Heart rate	Blood pressure	Analgesia	Nausea/vomiting	Dose (mg/kg)
Propofol	Decreased	Decreased	None	Decreased	2–2.5
Thiopental	Increased	Decreased	None	None	3–5
Ketamine	Increased	Increased	Yes	None	1–2
Etomidate	No change	No change	None	Increased	0.3
Narcotics	Decreased	Decreased	Yes	Increased	Drug dependent
Benzodiazepines	No change	Decreased	None	None	Drug dependent

* All dosages should be decreased for hypovolemic, elderly, or unstable patients.

arms, should be periodically repositioned during longer surgeries, and the anesthesia provider should be attentive to surgical maneuvers or changes in bed position that might put the patient at risk.

Postoperative Management

A common pitfall in emergency anesthesia care is the tacit assumption that the emergency patient will behave in similar fashion to a patient having the same operation on an elective basis: "a gallbladder is a gallbladder." This is frequently not the case. The patient undergoing elective laparoscopic cholecystectomy is far different physiologically from the patient presenting in septic shock. Myocardial reserve is decreased, anesthetic metabolism is prolonged, and fluid shifts will be more substantial. "Wind up" of the pain response may necessitate a higher dosage of analgesic medication to achieve the same degree of comfort. The time of day and the preoperative condition of the patient (intoxicated, head injured, full stomach) may be less conducive to emergence. The anesthesiologist and the surgeon, working together, must take these variables into consideration when determining both where the patient will go from the operating room (postanesthesia care unit [PACU] vs. intensive care unit [ICU]) and how quickly the patient is to be awakened and extubated.

The patient undergoing acute care surgery will typically emerge from anesthesia more slowly and will suffer more hemodynamic instability in the postoperative period than an elective patient. Reintubation in the PACU or ICU is a significant risk in this population, and conservative anesthesia practice is to send the patient out of the operating room still intubated and mechanically ventilated to allow for emergence and extubation on a delayed basis. When possible, informing the patient and family of this possibility in advance will help to relieve their anxiety. Our own practice is to transport the potentially unstable patient to the PACU still anesthetized and ventilated. Awakening is indicated by changes in the vital signs, overbreathing the ventilator, or movement and is initially treated with titrated doses of narcotic analgesics (usually morphine). The use of narcotics alone in this setting will provide adequate analgesia for the surgical wound, will suppress uncomfortable airway reflexes, and will avoid the sedating effects of benzodiazepines. For most patients, a sufficient narcotic load will allow for gradual, comfortable emergence. Because most muscle relaxants used for acute care surgery are short acting, there is not usually a need for reversal agents, although motor function must be clinically assessed before initiation of spontaneous ventilation. Ventilator support is weaned as tolerated based on the patient's respiratory rate, tidal volume, oxygen saturation, and end-tidal

TABLE 3.4. Extubation criteria following acute care surgery.*

- Adequate pain control
- Following commands or returned to baseline mental status
- Adequate pulmonary function (spontaneous respiratory rate 12–20; tidal volume >4mL/kg; $FiO_2 < 0.5$)
- Complete reversal of muscle relaxation (sustained head lift)
- Hemodynamic stability, not requiring rapid transfusion or bolus fluid therapy
- Normothermia
- Structurally adequate airway (air leak around endotracheal tube)
- No indication for surgery or other procedures that would benefit from continued intubation

*The patient must meet all of these criteria.

carbon dioxide levels. When minimal ventilator settings are achieved ($FiO_2 = 0.40$, pressure support of $10 cmH_2O$) we assess the patient for extubation using the criteria listed in Table 3.4.

The anesthesiologist and the surgeon share responsibility for completion of fluid resuscitation in the postoperative patient. Young patients, in particular, may achieve normal vital signs through compensatory vasoconstriction while still significantly hypovolemic. This "occult hypoperfusion syndrome"[6] is associated with an increased risk of subsequent organ system dysfunction and failure if not recognized and treated. Adequate systemic perfusion can be confirmed in a number of ways, including normalization of mixed venous oxygen saturation, maximization of cardiac output, and clearance of elevated serum lactate.[7]

Elderly patients, and those with known cardiovascular disease, present specific challenges in the postoperative period. Not only must adequate systemic oxygen delivery be ensured, but prophylaxis against myocardial ischemia should also be provided. It is reasonable based on current evidence to administer beta-adrenergic-blocking drugs to any elderly patient without specific risk factors throughout the perioperative period.[8] This is especially important in the 24 hours immediately following major surgery, when pain, shivering, and fluid shifts can all alter myocardial oxygenation for the worse.

Acute Care Situations

Intracranial Emergencies

Neurosurgical emergencies arise from conditions that increase intracranial pressure (ICP), reducing cerebral blood flow and thus brain tissue oxygenation. Elevated ICP will result in a decrease in the patient's level of consciousness and the potential for brain stem herniation and death if not promptly addressed. Trauma is the leading cause of increased ICP, as the result of epidural or subdural hemorrhage, intraparenchymal hemorrhage,

TABLE 3.5. Common neurosurgical emergencies.*

Case	Urgency	Duration	Blood loss	Postoperative pain	Potential for regional anesthesia
Subdural or epidural hematoma	1	2	2	3	2 (burr hole under local)
Intraparenchymal hemorrhage	2	4	1	3	4
Depressed skull fracture	3	3	2	3	4
Unstable cervical spine	2	3	3	2	4
Acute hydrocephalus	2	2	4	3	4

* Scale is from 1 to 4, with 1 being most urgent, shortest duration, least blood loss, greatest postoperative pain, and greatest potential for regional anesthesia.

or diffuse cerebral edema. Elevated ICP and the need for acute care surgery may also arise from spontaneous intracranial hemorrhage, intracranial malignancies, and impairment of cerebrospinal fluid circulation. Emergent craniectomy is indicated to correct the cause of increased ICP, and there is a strong time dependency of neurologic recovery on the speed with which surgery is performed. Table 3.5 lists the common neurosurgical emergencies.

In addition to the usual considerations outlined above, the anesthesiologist must initiate or continue maneuvers to improve cerebral oxygenation. These generally follow the guidelines of the Brain Trauma Foundation[9] and consist of the steps listed in Table 3.6. Application of these therapies depends on knowledge of the patient's intracranial physiology. This may be obtained from monitors of ICP (extradural catheters, intraparenchymal fiberoptic filaments, or ventricular catheters) and/or cerebral oxygenation (jugular venous bulb oxygen saturation, various investigational devices for measuring tissue perfusion). It is important for all anesthesiologists responsible for neurosurgical emergencies to have a working knowledge of the intracranial monitoring devices in use in their institution. This will allow for continued use during the perioperative period and will reduce the chance of iatrogenic complications (e.g., unintended closure of a ventriculostomy drain).

Pulmonary management should be directed toward aggressive support of cerebral oxygen delivery. Any patient with a deteriorating mental status should be promptly intubated, even before reaching the operating room. This is both to support ventilation and to avoid aspiration or sudden respiratory arrest during the cerebral CT that commonly precedes an acute care neurosurgery. Although it was once thought that increased levels of positive end-expiratory pressure (PEEP) would impair venous outflow from the brain, thus contributing to elevated ICP, it is now recognized that PEEP and other maneuvers to increase mean airway pressure are appropriate if they result in improved arterial oxygen saturation.[10] Hyperventilation acutely lowers ICP by vasoconstriction and reduction of cerebral blood flow. Because this therapy may exacerbate cerebral ischemia on the cellular level, it should be reserved for those

patients in imminent danger of herniation who are *en route* to acute care surgical decompression.[11] At all other times, the anesthesiologist should strive to maintain the patient's pCO_2 at normal levels.

Traditional teaching in neurosurgical emergencies was to limit fluid administration in an effort to reduce the development of cerebral edema. This approach is no longer recommended.[12] Volume restriction will lead to cerebral vasoconstriction and decreased cerebral blood flow, with disastrous consequences for brain tissue oxygenation. Brain trauma patients who experience even one episode of hypotension have substantially worse outcomes than those who do not.[13] Preservation of normal intravascular volume is the goal, which may require aggressive fluid administration to the patient with associated noncranial injuries. Placement of a pulmonary artery catheter or esophageal ultrasound probe to guide fluid volume therapy is appropriate in patients with severe neurologic conditions. Pressor or inotrope therapy may be necessary to support cerebral perfusion pressure, particularly for the patient requiring high-dose barbiturate therapy to reduce cerebral metabolism and ICP.

Although the acute care neurosurgical patient will typically have a depressed level of consciousness and may already have been intubated before reaching the operating room, normal anesthetic dosing is still appropriate. Analgesic therapy is important to minimize pain-mediated spikes in blood pressure and ICP. Muscle

TABLE 3.6. Maneuvers, in approximate order of application, to improve cerebral oxygenation.

- Optimization of systemic oxygenation
- Hemodynamic support
  - Fluid resuscitation to a euvolemic state
  - Pressor and/or inotropic therapy
- Elevation of the head and torso
- Adequate analgesia and sedation
- Drainage of cerebrospinal fluid via ventriculostomy
- Osmotic therapy
  - Mannitol
  - Hypertonic saline
- Barbiturate coma
- Decompressive craniectomy (controversial)
- Decompressive laparotomy (anecdotal/investigational)

relaxation, while not required for cranial exposure, is indicated as prophylaxis against sudden patient movement during delicate portions of the surgery, particularly if the patient's head has been secured in a rigid frame. Longer acting sedative/amnestic medications, such as benzodiazepines, should be avoided because they may cloud the assessment of neurologic status in the postoperative period. Inhaled volatile anesthetics are appropriate for intraoperative anesthesia; reduction in cerebral blood flow is more than counterbalanced by decreased metabolic demand at doses up to 1 MAC (minimum alveolar concentration).[14] Postoperatively, if an appropriate dose of analgesic has been administered, it should be possible to awaken and assess the patient without commitment to extubation. Even following the simplest of neurosurgical emergencies, such as relief of hydrocephalus or evacuation of an epidural hematoma, the patient will be slow to arouse. The anesthesiologist must recognize this and plan on continued postoperative mechanical ventilation until baseline neurologic function has recovered.

Neck Injury and Unstable Spine

Acute care spinal surgery is fortunately rare, as it is only indicated in patients with evolving neurologic deficits. Patients who are neurologically intact, and those with a complete spinal level unlikely to improve after surgery, are best treated on a scheduled basis, when it is easier to ensure the availability of the surgical specialist, the necessary instruments and hardware, and neurophysiologic monitoring. Emergent spinal surgery is commonly indicated for treatment of acute traumatic injuries, but can also be necessitated by an abscess or hematoma compromising the spinal canal. The common acute care procedures involving the neck or chest are listed in Table 3.7.

Airway management will be the first challenge for the anesthesiologist, as the potential exists for creating or worsening a spinal cord injury in the patient with an unstable cervical spine. Cooperative patients should receive an awake fiberoptic intubation following topical anesthesia of the upper airway and trachea, with general anesthesia withheld until confirmation of continued neurologic function after the patient has been positioned for surgery. Uncooperative patients or those with significant pulmonary compromise should undergo rapid-sequence intubation, with the diligent application of manual inline cervical stabilization throughout laryngoscopy and intubation.[15]

Hemodynamic instability may develop during surgery as the result of blood loss (more common with thoracic or lumbar fractures) or spinal shock (more common with cervical injuries). The anesthesiologist must first ensure that the patient has an adequate intravascular fluid volume (by TEE or pulmonary artery catheter monitoring) and should then add inotropic therapy in a titrated fashion to reverse the inappropriate vasodilation and negative inotropic state caused by the loss of sympathetic transmission.

The need for emergent neck exploration can arise following penetrating trauma or soft tissue infection. These cases will provide airway challenges similar to the patient with the unstable surgical spine and should be approached in a similar fashion. If time and patient cooperation allow, then fiberoptic examination and intubation of the airway under topical anesthesia and light sedation are desirable.[16] If the patient is in extremis, then a rapid-sequence approach is indicated, with a surgeon capable of emergent cricothyroidotomy standing by. Surgical debridement and drainage of a subpharyngeal or cervical abscess will usually be a short procedure, whereas exploration following penetrating trauma may lead to prolonged vascular or tracheal repairs. The anesthesiologist should have a sufficiency of monitoring and intravenous access to deal with all likely contingencies.

Extubation following either neck exploration or fixation of a cervical spine fracture should be approached with a great deal of trepidation, as edema and hematoma in the vicinity of the injury can produce rapid and lethal airway compromise following removal of the endotracheal tube.[17] In addition to the usual criteria for mental status, respiratory function, hemodynamic stability, and analgesia shown in Table 3.4, the anesthesiologist should also observe whether there is a leak of gas around the endotracheal tube when the cuff is deflated. Although not absolutely diagnostic, the presence of a leak around the

TABLE 3.7. Common emergencies involving the neck or chest.*

Case	Urgency	Duration	Blood loss	Postoperative pain	Potential for regional anesthesia
Threatened airway	1	1	4	3	2
Abscess	3	1	4	3	3
Penetrating neck injury	2	2	3	3	3
Traumatic aortic injury	2	3	1	1	4
Pulmonary hemorrhage	2	3	2	1	4
Bleeding after CT surgery	2	2	2	2	4

*Scale is from 1 to 4, with 1 being most urgent, shortest duration, least blood loss, greatest postoperative pain, and greatest potential for regional anesthesia.

tube is reassuring that the airway will not be critically compromised when the tube is removed.

Vascular Emergencies

The need for urgent vascular surgery may arise following blunt or penetrating trauma or as the result of atherosclerotic disease progression. Hemorrhagic disease (penetrating trauma to a large vessel, rupture of an aortic aneurysm) is an absolute emergency, whereas ischemic disease (trauma to a smaller vessel, thromboembolism) is urgent in proportion to the risk of infarction in the affected region of the body. Procedures to save a limb or organ threatened by end artery occlusion should be considered emergent.

Although elective vascular surgery patients have been shown to benefit from regional or combined regional and general anesthetic techniques,[18] this approach is less desirable in the emergency setting. Emergency procedures, especially those following trauma, are less predictable than elective cases and may take significantly longer than expected. The patient is also less well prepared and may be cold, acidotic, and vasoconstricted at the time of arrival in the operating room. Sympathetic blockade, while desirable in the long term, may cause significant short-term hypotension in the hypovolemic patient receiving a spinal or epidural anesthetic. Our own approach is to begin emergency cases with a careful general anesthetic. If the patient is likely to benefit from postoperative epidural analgesia, we will place the catheter at the conclusion of the procedure, following fluid volume resuscitation and normalization of coagulation parameters.

The need for systemic anticoagulation will complicate many acute care vascular procedures. This can be problematic for the patient who has multisystem injuries or who is already suffering dilutional coagulopathy secondary to hemorrhage and resuscitation. Close attention to coagulation studies is essential, as well as close communication with the surgeon to establish the degree of anticoagulation required.

Acute care vascular surgery patients will be at significant risk for perioperative myocardial ischemia and infarction. Although it may be tempting to delay surgery to pursue cardiac function studies such as dobutamine stress echocardiography, risk-benefit analysis rarely favors this approach.[19] First, it is unlikely that any cardiac intervention would be indicated before dealing with the acute care vascular condition. Second, it is appropriate to treat most acute care vascular surgery patients as the highest possible risk in any case. For the anesthesiologist this means a cardiac-friendly general anesthetic (generous narcotic administration, limited use of anesthetics with negative inotropic properties), perioperative beta-blockade, and the use of a specific cardiac function

monitor such as a pulmonary artery catheter or intraoperative TEE. Postoperative intensive care is usually indicated, and it is appropriate to plan for a gradual emergence from anesthesia with extubation only in the comfortable, resuscitated, and hemodynamically stable patient. Tachycardia is the most common risk factor for perioperative myocardial infarction, and any increase in heart rate should be aggressively treated with volume resuscitation, analgesia, and beta-blockade.[20]

Acute Abdomen

Abdominal emergencies include incarceration of hernias, acute appendicitis, diverticulitis, or cholecystitis, perforation of viscous organs, traumatic hemorrhage, bowel obstruction, and ectopic pregnancies. The suggestions for case prioritization presented above apply strongly to abdominal surgery cases, as does the recommendation for the attending anesthesiologist to personally see the patient as soon as possible. A brief visit can help to discriminate those patients who are well compensated and can afford to wait a short while from those who are septic, dehydrated, or otherwise severely compromised. In many situations rapid transportation to the operating room will facilitate intubation, placement of access and monitoring lines, and fluid volume resuscitation even before surgery begins. This is especially true if the patient is coming from an area of the hospital such as the emergency department where aggressive intensive care cannot be provided. Table 3.8 summarizes the common abdominal emergencies.

Beyond routine anesthetic concerns, successful facilitation of acute care abdominal surgery will generally depend on accurate management of the patient's cardiovascular system. Intraperitoneal hemorrhage arising from trauma or a perforated viscous can be rapidly life threatening, but is difficult to quantify until surgery begins. Nonhemorrhagic abdominal emergencies typically involve either acute sepsis (appendicitis, cholecystitis) or obstruction of the bowel. In either case acute inflammation, exacerbated by surgery, will lead to a rapid and profound "third-space" loss of intravascular fluid.[21] The anesthesiologist must be prepared for a large volume resuscitation, with adequate intravenous access and the ability to closely monitor the patient's circulation via central venous or pulmonary artery catheterization, TEE, or frequent laboratory analysis.

Postoperatively, caution is advisable in deciding to awaken the patient and wean them from mechanical ventilation. Although most patients undergoing straightforward appendectomy, cholecystectomy, or reduction of an incarcerated hernia can be extubated without difficulty (especially following laparoscopic surgery), patients undergoing more extensive surgeries should be allowed to emerge from anesthesia more gradually. Closure of the

TABLE 3.8. Common abdominal emergencies.*

Case	Urgency	Duration	Blood loss	Postoperative pain	Potential for regional anesthesia
Unstable blunt or penetrating trauma	1	3	1	1	4
Ruptured AAA	1	3	2	1	4
Perforated viscous	2	3	3	1	3
Stable penetrating trauma	2	3	3	2	3
Appendicitis	4	2	4	2	3
Acute cholecystitis	4	2	3	2	3
Bowel obstruction	3	3	3	1	3
Pelvic abscess	4	2	3	2	3
Tubal ectopic pregnancy	2	2	3	2	3
Testicular torsion	2	1	4	3	2
NASTI, septic shock	3	2	2	2	3

* Scale is from 1 to 4, with 1 being most urgent, shortest duration, least blood loss, greatest postoperative pain, and greatest potential for regional anesthesia. AAA, abdominal aortic aneurysm; NASTI, necrotizing acute soft tissue infection.

abdomen following major surgery may lead to increased intraperitoneal pressure, as injured and inflamed tissue continues to swell in the postoperative period. This abdominal compartment syndrome can significantly impair postoperative pulmonary function, even in the presence of attentive resuscitation,[22] Pressure on the diaphragm is less of a problem when the abdomen is left open, but fluid requirements will be substantial, and these patients are rarely stable enough for early extubation. Because muscle relaxation is required for abdominal exploration and subsequent closure, attention must be given to the adequacy of reversal at the end of the case. Acute care abdominal operations are also noteworthy for significant postoperative pain; for the patient who will not be taking oral medications, this leads to the use of intravenous patient-controlled analgesia for the first few postoperative days.[23]

Necrotizing Fasciitis, Soft Tissue Wounds, and Burns

Although usually not as exciting or dramatic as hemorrhagic or neurosurgical emergencies, soft tissue surgery occupies a large percentage of "off-hours" operating room time. Patients with open skin wounds require surgery for initial irrigation and debridement, follow-on surgeries for continued assessment, and an eventual definitive reconstruction and closure. The latter cases are clearly not emergent. Serial every-other-day irrigation and debridement procedures have a low urgency but cannot be completely disregarded because they are essential for moving the patient toward eventual closure and hospital discharge. Initial soft tissue surgeries have greater or lesser acuity depending on the patient's condition. Aggressive exploration and excision of dead tissue is an essential step in the treatment of the patient in septic shock from a necrotizing acute soft tissue infection (NASTI) and should be regarded as more urgent for patients who are less stable. Early fasciotomy of an extremity in a patient with compartment syndrome or a circumferential burn may be limb saving.[24] Early irrigation and sterile coverage of any skin defect will reduce the incidence and severity of subsequent infectious complications.[25]

The patient with an indication for emergent soft tissue surgery may be difficult to position on the operating room table and may require an intraoperative change in position to allow for complete surgical exposure. Because diabetes, obesity, and peripheral vascular disease are risk factors that predispose toward soft tissue infections (especially Fournier's gangrene), anesthetic management is usually not straightforward. General anesthesia is recommended for all but the most peripheral procedures, because surgical times are unpredictable, blood loss may be significant (particularly during the initial debridement), and the possibility of an active bacteremia is a contraindication to spinal or epidural needle placement. Once sepsis is controlled, an epidural catheter can facilitate both repeated operative procedures and ongoing analgesia.

Although uncontrolled arterial bleeding is unlikely, steady loss of blood from large areas of exposed fascia can quickly exsanguinate the soft tissue surgery patient. Large-bore intravenous access is recommended, along with the availability of cross-matched blood products and aggressive use of fluid and body warmers. The anesthesiologist should strive to maintain a reasonable hemoglobin concentration (8–10g/dL), adequate platelet count (>60,000), and normal coagulation factor function, particularly if the duration or extent of surgery is not clear. Especially during the initial, emergent, exploration and debridement it is wise to err on the side of overly vigorous resuscitation. Such patients will likely be getting sicker before they get better, while the requirement for multiple future surgeries will make it likely that any "over-transfused" blood products will simply delay the need for transfusion on another day. As with most acute care surgeries, the anesthesiologist should insist on adequate physiologic performance before considering an early extubation. Because the skin will usually not be closed, but simply covered with a vacuum or wet-to-dry dressing, soft tissue cases can end quickly. Allowing the patient some time in the PACU on mechanical ventilation to equilibrate fluids and fully recover from general anesthesia is often the wisest course of action.

The patient presenting in septic shock poses particular challenges. The patient will have a low systolic blood pressure because of both inappropriate vasodilation and myocardial depression induced by bacterial endotoxin. As for the hemorrhaging patient, anesthetic agents, particularly induction drugs, must be carefully titrated. An appropriate target level of anesthesia calculated to produce amnesia and analgesia should be selected, with fluids, inotropes, and vasopressors added as necessary to maintain perfusion pressure. It is difficult during the early stages of sepsis to discriminate hypotension due to vasodilation, which is best managed with fluid administration and judicious use of pressors, from hypotension due to myocardial dysfunction, which is best addressed with inotropes. The use of an intraoperative monitor of cardiac performance, such as a pulmonary artery catheter or TEE, is essential to guide fluid, drug, and anesthetic therapy.

Orthopedic Emergencies

Orthopedic operations account for a large percentage of unscheduled surgeries performed in most hospitals. Orthopedic emergencies—exsanguinating pelvic trauma or limb-threatening compartment syndrome—are rare, but urgent and acute orthopedic cases are common. The "urgent" category includes the treatment of open fractures of any bone and closed fractures of the long bones. Irrigation, debridement, and fixation of an open fracture is an urgent procedure, because the risk of osteomyelitis is directly related to the time interval between injury and definitive operative treatment.[26] Other orthopedic injuries may require urgent repair if they are associated with potentially reversible neurologic deficits, as discussed above for spinal surgery. Finally, dislocation of the hip, knee, shoulder, or elbow produces neurovascular compromise of the involved joint and is an indication for urgent sedation or general anesthesia to facilitate emergent reduction.[27] Table 3.9 lists the common orthopedic emergencies.

Early fixation of closed long-bone fractures is beneficial because it will facilitate patient mobilization and thus reduce the incidence of pulmonary complications.[28] Numerous retrospective studies have confirmed this finding, as summarized in the consensus statement of the Eastern Association for the Surgery of Trauma.[29] The benefits of early fixation must be weighed against the risks of aggravating other injuries, however, particularly for the patient with a significant traumatic brain injury (TBI). Some authors have found a worsening of outcome for patients with TBI undergoing early fracture fixation, whereas others have found no difference.[30,31] All of these studies agree, though, that early fixation is associated with an increased incidence of both hypotension and transient arterial desaturation in the operating room. Decisions regarding fluid resuscitation, anesthetic depth, and ventilator management may have a profound effect on the patient's ultimate outcome, meaning that close communication among the anesthesiologist, the operating surgeon, and the neurosurgical consultant is highly desirable. The decision to postpone or abbreviate indicated orthopedic procedures is not an easy one but may be necessary to avoid instability in a vulnerable patient who is not yet fully resuscitated.

The choice of anesthetic technique for the emergency orthopedic patient depends on the nature of the injury, the underlying health of the patient, and the duration of the intended surgery. Any patient with significant potential for hemodynamic instability should undergo a general anesthetic with endotracheal intubation, for the reasons listed earlier. Purely regional techniques should be reserved for patients with an appropriate mental status and degree of motivation, undergoing surgeries of predictable duration involving a single extremity (i.e.,

TABLE 3.9. Common orthopedic emergencies.*

Case	Urgency	Duration	Blood loss	Postoperative pain	Potential for regional anesthesia
Unstable spine	2	3	2	2	4
Unstable pelvis, shock	1	1	1	2	4
Open fracture	2	2	3	2	2
Closed long bone fracture	3	2	3	2	2
Acetabular fracture	3	3	3	1	2
Hip fracture	3	2	3	2	1
Reduction of dislocated joint	2	1	1	3	3

*Scale is from 1 to 4, with 1 being most urgent, shortest duration, least blood loss, greatest postoperative pain, and greatest potential for regional anesthesia.

isolated closed ankle fractures). However, the combination of regional and general anesthesia may provide the best of both techniques for patients undergoing extensive procedures. Use of epidural anesthesia for major orthopedic procedures of the femur, hip joint, and pelvis is associated with decreased intraoperative hemorrhage, decreased incidence of deep venous thrombosis, and improved postoperative analgesia.[32] Single-shot or catheter blockade of the brachial plexus can bring similar benefits to patients undergoing upper extremity or shoulder surgery.

Anesthetic challenges unique to orthopedic procedures include difficulty in finding sites for intravenous and arterial access, complex patient positioning to facilitate surgical exposure, and the physiologic changes produced by manipulation of unstable fractures. Transesophageal echocardiography has demonstrated that all patients undergoing internal medullary fixation of a femur fracture will experience embolization of fat and bone marrow.[33] The fat embolus syndrome (FES) occurs when this embolic challenge triggers an autoimmune reaction in the lungs.[34] The syndrome is characterized by the sudden onset of pulmonary hypertension, wheezing, hypotension, desaturation, petechiae, and disseminated intravascular coagulation. Treatment is supportive, beginning with the administration of intravenous fluids and epinephrine, and continuing with critical care management of acute respiratory distress syndrome, coagulopathy, and organ system failure. The ability to prophylax against FES with aggressive fluid volume administration before fracture manipulation has been proposed but not definitively confirmed.[35] There is no question, however, that the patient who is well resuscitated before the event will fare better during and after the onset of symptoms.

Pediatric Emergencies

Surgical emergencies in neonates are beyond the scope of this discussion, as they should be managed by specialty trained pediatric surgeons and anesthesiologists working in centers with the necessary experience and infrastructure to handle these cases well. Emergencies in older children, however, can present in almost any surgical or anesthetic practice. For the anesthesiologist, the key to successful management is a thorough understanding of

TABLE 3.10. Significant physiologic differences observed in pediatric patients undergoing acute care surgery.

- Reduced cooperation with procedures, especially with younger patients
- Reduced functional residual capacity, more rapid desaturation
- More compliant lungs and chest wall; usually easier to ventilate
- Lower baseline blood pressure and higher resting heart rate
- Increased compensation for hemorrhage; blood pressure decreases later than in adults
- More reliance on tachycardia to support cardiac output when stressed
- Increased heat loss
- Increased sensitivity to narcotics and sedatives

the differences between pediatric and adult physiology (Table 3.10). Although the goals of anesthesia are similar, the techniques by which they are achieved may need to be modified from the normal practice for adults. It is extremely important for the anesthesiologist to have knowledge of these differences, have all the equipment needed for pediatric cases, and be comfortable taking care of pediatric patients. Table 3.11 shows the three common emergencies presenting in older children.

The need for emergent surgery in children is most often precipitated by trauma, by airway compromise due to infection or foreign body aspiration, or by gastrointestinal tract compromise caused by appendicitis, hernia incarceration, or congenital abnormality. The acuity of the operation will vary as it will for an adult (as discussed earlier), but the practitioner must be wary of the rapid changes in vital signs that can occur in sick children when compensatory mechanisms for pulmonary or cardiovascular compromise are exhausted.

Children undergoing acute care surgery will require general anesthesia. Although anesthesia in elective pediatric patients is commonly induced by inhalation of a volatile gas and nitrous oxide before placement of an intravenous catheter, this approach may be more dangerous in the emergency setting. Although potentially traumatizing, placement of an intravenous catheter followed by rapid-sequence induction is the safest course for any child with the potential for hemodynamic instability. An exception to this rule is the child with an upper airway obstruction caused by epiglottitis or foreign body aspiration. Agitation may lead to the complete occlusion of a tenuous airway, meaning that the preferred approach

TABLE 3.11. Common pediatric emergencies.*

Case	Urgency	Duration	Blood loss	Postoperative pain	Potential for regional anesthesia
Aspirated foreign body	3	1	4	4	4
Epiglottitis	1	2	4	3	4
Fracture reduction	4	2	4	3	3

*Scale is from 1 to 4, with 1 being most urgent, shortest duration, least blood loss, greatest postoperative pain, and greatest potential for regional anesthesia.

is a gradual "breathe-down" induction until a deep enough level of anesthesia is reached that an intravenous catheter can be placed and the airway instrumented without a response from the patient.[36] Because of their smaller functional residual capacity and higher metabolic rate, apneic children will begin to desaturate much faster than apneic adults, even following adequate preoxygenation.

Once airway and intravenous access have been secured, successful anesthesia management in the pediatric patient is largely a matter of attention to detail. Temperature must be closely followed and the patient kept covered and actively warmed to the greatest degree possible. Blood loss must be carefully observed and adequate intravenous fluid therapy provided. Systemic narcotics will have a more profound effect on mental status than in adults and should be administered in a titrated fashion. Infiltration of the surgical site with a local anesthetic is highly recommended as an adjuvant to postoperative pain management. Most pediatric patients will emerge from anesthesia easily and should be extubated as soon as they are awake enough to support an open airway. Postoperative care should be in an age-appropriate unit.

Critique

This rapid onset of symptomatology in an otherwise healthy young man is malignant hyperthermia (MH) until proven otherwise. Although not highlighted in the vignette, hyperthermia would be associated with this presentation. Because MH is triggered by the use of volatile anesthetic agents in susceptible patients, the first step in treatment is a change in the anesthetic technique. Dantrolene sodium, a muscle relaxant, inhibits calcium release from the sarcoplasmic reticulum of the skeletal muscle, which is considered the key mechanism for this syndrome. Dantrolene sodium should be given intravenously (1–2.5 mg/kg). Although MH can make the patient rapidly unstable, immediate cessation of the operation will not always be practical and safe in the emergency setting.

Answer (D)

References

1. Egbert LD, Battit GE, Turndorf H, et al. The value of the preoperative visit by an anesthetist. JAMA 1963; 185:553.
2. Lubenow TR, Ivankovich AD, McCarthy RJ. Management of acute postoperative pain. In Barash PG, Cullen BF, Stoelting RK, eds. Clinical Anesthesia, 4th ed. Philadelphia: Lippincott, Williams & Wilkins, 2001: 1409–1410.
3. Horlocker TT, Abel MD, Messick JM, Jr, Schroeder DR. Small risk of serious neurologic complications related to lumbar epidural catheter placement in anesthetized patients. Anesth Analg 2003; 96:1547–1552.
4. Standards approved by the American Society of Anesthesiologists House of Delegates, October 1988, ASA Newsletter, December 1988.
5. Pagel PS, Schmeling WT, Kampine JP, et al. Alteration of canine left ventricular diastolic function by intravenous anesthetics in vivo: ketamine and propofol [published erratum appears in Anesthesiology 1992; 77:222]. Anesthesiology 1992; 76:419–425.
6. Blow O, Magliore L, Claridge JA, et al. The golden hour and the silver day: detection and correction of occult hypoperfusion within 24 hours improves outcome from major trauma. J Trauma 1999; 47:964–969.
7. Abramson D, Scalea TM, Hitchcock, et al. Lactate clearance and survival following injury. J Trauma 1993; 35:584–588.
8. Mangano DT, Layug EL, Wallace A, Tateo I. Effect of atenolol on mortality and cardiovascular morbidity after noncardiac surgery. Multicenter Study of Perioperative Ischemia Research Group. N Engl J Med 1996; 335:1713–1720.
9. Brain Trauma Foundation, American Association of Neurological Surgeons, Joint Section on Neurotrauma and Critical Care. Guidelines for the management of severe traumatic brain injury. J Neurotrauma 2000; 17:451–627.
10. McGuire G, Crossley D, Richards J, et al. Effects of varying levels of positive end-expiratory pressure on intracranial pressure and cerebral perfusion pressure. Crit Care Med 1999; 25:1059–1062.
11. Muizelaar JP, Marmarou A, Ward JD, et al. Adverse effects of prolonged hyperventilation in patients with severe head injury: a randomized clinical trail. J Neurosurg 1991; 75:731–739.
12. Frost EA. Perioperative management of the head trauma patient. Ann Acad Med Singapore 1994; 23:497–502.
13. Chestnut RM, Marshall LF, Klauber MR, et al. The role of secondary brain injury in determining outcome from severe head injury. J Trauma 1993; 134:216–222.
14. Todd MM, Drummond JC. A comparison of the cerebrovascular and metabolic effects of halothane and isoflurane in the cat. Anesthesiology 1984; 60:276.
15. Podolsky S, Baraff LJ, Simon RR, et al. Efficacy of cervical spine immobilization methods. J Trauma 1983; 23:461–465.
16. Desjardins G, Varon AJ. Airway management for penetrating neck injuries: the Miami experience. Resuscitation 2001; 48:71–75.
17. Epstein NE, Hollingsworth R, Nardi D, Singer J. Can airway complications following multilevel anterior cervical surgery be avoided? J Neurosurg 2001; 94:185–188.
18. Yeager MP, Glass DD, Neff RK, Brinck-Johnsen T. Epidural anesthesia and analgesia in high-risk surgical patients. Anesthesiology 1987; 66:729.
19. Chassot PG, Delabays A, Spahn DR. Preoperative evaluation of patients with, or at risk of, coronary artery disease undergoing non-cardiac surgery. BJA 2002; 89:747–759.
20. Mecca RS. Postoperative recovery. In Barash PG, Cullen BF, Stoelting RK, eds. Clinical Anesthesia, 4th ed. Philadelphia: Lippincott, Williams & Wilkins, 2001: 1382.

21. Buckley FB, Martay K. Anesthesia and obesity and gastrointestinal disorders. In Barash PG, Cullen BF, Stoelting RK, eds. Clinical Anesthesia, 4th ed. Philadelphia: Lippincott, Williams & Wilkins, 2001: 1044–1045.

22. Saggi BH, Sugerman HJ, Ivatury RR, Bloomfield GL. Abdominal compartment syndrome. J Trauma 1998; 45:597.

23. Smythe M. Patient-controlled analgesia: a review. Pharmacotherapy 1992; 12:132–143.

24. Mabee JR. Compartment syndrome: a complication of acute extremity trauma. J Emerg Med 1994; 12:651–656, 1994.

25. Haury B, Rodeheaver G, Vensko J, et al. Debridement: an essential component of traumatic wound care. Am J Surg 1978; 135:238.

26. Bednar DA, Parikh J. Effect of time delay from injury to primary management on the incidence of deep infection after open fractures of the lower extremities caused by blunt trauma in adults. J Orthop Trauma 1993; 7:532.

27. Kellam JF. Hip dislocations and fractures of the femoral head. In Levine AM, ed. Orthopaedic Trauma Association, American Academy of Orthopaedic Surgeons. Orthopaedic knowledge update: Trauma. Rosemont, IL: AAOS, 1996; 281–286.

28. Charash WE, Fabian TC, Croce MA. Delayed surgical fixation of femur fractures is a risk factor for pulmonary failure independent of thoracic trauma. J Trauma 1994; 37:667–672.

29. Dunham CM, Bosse MJ, Clancy TV, et al. Practice management guidelines for the optimal timing of long-bone fracture stabilization in polytrauma patients: the EAST practice management guidelines work group. J Trauma 2001; 50:958–967.

30. Jaicks RR, Cohn SM, Moller BA. Early fracture fixation may be deleterious after head injury. J Trauma 1997; 42:1–5.

31. Kalb DC, Ney AL, Rodriguez JL, et al. Assessment of the relationship between timing of fixation of the fracture and secondary brain injury in patients with multiple trauma. Surgery 1998; 124:739–744.

32. Holte K, Kehlet H. Effect of postoperative epidural analgesia on surgical outcome. Minerva Anestesiol 2002; 68:157–161.

33. Levy D. The fat embolism syndrome: a review. Clin Orthop Res 1990; 261:281.

34. Bulger EM, Smith DG, Maier RV, Jurkovich GJ. Fat embolism syndrome. A 10-year review. Arch Surg 1997; 132:435–439.

35. McDermott ID, Culpan P, Clancy M, Dooley JF. The role of rehydration in the prevention of fat embolism syndrome. Injury 2002; 33(9):757–759.

36. Gotta AW, Ferrari L, Sullivan C. Anesthesia for otolaryngologic surgery. In Barash PG, Cullen BF, Stoelting RK, eds. Clinical Anesthesia, 4th ed. Philadelphia: Lippincott, Williams & Wilkins, 2001: 996.

4
Fundamental Operative Approaches in Acute Care Surgery

David J. Ciesla and Ernest E. Moore

Case Scenario

A 55-year-old business woman is seen by the acute care surgeon for diffuse peritonitis. She is diaphoretic and hemodynamically labile. The patient stated that the onset of the sharp abdominal pain was abrupt and occurred 24 hours ago. Which of the following is the management approach of choice?

(A) Celiotomy
(B) Magnetic resonance imaging evaluation
(C) Computed tomography evaluation
(D) Laparoscopy
(E) Antimicrobial therapy and intensive care unit monitoring

Acute care surgical conditions present without warning and can encompass the entire field of surgery. Consequently, the acute care surgeon must be able to act decisively with incomplete information and unclear diagnoses. There is little time for preoperative preparation, and strategies often evolve as the operation progresses. Moreover, any anatomic region can present with an emergent condition, and multiple regions can be involved simultaneously. In preparation of this chapter, we reviewed all emergent operations performed at Denver Health Medical Center in 2002 and 2003. We excluded routine conditions such as appendicitis, cholecystitis, and superficial soft tissue infections with which all general surgeons are familiar. Trauma and nontrauma emergencies were categorized according to the anatomic region involved (Table 4.1). Although the abdomen was the most frequently involved region, the spectrum differed between trauma and nontrauma emergencies, with a greater proportion of trauma emergencies requiring attention outside the abdomen. Emergent cases were also classified according to the American Board of Surgery case reporting system (Table 4.2). The spectrum of surgical emergencies involves multiple aspects of general surgery that require thoracic and vascular expertise in addition to proficiency with alimentary and abdominal processes.

The aim of this chapter is to provide a standard operative approach to surgical emergencies based on anatomic regions. The ABCs of acute care resuscitation are well known as airway, breathing and circulation, but we also use this acronym to remind ourselves of the ABCs of acute care surgery. First, Assemble the team. Emergency conditions often require assistance from a myriad of services that not only includes operating disciplines such as anesthesia, neurosurgery and orthopedics but also ancillary services such as a blood bank and perfusionists. Next, Bring a book to the operating room. The nature of surgical emergencies does not allow much preoperative study, and it is critical to have a reference that reminds the acute care surgeon about the vital anatomic relationships in unfamiliar areas. Finally, Consider your protection. In emergent situations, the focus is usually on care of the deteriorating patient at the expense of personal safety. Moreover, actions often proceed much more rapidly than under nonemergent conditions, and there is greater potential for exposure to bodily fluids and contaminated sharps. Therefore, it is best to put on protective boots, eyewear, gloves, and gowns before assuming care of the patient rather than waiting until the situation reaches a crisis.

Patients requiring acute care surgery are in varying degrees of physiologic compromise. Metabolic derangements often require a damage control approach where the operation is suspended before definitive surgical therapy can be provided. Damage control can be applied to any anatomic region and is accomplished in three conceptual phases. The first phase involves abbreviated resuscitative surgery to control hemorrhage and contamination. Definitive reconstruction is deferred during this phase in favor of rapid measures to stem life-threatening

TABLE 4.1. Anatomic regions involved in acute care surgery.

Anatomic region	Trauma	Nontrauma
Neck	34 (10%)	3 (2%)
Chest	64 (19%)	21 (11%)
Abdomen and pelvis	191 (58%)	142 (75%)
Extremity	41 (12%)	23 (12%)

Source: Denver Health Medical Center, 2002–2003. From Ciesla DJ, Moore EE, Johnson JL, Moore JB, Cothren CC, Burch JM. The academic trauma center is the model for training the emergency surgeon. *J Trauma* 2005;58:657–662.

bleeding, restore perfusion where needed, and limit contamination. Wounds are closed temporarily, and the patient is transferred to the intensive care unit with the intent to return to the operating room under more favorable physiologic conditions. The second phase involves arresting of the "bloody viscious cycle" of acidosis, coagulopathy, and hypothermia by completing resuscitation in the intensive care unit. Adjunctive measures to refractory hemorrhage such as angiographic embolization are also carried out during this phase. The third phase consists of retuning to the operating room for definitive management of injuries and wound closure. Definitive wound closure is sometimes further delayed to allow reduction in tissue edema.

The decision to truncate the initial operation should be made when it appears likely that further operation is technically challenging without exceeding the patient's physiologic reserve. General indications include the inability to stop bleeding due to coagulopathy, an inaccessible major venous injury, and the need for prolonged operation in a patient with a suboptimal response to resuscitation.[1] Ideally, damage-control measures should be instituted as early as possible. Physiologic guidelines include a persistent base deficit of 10 or less, temperature of 33°C or less, and recalcitrant coagulopathy. The technical aspects of abridged surgery are dictated by the pattern of injuries. Procedures for expeditious vascular control include ligation of accessible blood vessels and selective arterial inflow occlusion using intravascular balloons and clamps. Temporary intraluminal shunts can be used to preserve distal tissue perfusion during resuscitation when there is extensive segmental vessel damage. Solid organ tamponade is achieved through gauze packing, circumferential mesh wrapping, and balloon catheter–type devices. Contamination from perforated intestine can be rapidly controlled by stapled closure or umbilical tape ligation. External tube drainage provides effective control of injuries to the biliary tree, pancreatic duct, and ureters. Once the goals of resuscitative surgery are met, wounds are temporarily closed with the aid of synthetic occlusive material. The specific approach to damage control is based on the anatomic region involved.

Key anatomic relationships and technical maneuvers are presented for each anatomic region. We focus on rapid exposure of key areas that allow surgical control, resection, and reconstruction of anatomic structures. Interfaces between traditional anatomic divisions such as the thoracic outlet and diaphragmatic hiatus often present difficult exposure problems (Figure 4.1). An approach to extending surgical incisions to expose an adjacent region is also provided. It is assumed that the reader is familiar with surgical principles and techniques on the level of a practicing general surgeon. The surgeon must be familiar with a versatile, self-retaining retractor that can be deployed rapidly. This is especially important where retraction is needed to expose the recesses of the abdomen such as the diaphragmatic hiatus and the pelvis.

Key Points

1. Assemble the team.
2. Bring an anatomy book to the operating room.
3. Begin communication with the anesthesiologist early in the case to gauge the physiologic state of the patient.
4. Consider damage control early.
5. Approach vascular injuries sequentially, starting with major arterial injuries and leaving contained hematomas for last.

TABLE 4.2. Spectrum of emergent operations.

Surgical emergencies	Trauma	Nontrauma
Alimentary tract	57 (17%)	88 (47%)
Stomach	7	16
Small bowel	23	33
Colon	27	39
Abdomen	101 (31%)	49 (26%)
General exploration	30	33
Abdominal decompression	7	11
Liver and biliary tract	35	0
Pancreas	9	5
Spleen	16	0
Abdominal wall	4	1
Vascular	87 (26%)	31 (16%)
Neck	9	1
Chest	11	3
Abdomen	26	4
Upper extremity	21	4
Lower extremity	20	19
Thoracic	53 (16%)	18 (10%)
Exploratory thoracotomy	6	16
Resuscitative thoracotomy	22	0
Repair diaphragm	9	0
Lung	5	1
Heart	11	1
Head and neck	25 (8%)	2 (1%)
Genitourinary	7 (2%)	1 (1%)
Total	330	189

Source: Denver Health Medical Center, 2002–2003. From Ciesla DJ, Moore EE, Johnson JL, Moore JB, Cothren CC, Burch JM. The academic trauma center is the model for training the emergency surgeon. *J Trauma* 2005;58:657–662.

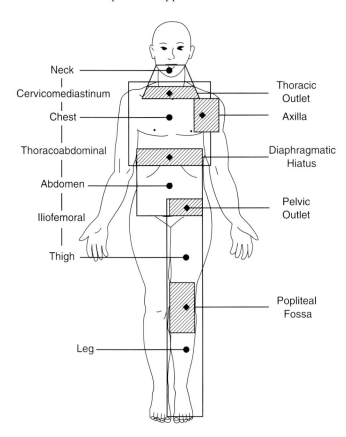

Neck — Cervicomediastinum — Chest — Thoracoabdominal — Abdomen — Iliofemoral — Thigh — Leg

Thoracic Outlet — Axilla — Diaphragmatic Hiatus — Pelvic Outlet — Popliteal Fossa

FIGURE 4.1. Interfaces between traditional anatomic divisions frequently present difficult surgical exposure problems.

Neck

Emergent Airway

Airway management is the first priority in the emergent setting. Surgical control of the airway is essential in the setting where orotracheal or nasotracheal intubation is contraindicated or impossible. The technique has been well described with minor variations. In brief, the cricothyroid membrane is identified by palpation between the thyroid and cricoid cartilage. A midline incision is made over the cricothyroid membrane to avoid injury to the anterior jugular veins and associated bleeding. Furthermore, a vertical incision can be extended superiorly or inferiorly if the cricothyroid membrane is initially misjudged. Confirmation of position is accomplished by palpation through the wound. The trachea is controlled by use of a trach-hook positioned on the inferior border of the thyroid cartilage. A transverse incision in the cricothyroid membrane is then made and enlarged bluntly. Finally, a 6-mm endotracheal tube is placed in the cricothyroidotomy under direct vision and secured to the neck. Relative contraindications to cricothyroidotomy include laryngotracheal separation, and patients less than eight years of age. In such cases, emergent tracheostomy may be necessary.

Alternatively, percutaneous transtracheal ventilation can be accomplished by inserting a large-bore intravenous catheter through the cricothyroid membrane, into the trachea, and attaching it with tubing to an oxygen source capable of delivering 50 psi or greater. A hole cut in the tubing allows for intermittent ventilation by occluding and releasing the hole. Adequate oxygenation can be maintained for greater than 30 minutes. However, because exhalation occurs passively, ventilation is limited; and carbon dioxide retention may occur.

Exposure

Exposure of the midline structures of the anterior neck is accomplished via a collar incision two finger breadths above the clavicles, extending laterally to the anterior boarder of the sternocleidomastoid muscle. The position of the skin incision can be varied according to the level of injury. An extension along the anterior boarder of the sternocleidomastoid muscle provides further lateral and superior neck exposure. Skin flaps deep to the platysma muscle raised superiorly to the thyroid cartilage and inferiorly to the suprasternal notch usually provide adequate exposure of anterior structures. Once exposed, the strap muscles are divided vertically in the midline to enter the pretracheal space. Complete mobilization of the sternothyroid muscles exposes the anterior trachea, thyroid, and bilateral carotid sheaths. The thyroid isthmus can be retracted superiorly or inferiorly or divided between clamps and suture ligated to expose the first three tracheal rings. The strap muscles can also be divided if more lateral exposure of the carotid sheath is required.

Unilateral neck exploration of the anterior triangle is accomplished via an incision along the anterior boarder of the sternocleidomastoid muscle from the mastoid process to the head of the clavicle (Figure 4.2). The omohyoid muscle crosses the anterior triangle of the neck deep to the sternocleidomastoid muscle and is retracted or divided as necessary. The carotid sheath is opened along the length of the incision to expose the carotid artery, jugular vein, and the vagus nerve. The facial vein, which marks the level of the carotid bifurcation, is divided and suture ligated. Lateral retraction of the jugular vein exposes the carotid artery. The ansa cervicalis, located within the carotid sheath, can also be divided without consequence.

Exposure of the distal carotid artery in zone three is difficult. The first step is division of the ansa cervicalis and mobilization of the hypoglossal nerve. Next, the portion of the posterior belly of the digastric is resected. Removal of the styloid process and attached muscles can be helpful. At this point, anterior displacement of the mandible becomes important. Some authorities have advocated division and elevation of the vertical ramus of the mandible. However, the parotid gland and facial

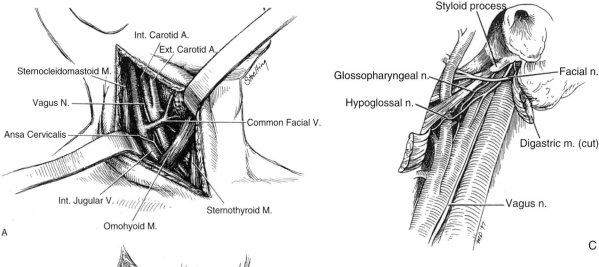

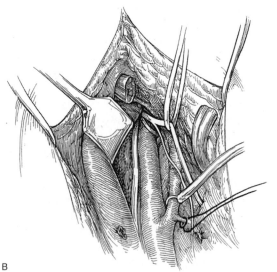

FIGURE 4.2. Vital Structures of the neck. **(A)** The relationship between the facial vein and the carotid bifurcation. The incision can be extended superiorly behind the ear for distal carotid exposure or inferiorly to a median sternotomy for proximal exposure. (Reprinted with permission from Ward RE. Injury to the cerebral vessels. In Blaisdell WF, Trunckey DD, eds. Trauma Management. New York: Thieme, 1986: 273.) **(B)** Key anatomic relationships of the distal internal carotid artery. The posterior belly of the digastric muscle has been divided and the mandible retracted anteriorly. Note the position of the hypoglossal and vagus nerves. (Reprinted with permission of Elsevier from Rutherford RB. Atlas of Vascular Surgery. Philadelphia: WB Saunders, 1993.) **(C)** Relative position of the facial, glossopharyngeal, and hypoglossal nerves to the internal carotid artery and styloid process. (Reprinted with permission of The McGraw-Hill Companies from Burch JM, Franciose RJ, Moore EE. Trauma. In Schwartz SI, Shires GT, Spencer FC, et al., eds. Principles of Surgery, 7th ed. New York: McGraw-Hill, 1999: 155–221.)

nerve prevent exposure of the internal carotid to the base of the skull. Excessive anterior traction on the mandible or parotid may damage the facial nerve; consequently, division of the ramus is seldom useful unless the surgeon is willing to resect the parotid and divide the facial nerve.

Proximal carotid, subclavian and vertebral arteries are approached through a supraclavicular incision located 1 cm above and parallel to the clavicle (Figure 4.3). The clavicular head of the sternocleidomastoid muscle is divided, the external jugular vein is divided and ligated, and the subclavian vein is retracted inferiorly. The anterior scalene muscle is then detached from the first rib to expose the second and third segments of the subclavian artery. Care must be taken to avoid transection of the phrenic nerve, which is surprisingly thin and traverses the surface of the anterior scalene muscle. This provides exposure of the subclavian artery, proximal vertebral artery, internal mammary artery, and thyrocervical trunk. The vagus nerve passes deep to the subclavian artery adjacent to the common carotid artery. Further exposure can be achieved by resection of the medial half of the

clavicle. Proximal injuries to the right subclavian artery sometimes require median sternotomy, whereas injuries to the proximal left subclavian artery are best approached through a left anterior lateral thoracotomy.

The cervical esophagus can be approached from either side thorough an incision along the anterior boarder of the sternocleidomastoid muscle. It is best to approach the distal cervical esophagus through a left neck incision. The sternocleidomastoid muscle is retracted laterally, and the omohyoid muscle is retracted or divided. The facial vein is ligated, allowing lateral retraction of the carotid sheath. When necessary, the inferior thyroid artery and the middle thyroid vein are divided and ligated. Medial retraction of the thyroid and trachea exposes the lateral esophagus. Care is taken to avoid injury to the recurrent laryngeal nerve, which lies in the tracheoesophageal groove. This is especially important if circumferential mobilization of the esophagus is required. Access to the space between the trachea and esophagus as well as the prevertebral space behind the esophagus is now possible.

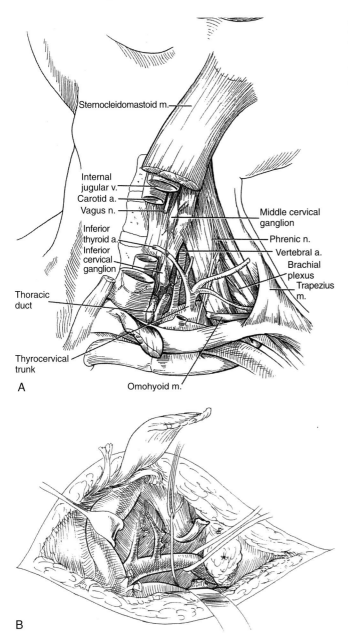

Sternocleidomastoid m.

Internal
jugular v.
Carotid a.
Vagus n.
Inferior
thyroid a.
Inferior
cervical
ganglion

Middle cervical
ganglion

Phrenic n.
Vertebral a.
Brachial
plexus
Trapezius
m.

Thoracic
duct

Thyrocervical
trunk

A   Omohyoid m.

B

FIGURE 4.3. **(A)** Vital structures of the proximal neck. **(B)** Retraction of the carotid sheath and scalene fat pad exposes the subclavian vessels and the anterior scalene muscles. The phrenic nerve is isolated, and the anterior scalene muscle is divided close to the scalene tubercle of the first rib. (A, B reprinted with permission from Wind GG, Valentine RJ. Anatomic Exposures in Vascular Surgery. Baltimore: Williams & Wilkins, 1991.)

Damage Control

The principles of damage control in the neck are to secure airway patency, stem blood loss, and control digestive tract contamination. The majority of airways are managed emergently by endotracheal intubation even with suspected tracheal violation. In cases of laryngotra-

cheal disruption or tracheal transection, the distal trachea has the potential for retraction into the mediastinum. Care must be taken to avoid airway occlusion by retraction of the wound edges during exposure while an endotracheal tube is placed into the distal trachea.

The initial maneuver to control active bleeding in the neck is direct pressure ideally using point control with the finger. Attempts at dissection, vessel identification, and clamping may worsen bleeding in an already unstable patient. Blind placement of clamps should specifically be avoided because of the risk of further injury to other vessels and nerves in close proximity. Difficult areas to control include the oropharynx and the base of the neck at the thoracic outlet. Intranasal packing or nasal placement of Foley catheter and balloon inflation can control profuse bleeding from the nose. Tight packing of the pharynx using laparotomy pads can usually control bleeding from the mouth. Endoluminal balloon occlusion using Fogarty-type catheters placed into the open end of a bleeding vessel or larger balloon-type catheters placed directly into the wound can provide effective control of bleeding and allow time for resuscitation or angiographic embolization. This technique is particularly useful for controlling vertebral artery injuries and carotid artery injuries near the skull base.[2] Distal perfusion past surgically accessible carotid injuries can be maintained temporarily using vascular shunts.

Esophageal contamination of neck wounds can result in lethal mediastinitis. Drainage of esophageal contamination can be temporarily controlled by placement of a nasogastric tube or a large T-tube directly into the esophagus through an esophageal wound. If more extensive drainage is required, a loop esophagostomy can be created, or the esophagus can be divided easily using an endoscopic stapler and the proximal end brought out through the wound as an end esophagostomy.

Key Points

1. Make a vertical incision and use a 6.0-mm endotracheal tube for emergent cricothyroidotomy.
2. For proximal exposure of major cervical vascular injuries, extend the cervical incision via a median sternotomy.
3. The facial vein lies directly superficial to the carotid bifurcation.
4. The hypoglossal nerve passes between the internal carotid artery and internal jugular vein then turns anteriorly across the lateral surface of the external carotid artery.
5. The recurrent laryngeal nerve is best found in the tracheoesophageal groove at the base of the neck.

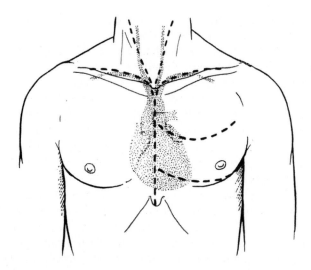

FIGURE 4.4. Incisions for thoracic emergencies. The choice of incision is based on the underlying injured vessel. Because the identity of the injured vessel is not always known, the surgeon must be prepared to extend the initial incision or perform additional incisions. (Adapted with permission of The McGraw-Hill Companies from Burch JM, Franciose RJ, Moore EE. Trauma. In Schwartz SI, Shires GT, Spencer FC, et al., eds. Principles of Surgery, 7th ed. New York: McGraw-Hill, 1999: 155–221.)

Chest

Incisions for thoracic emergencies are positioned according to the specific surgical emergency. In thoracic trauma, the identity of the injured vessel is not always known, and the emergency surgeon must be prepared to extend an incision or perform additional incisions (Figure 4.4).

Resuscitative Thoracotomy

Resuscitative thoracotomy is generically defined as that performed to revive patients from imminent or established cardiopulmonary arrest. Although this heroic procedure is most effective for penetrating cardiac wounds, it may be life saving for other exsanguinating intrathoracic injuries, pulmonary venous air embolism, or profound hypovolemic shock caused by massive hemorrhage from any source. The goals of emergency department thoracotomy are to (1) decompress pericardial tamponade, (2) control intrathoracic bleeding and air leak, (3) perform open cardiac massage, and (4) cross-clamp the descending thoracic aorta to redistribute blood flow to the heart and brain and to limit intraabdominal blood loss.

Successful resuscitative thoracotomy demands rapid entry into the chest. The skin incision is initiated at the sternal border and extended along the inframammary/pectoral crease to the midaxillary line. The incision is carried through the skin and chest wall muscles to the intercostals with a single continuous stroke. Placement of the incision directly on the body of a rib reminds the surgeon to curve the incision medially and laterally along the line of separation of an intercostal space. No attempt should be made to control chest wall bleeding until after resuscitative maneuvers are performed. The chest is entered laterally on top of the fifth rib with either knife to avoid injury to the heart. Two fingers are placed into the pleural space and the intercostal muscles divided between the fingers with scissors to protect the intrathoracic structures. The intercostal incision is extended medially to the sternum and posteriorly to the paraspinous muscles. Exposure can be enhanced by transecting the cartilaginous attachments of ribs above or below the intercostal incision at the left sternal border. A Finochietto retractor is then placed in the wound, with the rack toward the table in case an extension across the sternum is required (Figure 4.5).

The base of the left lung is elevated with the left hand, and the inferior pulmonary ligament is divided with a scissors. For profound hypovolemia, the descending thoracic aorta is cross-clamped just inferior to the left pulmonary hilum. Limited blunt dissection is generally

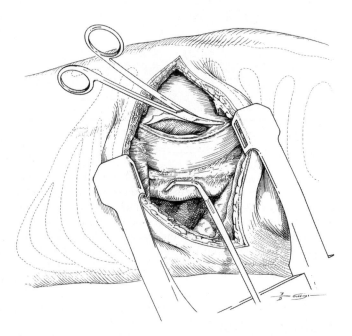

FIGURE 4.5. Open the pericardium anterior to the phrenic nerve. (Reprinted with permission of Elsevier from Moore EE. Emergency thoracotomy and aortic cross-clamping. In Moore EE, Eiseman B, Van Way CW, eds. Critical Decisions in Trauma. St. Louis: CV Mosby, 1984: 529.)

required to separate the esophagus from the aorta in the area of clamping. Proximal hilar injuries require prompt vascular control. After division of the inferior pulmonary ligament, the left pulmonary hilum is occluded between the fingers of the left hand. The right hand then places a Satinski clamp across the hilum from superior to inferior guided by the fingers of the left hand. An alternative is the hilar twist where the lung is torsed 180° about the pulmonary hilum after division of the inferior pulmonary ligament.

If there is evidence of intrapericardial blood or ineffective myocardial contraction, a generous vertical pericardiotomy is made anterior to the phrenic nerve large enough to deliver the heart for complete inspection or internal cardiac message. Open bimanual cardiac message is performed by placing the right hand behind the heart along the diaphragm and the left hand on the anterior surface of the heart. The heart is compressed with the flat of the hands over a large surface. Direct pressure with the fingertips must be avoided because of the potential for rupturing the ventricular wall.

Air embolism is a frequently overlooked lethal complication of pulmonary injury. The patient is placed in the Trendelenburg position to trap the air in the apex of the left ventricle. Emergency thoracotomy is followed by cross-clamping the pulmonary hilum on the side of the injury to prevent further introduction of air. Air is aspirated from the apex of the left ventricle with an 18-g needle and 50-cc syringe. Vigorous open cardiac massage is used to force the air bubbles through the coronary arteries. The highest point of the aortic root is also aspirated to prevent air from entering the coronaries or embolizing to the brain. Sometimes air can be aspirated directly from the right coronary artery. The patient should be kept in the Trendelenburg position and the hilum clamped until the pulmonary venous injury is controlled.

Anterolateral Thoracotomy

The left or right anterolateral thoracotomy is the most versatile incision for thoracic surgical emergencies. Because of the uncertain trajectory of bullets, it is the safest approach for gunshot wounds. Patients in extremis should remain in a supine position on the operating room table. Lateral positioning may limit access to the superior mediastinum or lesions in the opposite hemithorax, compromise ventilation of the dependent lung, or allow blood to spill over into the contralateral bronchial tree. A left anterolateral thoracotomy via the fifth intercostal space is preferred for resuscitation because this provides access for opening the pericardium, clamping the descending thoracic aorta or pulmonary hilum, and repair of most cardiac wounds.

Transsternal Anterior Thoracotomy

The left anterolateral thoracotomy, initially performed for resuscitation, is extended across the sternum through the right fifth intercostal space to provide access to right thoracic wounds or to improve exposure of the left chest. The transsternal incision is particularly important for controlling from the posterior mediastinum. The sternum is traversed with a Lebsche knife; the internal mammary arteries should be suture ligated following restoration of cardiac activity. Massive hemorrhage from pulmonary hilar wounds may be best controlled by intrapericardial ligation of the pulmonary veins as well as isolation of the main pulmonary artery.

The primary limitation of this incision is exposure of the superior thoracic aperture. For immediate vascular control of the aortic arch branches, the superior portion of the sternum should be opened with a Lebsche knife and the incision extended to the neck.

Left Book Thoracotomy

The left book or trap door thoracotomy is employed for access to the proximal left subclavian artery as it exits the posterior thoracic outlet, but its utility is controversial. The conceptual design is an en bloc left anterolateral thoracotomy, upper sternotomy, and left supraclavicular extension. Although the classic description consists of an initial third interspace incision, which entails an incision above the nipple traversing the breast or pectoralis major, we believe a standard submammary/pectoral skin incision with thoracic entry via the fourth intercostal space is preferable. The anterolateral thoracotomy is continued via the upper sternum and completed with a left supraclavicular incision, transecting the sternocleidomastoid and omohyoid muscles to disengage the trap door. The incision is technically challenging, and the underlying complex anatomy may be difficult to unravel within a large hematoma. Of note, the relatively small phrenic nerve should be isolated on the surface of the anterior scalene before this muscle is divided to access the subclavian artery distal to the thyrocervical trunk.

Under urgent conditions of free intrathoracic bleeding from a proximal left carotid or subclavian artery wound, median sternotomy with a left cervical extension may be done more expediently than the trap door configuration. Additionally, in cases where the left subclavian artery is injured outside the thoracic outlet, proximal subclavian control can be achieved through the anterolateral thoracotomy, and definitive repair can be achieved via separate supraclavicular incision without the intervening upper sternotomy.

Median Sternotomy

Median sternotomy has a relatively limited use for acute thoracic emergencies and is largely confined to anterior stab wounds to the heart or thoracic outlet injuries (Figure 4.6). Although a sternotomy provides an excellent view of the anterior surface of the heart, major injuries to the pulmonary hila may be difficult to manage, and posterior mediastinal structures are virtually inaccessible. The safety of median sternotomy can be ensured by preliminary blunt dissections of the retrosternal space via windows developed in the suprasternal notch and below the xiphoid process. The lungs should be deflated during sternal sawing to prevent violation of the pleural spaces. Finally, the initial separation of the sternal incision should be done slowly to avoid injury to the innominate vein, which is in close proximity to the upper sternum.

Median Sternotomy with Right or Left Cervical Extension

Rapid exposure of the proximal right subclavian, innominate, or proximal common carotid arteries is best achieved via a median sternotomy with appropriate cervical extension. A right supraclavicular incision is optimal to access the proximal right subclavian and innominate arteries, whereas carotid injuries in zone 1 of the neck are approached via extensions along the anterior border of the sternocleidomastoid muscle on the involved side. The strap muscles are divided to expose the proximal common carotid artery.

Left Posterolateral Thoracotomy

Posterolateral incisions also have a limited role in thoracic surgical emergencies. The conspicuous exception is an injury to the descending thoracic aorta, which is almost always due to blunt trauma. A large soft tissue incision is warranted under emergent conditions; the skin incision is begun under the left nipple and extended posteriorly below the tip of the scapula. The latissimus dorsi, serratus anterior, and trapezius muscles are divided to free the shoulder girdle. The typical blunt aortic injury occurs just distal to the left subclavian artery and is approached through the fourth interspace, whereas more distal injuries are approached through the sixth interspace. Transection of a rib posteriorly provides adequate exposure without the time required for rib resection.

Exposure

Great Vessels

The great vessels of the chest are best exposed through a median sternotomy or a bilateral anterolateral thoraco-

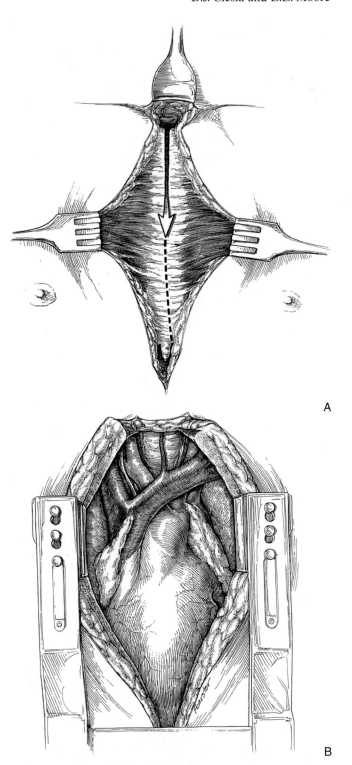

FIGURE 4.6. The median sternotomy. **(A)** The incision is made from the suprasternal notch to one side of the xiphoid process. **(B)** Final exposure of the great vessels through a median sternotomy. The thymus is not shown. (A, B reprinted with permission of Elsevier from Rutherford RB, Atlas of Vascular Surgery. Philadelphia: WB Saunders, 1993.)

tomy with transsternal division. Incision is made over the sternum in the midline from just below the suprasternal notch to below the xiphoid process. Blunt dissection beneath the sternum at the suprasternal notch and xiphoid process protects the underlying structures from injury during sternal division. The thymus is then divided in the midline to expose the anterior pericardium and great vessels. Proximal exposure of the aorta and superior vena cava requires opening the pericardium.

The left brachiocephalic vein can be dissected free and retracted to expose the origin of the innominate artery. Extension of a median sternotomy to a right neck incision along the anterior border of the sternocleidomastoid muscle exposes the innominate artery bifurcation, whereas extension to a right supraclavicular incision exposes the proximal right subclavian artery. This exposure requires lateral retraction of the internal jugular vein. Care must be taken to avoid injury to the phrenic nerve and the right vagus nerve, which passes over the anterior surface of the subclavian artery and the recurrent laryngeal nerve as it passes behind the subclavian artery.

The proximal left common carotid artery is somewhat more posterior than the innominate artery and is obscured by the left brachiocephalic vein. The innominate vein must be retracted inferiorly and the proximal internal jugular vein retracted laterally. Extension of the incision along the anterior border of the left sternocleidomastoid muscle provides exposure of the more distal left common carotid artery. Because the course of the aortic arch is anterior to posterior, it is difficult to reach the origin of the left subclavian artery through a median sternotomy. If a median sternotomy has been performed, the incision is extended to a trap door incision by transecting the sternum in the third or fourth intercostal space and adding a left supraclavicular incision. In hemodynamically unstable patients, initial control is achieved by applying pressure to the apex of the left chest through a left anterolateral thoracotomy. The superior lobe of the left lung is then retracted inferiorly to expose the aortic arch. The vagus nerve passes over the aortic arch just proximal to the origin of the left subclavian artery. The parietal pleura over the aortic arch is opened posterior to the vagus nerve.

Descending Thoracic Aorta

The descending thoracic aorta is exposed via a posterolateral thoracotomy in the fourth intercostal space. The left lung is deflated and retracted anteriorly. The aorta is then visible from the origin of the left subclavian artery to the diaphragmatic hiatus.

Esophagus

Surgical emergencies involving the thoracic esophagus (penetrating or barogenic perforation) usually involve the distal one third of the esophagus. The distal thoracic esophagus is approached through a left thoracotomy in the sixth intercostal space. The lung is retracted anteriorly after division of the inferior pulmonary ligament. The parietal pleura is then opened over the distal aorta, and the esophagus is dissected circumferentially. The area of esophageal injury is mobilized generously to ensure complete inspection of the injured segment and to allow easy manipulation. The distal esophagus and cardia of the stomach can be exposed by incision in the diaphragm at the esophageal hiatus and pulling the gastroesophageal junction into the chest. Because the aortic arch obscures the esophagus in the left chest, esophageal injuries proximal to the left pulmonary hilum are approached through the right chest. Division of the azygous vein at the superior aspect of the right pulmonary hilum is necessary for proximal exposure of the thoracic esophagus.

Pulmonary Hilum

The pulmonary hilum is optimally exposed through a posterolateral thoracotomy with the patient in the lateral decubitus position. However, most emergent operations begin with the patient in the supine position requiring an anterolateral thoracotomy. Placing extra padding under the involved side of the chest helps elevate the hilum with the patient in the supine position. The chest is entered through the fifth intercostal space because the critical anatomy of the lungs is at the hilar level. The intercostal muscles are divided in the rib space from the sternum to the transverse spinous processes. The key maneuver to exposing the hilar structures is traction on the lung to bring the hilar structures out from the mediastinum.

The anterior aspect of the pulmonary hilum is exposed by posterolateral retraction of the deflated lung. Dissection of the left pulmonary hilum is begun by incision in the pleura overlying the pulmonary artery. The soft tissue in the space bounded by the aortic arch, the vagus nerve, and the phrenic nerve is opened by sharp dissection. The main pulmonary artery is the most superior structure and is located just under the aortic arch. The superior pulmonary vein is the most anterior structure overlying the bronchus and pulmonary artery. The inferior pulmonary vein is identified within the medial aspect of the inferior pulmonary ligament. It is sometimes necessary to obtain control of the pulmonary veins from within the pericardium. The right pulmonary hilum is exposed in a similar fashion. The azygous vein courses over the superior margin of the right pulmonary hilum and can be divided for enhanced exposure of the right mainstem bronchus. The right pulmonary artery lies immediately anterior to the bronchus. The pulmonary veins are anterior and inferior to the pulmonary artery.

The posterior aspect of the pulmonary hilum is exposed by medial retraction of the lung. The bronchus is the most posterior structure in relation to the pulmonary artery and vein. The parietal pleura is incised at the transition of the chest wall to visceral pleura on the hilum. The pulmonary arteries lie anterior and lateral to the accompanying bronchus except for the left main pulmonary artery, which passes posterior to the left upper lobe bronchus. All pulmonary arteries are invested within a distinct perivascular sheath, which must be entered to be in the correct dissection plane. The pulmonary veins generally lie anterior and inferior to the artery and bronchus.

Damage Control

The quintessential damage-control maneuver in the chest is the resuscitative thoracotomy in the emergency department. The goal is to restore physiology by dramatic but temporary maneuvers so that the patient can survive transport to the operating room where definitive treatment is given. Once in the operating room, several damage-control techniques are used according to the injuries present. Exsanguinating abdominal injuries are addressed through a laparotomy with the aortic cross-clamp in place. Patients requiring cross-clamp times exceeding 30 minutes rarely survive. The damage-control maneuvers for thoracic injuries are slightly different from those for the abdomen. The emphasis in the chest is to provide rapid definitive treatment rather than suspend repair until after resuscitation in the surgical intensive care unit (SICU). This is because the physiologic requirements with respect to filling of the heart and expansion of the lungs do not tolerate packing as a method for controlling major bleeding.

Bleeding from cardiac wounds is initially controlled during resuscitative thoracotomy by digital pressure using a skin stapler directly on the myocardium. Once transported to the operating room, myocardial injuries are definitively repaired using large permanent sutures and pledgets on the right ventricle. Injuries to the great vessels and aorta are repaired primarily or with synthetic grafts. Placement of intravascular shunts maintains distal perfusion so that the operation can be suspended until resuscitation in the SICU is complete. In the dying patient, ligation of the carotid or subclavian arteries should be considered. Ligation of the subclavian artery is surprisingly well tolerated. If the patient survives, reconstruction using bypass grafts can be performed at a later operation.

Anatomic pulmonary resections are associated with a high mortality rate for patients with severe lung injury.[3] Nonanatomic resections and tractotomy using stapling devices provide for rapid exposure and control of parenchymal bleeding and air leaks.[4,5] Tractotomy is well tolerated because of the extensive collateralization of the lung.

Damage control of esophageal injuries is aimed at preventing mediastinal sepsis. Proximal esophageal drainage is accomplished by placement of an orogastric tube or creation of a cervical esophagostomy. Thoracic drainage is achieved by placement of chest tubes. Placement of gastrostomy or jejunostomy tubes can be delayed until later operation once resuscitation in the SICU is complete.

Thoracic incisions can be closed temporarily by using a large monofilament suture to approximate the skin. Laparotomy pads can be placed below the sternum to prevent the cut edges of the bone from injuring the heart. Occasionally, swelling of the postischemic myocardium and lungs as a result of resuscitation will prevent closure of the chest. In such cases, the wound is packed with laparotomy pads and closed with an adhesive impermeable surgical barrier (Ioban, 3M Corp.). Definitive closure is delayed until swelling resolves, usually within 23 to 48 hours.

Key Points

1. For hemodynamically unstable patients, begin with a transsternal left anterior thoracotomy and extend across the sternum if necessary.
2. Place the aortic cross-clamp below the left pulmonary hilum after dividing the inferior pulmonary ligament.
3. Open the pericardium anterior to the phrenic nerve.
4. Clamp the injured pulmonary hilum to control air embolism.
5. The pulmonary arteries are located anterior and lateral to the associated bronchus except for the left main pulmonary artery, which is posterior to the left upper lobe bronchus.
6. Avoid anatomic resections for penetrating trauma in favor of stapled pulmonary tractotomy.
7. Identify the phrenic nerve, which is surprisingly small, on the anterior scalene muscle when dissecting the proximal right subclavian artery.

Abdomen

The abdomen is the most frequently involved body region requiring acute care surgery (see Table 4.1). Although the general surgeon routinely performs abdominal operations, acute care surgery often requires exposure of structures not commonly encountered in elective procedures. This section focuses on rapid exposures of difficult areas of the abdomen. Anatomically, the abdomen is divided into three zones, the supramesocolic, containing the liver, spleen, and pancreas; the inframesocolic, containing the root of the mesentery; and the pelvis, containing the rectum and iliac vessels. Retroperitoneal structures include the pancreas, kidneys, aorta, and vena cava.

Incision

All emergent abdominal explorations in patients older than 6 years are performed using a midline incision because of its versatility (Figure 4.7). The ability to reach all parts of the abdomen and eviscerate the patient is mandatory. The midline laparotomy is easily extended with a transverse incision if enhanced exposure is required laterally or extended superiorly to a median sternotomy or across the costal margin into a rib space when pathology extends into the mediastinum or thorax. A transverse incision above the umbilicus extended well

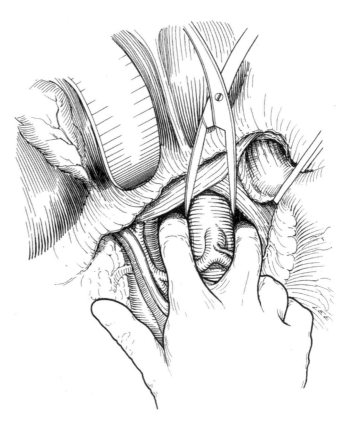

FIGURE 4.8. Control of the aorta at the diaphragmatic hiatus. (Reprinted with permission from Champion HR, Robbs JV, Trunkey DD. Rob and Smith's Operative Surgery, 4th ed. Trauma Surgery, Parts 1 and 2. London: Butterworths, 1989.)

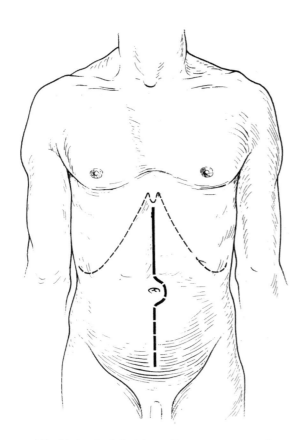

FIGURE 4.7. Abdominal incisions. Emergency procedures are performed through a midline laparotomy from the xiphoid process to the symphysis pubis. Additional exposure is achieved by extensions to median sternotomy, left thoracotomy, and unilateral or bilateral subcostal incisions. (Adapted with permission from Champion HR, Robbs JV, Trunkey DD. Rob and Smith's Operative Surgery, 4th ed. Trauma Surgery, Parts 1 and 2. London: Butterworths, 1989.)

onto the flanks may be appropriate for children under the age of 6 years. If the patient has been in shock or is currently unstable, no attempt should be made to control bleeding from the abdominal wall until major sources of hemorrhage have been identified and controlled. The incision should be made with a scalpel rather than with an electrosurgical unit because it is faster.

Liquid and clotted blood is rapidly evacuated with multiple laparotomy pads, and the aorta is palpated at the diaphragmatic hiatus to estimate blood pressure and a dialogue initiated with the anesthesiologist to determine the need for temporary aortic occlusion. If exsanguinating hemorrhage originates near the midline in the retroperitoneum, direct manual pressure is applied with a laparotomy pad and the aorta clamped at the diaphragmatic hiatus (Figure 4.8). The stomach and esophagus are retracted to the left to expose the right crus of the diaphragm. The posterior peritoneum is then divided between the right crus and the aorta. The index and middle fingers are placed on either side of the aorta as a guide to place a large curved vascular clamp parallel to the fingers pushed against the spine. Cephalad division of the median arcuate ligament and right crus can extend exposure over the lower thoracic aorta. The diaphragm is dissected laterally from the aorta into the posterior mediastinum. Although 5 to 7 cm of aorta can be exposed from this approach, more proximal control requires a left thoracotomy either by extension of the midline laparotomy or by separate incision. Circumferential dissection at this level is not recommended because of the presence of inferior phrenic and segmental arteries that are easily torn.

With massive ongoing bleeding, the source is addressed directly with fingers or by firm pressure of a laparotomy pad and fist while exposure is achieved. If the liver is the source of massive hemorrhage, the hepatic pedicle should immediately be clamped (Pringle maneuver) and the liver compressed by tightly packing several laparotomy pads between the injury and the underside of the anterior chest wall. In all other cases, a rapid palpation of the liver and spleen is performed, and, if injuries are confirmed, additional pads are placed in the respective upper quadrants.

For patients in cardiopulmonary arrest, closed cardiac message is ineffective in the presence of hypovolemia. Although the heart can be compressed by applying pressure to the underside of the diaphragm against the chest wall, opening the diaphragm and delivering the heart into the abdomen allows more effective open cardiac massage. An incision in the central tendon of the diaphragm to the left of the xiphoid process opens the inferior pericardium. Bimanual compression is then performed through the pericardiotomy. An exception is a suspected penetrating wound to the suprarenal aorta, in which case extension of the laparotomy across the left costal margin to a left thoracotomy is the preferred approach.

Exploration

Formal abdominal exploration should immediately follow control of life-threatening hemorrhage. A systematic evaluation of all abdominal contents is required to ensure that all pathology is identified at the initial operation. Although the sequence of exploration may vary with surgeon preference and the condition of the patient, exploration generally begins with evaluation of the liver and spleen. The root of the mesentery is inspected by retraction of the colon superiorly and evisceration of the small bowel to the right. The stomach, duodenum, small bowel, and colon are examined along with the mesentery. The posterior wall of the stomach can be visualized by entering the lesser sac through the anterior leaf of the gastrocolic omentum. Exploration of the retroperitoneal structures, including the kidneys, pancreas, aorta, and vena cava, is performed when clinically indicated and is described below.

Exposure

Supramesocolic Viscera

Suprarenal Aorta

Exposure of the supramesocolic aorta is accomplished by right medial visceral rotation that includes all abdominal contents to the left of the aorta (Figure 4.9). When the operation is initiated through a midline laparotomy, the left colon is mobilized along the lateral retroperitoneal attachments. The splenorenal and splenophrenic ligaments are divided, and the colon, spleen tail of the pancreas, and stomach are rotated medially. The left kidney and ureter can be left posterior or elevated with the adrenal gland and tail of the pancreas. This exposes the upper aorta at the diaphragmatic hiatus and includes exposure of the celiac axis, left renal artery, and origin of the superior mesenteric artery. The supraceliac abdominal aorta is exposed by dividing the left crus of the diaphragm. Dividing the celiac ganglion, which surrounds the celiac trunk at its origin on the aorta, exposes the celiac axis. Exposure of the thoracic aorta from within the abdomen is achieved by entering the left chest through circumferential incision in the diaphragm 3 cm from the intercostal margin. Alternatively, the left chest is entered by extending the midline laparotomy across the costal margin and performing a thoracotomy through an intercostal space. Control of the thoracic aorta is then accomplished by division of the left inferior pulmonary ligament and isolation of the aorta against the vertebral body. The distal abdominal aorta and proximal left iliac artery are exposed by medial reflection of the sigmoid colon and mesentery. Distal exposure of the left iliac artery and the right iliac artery is difficult with this approach and should be accomplished through an anterior transperitoneal approach.

Esophagus

Esophageal exposure is maximized by carrying the superior extent of the incision to the junction of the costal cartilages with the xiphoid process. This allows increased lateral retraction of the costal margin opening up the upper abdomen. The left lobe of the liver can usually be retracted superiorly and to the left, which, along with superolateral retraction of the left costal margin and inferior retraction of the stomach, exposes the esophageal hiatus. If the liver is large, division of the left triangular ligament allows retraction of the liver to the right. However, this can result in fracture of the cirrhotic or fatty infiltrated liver. To isolate the esophagus, the gastrohepatic ligament is divided over the caudate lobe of the liver and the lesser sac entered to the right of the lesser curve of the stomach. The gastroesophageal fat pad over the abdominal esophagus is taken off the stomach

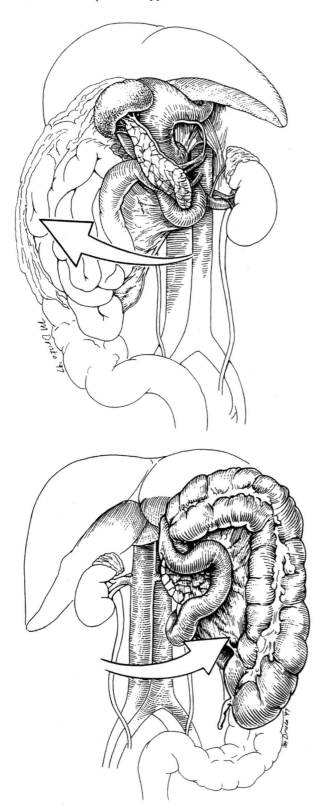

FIGURE 4.9. Right and left medial visceral rotations. (Reprinted with permission of The McGraw-Hill Companies from Burch JM, Franciose RJ, Moore EE. Trauma. In Schwartz SI, Shires GT, Spencer FC, et al., eds. Principles of Surgery, 7th ed. New York: McGraw-Hill, 1999: 155–221.)

and the phrenoesophageal ligament divided between the cardiac notch and the left crus of the diaphragm. Blunt finger dissection then defines the posterior esophagus from the left in conjunction with blunt dissection from the right through the lesser sac. Placement of an orogastric or nasogastric tube facilitates identification of the esophagus for blunt dissection.

Suprahepatic Inferior Vena Cava

The inferior vena cava exits the abdomen anterior and to the right of the esophagus and aorta. Exposure of the vena cava above the liver proceeds via midline laparotomy with firm traction of the costal margins superiorly. Extension to a median sternotomy greatly enhances exposure and allows control from inside the pericardium when necessary. The round, falciform, and coronary ligaments are divided to expose the bare area of the liver, and the liver is retracted inferiorly. The hepatic veins should be visible at this point and can be carefully dissected and encircled at their junctions with the vena cava. The suprahepatic vena cava is very short, and exposure is made difficult by the hepatic veins inferiorly and the diaphragm superiorly. If emergent control is required, the incision is extended to a median sternotomy, and the central tendon of the diaphragm is divided over the vena cava. Alternatively, the pericardium is opened vertically and the midline vena cava isolated just inferior to the right atrium.

Pancreas and Duodenum

Exposure of the head of the pancreas and the first and second portions of the duodenum usually proceeds simultaneously. A Kocher maneuver is performed by incision along the lateral peritoneal attachments of the duodenum sweeping the second and third portions of the duodenum medially to the inferior vena cava. This allows palpation of the head of the pancreas to the level of the superior mesenteric vessels and visual inspection of the anterior and posterior surfaces of the second and third portions of the duodenum. The Cattell and Braasch maneuver exposes the third and fourth portions of the duodenum by raising the mesentery of the terminal ileum and ascending colon from the posterior abdominal wall. Dissection begins at the lateral attachments of the cecum along the white line of Toldt and proceeds by elevating the mesentery of the ascending colon and ileum that contains the superior mesenteric artery and vein. The entire small bowel and ascending colon can then be reflected medially and superiorly out of the abdomen. Care must be taken to avoid injury to the right gonadal vessels and right ureter, which remain attached to the posterior abdominal wall. Alternatively, the fourth portion of the duodenum can be exposed by first performing a Kocher maneuver followed by division of the ligament of Treitz.

The ligament of Treitz is a fibromuscular fold of peritoneum suspended from the right crus of the diaphragm and attaches to the fourth portion of the duodenum. It represents the proximal attachment of the small bowel mesentery. Division of the ligament of Treitz allows rotation of the fourth portion of the duodenum from left to right behind the mesenteric vessels. Although this maneuver allows visualization of the anterior surface of the third portion of the duodenum, the posterior surface can be evaluated only by palpation.

Exposure of the pancreatic body and tail requires entering the lesser sac (Figure 4.10). Division of the gastrohepatic ligament will allow limited exposure to the head and superior border of the pancreas. Division of the gastrocolic ligament permits full inspection of the anterior surface of the pancreas along its length, including the inferior border. Division of the gastrocolic ligament is most commonly performed by transection of the anterior leaf of the greater omentum with ligation of the anterior epiploic arteries distal to the gastroepiploic arteries. The stomach is then reflected cephalad and the colon with attached greater omentum reflected caudally, thus opening the lesser sac. Wide exposure of the lesser sac occasionally requires extensive division of the gastrocolic ligament. Omental necrosis can result from the devascularization of the arc of Barkow by division of the right and left epiploic arteries along with the anterior epiploic arteries. An alternative approach to the lesser sac involves division of the posterior leaf of the greater omentum from the colon and ligation of the posterior epiploic arteries that variably arise from the transverse, dorsal, or great pancreatic arteries. Some posterior epiploic arteries also enter the colon directly or anastomose with the vasa recta of the middle colic circulation. The posterior leaf of the greater omentum is relatively avascular and is easily divided along the length of the transverse colon. With the stomach and attached greater omentum reflected cephalad and the transverse colon reflected caudally, the entire anterior surface of the pancreas is exposed. This also facilitates mobilization of the splenic flexure of the colon and division of the splenocolic and splenorenal ligaments. For suspected injuries to the pancreas, it is imperative to inspect the posterior pancreatic surface by incision of the peritoneum along the inferior border of the pancreas, taking care to avoid injury to the splenic vein.

The spleen is mobilized from lateral to medial to expose the posterior surface of the tail of the pancreas and the splenic hilum. This maneuver also exposes the posterior surfaces of the distal splenic artery and vein. The splenic vein can also be exposed by mobilization of the inferior boarder of the pancreas with superior retraction of the pancreatic body. Dissection of the vein proceeds by dissection along the posterior surface from lateral to medial to the junction with the superior mesen-

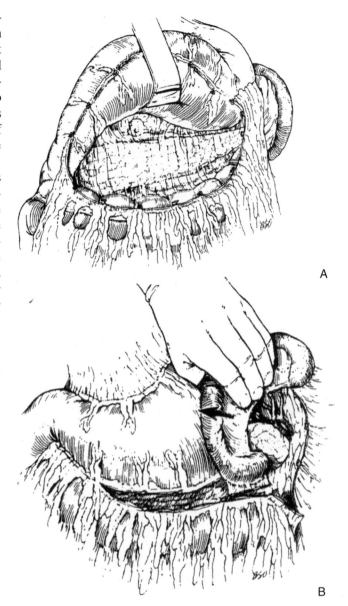

A

B

FIGURE 4.10. Exposure of the pancreas. **(A)** The gastrocolic ligament is opened and the stomach retracted superiorly to expose the head, neck, and body of the pancreas. **(B)** The spleen is mobilized and reflected medially, exposing the posterior aspect of the spleen and splenic vessels. (A, B reprinted with permission of Excerpta Medica Inc. from Asensio JA, Demetriades D, Berne JD, et al. A unified approach to the surgical exposure of pancreatic and duodenal injuries. Am J Surg 1997; 174:54–60.)

teric vein. The superior and anterior surface of the splenic vein contains multiple tributary veins that drain the pancreas. The inferior mesenteric vein may be encountered entering either the splenic vein or superior mesenteric vein. The splenic and superior mesenteric veins join to form the portal vein behind the neck of the pancreas. One should not hesitate to divide the neck of the pan-

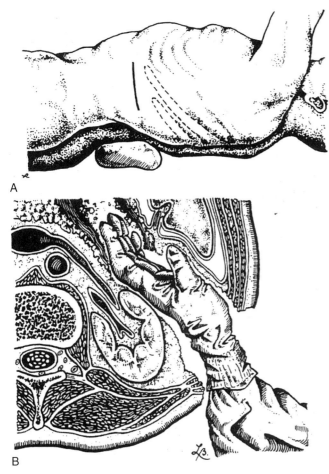

A

B

FIGURE 4.11. Posterior retroperitonostomy. **(A)** An incision is made 2 cm inferior to the twelfth rib through the muscle layers to the retroperitoneal space. **(B)** The incision is widened to allow exploration of the pancreatic region. (A and B reprinted with permission of Elsevier from Van Vyve et al.[6])

creas to expose these veins and control exsanguinating hemorrhage.

Access to the pancreatic tail is also achieved by a retroperitoneal peritonostomy (Figure 4.11).[6] An incision is made 2 cm inferior to the left twelfth rib with the patient in the right lateral decubitus position. After the muscles are severed, the pancreatic region can be reached by finger dissection of the exposed retroperitoneal space just above the renal fossa. The retroperitoneal opening is widened to allow exploration and extraction of necrotic pancreas and retroperitoneal fat.

Portal Structures

Emergent exposure of the porta hepatis is accomplished by retraction of the liver and gallbladder superolaterally and the hepatic flexure of the colon inferiorly. Exposure can be facilitated by lateral extension of the midline laparotomy and mobilization of the hepatic flexure. The gastrohepatic ligament is divided and the lesser sac entered over the caudate lobe of the liver. If necessary, a Pringle clamp is placed from left to right exiting the foramen of Winslow. The first and second portions of the duodenum are then mobilized by a Kocher maneuver that extends from the right edge of the hepatoduodenal ligament to the inferior vena cava below the right renal vein. Inferior traction of the duodenum improves exposure of the portal structures. The common bile duct and hepatic artery are anterior to the portal vein in the hepatoduodenal ligament. Isolation of the portal vein begins by incision along the right posterior boarder of the hepatoduodenal ligament with extension superiorly to the hilum of the liver and inferiorly to the head of the pancreas. The pyloric, duodenal, right gastric, and coronary veins enter the medial aspect of the portal vein near the head of the pancreas. The common bile duct is identified on the right side of the anterior surface of the portal vein. Following the cystic duct from the gallbladder leads to the common bile duct near the hilum of the liver. The course of the hepatic artery is followed from its origin at the celiac trunk by incision of the posterior peritoneum within the lesser sac and following the artery distally to the gastroduodenal artery, the first major branch.

Liver

The lower costal margins impair visualization and a direct approach to the liver. Exposure of the right lobe is improved by elevating the right costal margin with a large retractor. The right lobe is mobilized by dividing the right triangular and coronary ligaments. Following division of the right triangular ligament, the dissection is continued medially dividing the superior and inferior coronary ligaments. The right lobe is then rotated medially into the surgical field. Mobilization of the left lobe is accomplished in the same fashion. The superior surface is exposed by division of the round ligament between clamps followed by division of the falciform ligament over the surface of the liver to the hepatic veins. Care must be taken when dividing any of the coronary or falciform ligaments because of their proximity to the hepatic veins and retrohepatic vena cava.

Exposure of the retrohepatic vena cava requires firm superior retraction of the costal margins. Extension to a median sternotomy can greatly enhance retraction of the ribs and allow wider exposure. The right triangular ligament is then divided and the bare area of the liver exposed. The retroperitoneal attachments are divided as the right lobe of the liver is retracted medially. Several small hepatic veins enter the vena cava directly from the posterior surface of the right and caudate lobes of the liver and must be ligated and divided to avoid bleeding during mobilization of the right lobe. The right hepatic vein is identified as it enters the suprahepatic vena cava.

Inframesocolic Exposure

Root of the Mesentery

The anterior approach to the superior mesenteric artery and vein below the transverse mesocolon begins by reflection of the small bowel to the right and retraction of the transverse mesocolon anteriorly and superiorly. A transverse incision is made at the base of the transverse mesocolon from the fourth portion of the duodenum to the patient's right. The middle colic artery and vein are identified and traced proximally to their origins. The superior mesenteric artery lies to the left of the vein. Division of the ligament of Treitz and superior retraction of the inferior border of the pancreas allows limited exposure of the vessels. This approach allows rapid but limited exposure of the mesenteric vessels and is often appropriate for hemorrhage control or embolectomy. More proximal exposure requires dissection above the transverse mesocolon. Extensive exposure of the origin of the superior mesenteric artery and abdominal aorta is achieved by a right medial visceral rotation.

Infrarenal Aorta

The infrarenal aorta is exposed by retracting the transverse colon superiorly and the small bowel to the right. The posterior peritoneum is incised over the anterior aortic surface from the inferior border of the duodenum extending inferiorly to the right side of the aortic midline and onto the right common iliac artery at the aortic bifurcation. The iliac artery is controlled with a vascular clamp, taking care to avoid injury to the underlying iliac vein. No attempt should be made to separate the iliac artery from the vein. The right iliac artery crosses anterior to the left iliac vein just distal to the aortic bifurcation. The left common iliac artery is exposed by lateral retraction of the cut edge of the peritoneum and the artery controlled with a vascular clamp.

Inferior Vena Cava

Exposure of the inferior vena cava begins by dividing the lateral attachments of the right colon from the cecum to the hepatic flexure. The right colon is then reflected to the left. A Kocher maneuver is then performed, and the inferior vena cave is exposed from the caudate lobe of the liver to the iliac bifurcation. Circumferential dissection of the vena cava should be avoided in emergent operations because of the risk of injury to the lumbar veins, which enter the vena cava through the posterior wall. The right adrenal vein enters the vena cava above the right renal vein. The caudate lobe of the liver obstructs exposure of the suprarenal vena cava.

Pelvis

Superior displacement of the small bowel exposes the structures within the pelvis. Limiting the superior extent of the midline laparotomy facilitates packing of the small bowel within the abdomen. Mobilization of the sigmoid colon and rectum is straightforward and proceeds by incision of the posterior peritoneum along the left lateral attachments of the colon, continuing to the peritoneal reflection in the pelvis and to the right of the colon. The peritoneum is divided close to the bowel and dissection performed bluntly with care to avoid injury to the ureter. The presacral space is developed by blunt dissection posterior to the rectum in the sacral hollow. Anterior dissection between the uterus or prostate and the bladder is accomplished in a similar manner. If necessary, the lateral attachments containing the middle and inferior rectal vessels are divided for circumferential dissection of the rectum.

The iliac vessels are exposed by incision over the aortic bifurcation and sharp dissection along the anterior surface of the common iliac artery to its division into the external and internal iliac arteries. The right ureter crosses the iliac artery at its bifurcation and should be retracted laterally. The internal and external iliac veins lay posteromedial to the associated arteries. The injured right iliac vein is difficult to expose and may require temporary division of the overlying common iliac artery. The common iliac artery and its branches are exposed by retraction of the sigmoid colon and rectum to the right. The left ureter is retracted laterally and dissection carried out from the aortic bifurcation to the division of the common iliac artery.

Penetrating wounds to the aortic bifurcation and iliocaval confluence are difficult to control and are associated with a high mortality rate. The iliocaval confluence is exposed by first dividing the right common iliac artery between clamps and then developing the plane between the iliac artery and iliac vein to the aortic bifurcation (Figure 4.12). The aorta is rotated to the left and the underlying veins exposed.

Unilateral exposure of the iliac artery can be accomplished through an anterior oblique flank incision and retroperitoneal dissection. The incision is made at the lateral border of the rectus muscle approximately 3 cm superior and parallel to the inguinal ligament (Figure 4.13). The incision is extended to the midaxillary line and terminates midway between the iliac crest and tip of the twelfth rib. The external and internal oblique muscles are divided and the preperitoneal space entered through the transversus abdominus muscle and transversalis fascia. The preperitoneal space is then developed by blunt dissection over the iliac fossa, exposing the psoas and iliacus muscles. The ureter is retracted with the peritoneum away from the psoas muscle. The iliac vessels are located on the

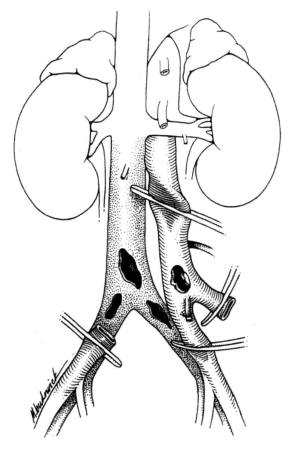

FIGURE 4.12. Exposure of the iliocaval confluence. The distal aorta and common iliac arteries are controlled with clamps. The right common iliac artery is divided between clamps and rotated to the left along with the aorta to expose the iliocaval confluence and the posterior wall of the aorta. (Reprinted with permission of Elsevier from Salam AA, Stewart MT. New approach to wounds of the aortic bifurcation and inferior vena cava. Surgery 1985; 98:105–108.)

medial aspect of the psoas muscle. Proximal exposure to the aortic bifurcation can be achieved with this approach. The external iliac artery can be exposed to the inguinal ligament with extension to a groin incision when necessary to expose the common femoral artery.

Damage Control

Liver

Perihepatic packing is capable of controlling hemorrhage from most hepatic injuries, and it has the advantage of freeing the surgeon's hands. The laparotomy pads should remain folded with two or three stacked together. The right costal margin is elevated, and the pads are strategically placed over and around the bleeding site. Additional pads should be placed between the liver, diaphragm, and anterior chest wall until the bleeding has been con-

trolled. Packing of injuries of the left lobe may not be as effective, because there is insufficient abdominal and thoracic wall anterior to the left lobe to provide adequate compression with the abdomen open. Because of the technical challenge and high mortality rate of hepatic vascular isolation, direct operative repair of retrohepatic venous injuries is avoided. If massive venous hemorrhage is seen from behind the liver and if reasonable hemostasis can be achieved with perihepatic packing, the patient can be transferred to the interventional radiology suite where hemorrhage from arterial sources are embolized and stents are placed to bridge venous injuries.

Perihepatic packing may not control hemorrhage from larger branches of the hepatic artery. The Pringle maneuver is used as an adjunct to packing for the temporary control of the arterial hemorrhage (Figure 4.14). The length of time that a Pringle maneuver can remain in place without causing irreversible ischemic damage to the

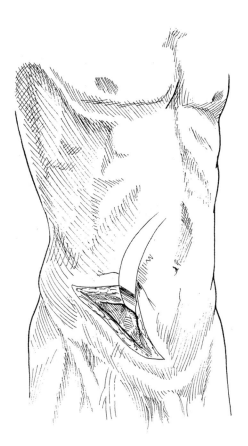

FIGURE 4.13. The iliac vessels can be approached through an incision 2 cm above and parallel to the inguinal ligament. The abdominal muscles are divided and the retroperitoneum elevated from lateral to medial. The incision can be extended inferiorly across the inguinal ligament over the femoral canal. (Reprinted with permission from Wind GG, Valentine R, Anatomic exposures in vascular surgery. Baltimore: Williams & Wilkins, 1991.)

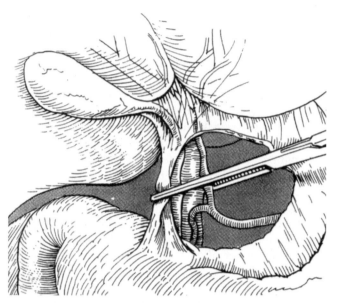

FIGURE 4.14. The Pringle maneuver. (Reprinted with permission of The McGraw-Hill Companies from Burch JM, Franciose RJ, Moore EE. Trauma. In Schwartz SI, Shires GT, Spencer FC, et al., eds. Principles of Surgery, 7th ed. New York: McGraw-Hill, 1999: 155–221.)

liver is unknown, but clamp times exceeding 60 minutes have been successful. Ligation of the right or left hepatic artery is appropriate for patients with recalcitrant arterial hemorrhage from deep within the liver. Its primary role is for injuries where application of the Pringle maneuver results in the cessation of arterial hemorrhage. Arterial ligation is a preferred alternative to a deep hepatotomy. When bilobar arterial bleeding persists, an intrahepatic balloon can be very effective. Our method is to tie a large Penrose drain to a hollow catheter and ligate the opposite end of the drain. The balloon is then inserted into the bleeding wound and inflated with soluble contrast media. If the control of the hemorrhage is successful, a stopcock or clamp is used to occlude the catheter and maintain the inflation. The catheter is left in the abdomen and removed at a subsequent operation 24 to 48 hours later. If recurrent hemorrhage occurs, selective embolization is usually effective.

Suturing of the hepatic parenchyma remains an effective hemostatic technique for persistently bleeding lacerations less than 5cm in depth. The preferred suture is 0 chromic attached to a large curved blunt needle. The large diameter of the suture helps prevent it form pulling through Glisson's capsule. A simple running technique is used to approximate the edges of shallow laceration. Deeper lacerations may be managed with interrupted horizontal mattress sutures placed parallel to the edge of the laceration. When tying the suture, tension is adequate when visible hemorrhage ceases or the liver blanches around the suture.

Most sources of venous hemorrhage within the liver can be managed with perihepatic packing. Even retrohepatic vena cava and hepatic vein injuries have been successfully tamponaded by closing the hepatic parenchyma over the bleeding vessel. Venous hemorrhage caused by penetrating wounds that traverse the central portion of the liver can be managed by suturing the entrance and exit wounds with horizontal mattress sutures.

For bleeding from minor lacerations that do not respond to compression, topical hemostatic techniques have been successful. Small bleeding vessels are usually controlled with the argon beam coagulator. Topical thrombin can also be applied to minor bleeding injuries by saturating either a gelatin foam sponge or a microcrystalline collagen pad and applying it to the bleeding site.

Spleen

Splenectomy is appropriate for significant splenic injuries in the patient with refractory coagulopathy. Bleeding from minor splenic injuries can be controlled by the argon beam coagulator or absorbable mesh splenorrhaphy in cases where the splenic capsule has been stripped. The mesh need not be sutured to the spleen but can be packed with laparotomy pads.

Kidney

Bleeding from moderate parenchymal injuries in the unstable patient usually responds to perirenal packing. For larger injuries, nonviable tissue is debrided, and surface vessels are ligated with absorbable sutures. Surface bleeding from capsular avulsion can be controlled by manual compression and argon beam coagulation. Prompt nephrectomy, however, is appropriate in the multiply injured patient with a major pedicle injury. Injuries to the ureter are not repaired in the unstable patient. Closed suction drains are placed in proximity to the injury for temporary drainage. The transected ureter can be temporarily ligated, preferably with placement of a nephrostomy tube or drained using an exteriorized ureteral stent. Bladder injuries are adequately managed with transurethral or suprapubic Foley catheters. More extensive injuries can be drained with bilateral stents passed retrograde through ureters and exteriorized through the abdominal wall.

Gastrointestinal Tract

Contamination from gastrointestinal perforations is contained by rapid closure using full-thickness running monofilament suture or stapling devices. Resection of devitalized tissue is accomplished rapidly by stapled division of the bowel and ligation of the mesentery. No attempt is made to restore gastrointestinal continuity in the unstable patient; reconstruction is delayed until re-operation following the completion of resuscitation. Biliary or pancreatic diversion is achieved by external tube drainage. Most injuries to the head of the pancreas can be managed by suture ligation of bleeding and packing. Severe injuries involving the ampulla can be managed by delayed pancreaticoduodenectomy.[7] The pylorus, pancreatic neck, and proximal jejunum are stapled and divided, the common bile duct is ligated, and biliary drainage is achieved by tube cholecystostomy.

Arteries

Larger arteries in the abdomen can often be repaired rapidly by lateral suture. Repair should always be attempted for injuries involving the aorta and the superior mesenteric, proper hepatic, and iliac arteries. When the artery is transected, distal perfusion can be preserved using intraluminal shunts. Placement occurs after achieving proximal and distal control of the injured vessel. The type of shunt used depends on the diameter of the injured artery. A critical step in shunt placement is securing the shunt within the vessel lumen; ligatures securing the shunt should be placed around uninjured segments of artery. Systemic heparinization is usually contraindicated because of bleeding from other injuries, but may be initiated in the SICU when resuscitation is complete and coagulopathy is resolved.

Veins

Ligation is the treatment of choice for venous injuries of the abdomen in the unstable patient. Ligation of the inferior vena cava, portal vein, superior mesenteric vein, and iliac veins is appropriate when the alternative is exsanguination. Ligation of the infrarenal vena cava and iliac veins may result in lower extremity venous hypertension, and prompt lower extremity fasciotomy should be considered. Ligation of the superior mesenteric and portal vein results in dramatic but transient bowel edema and requires aggressive fluid loading according to atrial filling pressures.

Wound Closure

Because the abdominal compartment syndrome can develop in the damage-control situation, the abdominal incision should not be closed. Damage control situations often result in significant bowel edema or require extensive abdominal packing. Many techniques of temporary abdominal closure using synthetic material have been described. The goal is to provide a tension-free closure that protects but does not irritate the bowel while accommodating the increased abdominal volume. We have adopted an abdominal closure using a fenestrated clear

plastic sheet placed over the bowel extending beneath the abdominal wall lateral to the wound edges. A surgical towel is placed over the drape to the wound edges over which two 10-mm suction drains are placed so that they exit the dressing superiorly. The abdomen is then covered with an adhesive surgical barrier (Ioban, 3M Corp.) to include the wound and surrounding skin. The drains are placed to wall suction to control draining abdominal fluid. The advantages of this closure are the rapidity with which it can be placed and the avoidance of suture damage to the skin edges.

Key Points

1. Make a big incision.
2. Extend the incision to a median sternotomy or laterally into the chest when more exposure is required.
3. Do not delay left medial visceral rotation for suspected injuries to the suprarenal aorta or its primary branches.
4. Apply a Pringle clamp early to control major bleeding from the liver.
5. Identify the common bile duct, common hepatic duct, and portal vein before dissecting the gastrohepatic ligament.
6. Divide the neck of the pancreas to expose the superior mesenteric and portal vein.
7. Do not circumferentially dissect the aorta, inferior vena cava, or the iliac vessels.

Extremities

Exposure

The principles of managing vascular emergencies are based on achieving proximal and distal control of the lesion and repair if possible or bypass when necessary. Immediate control is achieved by direct pressure over a bleeding wound or proximal control point. Inclusion of proximal and distal control points in the sterile field allows rapid control of life-threatening hemorrhage while direct pressure is applied to the wound. Tourniquets occlude collateral blood supply and should be used rarely. The uninjured lower extremity should be prepped in case autogenous vein grafts are required for vascular repairs. Although vascular emergencies often call for rapid exposure and restoration of limb perfusion, the procedure must be done carefully with proper vascular technique. Blind clamping may cause injury to adjacent nerves and should be avoided. Heparin should be used routinely unless contraindicated, and completion angiography should be performed unless normal palpable pulses are reestablished. The most significant risk factor for limb loss following injury is failed revascularization.[8]

Upper Extremity

The axillary artery is divided into three parts, the first extends from the first rib to the medial boarder of the pectoralis minor muscle, the second part lies under the pectoralis minor muscle, and the third extends from the lateral boarder of the pectoralis minor muscle distally. The axillary artery is approached through an incision 2 cm inferior and parallel to the clavicle centered over the deltopectoral triangle. The incision is extended laterally over the deltopectoral groove, which contains the cephalic vein that enters the subclavian vein at the deltopectoral triangle. The intramuscular groove between the pectoralis major and deltoid muscles is separated along the entire course of the wound. The pectoralis minor muscle is then divided below the coracoid process exposing the underlying neurovascular bundle. The axillary artery is most superficial at the deltopectoral triangle just medial to the coracoid process. The artery lies superior and deep to the axillary vein, which is retracted inferiorly. The nerves and brachial plexus lie deep to the first part of the axillary artery and must be identified to prevent clamp injury. Division of the pectoralis major muscle from its clavicular insertion can enhance exposure. The branches of the axillary artery are preserved because they provide collateral blood flow to the arm. The distal axillary and proximal brachial arteries are approached by extension of the incision over the lateral boarder of the pectoralis major muscle, following the course of the brachial artery in the grove between the biceps and triceps muscles. Separation of these muscles exposes the neurovascular bundle along its entire course to the bicipital aponeurosis.

The distal brachial artery is approached through an S incision at the antecubital fossa with the proximal extension positioned medially. The basilic vein is retracted medially, and the bicipital aponeurosis is divided to expose the median nerve and brachial artery. Isolation of the artery requires division of the flanking veins and communicating branches. Following the artery distally most easily identifies the brachial bifurcation. The ulnar artery passes medially deep to the pronator teres muscle. Isolation of the forearm arteries more distal to the brachial bifurcation requires distal counter incisions.

Lower Extremity

The common femoral artery begins at the inguinal ligament as a continuation of the external iliac artery. The artery is approached through a longitudinal incision over the femoral vessels such that the superior third of the incision is above the groin crease (Figure 4.15). The fascia

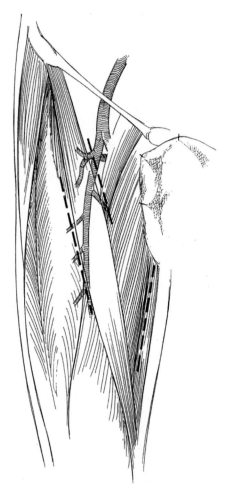

FIGURE 4.15. Approaches to the superficial femoral artery. Proximal exposure is achieved through an incision above the sartorius muscle, and distal exposure is achieved through an incision below the sartorius. Exposure of the distal profunda femoris artery is achieved through a medial incision and approach between the vastus medialis and adductor longus muscles. (Reprinted with permission of Elsevier from Rutherford RB, Atlas of Vascular Surgery. Philadelphia: WB Saunders, 1993.)

lata is opened inferior to the sartorius muscle and the femoral sheath exposed and opened. Care must be taken to avoid injury to the common femoral vein located medially. The profunda femoral artery arises laterally 3 to 5 cm distal to the inguinal ligament about the level at which the greater saphenous vein joins the common femoral vein. If more proximal control is needed, the incision is extended superiorly and laterally toward the anterior superior iliac spine with division of the inguinal ligament. Exposure of the distal superficial femoral artery is accomplished by extending the incision along the superior border of the sartorius muscle, which is retracted medially. This exposes the entire superficial femoral artery to the adductor hiatus.

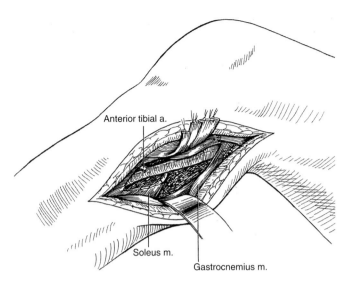

Anterior tibial a.

Soleus m.

Gastrocnemius m.

FIGURE 4.16. Exposure of the popliteal artery by division of the tibial attachments of the soleus and division of the tendons of the semitendinosus, gracilis, and sartorius muscles. (Reprinted with permission from Wind GG, Valentine RJ. Anatomic Exposures in Vascular Surgery. Baltimore: Williams & Wilkins, 1991.)

The popliteal artery is divided into three anatomic segments, the suprageniculate, midpopliteal, and infrageniculate. Medial approaches to the suprageniculate and infrageniculate sections provide rapid proximal and distal control to the popliteal artery and allow extension to expose the midpopliteal artery. The medial approach to the suprageniculate popliteal artery is through an incision positioned along the groove between the vastus medialis and sartorius muscles. The fascia over the sartorius is incised and the muscle retracted posteriorly. The adductor magnus tendon is separated from the semimembranous muscle to expose the popliteal vessels as they enter the adductor canal. The adductor magnus tendon can be divided to enhance exposure. The vein located laterally to the artery at this point may be paired and contains several bridging veins that must be divided to expose the artery. The collateral geniculate arteries should be preserved whenever possible to preserve collateral blood flow. Extension of the incision over the medial knee and division of the sartorius, semimembranous, semitendinosus, and gracilis muscles and the medial head of the gastrocnemius muscle exposes the midpopliteal artery (Figure 4.16). If divided, these muscles should be tagged with suture to facilitate reapproximation at the conclusion of the case.

The infrageniculate popliteal artery is approached through a longitudinal incision of the medial leg 1 cm posterior to the tibia from the medial tibial condyle inferiorly over the proximal third of the leg. The saphenous vein is located in this area and should be preserved. The fascia posterior to the tibia is divided superiorly to the insertion of the semitendinosus muscle and the gastrocnemius muscle retracted posteriorly. Division of the muscle attachments of the medial knee allows more proximal exposure as described earlier. Division of the tibial attachments of the soleus allows additional exposure. The popliteal vessels can usually be seen in the depths of the wound at this point, although the distal extent may be covered by the tibial attachments of the soleus muscle, which can be divided as necessary. The popliteal veins are paired at this level with numerous bridging veins that must be divided to provide adequate exposure of the artery. The anterior tibial artery passes through the interosseus membrane between the tibia and fibula. More distal exposure of this artery requires a separate incision through the anterior compartment of the leg. The tibioperoneal trunk and posterior tibial artery are exposed by distal extension of the soleus incision along the posterior surface of the tibia.

Fasciotomy

Forearm fasciotomy is performed through a volar incision that begins medial to the biceps tendon proximal to the elbow crease and extends toward the radial side of the arm following the medial boarder of the brachioradialis and continuing across the palm to the thenar crease (Figure 4.17). The fascia over the superficial flexor compartment is opened proximal to the elbow and extended distally across the carpel tunnel into the palm. The superficial radial nerve, radial artery, and brachial radialis are retracted laterally and the underlying muscles of the deep flexor compartment decompressed individually. Decompression of the deep flexor compartment is critical because forearm compartment syndromes most often affect this muscle group. If necessary, the dorsal forearm is decompressed through a straight incision beginning at the lateral epicondyle that extends to the midline of the wrist.

Decompression of the quadriceps compartment is accomplished through an anterolateral incision over the length of the thigh. The ileotibial band and fascia overlying the vastus lateralis is divided along its length.

The two-incision, four-compartment fasciotomy of the lower leg is performed through a medial incision positioned just posterior to the tibia and a lateral incision positioned just anterior to the fibula (Figure 4.18). The positions of the greater saphenous vein medially and peroneal nerve laterally must be considered when making the fasciotomy incisions. It is essential that all four compartments in the leg be released; thus the incisions should be long enough to afford complete longitudinal incision over the underlying compartments. The superficial posterior compartment is released through the medial incision by dividing the fascia between the tibia and

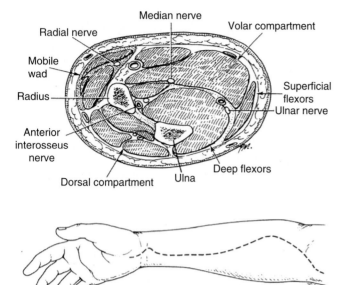

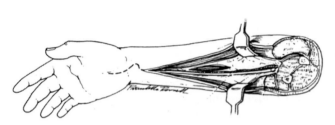

FIGURE 4.17. Forearm fasciotomy. A volar incision is made from the antecubital fossa to the mid palm with division of the transverse carpal ligament. The superficial and deep flexor compartments are then opened. (Reprinted with permission from Champion HR, Robbs JV, Trunkey DD. Rob and Smith's Operative Surgery, 4th ed. Trauma Surgery, Parts 1 and 2. London: Butterworths, 1989.)

Damage Control

When faced with surgical emergencies involving the extremities, one must always remember to preserve first the life and then the limb. In extreme circumstances, amputation may be the only option available to prevent death. When amputation is not possible, the dead extremity is packed in ice until the patient can tolerate the procedure. Examples include severe metabolic derangement resulting from reperfusion of an ischemic extremity, extensive necrotizing soft tissue infection, multisystem injuries with progressive shock, coagulopathy, and acidosis. Life-threatening hemorrhage from extremity injuries can usually be controlled by direct pressure, proximal and distal control of the bleeding vessel, or balloon catheter tamponade. Simple arterial or venous ligation is also a viable option when the physiologic condition of the patient will not allow definitive vascular repair. Distal perfusion can also be maintained during resuscitation by the use of intraluminal shunts.[9] Fracture stabilization is an important component in the treatment of complex extremity injuries. As with complex vascular injuries, definitive fracture fixation is often impossible because of the patient's physiologic state. The principles of damage control have been extended to orthopedic trauma.[10,11] Rapid external fixation of long bone and pelvic fractures can be accomplished in the emergency department, intensive care unit, and operating room. For multiply injured patients with femur fractures, damage-control orthopedic surgery minimizes the additional surgical impact induced by acute femoral stabilization.[12]

gastrocnemius. The deep posterior compartment is released by detaching the soleus muscle from the tibia, taking care not to injure the popliteal neurovascular bundle. The anterior and lateral compartments are released through the lateral incision centered between the tibia and fibula. The anterior intermuscular septum is identified by transverse incision over the two compartments. Two fasciotomy incisions are then made, one anterior and one posterior to the intermuscular septum along the length of the compartments.

Fasciotomy wounds are left open and dressed with application of bulky dressings. Local wound care and wet to dry dressings are applied on postoperative day 1. Primary wound closure is often possible, but split-thickness skin grafts may be required when ischemia-reperfusion–induced edema is significant or in crush injuries with extensive tissue destruction.

Key Points

1. Extend the inguinal incision across the inguinal ligament.
2. The profunda femoral artery arises on the lateral aspect of the common femoral artery.
3. Retract the sartorius anteriorly for proximal superficial femoral artery control and posteriorly for distal superficial femoral artery control.
4. Divide the semimembranous, semitendinosus, and sartorius muscles to expose the popliteal artery.
5. For combined injuries, place an arterial shunt first, repair the vein and then the artery, and perform a fasciotomy.
6. Use external skeletal fixation in the unstable patient.

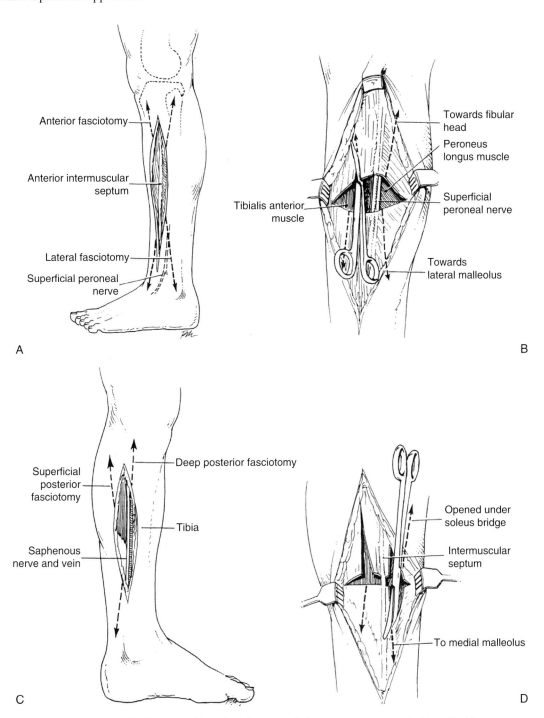

FIGURE 4.18. Four-compartment leg fasciotomy. **(A)** An incision is made 2 cm lateral to the tibia over the anterior intermuscular septum. **(B)** The anterior and lateral compartments are released by incision medial and lateral to the intermuscular septum while preserving the superficial peroneal nerve. **(C)** The superficial and deep posterior compartments are approached through an incision in the medial leg posterior to the saphenous vein. The intermuscular septum between the superficial and deep compartments is identified by a transverse incision. **(D)** The superficial compartment is decompressed by opening the fascia over the gastrocnemius muscles followed by decompression of the deep compartment by opening the soleus fascia. The fascial incisions must extend the entire length of the compartment. (A–D, reprinted with permission from Champion HR, Robbs JV, Trunkey DD. Rob and Smith's Operative Surgery, 4th ed. Trauma Surgery, Parts 1 and 2. London: Butterworths, 1989.)

Critique

With the abrupt onset of the patient's symptomatology, a perforated hollow viscus is the likely etiology. The 24-hour delay in definitive management has complicated this situation because this patient is now septic. Because the specific etiology is not known, the patient should be taken to the operating room and a midline, vertical incision (celiotomy) made to obtain the optimal exposure for the necessary exploration. This patient has secondary peritonitis, and there is no need for either intensive care unit monitoring or diagnostic evaluations in remote radiologic suites. Surgical intervention is the only option.

Answer (A)

References

1. Moore EE, Burch JM, Franciose RJ, Offner PJ, Biffl WL. Staged physiologic restoration and damage control surgery. World J Surg 1998; 22:1184–1190; discussion 1190–1191.
2. Firoozmand E, Velmahos GC. Extending damage-control principles to the neck. J Trauma 2000; 48:541–543.
3. Cothren C, Moore EE, Biffl WL, Franciose RJ, Offner PJ, Burch JM. Lung-sparing techniques are associated with improved outcome compared with anatomic resection for severe lung injuries. J Trauma 2002; 53:483–487.
4. Wall MJ, Jr, Hirshberg A, Mattox KL. Pulmonary tractotomy with selective vascular ligation for penetrating injuries to the lung. Am J Surg 1994; 168:665–669.
5. Wall MJ, Jr, Villavicencio RT, Miller CC, 3rd, et al. Pulmonary tractotomy as an abbreviated thoracotomy technique. J Trauma 1998; 45:1015–1023.
6. Van Vyve EL, Reynaert MS, Lengele BG, Pringot JT, Otte JB, Kestens PJ. Retroperitoneal laparostomy: a surgical treatment of pancreatic abscesses after an acute necrotizing pancreatitis. Surgery 1992; 111:369–375.
7. Eastlick L, Fogler RJ, Shaftan GW. Pancreaticoduodenectomy for trauma: delayed reconstruction: a case report. J Trauma 1990; 30:503–505.
8. Hafez HM, Woolgar J, Robbs JV. Lower extremity arterial injury: results of 550 cases and review of risk factors associated with limb loss. J Vasc Surg 2001; 33:1212–1219.
9. Porter JM, Ivatury RR, Nassoura ZE. Extending the horizons of "damage control" in unstable trauma patients beyond the abdomen and gastrointestinal tract. J Trauma 1997; 42:559–561.
10. Scalea TM, Boswell SA, Scott JD, Mitchell KA, Kramer ME, Pollak AN. External fixation as a bridge to intramedullary nailing for patients with multiple injuries and with femur fractures: damage control orthopedics. J Trauma 2000; 48:613–621; discussion 621–623.
11. Pape HC, Giannoudis P, Krettek C. The timing of fracture treatment in polytrauma patients: relevance of damage control orthopedic surgery. Am J Surg 2002; 183:622–629.
12. Pape HC, Grimme K, Van Griensven M, et al. Impact of intramedullary instrumentation versus damage control for femoral fractures on immunoinflammatory parameters: prospective randomized analysis by the EPOFF Study Group. J Trauma 2003; 55:7–13.

5
The Perioperative Management of the Acute Care Surgical Patient

Craig M. Coopersmith and Timothy G. Buchman

Case Scenario

In an apneic 70-year-man who is recovering in the intensive care unit after a protracted operative intervention 3 days ago, you notice that his ventilatory management is highlighted as follows:

(A) Volume-cycle ventilation
(B) FiO$_2$ is 60%
(C) PEEP is 15 cm H$_2$O
(D) Pressure support
(E) Endotracheal suctioning

Which of the above is the least appropriate?

Successful management of the acute care surgical patient requires comprehensive and complex physiologic monitoring and adaptive intervention that typically spans at least three venues: the emergency department, the operating room, and the intensive care unit. Coordinated care of the patient by emergency medicine physicians, anesthesiologists, and intensivists is as important in obtaining a favorable outcome as the judgment and skill of the operator. The purpose of this chapter is to frame a strategy for perioperative care of the acute care surgical patient in the intensive care unit. The point of view of this chapter is that of the intensivist, who has geographic responsibility for care of multiple patients in the intensive care unit yet must integrate effectively with the other venues that affect each acute care surgical patient in order to achieve optimal outcomes. It is common that the emergency surgeon plays the role of intensivist in the pre- and postoperative phases of care.

The use of the phrase "monitoring and adaptive intervention" and the allusion to a temporal sequence that brings the patient through multiple venues of care is not casual. It is intended to remind all caregivers that the physiologic response to stress—irrespective of whether the stress is traumatic, pathologic, or therapeutic (the stress of surgery)—has its own dynamics. The purpose of monitoring the patient is not to facilitate titration to a particular endpoint but rather to verify that the patient is on a safe physiologic trajectory. The purpose of adaptive intervention is not to make physiologic parameters "normal" but rather to ensure that care processes favor timely recovery.

A Perspective on Stress and Response

With rare exception, the indication for acute care surgery is a stressful event that triggers (and frequently overwhelms) compensatory mechanisms. Whatever the event—an obstructed loop of bowel, rupture of an abdominal aortic aneurysm, a juxtadiaphragmatic gunshot—there is a sequential and tripartite response. The three response phases are felicitously labeled with imperatives: escape, survive, and recover.

The escape phase invariably begins before medical intervention. The sympathetic nervous system is activated, releasing preformed epinephrine and norepinephrine that redirect blood flow toward vital organs (and limit hemorrhage when the stress involves bleeding). The release of cortisol initiates the process of metabolic reprogramming, mobilizing carbohydrate stores for immediate tissue use. Pain itself is attenuated. The teleologic explanation is to permit a traumatically injured animal to escape. What is important is not the teleology but rather the consequences that can confound initial evaluation. First, tachycardia, a relatively normal blood pressure, and a narrowed pulse pressure are frequent initial findings. Second, transient modest hyperglycemia (and consequent osmotic diuresis) may be physiologic but also deceptive—the patient appears to have adequate nutrients and hydration available. Third, pain is often obscured. In aggregate, the patient can initially appear to be better than the actual physiology. The importance of serial examination, especially of patients who appear to be relatively well, cannot be gainsaid.

Preoperative Care of the Acute Care Surgical Patient Following Initial Resuscitation

Acute care surgical operations may be immediate (e.g., abdominal gunshot wound with deep hypotension) or may follow an interval aimed at investigation (e.g., computed tomography scan of a tender abdominal mass) or may follow an attempt at nonoperative management (e.g., nasogastric suction to relieve a small bowel obstruction). Patients undergoing investigations and nonoperative management often receive care in the intensive care unit before operation. For this reason, initial resuscitation is operationally defined as that care required to transport the patient out of the emergency department irrespective of destination. Initial resuscitations that provide stability sufficient for transport are essential but often incomplete, and the intensive care unit often receives partially resuscitated patients who may require urgent or even emergent surgery.

Another common scenario is the inpatient who acutely deteriorates. The deterioration may be a complication of a prior operation (such as an anastomotic dehiscence or fascial dehiscence and evisceration). The deterioration may follow failed nonoperative management (such as "conservative" management of a splenic laceration with delayed hemorrhage). Although some limited resuscitation may occur on the wards, the intensivist is often called on to continue the resuscitation while the operating room is prepared.

These scenarios and sequences are important because the intensivist plays a pivotal role in advancing the completeness of the resuscitation and the readiness for operation. The frequent tension between "too sick to operate on" (i.e., needs further resuscitation) and "too sick not to operate on" (i.e., should be in the operating room now) is best addressed by rapid and systematic evaluation and intervention with specific attention to operative readiness and to projection of possible outcomes, including complications.

Physiologic Reassessment and the Second Phase of the Stress Response

The importance of serial reevaluation cannot be overemphasized. The most important reason to revisit the patient and the data is to evaluate the physiologic trajectory. That evaluation is grounded in familiarity with what happens to the physiology of stress following the escape phase, when survival becomes the priority.

Two major physiologic mechanisms—secretion of catecholamines and secretion of cortisol—persist, and global metabolic activity falls while blood is shunted away from nonessential tissues.[1] Temperature normally falls, so the "mildly febrile" patient is often "more inflamed"—more septic—than the absolute temperature suggests. Anorexia is common as internal nutrient consumption falls. Pain, discomfort, and general misery are prominent, and activity declines. In the absence of intravenous fluids, thirst is a common symptom. This period is decidedly hypometabolic—in its initial descriptions, this survival phase was called an "ebb" phase.[2] More than any other time in the clinical course, it is essential to inquire whether the patient perceives himself or herself to be "better, worse, or the same" since the prior examination. Patients who state that they are "the same"—as miserable as they were before receiving the ordinary interventions of intravenous fluids and pain medications that characterize initial care—are in fact becoming physiologically worse. These patients who are not responding to symptomatic management generally require accelerated evaluation and earlier definitive care.

Preoperative Actions

In this section, we assume that a diagnosis has been established, initial resuscitation is at least in progress, and plans have been made to take the patient to the operating room. Several preoperative actions have substantial effects on perioperative care, particularly if they are overlooked or omitted.

Relevant History

The urgency of acute care surgery often causes some elements of the history to go unasked or unanswered. Other elements are, in our experience, essential to safe perioperative management. These include the following:

- A complete list of current medications and food supplements. Lists can be obtained from patient, family, personal physician, pharmacy, or other health care agencies. The frequency with which important medications (such as thyroid replacement, corticosteroids, insulin, antiseizure agents) are omitted is matched by the failure to ascertain intake of over-the-counter drugs (such as antacids and salicylates) and diet supplements that contain highly active compounds. Although this information may have no bearing on the operation, it has great bearing on the perioperative period.

- Social history, with specific attention to alcohol consumption. Alcohol remains the most widely used drug to (self)-treat anxiety and depression, and unrecognized alcohol withdrawal syndromes are quite common. Because this may be the last time the patient will be awake enough to answer questions about substance use, it is imperative that the question be asked straightforwardly and answered accurately.
- Focused systems review. The focus should be on common postoperative complications. For example, asking about headaches is much less informative than asking about transient neurologic impairment that may not appear on physical examination. Whether the patient has ever had chest pain is probably less important than whether they have had arrhythmias or sustained a myocardial infarction. Whether the legs have ever had swelling is less important than whether the patient has ever had a deep venous thrombosis or pulmonary embolism. And so on.
- Functional status and reserve assessment. This is the most frequently overlooked aspect of the history that impacts perioperative care. Inquiry should be made about the patient's performance status just before the illness that is precipitating operation. Typical questions include exercise tolerance (e.g., climbing stairs and walking); assistance with activities of daily life (e.g., bathing and eating); and recovery time from recent illnesses such as a common cold. Verbatim descriptions of functional status are often more helpful than standard scales such as the New York Heart Association (NYHA) level, but both should be ascertained if at all possible.[3]
- Advance directives, including appointment of a personal representative. Many patients coming to acute care surgery are older and/or have little physiologic reserve. They should be advised that there may be some period—brief or prolonged—during the postoperative period that they may be too sleepy or weak to communicate reliably with medical staff. Even if the patient has not executed a legal document appointing a personal representative to make decisions when the patient is unable, identifying the patient's preferred surrogate in the medical record is often key to subsequent care. Similarly, it is always appropriate to ask whether the patient has advance directives and, if so, who has copies of the documents. It is a myth that patients and families are unduly frightened by this question: those who do not have directives will say so, and those who have prepared advance directives want the medical team to know about them.[4]

Pre-Illness Physiology

Acute care patients have physiology that is deranged from their ordinary status. Whether the usual (ordinary) status of a particular patient is "textbook normal" is another matter. It is therefore important to solicit whatever information is available about the patient's usual physiology—heart rate, blood pressure, breathing patterns (including use of home oxygen and external supports), temperature, weight, and physical activity. Recent electrocardiograms and blood studies are also helpful to understand the patient's physiology. As the population ages and acquires chronic illnesses such as diabetes mellitus, hypertension, and other cardiac and pulmonary diseases, individual parameters frequently change. For example, older obese patients with hypertension often are poorly controlled and "normally" run mean arterial pressures 20 torr or more above textbook values. They may require higher pressures to adequately perfuse vital viscera, and overzealous correction in the postoperative period can prolong and worsen the clinical course. Recent values are often known to patient and family; if not, records from the personal physician can (and should) be obtained.

Specific Signs and Symptoms

Surgical cases are usually undertaken emergently because there is immediate threat to life or limb. In many cases, the threat is some form of circulatory shock—hypovolemic, cardiogenic, or septic. Whereas the signs of hypovolemia are familiar, readily recognized by the surgeon and usually treated aggressively upon recognition, and whereas cardiogenic shock usually is identified and managed intraoperatively by the anesthesia team, the severity of sepsis is commonly obscured by survival stress responses, and therefore the physiologic impact is underappreciated by both surgeon and anesthesiologist. Failure to identify and aggressively treat sepsis in the preoperative and intraoperative phases of acute care surgical care can significantly prolong perioperative care and worsen outcomes. The following items should be considered during the preoperative evaluation of the patient:

- Is the mental status normal for this patient? Because the emergency surgeon usually has not encountered the patient before the preoperative evaluation, family and friends accompanying the patient (or other medical staff if the patient has been under medical care before consultation) should be consulted. Although hypoxia and hypoglycemia can cause altered mental status in acute care patients, sepsis is the more common cause of acute but mild mental status changes, assuming other parameters of perfusion (heart rate, blood pressure) are near normal.
- Is the patient tachypneic? Unless the patient has hypoxemia relative to his or her normal state, perhaps the most common cause for tachypnea in an acute care surgical patient is early sepsis. Other possibilities

include subclinical pulmonary embolism and diminished tidal volumes caused by pain or weakness.

- Is there mild jaundice? The picture is usually cholestatic. Scleral icterus may be hard to recognize, but a glance at the urine collecting in the urimeter often suggests that pigment is being spilled.
- Are the digits grey and cool? Acrocyanosis is a process, not an event. It begins with microvascular thrombosis that can be observed in fingers and toes. This is a manifestation of disseminated intravascular coagulation and can be one of the earliest signs of sepsis in patients with underlying microvascular disease, such as diabetes.
- Is there mild hyperglycemia? This often occurs just before the appearance of full-blown sepsis.
- Is there lactic acidemia? Small increases are common in early sepsis and signal mismatch between oxygen delivery and oxygen supply. High values (above 7 mmol/L) suggest (intraabdominal) catastrophe.
- Does the hemogram show an unexpectedly low value for platelets or absolute lymphocyte numbers? Both megakaryocytes and lymphocytes appear exquisitely sensitive to sepsis. Because many patients have had a complete blood count in the recent past, comparisons are often easy, and a decline in platelet count, absolute lymphocyte count, or both suggests sepsis in the appropriate clinical context.

The reason that the recognition of sepsis is important in the preoperative phase is that early, goal-directed resuscitation has been shown to improve outcome, and both the emergency surgeon and anesthesiologist should plan their care accordingly. Immediate administration of appropriately broad spectrum antimicrobial treatment is necessary but by itself insufficient. Adequate restoration of the erythron, timely use of sympathomimetic amines, and resuscitation to oxygen extraction goals (typically an SvO$_2$ >70%) must occur in parallel with acute care operation. Delaying resuscitation until arrival in the intensive care unit appears to result in sicker patients with prolonged recovery and worse outcomes, in both our hands and others'.[5]

Discussion of Perioperative Care Environments

Acute care surgery is associated with an unpredictable intraoperative course. Although most patients can have acute problems corrected and transfer to the general ward, a significant minority will require postoperative transfer to an intensive care unit. Advising the patient and family preoperatively that this is a common and even routine precautionary measure following acute care surgery will allow intensive care unit admission to be a reassurance as opposed to an unwelcome surprise.

Actions in the Operating Room

The acute care surgeon is properly concerned with providing the least risky operation that will set the stage for healing and recovery. Implementation of this "least risky" philosophy has led to several important advances, such as the damage-control laparotomy,[6] the open abdomen approach,[7] and planned second-look procedures,[8] discussed elsewhere in this book. With each of these approaches, the acute care surgeon acknowledges the therapeutic complementation of intensive care unit resuscitation and operative correction. A "least risky" approach also includes anticipating the types of supports that may be needed for prolonged perioperative care in the intensive care unit and providing the safest types of those supports. Considerations in the operating room should include the following:

- For patients who are undergoing emergency celiotomy, consideration should be given to placement of transabdominal enteral feeding access and, if appropriate, gastric decompression. Perioperative malnutrition is a common and vexing problem that translates into long intensive care unit stays, long ventilator runs, and increased complication rates (e.g., infection).[9] Although nasal gastric and small bowel catheters can be used to supply nourishment to many patients, they are uncomfortable and predispose to complications of their own, such as sinusitis and reflux/aspiration-related pulmonary infections. Surgical placement of a gastric tube with a small intestinal extension usually requires only a couple of extra minutes in the operating room but can allow for early and precise feeding while minimizing risks associated with gastroparesis and associated reflux.
- For all emergency patients, consideration should be given to early placement of a tracheostomy. Here, preoperative functional status can serve as an important guide to anticipating the need for prolonged mechanical ventilation. Patients who are dependent on home ventilatory supports (such as home oxygen or bilevel positive airway pressure [BiPAP]) and patients who are NYHA class IV and require major acute care surgery have a high probability of requiring prolonged ventilatory support. Tracheostomy facilitates many aspects of perioperative respiratory care in the intensive care unit and is often more comfortable for the patient, reducing agitation and thus simplifying sedation regimens as well. The above should not be construed as endorsement of indiscriminate performance of tracheostomy for the average acute care surgical patient but rather as recommendation for earliest possible placement of a tracheostomy where placement seems so likely as to be inevitable.

• Replacement of potentially contaminated vascular cannulae. Acute care surgical patients often require initial resuscitation under less than ideal conditions. This can lead to breaks in aseptic technique during insertion and maintenance of peripheral and central venous cannulae and of arterial cannulae. At the conclusion of an acute care surgical procedure, the various indwelling catheters should be inventoried and assessed for possible contamination. The exigency of the clinical situation may well preclude immediate replacement, but whenever possible critically ill acute care surgical patients should be given the benefit of properly aseptic cannulae.

Preparation of the Intensive Care Unit and its Team for Receipt of a Preoperative Patient

With increasing frequency (owing to the severity of illness, the ageing population, and the difficulties in finding an available operating room), the intensive care unit is notified by the emergency department that an acute care surgical patient requires ongoing resuscitation in the intensive care unit before operation. Safe transfer requires preparedness of the intensive care unit, which in turn requires specific communications. A minimum checklist includes the following:

1. Patient identifiers: name, date of birth, medical record number.

2. Illness leading to acute intensive care unit admission. This is more often descriptive than diagnostic, as in "distended abdomen and short of breath." An accurate description is nevertheless vital to care, because, although it could represent anything from a visceral perforation with pneumoperitoneum to acute intraabdominal hemorrhage, it points to the systems that are perceived to be most acutely compromised.

3. Life supports already in place. These may include ordinary endotracheal tubes and vasoactive infusions but may also include more exotic supports, such as Gardner-Wells tongs for patients who have sustained cervical spine trauma, high-frequency oscillating ventilators, and continuous venovenous filtration apparatus.

4. Monitors already in place. These may include bladder catheters and arterial and central venous catheters.

5. Timing of operation if known or planned. This is often omitted from the initial communication, yet essential—if the patient will spend only 30 minutes in the intensive care unit before operation, priorities are often altered and personnel often need to be redeployed to focus on immediate needs.

6. Known allergies. Although the general drug list can await the patient's arrival, knowing and apprising the team of any drug allergies can prevent serious complications.

7. Current vital signs, including temperature and pulse oximetry data.

Several preparations should be routinely made in anticipation of the arrival of an acute care surgical patient. Unless the patient is febrile, the room should be warmed. Whether the patient is intubated or not, an airway management kit and ventilator should be immediately available. At least one bag of a balanced salt solution (normal saline or lactated Ringer's) should be available: often there is an acute need to infuse fluids and administer critical drugs (paralytics, sedatives, vasoconstrictors) as the patient arrives in the intensive care unit. If the patient is hypovolemic, a rapid infusor should be prepared. The blood bank should be contacted by the intensive care unit team before the patient's arrival in order to determine whether a current blood specimen is available and, if so, what products have been made available for the patient. (It is insufficient to ask the staff of the emergency department or ward about blood products in readiness: they will report what they believe has been requested of the blood bank, not what is actually available.)

The Hand-Off

The intensive care unit team has two immediate tasks: (1) continue the resuscitation and (2) prepare the patient for operation. Often, both tasks must be accomplished concurrently and within a very short interval. Thus, it is important for all members of the intensive care unit team to remain focused on the tasks and to assume responsibilities that are complementary and not duplicative. Limiting the number of caregivers in the intensive care unit cubicle to those with assigned tasks is an important first step. We prefer to limit this number to five: the intensivist at the head of the bed; a respiratory therapist prepared to adjust the ventilator and (if necessary) assist with an emergency intubation; a nurse to tend to the monitoring needs of the patient; a nurse to tend to the treatment needs of the patient; and a scribe to enter the data onto the (paper or electronic) flow sheet. The transporting team bringing the patient to the intensive care unit is asked to help transfer (if necessary) the patient to the intensive care unit bed and then to step outside the cubicle so that the intensive care unit team can accomplish its tasks.

Patients frequently become unstable during transport. It is therefore important to assess the basics of airway, ventilation, and perfusion immediately upon arrival. An awake patient who, in response to a question, can identify himself or herself by voice has all three. Sedated and intubated patients must be immediately investigated by palpation of a pulse, a pulse oximetry signal, and verification that carbon dioxide is being exhaled. Verification of the presence of end-tidal CO_2 is strong evidence that the patient has both ventilation and perfusion.[11] For this reason, the CO_2 monitor is connected even before application of electrocardiographic leads and monitoring.

Provided that the patient is ventilating and perfusing, the seven items in the prearrival checklist should be reviewed next. Once these items are complete and there is understanding of the timing of the operation, the intensive care unit team should focus on the acute illness in the context of the patient's chronic health status. The duration and severity of the present illness are often reflected in the acute physiologic derangements. The chronic health status, including the roster of medications and treatments (the latter commonly including respiratory treatments such as BiPAP and renal treatments such as dialysis), provides insight into the extent to which current physiology represents a departure from normal. For example, a patient who is maintained on three antihypertensive drugs probably is inadequately resuscitated at a "normal" blood pressure of 120/80 torr. Finally, the complete record of resuscitative medications and treatments and the patient's responses should be reviewed. All of the above can usually be accomplished in about 3 minutes.

Ongoing Care in Anticipation of Operation

Almost as soon as the hand-off is complete, preparations must be made to transport the patient to the operating room. There is substantial risk that, unless attention is focused on the goals of resuscitation to minimize operative risk, some aspects of the patient's physiology can deteriorate through inattention. The single most useful tool to prevent inattention in this phase of care is to set explicit goals to be attained and maintained, with equally explicit statements for how these goals are to be achieved. For example, it is inadequate to simply state, "give the patient a fluid challenge." It is necessary to state, "administer 500 mL normal saline over 15 minutes, and report the effect of that challenge on heart rate, blood pressure, central venous pressure, and urine output over the subsequent 30 minutes." By explicitly listing the goals, the surgeon and intensivist can agree on the resuscitative endpoints. The intensivist should then identify and state the strategies to achieve these goals.

Postoperative Intensive Care

This section is organized into two intercalated parts. One describes the third phase of the stress response (recovery), and the other focuses on specific actions that must be taken at the bedside to minimize the risk that the patient falls off the recovery trajectory. This section is intended to be taken as a whole.

The Third Phase of the Stress Response

To recover from critical illness and the surgery required to control the source of that illness, local and remote tissues must be lysed and rebuilt. The plural "tissues" is used deliberately as a reminder that both high-turnover tissues (such as leukocytes) and slower turnover tissues (such as gut mucosa) and even very slow turnover tissues (such as lean muscle) are involved in these processes. It is the superposition of these processes that gives rise to fairly predictable dynamics and energetics.[12]

Early in the recovery phase, the patient remains deeply catabolic, mobilizing the building blocks necessary for repair. The clinical correlate is the appearance of nitrogen and potassium in the plasma, which are used for protein and cell assembly, respectively. Utilization of these moieties is less efficient than mobilization, and therefore they appear in urine waste. Generally this phase lasts about 4 days, provided that the emergency was readily controlled (e.g., simple appendicitis managed by appendectomy).

The *first transition* during the recovery phase is marked by more efficient use of potassium. Although nitrogen wastage continues, potassium losses in the urine return close to the patient's baseline. The endocrine correlate is the diminution of plasma levels of cortisol toward normal levels. This phase lasts about 3 days.

The *second transition* during recovery is marked by regain of control over nitrogen losses. The patient remains hypermetabolic—mild fever and tachycardia are still the norm. However, tissue repair accelerates, intestinal transit becomes normal, and the patient usually is well enough to be fully liberated from hospital supports (fluids, devices, incident-specific drugs) and plans made for discharge. It takes about 3 weeks for repair of the acutely injured tissue.

The *third* and generally final *transition* of the recovery phase involves rebuilding both lean muscle mass and fat stores. This lasts about 1 month.

In aggregate, recovery from surgical emergencies is typically a 2-month process. Depending on the chronic health status of the patient before the emergency, and the nature of the surgical emergency, this third phase of the stress response can be accelerated or delayed. Regardless, the three transitions must occur for recovery to continue to completion. When recovery stalls, there has typically been a failure to complete one of the three necessary transitions. Recognizing the transition failure as early as possible, creating a differential of possible causes, and removing whatever roadblock exists is essential to safe recovery.

To recognize transition failures, one must become conversant with the neuroendocrine events that are regulating the dynamics of tissue responses. Numbered and bolded are key ideas that illuminate milestones and problem points in the response to stress:

1. **Adrenocorticotropic hormone (ACTH).** The escape phase initiates central nervous system (CNS) coordination of the stress response.[13] Paraventricular neurons in the hypothalamus secrete corticotrophin-releasing hormone (CRH), thus initiating activation of the hypothalamic-pituitary-adrenal axis (HPA). The CRH arrives at the anterior pituitary gland to stimulate the secretion of ACTH from corticotrophic cells. Secretion of ACTH can be further upregulated by arginine vaopressin; however vasopressin has no intrinsic ACTH-releasing activity. Adrenocorticotropic hormone is not preformed. Rather, it is released proteolytically from a precursor molecule, proopiomelanocortin (POMC). (Another cleavage product of POMC is beta-endorphin, which is likely responsible, at least in part, for the blunted pain perception during the escape phase.) Once the ACTH reaches the general circulation and is transported to the adrenal cortex, it stimulates the latter to produce glucocorticoids, mineralocorticoids, and adrenal androgens. Collectively, ACTH levels are reserved and augmented early in acute stress. When they decline, it is because glucocorticoids—mostly cortisol—provide negative feedback to both the hypothalamus and the pituitary.

2. **Glucocorticoids.** These molecules have many effects. Skeletal muscle breaks down when they are in excess. Glucocorticoids modulate the stress response at the molecular level in at least three ways, ultimately inhibiting function of proinflammatory cytokines.[14] Glucocorticoids also affect growth and thyroid and reproductive functions in the context of acute stress. Their initial effects also promote secretion of growth hormone, suppress gonadotropin secretion (GnRH), and inhibit gonadal tissue. Although these effects might appear partially counterproductive (e.g., lysis of lean muscle) in the context of perioperative care, it must be constantly borne in mind that the stress response evolved to promote recovery following minor or moderate injury versus survival of major life threats.

3. **Autonomic nervous system (ANS).** While the HPA axis is marshalling the endocrine system, the peripheral autonomic system is also being activated. Because sympathetic (versus parasympathetic) activation is dominant early in the stress response, "sympathetic nervous system" (SNS) and "ANS" are often used synonymously. The stress causes rapid release of the catecholamines epinephrine and norepinephrine from the adrenal medulla into blood. This rise in catecholamine content is responsible for tachycardia and narrowed pulse pressure (via vasoconstriction and elevated diastolic pressure) that is

often seen following stress. However, the ANS does much more than merely mobilize catecholamines from stores. Efferent cholinergic preganglionic fibers project out from the interomediolateral column of the spinal cord to synapse in the sympathetic ganglia with projections to the smooth muscle of the vasculature, heart, gut, kidney, striated muscle, and fat. Autonomic nervous system function demonstrates dynamic compensation in the perioperative period.[15]

4. **Somatotropin (growth hormone).** Growth hormone (GH) comes from the pituitary gland. There are two hypothalamic regulators: a releasing hormone (GnRH) and an inhibitory hormone (somatostatin). Stress causes an initial rise in the average level of GH. Perhaps more important is a fundamental difference from the normal state—GH is continuously detectable. (In the normal unstressed state, GH is undetectable except for a couple of large amplitude diurnal pulses that last no more that a couple of hours.) The downstream effector of GH is principally insulin-like growth factor-1 (IGF-1), which instructs tissue to grow and divide. Insulin-like growth factor-1 is often measured in lieu of GH, because the former does not fluctuate nearly as much as GH itself and in fact can uncouple from GH under catabolic conditions.

5. **Aggregate effect.** The three axes—HPA, SNS, and somatotropin—are activated in concert at the onset of stress. Collectively, these affect nearly every bodily function, including—but not limited to—arousal, cardiac performance, vascular tone, ventilation, respiration, and urine production.

6. **Metabolic disequilibria.** The aggregate stress response also rebalances metabolic pathways. The key feature is mobilization of fuels for immediate use. The key hormone is glucagon, which is released as part of the ANS activation. Released from the pancreatic A cells, glucagons acts to raise blood glucose three ways: activation of lipolysis, glycogenolysis, and gluconeogenesis. Glucagon does not act alone—catecholamines and glucocorticoids assist with lipolysis; glucocorticoids assist with gluconeogenesis; and epinephrine triggers breakdown of glycogen. The one hormone that is involved with all three paths to mobilize sugar and free fatty acid for immediate use is glucagon.[17]

7. **Oxidation.** The fuels mentioned in the last section are not merely mobilized, they are oxidized in great quantity. This oxidation produces both carbon dioxide and heat, and the latter manifest as fever. Production of carbon dioxide nevertheless lags behind the prodigious oxygen consumption, with typical respiratory quotients of 0.7 for fat and 0.8 for carbohydrate.[18] The fact that the respiratory quotient is <1 should not be confused with the fact that total carbon dioxide production is elevated versus baseline.

8. **Muscle fate: proteolysis.** In starvation, synthesis is depressed, but there is no catabolism. The cells atrophy.

In stress, synthesis is augmented but overwhelmed by catabolism. The net process is proteolysis, not atrophy, and the clinical phenomenon is that of wasting—wasted energy and wasted tissue. In the absence of exogenous steroids, the resolution of stress-induced hypercortisolism correlates with abatement of proteolysis.[19]

9. **Signal blockade.** The stress response follows both actual injury and the perception of injury (pain). The hormonal variations characteristic of stress can be attenuated by preemptive sensory blockade using neuraxial anesthetics and analgesics. This blockade may be advantageous, especially for patients for whom the sudden release of catecholamines may have adverse consequences, such as tachycardia, vasoconstriction, and consequent increase in myocardial oxygen demand. New evidence suggests that neuraxial blockade may attenuate the catabolic response directly and improve substrate utilization.[20]

10. **Response simulation.** Re-creating the hormonal milieu of stress by infusion of a cocktail containing epinephrine, cortisol, and glucagons into unstressed animals or humans induces metabolic changes similar to those of authentic stress: metabolic rates increase, blood glucose concentration increases, muscle is lysed to release amino acids, and so on.[21]

11. **Why it happens: the counterregulation of insulin.** Recall that insulin's purpose is to extract building block molecules from the circulation—molecules such as sugars, fat, and amino acids—and place them into cells for storage. The response to stress is to make energy available immediately, so the stress hormones discussed so far—catecholamines, cortisol, and glucagons—must "counterregulate" insulin. This is the fundamental reason why critically ill surgical patients appear to be insulin resistant. This balance may help to explain why aggressive insulin therapy in the intensive care unit has improved outcomes[22]: the critically ill patient does not need the fuel to escape and survive, and pharmacologic doses of insulin may encourage an earlier shift back from catabolism toward an anabolic state.

12. **Why growth hormone was not mentioned in the previous paragraph.** The earliest descriptions of the counterregulatory response omitted the somatotropic axis, an error of omission. There is strong evidence that growth hormone secretion not only elevates in response to acute stress but shows more frequent pulsatility. Growth hormone's direct actions are lipolytic, insulin antagonizing, and immune stimulatory. But why do GH levels rise? Speculation abounds, but many believe that the stress state is one of growth hormone resistance just as it is one of insulin resistance. Recall that IGF-1 is the chief downstream effector in the somatotropic axis. Insulin-like growth factor-1, its growth hormone–dependent binding protein IGFBP-3, and its acid-labile subunit (ALS) all diminish along with growth hormone receptors. All of this

is consistent with a resistance state. (Unlike administration of exogenous insulin, which improves outcomes, the administration of exogenous growth hormone to further overcome peripheral resistance is associated with increased mortality in critical illness.[23])

13. **Thyroid hormone.** Within hours of the onset of stress, the active form of thyroid hormone (T_3) levels fall. Pituitary thyroid-stimulating hormone (TSH) sustains some ongoing release of the prohormone T_4 from the thyroid gland, but conversion in the periphery goes down the alternate pathway to produce "reverse T_3," which is metabolically inactive.[24] The teleology is that in the survival and earliest recovery stages following stress, there may be an advantage in conserving metabolic effort and directing what energy is available to local repair and not large-scale rebuilding. Perhaps equally important are the dynamics of TSH secretion. In health, the secretion is pulsatile. In acute critical illness, it remains pulsatile, but at a somewhat lower mean.

14. **Testosterone.** Within minutes of an acute stress, testosterone production by Leydig cells falls sharply.[25] Perhaps equally important are the dynamics of luteinizing hormone. The normal pulsatile release of this hormone is preserved (despite the fact that testosterone release is suppressed) in acute stress, just as TSH and GH pulsatilities are preserved.

15. **Prolactin.** This anterior pituitary hormone is secreted by lactotrophs. It enhances immune function, and, continuing the theme, its normally pulsatile secretion continues through acute stress.[26]

Actions and Considerations at the Bedside

With this insight into the hormonal events that accompany acute stress, one can begin to make sense of the routine processes of critical care.

Cardiac Monitoring and Care

All patients undergoing acute care surgical procedures receive continuous electrocardiogram (ECG) monitoring in the intraoperative and immediate postoperative setting. Typically, four to five limb and chest leads are monitored. This provides immediate feedback on the patient's heart rate and rhythm, allowing instantaneous detection of cardiac rate changes or rhythm abnormalities. Although multiple abnormalities may be picked up by ECG monitoring, the most common abnormality is tachycardia. Tachycardia, which reflects sustained ANS activity, is both a problem and a symptom.

Tachycardia may be a potent inducer of myocardial ischemia in patients at risk for heart disease.[27] Because 1% to 5% of unselected patients undergoing noncardiac surgery suffer cardiac complications, ranging from myocardial infarction to sudden death, controlling tachycardia is a potential life-saving maneuver. Treatment with beta-blockers has been shown in multiple prospective, randomized trials to decrease both morbidity and mortality in patients undergoing surgery.[28] Because tachycardia represents an increased hazard in patients with preexisting cardiac disease or myocardium "at risk," the benefit is most pronounced for patients undergoing vascular surgery and/or patients at high risk for perioperative cardiac events. Although the optimal timing and dosage of beta-blockade has not been conclusively determined, treatment is typically implemented in elective surgical patients before induction of anesthesia and should continue for at least the entire length of a patient's hospitalization. In the emergency setting, therapy often must be initiated and titrated in the intensive care unit. The optimal heart rate in a patient receiving beta-blockade is not clear, but many authorities recommend a target range of 50 to 65 beats per minute.[29] The role of beta-blockade for patients with congestive heart failure (CHF) is undefined—although this medication improves survival if given chronically to patients with CHF, it may exacerbate heart failure in the acute setting and usage for postoperative patients should be determined on a case by case basis. Because the predisposition to adverse effects of beta-blockade may not be known for any individual patient, and because acute care surgical patients often have deranged hepatic and renal physiologies, esmolol is often selected as the initial beta-blocking agent. Unlike other beta-blockers that require organ-based metabolism for clearance, esmolol is degraded by esterases present in blood, and its effects can be rapidly titrated by adjusting infusion rates.[30]

Tachycardia is generally a response to an acute underlying physiologic abnormality, and management involves not only beta-blocker prophylaxis but also identifying and treating the underlying cause. The most common etiologies for tachycardia in the perioperative period are pain and/or hypovolemia, and these must be either treated or ruled out expeditiously. The differential diagnosis for new-onset rapid heart rate is relatively broad and differs depending on whether a patient is in normal sinus rhythm. Sinus tachycardia precipitated by pain or hypovolemia generally responds quickly to specific therapy (analgesia and volume resuscitation, respectively). In contrast, atrial fibrillation with rapid ventricular response is generally a sign of a more complicated underlying process. It can be a sign of myocardial ischemia. It can be a sign of stretch on an overdistended atrium. All too frequently, however, it is the presentation of a pulmonary embolism. For this reason, the management of new-onset atrial fibrillation with rapid ventricular response requires not only immediate treatment to address the rhythm—typically with amiodarone and, if necessary, DC cardioversion to address a life-threatening tachycardia—but also a test to exclude pulmonary embolism such as a spiral CT scan.

A patient's preoperative age, symptomatic cardiac status, ECG, and magnitude of surgery all play a role in what type of cardiac monitoring patients need once they leave the operating room.[31] Typical intraoperative monitoring is not sensitive for detection of acute ST- or T-wave changes suggestive of myocardial ischemia.[32] Patients should have ECGs immediately postoperatively and daily for the first 2 days after surgery. Serial troponin levels should be drawn to rule out myocardial infarction immediately following surgery and every 12 hours for the first 24 hours as well as on postoperative day 4 or at hospital discharge (whichever is sooner) in acute care surgical patients with any cardiac history or who are over 40 years of age.[33] The decision to continue telemetry monitoring should be made on an individual basis, based on the patient's history and intraoperative course.

All acute care surgical patients require blood pressure (BP) monitoring. For most patients, automated BP devices in conjunction with continuous ECG monitoring and urine output adequately assess a patient's volume status. These devices can be set to measure the patient's BP every 5 to 15 minutes. For those patients in whom BP fluctuations may occur more frequently than these intermittent measurements can capture, additional monitoring may be needed with an invasive arterial catheter. Candidates for intraoperative arterial monitoring include patients who undergo operations longer than 4 hours in duration, who lose enough blood intraoperatively to cause hypovolemic shock, who need multiple blood draws, or who need precise BP control, such as patients with combined torso and neurotrauma. Patients with an anticipated postoperative need for constant BP monitoring, ventilator support, or inotropic support typically benefit from intraoperative arterial catheterization. Arterial catheters are preferentially placed in the radial artery, assuming good collateral flow is determined to be present, with minimal risk of occlusion, embolization, or infection.

When ECG and BP monitoring in conjunction with physical examination and urine output fail to delineate a patient's volume status, additional invasive monitoring will be needed. Central venous catheters allow measurement of the central venous pressure (CVP), an indirect approximation of volume status. Although measuring CVP is useful in many patients, right-sided filling pressures are an accurate estimation of left ventricular volume only if there is neither valvular disease nor pulmonary hypertension. If either of these conditions exists, CVP monitoring may lead to an inaccurate assessment of a patient's intravascular volume status and lead to inappropriate diuretic use or volume loading. If a central venous catheter is used to monitor CVP, the preferred site of insertion is the subclavian vein because the risk of infectious complications is lowest at this anatomic site.[34] If placement in the subclavian vein is contraindicated because of severe coagulopathy or likely need for chronic dialysis, the internal jugular vein is an acceptable alternative. Although internal jugular catheters have a twofold increase in infectious risk compared with subclavian catheters, they are preferable to femoral lines, which are associated with increased risk of deep venous thrombosis (DVT) in addition to bacteremia. (Where high-flow dialysis catheters are required, as for acute hemodialysis or continuous venovenous hemodiafiltration, the right internal jugular route is preferred.[35])

When a CVP is likely to be an inaccurate estimation of volume status or monitoring a patient's cardiac output is likely to be helpful (such as in a patient with severely decreased left ventricular ejection fraction), a pulmonary artery (PA) catheter may be beneficial. These catheters have the advantage of measuring left-sided heart pressures and may be more accurate in approximating left ventricular volume than CVP catheters. They also allow the intensivist to assess cardiac output when inotropic support might be necessary. When cardiac output will likely need to be continuously monitored, an oximetric PA catheter has the advantage of being able to measure continuous mixed venous saturation and is preferable to a standard PA catheter. Despite their theoretical advantages, a recent prospective randomized study of nearly 2,000 high-risk surgical patients showed no difference in outcomes between patients who received perioperative PA catheters and those who did not.[36] Although many believe that having extra physiologic data about a patient's cardiac and volume status is helpful in directing care, current literature does not support routine PA catheter placement, and a decision to place this invasive monitoring device in patients with unclear volume status, acute lung injury, or septic shock is generally made on a case-by-case basis.[37] If a PA catheter is placed, continuous monitoring of mixed venous oxygen saturation with fiberoptic oximetry is often helpful in ascertaining the effects of interventions and the adequacy of resuscitation.

Noninvasive cardiac output measurement is also available with the esophageal Doppler monitor (EDM).[38] The EDM is a soft 6-mm catheter that is placed into the esophagus. A Doppler flow probe at its tip allows monitoring of cardiac output, stroke volume, and flow time (a surrogate for intravascular volume) and may yield more accurate hemodynamic data than a PA catheter in patients with valvular lesions, septal defects, or pulmonary hypertension. Small-scale studies have shown EDM to be beneficial in perioperative management, but there is no evidence that it yields superior outcomes to PA catheters. Although its noninvasive nature avoids mechanical complications seen with PA catheters, it can be challenging to use because of difficulties in optimizing and analyzing the waveform generated.

Tonometers are another monitoring device designed to assess adequacy of fluid resuscitation.[39] Placed in either the stomach or sigmoid colon, tonometers measure intramucosal pH, which, along with tissue CO_2 to arterial CO_2 gradient, are theoretical surrogates of splanchnic perfusion. Proponents of tonometry believe it is valuable because mucosal ischemia is an early sign of impaired splanchnic perfusion, which is believed to be more sensitive than global indicators such as cardiac output or acidosis. Nonetheless, despite a decade of usage, no large study has demonstrated superior outcomes with the device, and, since it is difficult to use, expensive, and prone to dislodgement and errors of calibration, it has not gained widespread acceptance.

Pulmonary Monitoring and Care

Recall the core metabolic event in critical illness. Fuels are mobilized, carbon dioxide production rises, but oxygen consumption rises even faster. Getting oxygen to tissues becomes paramount, and oxygen delivery is the geometric product of cardiac output (discussed in the last section), hemoglobin concentration (discussed later), and oxygen saturation.

Because of its ability to detect slight decreases in arterial blood oxygen saturation almost instantaneously, pulse oximetry is monitored in all surgical patients in the immediate perioperative setting and selected patients after leaving the postanesthesia recovery room. In routine operations, monitoring is simple and can be performed using a detector on a patient's finger, earlobe, or forehead, where it estimates the difference in intensity between oxygenated and deoxygenated blood from the red and near-infrared regions of the spectrum and calculates the saturation of the arterialized blood. However, if the device cannot detect an arterial pulse, the waveform will be dampened and provide an inaccurate saturation estimation. Patients with hypothermia, hypotension, hypovolemia, or peripheral vascular disease or receiving vasoconstrictive medications may therefore have inaccurate pulse oximetry readings. Patients with elevated carboxyhemoglobin concentrations have falsely elevated saturation readings because carboxyhemoglobin is absorbed at the same wavelength as oxygenated hemoglobin.[41] Methemoglobinemia also leads to inaccurate readings by pulse oximetry, but interpretation is more complex because of the nonlinear relationship between SpO_2 and methemoglobin concentrations. Typically, patients with significant methemoglobinemia will register a saturation of 85% on pulse oximetry; in patients with a normal PaO_2 this leads the pulse oximeter to register falsely low saturations, although the saturation may actually be falsely elevated in the unusual patient with methemoglobinemia and severe hypoxia.

Postoperative pain and immobility may lead to decreased cough, clearance of secretions, and an inability to recruit alveoli. This, in turn, may lead to atelectasis, hypoxemia (especially in patients with preexisting pulmonary disease), and increased susceptibility to developing pneumonia. Appropriate pain control and early mobilization are therefore critical components in preventing pulmonary complications. Coughing and deep breathing exercises as well as incentive spirometer usage may also be useful adjuncts.

All patients who require mechanical ventilation benefit from capnography measurement. Capnography measures changes in the concentration of CO_2 in the ventilatory cycle by use of mass spectroscopy or infrared light absorption. The measurement typically obtained is end-tidal CO_2 ($ETCO_2$), a patient's peak CO_2 concentration that occurs at end expiration. $ETCO_2$ detection is a useful indicator of successful placement of an endotracheal tube, although it cannot be used as a sole indicator without concurrent physical examination and pulse oximetry monitoring because a stomach insufflated with air after esophageal intubation will yield detectable $ETCO_2$ on a portable monitor.[42] End-tidal CO_2 serves as a monitor of ventilation in patients on respirators. Once an $ETCO_2$—$PaCO_2$ gradient has been established by correlating a patient's monitored $ETCO_2$ with CO_2 concentration measured on an arterial blood gas (ABG), the need for further ABGs is minimized or abolished because both oxygenation and ventilation may be monitored non-invasively. Ventilated patients can typically be weaned and extubated by following the pulse oximeter and $ETCO_2$ in conjunction with other physiologic parameters.

The presence of $ETCO_2$ implies adequate ventilation and perfusion: delivered fuel has been oxidized, and the waste product is being brought to the lungs for excretion. An acute decrease in $ETCO_2$ is always a life-threatening emergency, representing a sudden decrease in one or both of these parameters. Frequent causes in the postoperative setting include a pulmonary embolus, low cardiac output state, or disconnection from the ventilator. A sudden decline in $ETCO_2$ requires immediate and undivided attention until the cause is ascertained and the problem rectified.

Neurologic Monitoring and Care

A brief but focused neurologic examination should follow every acute care surgical procedure as quickly as possible. The brain, which is only 2% of tissue weight, accounts for 20% of oxygen consumption. In general, patients should make rapid progress toward their preoperative level of consciousness and exhibit no lateralizing signs. In the immediate postoperative period, depressed mental status with nonfocal findings most commonly represents persistent anesthetic or drug effects or underresuscitation. However, it may also signify a problem with fuel delivery or regional utilization (i.e., a stroke). Immediate cessation of all sedative drugs (with the possible

exception of a very-low-dose opiate to manage pain) is the essential next step in management, and consideration should be given to benzodiazepine reversal with flumazenil. If improvement is not observed within minutes of these maneuvers, a prompt computed tomography scan of the head without intravenous contrast is indicated to exclude an intracranial hemorrhage, acute hydrocephalus, tumor enlargement, or other space-filling lesion. Localized weakness/paralysis may signify a stroke, a spinal cord lesion (such as an acute hematoma), or a pressure/traction injury on a peripheral nerve.

Critically ill acute care postoperative patients frequently accumulate opiates and sedative agents (such as propofol and midazolam) during their intensive care unit stay simply because these medications accumulate in tissues and cease to be "short acting" after just a few days' infusion. A popular method to prevent the continued effects of opioids and sedatives after they have been discontinued is a daily "wake up" where all sedatives are stopped until a patient becomes arousable.[43] Although data from critically ill medical patients demonstrate that this shortens intensive care unit length of stay, its effects have not been fully studied in postoperative patients, and this technique should be used with caution.

Special care should be exercised in the administration of morphine to acute care surgical patients predisposed to renal failure. Morphine is first glucuronidated in the liver. Morphine-6-glucuronide, ordinarily excreted by the kidney, is several times more potent than the parent compound. As a consequence, patients with deteriorating renal function can rapidly overdose on morphine.[44] Meperidine is also a poor choice for patients at risk for (or with) acute renal failure, because its metabolite accumulates and predisposes to seizures and other neurologic disturbances.[45]

Another problem that occurs late in postoperative patients is "polyneuropathy of critical illness," a syndrome of generalized weakness after prolonged intensive care unit stay. A recent study including surgical intensive care unit patients demonstrated that 25% of patients intubated greater than 1 week had severe muscle weakness (intensive care unit–acquired paresis) 7 days after they were awake off sedatives. This rises to 50% in patients who are septic.[46] Although multiple factors increase a patient's likelihood of developing this state, among the most important is the use of drugs that have a steroid nucleus, including corticosteroids themselves and several paralytic agents.[47] Unless there is a specific indication for neuromuscular blockade, deep sedation is preferable to mild sedation and chemical paralysis.

Renal Monitoring and Care

Patients who cannot take oral feedings require intravenous fluids. Except for patients with uncontrollable blood glucose, intravenous fluids should include dextrose, as the inclusion of this carbohydrate decreases obligate postoperative protein breakdown. For short operations that have minimal third spacing, hypotonic (0.45% normal saline) maintenance fluids containing 5% dextrose are typically adequate. Patients with high insensible losses, large operations resulting in third spacing, or increased catabolism above that normally caused by surgery (such as seen in sepsis) require additional fluids. In the immediate postoperative setting, fluid resuscitation is accomplished using an isotonic crystalloid solution such as 0.9% normal saline or lactated Ringer's. Additional fluid boluses may be given with either crystalloid or colloid. Although colloid solutions have the theoretical advantage of staying intravascular for a longer period of time, there is no convincing evidence demonstrating their superiority in postoperative resuscitation.

Monitoring serum electrolytes, blood urea nitrogen, and creatinine is necessary for patients with acute or chronic renal failure and those who have a large blood loss/fluid resuscitation intraoperatively. Basic metabolic profiles may also be helpful for patients not expected to be taking oral feeding for greater than 24 hours or who have excessive gastrointestinal losses measured through a nasogastric tube or an ostomy. Calcium levels also need to be checked in patients who receive massive transfusion intraoperatively.

Rapid fluid shifts (leading to periods of hypovolemia), nephrotoxic drugs, and intravenous dye loads can all lead to acute renal failure (ARF). Although no uniform diagnostic criteria exist for ARF, common definitions include an increase in serum creatinine level of 0.5 mg/dL or a 50% decrease in glomerular filtration rate. Although those with preexisting renal dysfunction are at higher risk, any surgical patient may develop ARF, and the incidence is as high as 20% in critically ill patients. Hypovolemia with relative hypotension is the single most common cause of decreased urine output in the immediate postoperative setting, and giving a fluid bolus is an appropriate first management step. If a patient has persistent oliguria and/or a rising serum creatinine level, additional workup must be performed, which may include a physical examination and urine electrolytes to determine whether the problem is prerenal (such as dehydration), postrenal (such as ureteral obstruction), or intrinsic (such as acute tubular necrosis). Invasive monitoring with a CVP or PA catheter may also be considered to clarify a patient's intravascular volume status and cardiac output.

With the stress of a major operation, the vasculature dilates and has increased permeability, leading to an accumulation of volume in the "third space." However, extravascular fluid accumulation does not perfuse the kidneys, and specific attention must be paid to intravascular volume, because a patient can have total body edema and still be functionally hypovolemic. The single best maneuver to prevent ARF is appropriate fluid resuscitation with maintenance of intravascular euvolemia. No pharmacologic agent has been demonstrated to prevent ARF. Although low-dose dopamine may improve urine output, there are convincing data from multiple trials that this drug neither improves renal function nor prevents ARF. Similarly, although high-dose diuretics may convert oliguric to nonoliguric renal failure, this does not alter the natural history of the disease and has even been associated with increased mortality in retrospective analyses.

Computed tomography scans with intravenous dye, a known nephrotoxin, are common in the perioperative period. Although hydration continues to be the single best preventative agent for postexamination acute tubular necrosis, n-acetylcysteine given 24 hours before and after the computed tomography scan has been demonstrated to result in a smaller dye-induced increase in serum creatinine level in patients with preexisting renal insufficiency compared with placebo, although it has not been shown to decrease the need for dialysis.[48] Alternatively, an infusion of sodium bicarbonate immediately before and after a dye load also appears to diminish contrast-induced nephropathy.[49]

Gastrointestinal Monitoring and Care

Patients requiring postoperative mechanical ventilation and those with preexisting peptic ulcer disease require stress ulcer prophylaxis, most commonly with H_2-blockers and more recently with proton pump inhibitors. Patients who are operated on for complications of ulcer disease should be treated instead with proton pump inhibitors as should intubated patients with bleeding despite receiving H_2-blockade. Although cytoprotective agents such as sucralfate are sometimes used for ulcer prophylaxis, they are associated with increased stress ulcer bleeding compared with other pharmacologic modalities and should not be used as first-line agents. Although the data are not as clear for extubated surgical patients who will not receive enteral nutrition for several days secondary to postoperative ileus, many surgeons choose to begin prophylaxis for these patients as well.

All patients with functional, intact gastrointestinal tracts should receive enteral nutrition. Although early enteral nutrition (within 12 to 24 hours) has been shown to be beneficial in burn patients, there are fewer data available to support use in the acute care surgical patient. Nevertheless, feeding is always preferable to starvation, and nutritional repletion represents an important component of care. Parenteral nutrition is typically not started unless a patient is expected to be without enteral nutrition for an aggregate of 7 days. Obviously, if the patient has had prolonged starvation because of either the acute surgical illness or chronic disease, parenteral nutrition should be instituted early as a bridge to enteral support. Provided the patient is not mechanically obstructed and provided that the intestinal circulation is not compromised by vasoactive infusions, enteral feeding can usually be initiated within a day of acute care surgery.

Multiple nutritional formulas exist based on a patient's renal function and volume status. Immune-enhanced formulas have been advocated for their potential ability to decrease infectious complications in the perioperative period and have been studied in multiple surgical populations. The most promising data demonstrate lower infection rates in malnourished cancer patients who undergo upper gastrointestinal surgery and receive pre- and postoperative immunonutrition. Preoperative but not postoperative immunonutrition has also been associated with decreased infection rates in patients with colorectal cancer. In contrast, immunonutrition is associated with increased mortality in septic patients and should not be given to critically ill septic patients. Although immunonutrition has been advocated for trauma patients, current data are conflicting and do not clearly demonstrate its efficacy or support its widespread use. Glutamine-supplemented formulas are probably safe for all patients, but formulas containing excess arginine may adversely affect patients with sepsis and should be used with caution.[50]

Hematologic Monitoring and Care

A complete blood count (CBC) and coagulation parameters should be obtained postoperatively for any procedure during which significant blood loss occurred. Follow-up CBCs should be obtained on an as-needed basis when there is concern for ongoing blood loss or fluid shifts likely to alter the hematocrit and to assess the white blood cell count for infectious concerns. The optimal perioperative hematocrit is uncertain. In the intensive care unit, prospective studies indicate that a hematocrit level of 21% 24% is acceptable (even in patients with mild coronary artery disease), and transfusing to achieve a higher blood count is potentially associated with a higher mortality rate, possibly related to the immunosuppressive effects of blood.[43] Patients with symptoms or signs of active myocardial ischemia or those with baseline severe ischemic cardiac disease (New York Heart Association class III or IV) typically should have their hematocrit kept above 30%. Although there is no direct evidence on goal hemoglobin in surgical patients who suffer a perioperative myocardial infarction, medical patients who are transfused to a hematocrit of 30% to 33% following a myocardial infarction have improved outcomes compared with those with lower levels.

All patients undergoing a major surgical procedure or who are at moderate or high risk should have mechanical and/or pharmacologic prophylaxis to prevent DVT and pulmonary embolism. Mechanical prophylaxis with graded compression stockings and intermittent pneumatic compression devices should be used for nearly all patients who will not be ambulatory immediately postoperatively and for whom there is no contraindication. For the simplest cases, unfractionated subcutaneous heparin should be used in addition. Unfractionated heparin does not alter the rate of major bleeding; however, it is associated with increased risk of minor bleeding and hematoma formation. For higher risk patients (i.e., when acute care surgery is performed in an elderly patient or with complications of cancer, or with polytrauma), low-molecular-weight heparin should be substituted for unfractionated heparin due to its increased efficacy in preventing DVT and/or pulmonary embolism. High-risk patients who are not candidates for prophylactic pharmacologic prophylaxis and patients who bleed while on anticoagulants should receive inferior vena caval filters.[52] Some of the newer filters can be removed within a couple of weeks of placement, an option that may be appropriate for a relatively young patient whose contraindication to anticoagulation is only temporary.

Endocrine Monitoring and Care

Hyperglycemia is common following acute care surgery. Hyperglycemia is associated with increased susceptibility to infection and polyneuropathy and to skeletal muscle wasting associated with prolonged mechanical ventilation in critically ill patients. Although the optimal blood glucose level in routine postoperative patients has not been identified, intensive insulin therapy to maintain blood glucose level in the range between 80 and 110 mg/dL is associated with a 34% decrease in hospital mortality rate compared with 180 to 200 mg/dL in surgical intensive care unit patients. Tight glucose control is also associated with substantial decreases in ARF, bloodstream infections, blood transfusions, and polyneuropathy compared with conventional treatment.[53]

Patients taking chronic corticosteroids for immunosuppression, adrenal insufficiency, or autoimmune disease need to have these continued in the postoperative setting. There is no evidence that perioperative "stress"-dose corticosteroids improve outcomes, and giving higher than usual corticosteroid doses should be discouraged.[54]

Adrenal insufficiency is a common problem in critically ill postoperative patients. Presentation varies widely from mild manifestations of Addison's disease to a hypotensive state identical to septic shock. Patients suspected of having adrenal insufficiency should have a corticotropin stimulation test. A recent prospective, randomized study demonstrates that septic patients with concurrent adrenal insufficiency (defined as a response of 9μg/dL or less) have markedly improved survival if treated for 1 week with hydrocortisone 50mg every 6 hours. Hydrocortisone has some mineralocorticoid effects, and supplemental fludrocortisone may not be required. However, if dexamethasone is used to replace glucocorticoid function, a daily dose of 50μg of fludrocortisone should be added. Once the decision is made to replace corticosteroids and supported by a corticotropin stimulation test, the replacement should continue for a minimum of 1 week before reassessment.[55]

Thyroid abnormalities are also commonly uncovered in the perioperative care of the acute care surgical patient. Although mild hypothyroidism is relatively well-tolerated and common in the general population (affecting 8% of women and 2% of men over 50 years), severe hypothyroidism is an infrequent and potentially fatal problem in the postoperative setting. Patients with myxedema coma may have hypothermia, delirium with slowed verbal response or unconsciousness, bradycardia, hypoventilation, hypotension, pleural and pericardial effusions, and otherwise diffuse edema. Typical laboratory findings indicative of hypothyroidism include both an elevated TSH concentration and a low or undetectable level of free T_4. Treatment includes daily thyroid replacement hormone as well as supportive care directed toward specific symptoms. Because critically ill postoperative patients have altered thyroid homeostasis, interpreting either TSH or free T_4 in isolation may lead to an inappropriate diagnosis of hypothyroidism in a patient who is "euthyroid sick," and therefore both tests should be sent when the diagnosis is considered.[56]

Infectious Disease Monitoring and Care

Measuring body temperature is an essential part of perioperative care. Hypothermia may contribute to coagulopathy, metabolic acidosis, myocardial dysfunction, arrhythmias, electrolyte imbalances, and an increased risk of surgical site infection. Hypothermia frequently develops in the operating room because of multiple factors, including exposure, evaporative losses, peripheral vasodilation caused by general anesthesia induction, and rapid fluid infusions. On the other hand, hyperthermia is frequent in the postoperative setting and can result in an increased metabolic rate associated with tachycardia and increased insensible fluid losses.

The most reliable method of measuring temperature is obtaining a core body temperature. This can be done in the operating room by an orally placed esophageal probe or via the thermistor tip of a PA catheter if one is present. At the bedside of a routine postoperative patient, core temperature can be estimated by an oral or rectal temperature or by use of a tympanic probe. Axillary temperatures may also be obtained but yield a less accurate approximation of core temperature.

Most fevers in the immediate postoperative setting are inflammatory in nature and will resolve with time and patient mobilization. Hyperthermia that persists beyond the third postoperative day is less usual and should yield further evaluation beyond a physical examination, which is always the first step in a fever workup. Because one third of nosocomial infections are preventable, strict adherence to basic tenets of infection control is important for the postoperative patient. Simple behaviors that decrease infection-associated morbidity and mortality include adequate hand hygiene, the presence of a multidisciplinary infection control team, adherence to contact isolation, use of adequate sterile barrier precautions when placing central venous catheters, and appropriate antibiotic prescribing patterns.

With a previously healthy patient and critical care as described in the preceding sections, most patients recover quickly, are readily weaned from various supports, and transferred out of the intensive care unit in short order. Those great successes are quickly forgotten as attention turns to the others who have fallen off the expected trajectory.

Sustained and Chronic Critical Illness

Recall what is supposed to happen in the perioperative period with respect to cortisol, potassium wasting, and nitrogen wasting. After the stress is resolved ("source control" and definitive repair), hypercortisolism, potassium wasting, and nitrogen wasting persist for a few days. As the hypercortisolism wanes, potassium is used more efficiently. Although ongoing potassium supplementation may be required—it is the major intracellular cation and is therefore necessary to rebuild cells—urine losses trail off. Within another few days, nitrogen wasting ceases. Like potassium, amino acids are still required to build new tissues and therefore nutrition that delivers up to 2 g/kg/day nitrogen are often administered, but the urine losses trail off.

In a significant minority of patients, the potassium and nitrogen losses continue. These patients, who remain hypermetabolic and catabolic for at least 10 days, form a new group of patients that can be viewed as chronically critically ill. They typically require multisystem support. Their metabolic picture deteriorates along a predictable course. They accumulate interstitial water but otherwise exhibit a wasting syndrome that cannibalizes skeletal and visceral protein, somewhere in the range of 100 g/day. Fatty acids are burned less efficiently and wind up in the pancreas, liver, and other viscera. Within cells, water and potassium are depleted. Hypoproteinemia is the norm. Insulin resistance persists. Triglycerides rise. The logical question, then, is what has happened to the secretion of the hypothalamic and pituitary hormones that orchestrated the stress response in the first place?[57]

The Hypothalamic-Pituitary-Adrenal Axis in Chronic Critical Illness

The secretion of cortisol persists despite falling ACTH. It may be that secretion of cortisol becomes autonomous. It may be that there are hitherto unknown secretagogues. However, in the absence of total adrenal failure, cortisol secretion persists even while adrenal androgens (DHEAS) and mineralocorticoids decline. Inspection of a biosynthetic pathway diagram suggests that an alteration in pregnenolone fate may underlie the divergent concentrations.

Growth Hormone and Thyroid Hormone in Chronic Critical Illness

Protracted critical illness is characterized by suppression of the normal pulsatile release of both growth hormone and thyroid hormone. The concentration of the downstream effectors of both decline: IGF-1 and the acid-labile subunit of the ternary complex decline alongside growth hormone, and peripheral T_4 and T_3 levels fall with TSH. The latter situation—low TSH, T_4 and T_3—is sometimes referred to as "euthyroid sick." Interestingly, both TSH and GH release in chronically critically ill humans can be reactivated by infusion of TRH and GHRH-2, which is a growth hormone–releasing peptide.[58] This observation suggests that chronic critical illness may have sustained effects on hypothalamic function.

Testosterone and Luteinizing Hormone in Chronic Critical Illness

As critical illness becomes chronic, peripheral testosterone levels become undetectable. Luteinizing hormone pulsatility tries to increase seemingly in response to the sustained testosterone deficiency, but the average value falls below threshold of detection. Echoing the theme of the previous paragraph, infusion of gonadotropin-releasing hormone (GnRH) along with TRH and GHRH-2 reactivates all three axes in men with chronic critical illness. Interestingly, the cocktail (all three releasing hormones) are required to activate all three axes—giving them separately is far less effective for each target axis.[59]

Prolactin in Chronic Critical Illness

Both prolactin levels and pulsatility diminish with prolonged critical illness. This may explain part of the anergy of critical illness, since immune health is at least partially dependent on prolactin. The declines in absolute prolactin level and in pulsatility are probably due in part to the effects of dopamine, a known suppressor of prolactin release. (This fact alone should raise doubts about the use of dopamine as a vasoactive agent in critical care.[60])

Conclusion

We conclude with the observation that chronic critical illness represents a physiologic trajectory quite different from acute illness and prompt recovery. The supportive interventions that form the mainstay of critical care—ventilation, feeding, and so on—neither reverse catabolism nor accelerate recovery in the chronically critically ill. Whether the changes in stress hormone physiology, especially the changes in anterior pituitary function ("up" in the acute response, "down" in chronic critical illness) simply represent casual association or whether there is causality is unknown at this time. If manipulation of anterior pituitary function by titrated administration of releasing hormones could even slightly attenuate and abbreviate chronic critical illness, there would be substantial benefit to patients, families, and caregivers.

Critique

More specifics regarding the patient are needed to fully determine if the above-mentioned ventilatory components are appropriate. However, this apneic patient clearly does not need pressure support, for this modality is used to facilitate weaning. For an apneic patient who is obviously unable to participate in weaning, the use of pressure support is absolutely superfluous.

Answer (D)

References

1. Woolf PD. Endocrinology of shock. Ann Emerg Med 1986; 15(12):1401–1405.
2. Cuthbertson DP. Second annual Jonathan E. Rhoads Lecture. The metabolic response to injury and its nutritional implications: retrospect and prospect. JPEN J Parenter Enteral Nutr 1979; 3(3):108–129.
3. Brozena SC, Jessup M. The new staging system for heart failure. What every primary care physician should know. Geriatrics 2003; 58(6):31–36.
4. Azoulay E, Pochard F, Chevret S, Adrie C, Bollaert PE, Brun F, Dreyfuss D, Garrouste-Orgeas M, Goldgran-Toledano D, Jourdain M, Wolff M, Le Gall JR, Schlemmer B. Opinions about surrogate designation: a population survey in France. Crit Care Med 2003; 31(6):1711–1714.
5. Baradarian R, Ramdhaney S, Chapalamadugu R, Skoczylas L, Wang K, Rivilis S, Remus K, Mayer I, Iswara K, Tenner S. Early intensive resuscitation of patients with upper gastrointestinal bleeding decreases mortality. Am J Gastroenterol 2004; 99(4):619–622.

6. Rotondo MF, Zonies DH. The damage control sequence and underlying logic. Surg Clin North Am 1997; 77:761–777.

7. Schein M, Saadia R, Decker GG. The open management of the septic abdomen. Surg Gynecol Obstet 1986; 163(6):587–592.

8. Lindblat B, Hakansson H. The rationale for "second look operation" in mesenteric vessel occlusion with uncertain intestinal viability at primary surgery. Acta Chir Scand 1987; 153:531–533.

9. Heys SD, Ogston KN. Peri-operative nutritional support: controversies and debates. Int J Surg Invest 2000; 2(2):107–115.

10. Freeman BD, Borecki IB, Coopersmith CM, Buchman TG. Relationship between tracheostomy timing and duration of mechanical ventilation in critically ill patients. Crit Care Med 2005; 33(11):2513–2520.

11. Weil MH, Bisera J, Trevino RP, Rackow EC. Cardiac output and end-tidal carbon dioxide. Crit Care Med 1985; 13(11):907–909.

12. Moore FD. Bodily changes in surgical convalescence. I. The normal sequence observations and interpretations. Ann Surg 1953; 137(3):289–315.

13. Udelsman R, Holbrook NJ. Endocrine and molecular responses to surgical stress. Curr Probl Surg 1994; 31(8):653–720.

14. Rhen T, Cidlowski JA. Antiinflammatory action of glucocorticoids—new mechanisms for old drugs. N Engl J Med 2005; 353(16):1711–1723.

15. Amar D, Fleisher M, Pantuck CB, Shamoon H, Zhang H, Roistacher N, Leung DH, Ginsburg I, Smiley RM. Persistent alterations of the autonomic nervous system after noncardiac surgery. Anesthesiology 1998; 89(1):30–42.

16. Gianotti L, Broglio F, Aimaretti G, Arvat E, Colombo S, Di Summa M, Gallioli G, Pittoni G, Sardo E, Stella M, Zanello M, Miola C, Ghigo E. Low IGF-I levels are often uncoupled with elevated GH levels in catabolic conditions. J Endocrinol Invest 1998; 21(2):115–121.

17. Exton JH, Friedmann N, Wong EH, Brineaux JP, Corbin JD, Park CR. Interaction of glucocorticoids with glucagon and epinephrine in the control of gluconeogenesis and glycogenolysis in liver and of lipolysis in adipose tissue. J Biol Chem 1972; 247(11):3579–3588.

18. Calzia E, Koch M, Stahl W, Radermacher P, Brinkmann A. Stress response during weaning after cardiac surgery. Br J Anaesth 2001; 87(3):490–493.

19. Weekers F, Van den Berghe G. Endocrine modifications and interventions during critical illness. Proc Nutr Soc 2004; 63(3):443–450.

20. Schricker T, Wykes L, Carli F. Epidural blockade improves substrate utilization after surgery. Am J Physiol Endocrinol Metab 2000; 279(3):E646–E653.

21. Bessey PQ, Watters JM, Aoki TT, Wilmore DW. Combined hormonal infusion simulates the metabolic response to injury. Ann Surg 1984; 200(3):264–281.

22. van den Berghe G, Wouters P, Weekers F, Verwaest C, Bruyninckx F, Schetz M, Vlasselaers D, Ferdinande P, Lauwers P, Bouillon R. Intensive insulin therapy in the critically ill patients. N Engl J Med 2001; 345(19):1359–1367.

23. Takala J, Ruokonen E, Webster NR, Nielsen MS, Zandstra DF, Vundelinckx G, Hinds CJ. Increased mortality associated with growth hormone treatment in critically ill adults. N Engl J Med 1999; 341(11):785–792.

24. Peeters RP, Wouters PJ, Kaptein E, van Toor H, Visser TJ, Van den Berghe G. Reduced activation and increased inactivation of thyroid hormone in tissues of critically ill patients. J Clin Endocrinol Metab 2003; 88(7):3202–3211.

25. Wang C, Chan V, Yeung RT. Effect of surgical stress on pituitary-testicular function. Clin Endocrinol (Oxf) 1978; 9(3):255–266.

26. Van den Berghe G, de Zegher F. Anterior pituitary function during critical illness and dopamine treatment. Crit Care Med 1996; 24(9):1580–1590.

27. Devereaux PJ, Goldman L, Cook DJ, Gilbert K, Leslie K, Guyatt GH. Related perioperative cardiac events in patients undergoing noncardiac surgery: a review of the magnitude of the problem, the pathophysiology of the events and methods to estimate and communicate risk. CMAJ 2005; 173(6):627–634.

28. Auerbach AD, Goldman L. Beta-blockers and reduction of cardiac events in noncardiac surgery: scientific review. JAMA 2002; 287(11):1435–1444.

29. Eagle KA, Berger PB, Calkins H, Chaitman BR, Ewy GA, Fleischmann KE, Fleisher LA, Froehlich JB, Gusberg RJ, Leppo JA, Ryan T, Schlant RC, Winters WL Jr, Gibbons RJ, Antman EM, Alpert JS, Faxon DP, Fuster V, Gregoratos G, Jacobs AK, Hiratzka LF, Russell RO, Smith SC Jr. American College of Cardiology/American Heart Association Task Force on Practice Guidelines (Committee to Update the 1996 Guidelines on Perioperative Cardiovascular Evaluation for Noncardiac Surgery). ACC/AHA guideline update for perioperative cardiovascular evaluation for noncardiac surgery—executive summary. A report of the American College of Cardiology/American Heart Association Task Force on Practice Guidelines (Committee to Update the 1996 Guidelines on Perioperative Cardiovascular Evaluation for Noncardiac Surgery). Circulation 2002; 105(10):1257–1267.

30. Wiest D. Esmolol. A review of its therapeutic efficacy and pharmacokinetic characteristics. Clin Pharmacokinet 1995; 28(3):190–202.

31. Kertai MD, Klein J, Bax JJ, Poldermans D. Predicting perioperative cardiac risk. Prog Cardiovasc Dis 2005; 47(4):240–257.

32. Landesberg G. Monitoring for myocardial ischemia. Best Pract Res Clin Anaesthesiol 2005; 19(1):77–95.

33. Chu WW, Dieter RS, Stone CK. Evolving clinical applications of cardiac markers: a review of the literature. WMJ 2002; 101(3):49–55.

34. Lorente L, Henry C, Martin MM, Jimenez A, Mora ML. Central venous catheter–related infection in a prospective and observational study of 2,595 catheters. Crit Care 2005; 9(6):R631–R635.

35. Canaud B, Desmeules S, Klouche K, Leray-Moragues H, Beraud JJ. Vascular access for dialysis in the intensive care unit. Best Pract Res Clin Anaesthesiol 2004; 18(1):159–174.

36. Sandham JD, Hull RD, Brant RF, Knox L, Pineo GF, Doig CJ, Laporta DP, Viner S, Passerini L, Devitt H, Kirby A, Jacka M. Canadian Critical Care Clinical Trials Group. A randomized, controlled trial of the use of pulmonary-artery

catheters in high-risk surgical patients. N Engl J Med 2003; 348(1):5–14.

37. Murphy GS, Nitsun M, Vender JS. Is the pulmonary artery catheter useful? Best Pract Res Clin Anaesthesiol 2005; 19(1):97–110.

38. Laupland KB, Bands CJ. Utility of esophageal Doppler as a minimally invasive hemodynamic monitor: a review. Can J Anaesth 2002; 49(4):393–401.

39. Theodoropoulos G, Lloyd LR, Cousins G, Pieper D. Intraoperative and early postoperative gastric intramucosal pH predicts morbidity and mortality after major abdominal surgery. Am Surg 2001; 67(4):303–308.

40. Webb RK, Ralston AC, Runciman WB. Potential errors in pulse oximetry. II. Effects of changes in saturation and signal quality. Anaesthesia 1991; 46(3):207–212.

41. Ralston AC, Webb RK, Runciman WB. Potential errors in pulse oximetry. III: Effects of interferences, dyes, dyshaemoglobins and other pigments. Anaesthesia 1991; 46(4):291–295.

42. Li J. Capnography alone is imperfect for endotracheal tube placement confirmation during emergency intubation. J Emerg Med 2001; 20(3):223–229.

43. Kress JP, Pohlman AS, O'Connor MF, Hall JB. Daily interruption of sedative infusions in critically ill patients undergoing mechanical ventilation. N Engl J Med 2000; 342(20):1471–1477.

44. Glare PA, Walsh TD. Clinical pharmacokinetics of morphine. Ther Drug Monit 1991; 13(1):1–23.

45. Seifert CF, Kennedy S. Meperidine is alive and well in the new millennium: evaluation of meperidine usage patterns and frequency of adverse drug reactions. Pharmacotherapy 2004; 24(6):776–783.

46. Garnacho-Montero J, Amaya-Villar R, Garcia-Garmendia JL, Madrazo-Osuna J, Ortiz-Leyba C. Effect of critical illness polyneuropathy on the withdrawal from mechanical ventilation and the length of stay in septic patients. Crit Care Med 2005; 33(2):349–354.

47. Hund E. Neurological complications of sepsis: critical illness polyneuropathy and myopathy. J Neurol 2001; 248(11):929–934.

48. Birck R, Krzossok S, Markowetz F, Schnulle P, van der Woude FJ, Braun C. Acetylcysteine for prevention of contrast nephropathy: meta-analysis Lancet 2003; 362(9384): 598–560.

49. Merten GJ, Burgess WP, Gray LV, Holleman JH, Roush TS, Kowalchuk GJ, Bersin RM, Van Moore A, Simonton CA 3rd, Rittase RA, Norton HJ, Kennedy TP. Prevention of contrast-induced nephropathy with sodium bicarbonate: a randomized controlled trial. JAMA 2004; 291(19):2328–2334.

50. Heyland DK, Samis A. Does immunonutrition in patients with sepsis do more harm than good? Intensive Care Med 2003; 29(5):669–667.

51. Hebert PC, Wells G, Blajchman MA, Marshall J, Martin C, Pagliarello G, Tweeddale M, Schweitzer I, Yetisir E. A multicenter, randomized, controlled clinical trial of transfusion requirements in critical care. Transfusion Requirements in Critical Care Investigators, Canadian Critical Care Trials Group. N Engl J Med 1999; 340(6):409–417.

52. Schuerer DJ, Whinney RR, Freeman BD, Nash J, Prasad S, Krem MM, Mazuski JE, Buchman TG. Evaluation of the applicability, efficacy, and safety of a thromboembolic event prophylaxis guideline designed for quality improvement of the traumatically injured patient. J Trauma 2005; 58(4):731–739.

53. Taylor JH, Beilman GJ. Hyperglycemia in the intensive care unit: no longer just a marker of illness severity. Surg Infect (Larchmt) 2005; 6(2):233–245.

54. Salem M, Tainsh RE Jr, Bromberg J, Loriaux DL, Chernow B. Perioperative glucocorticoid coverage: a reassessment 42 years after emergence of a problem. Ann Surg 1994; 219(4): 416–425.

55. Prigent H, Maxime V, Annane D. Clinical review: corticotherapy in sepsis. Crit Care 2004; 8(2):122–129.

56. Docter R, Krenning EP, de Jong M, Hennemann G. The sick euthyroid syndrome: changes in thyroid hormone serum parameters and hormone metabolism. Clin Endocrinol 1993; 39:499–518.

57. Van den Berghe G, de Zegher F, Bouillon R. Clinical review 95: acute and prolonged critical illness as different neuroendocrine paradigms. J Clin Endocrinol Metab 1998; 83(6):1827–1834.

58. Van den Berghe G, de Zegher F, Baxter RC, Veldhuis JD, Wouters P, Schetz M, Verwaest C, Van der Vorst E, Lauwers P, Bouillon R, Bowers CY. Neuroendocrinology of prolonged critical illness: effects of exogenous thyrotropin-releasing hormone and its combination with growth hormone secretagogues. J Clin Endocrinol Metab 1998; 83(2):309–319.

59. Van den Berghe G, Baxter RC, Weekers F, Wouters P, Bowers CY, Iranmanesh A, Veldhuis JD, Bouillon R. The combined administration of GH-releasing peptide-2 (GHRP-2), TRH and GnRH to men with prolonged critical illness evokes superior endocrine and metabolic effects compared to treatment with GHRP-2 alone. Clin Endocrinol (Oxf) 2002; 56(5):655–669.

60. Van den Berghe G, de Zegher F. Anterior pituitary function during critical illness and dopamine treatment. Crit Care Med 1996; 24(9):1580–1590.

6
The Hemodynamically Labile Patient: Cardiovascular Adjuncts and Assist Devices

Edward E. Cornwell III and Preeti R. John

Case Scenario

A 66-year-old retired teacher is being managed in the intensive care unit after having a myocardial infarction. The patient had no prior medical problems. The patient is hemodynamically labile and is refractory to volume support and all pharmacologic interventions. The patient is now in profound cardiogenic shock. Which of the following would most likely be the management of choice?

(A) Emergency cardiac catheterization
(B) Coronary artery bypass surgery
(C) Intraaortic balloon pump
(D) Continue inotropic support
(E) No further intervention is needed

New successes bring new challenges. Two dominant observations can be made regarding trends in the emergency care of the surgical patient over the last quarter century. An aging population and the increasing life expectancy present the ever-increasing specter of the geriatric patient developing medical problems that require emergency surgical and critical care. Improved anesthetic and perioperative techniques are responsible for many of these patients surviving acute care surgery and requiring postoperative critical care. Improvements in prehospital care, triage, and transport have led to many trauma systems achieving improved outcomes and presenting patients to trauma centers who decades earlier would not have survived. The result of these two observations is the trend toward the arrival in the surgical intensive care unit of more geriatric patients with comorbid cardiovascular diseases, as well as more critically ill and injured patients who in prior decades would not have

survived their traumatic injuries or major operations. The ultimate survival of these patients frequently depends on their being able to navigate a period of postoperative critical illness when hemodynamic support will be a mainstay of therapy. Accordingly, this chapter deals with cardiovascular adjuncts and assist devices that are available to the intensivist in the management of the hemodynamically labile patient.

Pharmacological Circulatory Support: Vasopressin

Vasodilatory shock caused by systemic inflammatory response syndrome (SIRS) sepsis is a common problem in critically ill patients. The typical hemodynamic pattern encountered is characterized by high cardiac output with low systemic venous resistance because of profound peripheral vasodilatation, resulting in end-organ hypoperfusion. Treatment includes appropriate antibiotics, expansion of intravascular volume, and inotropic agents.

Catecholamines are the first line of therapy for such patients; however, downregulation of adrenergic receptors has long been postulated to contribute to the progressive hemodynamic instability seen in septic shock. "Adrenergic hyposensitivity"—hypotension refractory to massive doses of adrenergic vasopressors—has been described[1] and is often responsible for that sinking, frustrating feeling feared by all experienced intensivists. In contrast, the phenomenon of "vasopressin hypersensitivity"—enhanced vasopressin sensitivity despite a relative arginine vasopressin (AVP) deficiency in septic shock—has also been described.[2]

Arginine vasopressin is an endogenous hormone secreted from the neurohypophysis (posterior pituitary) in response to an increase in serum osmolality or a

TABLE 6.1. Randomized controlled trials of arginine vasopressin (AVP).

Author and year	No. (controls, AVP)	Inclusion criteria	Dose	Outcome benefits	Comments
Dunser et al.,[5] 2003	48 (24, 24)	Catecholamine-resistant vasodilatory shock	4 U/hr	Lower HR, NE requirements, and incidence of new-onset tachyarrhythmias; higher MAP, CI, SVI, and LVSWI	GI perfusion (gastric tonometry) better preserved; bilirubin concentrations significantly higher in AVP-treated patients
Patel et al.,[6] 2001	24 (11, 13)	Septic shock that required high-dose vasopressor support	0.1 U/min <6 U/hr	NE infusion requirement decreased from 25 to 5.3 µg/min at 4 hr ($p < 0.001$)	Urine output and creatinine clearance increased in AVP patients
Malay et al.,[7] 1999	10 (5, 5)	Vasodilatory septic shock	0.04 Umin	Increased systolic arterial pressure (98 ± 5 to 125 ± 8 mm Hg, $p < 0.008$), systemic vascular resistance 878 ± 218 to 1,190 ± 213 dyne-scm, $p < 0.05$)	All AVP patients survived and had other catecholamine pressors withdrawn
Argenziano et al.,[8] 1997	10 (5, 5)	LVAD placement with post-bypass vasodilatory shock requiring catecholamine pressors	0.1 Umin	Increased mean arterial pressure (57 ± 4 to 84 ± 2 mm Hg, $p < 0.001$) and systemic vascular resistance 813 ± 113 to 1,188 ± 87 dyne-scm, $p < 0.001$) with decreased NE administration	Absolute vasopressin deficiency was observed in most patients

CI, cardiac index; GI, gastrointestinal; HR, heart rate; LVAD, left ventricular assist device; LVSWI, left ventricular stroke work index; MAP, mean arterial pressure; NE, norepinephrine; SVI, stroke volume index.

decrease in plasma volume and has little pressor effect in normal subjects. In arteriolar smooth muscle cells, stimulation of V1a receptors leads to an increase in cytoplasmic ionized calcium via the phosphatidyl-inositol-bisphosphonate cascade. This causes constriction of peripheral resistance vessels with resulting increased systemic vascular resistance. Vasopressin increases resistance in *efferent* glomerular arterioles but has virtually no effect on afferent glomerular arterioles. Hence it may result in increased glomerular perfusion pressure and flow and in elevated glomerular filtration rate. These vasopressor effects seem to be preserved during hypoxia and acidosis.

In contrast to hypovolemic and cardiogenic shock during which AVP concentrations increase substantially, it has been shown that most patients in vasodilatory septic shock are deficient in vasopressin.[3,4] Dysfunction of the baroreceptor reflex, inhibition of AVP production, and depletion of AVP stores during sustained hypotension (endotoxin is a potent vasopressin secretagogue) have been postulated as responsible mechanisms. Deficiency of endogenous AVP in septic shock may contribute to loss of vascular tone. Arginine vasopressin infusion may reverse this deficiency and restore endogenous vasopressor effects; there is emerging evidence of the effectiveness of AVP in this clinical scenario (Table 6.1).[5–8]

Mechanical Circulatory Systems

Extracorporeal Membrane Oxygenation

The first successful use of extracorporeal membrane oxygenation (ECMO) was reported by Hill et al.[9] in 1972, after a motorcycle accident victim was managed with venoarterial extracorporeal support for 3 days. For adults, ECMO has been used to provide postcardiotomy support, as a bridge to an implantable left ventricular assist device or a bridge to heart or lung transplantation, and to provide respiratory support.

Extracorporeal membrane oxygenation uses a modified heart lung machine to provide circulatory assistance. The circuit is similar in concept to cardiopulmonary bypass routinely used in the operating room; however, certain modifications to the circuit, particularly the inclusion of membrane oxygenators, permit extended periods of support (Figure 6.1). The extracorporeal circuit is heparin coated and consists of a centrifugal pump, a hollow-fiber oxygenator, an integrated heat exchanger, percutaneous arterial and venous femoral cannulas, and tubing.

Blood is removed from the patient, passed through an artificial membrane where gas exchange occurs, and then returned to the body by either the arterial (venoarterial) or the venous (venovenous) system. Cannulation for

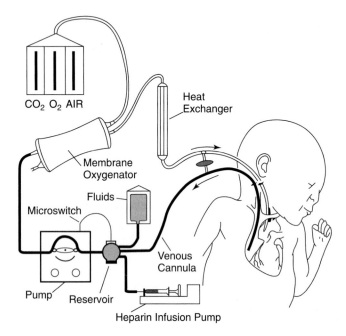

FIGURE 6.1. Extracorporeal membrane oxygenation. (Reprinted with permission from The McGraw-Hill Companies from Kern FH, et al. Extracorporeal circulation and circulatory assist devices in the pediatric patient. In Lake CL, ed. Pediatric Cardiac Anesthesia. Stamford, CT: Appleton & Lange, 1998.)

ECMO is variable and depends on the clinical situation and on whether a venoarterial or venovenous circuit is desired. It can be performed percutaneously using a modified Seldinger technique or an open technique.

Venoarterial circuits can be used for either cardiac or respiratory support. Venoarterial ECMO provides *cardiac* support by draining blood from the venous circulation, oxygenating it, and then returning it to the arterial circulation at physiologic perfusion pressures.

In venoarterial bypass, the right atrium is cannulated via the right internal jugular vein with a soft silastic or polyvinyl chloride catheter. Blood is siphoned passively by gravity drainage to a venous reservoir positioned below heart level. The blood is actively pumped from the reservoir by a roller head pump. This blood then circulates through the artificial lung, where gas exchange occurs against a filtered gas mixture of oxygen and carbon dioxide. The most common artificial lung used is a thin, gas-permeable silicone membrane that serves as a blood–gas interface, similar to the alveolar capillary membrane. Countercurrent flow of blood and gas on opposite sides of the membrane allows for effective diffusion of gases between the blood and gas phases. Oxygenation can be regulated by varying blood flow through the ECMO circuit to the extent that laminar flow will allow. The higher the volume of cardiac output diverted through the membrane lung, the better the oxygen deliv-

ery from the ECMO circuit. Blood is returned to the patient via a catheter positioned in the aortic arch through a right common carotid artery cannulation. Pressor support and vasodilators can usually be stopped while the patient is on venoarterial ECMO support, as perfusion pressure from the pump largely replaces cardiac output.

Venovenous ECMO maintains flow through the heart (unlike venoarterial ECMO) and has been the preferred method of *respiratory* support. Venovenous bypass precludes the need for arterial access. This technique involves draining desaturated blood from the right atrium and returning oxygenated blood through the right femoral vein. Advantages of venovenous bypass include avoidance of carotid artery cannulation and maintenance of pulmonary blood flow. The major disadvantage is that, unlike venoarterial bypass, venovenous ECMO does not provide cardiac support. Oxygen delivery in venovenous bypass remains dependent on native cardiac output.

Systemic anticoagulation therapy with heparin is administered for the duration of the bypass procedure to prevent clotting in the circuit and possible thromboembolization. Activated clotting times are measured hourly and are maintained within a certain range. Risks associated with ECMO are related to vessel cannulation, bleeding (heparinization, platelet dysfunction), thromboembolic phenomena, and infection.

Doll et al.[10] prospectively evaluated 219 adult patients (mean age 61.3 ± 12.1) in whom ECMO was used after cardiac surgery and concluded that it is an acceptable technique for short-term treatment of refractory postoperative low cardiac output. One hundred forty-four patients needed additional intraaortic balloon counterpulsation to improve coronary blood flow. Of 219 patients, 60% were successfully weaned from ECMO; of these, 24% were discharged from the hospital after approximately 30 days. Five-year follow-up was 96% complete: 74% of patients were alive with reasonable exercise capacity.

In a retrospective clinical study by Schwartz et al.,[11] 46 adults with underlying cardiocirculatory disease were supported with venoarterial cardiopulmonary bypass. They were placed emergently on ECMO because of prolonged cardiogenic shock or cardiopulmonary arrest. Results were encouraging, with 28 out of 46 (61%) weaned from cardiopulmonary bypass. Long-term survival was reported in 13 patients.

Ko and colleagues[12] reported the outcome of 76 adult patients who received ECMO support for postcardiotomy cardiogenic shock. Twenty-two received ECMO support, and 54 received concomitant intraaortic balloon pump (IABP) and ECMO support. Two were bridged to ventricular assist devices and two to heart transplantation. Twenty patients (26%) were eventually weaned off ECMO support and survived to hospital discharge; 20

were weaned off ECMO support but presented intrahospital mortality, and 30 died on EMCO support.

Intraaortic Balloon Pump

The IABP was first used clinically in 1968 for supporting patients with cardiogenic shock after acute myocardial infarction; it was reported by Kantrowitz et al.[13] that same year. Currently its principal indications for use in the cardiac surgical patient are for postoperative support (postcardiotomy heart failure), as an aid in weaning from cardiopulmonary bypass, and, more recently, for preoperative support of patients with unstable coronary syndromes and cardiogenic shock. It is the most commonly used assist device for temporary support of the failing ventricle after cardiac surgery.

The IABP is an intravascular, catheter-mounted, counterpulsation device with a polyurethane balloon (volume between 30 and 50 cc) connected to a driving system. The gas used is helium, because its low viscosity allows rapid movement and therefore fast inflation and deflation, which facilitates counterpulsation.

It is inserted percutaneously into the descending thoracic aorta via the common femoral artery and positioned in the descending thoracic aorta with the tip just distal to the left subclavian artery (Figure 6.2). It can also be introduced directly into the aorta if the chest is open (e.g., during heart surgery).

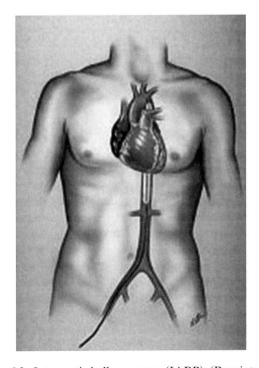

FIGURE 6.2. Intraaortic balloon pump (IABP). (Reprinted with permission of Abiomed, Inc., Danvers, MA.)

It works on the principle of counterpulsation, that is, it assists the heart in series synchronous with the patient's ECG and is timed to either the arterial pressure curve or to the ECG.

The balloon is inflated during cardiac diastole at the dicrotic notch of the arterial pressure waveform when monitoring aortic pressure. The diastolic rise in aortic root pressure augments coronary blood flow and increases coronary artery perfusion and myocardial oxygen supply.

Deflation occurs during cardiac diastole isovolumetric contraction of the left ventricle. The resulting reduction in afterload decreases peak left ventricular pressure and myocardial oxygen consumption. During systole the balloon is deflated, decreasing left ventricular afterload, which in turn decreases myocardial oxygen consumption and increases cardiac output. Proper balloon timing (inflation/deflation) improves the ratio between myocardial oxygen supply and demand.[14]

Stone et al.[15] conducted a large-scale study of IABP use in patients with acute myocardial infarction. Data were collected prospectively from a registry of 22,663 patients treated with aortic counterpulsation in 250 medical centers worldwide; 5,495 (24%) of the patients had an acute myocardial infarction (AMI). The following were indications for IABP use in patients with AMI: cardiogenic shock, hemodynamic support during catheterization and/or angioplasty before high-risk surgery, mechanical complications of AMI, and refractory postmyocardial infarction unstable angina as a bridge to angiography and revascularization.

In a series of small, randomized controlled trials from a single institution, a protective effect of preoperative IABP insertion in high risk patients was demonstrated.[16–19] Baskett et al.[14] conducted a prospective cohort study of IABP use in coronary artery bypass grafting over a 6-year time frame and across 10 tertiary care cardiac surgical centers in the United States and Canada. They demonstrated a marked increase in IABP utilization (46% increased rate) and also a substantial variation in indications for IABP use across the different centers.

Ventricular Assist Devices

Ventricular assist devices (VADs) are mechanical pumps that take over the function of the damaged ventricle and restore normal hemodynamics and end-organ blood flow. The term "ventricular assist device" describes any of a variety of mechanical blood pumps that are employed singly to replace the function of either the right or the left ventricle. The devices are designed to effectively unload either the right or the left ventricle while completely supporting the pulmonary or systemic circulation.

The LVADs support the left ventricle, and Thoractec's BiVAD can temporarily support both ventricles.

All LVADs have the same basic function: to improve cardiac output. Surgery involves implantation of the device into the left upper abdomen, either preperitoneally or intraabdominally (outside the chest wall), with an inflow canula attached to the left ventricle and an outflow canula anastomosed to the patient's ascending aorta. All the devices have a percutaneous lead or driveline with two channels: one channel connects the internal pump to an external controller, and the other channel acts as a vent to exchange air for activation of the device's diaphragm.

For *right* ventricular assistance, blood is withdrawn from the right atrium and returned to the main pulmonary artery. For *left* ventricular assistance, blood is withdrawn from either the left *atrium* or the apex of the left *ventricle*, passes through the LVAD, and is returned to the ascending aorta. Left *atrial* inflow cannulation is technically easier to perform but is thought to provide incomplete ventricular decompression. Left *ventricular* inflow cannulation provides very effective left ventricular decompression but requires a custom-designed canula. The reduction in myocardial oxygen demand is offset by the fact that left ventricular apical cannulation damages the myocardium, an important consideration for a patient with marginal ventricular function. For patients who receive mechanical circulatory support as a bridge to cardiac transplantation, ventricular recovery is not expected, and the apical canula is removed in its entirety at the time of recipient cardiectomy; a left ventricular apex cannula is ideally suited for these patients.

Bridge to Recovery

Left ventricular assist devices are used in patients who require ventricular assistance to allow the heart to rest and recover function, for example, in postcardiotomy shock. The device is a temporary measure until the patient's heart is able to function on its own: "ventricular reverse modeling."[20] In recent studies, LVAD use improved cardiac function in some patients to the extent that the devices were removed and the patients no longer required transplantation. The LVAD takes over cardiac function, and blood flow throughout the body increases. The heart itself benefits from this increase, which allows it to regain function. Possible physiologic changes responsible for reverse modeling include a decrease in myocardial stretch, profound volume and pressure unloading, increased myocardial perfusion, normalization of neurohormones, and reduced cytokine release.

The Food and Drug Administration (FDA) has approved two LVADs for short-term use in the intensive care unit to temporarily stabilize patients (Table 6.2):

TABLE 6.2. Comparison of ventricular assist devices (VADs).

VAD type	Advantages	Disadvantages
Centrifugal	Readily available Simple to use Relatively inexpensive	Nonpulsatile Systemic anticoagulation Constant supervision required Not FDA approved as a VAD

Pneumatic pulsatile	No blood trauma
	Anticoagulation +
	  Pulsatile flow
	Minimal supervision
	  required
		Limited patient mobility with
		  drive consoles
		Expensive

Electric pulsatile	Same as pneumatic pulsatile	Highly portable Hospital discharge permitted

Abiomed BVS 5000 (Abiomed, Danvers, MA) (Figure 6.3)
Biomedicus (Medtronic, Minneapolis)

Thoratec (pneumatic) is paracorporeal (outside the chest wall). It can be used in patients with small statures who, because of their size, would be unqualified to receive an LVAD. It can be removed without the patient undergoing heart transplantation because the heart has recovered enough to function on its own.

Bridge to Transplantation

Left ventricular assist devices are used in patients with end-stage heart disease or acute myocarditis who are not expected to recover adequate function and who require mechanical support prior to transplantation. Evidence shows that patients waiting for heart transplantation who have an LVAD implanted have a better outcome than medically managed patients waiting for transplantation.[21] Implantation of an LVAD before transplantation results in lower rates of morbidity and mortality after transplantation.[22]

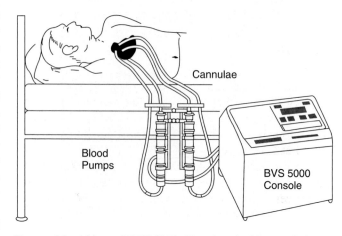

FIGURE 6.3. Abiomed BVS 5000. (Reprinted with permission of Abiomed, Inc., Danvers, MA.)

The FDA has approved the following models to be used as "bridge to transplantation":

Thoratec (pneumatic; can be used for either right or left ventricle. The biventricular assist device, BiVAD, supports both ventricles), Thoratec Laboratories
HeartMate (implanted pneumatic), Thoratec Laboratories
Novacor 100, Worldheart, Canada

Destination Therapy–Still in its Infancy

In 2002, the FDA approved the "FDA Circulatory System Devices Advisory Panel" recommendation that the HeartMate vented electric LVAD (Thoratec) be used as destination therapy for patients with end-stage heart failure who were ineligible for heart transplantation.[23-25]

The Randomized Evaluation of Mechanical Assistance for the Treatment of Congestive Heart Failure (REMATCH trial—marked the first trial of the devices as long-term therapy), conducted from May 1998 to July 2001 in 20 cardiac transplantation centers in the United States, compared the efficacy of two interventions for patients who had end-stage heart failure and were ineligible for transplantation because of age (older than 65 years) or comorbidity.[26,27] Patients were randomize to receive either an LVAD (specifically, a HeartMate vented electric device, manufactured by Thoratec, one of the study's sponsors) or medical therapy (drugs including beta-blockers, diuretics, digoxin, and angiotensin-converting-enzyme inhibitors). The REMATCH trial demonstrated that LVAD implantation resulted in substantially greater improvement in patient survival than medical therapy alone and could be used to replace cardiac function for extended periods. In this trial, 52% of the LVAD recipients survived, and 25% of the medical therapy patients survived. The median survival time among patients with LVADs was 408 days compared with 150 days for patients receiving medications alone. A clinically meaningful survival benefit and improved quality of life were demonstrated in the device group.

Critique

This patient has documented cardiogenic shock secondary to an acute myocardial infarction. With this patient being refractory to both volume and all pharmacologic interventions, the intraaortic balloon pump, the first "ventricular assistance" device, is the intervention of choice. The phased inflation, deflation of the balloon decreases the work of the heart and improves coronary blood flow. It can be a bridge to more definitive management.

Answer (C)

References

1. Chernow B, Rothl BL. Pharmacological manipulation of the peripheral vasculature in shock: clinical and experimental approaches. Circ Shock 1986; 18:141–155.
2. Landry DW, Levin HR, Gallant EM, et al. Vasopressin pressor hypersensitivity in vasodilatory septic shock. Crit Care Med 1997; 25(8):1279–1282.
3. Landry DW, Levin HR, Gallant EM, et al. Vasopressin deficiency contributes to the vasodilation of septic shock. Circulation 1997; 95:1122–1125.
4. Reid IA. Role of vasopressin deficiency in the vasodilation of septic shock. Circulation, 1997; 95:1108–1110.
5. Dunser MW, Mayr AJ, Ulmer H, et al. Arginine vasopressin in advanced shock: a prospective, randomized, controlled study. Circulation 2003; 107(18):2313–1319.
6. Patel BM, Chittock DR, Russell JA, et al. Beneficial effects of short-term vasopressin infusion during severe septic shock. Anesthesiology 2002; 96(3):576–582.
7. Malay MB, Ashton RC Jr, Landry DW, et al. Low-dose vasopressin in the treatment of vasodilatory septic shock. J Trauma 1999; 47(4):699–703.
8. Argenziano M, Choudhri AF, Oz MC, et al. A prospective randomized trial of arginine vasopressin in the treatment of vasodilatory shock after left ventricular assist device placement. Circulation 1997; 96(Suppl II):II-286–II-290.
9. Hill D, O'Brien TG, Murray JJ, et al. Extracorporeal oxygenation for acute post-traumatic respiratory failure (shock lung syndrome). Use of the Bramson membrane lung. N Engl J Med 1972; 286:629–634.
10. Doll N, Kiaii B, Borger M, et al. Five year results of 219 consecutive patients treated with extracorporeal membrane oxygenation for refractory postoperative cardiogenic shock. Ann Thorac Surg 2004; 77:151–157.
11. Schwarz B, Mair P, Margreikter J, et al. Experience with percutaneous venoarterial cardiopulmonary bypass for emergency circulatory support. Crit Care Med 2003; 31(3):758–764.
12. Ko WJ, Lin CY, Chen RJ, et al. Extracorporeal membrane oxygenation support for adult postcardiotomy cardiogenic shock. Ann Thorac Surg 2002; 73(2):538–545.
13. Kantrowitz A, Tjonneland S, Freed PS, et al. Initial clinical experience with intraaortic balloon pumping in cardiogenic shock. JAMA 1968; 203:113–118.
14. Baskett RJF, O'Connor GT, Hirsch GM, et al. A multicenter comparison of intraaortic balloon pump utilization in isolated coronary artery bypass graft surgery. Ann Thorac Surg 2003; 76:1988–1992.
15. Stone GW, Magnus Ohman E, Miller MF, et al. Contemporary utilization and outcomes of intra-aortic balloon counterpulsation in acute myocardial infarction. J Am Coll Cardiol 2003; 41:1940–1950.
16. Christenson JT, Simonet F, Badel P, et al. Optimal timing of preoperative intra-aortic balloon pump support in high-risk coronary patients. Ann Thorac Surg 1999; 68:934–939.
17. Christenson JT, Badel P, Simonet F, et al. Preoperative intra-aortic balloon pump enhances cardiac performance and improves the outcome of redo CABG. Ann Thorac Surg 1997; 64:1237–1244.

18. Christenson JT, Simonet F, Badel P, et al. Evaluation of preoperative intra-aortic balloon pump support in high risk coronary patients. Eur J Cardiothorac Surg 1997; 11(6): 1097–1103

19. Ohman EM, George BS, White CJ, et al. Use of aortic counterpulsation to improve sustained coronary artery patency during acute myocardial infarction. Results of a randomized trial. The randomized IABP study group. Circulation 1994; 90(2):792–799.

20. Madigan JD, et al. Time course of reverse modeling of the left ventricle during support with a left ventricular assist device. J Thorac Cardiovasc Surg 2001; 121(5):902–908.

21. Mehta SM, et al. Mechanical ventricular assistance: an economical and effective means of treating end-stage heart disease. Ann Thorac Surg 1995; 60(2):284–290.

22. Aaronson KD, et al. Left ventricular assist device therapy improves utilization of donor hearts. J Am Coll Cardiol 2002; 39(8):1247–1254.

23. Frazier OH, Reynolds M, Delgado M. Mechanical circulatory support for advanced heart failure. Where does it stand in 2003? Circulation 2003; 108:3064–3068.

24. Goldstein DJ, Oz MC, Rose EA. Implantable left ventricular assist devices. N Engl J Med 1998; 339(21):1522–1533.

25. Rose EA, Gelijns AC, Moskowitz AJ, et al. Long-term mechanical ventricular assistance for end-stage heart failure. N Engl J Med 2001; 15(20):1435–1443.

26. Rose EA, Moskowitz AJ, Packer M, et al. The REMATCH trial: rationale, design, and end points. Ann Thorac Surg 1999; 67:723–730.

27. Richenbacher WE, Naka Y, Raines NY, et al. Surgical management of patients in the REMATCH trial. Ann Thorac Surg 2003; 75(Suppl):S86–S92.

7
Principles and Practice of Nutritional Support for Surgical Patients*

Maheswari Senthil, Bobby Rupani, Jondavid H. Jabush, and Edwin A. Deitch

Case Scenario

You are asked to consult on a 75-year-old former school teacher who is in the intensive care unit for nutritional support. Since being admitted to the hospital 9 days ago, the patient has had a protracted hospital course and has had no nutritional support. The patient is receiving mechanical ventilation and is receiving antimicrobial therapy for a ventilator-associated pneumonia. She is septic and has necessitated pressor support in order to achieve hemodynamic goals. The patient now has a dedicated central line for parenteral nutrition. A feeding jejunostomy was placed several days ago. Which of the following is the most appropriate route for nutritional support for this patient?

(A) Central venous
(B) Jejunostomy
(C) Peripheral venous
(D) Gastric
(E) Do not initiate any nutritional support

The idea of acute care surgery conjures up visions of a spectrum of patients with diverse problems that cross many specialties. However, prolonged starvation or malnutrition worsens the outcome of all patients regardless of their diseases, and the development of acute malnutrition is especially common in the critically ill. Consequently, optimal nutritional support has become a key therapeutic aim in trauma patients and patients requiring acute care surgery. Recognition of the importance of nutritional therapy has led to a search for improved methods of nutritional support that promote wound healing and optimize host immune defenses. Unfortunately, impaired wound healing resulting in anastamotic leaks and wound-related problems as well as the development of septic complications and multiple organ failure still occurs.

Nonetheless, one potential way of reducing wound failure, muscle wasting, and sepsis-related morbidity and mortality is by limiting or preventing the adverse consequences of uncontrolled inflammatory-mediated hypermetabolism. Although immune and inflammatory dysfunction in these patients are multifactorial, the nutritional status of the patient clearly plays a major role in the ability to ward off an infectious challenge, and recent evidence suggests that the immune and inflammatory systems can be modulated by the use of specific means of nutritional support. Thus, this chapter focuses on nutritional support for the high-risk patient and emphasizes evidenced-based practice management (Figure 7.1).

Metabolism, Nutrition, and Infection

Understanding the basic biology of the metabolic response to injury and surgery as well as the role of nutrition in modulating this response is important, because the metabolic status of the patient influences muscle strength, various aspects of host defense against invading organisms, and wound healing. Although this section focuses primarily on the hypermetabolic response, the increased physiologic demands placed on the cardiac, pulmonary, renal, and other organ systems can complicate nutritional support and are noted.

The hypermetabolic response that occurs after a trauma, shock, or sepsis is characterized by a hyperdynamic circulatory state, fever, weight loss, and progressive skeletal muscle wasting, and it can remain elevated for weeks after healing is complete. The magnitude of the response parallels the extent of the injury/stress and

*This work was supported in part by NIH grant GM 59841 (to E.A.D.), Department of Surgery, UMDNJ–New Jersey Medical School, Newark, NJ 07103.

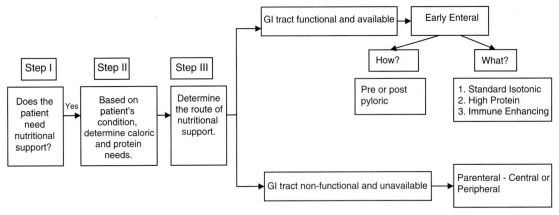

FIGURE 7.1. Schematic diagram illustrating a step-by-step approach to nutritional support. GI, gastrointestinal.

reaches a maximum of about twice normal (Figure 7.2).[1] Although the exact mechanisms that initiate and maintain the hypermetabolic response continue to be elucidated, multiple factors have been implicated as contributing to this hypermetabolic state. These include (1) immune and inflammatory-generated mediators, including interleukin-1 (IL-1), IL-6, tumor necrosis factor (TNF), prostanoids, and oxygen-free radicals and their products; (2) hormonal mediators, especially the counterregulatory hormones, catecholamines, cortisol, and glucagon;[2,3] and (3) the escape of bacteria or their products (endotoxin) from wounds[4] or intestine.[5] Although still being debated, the concept that gut- or wound-derived endotoxemia as one of the major triggers for the hypermetabolic response has gained attention, because loss of gut barrier function is relatively common after a major injury as well as in intensive care unit patients.[6] Additionally, endotoxin appears to induce fever by the same hypothalmic mechanisms as a major injury, and the hormonal and cytokine changes observed during endotoxemia are very similar to those observed after injury. Recently, the production of cytokines and other proinflammatory agents from the ischemic gut as well as the translocation of bacteria and endotoxin have been proposed to contribute to a prolonged systemic inflammatory and hypermetabolic response.[7,8] In this paradigm, stress states that lead to splanchnic ischemia result in the gut being a proinflammatory and cytokine-producing organ that exacerbates and/or perpetuates the systemic inflammatory and hypermetabolic responses. These facts, plus the observations that enteral nutrition preserves gut barrier function whereas parenteral nutrition is associated with gut atrophy and increased gut permeability,[9] have led to the principle that enteral nutrition is superior to parenteral nutrition and should be administered whenever possible.

Metabolically, a major injury or stress state is characterized by increased skeletal muscle proteolysis, lipolysis, and gluconeogenesis. The amino acids released from skeletal muscle are shunted to the liver, where they are used in gluconeogenesis and for the synthesis of acute-phase reactants. Newly synthesized glucose leaves the liver and reaches the injured tissues, where it is metabolized to lactate. The wound-generated lactate returns to the liver, where it is converted back to glucose (the Cori cycle). The oxidation of fat provides the majority of energy required to fuel these metabolic processes. Thus, through a process of "autocannibalism" the body liberates protein stored in the muscle to serve as substrate for

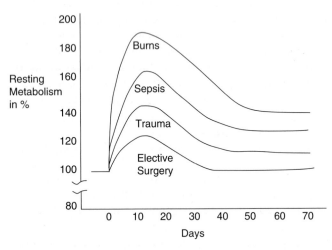

FIGURE 7.2. Chart illustrating an increase in resting energy expenditure over baseline for elective surgery, skeletal trauma, sepsis/peritonitis, and burn patients. The persistence of a hypermetabolic state for several days after initial injury is also depicted. (Adapted from Long CL, Schaffel N, Geiger JW, Schiller WR, Blakemore WS. Metabolic response to injury and illness: estimation of energy and protein needs from indirect calorimetry and nitrogen balance. J Parenter Enteral Nutr 1979; 3(6):455, with permission from the American Society for Parenteral and Enteral Nutrition (A.S.P.E.N.). A.S.P.E.N. does not endorse the use of this material in any form other than its entirety.)

the synthesis of proteins and glucose that are important in wound healing and antibacterial defense. In fact, the development of a hypermetabolic response appears to be essential for survival after major injury. However, because the hypermetabolic response continues until wound healing is complete, these patients require increased levels of calorie and nitrogen support. If these increased metabolic needs are not met, visceral protein loss, impaired antibacterial host defenses, muscle weakness, and delayed wound healing result.

One of the greatest threats to survival in successfully resuscitated patients requiring urgent surgery is infection, with intensive care unit pneumonia or the inability to successfully eradicate or control an initial infectious focus being leading causes of death. Because of the relationship between nutrition, immunity, and wound healing,[10] optimal nutritional support assumes major importance for these patients. Not only does inadequate nutritional support impair host immune defenses, but it will potentiate muscle weakness and retard wound healing. Likewise, it is those patients in whom the hypermetabolic response is greatest who are at the highest risk of developing an infection. For example, it is well known that patients sustaining major injuries develop numerous defects in their immune systems that predispose them to an increased risk of infection.[11] These changes include alterations in essentially every aspect of the innate and acquired host immune defense systems, and, for many components of the immune system, the degree of the immunosuppression correlates directly with the magnitude of the injury. This relationship is documented most easily in the burn patient, where there is a direct association between burn size and the risk of infection, with the incidence of infection being increased markedly in patients with burns involving more than 40% of the body surface area. Furthermore, once an infection has occurred, the ability of a patient to survive that infectious episode is inversely related, at least in part, to the severity of the injury or stress state. Thus, it is in those patients with the most severe injuries or severe diseases that the need for nutritional support is greatest.

In addition to impairing the innate and acquired immune systems, catabolic states promote profound muscle wasting through accelerated proteolysis. The resultant muscle weakness predisposes to pneumonia by limiting the ability of the host to cough and clear secretions. In this light, it is not hard to visualize why optimal nutritional support (through its wound healing, muscle sparing, and immune-enhancing effects) is a critical component of the care of the high-risk surgical patient and that careful attention to nutritional needs is an essential part of the infection control process. Thus, although the initial metabolic response to stress, injury, or sepsis is an adaptive response by the body to mobilize energy substrates and protein to meet acute physiologic challenges

and maintain essential body functions, prolonged persistence of this response ultimately becomes maladaptive and contributes to morbidity and mortality.

Goals of Nutritional Support

Although there is clinical evidence that aggressive nutritional support improves outcome parameters in trauma, burn, and intensive care unit patients,[12–14] the optimal clinical approach to the nutritional support of these patients continues to evolve, and some controversies remain. Before addressing the controversies or going into detail about the who, when, what, how, and why of nutritional support of the high-risk patient, the basic goals of nutritional support are briefly summarized. The first set of goals is to prevent starvation and specific vitamin or nutrient deficiencies and to avoid or minimize the complications associated with enteral or parenteral alimentation. The second set of goals is to provide the correct amount and mix of nutrients, which will prevent, limit, or modulate disease-related adverse physiologic effects and complications. These goals of optimal nutritional support will be met only when the appropriate patient receives the right amount of the correct nutrient mix in the safest manner possible.

The achievement of these goals presupposes several assumptions. It assumes that the clinician can determine the patient's nutritional requirements and knows how much of the ordered nutritional support that the patient is receiving and is able to assess the effectiveness of the specific nutrient support being administered. Yet these assumptions cannot always be met. For example, although numerous parameters have been shown to aid in assessing nutritional status in patients undergoing elective surgery, monitoring of the nutritional status of the trauma and intensive care unit patients is difficult, because traditional serum (albumin or transferrin levels) and immunologic (skin test reactivity or total lymphocyte count) markers of nutritional status are all directly altered by infection, injury, and inflammation and thus are not fully accurate predictors or markers of the patient's nutritional status. Similarly, daily weights and nitrogen balance studies are fraught with error in these patients. Daily weights are frequently inaccurate because of the presence of dressings and the occurrence of fluid shifts, and nitrogen balance studies are confounded by the fact that large amounts of protein may be lost through drainage tubes and soft tissue wound. Yet, with limited objective means to assess nutritional status or the response to nutritional therapy, these patients must be kept in as positive a nutritional balance as physiologically possible.

In fact, the use of traditional methods of monitoring nutritional support has been recently questioned by

Jeejeebhoy,[15] who concluded that changes in muscle function correlate much better with patient outcome than traditional measurements of nitrogen balance or total body protein levels. He states that the important relationship between exercise (or the lack thereof) and muscle mass is frequently ignored in assessing the nutritional needs as well as the response of critically ill patients to nutritional support. Undoubtedly, studies directed at developing and validating functional tests to guide nutritional assessment and support will emerge in the future, and these tests are likely to significantly contribute to the care of the high-risk patient. In the interim, the most practical approach is to estimate the daily caloric and protein needs and make certain they are delivered. The use of daily flow sheets to monitor and quantify the total amounts of delivered nutrients and their composition (carbohydrates, fats, and proteins) are helpful to avoid under- or overfeeding.

Nutritional Support: Who, How Much, and What

Although, to some extent, controversy still exists concerning the optimal amount and composition of the nutritional regimen necessary for an optimal clinical outcome, some points are clear (see Figure 7.1). These patients require increased amounts of both calories and protein. Glucose is important because wounds and the cellular components of the immune and inflammatory systems are obligate glucose consumers, and the administration of carbohydrate decreases proteolysis. Thus, about 60% to 70% of the calories administered should be carbohydrate calories. Although the administration of large carbohydrate loads is necessary, it is equally important not to exceed the patient's ability to metabolize the administered glucose. In this regard, the now classic studies by Burke et al.[16] indicate that the maximal amount of glucose that can be metabolized in most patients ranges between 5 and 7 mg/kg body weight per minute (this represents 1,800 to 2,200 cal/day for the average adult). If the rate of glucose administration exceeds glucose metabolism, the following metabolic consequences are likely to occur: glucose intolerance, increased carbon dioxide production, increased fat synthesis, and the development of a fatty liver. Furthermore, because fat synthesis is an energy-requiring process, overfeeding glucose is energetically inefficient. The potential dangers of hyperglycemia have been recently highlighted in a prospective, randomized, controlled trial of 1,548 ventilated surgical intensive care unit patients randomized to receive insulin to maintain tight glucose control (blood glucose levels kept between 80 and 110 mg/dL) versus patients treated conventionally (insulin only administered if glucose level is

>215 mg/dL).[17] The group randomized to tight glucose control had a 50% reduction in mortality compared with the patients receiving conventional glucose control. This study further emphasizes the importance of euglycemia and the potential dangers of overfeeding.

Protein administration is important, because severely stressed or septic patients receiving a high-protein diet have improved outcomes compared with patients receiving a more standard diet, especially when the nutrient mix is administered enterally. The importance of a high-protein enteral diet was first documented over 20 years ago in a randomized controlled study[12] showing improved survival in thermally injured children who were administered high-protein diets with a calorie-to-nitrogen ratio of 100:1 versus comparably burned children receiving a more standard diet with a calorie-to-nitrogen ratio of 150:1. This was true even though the children receiving the high-protein diet received less total calories. In healthy individuals, normal protein intake is approximately 0.8 to 1.0 g/kg/day, with each gram of protein providing 4.0 kcal. In most stressed patients, utilization of exogenous protein for synthetic purposes levels off at approximately 1.5 g/kg/day, and provision of protein in excess of 2.0 g/kg/day generally contributes little to the restoration of nitrogen balance and can lead to significantly elevated blood urea nitrogen levels.[18]

Dietary supplementation with lipids and fats is important, because the prolonged absence of adequate lipid supplementation can lead to a number of problems. However, it is equally clear that certain exogenous fats, such as the omega-3 fatty acids, can have profound suppressive effects on both the production of cytokines and selective components of the immune system.[19] Additionally, excessive parenteral fat administration can lead to hyperlipidemia, hypoxia, and increased risk of infection and, in some studies, a higher postoperative mortality rate.[20] On the other hand, fat has been shown to have protein-sparing effects similar to (but not as effective as) that of glucose. As a result, the provision of 30% of nonprotein calories as fat, especially when provided enterally, may be helpful in minimizing the problems associated with high glucose loads by reducing the amount of carbohydrate that must be administered to meet the patient's energy needs. Furthermore, because the adverse effects of dietary lipids appear to be dose dependent, to avoid complications intravenous lipid preparations, when given, should be infused slowly and lipid clearance monitored to ensure that the serum triglyceride levels do not rise to more than 10% to 20% over baseline. Severe hypermetabolic states and multiple organ failure may profoundly impair the metabolism of intravenously administered lipids, necessitating their discontinuance. However, because enterally administered lipids appear to be tolerated better than intravenously administered lipids and appear to be associated with a lower incidence of side effects, enteral lipids can be administered safely to most patients. Currently, the optimal amount and composition of dietary fats for the stressed or intensive care unit surgical patient has not been determined and is an area of active investigation. Nonetheless, for the reasons listed above, it appears important to administer lipids enterally as well as to limit the amount of lipid to 20% to 30% of the patient's estimated nonprotein calorie requirements.

There are numerous methods of estimating nutritional requirements, and they all have their strengths and weaknesses. One common method is to calculate basal energy expenditure (BEE) and then apply a correction factor based on the predicted level of hypermetabolism to arrive at a value for total energy expenditure (TEE). A second approach is to use indirect calorimetry to quantify the metabolic needs of the patient. With indirect calorimetry, a metabolic cart is used to estimate energy requirements by determining oxygen consumption and carbon dioxide production via analysis of inspired and expired gases. The accuracy of indirect calorimetry is good when measurements are taken under strictly controlled conditions. However, this method is expensive and may pose difficulty in obtaining accurate results for patients who are not intubated as well as intubated patients on high inspired oxygen levels.[21] Furthermore, although indirect calorimetry may accurately reflect the energy requirements over the 20- to 30-minute period of the study, it is not clear that these values can be extrapolated to the entire 24-hour period. Interestingly, some studies comparing indirect calorimetry to formula-derived estimates of caloric needs indicate that formula-derived values may be too high.[22] However, this problem can be minimized by using the patient's ideal rather than actual body weight in calculating basal caloric needs. By using ideal body weight, the calculated nutritional values should more closely reflect the mass of metabolically active tissue (lean body mass) rather than the fat mass or extra body water. Thus, we recommend the following approach to the nutritional support of the high-risk patient, as outlined in Figure 7.3.

The amount of calories to be administered is estimated initially using the Harris-Benedict equation (based on ideal body weight) to calculate basal energy expenditure.[23] This number is then multiplied by a stress factor that is related to the condition and disease process of the patient (see Figures 7.2 and 7.3). Once the total caloric requirements to meet the patient's metabolic needs have

Basal Energy Expenditure (BEE) per Harris – Benedict Equation

Male: BEE = $66 + (13.7 \times Wt) + (5 \times Ht) - (6.8 \times age)$
Female: BEE = $665 + (9.6 \times Wt) + (1.8 \times Ht) - (4.7 \times age)$

Weight (Wt) in kilograms; Height (Ht) in centimeters;

Conditions	Energy Requirement	Approximate caloric requirement Kcal/kg/day	Protein gm/kg/day	NPC:N*
Elective Surgery	1.00–1.25 × BEE	25–30	1.0–1.2	150:1
Multiple Trauma	1.25–1.5 × BEE	30–35	1.4–1.5	120:1
Sepsis/Peritonitis	1.5 × BEE	30–35	1.4–1.8	90–120:1
Massive Burns (> 50% TBSA)	1.75–2.0 × BEE	35–40	1.8–2.0	80–100:1

BEE – Basal Energy Expenditure; NPC:N – Non protein calorie to nitrogen ratio; TBSA – Total body surface area;
*6.25 gm of protein = 1 gm of nitrogen

Example: Consider a 5 ft 6 in tall, 60-year-old male weighing 65 kg, who is undergoing emergency laparotomy for perforated viscus.
Step I: Based on the Harris-Benedict equation, his BEE = 1353 kcal which is 21 kcal/kg/day.
Step II: Multiplied with a stress factor of 1.5 his estimated caloric needs = 2030 kcal which is 31 kcal/kg/day.
Step III: Protein requirement of 1.5 g/kg/day = 98 g/day
NPC:N = 120:1

FIGURE 7.3. Calculating the caloric and protein needs of surgical patients. Step I: Calculate the basal energy expenditure using the Harris-Benedict equation. Step II: Based on patient's condition, multiply the BEE with a stress factor to derive the total caloric needs. Step III: Multiply the recommended protein (g/kg) for each subgroup of patient population with the patient's weight to derive the total protein required/day.

been estimated, protein requirements are determined. This can be done in a number ways. For example, the amount of protein can be based on a specific nonprotein calorie to nitrogen ratio, on body weight, or by estimating protein needs as being 15% to 20% of total calories. Whether one uses a nonprotein to calorie ratio of 100:1, grams of proteins/kg, or 15% to 20% of total calories as protein, one gets very similar results, as shown by the following clinical example.

Consider a 5 ft 6 in tall, 60-year-old male weighing 65 kg who is undergoing acute care laparotomy for a perforated viscus. Based on the Harris-Benedict equation, his BEE would be 1,353 kcal. His estimated caloric needs would be about 2,030 kcal if his calculated BEE is multiplied with a stress factor of 1.5. If 20% of his nutrition support regimen consisted of protein calories (406 kcal), he would receive about 101 g of protein or 16 g of nitrogen and 1,624 nonprotein calories (25 kcal/kg). This would be equivalent to 1.5 g protein/kg body weight and a nonprotein calorie to nitrogen ratio of approximately 100:1.

Overfeeding during critical illness may actually be more hazardous than underfeeding in some circumstances (Table 7.1). This idea is supported by the fact that overfed animals have a higher mortality rate and an increased susceptibility to infection than underfed or normally nourished animals. Additionally, in a study of postoperative patients, overfeeding of parenteral carbohydrate (manifest as a respiratory quotient >0.95) was associated with a significantly higher incidence of septic complications and mortality than a similar group of patients whose respiratory quotient was <0.95.[20] Thus, although less attention has been focused on overfeeding than underfeeding, it is becoming increasingly clear that overfeeding as well as underfeeding can be harmful. Thus, it is critical to avoid the dangers of overfeeding and to keep in mind that stress-based hypermetabolism cannot be reversed by overfeeding as long as the physiologic signals that induced the stress response are present.

It is important to remember that nutritional needs may change during the patient's hospital stay. For example,

TABLE 7.1. Adverse effects of overfeeding.

Substance	Adverse effects
Glucose	Respiratory insufficiency due to increased CO_2 production
	Hepatic steatosis/fatty liver
	Impaired neutrophil function
	Energy substrate for support of bacterial overgrowth
Protein	Azotemia
	Potentiates encephalopathy
Lipid	Impaired immune function and increased susceptibility to infection
	Impaired pulmonary function
	Reticuloendothelial blockade

placing a patient on mechanical ventilation reduces the energy spent on the work of breathing and may result in up to a 20% reduction in energy expenditure.[24] In contrast, energy and protein requirements may increase during the recovery period when the patient's activity level increases and the catabolic response is replaced by anabolism. Thus, it is frequently important to continue nutritional support throughout the patient's hospital course. Additionally, for nutritional support to be most effective in restoring muscle mass and strength, as the patient's activity level progresses, nutritional support should be combined with a progressive exercise program. It is also important to keep in mind that many factors besides the magnitude of the injury affect the degree of hypermetabolism and hence nutritional needs. One factor, which is often ignored, is the ambient temperature of the patient's environment. Recognition that the relationship between thermogenesis and energy expenditure is U shaped and that there is a specific temperature range (zone of thermal neutrality) at which energy expenditure is minimal is of clinical significance. In healthy individuals, the zone of thermal neutrality is between 27° and 29°C (80° to 84°F). Injured patients, especially burn patients, will increase their zone of neutrality to as high as 32°C. Because temperatures above or below this zone of neutrality are associated with increased energy expenditure, total energy expenditure can be reduced by maintaining the patient in an optimal thermoneutral environment, which is in the range of 27° to 30°C.[25] Other factors commonly experienced by these patients, such as pain, anxiety, and stress, also increase the metabolic rate. Thus, it is important to limit these factors to the extent possible. In contrast, although fever increases the metabolic response, because fever has significant beneficial effects on the host's ability to fight infection, attempts to normalize body temperature in these patients just because it is elevated are not indicated.

Diet-induced thermogenesis is a less-recognized but potentially important cause of increased energy expenditure. If substrate is provided in amounts greater than needed for energy requirements, energy expenditure may be increased by 20% or more. Using carbohydrate metabolism as an example, this point is easily illustrated. If administered carbohydrate is immediately used, energy expenditure changes by about 1%; but, if carbohydrate is converted or stored as glycogen or adipose tissue, energy expenditure increases by 5% and 22%, respectively. There is also experimental evidence to suggest that enterally provided nutrients are associated with less energy expenditure than parenteral infusion of the same nutrients, presumably because of the better preservation of intestinal barrier function by enteral than parenteral nutrition.[26]

To summarize, many patients requiring urgent surgery will benefit from aggressive nutritional support as well as maneuvers to limit the stress state. The composition and level of nutritional support will vary based on age and body surface area as well as on the magnitude of the stress state. As is discussed in the next section, as much of a patient's nutritional requirements should be delivered enterally as possible. Consequently, our approach to the nutritional support of the high-risk, compromised patient is based on the institution of very early enteral feeding of a high-protein diet.[27] Finally, efforts are made to control pain and anxiety, avoid overfeeding, and maintain these patients in an optimal thermal environment to prevent exacerbation of the hypermetabolic response.

Nutritional Support: Route and Timing

Having decided on the basic amount and composition of the nutrient mix, it is next time to decide on the route and timing of nutritional support prior to choosing the exact nutrient strategy to employ. Although total parenteral nutrition (TPN) has and continues to benefit select critically ill patients, in circumstances where either enteral or parenteral nutrition can be administered, enteral nutrition is preferable for several biologic reasons in addition to its superiority in terms of cost, safety, and convenience. For example, there currently exists an ever enlarging body of clinical and experimental evidence documenting that TPN may impair host immune defenses.[9] The experimental studies indicating that TPN itself impairs host defenses are consistent with the findings of randomized clinical trials of TPN in multiple patient populations, which have documented that the administration of TPN increases the incidence of infectious complications in all but the most severely malnourished patients (Table 7.2).[28,29] In contrast to TPN, enteral alimentation appears to preserve host immune function. Numerous experimental studies have documented that antibacterial host defenses, such as lymphocyte, neutrophil, and gut-associated immune function, are better preserved in enterally fed than in parenterally

fed humans and animals.[9] Furthermore, enterally fed animals tolerate an infectious challenge far better, and with a significantly lower mortality rate, than animals fed the identical diet parenterally.

As previously mentioned, as early as 1980[12] it was conclusively demonstrated that high-protein enteral feedings would improve outcome in a prospective randomized trial of burned children. In this study, high-protein enteral feedings were associated with significantly less impairment of systemic immunity, fewer septic complications, and a marked increase in survival. Similar results have been documented in burned adults[30] as well as by a number of randomized, prospective trials of enteral versus parenteral alimentation in trauma patients.[13] These studies have also documented a significantly decreased incidence of infectious complications in enterally fed patients versus those receiving TPN, although survival was not improved (Table 7.3).

Investigations into the potential mechanisms underlying the protective effects of enteral alimentation have produced some interesting observations. For example, the observation that enteral but not parenteral feedings immediately after a burn injury will markedly attenuate the hypermetabolic response was first made experimentally 20 years ago.[31] On the basis of this study and early studies of bacterial translocation,[5] it was postulated that early enteral feeding may attenuate the hypermetabolic response by preserving the intestinal mucosal barrier and thereby preventing the translocation of bacteria or endotoxin from the gut to the portal or systemic circulations. Since then, confirmatory clinical studies of burn patients have documented that the barrier function of the intestine is lost immediately after thermal injury, mechanical trauma, in intensive care unit patients, and during episodes of sepsis.[32] Additionally, studies of human volunteers demonstrated impaired neutrophil function[33] and an exaggerated response of glucagon, epinephrine, and cytokine production[34] after endotoxin challenge in subjects receiving TPN and complete bowel rest for 7 days

TABLE 7.2. Prospective randomized trials comparing TPN versus intravenous fluids, showing increased infectious complications with TPN.

Study	Patient population	Total No. of trials/patients	Outcome	
			Infection	Mortality
McGeer et al.,[28] 1990 Meta-analysis	Cancer patients undergoing chemotherapy	12 RCT	Increased in TPN Odds ratio = 3.1 $p < 0.001$	Increased in TPN Relative risk = 0.81 $p = 0.06$
Veteran's Cooperative Study,[29] 1991 PRCT	Malnourished patients requiring laparotomy or noncardiac thoracotomy	395 patients TPN = 192 Control = 203	Increased in TPN[†] 14.1% vs. 6.4% $p = 0.01$	NS 10.9% vs 9.4%

NA, not available; NS, not statistically significant; PRCT, prospective randomized controlled trial; TPN, total parenteral nutrition.

[†]Increased rate of infection was confined to borderline or mildly malnourished. Severely malnourished patients had a significant decrease in noninfectious complications with no concomitant increase in infectious complications.

TABLE 7.3. Meta-analysis of prospective randomized trials comparing enteral diet versus parenteral nutrition.

Study	Patient population	Total No. of trials/patients	Infections/septic complications (TEN vs. TPN)			Survival at 10 and 30 days
			All patients	Excluding catheter-related sepsis		
				All patients	Trauma patients*	
Moore et al.,[13] 1992 Meta-analysis	High-risk surgical and trauma patients	8 PRCT (n = 230) TEN = 118 pts TPN = 112 pts	Decreased in TEN (18% vs. 35%) $p = 0.01$	Decreased in TEN (16% vs. 29%) $p = 0.03$	Decreased in TEN (19% vs. 33%) $p = 0.04$	No difference between two groups

PRCT, prospective randomized controlled trial; pts, patients; TEN, total enteral nutrition (Vivonex was started within 72 hours of operation); TPN, total parenteral nutrition.

*Trauma patients with abdominal trauma index = 15 to 40, injury severity score = 9 to 40.

compared with subjects receiving enteral feedings. The human volunteers fed parenterally also manifested an enhanced acute-phase protein response, increased peripheral amino acid mobilization, and increased peripheral lactate production. Thus, in addition to causing immune suppression, it appears that TPN may exacerbate the metabolic derangements seen in sepsis through an enhancement of cytokine production, as well as through an exaggerated metabolic response mediated by the counterregulatory hormones. Therefore, because TPN is less effective in maintaining the gut barrier and host immune function than enteral feeding, the indiscriminate use of TPN in the face of a functioning gut is not justified.

Although it is clear that enteral nutrition is preferable to parenteral nutrition for patients with a functioning gastrointestinal tract, simply providing nutrients via the gut does not guarantee normal gut barrier function. The role of selective intestinal malnutrition in the evolution of gut failure and gut-related systemic inflammation has received increasing attention since the late 1980s, when several groups identified the concept that gut barrier failure may occur in critically ill patients because standard parenteral nutritional formulas do not fully support intestinal mucosal function and structure.[35–37] Furthermore, based on a series of studies documenting that

certain factors not present in TPN, such as fiber and glutamine, are essential for the maintenance of normal intestinal barrier function, it has become clear that the gut must be fed as well as the rest of the body.[9] Thus, it has become increasingly evident over the past decade that specific components of the diet may be just as important as the route by which it is administered and that nutritional support of the patient must include nutritional support of the gut as well as other organs. To this end, the most effective method for the prevention and treatment of gut barrier failure is early enteral feeding of a high-protein, fiber-containing diet containing specific nutrients. This notion that specific nutrients can exert beneficial physiologic effects beyond those traditionally associated with nutrient administration has led to the concept of nutrient pharmacology and the development of immune-enhancing diets.

These immune-enhancing diets contain factors (glutamine, fiber, omega-3 fatty acids, nucleosides, and high levels of arginine) that support immune function as well as enterocyte growth and function. Two meta-analyses of randomized controlled trials comparing patients receiving standard enteral nutrition with patients receiving commercially available (Immun-Aid, Impact) immune-enhancing diets was recently reported (Table 7.4).[14,38]

TABLE 7.4. Prospective randomized controlled trials comparing immune-enhancing enteral diets versus standard enteral diets.

Study	Patient population	Total No. of trials/patients	Outcome (IED vs. standard)		
			Infection	LOS	Mortality
Beale et al.,[14] 1999 Meta-analysis	ICU patients	12 PRCT	Decreased in IED $p = 0.005$	Decreased in IED $p = 0.0002$	No difference between two groups $p = 0.76$
Heyland et al.,[38] 2001 Meta-analysis	Surgical and critically ill patients	22 PRCT	Decreased in IED $p < 0.001$*	Decreased in IED $p < 0.001$	No difference between two groups $p = 0.54$
Galban et al.,[39] 2000 PRCT	Septic ICU patients with APACHE II score >10	IED = 89† Standard = 87†	Decreased in IED (8% vs. 22%) $p = 0.01$	NS (18.1 vs. 17.7 days)	Decreased in IED (19% vs. 32%) $p < 0.05$

ICU, intensive care unit; IED, immune-enhancing diet; LOS, length of stay; NS, not statistically significant; PRCT, prospective randomized controlled trial.

*Decrease in infection was significant only in elective surgical patients, not in critically ill.

†Enteral nutrition started within 36 hours of diagnosis of sepsis.

Although there was no statistically significant beneficial effect on mortality, the patients fed the immune-enhancing diets had a significant reduction in the rate of infection, days on the ventilator, and hospital stay. Additionally, a recently published prospective randomized multicenter clinical trial has shown that the administration of an immune-enhancing diet resulted in a significant reduction in mortality as well as in the infection rate in septic intensive care unit patients.[39] Based on these studies, it appears that all intensive care unit patients as well as significantly stressed patients should receive a high-protein enteral diet, with the use of immune-enhancing diets being reserved for those patients who are septic or at highest risk of becoming septic (Figure 7.4).

The timing of the initiation of enteral feeding may also be important. There are several reasons to believe that a policy of immediate/early enteral feeding will be superior to delayed enteral feeding, even though only limited amounts of enterally administered nutrients may be absorbed during the first few days after insult. This concept is based on the observation that even short periods of starvation or TPN use can lead to atrophy of gut tissue out of proportion to that seen in other organs and that intraluminal nutrients play a major role in the maintenance of gut structure and function. Furthermore, clinically, the transition to an oral diet after a period of TPN or prolonged starvation is often associated with diarrhea and malabsorption, which is believed to be a direct result of mucosal atrophy. This diarrheal state, by impairing the ability of the patient to tolerate enteral feeding, may result in further limitation of enteral intake and thus promote further mucosal atrophy. Therefore, it is easy to visualize a potential cycle where starvation or TPN, by causing mucosal atrophy, predisposes to malabsorption and diarrhea and thereby impairs the ability of the patient to tolerate subsequent enteral feedings. In fact, a recent prospective randomized clinical trial documented that early enteral nutrition, started within 6 hours of injury and shock, reduced the incidence of organ failure and largely prevented injury-induced increases in gut permeability when compared with patients whose enteral feedings were begun 24 or more hours postinjury.[40]

Although there is experimental and some clinical evidence that early enteral feeding is beneficial,[8,27,40] especially if begun shortly after injury, early enteral feeding is only now beginning to gain more widespread clinical acceptance. This reluctance to institute enteral feedings until after the acute injury phase is over and gastrointestinal function has returned to normal is related largely to the fear that immediate feeding will result in a higher rate of complications than delayed feeding, such as aspiration of gastric contents. Based on studies in burn and trauma patients,[27,40] this fear seems to be largely unfounded. Although there have been a few case reports of very early enteral (jejunostomy) feeding being associated with intestinal ischemia in underresuscitated trauma

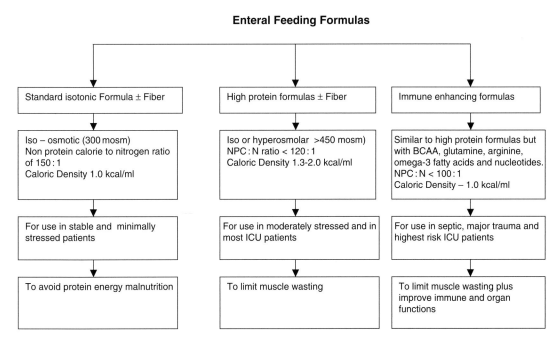

FIGURE 7.4. Categories of enteral feeding formulas: major categories of enteral formulas and their compositions, indications, and uses for specific patient populations. BCAA, branched chain amino acids; ICU, intensive care unit; NPC:N ratio, non-protein calorie to nitrogen ratio.

patients, the incidence of this complication is significantly less than 1%, and, in a recent review of the literature on this issue, the authors found a similar incidence of bowel necrosis in nonenterally fed high-risk patients.[41] Nonetheless, it appears prudent to establish hemodynamic stability and ensure that the patient is out of shock before the initiation of enteral feeding. On the other hand, clinical experience with patients suggests that enteral feeding *after* an episode of hypotension may prevent or reduce the extent of small bowel ischemia.[40,42]

Having decided to use enteral nutrition and having established which category of enteral formula to use for a specific patient (see Figure 7.4), it is now time to determine whether the patient should be fed into the stomach or the jejunum. Despite the rhetoric and debate over whether intragastric or postpyloric feeding is superior, in most cases this is a dealer's choice. Because of convenience, we believe that intragastric feedings should be attempted in most patients and if tolerated then continued. The advantages of intragastric feeding are that hyperosmolar as well as isoosmolar solutions can be administered and bolus feedings can be given. In contrast, hyperosmolar jejunal feedings are not as well tolerated and are more likely to cause distension, cramping, and diarrhea than gastric feedings. Additionally, a continuous feeding regimen must be used with the jejunal administration of nutrients. The main disadvantage of intragastric feeding is the risk of aspiration and the failure to administer adequate nutritional support in patients with gastric ileus. Whether feeding into the stomach or the jejunum, a similar nutrient administration strategy can be applied. Feedings are started at a rate of 25 to 30 mL/hr and advanced slowly over the next 36 to 72 hours to meet caloric and nutrient goals. If gastric bolus feeding is used, then approximately 100 mL of the enteral formula is given and the nasogastric tube is clamped. Gastric residuals are then measured 4 hours later just before the next scheduled bolus feeding. As long as the gastric residuals remains less than 100 to 150 mL, the next bolus feeding is given, the tube clamped, and the process continued. The strategy of measuring gastric residuals every 4 hours should also be used when continuous intragastric feedings are administered to decrease the risk of the patient developing high gastric residuals and hence the increased possibility of pulmonary aspiration. During the initiation and early days of enteral feeding, the patient should be monitored closely for signs of feeding intolerance, such as distension, diarrhea, cramping, or increased gastric residuals. In some patients with borderline gastric ileus, the use of prokinetic agents or erythromycin may be helpful.

For patients who have nasogastric or nasojejunal tubes and who are likely to require prolonged enteral nutrition (>30 days), the tubes should be replaced with a feeding gastrostomy or jejunostomy for patient comfort and for ease of nutrient administration. For most patients, placement of a percutaneous gastrostomy is preferred over a jejunostomy, because operative jejunostomies have a low but significant complication rate of 2% to 3%,[43,44] and they are more difficult to use and maintain than gastrostomies. Additional details on feeding tube–related complications as well as the management of specific side effects of enteral feeding are well covered in several recent reviews.[44,45]

Nutrient Pharmacology

Nutrient pharmacology is based on the concept that specific nutrients and growth factors can improve the clinical outcome of critically ill patients by functioning as organ- and tissue-specific fuels or stimulants. In this capacity, these specific nutrients and growth factors support the physiologic function and repair of certain organs and tissues as well as augment the immune system and promote wound healing. These factors include the specific nutrients added to the immune-enhancing diets as well as anabolic agents. Research in this area has been intense, because even immune-enhancing nutritional diets are only partially capable of reversing stress, sepsis, or injury-induced hypercatabolism or ameliorating impaired tissue repair processes and immune as well as organ dysfunction.

One novel area of research involves the use of hormones to improve wound healing, improve immune function, and support organ function in addition to limiting the hypermetabolic response. This approach was thought likely to be ultimately successful based on initial clinical studies performed in the mid-1990s showing that growth hormone (GH) accelerates wound healing[46] and insulin-like growth factor-1 (IGF-1) may preserve lean body mass[47] in patients with major burns. Since then, both GH and IGF-1 have been shown to limit muscle wasting and promote anabolism in a large number of patient populations, including patients who sustained mechanical or thermal trauma as well as those with sepsis, with pancreatitis, or undergoing major gastrointestinal operations.[48,49] Because IGF-1 appears to be the mediator of the anabolic effects of GH, the risk of side effects (especially hyperglycemia) is higher with GH, and GH resistance has been documented in septic patients, IGF-1 is a conceptually more attractive candidate hormone than GH. Furthermore, IGF-1 has been shown to limit catabolism as well as gut atrophy and bacterial translocation, indicating that it may be useful in preserving gut function as well as muscle mass. Further concerns were raised about the safety of GH by a recent large prospective randomized trial showing that septic patients and patients with MODS who were randomized to the high-dose GH arm of the study had higher morbidity and mortality rates.[50]

Like IGF-1, other hormones, such as bombesin,[51] neurotensin,[52] epidermal growth factor,[53] and even basic fibroblast growth factor,[54] have also been shown to have beneficial effects on gut structure and function, illustrating the concept that the gut response to dietary manipulations and injury can be hormonally modulated.

Vitamin and mineral supplementation are also areas of intense investigation, because these substances have been found to exert a number of important protective effects. Collectively they are called "micronutrients," as they are found in extremely small amounts in the body. Micronutrients play a key role in cellular function and are critical for wound healing, antioxidant production, and immune function. For example, vitamins C and E are important nutrient antioxidants, vitamins A and C are important in wound healing, and vitamins A, D, C, and E as well as zinc and selenium are important in wound healing. Other potentially beneficial effects of micronutrients and antioxidants are being continuously uncovered. For example, three clinical trials of critically ill surgical patients, two of which were prospective randomized clinical trials, showed that early splanchnic-directed antioxidant therapy was effective in decreasing organ failure and shortening intensive care unit stays.[55–57] These studies were based in large part on the idea that splanchnic blood flow is decreased after injury or during shock, resulting in the subsequent development of ischemia-reperfusion–mediated gut injury and inflammation.

Although frequently overlooked, deficiencies of specific trace minerals, such as copper, selenium, zinc, and chromium, can result in impaired wound healing, depressed cellular immunity, and augmented oxidant-mediated tissue damage. Thus, each of these minerals is briefly discussed. The critical nature of these trace minerals is based on their key roles as cofactors in important cellular pathways and defenses. For example, copper is a cofactor for a number of key enzymes, such as superoxide dismutase, cytochrome C oxidase, and lysyl oxidase, and thus is involved in antioxidant defenses, metabolism, and wound healing. The recommended dose of copper is 1.5 to 3 mg/day for critically ill patients.[58] Like copper, selenium also plays a key role in antioxidant defenses, as it is an integral part of the antioxidant enzyme glutathione peroxidase.[59] Selenium deficiency has been reported with acute illness,[60] low oral intake,[61] malnutrition,[62] and long-term TPN use.[63] Once established, selenium deficiency is associated with oxidant-induced disorders such as cardiomyopathy[63] and myositis.[64] At present, the recommended dose of selenium for critically ill patients is 100 μg/day.

Chromium in its organically complex form, also know as "glucose tolerance factor," potentiates the action of insulin on carbohydrate and lipid metabolism, thereby fostering an anabolic state.[65] Chromium deficiency has been reported with long-term TPN use and is associated with the development of new-onset hyperglycemia.[66] The recommended dose of chromium is 50 to 200 μg/day, but higher doses might be needed for hypermetabolic patients.

Zinc is an essential nutrient for rapidly proliferating cells because it is an integral component of DNA and RNA polymerase. Additionally, zinc is a key cofactor of superoxide dismutase and thus is an important component of the body's antioxidant defenses and is also required for optimal wound healing.[67,68] Finally, not only is zinc deficiency relatively common in critically ill patients but it also has been documented to lead to impaired cellular immunity.[69] The recommended zinc dose for critically ill patients is 25 mg/day. Most enteral formulas provide the recommended daily doses of these essential micronutrients; however, patients receiving long-term TPN would require intravenous supplementation to avoid deficiency.

Avoiding a deficiency of micronutrients in critically ill patients is vital in decreasing complications and promoting positive outcomes. On the other hand, although a decrease in circulating iron is a constant feature of major injuries[70] and was once thought to be an abnormality requiring correction, there is abundant evidence documenting that hypoferremia is actually an important part of the host's immune antibacterial defenses.[71] That is, because microorganisms require iron for cell replication and multiple metabolic functions, the hypoferremic response to injury appears to be a protective response that aids the host by decreasing the availability of iron for use by invading microorganisms. Studies documenting that iron replacement therapy increases the risk of severe infections as well as mortality in both human and animal studies confirm the protective effects of hypoferremia against infection. Consequently, because iron replacement therapy for stressed patients predisposes to infectious complications and deaths, iron replacement therapy is not indicated.

In summary, a highly sophisticated "nutrient pharmacology" appears to be evolving, based on which specific nutrients will be given or withheld in order to modulate specific physiologic processes.

Anabolic Agents

Despite the fact that optimal nutritional regimens decrease the rate of catabolism, limit muscle wasting, and improve immune function and wound healing, nutritional support alone is not sufficient to completely limit muscle wasting or compensate for the increased catabolic response observed in septic or severely stressed patients. Consequently, the strategy of using anabolic agents in concert with high-protein diets has been employed to further limit muscle wasting. Anabolic agents tested include growth hormone and IGF-1 (discussed in the previous section on nutrient pharmacology) as well as testosterone, testosterone analogs, oxandralone, insulin, and most recently the beta-blocker propanolol. Testosterone and testosterone analogues are not considered here, because they have a significant risk of causing hepatotoxicity, can have masculinizing effects, and have been found to be less effective in limiting muscle wasting than other agents. Emphasis on the other anabolic agents is appropriate.

Oxandralone is an oral synthetic testosterone analog that has minimal virilizing activity and little hepatotoxicity when compared to testosterone. Several prospective controlled trials have shown that oxandralone combined with a high-protein diet increases lean body mass and limits muscle protein wasting in acute and rehabilitating burn patients by increased protein synthesis.[72,73] It has also been used successfully in a variety of catabolic populations, including people with hepatitis and acquired immunodeficiency syndrome wasting myopathy.[74,75] More recently, a prospective randomized controlled trial with burn patients showed that oxandralone increases constitutive proteins such as albumin, prealbumin, and retinol-binding protein and reduces acute-phase protein levels.[76] When compared with human growth hormone or testosterone, the advantages of oxandralone are that it is orally administered, cost effective with comparable and/or better anabolic effect, and less toxic.[77–79] Although the data are limited and most studies showing efficacy in *acutely* hypercatabolic patients were performed with burn patients, because of its favorable risk-benefit ratio, there is much to recommend the use of oxandralone for the high-risk surgical patient. In fact, oxandralone is approved by the FDA for use as an anabolic agent in trauma and severely stressed patients. The dose of oxandralone is 20 mg/day given as two 10-mg oral doses, and it can be safely administered by mouth or via a nasogastric tube. Because of its well-documented beneficial effects on restoring lost muscle mass during the recovery and rehabilitation phases, oxandrolone should be continued until muscle mass is largely restored in patients who have had prolonged episodes of hypercatabolism and lost significant muscle mass.

Insulin, apart from its effect on blood glucose, also appears to have anabolic effects by increasing skeletal muscle glucose uptake and net protein synthesis.[80] This anabolic effect of insulin was initially reported using a very high dose of continuous insulin infusion (mean of 32 U/hr) for severely burned children. At this high dosage of insulin, concomitant glucose infusions were required to prevent significant hypoglycemic events. Since then, further studies with burned children have shown that doses of insulin as low as ~5–10 U/hr are sufficient to promote muscle anabolism without the drawback of hypoglycemia associated with the higher dose insulin

regimen.[81,82] Although insulin was given for up to 4 weeks in these studies and was found to limit muscle wasting in the early post-burn period and to promote positive nitrogen balance and reconstitution of lean muscle mass in the later stages of injury, there is almost no information on its effectiveness as an anabolic agent for non-burn patients or adults. This lack of data outside of the burn patient population makes its use for adult surgical patients problematic. On the other hand, the use of continuous insulin therapy to maintain tight plasma glucose control (80 to 110 mg/dL) has been recently shown in a prospective randomized controlled trial to reduce the mortality rate of ventilated surgical intensive care unit patients by almost 50%.[17] Until more clinical data accrue on the effectiveness of insulin in various populations of high-risk surgical patients, its routine use cannot be unequivocally recommended.

Another area of active research is the use of beta-blockers in attenuating the stress- or injury-induced hypermetabolic response. The rationale for the use of beta-blockers for hypermetabolic patients is based on the fact that catecholamines are increased severalfold after injury or during stress states, and they have been documented to significantly contribute to the hypercatabolic response as well as increased energy needs. Although the data on beta-blockers for patients with acute surgical illness are still very limited, two recent prospective randomized trials in severely burned children documented that propranolol attenuated the acute hypermetabolic response and reversed muscle protein catabolism by decreasing heart rate and resting energy expenditure as well as increasing muscle protein synthesis.[83,84] In these studies, propanolol was administered at a dose sufficient to decrease the heart rate of these burned children by 15% to 20%. As for insulin, there are no studies with adult or non-burn patients testing propanolol as an anabolic agent. However, the ability of beta-blockade to reduce the mortality of patients with cardiovascular disease undergoing surgery is well established.[85] In this second scenario, beta-blockade to a heart rate of 80 is thought to improve survival by limiting postoperative cardiac complications. For this reason, the use of beta-blockers, for at least certain subgroups of high-risk patients, appears beneficial.

It is well recognized that hypercatabolism and muscle wasting is a serious consequence of sepsis, trauma, or severe stress states and that, once 10% to 15% of the muscle mass is lost, immune function decreases, wound healing is impaired, and the risk of nosocomial infections, especially pneumonia, is increased. Consequently, providing optimal nutritional support of the high-risk surgical patient is a priority. Accomplishing this goal requires a thorough knowledge of the metabolic response to injury and stress as well as recognition of the various nutritional options available.

Critique

Having been in the hospital for 9 days, this patient definitely needs nutritional support. Unfortunately, the enteral route (gastric or postpyloric) is the preferred conduit for nutrition; however, hemodynamic instability is a contraindication for enteral feeding. Because this patient requires pressor support, she cannot be considered hemodynamically stable. Therefore, the route for nutritional support, in this setting, is parenteral (central).

Answer (A)

References

1. Long CL. Metabolic response to injury and illness: estimation of energy and protein needs from indirect calorimetry and nitrogen balance. J Parenter Enteral Nutr 1979; 3:452–456.
2. Hill AG, Hill GL. Metabolic response to severe injury. Br J Surg 1998; 85:884–890.
3. Bessey PQ, Watters JM, Aoke TT, et al. Combined hormonal infusion stimulates the metabolic response to injury. Ann Surg 1984; 200:264–281.
4. Aulick LH, Wroczyski FA, Coil JA, et al. Metabolic and thermoregulatory responses to burn wound colonization. J Trauma 1989; 29:478–483.
5. Deitch EA. Bacterial translocation of the gut flora. J Trauma 1990; 30:S184–S190.
6. Deitch EA. Multiple organ failure: pathophysiology and potential future therapies. Ann Surg 1992; 216:117–134.
7. Deitch EA, Xu DZ, Franko L, et al. Evidence favoring the role of the gut as a cytokine generating organ in rats subjected to hemorrhagic shock. Shock 1994; 1:141–146.
8. Deitch EA. Role of the gut lymphatic system in multiple organ failure. Curr Opin Crit Care 2001; 7:92–98.
9. Mainous MR, Block EF, Deitch EA. Nutritional support of the gut: how and why. New Horiz 1994; 2:193–201.
10. Hulsewe KWE, van Acker BAC, von Meyenfield MF, et al. Nutritional depletion and dietary manipulation: effects on the immune response. World J Surg 1999; 23:536–544.
11. Deitch EA. Infection in the compromised host. Surg Clin North Am 1988; 68:181–197.
12. Alexander JW, MacMillan BG, Stinnett JD, et al. Beneficial effects of aggressive feeding in severely burned children. Ann Surg 1980; 192:505–517.
13. Moore FA, Feliciano DV, Andrassy RJ, et al. Early enteral feeding, compared with parenteral, reduces postoperative septic complications: the results of a meta-analysis. Ann Surg 1992; 216:172–183.
14. Beale RJ, Bryg DJ, Bihari DJ. Immunonutrition in the critically ill: a systematic review of clinical outcome. Crit Care Med 1999; 27:2799–2805.
15. Jeejeebhoy KN. How should we monitor nutritional support: structure or function? New Horiz 1994; 2:131–138.
16. Burke JF, Wolfe RR, Mullany CS, et al. Glucose requirements following burn injury. Ann Surg 1979; 190:274–285.
17. Van Den Berghe G, Wouters P, Weekers F, et al. Intensive insulin therapy in critically ill patients. N Engl J Med 2001; 345:1359–1367.
18. Greig PD, Elwyn DH, Askanazi J, et al. Parenteral nutrition in septic patients: effect of increasing nitrogen intake. Am J Clin Nutr 1987; 46:1040–1047.
19. Endres S, Ghorbani R, Kelly VE, et al. The effect of dietary supplementation with n-3 polyunsaturated fatty acids on the synthesis of interleukin-1 and tumor necrosis factor by mononuclear cells. N Engl J Med 1989; 320:265–271.
20. Nghia MV, Waycaster M, Acuff RV, et al. Effects of postoperative carbohydrate overfeeding. Am Surg 1987; 53:632–635.
21. Campbell SM, Kudsk KA. "High tech" metabolic measurements: useful in daily clinical practice? J Parenter Enteral Nutr 1983; 12:610–612.
22. Klein S, Kinney J, Jeejeebhoy K, et al. Nutrition support in clinical practice: review of the published data and recommendations for future research directions. J Parenter Enteral Nutr 1977; 21:133–156.
23. Harris J, Benedict F. A Biometric Study of Basal Metabolism in Man. Washington, DC: Carnegie Institute, 1919.
24. Weissman C, Kemper M, Askanazi J, et al. Resting metabolic rate of the critically ill patient: measured versus predicted. J Anesthesiol 1986; 64:673–679.
25. Wilmore DW, Mason AD Jr, Johnson DW, et al. Effect of ambient temperature on heat production and heat loss in burn patients. J Appl Physiol 1975; 38:593–597.
26. Saito H, Trocki O, Alexander JW, et al. The effect of route of nutrient administration on the nutritional state, catabolic hormone secretion and gut mucosal integrity after burn injury. J Parenter Enteral Nutr 1987; 11:1–7.
27. McDonald WS, Sharpe CW Jr, Deitch EA. Immediate enteral feeding in burn patients is safe and effective. Ann Surg 1991; 213:177–183.
28. McGeer AJ, Detsky AS, O'Rourke K. Parenteral nutrition in cancer patients undergoing chemotherapy: a meta-analysis. Nutrition 1990; 6:233–2340.
29. The Veterans Affairs Total Parenteral Nutrition Cooperative Study Group: Perioperative total parenteral nutrition in surgical patients. N Engl J Med 1991; 325:525–532.
30. Herndon DN, Barrow RE, Stein M, et al. Increased mortality with intravenous supplemented feeding in severely burned patients. J Burn Care Rehabil 1989; 10:309–313.
31. Mochizuki H, Trocki O, Dominioni L, et al. Mechanism of prevention of postburn hypermetabolism and catabolism by early enteral feeding. Ann Surg 1984; 200:297–310.
32. Deitch EA, Sambol JT. The gut-origin hypothesis of MODS. In Deitch EA, Vincent JL, Windsor A, eds. Sepsis and Multiple Organ Dysfunction. Philadelphia: WB Saunders, 2002: 105–116.
33. Meyer J, Yurt RW, Duhaney R, et al. Differential neutrophil activation before and after endotoxin infusion in enterally versus parenterally fed human volunteers. Surg Gynecol Obstet 1988; 167:501–509.
34. Fong Y, Marano MA, Barber A, et al. Total parenteral nutrition and bowel rest modify the response to endotoxin in humans. Ann Surg 1989; 210:449–456.

35. Wilmore DW, Smith RJ, O'Dwyer ST, et al. The gut: a central organ after surgical stress. Surgery 1988; 104:917–923.

36. Speath G, Berg RD, Specian RD, Deitch EA. Food without fiber promotes bacterial translocation from the gut. Surgery 1990; 108:240–247.

37. Alverdy JC, Aoys E, Moss GS. Total parenteral nutrition promotes bacterial translocation from the gut. Surgery 1988; 104:186–190.

38. Heyland DK, Novak, F, Drover, J et al. Should immunonutrition become routine in critically ill patients?: a systematic review of evidence. JAMA 2001; 286:944–953.

39. Galban C, Montejo JC, Mesejo A, et al. An immune enhancing enteral diet reduces mortality rate and episodes of bacteremia in septic intensive care unit patients. Crit Care Med 2000; 28:643–648.

40. Kompan L, Kremzar B, Gadzijev E, et al. Effects of early enteral nutrition on intestinal permeability and the development of multiple organ failure after multiple injury. Intensive Care Med 1999; 25:157–161.

41. Zaloga GP, Roberts PR, Marik P. Feeding the hemodynamically unstable patient: a critical evaluation of the evidence. Nutr Clin Pract 2003; 18:285–293.

42. McClave SA, Chang WK. Feeding the hypotensive patient: does enteral feeding precipitate or protect against ischemic bowel? Nutr Clin Pract 2003; 18:279–284.

43. Sarr MG. Appropriate use, complications and advantages demonstrated in 500 consecutive needle catheter jejunostomies. Br J Surg 1999; 86:557–561.

44. Tapia J, Murguia R, Garcia G, et al. Jejunostomy techniques, indications and complications. World J Surg 1999; 23:596–602.

45. American Gastroenterological Association Medical Position Statement: guidelines for the use of enteral nutrition. Gastroenterology 1995; 108:1280–1301.

46. Gilpin DA, Barrow RE, Rutan RL, et al. Recombinant human growth hormone accelerates wound healing in children with large cutaneous burns. Ann Surg 1994; 220:19–24.

47. Cioffi WG, Gore DC, Rue LW, et al. Insulin-like growth factor-1 lowers protein oxidation in patients with thermal injury. Ann Surg 1994; 220:310–316.

48. Wilmore DW. The use of growth hormone in severely ill patients. Adv Surg 1999; 33:261–274.

49. Gibson FAM, Hinds CJ. Growth hormone and insulin-like growth factors in critical illness. Intensive Care Med 1997; 23:369–378.

50. Takala J, Ruokonen E, Webster NR, et al. Increased mortality associated with growth hormone in critically ill adults. N Engl J Med 1999; 341:785–792.

51. Haskel Y, Xu D, Lu Q, et al. Elemental diet-induced bacterial translocation can be hormonally modulated. Ann Surg 1993; 217:634–642.

52. Evers BM, Izukura M, Townsend CM, et al. Neurotensin prevents intestinal mucosal hypoplasia in rats fed an elemental diet. Dig Dis Sci 1992; 37:426–431.

53. Jacobs DO, Evans DA, Mealy K, et al. Combined effects of glutamine and epidermal growth factor on the rat intestine. Surgery 1988; 104:358–364.

54. Gianotti L, Alexander JW, Fukishima R, et al. Reduction of bacterial translocation with oral fibroblast growth factor and sucralfate. Am J Surg 1993; 165:195–200.

55. Barquist E, Kirton O, Windsor J, et al. The impact of antioxidant and splanchnic-directed therapy on persistent uncorrected gastric mucosal pH in the critically injured trauma patient. J Trauma 1998; 44:355–360.

56. Porter JM, Ivatoury RR, Azimuddin K, et al. Antioxidant therapy in the prevention of organ dysfunction syndrome and infectious complications after trauma: early results of a prospective randomized study. Am Surg 1999; 65:478–483.

57. Nathens AB, Neff MJ, Jurkovich GJ, et al. Randomized, prospective trial of antioxidant supplementation in critically ill surgical patients. Ann Surg 2002; 236:814–822.

58. Demling RH, Debiasse MA. Micronutrients in critical illness. Crit Care Clin 1995; 11:651–673.

59. Rotruck J, Pope A, Ganther H, et al. Selenium: biochemical role as a component of glutathione peroxidase. Science 1979; 179:588–590.

60. Haeker F, Stewart P. Effects of acute illness on selenium homeostasis. Crit Care Med 1990; 18:442–449.

61. McKenzie RL, Rea HM, Thomson CD, et al. Selenium concentration and glutathione peroxidase activity in blood of New Zealand infants and children. Am J Clin Nutr 1978; 31:1413–1418.

62. Levine RJ, Olson RE. Blood selenium in Thai children with protein calorie malnutrition. Proc Soc Exp Biol Med 1970; 134:1030.

63. Fleming CR, Lie JT, Mc Call JT, et al. Selenium deficiency and fatal cardiomyopathy in a patient on home parenteral nutrition. Gastroenterology 1982; 83:689–693.

64. Brown MR, Cohen HJ, Lyons JM, et al. Proximal muscle weakness and selenium deficiency associated with long term parenteral nutrition. Am J Clin Nutr 1986; 43:549–554.

65. Anderson RA, Polansky MM, Bryden NA, et al. Supplemental–chromium effects on glucose, insulin, glucagon and urinary chromium losses in subjects consuming controlled low chromium diets. Am J Clin Nutr 1991; 54:909–916.

66. Brown RO, Forloines-Lynn S, Cross RE, et al. Chromium deficiency after long term parenteral nutrition. Dig Dis Sci 1986; 31:661–664.

67. Kohn S, Kohn D, Schiller D. Effect of zinc supplementation on epidermal Langerhans cells of elderly patients with decubitus ulcers. J Dermatol 2000; 27:258–263.

68. Rostan EF, DeBuys HV, Madey DL, et al. Evidence supporting zinc as an antioxidant for skin. Int J Dermatol 2002; 41:606–611.

69. Bogden JD. Influence of zinc on immunity in the elderly. J Nutr Health Aging 2004; 8:48–54.

70. Deitch EA, Sittig KM. A serial study of the erythropoietic response to thermal injury. Ann Surg 1993; 217:293–299.

71. Weinberg ED. Iron depletion: a defense against intracellular infection and neoplasia. Life Sci 1992; 50:1289–1297.

72. Demling RH, Desanti L. Oxandralone, an anabolic steroid, significantly increases the rate of weight gain in the recovery phase after major burns. J Trauma 1997; 43:47–51.

73. Wolf SE, Thomas SJ, Dasu MR, et al. Improved net protein balance, lean mass and gene expression changes with

oxandralone treatment in the severely burned. Ann Surg 2003; 237:801–811.

74. Mendenhall CL, Moritz TE, Roselli GA, et al. A study of oral nutritional support with oxandralone in malnourished patients with alcoholic hepatitis: results of a Department of Veterans Affairs cooperative study. Hepatology 1993; 17:564–570.

75. Berger J, Poll L, Hall C, et al. Oxandralone in AIDS wasting myopathy. AIDS 1996; 10:1657–1662.

76. Thomas S, Wolf SE, Murphy KD, et al. The long term effect of oxandralone on hepatic acute phase proteins in severely burned children. J Trauma 2003; 56:37–44.

77. Demling RH. Comparison of the anabolic effects and complications of human growth hormone and the testosterone analog, oxandralone, after severe burn injury. Burns 1999; 25:215–221.

78. Fox M, Minor A, et al. Oxandralone: a potent anabolic steroid. J Clin Endocrinol Metab 1962; 22:921–923.

79. Karim A, Ranney RE, Zagarella BA, et al. Oxandralone disposition and metabolism in man. Clin Pharmacol Ther 1973; 14:862–866.

80. Sakurai Y, Aarsland A, Herndon DN, et al. Stimulation of muscle protein synthesis by long- term insulin infusion in severely burned patients. Ann Surg 1995; 222:283–297.

81. Ferrando AA, Chinkes DL, Wolf SE, et al. A submaximal dose of insulin promotes net skeletal muscle protein synthesis in patients with severe burns. Ann Surg 1999; 229:11–18.

82. Thomas SJ, Morimato K, Herndon DN, et al. The effect of prolonged euglycemic hyperinsulinemia on lean body mass after severe burn. Surgery 2002; 132:341–347.

83. Herndon DN, Hart DW, Steven EW, et al. Reversal of catabolism by beta-blockade after severe burns. N Engl J Med 2001; 345:1223–1229.

84. Hart DW, Wolf SE, Chinkes DL, et al. B-blockade and growth hormone after burn. Ann Surg 2002; 236:450–457.

85. Poldermans D, Boersma E, Bax JJ, et al. The effect of bisoprolol on perioperative mortality and myocardial infarction in high risk patients undergoing vascular surgery. N Engl J Med 1999; 341:1789–1794.

8
The Intensive Care Unit: The Next-Generation Operating Room

Philip S. Barie, Soumitra R. Eachempati, and Jian Shou

Case Scenario

A 39-year-old man is in his seventh day in the intensive care unit on ventilatory support (transoral–translaryngeal endotracheal intubation) after having acute care surgery for a ruptured abdominal aortic aneurysm. Although the patient has brain stem function and is hemodynamically stable, he is unresponsive to voice. The current ventilator settings are as follows:

IMV = 12 breaths/min P_aO_2 = 120 mmHg
FiO_2 = .40 PCO_2 = 37 mmHg
PEEP = 5 cm H_2O pH = 7.39

The nurse notes that the patient has no spontaneous breathing and requires frequent suctioning. He has had recent temperature spikes. Chest x-ray demonstrates no atelectasis. Which of the following is the airway management of choice at this time?

(A) Transnasal–translaryngeal endotracheal intubation
(B) Continue transoral–translaryngeal endotracheal intubation
(C) Percutaneous tracheostomy
(D) Independent lung ventilation
(E) Inverse: E ratio ventilation

Demands upon the operating room (OR) are a fixture of modern health care. Operating room time is expensive and scarce and is often allocated in advance in "blocks" to busy surgeons. Timely completion of the elective surgical schedule is important for prudent hospital fiscal management and also for patient and surgeon satisfaction. Surgical emergencies demand priority access to the OR and, because of their inherent unpredictability, are disruptive to the OR schedule. It can be difficult to schedule a nonemergency case on short notice.

For many reasons, the intensive care unit (ICU) is viewed increasingly as an OR itself, a bona fide, convenient alternative to scheduling a case in the main OR. The scope of surgical procedures that can be undertaken at the bedside is broad. For acute care surgical procedures or urgent procedures on critically ill patients who are too unstable for intrahospital transport to the OR, operating at the bedside is plausible. However, no matter how careful the planning or exigent the need, using the ICU cubicle as an OR has inherent limitations not easily overcome. The risks of intrahospital transport for most patients may be overstated. The patient may not be moved, but almost everyone and everything required to perform surgery in the ICU must be brought to the bedside. Space at the immediate bedside is constrained in almost all ICUs, and it may be difficult to place everything in the immediate vicinity. Importantly, infection control practices that are the standard of care in the OR cannot be replicated in the ICU. That which can be accomplished surgically in the ICU, effectively and safely, and under what conditions and constraints, is the subject of this review. Unfortunately, there is little Class I evidence in this subject area; therefore, much of this chapter is based by necessity on retrospective data and expert opinion.

Rationale

All things considered, operations should be performed in the OR. The modern OR has evolved to become a bastion of integrated special-purpose high technology. Integrated OR teams can support unstable critically ill or injured patients for protracted periods during complex operations in an environment where considerations of patient safety are paramount. Almost any pharmaceutical that can be administered in the ICU is available for administration in the OR. Inhalational anesthetics can be given, which is impossible elsewhere. Drugs to manage rare complications of anesthesia, such as malignant hyperthermia syndrome, are readily available only in the OR. Monitors and anesthesia ventilators are nearly as sophisticated as those used in ICUs. Overhead lighting is designed for the purpose. Room temperature can be controlled. A dropped instrument can be retrieved, cleaned, resterilized, and returned to the field within 5 minutes. Supplies or instruments not requested in advance are immediately at hand, minimizing costly delays.

Yet operations are performed at the bedside, and increasingly often. The reasons are several. Some acute care operations cannot wait. Operating room time may not be available within a reasonable time frame; neither can some surgeons wait. Other procedures are sufficiently minor that mobilization to take the patient to the OR constitutes a waste of resources. The resources in personnel and portable monitoring equipment necessary for transport of the patient to the OR are substantial and often unjustifiable for performance of a brief, minor operation. However, every "road trip" must be assessed not only from as risk-benefit perspective but also from a cost-benefit perspective.[1] Those patients who should travel are those who must, and no others.

Published guidelines[2] for intrahospital transport indicate that, at a minimum, the ICU patient's respiratory therapist and nurse should accompany the patient out of the ICU for the duration of the transport, but to do so might require juggling the ICU staff on the fly to accommodate the departure, or it might be impossible if the patient does not have one-to-one nursing (a rarity). Physician accompaniment is a poor substitute in that the physician is often a junior one with limited familiarity with the patient's case and has limited skills for troubleshooting the myriad things that can go wrong with infusion pumps, intravenous tubing, and the like. However, the putative lack of safety of the intrahospital "road trip" is probably overstated. Szem et al. observed a cohort of critically ill, mechanically ventilated surgical patients on intrahospital transports and stratified the transports in terms of risk (number of vasoactive drugs infusing and use of therapeutic positive end-expiratory pressure [PEEP]). Transports were less common to the OR than to the radiology suite (where monitoring and support capabilities are often rudimentary in contrast to those available in the OR). Despite the high severity of illness and the high-risk nature of the most common destination, the incidence of transport-related mishaps was only 5%, all of which were minor (e.g., tangled intravenous tubing, low battery). Stevenson et al.[4] noted that even the sickest ICU patient can be transported safely if risk and benefits are weighed carefully, patients are stabilized insofar as possible before the transport is undertaken, and monitoring is continuous throughout. All members of the transport team must be educated in patient evaluation; potential risks, complications, and interventions; and equipment operation and troubleshooting. All members of the transport team must understand their roles and responsibilities in detail and must communicate effectively. Written policies are useful to define the levels of personnel, training, and support and the equipment necessary for safe patient transport. The same can be said for the roles and responsibilities of the members of the operating team at the bedside.

The issues with respect to intrahospital transport of critically ill children have also been examined.[5] Transportation of critically ill children may be more hazardous than for adults. In a prospective observational study by Wallen et al.,[5] only 24% of transports were uneventful. Physiologic perturbation occurred in 72% of transports, and an equipment-related mishap occurred in 10% of transports. At least one "major" intervention was required in 14% of transports (34% for mechanically ventilated patients vs. 10% for nonventilated patients); however, neither cardiac arrest nor death was observed. Notably, 11% of pediatric patients became hypothermic during the transport episode. Whereas both the intensity of pretransport of therapy (as measured by the Therapeutic Intensity Scoring System, TISS) and the duration of transport were independent risk factors for physiologic deterioration and the need for intervention, equipment malfunction was predicted only by the duration of transport.[5]

What Resources Are Needed?

Preparation of the Unit and Staff

First and foremost, the staff of the ICU must be familiar and comfortable with the use of the ICU as an OR.[6] If the staff is experienced, the chance of procedure-related complications is much reduced. If the staff is not familiar with the roles and responsibilities they will be asked to assume in the ICU/OR, then an intensive, comprehensive educational program that addresses all common and many less common bedside operations must be implemented. The "learning curve" for physicians of the first few procedures might best be addressed by performing the operation in the OR under conditions that reproduce those expected to prevail in the ICU, but such precautions do not address the educational and training needs of the bedside nurse or respiratory therapist in the ICU.

The operations performed at the bedside will vary from ICU to ICU based on the specialty orientation and case mix of the particular unit. An example of procedures performed in a trauma ICU is shown in Table 8.1.[7] Among trauma patients, laparotomy in several guises was more common than either tracheostomy or access procedures for enteral feeding.[7]

TABLE 8.1. Scope of procedures performed at the bedside in the
ICU at a level I trauma center.

Laparotomy (in 13 patients)	43
Irrigation after drainage of abscess	15
Removal of packs	13
Removal and replacement of packs	10
Drainage of abscess	4
Jejunostomy	1
Tracheostomy	24
Open	16
Percutaneous	8
Percutaneous endoscopic gastrostomy	10
Fasciotomy, lower extremity	2

Source: Data from Porter et al.[7]

Detailed protocols that define roles and responsibilities, medications, monitoring equipment, disposable supplies, and surgical instruments to be needed for each procedure are desirable in part because most of what is required, including nursing services that exceed what the patient's primary nurse can provide, will need to be brought to the bedside in advance of the procedure. All needed equipment (and reasonably anticipated needs) must be at the bedside before the start of the procedure. Unfortunately, such protocols probably exist in few ICUs. Communication is essential so that if additional nursing personnel will need to be at the bedside for the procedure, adequate coverage for the other patients is ensured. Particular consideration should also be given to whether an anesthesiologist or nurse anesthetist should be part of the bedside team for the procedure.

Co-administration of a narcotic, a benzodiazepine, and a neuromuscular blocking agent may constitute full general anesthesia, depending on dosage; administration, monitoring, and available airway management skills must be equivalent in all practice venues. All patients must be monitored adequately, commensurate with the magnitude of the procedure. Continuous pulse oximetry, electrocardiograph tracing, and blood pressure measurement together represent a minimum standard for every procedure, no matter how minor. Invasive hemodynamic monitoring or end-tidal CO_2 monitoring may be required for more complex undertakings.

Preparation of the Patient

Informed consent must be obtained from the patient or the designated representative according to local norms unless the intervention is for an immediately life-threatening condition. Renal and hepatic function should be ascertained for proper dosing of medications (see below) (Table 8.2). The coagulation system should also be assessed to determine the risk of bleeding and the need to administer coagulation factors or platelets before surgery. It must be remembered that the platelet count does not reflect platelet function and that conventional tests of platelet function are either unreliable (e.g., template bleeding time) or not immediately available (e.g., thromboelastography). Patients who have received aspirin or another nonsteroidal antiinflammatory agent should be considered for transfusion of platelets to "cover" the procedure, but specific guidelines do not exist. Patients with renal dysfunction (blood urea nitrogen concentration above ~70 mg/dL) also have platelet dysfunction and can receive either cryoprecipitate or D,D-arginine vasopressin for short-term stabilization of platelet function. Enteral feedings should be held for up to 6 hours before the procedure unless it is very minor and positioning will not increase the risk of aspiration. Preoxygenation (with pure oxygen) of all patients for about 15 minutes before the procedure may also be beneficial.

A Culture of Safety and Accountability

The hazards of accidental injury by sharps (e.g., needles, scalpel blades) and the risks of blood-borne transmission of etiologic agents are real. Policies and procedures have been changed in virtually every OR to minimize the risk, which fortunately has been decreasing.[8] Overall annual percutaneous injury rates decreased from 21/100 beds to 16.5/100 beds between 1997 and 2001 in a nine-hospital midwestern U.S. hospital system whose facilities, urban and rural, ranged from 113 to 1,400 beds.[8] Average annual injury rates were higher in large hospitals, but smaller hospitals had significantly higher proportions of injury in the emergency department, OR, and ICU (12.3% vs. 9.4% for the ICU setting). Intensive care units in teaching hospitals also had higher proportions of percutaneous injuries than did nonteaching hospitals (11.4% vs. 7.8%).

In the OR, particular attention is paid to communication among team members, protocols for passing sharp instruments to and from the operative field and instrument table, and meticulous accounting of sharps throughout the operation. Similar attention to detail is mandatory if surgery at the bedside in the ICU will be made as safe as possible for the patient and the operating team. Sterile gowns, sterile double gloves, masks, caps, and eye protection should be used for any bedside procedure where the possibility exists of splashing blood or bodily fluids.

In particular, accounting for the whereabouts of sharps at the bedside remains an issue in the authors' estimation. The mattress must never be used as a "pincushion" for needles. The period of highest risk to practitioners appears to be during "clean up" in the aftermath of minor procedures, when the accounting process for sharps is informal and, indeed, often haphazard. When drapes are collected for disposal at the end of the procedure (usually by the person who performed the procedure, who may

TABLE 8.2. The formulary for analgesia, anesthesia, and sedation in the ICU.

Agent	Initial IV adult dose	Comments
Induction agents		
Etomidate	6 mg or more	Maintains CO and BP. Reduces ICP but maintains CPP. Short $T_{1/2}$; use infusion for maintenance. Possible adrenal suppression.
Ketamine	1–2 mg/kg	Rapid-onset, short-duration agent for induction of anesthesia. Can be given by continuous infusion for maintenance and at lower dose for sedation without anesthesia. Transiently increases BP and HR. Raises ICP and intraocular pressure. Usually does not depress respiration. Crosses the placenta, but generally safe in pregnancy and for neonates and children. Concurrent narcotics or barbiturates may prolong recovery. Can cause anxiety, disorientation, dysphoria, and hallucinations, which may be reduced by a short-acting benzodiazepine during emergence. Atropine pretreatment is recommended to decrease secretions but may increase incidence of dysphoria. Hepatic metabolism.
Propofol	1.5–2.5 mg/kg	Provides no analgesia. Potent amnestic effect. Causes apnea and loss of gag reflex. Can cause marked low BP. Infuse at 0.05–0.3 mg/kg/min for prolonged sedation. Minimal accumulation (hepatic insufficiency) facilitates rapid elimination. Account for 1 kCal/mL (lipid infusion) in nutrition prescription. Use of same vial >12 hr associated with bacteremia. Safety for children still debated.
Thiopental	1–5 mg/kg	Used rarely, now mostly for TBI management. Reduces BP and CPP. Accumulates with prolonged use or infusion, especially with hepatic insufficiency.
Intravenous sedatives/analgesics		
Midazolam	0.5–4 mg	Short $T_{1/2}$, but accumulates during infusion owing to active metabolites. Only benzodiazepine with potent amnestic effect. Can cause low BP and loss of airway. Primarily used for short-term sedation for ICU procedures. Renal elimination.
Diazepam	2.5–5.0 mg	Long $T_{1/2}$ limits usefulness in ICU except rare cases when very long-term sedation is required. Terminates epileptiform activity effectively. Hepatic elimination.
Lorazepam	1–4 mg	Effective anxiolytic. Preferred agent for continuous infusion of benzodiazepines (starting dose, 1 mg/hr). Can cause low BP, especially with hypovolemia, and paradoxical agitation. Hepatic elimination.
Morphine	2–10 mg	Analgesic and sedative effects. Can cause low BP, CO, and apnea. Tolerance and withdrawal possible after long-term use. Can be given as IV infusion or by PCA for analgesia or to facilitate prolonged mechanical ventilation or withdrawal of care. Hepatic elimination.
Hydromorphone	0.5–2.0 mg	Hydrated ketone of morphine with similar use and risk profiles. Approximately eightfold more potent than morphine. Hepatic elimination.
Fentanyl	50–100 mcg	Approximately 50-fold potency compared with morphine, but less likely to cause low BP in appropriate dosage (less histamine release). Versatile for ICU use given IV or by epidural infusion or PCA. Less potent than local anesthetics for epidural analgesia or abrogation of surgical stress response. Can cause truncal rigidity and apnea with inability to ventilate by hand (use neuromuscular blockade to facilitate intubation in that setting). Hepatic elimination.
Meperidine	25–100 mg	Of little use in the ICU. Low doses cause postoperative shivering, which increases VO_2 and HR. Accumulates even in mild renal insufficiency and can cause seizures. Contraindicated with monoamine oxidase inhibitors (hyperthermia, death).
Neuromuscular blocking agents		
Succinylcholine	0.75–1.5 mg/kg	Only depolarizing NBMA (occupies ACh receptor). Rapid onset, effect dissipates within 10 min of single dose. Causes hyperkalemia. Can precipitate malignant hyperthermia syndrome. Increases ICP and intraocular pressure. Contraindicated in TBI, spinal cord injury, neuromuscular disease, and burns. Metabolized by plasma cholinesterase, absence of enzyme (relatively common) causes prolonged paralysis.
Atracurium	0.2–0.5 mg/kg	Short-acting, non-depolarizing NMBAs (competitive inhibitors of Ach). Relatively slow in onset
Cisatracurium	0.2–0.5 mg/kg	compared with other agents in class. The drugs are similar, except atracurium causes histamine release and can cause high HR, low BP. Cisatracurium now used preferentially; short acting and requires IV infusion for prolonged effect. Effect potentiated by hypokalemia. Many drug interactions. Elimination by Hoffman elimination and ester hydrolysis; thus can be used for patients with renal/hepatic insufficiency.
Mivacurium	0.15 mg/kg	Non-depolarizing NMBA with slow onset and moderate duration of action. Can be given by continuous infusion. Releases histamine; causes bronchospasm. Can cause decreased or increased HR and cardiac dysrhythmias. Faster onset and recovery in children ages 2–12 years. Enhanced blockade in pregnant patients given magnesium for preeclampsia. Inactivated by plasma cholinesterases; prolonged paralysis possible in enzyme-deficient patients.
Pancuronium	0.05–0.1 mg	Rapid onset, prolonged effect. Causes hypertension and tachycardia. Used for induction of neuromuscular blockade, but should be converted to a drug such as continuously infused cisatracurium for maintenance. Eliminated by kidneys and liver, resulting in accumulation with repeated doses.

TABLE 8.2. *Continued*

Agent	Initial IV adult dose	Comments
Rocuronium	0.6 mg/kg	Nondepolarizing NMBA with rapid onset and moderate duration of action. Some potential for histamine release; can cause bronchospasm. Can cause decreased or increased HR and cardiac dysrhythmias. Children less than 1 year of age are more susceptible to the drug. Metabolized by liver.
Vecuronium	0.08–0.10 mg/kg	Nondepolarizing NMBA with rapid onset and short duration of action. Less potential for histamine release. Can cause malignant hyperthermia syndrome. Metabolized by liver.
Miscellaneous agents		
Droperidol	0.625 mg	Potent antiemetic effect but used rarely in the ICU. Sedative effects. Can cause low BP, especially in conjunction with vasodilators. Antidopaminergic properties contraindicate use in Parkinson's disease. Can cause extrapyramidal effects. Hepatic elimination.
Haloperidol	2–5 mg	Used commonly for anxiolysis (often preferred to lorazepam), especially when respiratory depression is undesirable. Not FDA-approved for IV administration, but IV route is commonplace in practice. Antidopaminergic properties contraindicate use in Parkinson's disease. Can cause Extrapyramidal effects. Hepatic elimination.
Ketorolac	0.5–1.0 mg/kg	Parenteral NSAID used in lieu of opioids o, for opioid-sparing effect in combination. Interferes irreversibly with platelet function and can cause incisional or GI hemorrhage and acute renal failure. Use strictly limited to less than 5 days in postoperative period.
Reversal agents		
Flumazenil	0.1–0.2 mg	Benzodiazepine antagonist. Rapid onset and short duration. Adverse effect of benzodiazepine can persist after drug wears off. Repeated doses of up to 0.8 mg can be used. Abrupt antagonism of chronic benzodiazepines use can precipitate seizures.
Naloxone	Up to 0.4 mg	Opioid antagonist. Rapid onset and short duration. Often diluted 0.4 mg/10 mL and titrated 0.04–0.08 mg at a time to reverse undesirable side effects while preserving analgesia. Repeated doses of up to 0.4 mg or continuous IV infusion can be used. Abrupt antagonism of opioid use can precipitate hypertension, increased HR, pulmonary edema, or myocardial infarction.
Edrophonium with Atropine	0.5–1.0 mg/kg 0.007–0.014 mg/kg	Edrophonium is an anticholinesterase inhibitor with antidysrhythmic properties. Rapid onset, short duration; therefore, used usually in concert with atropine, which counteracts the increased secretions, decreased HR, and bronchospasm. Not effective for reversal of neuromuscular blockade caused by depolarizing agents. Renal and hepatic elimination (edrophonium). Atropine may cause fever.
Neostigmine with Glycopyrrolate	0.5–2.0 mg 0.1–0.2 mg	Cause salivation and severe bradycardia. May cause bronchospasm or laryngospasm. Metabolized by kidneys. Not effective for reversal of neuromuscular blockade caused by depolarizing agents. Because of profound low HR response, given in same syringe with glycopyrrolate (or sometimes atropine). Glycopyrrolate counteracts low HR and unopposed causes increased HR. May cause fever. Glycopyrrolate is contraindicated in GI ileus/obstruction and in neonates.

Ach, acetylcholine; BP, blood pressure; CO, cardiac output; CPP, cerebral perfusion pressure; FDA, U.S. Food and Drug Administration; GI, gastrointestinal; HR, heart rate; ICP, intracranial pressure; ICU, intensive care unit; IV, intravenous; NBMA, neuromuscular blocking agent; NSAID, nonsteroidal antiinflammatory drug; PCA, patient-controlled analgesia; $T_{1/2}$, elimination half-life; TBI, traumatic brain injury, VO_2 oxygen consumption.

have been working only with the patient's primary nurse), it is easy to overlook an unsecured sharp lurking within the folds of the drape. Even if no injury occurs at the bedside, if a sharp is discarded inadvertently in the trash rather than the ubiquitous "sharps containers," untold numbers of hospital workers and sanitation workers are placed at risk.

Infection Control

Intensive care units are bastions of health care–acquired infections and multidrug-resistant bacterial pathogens. There is substantial foot traffic in the unit and at the bedside, making the environment strikingly different from that of the OR. For these and other reasons, infection control can be difficult to maintain in the ICU, although adherence is crucial for the safe performance of procedures and operations at the bedside. The application of the principles of infection control and the implementation of preventive strategies is simple and should not be considered as constraining or controlling, if implemented and adhered to as an integral part of the behavior of all staff members who provide direct patient care.[9] Specific measures, including hand washing, barrier precautions, pulmonary toilet, positioning, early removal of catheters and drains, and the control of antibiotic use should be integrated fully into the continuous process of improvement of the quality of care. As one example, Jacobs et al.[10] observed a 32% infection rate after percutaneous tracheostomy and associated it with a 34%

incidence of "inappropriate" administration of antibiotics for therapy of nosocomial pneumonia. After instituting an antibiotic administration protocol that decreased the incidence of inappropriate antibiotic administration to 4%, the incidence of infection complicating percutaneous tracheostomy was reduced significantly to 11%.

Anesthesia, Analgesia, and Sedation

Almost every bedside procedure requires analgesia, sedation, or anesthesia, alone or in some combination. Published guidelines describe in detail the sustained use of these agents for indications such as prolonged mechanical ventilation or control of increased intracranial pressure.[11] Aranda and Hanson[12] have described a systematic approach to the use of these agents in the ICU setting.

The critical care team should review the anesthesia record as soon as all postoperative patients are admitted to the ICU, looking in particular for signs of allergy, drug interactions, or destabilizing adverse effects that may inform future decision making. A panoply of agents is available for use during bedside procedures and operations (see Table 8.2), and the choice must be based on several factors. Is the patient intubated? Are the patient's hemodynamics stable and normal? Will the procedure require general anesthesia, or will local anesthesia suffice? If general anesthesia is required, for how long must it be effective? Will neuromuscular blockade be needed? If sedation is planned, will it be conscious sedation or maintained at a deeper level? Will repetitive administration be required for multiple procedures? Will the agents require reversal, or will they be allowed to "wear off"? Will metabolism of the agents be impaired by abnormal organ function? Will the personnel available be able to manage the agent(s) chosen?

For children, sedation or anesthesia may be necessary for performance of bedside procedures that may only require local anesthesia when performed in adults. The combination of intravenous midazolam analgesia and ketamine anesthesia is safe and effective for bedside procedures in children, including lumbar puncture, bone/bone marrow aspiration/biopsy, central venous catheter placement, liver biopsy, and thoracentesis.[13] Among 127 patients who underwent a total of 295 monitored procedures reviewed by Slonim and Ognibene,[13] only 9 complications were noted. In particular, the dysphoric emergence phenomenon that is characteristic of ketamine administration to adults was observed only once.

There has been ongoing concern regarding the safety of administration of propofol to children, specifically relating to the risk of lactic acidosis. Wheeler et al.[14] reviewed 91 children who received propofol for 110 bedside procedures in a pediatric ICU, some of whom were not critically ill and were moved to the ICU for the express purpose of the procedure. Adequate sedation was achieved in all cases, at a mean total dose of 4.23 mg/kg. The mean duration of the ICU stay was 108 minutes. Three patients had hypotension, and three patients had arterial oxygen desaturation, but no instance required endotracheal intubation or therapy other than the administration of fluid.

Ultrasound

Ultrasound has become almost indispensable in the armamentarium of the surgeon at the bedside.[15] With real-time imaging, the information obtained can augment the physical examination, refine the differential diagnosis, or guide an intervention. Although surgeon-performed ultrasound was developed for rapid evaluation of the abdomen of the hypotensive trauma patient, ultrasound can also increase the safety of central venous catheterization, assess the presence, depth, and extent of an abscess, guide and confirm the aspiration of a fluid collection or the gallbladder, or diagnose wound dehiscence before it is apparent on physical examination. The use of ultrasound imaging to detect a pleural effusion has essentially supplanted the lateral decubitus chest radiograph. Moreover, thoracentesis and central venous catheter insertion are facilitated and made safer. As surgeons become more facile with ultrasound imaging, other uses will develop for the assessment of patients in the acute setting.

Bedside Neurologic Surgery

Intervention at the bedside may be required for evaluation and management of increased intracranial pressure (ICP). Maintenance of cerebral perfusion is important for management of patients with traumatic brain injury, and determination of both ICP and cerebral perfusion pressure is central to management. Intracranial pressure can be assessed by extradural pressure transduction (e.g., the "bolt"), by parenchymal placement of a fiberoptic catheter, or by placement of a catheter into a lateral cerebral ventricle (e.g., ventriculostomy) via a twist-drill craniotomy (burr hole). The value of the information gained justifies performance of this highly invasive procedure despite the high incidence of complications, including hemorrhage, malposition, occlusion, and an 8% incidence of infection (ventriculitis).

Invasive placement of intracranial monitoring devices has traditionally been by neurosurgeons at the bedside in the ICU rather than in the trauma bay or the OR. Infection control is paramount for ventriculostomy catheter insertion, because, although prolonged catheterization increases the risk of infection, neither antibiotic prophylaxis nor scheduled catheter changes reduce the risk.[16,17]

However, a dearth of neurosurgical coverage for trauma in many areas has increased interest in the placement of these devices by non-neurosurgeons. In a review of 157 parenchymal ICP monitors placed in 146 patients with intracranial injury, surgical residents placed 87 ICP monitors without attending supervision and 43 with immediate supervision by either general surgeons or neurosurgeons.[18] Neurosurgeons placed 26 monitors without the participation of residents. No major technical complications, episodes of catheter-induced intracranial hemorrhage, or infectious complications were reported. Protocols have also been described to train non-neurosurgeons in the safe placement of ventriculostomy catheters.[19]

Drainage of chronic subdural hematoma at the bedside has also been described,[20] using twist-drill craniotomy under local anesthesia. In a prospective observational trial, Reinges et al.[20] followed 118 adult patients, 19 of whom had bilateral lesions. Treatment of unilateral chronic subdural hematoma was 92% successful, albeit after a mean of 3.2 taps (0–5) for drainage. Treatment of bilateral hematomas was equally successful but required up to 10 taps for success. The failure rate was 9%, owing to hemorrhage (n = 2), identification of subdural empyema (n = 2), or inadequate drainage (n = 7). A preoperative computed tomography (CT) scan that demonstrated septation of the hematoma was a significant predictor of treatment failure.

Bedside Surgery of the Head and Neck

In a review of 1,268 cases, Abbas et al.[21] found 10 cases (incidence, 0.8%) for reopening of cervical incisions following thyroid or parathyroid surgery, usually for hemorrhage. In only two instances was emergency reopening at the bedside necessary, but tracheostomy was required for one of those two cases. Notably, the median time interval from the completion of surgery to the intervention for cervical hematoma was 16 hours (range, 2–48 hours).

Several anecdotal reports attest to the efficacy of fine-needle aspiration or percutaneous drainage for the management of fluid collections in the neck following surgery or trauma. Fritscher-Ravens et al.[22] reported three critically ill patients who underwent successful fine-needle aspiration at the bedside in the ICU, two of whom had a therapeutic intervention. A mediastinal abscess after percutaneous tracheostomy was aspirated in one patient, leading to appropriate antibiotic therapy and complete recovery. A paratracheal hematoma compressing the airway was aspirated in another patient with multiple trauma, thereby avoiding tracheostomy. Yeow et al.[23] reviewed 34 patients who had 41 fluid collections drained percutaneously after major head and neck oncologic

surgery. Prior fine-needle aspiration had been "successful" in only 56% of patients, which increased to 91% after closed-suction percutaneous drainage for a mean of 9 days. The collections were approached through the ipsilateral posterior triangle, and no complications were noted.

The Cervicothoracic Interface: Tracheostomy

Tracheostomy is perhaps the most commonly performed "real" operation at the bedside in the ICU, but what does reality reflect, given that tracheostomy is increasingly performed using a percutaneous technique through an incision that is less than 1 cm in length? Some tracheostomies are best performed in the OR even now, although some debate persists as to whether bedside open or percutaneous tracheostomy is preferable. Reflecting its commonplace performance, tracheostomy is the area in this review where good-quality data are ample to answer most, if not all, questions. The most common indication of tracheostomy is acute respiratory failure that transitions into ventilator dependence (Table 8.3),[24] followed by airway "protection" for the patient who is obtunded or whose gag reflex is impaired or absent. The third most common indication for tracheostomy is maxillofacial trauma.

Large series of open tracheostomies at the bedside have been reported with morbidity rates comparable to tracheostomy performed in the operating room.[25] For adult patients with difficult anatomy, cricothyroidostomy is a safe long-term alternative to a conventional infrathyroid tracheostomy.[26] On the other hand, percutaneous tracheostomy is advocated as a safe, cost-effective bedside procedure, especially when performed with attention to detail (Table 8.4) under direct airway visualization by fiberoptic bronchoscopy,[27] although the necessity of bronchoscopy has been questioned owing to a paucity of supporting data. As with the introduction of

TABLE 8.3. Indications and patient selection criteria for 71 bedside percutaneous tracheostomies in a surgical ICU.

Indications	
Acute respiratory failure	58%
Airway protection	37%
Maxillofacial trauma	5%

Selection criteria
Positive end-expiratory pressure (PEEP) <10 cm H_2O
No previous tracheostomy
No anatomic distortion of the cervical region
No other indication to go to the operating room

Source: Data from Mittendorf et al.[24]

TABLE 8.4. Technical issues to consider in the performance of percutaneous dilational tracheostomy.

1. Use well-defined patient selection criteria. If percutaneous tracheostomy is contraindicated, go to the operating room.
2. The tracheostomy tube should be checked and ready on the operative field before the procedure is started.
3. Insert a tracheostomy tube of the largest possible size to minimize the work of breathing and facilitate pulmonary toilet. For most adults, an 8-F tube can be placed without difficulty.
4. Use a single cannula flexible tracheostomy tube or a longer tracheostomy tube when indicated; this pertains especially to obese patients who are likely to have a "deep" trachea and to those who have developed tracheomalacia from prolonged endotracheal intubation and have an air leak around an intact, properly positioned balloon.
5. Tracheostomy and intubation trays must be immediately available in anticipation of complications.
6. A vertical skin incision is less likely to encounter bleeding from the anterior cervical veins.
7. Ensure that the skin incision is of sufficient size to permit the unimpeded transcutaneous passage of the size of tracheostomy tube that is chosen. Palpation of the tracheal rings is also facilitated.
8. Ensure that the patient is sedated adequately and that infiltrative local anesthesia is used liberally. Intratracheal lidocaine may suppress the cough reflex effectively for the duration of the procedure. Neuromuscular blockade is optional; if used, personnel with advanced airway management skills must be present.
9. Monitor vital signs, oxygen saturation, and end-tidal CO_2 concentration continuously throughout the procedure.
10. Deflate the endotracheal tube cuff, remove the tape securing the endotracheal tube, and ventilate with pure oxygen at increased tidal volume on the ventilator to compensate for decreased minute ventilation.
11. Performance of the procedure under the guidance of fiberoptic bronchoscopy is strongly recommended.
12. Withdraw the endotracheal tube sufficiently so that the finder needle does not transit the endotracheal tube. Direct vision of the airway lumen facilitates this greatly.
13. Do not direct the cannula needle cranially so as to minimize the possibility that the guidewire will pass toward the pharynx rather than the carina.
14. The heavily calcified trachea may require more force for passage of the tube than may be anticipated at the outset.
15. Confirm intratracheal position of the endotracheal tube immediately, ideally by both capnography and bronchoscopy. Immediate postprocedure bronchoscopy also confirms intratracheal hemostasis and evacuates blood and subglottic secretions that may have entered the lower airway during the procedure.
16. Secure the tube carefully (and redundantly) to prevent dislodgement.
17. Use flexible tubing and a double swivel connection to connect the patient to the ventilator to lessen trauma to the stoma.
18. Provide postoperative and ongoing facial and oral care to the patient as soon as circumstances permit.

any "new" procedure, there is a "learning curve" before proficiency is achieved; Massick et al.[28] estimated that the institutional learning curve for percutaneous tracheostomy is about 20 cases. It is recommended that percutaneous tracheostomy at the bedside should always be performed with skilled people and with instrumentation available immediately for conversion to open tracheostomy.

Dulguerov et al.[29] performed a meta-analysis of percutaneous or surgical tracheostomy, although their conclusions are limited by the lack of head-to-head comparisons in the literature at the time of their analysis and the nonrigorous design of earlier studies. The authors concluded that although overall tracheostomy complication rates have decreased, mortality (0.4%) and early complications are more common after percutaneous tracheostomy, whereas late complications are more common after open tracheostomy. Freeman et al.[30] reported a meta-analysis of five trials (236 patients) that compared the procedures directly (Table 8.5). Operative time was 7.8 to 10.9 minutes shorter for percutaneous tracheostomy. The incidences of bleeding and stomal infections were lower for percutaneous tracheostomy, whereas the overall complication rate and mortality rate were comparable. Freeman et al.[31] followed their meta-analysis with their own randomized, prospective, single-center, multi-ICU (medical, surgical, coronary care) trial of open tracheostomy (in the OR) versus percutaneous tracheostomy (at the bedside). They found that percutaneous tracheostomy was associated with comparable outcomes at lower cost. However, Grover et al.[32] estimated that open tracheostomy at the bedside was $180 less costly and resulted in lower charges by $658 when compared with percutaneous tracheostomy, even ignoring the professional fee for fiberoptic bronchoscopy, which would have magnified the cost advantage of the open procedure.

Tracheostomy in children has been regarded as a technically demanding procedure, best performed in the OR. There has been historical reluctance to perform percutaneous tracheostomy for children, owing to technical concerns relating to the small size of the airway and the skills required for acute care endotracheal intubation of the pediatric airway. Prospective comparative data have not been published. In a retrospective analysis of open

TABLE 8.5. Meta-analysis of five comparative trials (236 patients) of open versus percutaneous tracheostomy in critically ill patients.

Parameter	Odds ratio in favor of percutaneous tracheostomy	95% confidence interval
All complications	0.73	0.05–9.37
Postoperative complications	0.14	0.07–0.29*
Perioperative bleeding	0.14	0.02–0.39*
Postoperative bleeding	0.39	0.17–0.88*
Stomal infection	0.02	0.01–0.07*
Death	0.63	0.18–2.00

* Statistically significant result.
Source: Data from Freeman et al.[30]

tracheostomy in the OR (n = 300) versus bedside percutaneous tracheostomy in the pediatric ICU for patients aged 15 days to 8 years, safety was comparable (overall incidence of complications, 9%), and hospital charges related to the percutaneous procedure were nearly $1,500 less.[33] However, most of the procedures were performed for chronic illnesses (e.g., laryngotracheal disorders, bronchopulmonary dysplasia, neurologic disorders) where hypoxemia was less of an issue.

Open tracheostomy has also been implicated historically to be associated with higher rates of sternal wound infection and mediastinitis following median sternotomy. Comparative data for open versus percutaneous tracheostomy in this setting have not been reported, but Byhahn et al.[34] reported a prospective series of median sternotomy patients who underwent percutaneous tracheostomy within the first 2 weeks postoperatively. Systematic surveillance cultures of the tracheostomy and sternotomy sites were performed. No patient developed a tracheostomy infection, whereas four patients (2.8%) developed a sternal wound infection. In only two of the four patients was there microbiologic concordance (methicillin-resistant *Staphylococcus aureus*), leading the authors to conclude that percutaneous tracheostomy is safe, even in the immediate aftermath of median sternotomy.

The timing of tracheostomy remains controversial. Proponents of early tracheostomy (generally within 7 days as opposed to after 14 days) believe that the provision of pulmonary toilet is enhanced and that the result should be a lower incidence of pneumonia and shorter durations of mechanical ventilation and care in the ICU. Detractors maintain that the putative benefits of early tracheostomy remain unproved. Several prospective trials have been published, but one suffers from acknowledged enrollment bias.[35] Neither of the two studies performed with trauma patients showed any benefit from early tracheostomy.[35,36] However, Rumbak et al.,[37] studying critically ill medical patients, found significantly lower incidences of unplanned extubation (0 vs. 6), pneumonia (32% vs. 62%), and mortality (5% vs. 25%) following early tracheostomy. The length of stay in the ICU was shorter after early tracheostomy (5 vs. 16 days), as was the duration of mechanical ventilation (8 vs. 17 days).

Bedside Thoracic Surgery

Procedures upon the thorax at the bedside are common, but most are either thoracentesis or tube thoracostomy. Thoracotomy is performed rarely and only for patients in extremis, with one notable exception. Opening the pleural cavity has implications for oxygenation, ventilation, hemodynamics, and gas exchange that can be profound. Major thoracic surgery requires ventilatory support (e.g., split-lung ventilation) that is difficult to provide at the bedside.

Pleural effusion is common following surgery, usually reflecting fluid overload and hypoalbuminemia, or a sympathetic effusion from an inflammatory process on either side of the diaphragm, but sometimes reflecting post-traumatic or parapneumonic effusion or empyema. Less common causes of pleural effusion include liver disease and migration of central venous catheters.[38] The incidence of pleural effusion identified by physical examination or portable chest radiography among ICU patients is approximately 8%, but, if screened for by routine ultrasonography, the incidence of pleural effusion may exceed 60%. Thoracentesis is usually necessary for diagnosis or treatment because no clinical parameter excludes the possibility of infection and is safe for patients on mechanical ventilation.[38] In a longitudinal prospective observational study of pleural effusions among 1,351 critically ill medical ICU patients, 113 effusions were identified and 81 patients underwent unguided thoracentesis.[39] An infection was identified in 43% of patients, including 14 cases of empyema thoracis. An improvement in diagnosis or therapy was realized by 56 patients, whereas the incidence of pneumothorax was 7%.

Ultrasound-guided thoracentesis may increase further both the yield and the safety of thoracentesis.[40] In a prospective study of 40 mechanically ventilated patients who underwent 45 image-guided procedures, fluid was obtained with 44 procedures, despite being apparent by portable radiography in only 60% of cases.[40] The incidence of complications was zero. In another report, Mayo et al.[41] reported the incidence of pneumothorax to be only 1.3% for ultrasound-guided thoracentesis in mechanically ventilated patients.

Tube thoracostomy may be necessary for patients with large, recurrent, or loculated pleural effusions or for the management of empyema thoracis. Talmor et al.[42] reported that unilateral or bilateral tube thoracostomy may improve oxygenation substantially for patients with acute respiratory distress syndrome (ARDS) that is refractory to ventilation with PEEP. Tube thoracostomy was undertaken for 19 patients (10%) with ARDS who did not respond to application of a mean PEEP of 16 cm H_2O. Oxygenation improved immediately for 17/19 patients and remained improved in all responders at 24 hours after chest tube insertion.

In some cases of loculated pneumothorax, routine tube thoracostomy may not succeed in decompression. Although there is no inherent reason why ultrasound at the bedside cannot be used to support the directed percutaneous placement of a pleural drainage catheter, that technique has not been reported, whereas CT-guided drainage of loculated pneumothorax has been reported.[43] Chon et al.[43] described the CT-guided placement of 17 catheters into nine mechanically ventilated patients with loculated thoracic air collections where tube thoracostomy had failed or the collection was deemed inaccessible. The catheter size ranged from 7 to 28 French. All but one collection was evacuated definitively; there were no complications and one death that was unrelated to the procedure. Clinical improvement (improved oxygenation) was occasioned by the procedure approximately 60% of the time.

Reopening of the sternotomy incision may be indicated following cardiac arrest in the aftermath of cardiac surgery, usually for mediastinal hemorrhage and cardiac tamponade. In the immediate postoperative period, the only instrumentation required for reopening of a sternotomy is a wire cutter and a retractor, but the surgeon should be prepared for substantial bleeding. Mackay et al.[44] reviewed the reopening of a chest incision for cardiac arrest in 79 surgical patients, 58 of which were opened in the ICU and 19 on the ward. Overall survival to hospital discharge was 25%. Patients were more likely to survive if the arrest and reopening of the chest occurred in the ICU within 10 minutes of the arrest (33%) or if the arrest occurred within the first 24 hours after surgery.

Fiser et al.[45] examined cardiac reoperation retrospectively in the ICU but specifically excluded from their analysis patients who had had a cardiac arrest. Among 6,908 patients over a 9-year period, 340 (4.9%) underwent reoperative cardiac surgery in the ICU, with a survival rate of 85%. The incidence of surgical site infection, 2.1%, was not different from the 1.9% incidence noted in the patients who did not undergo reoperation.

Ligation of a patent ductus arteriosus (PDA) is indicated in the unusual circumstance when infusion of indomethacin fails to achieve closure medically. The operation is not demanding technically but, owing to the hypoxemia inherent, is considered a high-risk procedure. Increasingly, PDA ligation is performed at the bedside in the neonatal ICU. Gould et al.[46] reviewed 72 PDA ligations, 38 of which were performed in the neonatal ICU of a pediatric specialty hospital. The other 34 procedures were performed by a team of professionals (attending cardiac surgeon, cardiac surgical fellow, attending pediatric cardiac anesthesiologist, certified registered nurse anesthetist, cardiac operating room nurses) at one of six referring hospitals without pediatric cardiac surgical capability. The incidences of complications were similar regardless of locale (pneumothorax [n = 3] and a single case each of bleeding, chylothorax, and pleural effusion), as were the rates of mortality (overall, 9.7%, with none within 96 hours after surgery or attributed to either surgical or anesthetic complications).

Bedside Abdominal Surgery

A variety of bedside procedures may be performed in the ICU relating to the abdomen or abdominal pathology. Some of the procedures may be performed by residents or by fellows undergoing training in critical care, whereas others will require the expertise of specialty physicians. The procedures can range from being minimally invasive, requiring only local anesthetic, to major procedures requiring full general anesthesia with neuromuscular blockade. Because all of these procedures are invasive to some degree, contraindications to all of them include coagulopathy, refusal by patient or surrogate, and lack of adequate supervision.

Paracentesis

Ascites is a common development in critically ill patients.[47] Risk factors for ascites include liver failure, renal failure, congestive heart failure, and anasarca. Most often, ascites is a benign concomitant condition to a related, more severe disease process. Occasionally, the presence of ascites warrants removal by paracentesis for either diagnosis or therapy. Among the common indications for paracentesis is severe patient discomfort. Sometimes, 4 to 6 L of ascites is removed. The procedure is most commonly performed in patients with severe cirrhosis and may have to be performed repeatedly. Frequent reaccumulation of the fluid may require the creation of a permanent peritoneovenous shunt. Other patients may need paracentesis in anticipation of liver transplantation. Another therapeutic indication for paracentesis is decompression of abdominal compartment syndrome (ACS). In this case, the fluid usually has accumulated rapidly as a result of massive fluid resuscitation,[48] but ACS caused by malignant ascites has been reported.[49] Signs of ACS include oliguria, increased bladder pressure, increased airway pressures, hypotension, and acidosis. If ascites is a major component of the abdominal contents in ACS, a catheter may be placed to allow continuous pressure monitoring and fluid removal and to prevent rapid reaccumulation of the fluid. Sometimes, paracentesis is used to evaluate ascitic fluid for diagnosis. In these cases, the fluid should be sent for cell count with differentiation, amylase concentration, cytology, bacterial Gram stain and culture, and culture for mycobacteria, viruses, and fungi. The presence of bacteria in ascitic fluid may indicate that the patient has an undetected intestinal perforation or a condition called "primary (spontaneous) bacterial peritonitis" in which ascitic fluid can become infected without visceral perforation or manipulation.

Specific contraindications to paracentesis include a previous abdominal operation (relative), an indication for laparotomy for an abdominal condition such as intestinal ischemia, and the presence of dilated intestine such as in intestinal obstruction or paralytic ileus.[50] Other contraindications include the presence of diffuse abdominal wall pathology that would preclude a safe sterile needle puncture into the abdominal cavity, such as extensive abdominal wall burns, large open abdominal wounds with infection, or extensive *caput medusae* from portal hypertension.

Several techniques of paracentesis have been described. Ultrasound can be performed at the bedside in the ICU to determine the presence and location of ascites; this can be essential for successful paracentesis when the volume of ascites is small. For most paracentesis procedures and especially those involving smaller volumes of intraperitoneal fluid, gastric and bladder decompression is recommended, which often preexists in the ICU. The authors' preferred technique of paracentesis is to position the patient at 45 degrees upright in partial left decubitus position. A point at the midline between the umbilicus and the anterior superior iliac crest is prepared into a sterile field and anesthetized with 1% lidocaine. An 18-gauge needle suffices for diagnostic paracentesis, whereas a larger needle is needed when a drainage catheter may need to be placed; central venous catheterization kits are convenient for the purpose. The needle is advanced holding negative pressure until fluid is aspirated.

Serious complications of paracentesis include local or intraperitoneal hemorrhage or bowel perforation. The abdominal examination and blood count should be monitored after the procedure. Hypotension may occur after large- volume paracentesis; restitution of intravascular fluid volume with crystalloid or colloid approximating the oncotic constitution of the removed fluid is restorative. Persistent drainage (ascitic fistula) may ensue after reaccumulation of tense ascites but is managed easily by placement of sutures in the abdominal wall.

Peritoneal Dialysis Catheter Placement

Peritoneal dialysis catheter placement can be performed under local anesthesia in the ICU. The primary indication for this procedure remains acute renal failure and is most performed in the pediatric population. For adults, the preferred method of renal replacement therapy is hemofiltration.[51] Another described indication for peritoneal dialysis includes necrotizing pancreatitis with continuous irrigation,[52] but it is now rare in practice because of questionable benefit. The placement of peritoneal dialysis catheters can be theoretically anywhere on the anterior abdominal wall. Cuffed or noncuffed catheters for peritoneal dialysis can be used depending on the permanency of the need for the catheter.

Percutaneous Cholecystostomy

In critically ill patients, acute cholecystitis may develop in the absence of gallstones. Rare before 1950, acute acalculous cholecystitis has been increasingly noted over the past 15 years as a source of acute pathology in ICU patients.[53] Risk factors include sepsis, diabetes mellitus,

abdominal vasculitis, systemic lupus erythematous, congestive heart failure, shock, renal disease, acquired immunodeficiency syndrome, total parenteral nutrition, trauma, burns, and hypovolemia. This disease process is characterized by abdominal pain (if the patient can communicate), fever, leukocytosis, jaundice from cholestasis, and gallbladder ischemia.

The diagnosis of acute acalculous cholecystitis may be difficult because most patients are critically ill, possibly intubated with sedation. Additionally, the gallbladder may be only one source of sepsis in these patients. Consequently, diagnosis is most frequently accomplished by gallbladder imaging in the proper clinical context. Ultrasound is preferred, as it may be brought to the bedside, and pathognomonically reveals a gallbladder wall thickness of ≥3.5mm with pericholecystic fluid. Computed tomography is equally accurate for the same findings.

The treatment for acute acalculous cholecystitis is increasingly a cholecystostomy tube. For patients with diffuse peritonitis suggesting perforation, or if the diagnosis is insecure, abdominal exploration is indicated. However, most patients have a condition amenable to placement of a percutaneous cholecystostomy tube at the bedside or in the interventional radiology suite. For most patients in the ICU, percutaneous cholecystostomy is the preferred method of cholecystostomy.[54] After local anesthetic infiltration, the gallbladder is punctured under ultrasound guidance. By Seldinger technique, an 8-F pigtail catheter is placed into the gallbladder.

Complications of the procedures include bleeding and, rarely, visceral perforation. A more common complication can be the spillage of infected bile into the peritoneal cavity either at the time of the procedure or alongside the cholecystostomy tube. Consequently, if the patient worsens or fails to improve, the patient should be imaged to ensure that the catheter is patent, that bile has not leaked into the abdomen, and that no other diagnosis is possible. After the patient improves, a tube cholecystogram should confirm the absence of gallstones; if absent, the tube may be removed without interval cholecystectomy.

Open cholecystostomy can also be performed at the bedside and is an option if image guidance is unavailable or unsuccessful. In this procedure, an incision is placed over the gallbladder in the right upper quadrant, and the dissection is taken down to the peritoneal cavity. A 2-0 silk pursestring suture is placed in the dome of the gallbladder, and a 16- or 20-Fr Malecot catheter is placed in the gallbladder and exteriorized.

Enteral Feeding Access

The advantages of enteral nutrition for the critically ill patient have been well established, including a decreased risk of infection. Either gastric/duodenal or small intestinal feeding tubes can be placed; either can be temporary or permanent. Ideally, feeding tubes can be placed in the operating room when the patient is being operated on for another indication. However, some patients, especially those who have not undergone abdominal surgery, may require placement of a feeding tube in the ICU.

Gastric feeding can occur in the majority of patients but has been believed by some to be associated with increased rates of aspiration, pneumonia, and feeding intolerance. Nonetheless, many patients have successfully received gastric feeding in the ICU setting with no complications. Head-up positioning and use of promotility agents such as erythromycin may facilitate successful gastric feedings.[54,55] The amount of residual solution that is considered inordinately high for subsequent feeding, as determined by regular aspiration of the tube, can be an absolute volume (e.g., 100–150 mL) or a volume related to the rate of feeding (e.g., four times the hourly infusion rate). Many clinicians prefer to use a soft, narrow-gauge feeding tube (e.g., Dobhoff tube) instead of a conventional nasogastric tube to reduce the long-term effects of prolonged nasogastric intubation (e.g., sinusitis).

Permanent gastric feeding tubes can be placed by either open or percutaneous technique. Open technique is typically performed in the operating room with general anesthesia. Most commonly, percutaneous gastric tubes are placed in the ICU by surgical endoscopists or gastroenterologists. The technique of percutaneous endoscopic gastrostomy (PEG) is well described.[56,57] A gastroscope is introduced into the stomach with the patient in the supine position, and the stomach is insufflated with air. Using abdominal wall ballotment with a single digit, the most ventral area of the stomach is located with endoscopic visualization. Generally, this area is approximately 2 to 3 cm lateral to and below the xiphoid process. A percutaneous needle catheter is placed into the stomach, and a flexible guidewire is placed in the stomach and grasped from above by a snare from the gastroscope. The wire is brought out through the mouth and attached externally to the tube, which is then brought up through the abdominal wall via the mouth, esophagus, and stomach and secured. Repeat endoscopy is recommended to ensure that the tube is positioned satisfactorily in the stomach. If too tight, ischemic necrosis of either the gastric or the abdominal wall may lead to a serious infection.[58,59] Some clinicians prefer a "G-J" tube that is placed similarly, but the device has a distal limb as well as a gastric balloon so that gastric aspiration and duodenal feeding can occur simultaneously.

Small intestinal tubes are most popular for patients with poor tolerance of gastric feeding and can be placed open in the operating room, by laparoscopy, or by a "closed" method in the ICU. Small intestinal tubes can be placed in the proximal duodenum or in the jejunum distal to the ligament of Treitz. In the ICU, temporary tubes can be placed in either of these two sites by a variety of methods, including the use of a weighted catheter followed by positional changes, the use of gastric motility agents, magnetic guidance, a pH probe, and ultrasound guidance. Recently, endoscopic placement of a jejunal feeding catheter by a "push" technique has been described. In this method, a 7-Fr nasobiliary tube is placed via the biopsy channel of the gastroscope into the jejunum after endoscopic visualization of the jejunum.[60]

Some clinicians believe that enteral feedings distal to the stomach are preferable. Higher volumes of feeding solution can be administered sooner and infection rates may be lower, but overall outcomes appear not to be affected.[61]

Other Uses of Bedside Endoscopy

Bedside endoscopy may be performed in critically ill patients in several other therapeutic and diagnostic settings, including gastrointestinal bleeding or the diagnosis of bowel viability.[62] Generally, these procedures are performed in the ICU with sedation. In many cases, these patients are already intubated for airway protection or factors related to their critical illness.

Causes of upper gastrointestinal bleeding include peptic ulcer disease, gastritis, portal hypertension, esophagitis, and malignant disease.[63] A variant of gastritis particular to critically ill patients is stress-related gastric mucosal hemorrhage (SRGMH) caused by gut barrier disruption that results from ischemia-reperfusion injury of the stomach. Risk factors of SRGMH include burns, head injury, solid organ transplantation, renal failure, use of nonsteroidal antiinflammatory agents, mechanical ventilation, and coagulopathy, with the latter two factors of particular importance. Suggested methods of prophylaxis to prevent the complication of SRGMH include H_2-receptor blockade and proton pump inhibition, with barrier protection (e.g., sucralfate) and misoprostil probably less effective.

Causes of lower gastrointestinal bleeding in critically ill patients include malignant disease, polyps, diverticulosis, and angiodysplasia, as well as profuse upper gastrointestinal bleeding. Another important manifestation of lower gastrointestinal hemorrhage includes the various forms of ischemic enteritis. Whereas small bowel ischemia can occur acutely from an arterial embolus or low-flow state, the development of colonic ischemia may result from gut barrier disruption or surgical interruption of blood flow to the colon (e.g., aortic aneurysm surgery). Ischemic colitis can be acute or chronic and can manifest a wide spectrum of involvement and severity. Initial investigation of ischemic colitis includes colonoscopy, but importantly only the mucosa can be evaluated in this manner. The presence of full-thickness necrosis is not generally discernible from colonoscopy. No data exist supporting the use of antibiotics for ischemic colitis before full-thickness necrosis, although antibiotics are used frequently for this indication. Clinicians have observed that, when surgery is indicated, ischemic colitis can have a mortality rate up to 80%.

Bedside Laparotomy

In general, laparotomy in the operating room is preferred because of optimization of anesthetic support, nursing support, operating instruments, and lighting and to facilitate operative exposure. However, certain patients may be too unstable for transport or may need immediate laparotomy in the ICU.

The most urgent indication for bedside laparotomy may be for decompressive treatment of ACS.[64,65] In this syndrome, the patient may have a potentially lethal constellation of symptoms, including hypoventilation, arterial desaturation, acidosis, oliguria, hypotension, increased abdominal (intravesical) pressures, and increased airway pressures. The causes of ACS include large-volume resuscitation, massive blood loss, large burns, small bowel obstruction, ischemia-reperfusion injury, abdominal packing, and hemoperitoneum. When ACS presents acutely, the patient may be unable to be ventilated; midline laparotomy in the ICU may be a life-saving maneuver.

Other reasons for bedside abdominal exploration include changing of abdominal dressings after previous abbreviated laparotomy for decompression of ACS or treatment of diffuse abdominal infection.[66] For patients who require multiple abdominal washouts for tertiary peritonitis, bedside laparotomy has become an excellent manner to achieve source control of infection and minimize patient morbidity. Abdominal operations that require intestinal anastomoses, ostomy creation, or definitive control of hemorrhage are better performed in the operating room. However, for patients who need a change of abdominal packing or a "washout" of infected fluid, bedside laparotomy is often an excellent option.

Critically ill trauma patients may be the patient population in whom the largest numbers of bedside laparotomies are performed. Diaz et al.[66] reviewed 75 patients who underwent 95 bedside laparotomies over a 4-year period. The most common indications for bedside laparotomy included ACS (49.5%), exploration for infection (19%), and washout/pack removal (14.7%). These authors performed bedside fascial closure in 12.6% of patients. In this study, the mortality rate approximated 50%; other reported complications included fistula formation (10.9%) and intraabdominal abscess formation (6.5%).

Several methods of managing the fascial layer of the "open abdomen" are options at the bedside.[67] When the patient is in extremis, simple placement of a sterile towel followed by a sterile sheet may temporize the closure. In cases where the patient's physiology allows a more definitive closure, more options are open, including a "vacuum pack," absorbable mesh, nonabsorbable mesh with a "zipper," or other reclosable prosthetic devices[68,69] When the tissue on the surface has become clean granulation tissue and the fascia is not amenable to primary closure, some surgeons prefer skin grafting on the surface, whereas others prefer long-term wound care with a non-adhesive surface such as petrolatum gauze dressings. Quite often, these patients are left long-term with a ventral hernia independent of the method of abdominal wall management during the time of the open abdomen.[70] These hernias should usually be repaired after at least 6 months to allow closure of the initial wound and restitution of the patient's functional status.

Bedside Laparoscopy

Bedside laparoscopy, or "peritoneoscopy," has been described in both critical care and emergency department settings.[71] Indications for this procedure include the diagnosis of bowel viability, intestinal perforation, or depth of traumatic injury. This procedure has been performed with a variety of methods.[72] Either general or local anesthesia may be used. For patients receiving local anesthesia, a smaller port is used (3 or 5 mm), and nitrous oxide may be used for insufflation instead of carbon dioxide. For critically ill patients, major operative therapy generally should not be undertaken during bedside laparoscopy. Patients requiring larger procedures should be taken to the operating room or receive bedside laparotomy. Contraindications to the procedure at the bedside include a patient unable to tolerate the procedure, previous abdominal surgery, inadequate personnel available to perform laparotomy, and need for immediate laparotomy. As experience increases with bedside laparoscopy, consensus indications for the procedure will be reported.[73]

Bedside Extremity Surgery

Extremity pathology and complications can develop or become exacerbated in ICU patients. These pathologies can be overlooked easily despite extensive monitoring in the critical care setting. Common lower extremity pathologies in ICU patients that may require surgical intervention include severe soft tissue infection (necrotizing fasciitis [NF]), joint and bone infection, deep vein thrombosis/pulmonary embolism, and extremity compartment syndrome. The related surgical procedures are debridement of necrotic soft tissue, arthrocentesis, inferior vena cava (IVC) filter placement, lower extremity compartment pressure measurement, fasciotomy, and escharotomy. On many occasions, these procedures can be performed at the ICU bedside. Upper extremity surgery is less common in the ICU, but notably may include phlebectomy for suppurative thrombophlebitis or surgery to control other infections.

Surgical Debridement for Necrotizing Fasciitis

Necrotizing fasciitis (NF) is a life-threatening infection resulting in necrosis of skin, subcutaneous tissue, and fascia. Mortality rates average about 25%.[74] Extremity NF can result in a high rate of limb loss. Predisposing conditions include traumatic and surgical wounds, diabetes mellitus, and immunosuppression.[75] In hospitalized patients, NF of extremities often arises at surgical wound and intravenous (IV) sites.

Necrotizing fasciitis may be caused by a variety of aerobic and anaerobic microorganisms.[76] Infections caused by mixed flora constitute about 80% of all infections, whereas group A streptococcal infections constitute about 20% of cases. Pain that is disproportionate to other physical findings is a hallmark of the diagnosis. Cutaneous findings include diffuse erythema and edema that may progress to necrosis and hemorrhagic bullae.[74] Crepitus and radiographic signs of tissue gas are not reliably present. In rare cases the NF can lead to extremity compartment syndrome.[77] Because of rapid progression, early diagnosis and treatment are crucial determinants of outcome.[74] Additional studies such as ultrasonography, plane radiography, CT scan, or magnetic resonance imaging (MRI) to look for soft tissue gas and inflammation may help diagnosis, provided that definitive surgical debridement is not delayed. In some cases, biopsy with a frozen section of affected soft tissue may be necessary to establish the diagnosis,[78] again provided that definitive therapy is not delayed. This biopsy procedure can be done safely in the ICU setting. Treatment includes early surgical debridement, broad-spectrum antibiotics, nutritional support, and hemodynamic support.[74,75] Early surgical debridement is the key to avoid loss of limb or life.[79] Wounds should be left open, and subsequent debridement is often needed.[80]

Bedside Arthrocentesis

Arthrocentesis is performed rarely in the ICU, but it is an effective means to diagnosis post-traumatic hemarthrosis, septic arthritis, and gout. Intraarticular injection can be performed for local antibiotic therapy. Contraindications include overlying skin cellulitis and coagulopathy; particularly, hemophilia is an absolute contraindication.

The patient is placed supine. For knee arthrocentesis, after sterile preparation and draping of the entire joint, 1% lidocaine is injected subcutaneously at the level of the lateral superior pole of patella. The needle is directed slightly inferior toward the posterior surface of the patella and advanced into the joint. For ankle arthrocentesis, the needle is inserted at 2.5 cm proximal and 1.3 cm medial to the tip of the lateral malleolus. The joint may be irrigated with saline, and drugs may be injected into the joint as indicated. Complications include puncture site skin infection and infection of the joint caused by contamination by the arthrocentesis. Most cases of postprocedure bleeding are caused by coagulopathy. Treatment includes compression dressing and specific correction of the coagulopathy.

Lower Extremity Compartment Pressure Measurement, Bedside Fasciotomy, and Escharotomy

Extremity compartment syndrome exists when compartment pressure (usually below the knee, but possible in the thigh as well) exceeds the microvascular perfusion pressure, resulting in ischemia of nerve and muscle. Secondary edema elevates the compartment pressures further. Delayed diagnosis and treatment of compartment syndrome results in permanent neuromuscular damage, necrosis of muscle and other soft tissue, and even loss of the extremity. Lower extremity compartment syndrome may develop following crush injury, tibia/fibula fracture, prolonged arterial occlusion with reperfusion injury, acute obstruction of venous return, excessive external pressure as may occur with extensive, circumferential third-degree burns, prolonged use of military antishock trousers (MAST), and intramuscular or intracompartmental bleeding. Lower extremity compartment syndrome has also been reported after routine pelvic surgery,[81] laparoscopic gastric bypass surgery for obesity,[82] malignant hyperthermia,[83] diabetes mellitus,[84] and coronary artery bypass grafting.[85] Because of its higher sensitivity to ischemia, the peripheral nerve is affected first; therefore, the earliest presentation is pain and paresthesia. Paralysis and pulselessness are late signs of compartment syndrome that may not be reversible with decompression.

The early diagnosis of compartment syndrome depends mainly on clinical vigilance and careful physical examination. For unconscious and pediatric patients, diagnosis can be difficult. Adjunctive testing can be helpful in the diagnosis of suspected cases. Compartment pressures can be measured at the bedside with either specific devices or a 22-g needle connected to a pressure transducer, remembering that pressures must be measured in all four fascial compartments among tibia, fibula, and deep fascia in the lower extremity.

Compartment pressures of less than 20 mm Hg are considered normal, whereas pressures higher than 30 mm Hg are abnormal and an indication of compartment syndrome if consistent with clinical findings. Because the consequences of compartment syndrome are serious, including limb loss, early aggressive treatment is indicated when clinical suspicion is established. The main treatment for compartment syndrome is fasciotomy, which can be performed at the bedside in the ICU if necessary.[86]

Under deep IV sedation and local anesthesia, the diseased leg is prepared and draped below the inguinal ligament to the toes. Two incisions are made, one lateral to the tibia between the tibia and fibula and the other medial to the tibia. Skin incisions are made preferentially with the scalpel to minimize thermal injury to the skin. Subcutaneous tissue is divided, including the investing deep fascia with cautery. The greater saphenous vein should be avoided. The anterior and lateral compartments are opened through the lateral incision, and the two posterior compartments are opened through medial incision. The fascial incisions should be extended to the full length of the compartment to fully release the compartment. Muscle viability in the compartment should be evaluated, and any nonviable tissue should be debrided. Wet-to-dry dressing is finally applied. The leg should be placed in the position of function, with the knee flexed slightly and the ankle in neutral position. Frequent dressing changes, and reassessment of muscle viability and vascular status are mandatory.

In burn patients, circumferential third-degree burns can cause severe external compression to the extremity that can induce compartment syndrome. The tissue edema associated with burn injury or resuscitation will further contribute the elevation of compartment pressures. This could be overlooked due to burn-related change of skin appearance or severe pain caused by surrounding second- or first-degree burn. If compartment syndrome is suspected, emergent escharotomy is indicated,[87] in the ICU if necessary.

The patient should be maintained on proper life support, and resuscitation should continue as indicated. The escharotomy sites need sterile preparation and sterile draping, but anesthesia is not necessary because the eschar is insensate (see below). Electrocautery may be used to make the incision through the non-viable eschar. The length of incision should be adjusted to the length of the wound, usually extending the eschar into uninjured skin proximally and distally, where local anesthesia must be used. This will ensure no residual band of eschar capable of impeding capillary blood flow as the tissue edema progresses. The incision should be deep enough into subdermal fat to release completely the compression caused by the circular eschar, but, in contrast to fasciotomy, usually does not need to extend that deep.

The postescharotomy patient should be observed closely for signs of extremity ischemia. Incomplete escharotomy should be identified early and followed by completion of the escharotomy. Some data suggest that noninvasive near-infrared spectroscopy might be of help to diagnose and monitor compartment syndrome.[88]

Bedside Inferior Vena Cava Filter Placement

Deep venous thromboembolism (DVT) is often silent, yet potentially fatal. When symptoms do occur, they are often nonspecific, but the first manifestation may be life-threatening, including pulmonary embolism (PE). Ultrasound has been used for routine screening for DVT, but the yield is low and the technique is not cost effective.[89] Therefore, identification of at-risk patients and an optimal method of prophylaxis are vital. Most cases of DVT/PE arise from the lower extremity. Routine prophylaxis includes pneumatic compression devices or heparinoids. Systemic anticoagulation is the standard therapy for DVT and prevention of PE. In certain clinical situations these modalities may be ineffective or contraindicated (e.g., pneumatic compression devices may be contraindicated with lower extremity fractures or compartment syndromes, whereas heparin may be contraindicated for patients with traumatic brain injury).

The alternative is placing a filter in the IVC to prevent dislodged thrombus from the lower extremity or pelvic veins from embolizing to the pulmonary artery. The indications for IVC filter placement are recurrence of DVT or development of PE despite adequate anticoagulation, hemorrhage, thrombocytopenia, and, controversially, prophylaxis of patients at high risk for DVT and PE. The largest population receiving IVC filters for a prophylactic indication include trauma patients who have contraindications to anticoagulation, such as closed head injury or the need for multiple procedures. Other patient populations who are considered very "high risk" for pulmonary embolism, such as those with major pelvic fracture or spinal cord injury, also sometimes receive prophylactic IVC filters, as do patients unable to wear pneumatic compression devices (e.g., lower extremity fractures or dressings). Patients with a contraindication to anticoagulation include those with traumatic brain injury, complex pelvic fracture, multiple long bone fractures, nonambulating patients with severe multiple trauma, or a large free-floating thrombus.

The ideal position of a vena cava filter is just below the renal veins; therefore, knowledge of each patient's renal vein anatomy is important for proper placement of the filter. Technology has emerged that allows sufficient resolution of anatomic detail to permit placement of IVC filters safely and accurately at the bedside. Sing et al.[90] demonstrated the safety and efficacy of bedside venogram and IVC filter insertion in a prospective observational study of 158 IVC filter insertions for severe trauma patients at the ICU bedside. Visualization and resolution of venous anatomy using transcutaneous or intravascular ultrasound has been demonstrated to be safe and cost effective[91]; iodinated contrast or CO_2 gas (visible by ultrasound) appear to be comparable.[92–94] The incidences of filter misplacement, access thrombosis, filter migration, and IVC occlusion are less than 1% each, which is comparable with the traditional method. Failures of visualization by duplex untrasound are due mainly to extreme obesity, unusual anatomy, and bowel gas interference. Intravascular ultrasound may mitigate those shortcomings.[95] Garrett et al.[95] used bedside intravascular ultrasound in 28 patients when transabdominal ultrasound yielded inadequate visualization of the IVC and were able to visualize the IVC adequately to place the IVC filter in 26 patients (93%). Postprocedure abdominal radiographs confirmed proper placement, based on bony landmarks, in 24 of 26 patients (92%).

Recently, the placement of temporary IVC filters has been described, which can be deployed in the ICU setting as well. However, prophylactic IVC filter placement after trauma is controversial, because Class I data are lacking, although safety is established.[96] Whether the increasing availability of removable filters changes the indications remains to be determined.[97] Case series report that "removable" filters are indeed removed successfully more than 90% of the time when attempted,[97] but the likelihood decreases substantially when attempted more than 14 days after insertion.

The intensive care unit will likely be the next-generation operating room. The acute care surgeon must play a pivotal role in the ICU setting. In fact, proposed curriculum for this specialty includes the requirements (Accreditation Council of Graduate Medical Education and American Board of Surgery) for critical care certification.

Critique

With respect to optimal airway management, the recommmendation for this patient would be establishment of a surgical airway to facilitate pulmonary toilet and lessen the chance of periglottic complications (e.g., stricture). Currently, most tracheostomies at many of the tertiary centers are being done at the bedside (percutaneous tracheostomy), obviating the need for such patients to be transported to the OR.

Answer (C)

References

1. Braxton CC, Reilly PM, Schwab CW. The traveling intensive care unit patient. Road trips. Surg Clin North Am 2000; 80:949–956.

2. Warren J, Fromm RE Jr, Orr RA, et al. American College of Critical Care Medicine. Guidelines for the inter- and intrahospital transport of critically ill patients. Crit Care Med 2004; 32:256–622.

3. Szem JW, Hydo LJ, Fischer E, et al. High-risk intrahospital transport of critically ill patients: safety and outcome of the necessary "road trip." Crit Care Med 1995; 23:1660–1666.

4. Stevenson VW, Haas CF, Wahl WL. Intrahospital transport of the adult mechanically ventilated patient. Respir Care Clin North Am 2002; 8:1–35.

5. Wallen E, Venkataraman ST, Grosso MJ, et al. Intrahospital transport of critically ill pediatric patients. Crit Care Med 1995; 23:1588–1595.

6. Barba CA. The intensive care unit as an operating room. Surg Clin North Am 2000; 80:957–973.

7. Porter JM, Ivatury RR, Kavarana M, Verrier R. The surgical intensive care unit as a cost-efficient substitute for an operating room at a level I trauma center. Am Surg 1999; 65:328–330.

8. Babcock HM, Fraser V. Differences in percutaneous injury patterns in a multi-hospital system. Infect Control Hosp Epidemiol 2003; 24:731–736.

9. Eggiman P, Pittet D. Infection control in the ICU. Chest 2001; 120:2059–2093.

10. Jacobs S, Al Rasheed AM, Abdulsamat W, et al. Effects of a simple protocol on infective complications in intensive care unit patients undergoing percutaneous dilatational tracheostomy. Respir Care 2003; 48:29–37.

11. Jacobi J, Fraser GL, Coursin DB, et al. Clinical practice guidelines for the sustained use of sedatives and analgesics in the critically ill adult. Crit Care Med 2002; 30:119–141.

12. Aranda M, Hanson CW III. Anesthetics, sedatives, and paralytics. Understanding their use in the intensive care unit. Surg Clin North Am 2000; 80:933–947.

13. Slonim AD, Ognibene FP. Sedation for pediatric procedures, using ketamine and midazolam, in a primarily adult intensive care unit: a retrospective evaluation. Crit Care Med 1998; 26:1900–1904.

14. Wheeler DS, Vaux KK, Ponaman ML, Poss BW. The safe and effective use of propofol sedation in children undergoing diagnostic and therapeutic procedures: experience in a pediatric ICU and a review of the literature. Pediatr Emerg Care 2003; 19:385–932.

15. Rozycki GS, Cava RA, Tchorz KM. Surgeon-performed ultrasound imaging in acute surgical disorders. Curr Probl Surg 2001; 38:141–212.

16. Rebuck JA, Murry KR, Rhoney DH, et al. Infection related to intracranial pressure monitors in adults: analysis of risk factors and antibiotic prophylaxis. J Neurol Neurosurg Psychiatry 2000; 69:381–384.

17. Wong GK, Poon WS, Wai S, et al. Failure of regular external ventricular drain exchange to reduce cerebrospinal fluid infection: result of a randomised controlled trial. J Neurol Neurosurg Psychiatry 2002; 73:759–761.

18. Harris CH, Smith RS, Helmer SD, et al. Placement of intracranial pressure monitors by non-neurosurgeons. Am Surg 2002; 68:787–790.

19. Ko K, Conforti A. Training protocol for intracranial pressure monitor placement by nonneurosurgeons: 5-year experience. J Trauma 2003; 55:480–483.

20. Reinges MH, Hasselberg I, Rohde V, et al. Prospective analysis of bedside percutaneous subdural tapping for the treatment of chronic subdural haematoma in adults. J Neurol Neurosurg Psychiatry 2000; 69:40–47.

21. Abbas G, Dubner S, Heller KS. Re-operation for bleeding after thyroidectomy and parathyroidectomy. Head Neck 2001; 23:544–546.

22. Fritscher-Ravens A, Sriram PV, Pothman WP, et al. Bedside endosonography and endosonography-guided fine-needle aspiration in critically ill patients: a way out of the deadlock? Endoscopy 2000; 32:425–427.

23. Yeow KM, Liao CT, Tsay PK, et al. US-guided catheter drainage of postoperative head and neck fluid collections. J Vasc Interv Radiol 2003; 14:589–595.

24. Mittendorf EA, McHenry CR, Smith CM, et al. Early and late outcome of bedside percutaneous tracheostomy in the intensive care unit. Am Surg 2002; 68:342–346.

25. Upadhyay A, Maurer J, Turner J, et al. Elective bedside tracheostomy in the intensive care unit. J Am Coll Surg 1996; 183:51–55.

26. Francois B, Clavel M, Desachy A, et al. Complications of tracheostomy performed in the ICU: Subthyroid tracheostomy vs. surgical cricothyroidostomy. Chest 2003; 123:151–158.

27. Barba CA, Angood PB, Kauder DR, et al. Bronchoscopic guidance makes percutaneous tracheostomy a safe, cost-effective, and easy-to-teach procedure. Surgery 1995; 118:879–883.

28. Massick DD, Powell DM, Price PD, et al. Quantification of the learning curve for percutaneous dilatational tracheotomy. Laryngoscope 2000; 110:222–228.

29. Dulguerov P, Gysin C, Perneger TV, Chevrolet JC. Percutaneous or surgical tracheostomy: a meta-analysis. Crit Care Med 1999; 27:1617–1625.

30. Freeman BD, Isabella K, Lin N, Buchman TG. A meta-analysis of prospective trials comparing percutaneous and surgical tracheostomy in critically ill patients. Chest 2000; 118:1412–1418.

31. Freeman BD, Isabella K, Cobb JP, et al. A prospective, randomized study comparing percutaneous with surgical tracheostomy in critically ill patients. Crit Care Med 2001; 29:926–930.

32. Grover A, Robbins J, Bendick P. Open versus percutaneous dilatational tracheostomy: efficacy and cost analysis. Am Surg 2001; 67:297–301.

33. Klotz DA, Hengerer AS. Safety of pediatric bedside tracheostomy in the intensive care unit. Arch Otolaryngol Head Neck Surg 2001; 127:950–955.

34. Byhahn C, Rinne T, Halbig S. Early percutaneous tracheostomy after median sternotomy. J Thorac Cardiovasc Surg 2000; 120:329–334.

35. Sugerman HJ, Wolfe L, Pasquale MD, et al. Multicenter, randomized, prospective trial of early tracheostomy. J Trauma 1997; 43:741–747.

36. Barquist E, Amortegue J, Cohn SM, et al. A randomized prospective study of early vs. late tracheostomy in trauma patients. Presented at the Annual Meeting of the American Association for the Surgery of Trauma, Maui, Hawaii, September 29, 2004.

37. Rumbak MJ, Newton M, Truncale T, et al. A prospective, randomized, study comparing early percutaneous dilational tracheotomy to prolonged translaryngeal intubation (delayed tracheotomy) in critically ill medical patients. Crit Care Med 2004; 32:1689–1694.

38. Azoulay E. Pleural effusions in the intensive care unit. Curr Opin Pulm Med 2003; 9:291–297.

39. Fartoukh M, Azoulay E, Galliot R, et al. Clinically documented pleural effusions in medical ICU patients: how useful is routine thoracentesis? Chest 2002; 121:178–184.

40. Lichtenstein D, Hulot JS, Rabiller A, et al. Feasibility and safety of ultrasound-aided thoracentesis in mechanically ventilated patients. Intensive Care Med 1999; 25:955–958.

41. Mayo PH, Goltz HR, Tafreshi M, Doelken P. Safety of ultrasound-guided thoracentesis in patients receiving mechanical ventilation. Chest 2004; 125:1059–1062.

42. Talmor M, Hydo L, Gershenwald JG, Barie PS. Beneficial effects of chest tube drainage of pleural effusion in acute respiratory failure refractory to positive end-expiratory pressure ventilation. Surgery 1998; 123:137–143.

43. Chon KS, van Sonnenberg E, D'Agostino HB, et al. CT-guided catheter drainage of loculated thoracic air collections in mechanically ventilated patients with acute respiratory distress syndrome. AJR Am J Roentgenol 1999; 173:1345–1350.

44. Mackay JH, Powell SJ, Osgathorp J, Rozario CJ. Six-year prospective audit of chest reopening after cardiac arrest. Eur J Cardiothorac Surg 2002; 22:421–425.

45. Fiser SM, Tribble CG, Kern JA, et al. Cardiac reoperation in the intensive care unit. Ann Thorac Surg 2001; 71:1888–1892.

46. Gould DS, Montenegro LM, Gaynor JW, et al. A comparison of on-site and off-site patent ductus arteriosus ligation in premature infants. Pediatrics 2003; 112:1298–1301.

47. Gines P, Cardenas A, Arroyo V, Rodes J. Management of cirrhosis and ascites. N Engl J Med 2004; 350:1646–1654.

48. Sharpe RP, Pryor JP, Gandhi RR, et al. Abdominal compartment syndrome in the pediatric blunt trauma patient treated with paracentesis: report of two cases. J Trauma 2002; 53:380–382.

49. Etzion Y, Barski L, Almog Y. Malignant ascites presenting as abdominal compartment syndrome. Am J Emerg Med 2004; 22:430–431.

50. Aslam N, Marino CR. Malignant ascites: new concepts in pathophysiology, diagnosis, and management. Arch Intern Med 2001; 161:2733–2737.

51. Phu NH, Hien TT, Mai NT, et al. Hemofiltration and peritoneal dialysis in infection-associated acute renal failure in Vietnam. N Engl J Med 2002; 347:895–902.

52. Platell C, Cooper D, Hall JC. A meta-analysis of peritoneal lavage for acute pancreatitis. J Gastroenterol Hepatol 2001; 16:689–693.

53. Barie PS, Eachempati SR. Acute acalculous cholecystitis. Curr Opin Gastroenterol 2003; 5:302–309.

54. Booth CM, Heyland DK, Paterson WG. Gastrointestinal promotility drugs in the critical care setting: a systematic review of the evidence. Crit Care Med 2002; 30:1429–1435.

55. Berne JD, Norwood SH, McAuley CE, et al. Erythromycin reduces delayed gastric emptying in critically ill trauma

patients: a randomized, controlled trial. J Trauma 2002; 53:422–425.

56. Dharmarajan TS, Unnikrishnan D, Pitchumoni CS. Percutaneous endoscopic gastrostomy and outcome in dementia. Am J Gastroenterol 2001; 96:2556–2663.

57. Dwyer KM, Watts DD, Thurber JS, et al. Percutaneous endoscopic gastrostomy: the preferred method of elective feeding tube placement in trauma patients. J Trauma 2002; 52:26–32.

58. MacLean AA, Miller G, Bamboat ZM, Hiotis K. Abdominal wall necrotizing fasciitis from dislodged percutaneous endoscopic gastrostomy tubes: a case series. Am Surg 2004; 70:827–831.

59. Lang A, Bardan E, Chowers Y, et al. Risk factors for mortality in patients undergoing percutaneous endoscopic gastrostomy. Endoscopy 2004; 36:522–526.

60. Reed RL, Eachempati SR, Russell M, et al. Endoscopic placement of jejunal feeding catheters in critically ill patients by a "push technique." J Trauma 1998; 45:285–289.

61. Montecalvo MA, Steger KA, Farber HW, et al. Nutritional outcome and pneumonia in critical care patients randomized to gastric versus jejunal tube feedings. The Critical Care Research Team. Crit Care Med 1992; 20:1377–1387.

62. Cappell MS, Friedel D. The role of sigmoidoscopy and colonoscopy in the diagnosis and treatment of lower gastrointestinal disorders: technique, indications, and contraindications. Med Clin North Am 2002; 86:1217–1252.

63. Savides TJ, Jensen DM. Therapeutic endoscopy for nonvariceal gastrointestinal bleeding. Gastroenterol Clin North Am 2000; 29:465–487.

64. Ivatury RR, Porter JM, Simon RJ, et al. Intra-abdominal hypertension after life-threatening penetrating abdominal trauma: prophylaxis, incidence, and clinical relevance to gastric mucosal pH and abdominal compartment syndrome. J Trauma 1998; 44:1016–1021.

65. Rotondo MR, Schwab CW, McGonigal MD, et al. "Damage control": an approach for improved survival in exsanguinating penetrating abdominal injury. J Trauma 1993; 35:375–382.

66. Diaz JJ, Mauer A, May AK, et al. Bedside laparotomy for trauma: are there risks? Surg Infect 2004; 5:15–20.

67. Sriussadaporn S, Pak-Art R, Bunjongsat S. Immediate closure of the open abdomen with bilateral bipedicle anterior abdominal skin flaps and subsequent retrorectus prosthetic mesh repair of the late giant ventral hernias. J Trauma 2003; 54:1083–1089.

68. Losanoff JE, Richman BW, Jones JW. Adjustable suture-tension closure of the open abdomen. J Am Coll Surg 2003; 196:163–164.

69. Kafie FE, Tessier DJ, Williams RA, et al. Serial abdominal closure technique (the "SAC" procedure): a novel method for delayed closure of the abdominal wall. Am Surg 2003; 69:102–105.

70. Jernigan TW, Fabian TC, Croce MA, et al. Staged management of giant abdominal wall defects: acute and long-term results. Ann Surg 2003; 238:349–355.

71. Rosin D, Haviv Y, Kuriansky J, et al. Bedside laparoscopy in the ICU: report of four cases. J Laparoendosc Surg 2001; 11:305–309.

72. Kelly JJ, Puyana JC, Callery MP, et al. The feasibility and accuracy of diagnostic laparoscopy in the septic ICU patient. Surg Endosc 2000; 14:617–621.

73. Branicki FJ. Abdominal emergencies: diagnostic and therapeutic laparoscopy. Surg Infect 2002; 3:269–282.

74. Barie PS, Eachempati SR. Necrotizing soft tissue infections. In Dries D, ed. Fifth Critical Care Refresher Course. Anaheim, CA: Society of Critical Care Medicine, 2001; 193–201.

75. Trent JT, Kirsner RS. Necrotizing fasciitis. Wounds 2002; 14:284–292.

76. Bisno AL, Stevens DL. Streptococcal infections of skin and soft tissues. N Engl J Med 1996; 334:240–244.

77. Miron D, Lev A, Coodner R, Merzel Y. *Vibrio vulnificus* necrotizing fasciitis of the calf presenting with compartment syndrome. Pediatr Infect Dis J 2003; 22:666–668.

78. Majeski J, Majeski E. Necrotizing fasciitis: improved survival with early recognition by tissue biopsy and aggressive surgical debridement. South Med J 1997; 90:1065–1068.

79. Bilton BD, Zibari GB, McMillan RW, et al. Aggressive surgical management of necrotizing fasciitis serves to decrease mortality: a retrospective study. Am Surg 1998; 64:397–400.

80. Barillo DJ, McManus AT, Cancio LC, et al. Burn center management of necrotizing fasciitis. J Burn Care Rehabil 2003; 24:127–132.

81. Raza A, Byrne D, Townell N. Lower limb (well leg) compartment syndrome after urological pelvic surgery. J Urol 2004; 171:5–11.

82. Gorecki PJ, Cottam D, Ger R, et al. Lower extremity compartment syndrome following a laparoscopic Roux-en-Y gastric bypass. Obes Surg 2002; 12:289–291.

83. Johnson IA, Andrzejowski JC, Currie JS. Lower limb compartment syndrome resulting from malignant hyperthermia. Anaesth Intensive Care 1999; 27:292–294.

84. Smith AL, Laing PW. Spontaneous tibial compartment syndrome in type I diabetes mellitus. Diabet Med 1999; 16:168–169.

85. James T, Friedman SG, Scher L, Hall M. Lower extremity compartment syndrome after coronary artery bypass. J Vasc Surg 2002; 36:1069–1070.

86. Hyde GL, Peck D, Powell DC. Compartment syndromes: early diagnosis and a bedside operation. Am Surg 1983; 49:563–568.

87. Li X, Liang D, Liu X. Compartment syndrome in burn patients: a report of five cases. Burns 2002; 28:787–789.

88. Giannoti G, Cohn SM, Brown M, et al. Utility of near-infrared spectroscopy in the diagnosis of lower extremity compartment syndrome. J Trauma 2000; 48:396–399.

89. Knudson MM, Ikossi DG. Venous thromboembolism after trauma. Curr Opin Crit Care 2004; 10:539–548.

90. Sing RF, Jacobs DG, Henifird BT. Bedside insertion of inferior vena cava filters in the intensive care unit. J Am Coll Surg 2001; 192:570–576.

91. Conners MS, Becker S, Guzman RJ, et al. Duplex scan-directed placement of inferior vena cava filters: a five-year institutional experience. J Vasc Surg 2002; 35:286–291.

92. Holtzman RB, Lottenberg L, Bass T, et al. Comparison of carbon dioxide and iodinated contrast for cavography prior to inferior vena cava filter placement. Am J Surg 2003; 185:364–368.

93. Ashley DW, Gamblin TC, Burch ST, et al. Accurate deployment of vena cava filters: comparison of intravascular ultrasound and contrast venography. J Trauma 2001; 50:975–981.

94. Ashley DW, Gamblin TC, McCampbell BL, et al. Bedside insertion of vena cava filters in the intensive care unit using intravascular ultrasound to locate renal veins. J Trauma 2004; 57:26–31.

95. Garrett JV, Passman MA, Guzman RJ, et al. Expanding options for bedside placement of inferior vena cava filter with intravascular ultrasound when transabdominal duplex ultrasound imaging is inadequate. Ann Vasc Surg 2004; 18:329–334.

96. Greenfield LJ, Proctor MC, Michaels AJ, Taheri PA. Prophylactic vena caval filters in trauma: the rest of the story. J Vasc Surg 2000; 32:490–495.

97. Stein PD, Alnas M, Skaf E, et al. Outcome and complications of removable inferior vena cava filters. Am J Cardiol 2004; 94:1090–1093.

9
Burns

Basil A. Pruitt, Jr., and Richard L. Gamelli

Case Scenario

A 50-year-old woman is involved in a house fire and sustains third-degree partial- and full-thickness burns to the torso and upper extremities. After 24 hours of fluid resuscitation, the amount of fluid substantially exceeds what was calculated using the Parkland formula. The patient had no associated blunt trauma. Which of the following is the most likely reason for the increased fluid requirement?

(A) Occult blunt trauma injury
(B) Inhalation injury
(C) Miscalculation of the amount of fluid required
(D) Miscalculation of cutaneous burns
(E) The amount of fluid resuscitation is not needed

The frequency of burn injury and its omnisystem effects make the treatment of burn patients a commonly encountered management challenge for the emergency/trauma surgeon. The biphasic pathophysiologic organ system changes evoked by burn injury represent the stereotypic response to injury and make the burn patient the universal trauma model (Table 9.1). The acute care surgery components of initial burn care include fluid resuscitation and ventilatory support as well as preservation and restoration of function of the other organ systems. Following resuscitation, burn patient management is focused on wound care and provision of the necessary metabolic support. The involvement of the emergency/trauma surgeon in burn wound management is depends on the extent of the wound, depth of the wound, and site of care (i.e. a general hospital in which an emergency/trauma surgeon might provide definitive wound care for a patient with burns of limited extent as opposed to a burn center where the wound care of a patient with extensive burns would be provided by a burn surgeon). The emer-

gency/trauma surgeon must be able to identify those patients who are best cared for at a burn center and ensure the safe and expeditious transport of those patients requiring transfer.

Epidemiology

The precise number of burns that occur in the United States each year is unknown because only 21 states mandate the reporting of burn injury, and in 9 of those states only specific burns defined by etiology or extent must be reported. An estimated total number of burns has been obtained by extrapolation of those data collected in less than half of the states to the entire population. At present, 1.25 million is regarded as a realistic estimate of the annual incidence of burns in the United States.[1] The vast majority (more than 80%) of those burns involve less than 20% of the total body surface, and only 190 to 263 patients per million population are estimated to require admission to a hospital for burn care each year.[2] Statewide hospital discharge data for 1994 in Pennsylvania identified three distinct age-related peak hospital discharge rates for burns: less than 5 years, 25 to 39 years, and 65 years and older.[3] Scalds and hot substances caused the burn injury in 58% of patients, and fire and flame sources caused the burn in 34%. Personal assault and self-inflicted injuries each accounted for 2% of the burns.

Within the population of burn patients requiring hospital care, there is a smaller subset each year of approximately 20,000 burn patients who, as defined by the American Burn Association (Table 9.2), are best cared for in a burn center.[4] This subset consists of 42 patients per million population with major burns and 40 patients per million population having lesser burns but a complicating cofactor. These patients are typically cared for in the 132 self-designated burn care facilities in the United States and the 14 similar facilities in Canada, the

TABLE 9.1. Organ system response to burn injury.

Organ system	Early change	Later response
Cardiovascular	Hypovolemia	Hyperdynamic state
Pulmonary	Hypoventilation	Hyperventilation
Endocrine	Catabolism	Anabolism
Urinary	Oliguria	Diuresis
Gastrointestinal	Ileus	Hypermotility
Skin	Hypoperfusion	Hyperemia
Immunologic	Inflammation	Anergy
Central nervous system	Agitation	Obtundation

geographic distribution of which correlates closely with population density.[5] This distribution may necessitate the use of aeromedical transfer by either fixed wing or rotary wing aircraft to transport burn patients to these facilities from remote areas.

There are identifiable populations at high risk for specific types of injuries that will require treatment by the emergency/trauma surgeon. Scald burns, which cause over 100,000 patients to seek treatment in hospital emergency departments annually, are the most frequent form of burn injury overall.[6] Sixty-five percent of children aged 4 years and under who require in-hospital burn care have scald burns, the majority of which are due to contact with hot foods and liquids. In children of all ages treated in emergency rooms for burns, thermal burns outnumber scald burns by more than a factor of 2.[7] The occurrence of tap water scalds can be minimized by adjusting the temperature settings on hot water heaters or by installing special faucet valves that prevent delivery of water at unsafe temperatures.

For adults, flames and the ignition of flammable liquids are the most common causes of burns. In the octogenar-

TABLE 9.2. Burn center referral criteria.

I. Partial-thickness burns involving more than 10% of the total body surface area
II. Full-Thickness burns involving 1% or more of the total body surface area
III. Less extensive burns involving face, hands, feet, genitalia, perineum, or major joints
IV. Significant electric burns, including lightning injury
V. Significant chemical burns
VI. Significant inhalation injury
VII. Lesser burns in patients with preexisting medical conditions that can complicate management, prolong recovery, or affect mortality
VIII. Lesser burns in association with concomitant trauma sufficient to influence outcome*
IX. Any size burn in a child in a hospital without qualified personnel or the equipment needed for the care of children
X. Any size burn in a patient who will require special social or psychiatric intervention or long-term rehabilitation

* If the mechanical trauma poses the greater immediate risk, the patient may be stabilized and receive initial care at a trauma center before transfer to a burn center.

ian population, scalds and flames each cause approximately 30% of burn injuries. In this elderly group of patients, preexisting disease contributes to the injury event in approximately two-thirds of patients, and their morbidity and mortality rates are higher than those of younger patients.[8]

One-fifth to one-quarter of all serious burns are employment related. Kitchen workers are at relatively high risk for scald injury, and roofers and paving workers are at greatest risk for burns caused by hot tar. In 1988, there were 236,200 patients treated in emergency rooms for chemical injuries.[9] Employees involved in plating processes and the manufacture of fertilizer are at greatest risk for injury caused by strong acids, and people involved with soap manufacturing and the use of oven cleaners are at greatest risk of injury from strong alkalis. Employment also defines those at greatest risk to injuries by phenol, hydrofluoric acid, anhydrous ammonia, cement, and petroleum distillates.

Injuries caused by white phosphorus and mustard gas are most frequent in military personnel. Civilian recreational explosive devices, fireworks, are a seasonal cause of burn injury. The highest incidence of firework injuries occurs during the Fourth of July holiday in the United States and during religious celebrations in countries such as India.[7]

Electric current causes approximately 1,000 deaths per year.[10] One-quarter of electric injuries occur on farms or industrial sites, and one-third occur in the home. Young children have the highest incidence of electric injury caused by household current as a consequence of inserting objects into an electrical receptacle or biting or sucking on electric cords and sockets. Adults at greatest risk of high-voltage electric injury are utility company employees, electricians, construction workers (particularly those manning cranes), farm workers moving irrigation pipes, oil field workers, truck drivers, and individuals installing antennae. National death certificate data document an average of 107 lightning deaths annually.[11] The vast majority (92%) of lightning-associated deaths occur during the summer months, when thunderstorms are most common. Slightly more than one-half of patients killed by lightning were engaged in outdoor activities such as golfing or fishing, and one-quarter of patients who died from lightning injury were engaged in employment-related activities.[12]

Child abuse is a special form of burn injury, typically inflicted by parents but also perpetrated by siblings and child care personnel. The most common form of thermal injury abuse in children is caused by intentional application of a lighted cigarette. Burning the dorsum of a hand by application of a hot clothing iron is another common form of child abuse. The burns on abused children who require in-hospital care are most often caused by immersion in scalding water, with the injury typically involving

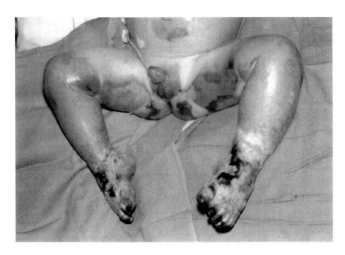

FIGURE 9.1. The burns on this abused child show the typical distribution (feet, legs, posterior thighs, buttocks, and genitalia) of injury caused by intentional immersion scalding. Note the pink to red color and moist surface of the partial-thickness injuries on the proximal legs and distal thighs. The pallor, hemorrhagic discoloration, and eschar caseation of the full-thickness injuries of the feet and distal legs are characteristic of third-degree burns that required skin grafting for closure.

the feet, posterior legs, buttocks, and sometimes the hands (Figure 9.1). It is important that the emergency/trauma surgeon identify and report child abuse, because, if abuse is undetected and the child is returned to the abusive environment, repeated abuse is associated with a high risk of fatality. In recent years, elder abuse has become more common, and it too should be reported and the victim protected.

Pathophysiology

Local Effects

The cutaneous injury caused by a burn is related to the temperature of the energy source, the duration of the exposure, and the tissue surface involved. At temperatures less than 45°C, tissue damage is unlikely to occur in either adults or children even with an extended period of exposure. In the adult, exposure for 30 seconds when the temperature is 54°C will cause a burn injury.[2] In the child with relatively thinner skin, exposure to the same temperature for 10 seconds produces a significant degree of tissue destruction. When the temperature is elevated to 60°C, a not uncommon setting for home water heaters, tissue destruction can occur in less than 5 seconds in children. At 71°C, a full-thickness burn can occur in a near-instantaneous manner. It is no surprise that when patients come in contact with boiling liquids, live flames, or are injured in industrial accidents where temperatures can exceed 1,000°C, significant depths of injury occur. The systemic consequences of the injuries are related to the

depth and the extent of the body surface area involvement as well as the patient's underlying physiologic status and whether any other associated traumas occurred. The combination of the variables of tissue involved, intensity of the heat source, and duration of exposure will determine whether the patient has a full-thickness injury or a partial-thickness injury.

The burn injury can cause three zones of damage. Centrally located is the zone of necrosis. Surrounding this is an area of lesser cell injury, the zone of stasis, and surrounding that an area of minimally damaged tissue, the zone of hyperemia, which abuts undamaged tissue. In a full-thickness burn, the zone of coagulation involves all layers of the skin extending down through the dermis and into the subcutaneous tissue. In partial-thickness injuries, this zone extends down only into the dermis, and there are surviving epithelial elements capable of ultimately resurfacing the wound. In the zone of stasis blood flow is altered but is restored with time as resuscitation proceeds. If thrombosis were to occur in a patient who is not adequately resuscitated, the zone of stasis can be converted to a zone of coagulation. The zone of hyperemia is best seen in patients with superficial partial-thickness injuries as occur with severe sun exposure.

Along with the changes in wound blood supply there is significant formation of edema in the burn-injured tissues. Release of local mediators from the burned tissue as well as from leukocytes causes alterations in local tissue homeostasis. Factors elaborated in the damaged tissues include histamine, serotonin, bradykinin, prostaglandins, leukotrienes, and interleukin-1. Complement is also activated, which can further modify transcapillary fluid flux. The changes in tissue water content have been ascribed to increased capillary filtration as well as changes in interstitial hydrostatic pressure.[13–16] The net effect of these various changes is significant movement of fluid into the extravascular fluid compartment. The ongoing development of edema fluid in the burn-injured tissue conceptually represents increased vascular permeability. Subsequent changes in lymph flow from burned tissue have been ascribed to changes in lymphatic vessel patency, with obstruction occurring because of serum proteins that have transmigrated from the damaged capillaries.[17] Maximum accumulation of both water and protein in the burn wound occurs at 24 hours postinjury.[18] This accumulation in tissues can remain beyond the first week postburn. In addition to the changes in transcapillary fluid movement within the burn-injured tissues, patients who have more than a 20% to 25% body surface burn have similar fluid movement in undamaged tissue beds. This may in part be related to the changes in transcapillary fluid flux or be a response to the volume of resuscitation fluids administered.[19,20]

The injuries that will be apparent on examination are the consequences of the level of tissue destruction

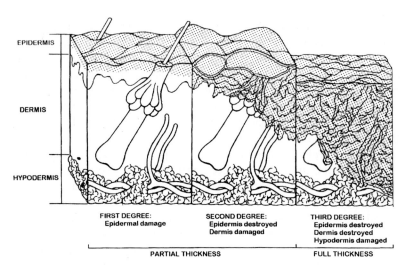

EPIDERMIS

DERMIS

HYPODERMIS

FIRST DEGREE:
Epidermal damage

SECOND DEGREE:
Epidermis destroyed
Dermis damaged

THIRD DEGREE:
Epidermis destroyed
Dermis destroyed
Hypodermis damaged

PARTIAL THICKNESS   FULL THICKNESS

FIGURE 9.2. Diagram of the skin, adnexa, and subcutaneous tissue showing, by stippled shading, the depth of tissue injury that defines both first-degree and second-degree partial-thickness burns and third-degree full-thickness burns.

(Figure 9.2). When the wounds are superficial they are associated with hyperemia, fine blistering, increased sensation, and exquisite pain upon palpation. The wounds are hyperemic and warm and readily blanch. These types of injuries represent first-degree burns or, alternatively, are termed "superficial partial-thickness injuries." With a second-degree, or deeper partial-thickness, burn the wound presents with intact or ruptured blisters or is covered by a thin coagulum termed "pseudoeschar." The key physical finding is preservation of sensation in the burned tissue, although it is reduced (Table 9.3). With proper care, superficial and even deeper partial-thickness injuries are capable of healing. Burn blister fluid represents a near pure acellular filtrate of plasma. Interestingly, when studied, this fluid is not necessarily found to promote wound healing.[21] Infection risk in deep partial-thickness wounds is significant, and, if an infection develops, it can lead to a greater depth of skin loss.

When the injury penetrates all layers of the skin or extends into the subcutaneous or deeper tissues, the wound will appear pale or waxy, be anesthetic, dry, and inelastic, and contain thrombosed vessels (see Figure 9.2). Occasionally in children or young women, the initial appearance of a wound may be more that of a brick red coloration. Such wounds will have significant edema, are inelastic, and are insensate. Over the subsequent days the extravasated hemoglobin, which is still fully oxygenated immediately postinjury and is responsible for the wound color, undergoes reduction, and the wound appearance is more characteristic of that of a full-thickness wound. Full-thickness wounds are infection prone wounds, as they no longer provide any viable barrier to invading organisms and if left untreated become rapidly colonized and a portal for invasive burn wound sepsis.

Systemic Response

The organ system response to a major burn injury results in some of the most profound physiologic changes that a person is capable of enduring. The magnitude of the response is proportional to the burn size, reaching a maximum at about a 50% body surface area burn. The

TABLE 9.3. Clinical characteristics of burn injuries.

	Partial thickness		Full thickness, third degree
	First degree	Second degree	
Cause	Sun or minor flash	Higher intensity or longer exposure to flash	Higher intensity or longer exposure to flash
		Relatively brief exposure to hot liquids, flames	Longer exposure to flames or "hot" liquids
			Contact with steam or hot metal
			High-voltage electricity
			Chemicals
Color	Bright red	Mottled red	Pearly white
			Translucent and parchment-like
			Charred
Surface	Dry	Moist	Dry, leathery, and stiff
	No bullae	Bullae present	Remnants of burned skin present
			Liquefaction of tissue
Sensation	Hyperaesthetic	Pain to pin prick inversely proportional to depth of injury	Surface insensate
			Deep pressure sense retained
Healing	3–6 days	Time proportional to depth of burns: 10–35 days	Requires grafting

duration of the changes is related to the persistence of the burn wound and resolves with wound closure. The organ-specific response follows the pattern that occurs with other forms of trauma, with an initial level of hypofunction followed by the hyperdynamic flow phase. The changes in the cardiovascular response are some of the more critical ones and directly impact the initial care and management of the burn patient. Following burn injury there is a transient period of decreased cardiac performance in association with elevated peripheral vascular resistance. This can be further compounded by failure to replace adequately the patient's intravascular volume loss, leading to further impairments of cardiac filling, decreased cardiac output, and worsening organ hypoperfusion. Systemic hypoperfusion can result in further increases in systemic vascular resistances and reprioritization of regional blood flow. The idea that the burn is responsible for causing a myocardial depressant to appear in circulation or whether the impaired cardiac performance is simply a consequence of inadequate volume restoration remains an open question.

What seems to be clear from experimental studies is that when there is a failure to resuscitate a burn patient adequately there is substantially impaired myocardial performance.[22] Conversely, the provision of adequate resuscitation volumes can preserve cardiac performance.[23] Patients receiving appropriate volume restoration during the course of their resuscitation develop normal cardiac performance values within 24 hours of injury, and by the second 24 hours these values further increase to supranormal levels. It is not uncommon to see adult patients with cardiac outputs in excess of 10 L/min. In association with changes in cardiac output, there is a reduction in the systemic vascular resistance to 30% to 40% of normal values. The patient at this juncture is in a hyperdynamic flow phase as part of the hypermetabolic response to the injury, which will revert back to more normal levels with wound closure. However, there may be some element of increase present in major burn victims for months after recovery until the wound is fully mature.

Pulmonary changes following burn injury are the consequences of direct parenchymal damage as occurs with inhalation injury and of the changes that occur solely related to the burn injury. With isolated burn injury neutrophil sequestration occurs in the lungs and may mediate lung injury. One potential mediator of this response may be platelet-activating factor, which serves to prime neutrophils.[24] The changes in the pulmonary vascular response parallel those of the peripheral circulation, although the increase may be to a greater degree and with a longer duration of change.[25] Capillary permeability in the lung appears to be mostly preserved following burn injury, with the primary change being an increase in the lung lymph flow but no change in the

lymph to plasma protein ratio.[26] Lung ventilation increases in proportion to the burn size, with the patient having an increase in both respiratory rate and tidal volume. The increases are primarily related to the overall hypermetabolic response to the burn injury. Further perturbations in the patient's ventilatory status not related to the presence of an inhalation injury would indicate a supervening process. Such common events include fever, sepsis, pneumonia, occult pneumothorax, pulmonary embolism, congestive heart failure, and an acute intraabdominal process. In patients without these events, pulmonary gas exchange is relatively preserved, and there is relatively little change in pulmonary mechanics.

The renal response to burn injuries is largely orchestrated by the cardiovascular response. Although initially there may be a reduction in renal blood flow, this is restored with resuscitation. If the resuscitation is delayed or the fluid need underestimated, renal hypoperfusion will occur with early-onset renal dysfunction secondary to renal ischemia. If the patient also experiences myoglobinuria or hemoglobinuria, which are capable of causing direct tubular damage, sequential injury can occur, leading to further impairment of renal function. The changes in renal blood flow following burn injury require that the doses of certain medications such as aminoglycoside antibiotics be adjusted to attain therapeutic levels. For patients who are receiving nutritional support, large doses of carbohydrates can cause glycosuria, resulting in an inappropriate osmotic diuresis necessitating therapeutic intervention (i.e., reduction of glucose load and/or administration of insulin). Daily urinary outputs of burn patients who are receiving protein loads greater than normal need to be relatively greater than those of nonburn patients in order to excrete the increased solute load.

Burn-induced changes in gastrointestinal (GI) tract motility and a reduced capacity to tolerate early feedings previously had been thought to preclude the use of the GI tract as the primary route for nutritional support. With near-immediate institution of enteral feedings via nasogastric or nasoduodenal tubes, GI motility can be preserved, mucosal integrity protected, and effective nutrient delivery achieved. It seems that delay in the initiation of enteral feeding is associated with the onset of ileus, which can also occur when the burn resuscitation has been complicated. Patients who are underresuscitated will have alterations in GI tract motility and mucosal integrity as a consequence of intestinal hypoperfusion. Patients who have received massive resuscitation volumes will have significant edema of the retroperitoneum, bowel mesentery, and bowel wall leading to a paralytic ileus. In patients who are intoxicated at the time of their burn injury, there may be further alterations in the GI tract with changes in the mucosal barrier function and alterations in local immunity.[27] In the past, the major GI complications following burn injuries were related to upper GI ulceration and bleeding. However, there has been a relative shift in the site of postburn GI complications, with the small bowel and colon now being more often affected.[28]

Burn injury results in an elevated hormonal and neurotransmitter response similar in magnitude to that of the "fight or flight" response.[29] The duration of the neurohumoral response is prolonged, and it can be further increased with surgical stress. This can adversely impact the burn-induced metabolic changes and immune response. The increases in glucocorticoids and catecholamines correctly support the stress response of the injured patient except when this response becomes dysfunctional. In pathologic studies of humans as well as of animals, when there is an insufficient stress hormone response an otherwise survivable insult becomes fatal. Many of the multisystem changes occurring postburn can be related in part to the alterations in catecholamine secretion, particularly the changes in resting metabolic expenditures, substrate utilization, and cardiac performance. As wound closure is accomplished, the altered neurohumoral response abates as the catabolic hormones recede and the anabolic hormones become predominant.

Burn injury results in the loss of balance in both leukocyte and erythrocyte production and function. Burns of greater than 20% total body surface area are associated with alterations in red cell production resulting in anemia.[30] Patients with major thermal injuries may lose up to 20% of their red cell mass in the first 24 hours due to thermal destruction of red cells in the cutaneous circulation. Such loss can be further compounded by frequent blood draws, blood loss related to surgical procedures, hemodilution with resuscitation, and transient alterations in erythrocyte membrane integrity. Longer term changes appear to be related to hyporesponsiveness of the erythroid progenitor cells in the bone marrow to erythropoietin.[31] Burn patients manifest increased circulating levels of erythropoietin following injury, and attempts to augment these levels to improve red cell production have met with little success. During the early stages of resuscitation, reductions in platelet number, depressed fibrinogen levels, and alterations in coagulation factors return to normal or near-normal values with appropriate resuscitation. Subsequent changes if they occur may be related to a septic process or, in the case of platelets, heparin-induced platelet antibodies if heparin flushes are used as part of the maintenance protocol for intravascular devices. Changes in white cell number occur early with an increase in neutrophils due to demargination and accelerated bone marrow release. With uncomplicated burn injury, bone marrow myelopoiesis is relatively preserved.[32] With a septic complication there appears, based on experimental evidence, to be a reduction in granulocyte formation

and a relative shift to monocytopoiesis.[33] This defect appears not to be related to a lack of granulocyte colony–stimulating factor but is a growth arrest within the bone marrow of granulocyte precursor cells.[34,35]

In addition to the changes occurring in the bone marrow and the nonspecific aspects of the host defense mechanisms, there are significant further depressions in the immune response. Burn injury causes a global impairment in host defense mechanisms. Alterations of the humoral immune response include reductions in immunoglobulins G (IgG) and M (IgM) secretion, decreased fibronectin levels, and increases in complement activation. Cellular changes include alterations in T-cell responsiveness, changes in the T-cell subpopulations favoring the cytotoxic/suppressor T cell, alterations in antigen processing and presentation, reductions in interleukin-2 (IL-2) release, and impairment of delayed-type hypersensitivity reactions. In addition to the changes noted in granulocytes and monocytes and their release from the bone marrow, there are corresponding functional changes. Granulocytes have been noted to have impaired chemotaxis, decreased phagocytic activity, decreased antibody-dependent cell cytotoxicity, and a relative impairment in their capacity to respond to a second challenge.[36] The relative shift to monopoiesis is associated with an increase in secretion of prostaglandin E_2 (PGE_2).[37] More recently, dendritic cells, a critical component in the immune response, have been found to be significantly altered following burn injury with infection.[38] The clinical importance of these observations is that the burn patient is at significant risk for postburn infectious complications. This mandates the strictest adherence to aseptic technique in the management of the wounds and the insertion of intravascular devices, the judicious use of antimicrobial agents, aggressive nutritional support, and the achievement of rapid wound closure.

Resuscitation Priorities

In the immediate postburn period the changes induced in the cardiovascular system by burn injury receive therapeutic priority. If the early postburn plasma volume loss is unreplaced, burn shock may occur accompanied by kidney and other organ failure and even death. In all patients with burns of more than 20% of the total body surface area and those with lesser burns in whom physiologic indices indicate a need for fluid infusion, a large-caliber intravenous cannula should be placed in an appropriately sized peripheral vein underlying unburned skin. If no such sites are available, a vein underlying the burn wound may be cannulated. If there are no peripheral veins available, the cannula can be placed in a femoral, subclavian, or jugular vein. Lactated Ringer's solution should be infused at an initial rate of 1 L/hr in the adult and 20 mL/kg/hr for children who weigh 50 kg or less. That infusion rate is adjusted following estimation of the fluid needed for the first 24 hours following the burn.

Fluid Administration

Resuscitation fluid needs are proportional to the extent of the burn (combined extent of partial- and full-thickness burns expressed as a percentage of total body surface area) and are related to body size (most readily expressed as body weight) and age (the surface area per unit body mass is greater in children than in adults.) The patient should be weighed on admission and the extent of partial- and full-thickness burns estimated according to standard nomograms (Figure 9.3) or, for the adult, by

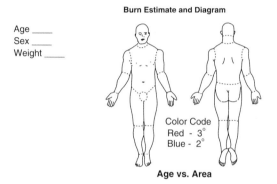

Burn Estimate and Diagram

Age ____
Sex ____
Weight ____

Color Code
Red - 3°
Blue - 2°

Age vs. Area

Area	Birth 1 yr	1–4 yr	5–9 yr	10–14 yr	18 yr	Adult	2°	3°	Total	Donor Area
Head	19	17	13	11	9	7				
Neck	2	2	2	2	2	2				
Ant. Trunk	13	13	13	13	13	13				
Post. Trunk	13	13	13	13	13	13				
R. Buttock	2½	2½	2½	2½	2½	2½				
L. Buttock	2½	2½	2½	2½	2½	2½				
Genitalia	1	1	1	1	1	1				
R.U. Arm	4	4	4	4	4	4				
L.U. Arm	4	4	4	4	4	4				
R.L. Arm	3	3	3	3	3	3				
L.L. Arm	3	3	3	3	3	3				
R. Hand	2½	2½	2½	2½	2½	2½				
L. Hand	2½	2½	2½	2½	2½	2½				
R. Thigh	5½	6½	8	8½	9	9½				
L. Thigh	5½	6½	8	8½	9	9½				
R. Leg	5	5	5½	6	6½	7				
L. Leg	5	5	5½	6	6½	7				
R. Foot	3½	3½	3½	3½	3½	3½				
L. Foot	3½	3½	3½	3½	3½	3½				
						Total				

FIGURE 9.3. Example of a form used to document extent of burn. Figure outlines are filled in with a blue pencil and a red pencil to indicate distribution of partial-thickness and full-thickness burns, respectively. Note the columns indicating how the percentage of total body surface area represented by body part surface changes with time. (*Source:* Adapted courtesy of the U.S. Army Burn Center, Fort Sam Houston, Texas.)

the use of the rule of nines, which recognizes the fact that the surface area of various body parts represents 9% or a multiple thereof of the total body surface area (i.e., each upper limb and the head and neck 9%; each lower limb, posterior trunk and buttocks, and anterior trunk 18%; and the perineum and genitalia 1%). These surface area relationships differ in children, whose head and neck represent 21% of the total body surface area and each lower limb 14% at age 1 year. The fraction of the total body surface area represented by the head decreases progressively, and that represented by the lower limbs increases progressively to reach adult proportions at age 16 years. The fact that the palmar surface of the patient's hand (palm and digits) represents 1% of his or her total body surface can be used to estimate the extent of irregularly distributed burns (i.e., the number of the patient's "hands" needed to cover the patient's burn wounds).[39]

The fluid needs for the first 24 hours can be estimated on the basis of the Advanced Burn Life Support and Advanced Trauma Life Support consensus formulas[40]:

$$\text{Adults} = 2–4\,\text{mL LR}/\%\,\text{TBSAB}/\text{kg, BW}$$
$$\text{Children} = 3–4\,\text{mL LR}/\%\,\text{TBSAB}/\text{kg, BW,}$$

where TBSAB is total body surface area burned, LR is lactated Ringer's, and BW is body weight. Because of the greater surface area per unit body mass in children, the volume of fluid required for the first 24 hours is relatively greater than that for an adult. One of the authors (B.A.P.) prefers to make the estimate using 2 mL/% TBSAB/kg BW for an adult and 3 mL/% TBSAB/kg BW for children to minimize volume and salt loading. The infused volume is increased only as needed to achieve adequate resuscitation. The other author (R.L.G.) makes the estimate using 4 mL/% TBSAB/kg BW for all burn patients out of concern about delayed initiation of infusion. One-half of the estimated volume should be administered in the first 8 hours after the burn. If the initiation of fluid therapy is delayed, the initial half of the volume estimated for the first 24 hours should be administered in the hours remaining before the eighth postburn hour. The second half of the fluid is administered over the subsequent 16 hours.

The limited glycogen stores in a child may be rapidly exhausted by the marked stress hormone response to burn injury. Serum glucose levels in the burned child should be monitored and 5% dextrose in 2 normal saline administered if serum glucose decreases to hypoglycemic levels. In the case of small children with small burns, the resuscitation fluid volume as estimated on the basis of burn size may not meet normal daily metabolic requirements. In such patients, maintenance fluids should be added to the resuscitation regimen.

The infusion rate is adjusted according to the individual patient's response to the injury and the resuscitation regimen. The high circulating levels of catecholamines evoked by the burn and the progressive edema formation in burned and even unburned limbs commonly make measurements of pulse rate, pulse quality, and even blood pressure difficult and unreliable as indices of resuscitation adequacy. Because the hourly urinary output is a generally reliable and readily available index of resuscitation adequacy, an indwelling urethral catheter should be placed and the urinary output measured and recorded each hour. The fluid infusion rate is adjusted to obtain 30 to 50 mL of urine per hour in the adult and 1 mg/kg body weight per hour in children weighing less than 30 kg. To avoid excessive fluctuation of the infusion rate, the administration of fluid is increased or decreased only if the hourly urinary output is one-third or more below or 25% or more above the target level for 2 or 3 successive hours. If for either adults or children the resuscitation volume infused in the first 12 hours to achieve the desired urinary output or other indices of resuscitation adequacy exceeds estimated needs by more than twofold or will result in administration of 6 mL or more per percent body surface area burned per kilogram body weight in the first 24 hours, human albumin diluted to a physiologic concentration in normal saline should be infused and the volume of crystalloid solution reduced by a comparable amount. Inasmuch as functional capillary integrity is gradually restored during the first 24 hours postburn, such use of colloid-containing fluid is best reserved for the latter half of the first postburn day.

Restoration of functional capillary integrity and the establishment of a new transvascular equilibrium across the burn wound are manifested by the fact that both protein and water contents of the burn-injured tissue reach maxima at or near 24 hours after injury.[18] Consequently, the volume of fluid needed for the second 24 hours postburn is less, and colloid-containing fluids can be infused to reduce further volume and salt loading. Human albumin diluted to physiologic concentration in normal saline is the colloid-containing solution infused in a dosage of 0.3 mL per percent burn per kilogram body weight for patients with 30% to 50% burns; 0.4 mL per percent burn per kilogram body weight for patients with 50% to 70% burns; and 0.5 mL per percent burn per kilogram body weight for patients whose burns exceed 70% of the total body surface area. Electrolyte-free, 5% glucose in water is also given in the amount necessary to maintain an adequate urinary output. The colloid-containing fluids for the second 24 hours for burned children are estimated according to the same formula, but half-normal saline is infused to maintain urinary output and avoid inducing physiologically significant hyponatremia by infusion of large volumes of electrolyte-free fluid into the relatively small intravascular and interstitial volume of the child.

During the second 24 hours after injury, fluid infusion "weaning" should be initiated to minimize further volume loading. For the patient who is assessed to be adequately resuscitated, the volume of fluid infused per hour should be arbitrarily decreased by 25% to 50%. If urinary output falls below target level, the prior infusion rate should be resumed. If urinary output remains adequate, the reduced infusion rate should be maintained over the next 3 hours at which time another similar fractional reduction of fluid infusion rate should be made. This decremental process will establish the minimum infusion rate that maintains resuscitation adequacy in the second postburn day.

As resuscitation proceeds and edema forms beneath the inelastic eschar of encircling full-thickness burns of a limb, blood flow to underlying and distal unburned tissue may be compromised. Circulatory compromise can occur in limbs with mixed depth partial-thickness burns and on occasion in limbs with less than completely circumferential burns. Edema and coolness of distal unburned skin on a burned limb are normal accompaniments of the injury and are not indicative of circulatory compromise requiring surgical release. Cyanosis of distal unburned skin and progressive parasthesias, particularly unrelenting deep tissue pain, which are the most reliable clinical signs of impaired circulation, may become evident only after relatively long periods of relative or absolute ischemia. Those limitations can be overcome by scheduled (q 1–2 hours) monitoring of the pulse signal in the palmar arch vessels and the posterior tibial artery using an ultrasonic flowmeter. In an adequately resuscitated patient, absence of pulsatile flow or progressive diminution of the pulse signal on repetitive examinations is an indication for escharotomy. Because the full-thickness eschar is insensate, the escharotomy can be performed as a bedside procedure without anesthesia using a scalpel or an electrocautery device. On an extremity, the escharotomy incision, which is carried only through the eschar and the immediately subjacent superficial fascia, is placed in the midlateral line and must extend from the upper to the lower limit of the burn wound (Figure 9.4). The circulatory status of the limb should then be reassessed. If that escharotomy has not restored distal flow, another escharotomy should be placed in the midmedial line of the involved limb. A fasciotomy may be needed when there has been a delay in restoring the patient's limb circulation and in particular if the patient is receiving a massive fluid load. Mistakes in the performance of escharotomies include injuries to extensor tendons and digital neurovascular bundles, insufficient depth and length of the incision, and delay in performing the escharotomy. Additionally, delayed bleeding from previously thrombosed vessels transected during the escharotomy should be promptly controlled. Continuous elevation and active exercise of a burned extremity for 5 minutes every hour limits edema formation and may eliminate the need for escharotomy.[41]

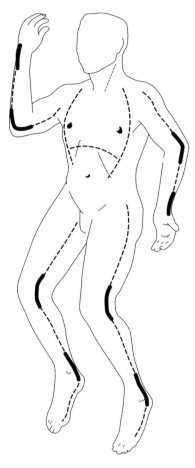

FIGURE 9.4. The dashed lines indicate the preferred sites of escharotomy incisions for the limbs (midlateral and midmedial lines), thorax (anterior axillary lines and costal margin), and neck (lateral aspect). The thickened areas of the lines on the limbs emphasize the importance of carrying the incisions across involved joints.

Edema formation beneath encircling full-thickness truncal burns can restrict the respiratory excursion of the chest wall. If the limitation of chest wall motion is associated with hypoxia and progressive increase in the work of breathing and peak inspiratory pressure, escharotomy is indicated to restore chest wall motion and improve ventilation. These escharotomy incisions are placed in the anterior axillary line bilaterally, and, if the eschar extends onto the abdominal wall, the anterior axillary line incisions are joined by a costal margin escharotomy incision (Figure 9.4). Rarely, encircling full-thickness burns of the neck or penis will require release by placement of an escharotomy incision in the midlateral line(s) of the neck or the dorsum of the penis.

Fluid management after the first 48 hours postburn should permit excretion of the retained fraction of the water and salt loads infused to achieve resuscitation, prevent dehydration and electrolyte abnormalities, and allow the patient to return to preburn weight by the eighth to tenth postburn day.[39] Infusion of the large volumes of lactated Ringer's required for resuscitation commonly produces a weight gain of 20% or more and a reduction of serum sodium concentration to approximate that of lactated Ringer's (i.e., 130 mEq/L). Such patients do not need additional sodium and, in fact, have an elevated total body sodium mass in association with increased total body water. Correction of that relative hyponatremia is facilitated by the prodigious evaporative water loss from the surface of the burn wound, which is the major component of the markedly increased insensible water loss that is present following resuscitation. Insensible water loss, which must be taken into account in postresuscitation fluid management, can be estimated according to the following formula[42]:

$$\text{Insensible water loss (mL/hr)} = (25 + \% \text{ TBSAB}) \times \text{TBSA in m}^2,$$

where TBSAB is total body surface area burned and TBSA is total body surface area. The water loss should be replaced only to the extent that will permit a daily loss of 2% to 2.5% of the resuscitation-associated weight gain (as measured 48 hours after the burn) until preburn weight is attained. Inadequate replacement of insensible water loss makes hypernatremia the most commonly encountered electrolyte disturbance in the extensively burned patient following resuscitation. Such hypernatremia should be managed by provision of sufficient electrolyte-free water to allow excretion of the increased total body sodium mass and replace insensible water loss to the extent needed to prevent hypovolemia.

During resuscitation hyperkalemia is the most frequently encountered electrolyte disturbance and is typically a laboratory sign of hemolysis and muscle destruction by high-voltage electric injury or a particularly deep thermal burn. Hyperkalemia may also occur in association with acidosis in patients who are grossly underresuscitated. Hyperkalemia in the burn patient is treated as in any other surgical patient. In the case of patients with high-voltage electric injury, acute care debridement of nonviable tissue and even amputation may be necessary to remove the source of the potassium. Hypokalemia may occur after the resuscitation period in association with alkalosis as a consequence of hyperventilation and may also accompany postresuscitation muscle wasting. Potassium losses are increased by the kaluretic effect of the mafenide acetate in Sulfamylon burn cream and, as noted below, by transeschar leaching in patients treated with 0.5% silver nitrate soaks.

Significant depression of ionized calcium levels is uncommon, but total calcium levels may be depressed if calcium binding proteins such as albumin decrease as may happen in patients receiving a high volume of resuscitation fluid. In extensively burned children, hypocalcemia has been associated with hypoparathyroidism and renal resistance to parathyroid hormone.[43] Symptomatic acute hypocalcemia should be treated with intravenous calcium (90 to 180 mg of calcium infused over 5 to 10 minutes) to control cardiac dysfunction and neuromuscular hyperactivity. Prolonged administration of parenteral nutrition and/or failure to supply sufficient phosphate to meet the needs of tissue anabolism following wound closure may cause hypophosphatemia. Administration of large volumes of antacids for stress ulcer prophylaxis is an infrequent cause of hypophosphatemia now that acid secretion inhibitors are used for that purpose. Hypophosphatemia can be prevented and treated by appropriate dietary phosphate supplementation.

The timely administration of adequate fluid as detailed above has essentially eliminated acute renal failure as a complication of inadequate resuscitation of burn patients. In a recent 10-year period, at the U.S. Army Burn Center, only 2 out of 2,132 burn patients treated developed early renal failure, and those patients had established anuria when they were received in transfer from other institutions.[44] Far more common today are the complications of excessive resuscitation (i.e., compartment syndromes and pulmonary compromise. Compartment syndromes can be produced in the calvarium, muscle compartments beneath the investing fascia, and the abdominal cavity. Cerebral edema, which can efface the epidural space and compress the ventricular system, is most apt to occur in burned children and is manifested by obtundation and changes evident on computerized tomographic scans. Such changes should be addressed by maintaining cerebral perfusion pressure and minimizing further edema formation by reducing fluid infusion rate and inducing diuresis. Anterior ischemic optic neuropathy, manifested by visual field defects and even blindness, is another complication of excessive fluid infusion. It has typically occurred in association with other compartment syndromes and anasarca in critically ill patients, particularly in those who are nursed in a prone position. Consequently, prone positioning should be avoided for severely injured, critically ill burn patients requiring large volumes of parenteral fluids. The occurrence of visual field defects should prompt alteration of fluid therapy and induction of a diuresis.[45]

Excessive fluid administration may also cause formation of enough ascitic fluid and edema of the abdominal contents to produce intraabdominal hypertension. The abdominal compartment syndrome represents progression of intraabdominal hypertension to the point of organ dysfunction (i.e., typically oliguria and/or altered pulmonary mechanics). Infusion of resuscitation fluid volumes in excess of 25% of body weight has been associated with a high incidence of abdominal compartment syndrome.[46] For all patients who have received that volume of resuscitation fluid, hourly monitoring of intra-

cystic pressure should be instituted. Elevation of intracystic pressure above 25 mm Hg, as measured through a urethral catheter, should prompt therapeutic intervention, beginning with adequate sedation, reduction of fluid infusion rate, diuresis, and paracentesis. If organ failure becomes, evident a midline abdominal incision should be made to reduce the elevated intraabdominal pressure. This incision can be temporarily closed with a polyethylene "bag" or a vacuum-assisted closure device. The abdomen can be definitively closed as soon as visceral edema resolves.

Compartment syndromes may also occur in the muscle compartments underlying the investing fascia of the limbs of burn patients, even in limbs that are unburned. To assess compartment pressure, the turgor of the muscle compartments should be assessed on a scheduled basis by simple palpation. A stony hard compartment is an ominous finding that should prompt further evaluation. The adequacy of arterial flow in all limbs of a burn patient should be monitored on a scheduled basis using the ultrasonic flowmeter. Ultrasonic detection of pulsatile flow is reassuring, but the ultrasonic flow signals can be misleading because flow in large vessels may be maintained even though microcirculatory flow is severely compromised within a muscle compartment. Direct measurement of intracompartmental pressure using either a wick or a needle catheter is much more reliable. A muscle compartment pressure of 25 mm Hg or more necessitates performing a fasciotomy of the involved compartment in the operating room using general anesthesia.

Edema causing airway obstruction, in the absence of inhalation injury, has also been attributed to excessive resuscitation fluid. This complication, which necessitates endotracheal intubation, has been of particular concern in small children with extensive scald burns who have received in excess of 6 mL of lactated Ringer's per percent body surface area burned per kilogram body weight. Pulmonary edema is rare during the initial 48-hour resuscitation period but may occur in patients with extensive burns following resuscitation when the edema fluid is being resorbed and the protective early postburn pulmonary vascular changes have dissipated. The treatment of pulmonary edema in the burn patient is the same as for other patients.

Ventilatory Support and Treatment of Inhalation Injury

Pathophysiology

Patients suffering both inhalation injuries and thermal burns have a significantly increased incidence of complications and probability of death. Although an inhalation injury alone carries a mortality rate of 5% to 8%, a combination of a thermal injury plus inhalation injury can easily result in a mortality rate 20% above that predicted on the basis of age and burn size. Patients who have an otherwise survivable injury may succumb to their burn as a consequence of their inhalation injury and the complications that occur, particularly a Gram-negative pneumonia.[47] Injuries to the airway are due to the direct damage of inhaled products of combustion or pyrolysis that cause inflammation and edema. Damage to the airway, while in part related to the heat content of the inhaled material in the oropharynx, is, in the more distal airways, principally related to the particulate material contained within the smoke and the chemical composition of inhaled materials. Moist heat, which occurs with steam, has 4,000 times the heat-carrying capacity of dry smoke and is capable of causing more extensive thermal damage of the tracheobronchial tree.[48]

Presenting patient signs and symptoms are stridor, hypoxia, and respiratory distress.[49] The probability that a patient has suffered an inhalation injury is highly correlated with being burned in an enclosed space, having burns of the head and neck, and having elevated carbon monoxide levels. The extent and severity of the inhalation injury are directly related to the duration of exposure and to the various toxins contained within the smoke. Injury caused by heat is typically confined to the upper airway and supraglottic structures.[50] Particulate material within smoke is the vehicle by which the toxic materials are carried to the distal airway. Particles of less than 5 μm in size can reach the terminal bronchi and the alveoli. Upper airway injuries involve the mucous membranes, nasopharynx, hypopharynx, epiglottis, glottis, and larynx. The lining mucous membranes as well as the cartilage of the glottis are easily damaged and can cause acute airway compromise.[50] Direct thermal injury to the lower airway is uncommon as rapid dissipation of heat occurs as the gases move through the upper airway. Injury to the tracheobronchial structures and pulmonary parenchyma is related to the toxins in the inhaled smoke and to the ensuing host inflammatory response. Activation of the inflammatory cascade results in the recruitment of neutrophils and macrophages, which propagate the injury.[51] Cellular damage is perpetuated by those cells that further the inflammatory response, which in turn leads to progressive pulmonary dysfunction.[52] Altered surfactant release causes obstruction and collapse of distal airway segments.[53] As part of the response to injury there is a marked and near-immediate change in bronchial artery blood flow, which can increase by up to 20-fold.[50] These changes in bronchial blood flow are also associated with marked alterations in vascular permeability within the lung and are thought to play an important role in the pathophysiologic response to inhalation injuries.[54] The net effect is that extensive destruction and inflammation reduce pulmonary compliance and impair gas exchange, resulting in altered pulmonary blood flow patterns and ventilation perfusion mismatches.[55]

Asphyxiants

Carbon monoxide and cyanide gases are present in smoke and when inhaled are rapidly absorbed and cause systemic toxicity as well as impaired oxygen utilization and delivery. Carbon monoxide is an odorless, nonirritating gas that rapidly diffuses into the bloodstream and rapidly binds to the iron moiety of the hemoglobin molecule. Carbon monoxide has a 240 times greater affinity for hemoglobin than does oxygen; thus, it easily displaces oxygen. Carbon monoxide directly impairs the ability of hemoglobin to deliver oxygen to the tissues. Carbon monoxide also binds to enzymes within the mitochondria involved in intracellular oxygen utilization and cellular energetics.[56] Signs and symptoms of carbon monoxide poisoning are typically mild to none when carbon monoxide-hemoglobin (carboxyhemoglobin) levels are 10% or less. When carboxyhemoglobin levels are between 10% and 30%, symptoms are present and often manifested by headache and dizziness. Severe poisoning is seen in patients with carboxyhemoglobin levels of greater than 50%, which can be associated with syncope, seizures, and coma.

The diagnosis of carbon monoxide poisoning is made in a patient with burns on the basis of circumstances of injury, physical findings, and the measurement of blood carboxyhemoglobin level. It is important to note that pulse oximetry values do not differentiate between carboxyhemoglobin and oxyhemoglobin. Patients with significant carbon monoxide intoxication can have elevated oxygen saturations but will not have satisfactory blood oxygen contents. The primary treatment modality for carbon monoxide intoxication is provision of increased levels of inspired oxygen. The carbon monoxide half-life will decrease from 6 to 8 hours with room air to 40 to 80 minutes with 100% of FiO$_2$. Administration of oxygen in a hyperbaric chamber can further decrease the half-life to 15 to 30 minutes.[57] In a recently reported randomized trial, Weaver and colleagues[58] found that hyperbaric oxygen therapy significantly benefitted patients with acute carbon monoxide poisoning. The utility of this for patients suffering major burns in association with carbon monoxide poisoning is yet to be demonstrated. It is a significant practical question whether a patient can safely undergo treatment with hyperbaric oxygen therapy when there are other life-saving treatments that are needed. An approach that has worked well is to maintain the patient on 100% FiO$_2$ until carboxyhemoglobin levels are less than 15% and then to maintain this level of increased oxygen for an additional 6 hours at which time weaning of the FiO$_2$ can be initiated and conducted in accordance with standard criteria.

TABLE 9.4. Toxic agents in smoke.

Irritant	Characteristics	Mechanism of toxicity
Acrolein	Lipophilic	Direct epithelial damage
Hydrogen chloride	Water soluble	Forms free radicals
Phosgene	Low solubility	Causes the release of arachidonic acid metabolites
Ammonia	Water soluble	Forms hydroxyl ions and causes liquefactive necrosis
Nitric oxide	Lipid soluble	Causes lipid peroxidation
Sulfur dioxide	Water soluble	Causes lipid peroxidation

Cyanide poisoning, which can occur in combination with carbon monoxide intoxication, further disrupts normal cellular utilization of oxygen by binding to the cytochrome oxidase, resulting in cellular lactic acid production and greater cellular dysfunction.[59] Blood concentrations of cyanide greater than 0.5 mg/L are toxic. Treatment of cyanide poisoning includes the administration of oxygen as well as decontaminating agents such as amyl and sodium nitrates. These compounds induce the formation of methemoglobin, which can act as a scavenger of cyanide.[60] Sodium thiosulfate, which can be administered intravenously, enhances the enzymatic detoxification of cyanide to thiocyanate but acts slowly. Hydroxycobalamin, which acts more rapidly and has few side effects, is the antidote of choice.

Smoke can also contain a variety of toxic compounds that cause or initiate further damage to the airway (Table 9.4). The composition of each fire is different, adding to the difficulty in caring for these patients. Such additional products in smoke include acrolein, hydrogen chloride, phosgene, ammonia, nitric oxide, and sulfur dioxide all of which are capable of causing significant injury.

Airway Management

The most critical factors in the initial assessment of a burn patient are the patency of the airway and the ability of the patient to maintain and protect the airway. Standard criteria should be used to determine the need for mechanical stabilization of the airway, also keeping in mind the systemic response to a major burn and the local response to an airway injury, which can combine to cause progressive airway swelling and edema that will impair air flow. In an adult trachea of 14 mm, 1 mm of edema will result in a 25% reduction in cross-sectional area. A similar degree of swelling in a 6-mm trachea of a child will result in greater than a 50% reduction in cross-sectional area. Circumferential torso burns will further impair the ability of the patient to respire. Allowing airway compromise to proceed to a critical state before intubating the patient and stabilizing the airway is not appropriate care. The safest approach when there is

concern about the airway, particularly in a patient needing transport for definitive care, is to perform early intubation.

Part of the initial management of the patient with inhalation injury should include a thorough evaluation of the airway, including bronchoscopy. The clinical findings of an inhalation injury on bronchoscopy include airway edema, inflammation, increased bronchial secretions, presence of carbonaceous material that can diffusely carpet the airway, mucosal ulcerations, and even endoluminal obliteration caused by sloughing mucosa, mucous plugging, and cast formation (Figure 9.5). Signs of gastric aspiration may also be evident. Repeat bronchoscopy can be performed for removal of debris and casts as well as surveillance for infection.[61]

Direct airway treatment has been attempted but with variable responses. Nakae and colleagues[61] conducted an open-label trial of the use of aerosolized heparin and n-acetylcysteine in children with inhalation injuries. The treated patients had an improved outcome compared with an untreated cohort.[61] As of yet, a randomized prospective study has not yet been performed to confirm the utility of this approach particularly for adults. One noticeable effect with the empiric use of aerosolized heparin is the rapid clearing of particulate material and carbonaceous deposits from the airway. Inasmuch as the development of pneumonia in patients with inhalation

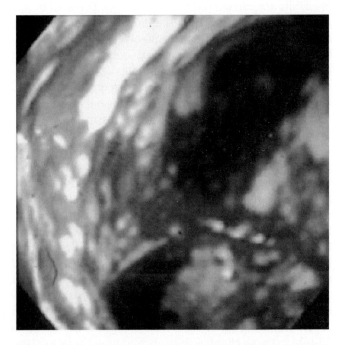

FIGURE 9.5. Endoscopic view of a bronchus in a patient with severe inhalation injury. Note bright white areas reflecting light from edematous mucosa, erythema, and focal ulceration of other areas of the mucosa and the extensive black carbonaceous material from the smoke deposited on the endobronchial surface.

injuries negatively impacts outcome, it is disappointing that prophylactic antibiotics have not been effective.[62] As a practical matter, it is best to culture these patients early to identify the organisms that have colonized their airways as a consequence of their injury and urgent airway manipulation. This information can guide therapy should the patient develop the signs and symptoms of early-onset pneumonia. Steroids are not recommended for patients suffering inhalation injuries.[63]

Mechanical Ventilation

The critical feature in the management of patients suffering inhalation injuries is to minimize further damage to the airway and lung parenchyma while providing adequate gas exchange.[64] A critical feature in the management of patients with inhalation injuries is to control airway pressures and thereby limit ventilation-induced barotraumas.[49,65] It is important to recognize that lung damage is not homogenous but patchy in distribution and requires that the level of positive end-expiratory pressure (PEEP) used to maximize airway recruitment be limited to avoid ventilator-associated lung injury.[66,67] In states of severe lung injury, mechanical ventilation can lead to increases in sheer forces and changes in pulmonary blood flow. This in association with reductions in elasticity and alterations in lung compliance results in further lung injury and ventilation perfusion abnormalities.[68,69]

Using a standard volume mode of ventilation does not represent the best management of the damaged airway. Inverse ratio ventilation provides a strategy one can use in an attempt to counteract these changes and allow reductions in the level of PEEP and respiratory pressures to improve oxygenation.[70] Unfortunately, a clear advantage of inverse ratio ventilation over standard approaches has not been consistently shown.[71] An alternative strategy is high-frequency ventilation in which rapid respiratory rates and small tidal volumes are used to achieve adequate oxygenation and ventilation while minimizing barotrauma.[72] The three major types of high-frequency ventilation are high-frequency interrupted flow positive pressure ventilation, high-frequency jet ventilation, and high-frequency oscillation. High-frequency interrupted flow positive pressure ventilation delivers small tidal volumes (4 mL/kg) at flow rates of 250 L/min with a frequency of 100 breaths per minute. In this mode, expiration is passive and thus there is an increased risk of air trapping and overdistention. High-frequency jet ventilation employs small tidal volumes and high respiratory rates, with the volumes determined by jet velocity and duration of flow. High-frequency oscillation maintains lung volumes by applying a constant airway pressure but does not allow for patient-triggered inspiratory flow. With this mode of ventilation, inspiration and expiration are active processes, and air trapping is reduced.

Patient oxygenation is maintained by increasing the mean airway pressure until an adequate oxygen level is achieved, whereas ventilation is achieved by oscillating airway pressure through electromagnetically driven pistons that deliver cyclic tidal volumes and facilitate ventilation. There has been limited experience with the use of extracorporeal membrane oxygenation in the management of inhalation injuries in selected centers.[73]

An approach that has worked well with many patients with inhalation injuries has been to identify promptly the presence of airway compromise and ensure that the patient is intubated with a properly sized endotracheal tube. Currently, it is our preference for the pediatric population to use a cuffed tube that may need to be inflated to achieve maximum ventilatory efficiency. For those patients who are seen to have signs of inhalation injury on bronchoscopy, there is aggressive management of retained secretions with the use of bronchodilators and mucolytic agents along with aerosolized heparin. Meticulous control of airway pressure is practiced with the early performance of torso escharotomies and prompt treatment of an abdominal compartment syndrome particularly in the burned child. Mean airway pressures are maintained at less than 32 to 34 cm H_2O, and ready use is made of chemical paralysis of the patient with a low threshold for conversion to pressure-controlled ventilation with titration of tidal volumes to lessen further the risk of ventilator-associated barotrauma. This may require the acceptance of smaller than usual tidal volumes and permissive hypercapnia, which is acceptable as long as arterial blood pH is above 7.26 and the patient is hemodynamically stable. These approaches along with a tightly controlled fluid resuscitation will in most circumstances avoid the need for alternative ventilator strategies in the care of these patients. Others, including one of the authors (B.A.P.), prefer to use high-frequency interrupted flow positive pressure ventilation (HFIFPP) prophylactically. For all patients with inhalation injury, HFIFPP ventilation is initiated on admission to minimize airway obstruction, maintain lung volume, and reduce the risk of pneumonia.

Other Organ System Support

Pain Control

The pain experienced by patients suffering from acute thermal injuries is a complex integration of the objective neurologic input from the damaged tissue and the patient's fear and anxiety resulting from the traumatic event. The patient's pain is compounded further by wound care and the therapy required to maintain functional status. If the patient begins to perceive that there is no escape from the situation, his or her fear and anxiety will be amplified and may be magnified further by the appearance and expression of concern by family and friends. Furthermore, as the burn begins to heal, there may be increased wound sensitivity during dressing changes and therapy sessions. This can further distress patients, as they perceive that, instead of the pain improving with recovery it seems to be worsening. Pain is a fifth vital sign, and it should be monitored, its level documented, and treatment be properly planned. Appropriate therapeutic options must be available to provide patients with pain control.

For patients who are hospitalized for on-going care or require surgery, it is best to initiate long-acting oral narcotic agents for background pain control and administer shorter acting narcotics either orally or parenterally, along with anxiolytic agents, for procedure-related pain. For an acutely injured patient undergoing a procedure in the ICU or ward, intravenous morphine remains the mainstay for analgesia along with oral compounds such as hydrocodone, which is preferable to oxycodone, which has a greater propensity for abuse. Clonidine can also be added to the pain regimen for patients who are having an initial poor response to narcotics and anxiolytic agents.[74] For patients who are intubated and being maintained on mechanical ventilation, the continuous administration of intravenous morphine and diazepam or propofol and fentanyl are two commonly used regimens to achieve pain control and sedation and prevent unplanned extubation. In the postoperative care of patients having skin graft procedures, the most painful wound is often not the burn wound but the donor site. Jellish et al.[75] have reported that the treatment of the skin graft harvest site with local anesthetic agents significantly improved the patient's pain score postoperatively. Patient-controlled analgesia is also a very effective strategy for patients who understand and can manipulate the delivery system. An important factor leading to effective pain control is to have established protocols that all members of the team understand and can use safely. There must be flexibility in the medication regimen, and the patients must be fully informed that every attempt will be made to provide them the greatest comfort within the context of safe and compassionate care.

Neurologic Deficits

Immediately following burn injury the patient with an altered mental status needs to undergo a careful evaluation for injuries occurring during and prior to the time of the fire. Additionally, the patient's preinjury neurologic status needs to be determined for any prior impairment. For patients who are obtunded, the primary concern is central nervous system injury caused by hypoxia and carbon monoxide poisoning. The use of alcohol or drugs during the time leading up to the burn injury can con-

found the assessment of the burn-injured victim. Testing for alcohol and drugs aids in the evaluation of such patients.[76] This is particularly important because the impact of alcohol appears to significantly modify the patient's chance for survival. The patient, particularly an elderly patient, should also be evaluated for a primary central nervous system event that might have precipitated the injury, such as a seizure, stroke, or intracranial hemorrhage. The possibility of an assault must always be foremost in one's thoughts, particularly for children, when the history of the injury does not match the findings. It is not uncommon that a burn is a signal finding for child abuse.[77] This can also be the case for adults when the initial event was an assault and the burn is an attempt to disguise the physical attack.

Patients presenting with agitation must be rapidly evaluated for hypoxia and treated. The initial management of a patient who has a deteriorating mental status is a review of the medications and medication doses that have been administered to determine whether reversal agents should be given. In the treatment of children, the doses should be age and weight appropriate and carefully titrated to the patient's need. Later in the course of a burn patient's care, changes in mental status require a detailed review of medications for pain and sedation, measurement of serum electrolyte values particularly sodium, and evaluation for a septic process and the onset of renal or hepatic failure. Patients with impaired mental status either early or late must always be assessed for the status of their airway, their ability to maintain a patent airway, and the need for tracheal intubation.

Gastrointestinal Responses and Complications

Impaired GI motility and focal gastric mucosal ischemia occur in virtually all patients with burns involving more than 25% of the total body surface, with the severity of change proportional to the extent of the burn.[78] The resulting ileus necessitates nasogastric intubation to prevent emesis and aspiration. If the mucosa is unprotected by instillation of antacid or treatment with an H_2 histamine receptor antagonist, ischemic erosions in the mucosa may progress to frank ulceration with associated bleeding or even perforation. Sufficient antacid (typically 30 mL, but 60 mL may be needed) should be instilled each hour to maintain the pH of the gastric contents above 5. At present, a histamine H_2 receptor antagonist (e.g., 400 mg of cimetadine given intravenously every 4 hours) or proton pump inhibitors are more commonly used for stress ulcer prophylaxis. When GI motility returns, enteral feeding should be initiated, and the antacid therapy (e.g., a 1,200–2,400 mg daily dose of cimetadine) can be added to enteral feeds. A randomized study comparing antacid prophylaxis and nonacid buffering sucralfate prophylaxis showed no difference in recovery of

Gram-negative organisms from the upper GI tract and no difference in the occurrence of Gram-negative pneumonia, but lesser gastric mucosal protection and a higher incidence of Gram-positive pneumonia in the sucralfate-treated group.[79]

Wound Care

Initial Wound Care

Initial wound care is focused on preventing further injury. Immediately upon removal of the burn victim from the site of injury, attention should be given to removing burning clothing, disrupting contact with metal objects that may retain heat, and cooling of any molten materials adherent to the skin surface. Attempted cooling of burn wounds must be done with caution as local vasoconstriction can impair wound blood flow and extend the depth of the injury. The use of surface cooling of the burn is limited to patients with small burns typically not requiring hospitalization. Hypothermia can rapidly occur in children as well as adults, particularly elderly patients, if they are placed in cool or wet dressings. Patients being prepared for transport or admitted for definitive care should be placed in sterile or clean dry dressings and be kept warm. Prolonged exposure of the burn victim's wounds leads to cooling and further impairs the patient's response to the injury. Items of clothing or jewelry that may impair circulation should be removed before the onset of burn wound edema to prevent further compromise of the circulation. In cases of chemical injury, removal of contaminated clothing with copious water lavage of liquid chemicals and removal by brushing of powdered materials at the scene can limit the extent of the resultant burn injury. The ability to perform these maneuvers at the scene must be balanced against the patient's associated injuries that would mandate immediate transport for the care of life-threatening injuries. No attempt should be made at chemical neutralization of the suspected chemical agent, as such treatment would result in an exothermic reaction and cause additional tissue damage. The care provider must exercise extreme caution when working with victims of chemical injury to prevent self-contamination and personal injury. In all circumstances, the individuals caring for burn patients should wear personal protection devices

After admission to the hospital and as soon as resuscitative measures have been instituted the patient should be bathed and the burn wounds cleansed with a detergent disinfectant. Chlorhexidine gluconate is a cleansing agent with an excellent antimicrobial spectrum. During cleansing of the wound the patient must not be allowed to become hypothermic. The treatment area and the cleansing fluids should be warm, and the procedure should be done expeditiously. Materials that are densely adherent to the wound, such as wax, tar, plastic, and metal, should be gently removed or allowed to separate during the course of subsequent dressing changes. Sloughing skin, devitalized tissue, and ruptured blisters should be gently trimmed from the wound. No formal attempt is made to remove the burned tissue during these wound-dressing debridements. Patients may experience considerable pain and apprehension during these dressing changes and should receive adequate pain medication. For the patient on whom blisters are present, whether to remove them or allow them to remain is a matter of opinion. Blisters that are intact, particularly thick blisters on the palm of a hand, maybe left intact.[80] Intact blisters must be closely monitored for signs of infection or rupture at which time they should be debrided and the wound treated. If a blister can be kept intact, wound healing should be complete in less than 3 weeks. The idea that intact blisters are an effective biologic dressing has been called into question, and some authors recommend removing all blisters and treating the burn as an open wound.[21,81,82] Careful wound cleansing should be done at each dressing change, with serial debridement of devitalized tissue performed as necessary. The wound should be monitored for signs of infection and change in depth from the initial assessment. It is not uncommon for the initial wound depth to have been underestimated in children and young women. Additionally, the extent of body surface involvement should be recalculated to ensure that the initial burn size determination was accurate.

Topical Antimicrobial Therapy

The burn injury sets in progress a series of events leading to impaired local and systemic immunity. The damaged skin surface can serve as the portal for microbial invasion if it becomes progressively colonized. As microbial numbers increase within the wound to levels of 100,000 organisms per gram of tissue, an invasive wound infection and ultimately systemic sepsis may occur. Topically applied antimicrobial agents, which penetrate the burn eschar, are capable of achieving sufficient levels to control microbial proliferation within the wound. Systemic antibiotics do not achieve sufficiently high concentrations in the wound to achieve therapeutic levels, as the eschar is in large part avascular. These concepts form the basis for the use of topical antimicrobial agents in the prophylactic treatment of the burn wound and as a part of the management of burn wound infections.[83] Topical agents per se do not heal the wound but prevent local burn wound infection from destroying viable tissue in wounds capable of spontaneous healing. For burns that will require excision and grafting, control of the burn wound microbial environment prevents the development of systemic sepsis secondary to invasive burn wound sepsis. The utility of topical agents is most clearly apparent in improving patient outcome in burns of greater than 30% total body surface area. The need for topical antimicrobial compounds in the management of small burns has never been demonstrated, and these injuries can be effectively managed with a petroleum-based dressing.[84-87] That being said, it has become common practice to apply topical antimicrobial agents even to small burn wounds despite the fact that there are no data to support this approach. Topical antimicrobial burn wound agents include cream, ointment, and liquid-based products that require daily to twice daily dressing changes and reapplication. Also available are materials impregnated with antimicrobial compounds that typically are changed following a several-day period of application.

Silver sulfadiazine, the most widely used agent, is available as a 1% suspension in a water-soluble micronized cream base. The cream is easily applied, causes little or no pain on application, and can be used open or as a closed dressing. As a closed dressing, the cream can be directly applied to the wound as a continuous layer and then covered over with a dressing or be impregnated into the dressing, which is then applied to the wound. At each dressing change the cream should be totally removed and not allowed to form a caseous layer that will obscure the wound bed. When silver sulfadiazine is used in the management of superficial partial-thickness burns, the dressing becomes discolored, the wound exudate appears infected, and the wound develops a yellow-gray pseudoeschar that is easily removed. The ability of silver sulfadiazine to penetrate an eschar and prevent wound infectious complications in burns of more than 40% to 50% total body surface area is thought to be poor. However, wound cleansing with chlorhexidine as a part of the wound management along with silver sulfadiazine has proved to be a very effective combination for patients with larger burns. The most common toxic side effect of silver sulfadiazine is a transient leukopenia, which, when it does occur in up to 15% of treated patients, resolves spontaneously without discontinuation of the drug.[88] The proposed mechanisms for this response have ranged from leukocyte margination in the wound (not drug related) to a direct cytotoxic effect of the drug on the bone marrow granulocyte and macrophage progenitor cells.[89] Silver sulfadiazine is active against a wide range of microbes, including *Staphylococcus aureus*, *Escherichia coli*, *Klebsiella* species, many but not all *Pseudomonas aeruginosa* infections, *Proteus* species, and *Candida albicans*.

Mafenide acetate was one of the first effective topical agents introduced for the management of the burn wound. It was initially available as Sulfamylon burn cream (an 11.1% suspension in a vanishing cream base). It is commonly used on exposed wounds treated by the open technique, although it is possible to use it under a light dressing. Mafenide acetate is highly effective against Gram-positive and Gram-negative organisms but provides little antifungal activity.[90] Mafenide acetate readily diffuses into the eschar and is the agent of choice for significant burns of the ears because it is also capable of penetrating cartilage. Drawbacks with the use of mafenide acetate include pain on application to partial-thickness burns and limited activity against methicillin-resistant *S. aureus*. Mafenide acetate also inhibits carbonic anhydrase, which increases urinary loss of bicarbonate, which may cause hyperchloremic acidosis and accentuate postburn hyperventilation. Fortunately, this effect is time limited, because the kidney typically escapes from such inhibition in 8 to 10 days. Mafenide acetate has more recently become available as a 5% aqueous solution and is an excellent agent to use on freshly grafted wounds and is not associated with the problems found with the cream formulation.

Silver nitrate as a 0.5% solution has been available since the 1960s and is effective against Gram-positive and Gram-negative organisms. The silver moiety is deposited on the burn wound and does not penetrate the eschar to any great extent. Silver nitrate soak solution leaches sodium, potassium, chloride, and calcium from the wound in association with transeschar water absorption, which can result in mineral deficits, alkalosis, and water loading. These side effects can be minimized by giving sodium and other mineral supplements and by modifying fluid therapy. These problems and the labor required to use silver nitrate effectively limit its routine use currently, and most see silver sulfadiazine as a highly acceptable alternative.

Silver-impregnated dressings consisting of a polyethylene mesh coated with a nanocrystalline film of pure silver ions bonded to a flexible rayon-polyester sheet have recently become available for clinical use (Figure 9.6).[91] When the fabric base is in contact with wound fluids, the silver is released continuously and serves as the antimicrobial agent deposited onto the wound. The treatment interval with such a composite may extend up to several days, depending on the fabrication design, with dressing changes needed only once or twice per week. This approach approximates the therapeutic utility of silver nitrate and has not been associated with the problems found with silver nitrate. However, one must know that the wound has not become compromised during the extended treatment periods. It is not advisable to use this approach in the care of perineal wounds, particularly in small children with frequent bowel movements or wounds with excessive drainage or difficulty in maintaining contact between the dressing and the burn wound surface. The effectiveness of this membrane in treating extensive full-thickness burns is unconfirmed, and at present it is used to treat partial-thickness burns.

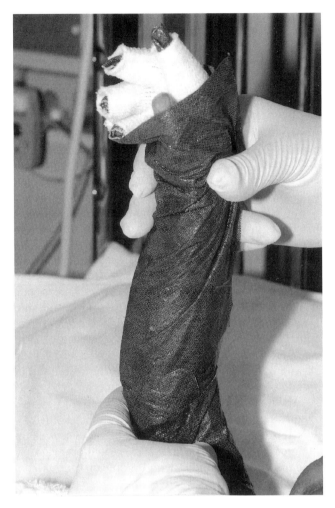

burn team to make a precise assessment of the extent of the burn and the depth of injury. In addition to burn wound evaluation, the burned child must be inspected for any signs of abuse, which includes a detailed examination of the entire skin surface. Unless there will be an extended period of time before patient transfer to a burn center, placing the patient in a dry dressing, particularly if it is one with a nonadherent lining, and keeping the patient warm is the preferred initial management.

The sterilely gloved hand is used to apply the burn cream of choice in a thickness sufficient to obscure the surface of the burn (Figure 9.7). The wounds are then either left exposed or covered by a light occlusive dressing. Twelve hours later the topical agent is reapplied to the entirety of the burn wound. If a dressing is used over the topical agent, it is removed before reapplication of the topical agent, following which a new dressing is applied. To optimize antimicrobial coverage and

FIGURE 9.6. Microbial control can be achieved in partial-thickness burn wounds by application of a polyethylene mesh coated with a nanocrystalline film of pure silver ions as shown here. When in contact with wound fluids, the silver is released continuously to limit bacterial proliferation on and in the wound.

For superficial partial-thickness burns the use of bacitracin ointment represents a satisfactory alternative particularly for patients with a known sulfa allergy. It may be used open, especially with superficial facial burns, or as a component of a closed dressing. Other topical agents include antibiotic combinations such as triple antibiotic ointment (neomycin, bacitracin zinc, and polymyxin B) and polysporin (bacitracin zinc and polymyxin B). In the case of methicillin-resistant staphylococci, mupirocin is a useful agent.[92] These agents are also capable of being used with open or closed dressing techniques.

The application of topical antimicrobial agents to the burns of patients who will be transferred to a burn center may preclude the use of biologic membrane dressings that must adhere to the wound surface to be effective. Additionally, upon admission to a burn center, any previously placed dressing must be removed to permit the

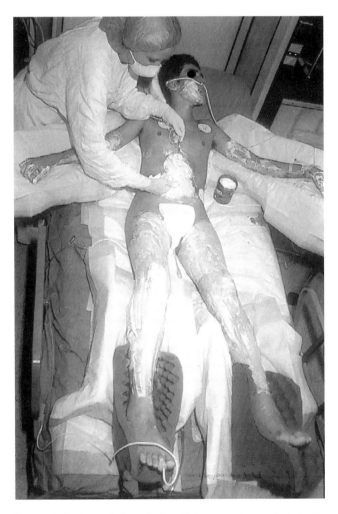

FIGURE 9.7. A topical antimicrobial cream is applied to the entirety of the burn wound as shown here after the daily wound cleansing and inspection procedure. The topical agent is reapplied 12 hours later to maintain microbial control.

minimize side effects, one can alternate topical agents (i.e., apply Sulfamylon burn cream after the morning cleansing and apply Silvadene burn cream in the evening).[93] If 0.5% silver nitrate soaks are used for topical wound care (as may be necessary for a patient allergic to sulfonamides), they should be changed two or three times a day and kept moist between changes by infusing additional soak solution every 2 hours. All environmental surfaces and equipment as well as the clothing and exposed skin of attending personnel must be protected from contact with the silver nitrate solution, which will cause dark-brown discoloration of virtually anything with which it comes in contact.

Each day the topical agent is totally removed in the course of the daily cleansing, and the entirety of the burn wound is examined to detect any signs of infection. If signs of infection are identified, a biopsy specimen of the eschar and the underlying viable tissue should be obtained from the area of the wound suspected of harboring infection. The biopsy sample is subjected to histologic examination and should also be cultured to determine predominant organisms. Histologic confirmation of invasive infection (the presence of bacteria or fungi in viable tissue underlying or adjacent to the burned tissue) necessitates a change to Sulfamylon burn cream topical therapy (mafenide acetate can diffuse into nonviable tissue to limit microbial proliferation), subeschar antibiotic infusion, physiologic fine tuning of the patient, and prompt surgical excision of the infected tissue.[94]

Burn Wound Excision and Grafting

Excision of the burned tissue and grafting is required for wounds that are full thickness in depth and is now considered to be the optimum management of wounds with a mixed depth of injury. Wounds that are capable of spontaneous closure within 2 to 3 weeks postinjury can be managed expectantly provided the cosmetic and functional outcomes will be acceptable. Wounds that will require a longer period of time to close, in general, develop significant scarring, painful or unstable scars, intense pruritus, and, in areas of function, delayed return or even loss of functional capacity. Many such wounds will require revision at a later time, with the patient having needlessly been denied the appropriate care. Wounds that are assessed as needing excision and closure should undergo removal as soon as possible. Jackson and associates[95] demonstrated in the 1950s the feasibility of burn wound excision and closure in wounds of up to 30% total body surface area. Present-day management of burn patients has extended this approach to all but the most massive of burn injuries.

If the patient is otherwise stable, burn wound excision can be carried out within a matter of hours postinjury. For the patient with a small burn, delay is often related to scheduling of the operating room and the surgical team. Timely excision for the patient with a small burn reduces the period of disability and the overall cost of the injury. For patients with a large burn wound, the timing and extent of the surgery are based on the patient's relative physiologic stability and capacity to undergo a major operative procedure. Early burn wound excision and closure in patients with large wounds shortens the length of hospitalization, reduces cost, and favorably impacts overall burn mortality.[96,97] The presence of the burn wound is the primary stimulus for the ongoing problems facing the burn patient. Closure of the burn serves to ameliorate much of the postburn pathophysiology and is one of the most effective means by which to improve a burn patient's outcome.

Wounds that are small in size or linear in shape can be managed by excision of the burn and primary wound closure. This is useful for burns of the upper inner arm in the elderly, localized burns of a pendulous breast, abdominal burns, buttock injuries, and thigh burns. Primary wound closure can also be achieved in some wounds with local tissue transfer techniques. This approach works quite well when these wounds are excised early, before significant microbial colonization of the wound occurs. In such cases, the burn is transformed into a healing surgical incision and creation of a skin graft donor site is avoided.

For selected cases the injury may be of such a nature that amputation of the burned part is the most appropriate plan. For the patient with significant multisystem trauma, the expeditious removal of the burn injury might be seen as the best option for the patient's overall survival. In a recent study, Santaniello and associates[98] found that the mortality rate for trauma victims with significant burn injuries and trauma was 28.3%, whereas for patients with burns only it was 9.8% and for patients with trauma only it was 4.3%. The management of these challenging patients requires a coordinated, well-conceived plan of care that accounts for all of the patient's injuries and integrates the treatment needs of each injury to achieve an overall satisfactory outcome. A mangled extremity, which has also suffered a severe burn that is deemed nonsalvageable, should undergo early amputation. It is not necessary to extend the amputation to a level that allows closure with unburned tissue. If viable muscle is available to close the amputation site, the wound bed can be resurfaced with an autogenous skin graft. A grafted amputation site can, with a modern prosthesis, function as a durable stump. For a patient who is paraplegic and suffers an extensive deep lower extremity burn injury, amputation can be a viable alternative to excision and grafting.

A similar option may need to be considered for the patient in whom significant preexisting peripheral vascular disease makes the likelihood of a healed and functional extremity highly unlikely. This unfortunately has become an all too frequent occurrence in the care of elderly burn patients who have progressive complications from long-standing diabetes mellitus. The amputation level should be that which will maintain maximum function. This might be a transmetatarsal or Chopart-type amputation for patients with injuries of the distal foot. For patients confined to a wheelchair who have injuries to the leg, a through-knee amputation as opposed to an above-knee amputation provides a weight-bearing platform for sitting. For the patient in whom the initial insult represents a deep composite injury, repeated failed attempts at salvage are not in the patient's ultimate best interest. Such wounds often become infected, and tissue that could have been preserved now must in the end be sacrificed with the functional end result less than that which would have occurred with early amputation.

Excision and grafting will be required for wounds not amenable to primary closure. The extent of the procedure that a patient can undergo is related to the patient's age and physiologic status and to the skill of the operating team. A 17% surface area burn should be a universally survivable injury for a 17-year-old patient, whereas for a patient in the eighth decade of life the mortality rate can easily be 50%. An otherwise healthy individual with available donor sites can well tolerate a 20% to 25% total body burn excision and autografting in one procedure. Implicit in this approach is the use of experienced operating teams, an anesthesiologist who thoroughly understands the unique problems of the patient with a major body surface area burn, and an operating room fully equipped to treat such a patient, as well as ready availability of blood products and the capacity to care for the patient postoperatively. A patient having this extent of surgery in essence undergoes a doubling of the surface area of "injury"—the now excised and grafted wound along with the partial-thickness wound produced by the donor site. For patients with wounds of a larger size (>30% total body surface area) or those who cannot tolerate a single procedure to achieve closure, staged excision of burned tissue is performed, and the resulting wounds are closed with available cutaneous autografts or a biologic dressing.[99]

The technique of burn wound excision is based on the depth of the wound and anatomic site to be excised. Excision of deep partial-thickness wounds to the level of a uniformly viable bed of deep dermis, by the tangential technic pioneered by Janzekovic,[100] and immediate coverage with cutaneous autograft results in rapid wound closure with a typically excellent result. This can be done with an unguarded Weck knife, a Goulian-guarded Weck knife, a handheld dermatome, or a powered dermatome set at 0.0016 to 0.0030 of an inch, depending on the area to be excised and the age and gender of the patient. Optimally, the desired wound bed is achieved in one pass of the knife as evidenced by diffuse bleeding. If this endpoint is not realized, another pass of the knife will be

needed. A frequent error is attempting this technique in wounds of an inappropriate depth and assuming that punctuate bleeding indicates a viable bed. Such wounds will heal with a poor take of the grafted skin as the bed contains marginally viable tissue incapable of supporting the cutaneous autograft. These wounds at the initial graft dressing change may appear to be doing well only to fail at 5 to 10 days postoperatively. Tangential excision as originally reported was employed early in the first week postburn; however, it can be successfully applied any time to a wound that is not infected or heavily colonized. During the performance of this procedure, the amount of blood loss can be minimized with the use of a tourniquet on extremity burns or subeschar clysis containing epinephrine. The decision that the depth of the excision is satisfactory with these adjuncts will be based primarily on the appearance of the wound, an appreciation of which most experienced burn surgeons have had to learn to some degree through trial and error.

A modification of tangential excision is wound excision via layered escharectomy. With this technique, the wound is sequentially excised to a viable bed of subcutaneous tissue and elements of deep dermis particularly at the wound margin. This allows relative preservation of body part contour, a graft with ultimately more pliability, decreased limb edema, and a cosmetically more acceptable transition at the juncture of the grafted wound with the unburned skin of the wound margins.

An alternative to layered excision is to excise the wound with a scalpel or electrocautery. Using knife excision, the wound is excised to the muscle fascia or to viable deep subcutaneous tissue. Bleeding can be significant with such procedures; therefore, the excision and control of bleeding must be done efficiently. The use of electrocautery to perform the dissection limits the blood loss without compromising the recipient graft site. Imperative with electrocautery excision into the deep fat is avoidance and limitation of thermal injury to the wound bed, which will compromise the "take" of the applied skin graft. The use of the cutting mode with rapid dissection is necessary. When excision to fascia has been performed, the viability of the fascia should be assessed. The surgeon must determine if the fascia requires removal and the underlying muscle used as the graft bed. In the performance of fascial excisions caution should be exercised during the dissection to avoid entrance into a joint or bursa and injury of extensor tendons in the hand or the Achilles' tendon at the ankle.

The blood loss occurring with burn wound excision is related to the time of excision postburn, the area to be excised, the presence of infection, and type of excision (i.e., fascial or tangential). Donor sites can also represent a significant portion of the blood loss. The use of the scalp or previously harvested donor sites is associated with increased bleeding. The quantity of blood loss has been estimated to range from 0.45 to $1.25\,mL/cm^2$ burn area excised.[101] Adjunctive measures that can be used to control blood loss include elevation of limbs undergoing excision, applications of topical thrombin and/or vaso-constrictive agents in solutions to the excised wound and donor site, clysis of skin graft harvest sites and/or the eschar prior to removal, and application of tourniquets. Spray application of fibrin sealant can also reduce bleeding from the excised wound after release of the tourniquet. Blood loss will be compounded if the patient has become coagulopathic, hypothermic, or acidotic during the procedure. Perioperative cold stress, which may induce hypothermia, can be reduced by maintaining the temperature of the operating room between 30° and 32°C and by using warmed fluids for wound irrigation. The harvest, application, and postoperative care of split-thickness skin grafts and skin graft donor sites are the same as for any other surgical patient.

Grafting of the burn wound is usually done at the time of excision. However, there are instances when it is advisable to stage the skin-grafting procedure. The surgeon must be aware of the patient's status throughout the surgical procedure and if necessary reassess the extent of the planned procedure. It may be best to perform the excision only and to stage the timing of skin graft application. Additionally, if the wound bed is suspect as to its viability, then only excision should be performed. The wound can be dressed with a 5% Sulfamylon solution dressing or covered with allograft skin or any of several biologic dressings and subsequently reevaluated. The cutaneous allograft is a very useful approach when excising facial burns where the goal is to preserve all possible elements and perform the definitive grafting procedure on a "tested" recipient bed. When an infected wound is being excised, no attempt at placing autograft skin should be considered until the infection has been resolved following treatment with topical and systemic antimicrobial agents as determined by culture results and inspection of the wound.

The choice of the donor site for the performance of a cutaneous autograft will in some patients be limited to those skin sites that have not been injured with burns. When there is a choice of donor sites, the requirements of the recipient site and the potential for donor site morbidity should be factored into selecting the site of graft harvest. In the grafting of facial burns, color match is an important consideration, and obtaining a graft from a site above the clavicles or the inner aspect of the thigh will provide the best result. For children, harvest of a graft from the scalp results in a donor site that is not particularly painful postoperatively and has no long-term cosmetic consequences. The harvest of grafts from posterior body surfaces provides, in general, a more acceptable wound for most patients. Although the anterior thigh is an often-selected site, it can heal with significant hyper-

trophic change and cause a patient more problems and distress than the grafted burn.

The use of sheets of autograft skin for resurfacing the burn represents the gold standard. This is the only acceptable approach for burns of the face and neck and the best choice in grafting of the hands and breast. Every attempt should be made to use such autografts in children, because they provide the best long-term results. It may not be possible to achieve these objectives for patients with extensive burns or for those in whom the pattern and location of the injury limits donor site availability. The use of meshed cutaneous autografts allows the surgeon to increase the area covered. Skin graft meshing devices of various design and manufacture are available with expansion ratios from 1:1 to 1:9. The wider the mesh, the greater the wound area covered; however, it will take the wound longer to close by ingrowth from the margins of the mesh reticulum to fill the open interstices during which time there is the very real potential for graft loss and wound infection to occur. Additionally, widely meshed autografts have a greater propensity to form hypertrophic burn scars and may provide a skin surface with unsatisfactory mechanical stability, inadequate pliability, permanently poor cosmetic appearance, and restricted joint mobility. Despite these potential limitations, the use of meshed cutaneous autografts is an important strategy and potentially life-saving approach for patients with extensive body surface area burns.

The technique of skin graft harvesting would seem to be a relatively simple procedure, yet it is often not done well. As noted earlier, the harvest site should be the one that will yield a graft with the desirable characteristics and the least donor site morbidity. Grafts should be of sufficient size to achieve wound closure with a minimum of intergraft seams. Powered dermatomes are available with up to 6-inch cutting widths that provide excellent sheets of skin for facial grafts or when meshed, can cover a significant burn area. Donor site preparation is essential to obtain a uniform graft. Powered clysis, can rapidly be accomplished over an extensive harvest site using an air-powered surgical wound irrigating system equipped with a 14- or 16-gauge needle attached to 3-L bags of normal saline. This provides a stable, uniform surface for graft harvest and limits the difficulties encountered when harvesting over contoured surfaces or bony prominences. The thickness of the harvested graft should be related to the site to be grafted, whether the graft is to be meshed, the mesh ratio, and, to some degree, surgeon preference. The desired thickness of the graft also influences donor site selection (i.e., a "thick" graft should be harvested from an area of "thick" skin). Harvest of a "thick" graft from an area of "thin" skin (i.e., the inner arm) can produce a full-thickness wound that will have to be grafted.

Skin grafts through which one can read printed material are primarily epithelial autografts with a minimal amount of dermis (0.004–0.006 inch), whereas those that are more opaque contain a variably greater amount of dermis (0.008–0.012 inch). Thinner grafts yield a better donor site and function well on a dermal wound bed but may not do well when placed on a wound excised to fascia. For elderly patients, thin grafts that contain insufficient numbers of keratinocyte progenitor cells are considered the cause of melting graft syndrome and prolong the time of reepithelialization. Thicker grafts are more pliable, heal with less contraction, and will do better than thin grafts when meshed. The thicker grafts may result in donor site scarring and delay in donor site closure, especially in the elderly patient.

The harvested graft should be placed on the prepared burn wound parallel to the major flexion creases and can be attached mechanically with staples or sutures or secured with tissue adhesives such as fibrin glue. A properly placed set of grafts on an extremity should at the end of the operation be able to remain in place as the extremity is put through a gentle range of motion. One of the most important aspects of a skin-grafting procedure is the application of a proper dressing. A highly successful approach is to use multiple layers of a nonadherent linen dressing moistened with a 5% solution of mafenide acetate applied circumferentially to the excised and grafted wounds on an extremity. A bolster produced by using net dressings drawn tightly over the burn dressings and stapled to the skin is used to "fix" the grafts on torso wounds. Graft failure occurs as a result of inadequate excision, inadequate hemostasis, infection, subgraft seroma formation, mechanical sheering during postoperative care, or, rarely, "upside down" application. The first dressing change is typically done 48 to 72 hours postoperatively. If a sheet graft is well intact at that time, a nonadherent dressing is reapplied to protect the wound. In the case of meshed autografts, the moist dressings of mafenide acetate solution, changed daily or more often as required, are continued until the mesh is closed.

Skin Substitutes

Although split-thickness cutaneous autografts are the usual method of wound closure, there is often the need for a skin substitute. Alternative wound coverings are used to achieve wound closure when the available donor surface area is not sufficient, when there is a need to test the wound bed, or for primary management of selected partial-thickness wounds. The goal with a skin substitute is to obtain temporary physiologic wound closure and protect the wound from bacterial invasion. The two most commonly used naturally occurring biologic dressings are human cutaneous allograft and porcine cutaneous xenograft. Human allograft skin is commercially available as split-thickness grafts in either fresh viable or cryopreserved form. Both of these preparations are capable of becoming vascularized; however, this best occurs with fresh allograft skin. Allograft skin can provide wound coverage for 3 to 4 weeks before rejection.[102] Xenograft tissue is available as reconstituted sheets of meshed porcine dermis or as fresh or prepared split-thickness skin. Porcine skin impregnated with silver ions to suppress wound colonization is also available. Xenograft skin can be used to cover partial-thickness injuries or donor sites, which reepithelialize beneath the xenograft.[103]

Various synthetic membranes have been developed that provide wound protection and possess vapor and bacterial barrier properties. Biobrane™ (Dow-Hickham, Sugarland, TX), is one such product that has been used in the management of partial-thickness and donor site wounds.[104] This bilaminate membrane consists of a collagen gel adherent to a nylon mesh as the dermal analog to promote fibrovascular ingrowth and a thin outer silastic film as the epidermal analog to provide barrier properties. Biobrane has also been used as the scaffold for the growth of allogenic fibroblasts that secrete, while in culture, various growth factors along with other mediators. The fibroblasts are then removed by freezing to complete preparation of the membrane. These membranes are currently approved for use in fully excised wounds, donor sites, and superficial partial-thickness burns.[105]

Another collagen-based skin substitute is the dermal replacement developed by Burke and Yannas, presently in use as Integra™ (Integra LifeScience Corporation, Plainsboro, NJ). This membrane consists of an inner layer of collagen fibrils with added glycosaminoglycan and an outer barrier membrane of polysiloxane. It is placed over freshly excised full-thickness wounds, and, once fully vascularized, the epidermal analog is removed and the vascularized "neodermis" covered with a thin split-thickness cutaneous autograft.[106] A permanent skin substitute for burn care victims represents the search for the Holy Grail. Presently, cultured epithelial autografts are commercially available but are limited in their use because of suboptimal graft take, fragility of the skin surface, and high cost.[107]

Use of any biologic dressing requires that the excised wound and the dressing that has been applied be meticulously examined on at least a daily basis. Submembrane suppuration or the development of infection necessitates removal of the dressing, cleansing of the wound with a surgical detergent disinfectant solution, and even reexcision of the wound if residual nonviable or infected tissue is present. Following such wound care, the biologic dressing can be reapplied, and, if it remains adherent and intact for 48 to 72 hours without suppuration, that biologic dressing can be removed and the wound closed definitively with cutaneous autografts.

The proper management of the patient's burn wounds is critical to achieve the optimum cosmetic and functional outcome and the timely return of the patient to full activity. For patients with major burns, the wound must be properly cared for and closure achieved expeditiously to lessen the level of physiologic disruption that accompanies a major burn. Failure to do so can result in invasive wound infection, chronic inflammation, erosion of lean body mass, progressive functional deficits, and even death.

The Treatment of Special Thermal Injuries

Electric Injury

This topic is dealt with in Chapter 10.

Chemical Injuries

A variety of chemical agents can cause tissue injury as a consequence of an exothermic chemical reaction, protein coagulation, dessication, and delipidation. The severity of a chemical injury is related to the concentration and amount of chemical agent and to the duration with which it is in contact with tissue.[108] Consequently, initial wound care to remove or dilute the offending agent takes priority in the management of patients with chemical injuries (Figure 9.8). Immediate copious water lavage should be instituted while all clothing, including gloves, shoes, and underwear, exposed to the chemical are being removed.

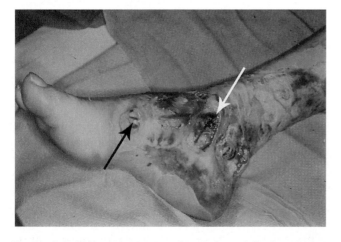

FIGURE 9.8. Failure to remove footwear and institute water lavage to dilute and remove concentrated lye, which had spilled into the boot of this patient, resulted in severe tissue injury during transportation to the hospital. Note extensive liquefaction of tissue, thrombosed vessels (white arrow), and edema of the extensor tendons exposed at the midmetatarsal level on the dorsomedial aspect of the foot (black arrow).

The lavage is continued for at least 30 minutes or until dilution has lowered the concentration of the agent below that which will cause tissue damage or until testing the involved surface with litmus paper confirms that the agent has been removed. For patients in whom extensive surface injury has occurred, the irrigation fluid should be warmed to prevent the induction of hypothermia. Although seldom needed, if a patient with concentrated alkali injuries requires prolonged irrigation and is hemodynamically stable, the patient can be cared for while sitting in a chair under a shower.

The appearance of skin damaged by chemical agents can be misleading. In the case of patients injured by strong acids, the involved skin surface may have a silky texture and a light brown appearance that can be mistaken for a sunburn rather than the full-thickness injury that it is. Skin injured by delipidation caused by petroleum distillates may be dry, show little if any inflammation, and appear to be undamaged but found to be a full-thickness injury on histologic examination.

Variable degrees of pulmonary insufficiency may occur in patients with cutaneous injuries caused by volatile chemical agents that can also be inhaled, such as anhydrous ammonia, the ignition products of white phosphorus, mustard gas, chlorine, and even the vapors of strong acids. Additionally, pulmonary insufficiency may be caused by the inhalation of the gaseous products of petroleum distillates as may occur in patients who sustain delipidation injuries due to partial immersion in gasoline and other petroleum products.

In the case of patients with anhydrous ammonia injury, any powdery condensate adherent to the skin should be brushed off before irrigation. Hydrofluoric (HF) acid injury is most common in those involved in etching processes; the cleaning of air-conditioning equipment, patio grills, and other metallic objects with spray products containing HF; and petroleum refining. After contact with HF acid, there is a characteristic pain-free interval of variable duration with subsequent appearance of focal pallor that progresses to penetrating necrosis, typically accompanied by severe pain. Immediately after injury, calcium gluconate gel should be applied topically or prolonged irrigation with a solution of benzalkonium chloride instituted. The persistent severe pain that may occur in digits injured by HF acid can be relieved by injecting 10% calcium gluconate into the artery supplying that finger. Local tissue injection of calcium gluconate is an alternate route of delivery but may in itself compromise the blood supply of the involved digit. Persistent pain caused by subungual HF acid is best treated by removal of the nail under digital block anesthesia. The pain typically relents and the nail grows back with little or no deformity. If these measures fail to control pain, local excision and skin grafting will be needed to remove the damaged tissue and achieve pain relief.[109] Extensive HF acid injury may induce systemic hypocalcemia, which is treated by intravenous infusion of calcium.

Burns caused by phenol should be treated with immediate water lavage to remove, by physical means, the liquid phenol on the cutaneous surface. Following that lavage, the involved area should be washed with a lipophilic solvent such as polyethylene glycol to remove any residual adherent phenol that is only slightly soluble in water.[110] Intensive systemic support is required for patients with extensive phenol burns, in whom absorption of the agent can cause central nervous system depression, hypothermia, hypotension, intravascular hemolysis, and even death.

Injuries caused by white phosphorus are usually discussed with other chemical injuries but are actually conventional thermal burns caused by the ignition of the particulate phosphorus. These injuries are most commonly encountered in military personnel injured by explosive antipersonnel devices (grenades), which can cause mechanical tissue damage and drive fragments of white phosphorus into the soft tissues. All wounds containing white phosphorus particles should be covered with a wet dressing that is kept moist to prevent ignition of the particles by exposure to air. If the interval between injury and definitive wound care will be so long as to permit dessication of the wet dressings, the wounds can be briefly washed with a freshly mixed dilute 0.5% to 1% solution of copper sulfate followed by copious rinsing. Such treatment generates a blue-gray cupric phosphide coating on the retained phosphorous particles that both impedes ignition and facilitates identification.[111] Whatever form of topical treatment is employed, the wound should be debrided and all retained phosphorous particles, which can be readily identified with an ultraviolet lamp, removed. The removed particles should be placed under water to prevent them from igniting and causing a fire in the operating room.

Strong acids and alkali can cause devastating ocular injuries and must be treated immediately, even before leaving the scene of the injury, by irrigation with water, saline, or phosphate buffer. In the hospital, eye irrigation must continue until the pH of the eye surface returns to normal. The rapid penetration of ocular tissue by strong alkalis necessitates prolonged irrigation (12 to 72 hours). Such irrigation is best carried out with a modified scleral contact lens with an irrigating side arm. The effects of iritis induced by chemical ocular injury are minimized by installation of a cycloplegic such as 1% atropine following irrigation. If irrigation and removal of the offending agent is delayed, the entire globe may be so damaged as to lose turgor and all visual function. Even with early irrigation, corneal damage can be severe, and late complications of symblepharon and xerophthalmia may occur. An ophthalmologist should be involved in the care of such patients from the time of admission.

Bitumen Burns

Bitumen injuries are commonly caused by hot tar coming in contact with the skin. The injury that results is a thermal contact burn, which is not associated with any significant component of a chemically mediated injury. There is no significant absorption of materials unless the patient is in an explosion and has ingested or inhaled the material. The primary initial treatment is urgent cooling of the molten material with no attempt made to remove the tar. By cold application, the transfer of heat can be limited and the degree of tissue damage minimized. There are various agents that have been advertised as being effective for the removal of tar and asphalt products. These have varied from mayonnaise to simple petroleum-based jellies and seem to be similar in terms of efficacy. Considering that the initial temperature of liquid tars and asphalts are typically in excess of 600°F, early concerns about infection would seem to be unfounded and offer no support for urgent removal with potential destructive consequences to underlying otherwise viable tissue. It is preferable to apply an emulsifying petroleum-based ointment and allow the tar to separate during the first day or two after admission.[108]

Cold Injuries

Injuries occurring secondary to environmental exposure can result in local injuries, frostbite, or systemic hypothermia. During the wintertime in urban environments, the most common mechanism of injury involves homeless persons or an elderly patient who has become disoriented and wandered from home. The pathophysiology of the local injuries consists essentially of crystal formation caused by freezing of both extracellular and intracellular fluids. Consequently, the cells dehydrate and shrink, and blood flow is altered to the exposed area resulting in tissue death. During the thawing of damaged tissues, microemboli that have formed further occlude the microvascular circulation, adding insult to injury.[112] It is important to note that the initial clinical presentation of the patient is not likely representative of the ultimate degree of tissue loss. Patients presenting with frostbite will have coldness of the injured body part with loss of sensation and proprioception. On initial examination, the limb may well appear pale or cyanotic or have a yellow-white discoloration. During rapid rewarming at 40° to 42°C in water for 15 to 30 minutes, hyperemia will occur followed by pain, paresthesias, and sensory deficits. Over the subsequent 24 hours, edema and blistering will develop, and it may be the better part of a week before one can determine the true depth and extent of the injury.

In the initial management of the patient, rewarming is critical, but it must be done only when there is no chance for an episode of refreezing. If blisters appear, the question of whether they should be preserved or debrided has proponents of both sides of the answer. Some authors suggest that white blisters can be debrided whereas purplish blue blisters should be left intact. The injured extremity should be elevated in an attempt to control edema and padded to avoid pressure-induced ischemia as a secondary insult. Administration of pain medication is based on the patient's response. Frostbite wounds are tetanus-prone wounds, and therefore tetanus toxoid should be administered based on the patient's immunization status.

Before any definitive plans are made for surgical intervention, sufficient time should be allowed to pass so that a clear demarcation between viable and nonviable tissue is apparent (Figure 9.9). However, it is not in the patient's best interest to follow the adage of "freeze in January and amputate in June."[113] Although it will take some time for definitive delineation of the depth of the injury, once the wounds have begun to mummify the thought that there will be tissue salvage seems more than naive. Patients suffering frostbite injuries should be evaluated for other potential trauma and treated for systemic hypothermia if it is present. The posthospitalization disposition of cold injury patients requires a clear understanding of their preexisting health status and the factors that predisposed them to injury, such as dementia or major psychological disease.[114]

Radiation Injury

Radiation exposure secondary to the detonation of a thermonuclear device is not as likely as is exposure from an industrial or medical accident, misuse of radiation materials, or acts of terrorism. The dispersal of radioactive substances can take several forms, including accidents during storage and mishandling, accidents during transportation of radioactive materials, intentional dispersal either alone or in combination with other agents, and intentional dispersal through an explosive device. In both storage and transport accidents, the dispersal and subsequent exposure to radioactive materials is usually limited to the people immediately involved and is well contained geographically once the event is recognized. It is typically difficult to expose large numbers of individuals to significant doses of radiation at any given time, and the risks are limited to those involved in a given incident. Small-dose radiation exposure does not affect health for many years and is associated with few acute problems, although it is still a significant health risk. In the event of intentional radiation dispersal, the risk of exposure and injury as well as the source involved need to be evaluated. The risk of trauma is related to the primary explosive device itself as well as trauma related to the secondary effects of the explosion, such as shell fragments, structure collapse, or injury from debris. Psychological trauma from witnessing the primary event or from the experience of living through the event, with the associated physical manifestations, may pose a further problem in the handling of a significant number of injured victims.

Exposure risk is related to primary contamination from the particles released from the explosive device, secondary contamination from particles that have become mixed with debris, debris dust, and fallout, and tertiary contamination from exposure to particles in contact with patients. Ionizing radiation is composed of two types: radiation that has mass and radiation that is energy only. Exposure to alpha particles, which are relatively large, highly charged particles, slow moving, and penetrate only a few microns into tissue, can be effectively shielded with

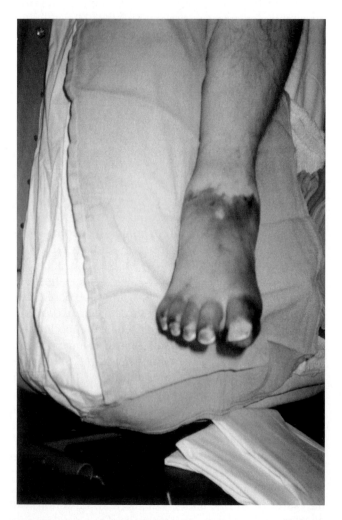

FIGURE 9.9. Spontaneous healing of frostbite injury proximal to the discolored skin on the dorsum of this foot is indexed by decreased hair growth in that area. The demarcation of nonviable tissue shown here permitted amputation at a midfoot level and salvaged the heel pad.

ordinary substances such as paper, cardboard, or clothing. Alpha particles can be a source of secondary and tertiary contamination. Beta particles, made up of either positively or negatively charged species, have greater energy, can penetrate more deeply into tissues, require shielding with material such as aluminum to prevent exposure. Both alpha and beta particles result from the decay of a radioactive source. Gamma and x-rays are produced by radioactive decay or an x-ray source; they have neither mass nor charge; however, they penetrate deeply, and shielding requires the use of such materials as lead, steel, or thick cement. Following removal from the source of radiation, no further exposure occurs, and the patient poses no danger to those providing care. Radiation caused by neutrons requires special consideration. Nuclear reactors are the major source of neutron emission and create radiation that penetrates deeply, causing widespread damage to underlying tissues.

Radiation exposure of 2 to 4 gray (Gy) can cause nausea and vomiting, hair loss, and bone marrow injury leading to death from infection up to 2 months after exposure. Exposures of 6 to 10 Gy result in the destruction of the bone marrow and injury to the GI tract with a mortality rate approaching 50% within 1 month. When the exposure is 10 to 20 Gy there is severe injury to the GI tract, and death can occur in as little as 2 weeks. When exposure is above 30 Gy, cardiovascular and nervous system damage occur primarily as a result of hypotension and cerebral edema. There is almost immediate nausea, vomiting, prostration, hypotension, ataxia, and convulsion, and death can occur in a matter of hours. At present there appears to be no effective treatment following radiation exposure. For treatment to be effective, it would need to be given before the exposure. In cases of accidental exposure, treating bone marrow suppression, although successful, has not prevented death, which usually occurs from radiation pneumonitis, GI tract injury, and hepatic and renal failure.[115,116]

The burn injuries resulting from radiation exposure are usually localized and represent a high radiation dose to the skin. They appear identical to a thermal burn and may present with erythema as with a first-degree burn, which will heal following some sloughing of the skin. With higher dose exposures, blisters may occur as with a partial-thickness burn, and healing occurs in a similar manner. When the radiation exposure has been significant, such as 20 Gy, radionecrosis occurs. If the event leading to the radiation exposure causes surface contamination, decontamination needs to be done before dealing with the wound. This consists of saline irrigation of the wound and treatment with standard aseptic techniques. It is not necessary to excise the wound urgently unless it is contaminated with long-life radionuclides such as alpha-emitting particles. Patients who have greater than a 1 Gy whole-body exposure should be considered for early wound closure so that the wound itself does not become the site of a lethal infection.[117]

To manage radiation-exposed victims effectively, a hospital must have a well-organized plan in place and the appropriate decontamination facility within the emergency room. The goals are to save the patient's life and to prevent further injury. The decontamination must be done so that the personnel providing care to the patient do not become exposed. All contaminated materials must be carefully handled to prevent contamination of the hospital and its facilities and the public sewage system.

Toxic Epidermal Necrolysis

Toxic epidermal necrolysis (TEN) is a rare, life-threatening mucocutaneous form of exfoliative dermatitis that is often secondary to drug sensitivity. The incidence of TEN has been estimated at 0.4 to 1.2 cases per million population per year.[118] These patients may give a history of sore throat, burning eyes, fever, and malaise and present with systemic toxicity. Physical findings can include rash, bullae, and diffuse exfoliation, with the large areas of separation having the appearance of a partial-thickness burn. When lateral stress is applied to the involved skin it separates at the dermal-epidermal junction, Nikolsky's sign. The resulting wounds give the appearance of a wet surface as seen in a second-degree burn.

The mechanism of injury is thought to be keratinocyte apoptosis induced by interactions between the cell surface death receptor Fas and its receptor FasL or CD95L.[119] Lyle in 1956 was the first to describes two entities in the initial description of TEN consisting of staphylococcal scalded skin syndrome (SSS) and what today is recognized as TEN.[120] Staphylococcal scalded skin syndrome is a generalized exfoliative dermatitis due to infections with staphylococcal organisms. In SSS, the lesion is at the intraepidermal layer with blister formation followed by desquamation of large sheets of skin with relatively rapid reepithelialization over 7 to 10 days. The outcome in patients with SSS is significantly better than that in TEN patients. In TEN, there is necrosis of all layers of the skin and a mortality rate between 30% and 40%, whereas with SSS it is 3% to 4%.

Stevens-Johnson syndrome (SJS) is an entity in which there is also extensive epidermolysis, often presenting with target-shaped skin lesions with differentiation from TEN related to the extent of cutaneous involvement. One current delineation classifies patients with less than 10% to 30% cutaneous involvement as SJS and those with greater than 10% to 30% as TEN, particularly if it involves oral-genital and ocular mucosae.[121] Whether SJS and TEN represent the same process, differing only in the extent of cutaneous involvement and sites affected, or are pathologically distinct entities has not been determined with any degree of certainty.

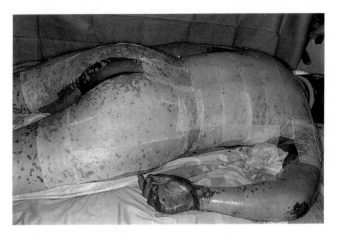

FIGURE 9.10. The back, buttocks, and upper thighs of this patient with toxic epidermal necrolysis (TEN) have been covered with a translucent collagen-based skin substitute, Biobrane, following cleansing with saline and gentle debridement of exfoliated epidermis. Note focal areas of adherent darkly pigmented epidermis that were left in place and covered with the bilaminate membrane, which provides barrier function, reduces pain, and prevents dessication of the exposed dermal surface to promote healing. The undressed wounds of the arms and legs were covered with Biobrane after this photo was obtained.

Patients with TEN have wound care needs identical to those of patients with extensive second-degree wounds. They exhibit significant fluid losses and have specialized nutritional needs. Care of these patients in a burn center by experienced surgeons has resulted in a significant improvement in outcome.[122] General principles of management of these patients include the cessation of potential precipitating drugs, the discontinuance of systemic steroids if recently initiated, ophthalmologic evaluation, and skin biopsy confirmation of the diagnosis.[123] Additionally, systemic antibiotics should be reserved for those cases in which infection is highly likely. Replacement of fluid and electrolytes and provision of nutritional support and aggressive wound care are critical elements in the care of these patients. Wound care may consist of the application of a biologic dressing once all of the nonviable tissue is fully debrided or the use of silver-impregnated dressings (Figure 9.10). The most frequent mistakes in the care and management of these patients are underestimating the extent of the cutaneous involvement, airway compromise, and not understanding how rapidly these patients can become critically ill. To date, the results of studies of various modalities that can be employed to control the degree of skin slough have been too inconsistent to recommend their general use.[124]

Mechanical Injury

The combination of burn injury and multisystem trauma occurs in up to 4% to 5% of all burn patients.[125,126]

Patients suffering combination injuries are typically male, with their injuries having occurred from a flame ignition during an assault or motor vehicle crash. Victims suffering a combination of burns and trauma tend to have a higher incidence of inhalation injury, higher mortality rate, higher injury severity score (ISS), and longer length of stay, despite no differences in total body surface area burned, than patients with only burns. Trauma victims with burns with an inhalation injury have a near threefold increase in their mortality rate.[98] Those victims not surviving their injuries typically are significantly older and have a higher ISS and a larger body surface area burn than trauma victims with burns who survive their injuries. The management priorities for patients suffering burns plus trauma must be as for patients with trauma. Understanding the mechanism of injury is vital in determining the probability of associated injuries and provides a guide for the workup of the patient. A formal trauma evaluation should be performed for all burn victims when the history of the event points to the possibility of combined mechanisms of injury.

Life-threatening injuries must be promptly treated and fractures immobilized, and the resuscitation fluid needs of the patient should be calculated to include the burn wound–mandated needs and those of the associated trauma. Blood is not part of the initial resuscitation for patients with only burn injuries, but when there is multiple trauma blood transfusions may be necessary in the early management of the patient. Often the presence of a major burn wound results in the patient being viewed as having only a burn, and the standard assessment of a trauma patient is not done. Patients with impaired neurologic status should undergo a computerized axial tomographic scan to rule out intracranial pathology along with evaluation for a spinal injury. This is particularly important if the patient jumped from a burning building to escape the fire, was injured in an industrial accident, or was involved in a motor vehicle crash. Potential thoracic, abdominal, or pelvic injuries should be evaluated with chest, abdominal, and pelvic roentgenograms as well as with abdominal computed tomography and FAST (focused abdominal sonography in trauma) examinations. Diagnostic peritoneal lavage may also be used for the unstable patient to verify the presence of an injury requiring exploratory laparotomy. The nonoperative management of significant injuries of the spleen or liver requires thoughtful consideration for patients with a major burn, and it maybe prudent to opt for surgical management particularly if the abdominal wall is extensively burned. For patients with major long bone injuries, early operative intervention with stabilization will facilitate their overall management as well as that of the burn. In selected circumstances, early burn excision with skin graft wound closure may be the best approach to facilitate the operative management of the orthopedic injury.

The management of patients with significant burn injuries in conjunction with mechanical trauma requires a highly coordinated plan of care. The patient must be continuously reassessed to avoid missing an injury, and the surgeon must be vigilant to the development of trauma-related complications.

Metabolic and Nutritional Support

Estimation and Measurement of Metabolic Rate

Burn injury alters central and peripheral thermoregulatory mechanisms, the predominant route of heat loss, the distribution and utilization of nutrients, and metabolic rate. All of these postburn metabolic changes must be considered when planning the metabolic support and nutritional management of the hypermetabolic burn patient necessary to minimize loss of lean body mass, accelerate convalescence, and restore physical abilities. Metabolic support includes patient care procedures and environmental manipulations in addition to the provision of adequate nutrition.

The perceived temperature of comfort of burn patients (on average 30.4°C) is higher than that of unburned control patients and necessitates maintaining the ambient temperature at that level in the patient's room to prevent the imposition of added cold stress, which would exaggerate an already elevated metabolic rate.[127] Physical therapy with active motion to the extent possible and passive motion to stretch muscles in the absence of spontaneous motion is instituted on admission to minimize muscle wasting secondary to disuse. Analgesic and anxiolytic agents should be used as needed to prevent pain and anxiety-related increases in circulating catecholamine levels, which can further increase metabolic rate. Assiduous monitoring is necessary to facilitate early diagnosis and prompt treatment of infections and thereby reduce their metabolic impact. The importance of excision and grafting of the burn wound has been emphasized by recent studies showing that such treatment reduces resting energy expenditure in burn patients, even if the entire wound cannot be excised and grafted at a single sitting.

Even though metabolic rate can be reduced by pharmacologic means, studies indicating that the hypermetabolic response to burn injury is wound directed speak for meeting caloric needs rather than reducing nutrient supply to the burn wound by pharmacologic intervention. One must determine the resting energy expenditure in order to calculate the nutrients required to meet the patient's needs. Bedside indirect calorimetry is the most accurate means of determining metabolic rate, but a bedside metabolic cart may not always be available. A number of formulas permit one to make close approximations of daily energy expenditure in a variety of surgical patients. A formula based on studies of extensively burned patients is useful in estimating burn patient calorie needs.[128]

$$EER = [BMR \times (0.89142 + 10.01335 \times TBS)] \times m^2 \times 24 \times AF,$$

where EER is estimated energy requirements, BMR is basal metabolic rate, TBS is total burn size, m^2 is total body surface area in square meters, and AF is activity factor of 1.25 for burns. A rule of thumb estimate for nutritional needs of patients whose burns involve more than 30% of the body surface is 2,000 to 2,200 kilocalories and 12 to 18 grams of nitrogen per square meter of body surface per day.[39]

Nutritional Support

Meeting the metabolic needs of the burn patient can be accomplished by providing nutritional support via the GI tract or by the intravenous route. After determining what the metabolic needs will be for an individual burn patient, the next question is will the patient be capable of meeting the needs by oral intake? For patients who can eat, it is not likely that a standard hospital diet will meet the calculated needs, and it is often necessary to supplement the patient's intake with various nutritional supplements. A calorie count should be recorded to verify that the patient is capable of consistently meeting the daily nutrient intake goal. For the patient who is incapable of achieving the necessary nutrient intake or who cannot eat, one must decide how to deliver the feedings. Total parenteral nutrition in the past provided a way by which patients could receive the majority or all of their calorie and protein needs but at present has largely been supplanted by the use of enteral nutritional support. Compared with total parenteral nutrition, enteral nutritional support is technically easier to accomplish, lower in cost, supports the health of the GI tract, and ameliorates the systemic inflammatory response syndrome.[129–133]

At the time of admission, a patient who will require specialized nutritional support should have either a nasogastric or nasoduodenal tube placed. Patients can safely and effectively be fed by either of these routes with appropriate precautions. It is not required that one use custom-made feedings to meet the patient's nutrient needs. It is possible by using combinations of currently available commercial products to obtain the necessary blend of nutrients, feeding density, water, and protein requirements while avoiding the cost of compounding specialized enteral feedings. It is preferable to start enteral feedings soon after the patient is admitted. The patient should be fed with the head of the bed elevated to 30°, with feeding residuals checked frequently to avoid gastric distention and possible aspiration. A potential advantage of early enteral feedings is modulation of the hypermetabolic response, although the actual ability of early feedings to achieve this goal has been called into question.[134–136] When feedings are initiated early postinjury, the desired rate of administration can typically be reached within 24 to 48 hours of admission. There are multiple recommendations regarding the initial concentration, rate, incremental increase, and frequency of the increases. Starting a tube feeding of standard concentration at 20 to 40 mL/hr and advancing the rate a similar amount every 4 hours works well for most patients. The most important issues are that the nursing staff understands the goals, knows how to monitor for feeding intolerance, and appreciates the attention to detail necessary to achieve consistent delivery of the feedings.

If a patient is intolerant of gastric feedings and gastric aspirate volume exceeds the total of two hourly feedings, the administration of metoclopramide will often resolve the problem. If the patient fails to respond to metoclopramide, an attempt should be made to place either a nasoduodenal or nasojejunal feeding tube, which will minimize this feeding difficulty and lessen the risk of aspiration. Patients who become septic will often manifest changes in feeding tolerance along with new-onset hyperglycemia or changes in insulin needs as early signs pointing to this problem. For patients receiving central vein alimentation, the risk of catheter sepsis must be evaluated as an etiology for the patient's septic process. For patients who become intolerant of enteral feedings or develop GI complications that prevent use of the GI tract, total parenteral nutrition will be required. However, with careful attention to detail and a well-designed, patient-specific enteral feeding protocol, this should rarely be needed in the care of a burn patient.

Monitoring

The complications associated with the use of enteral or parenteral support in the burn patient are in large part similar. Burn injury induces insulin resistance, which may lead to hyperglycemia. The maintenance of blood glucose values with aggressive insulin replacement has a favorable impact on the outcome of critically ill patients.[137] For critically ill patients the preferable route of administration of insulin is intravenously, with the goal of maintaining plasma glucose values between 80 and 110 mg/dL. There is a well-recognized limit to the caloric load that a critically ill patient can tolerate from carbohydrates, and for the 70-kg patient this is approximately 1,800 kCal per day from glucose.[138] Excessive amounts of glucose can result in respiratory quotient (RQ) values >1, which may cause hepatic steatosis and complicate ventilatory management.

Sufficient protein to meet metabolic demands must be provided. To estimate protein needs, 24-hour urine urea

nitrogen is measured to which an additional 0.1 to 0.2 g of nitrogen per percent total body surface area burn remaining is added. These determinations can be done on a weekly basis unless there is a special need to perform them more frequently. Numerous studies have been done to determine precise protein needs and the optimum balance of protein to nonprotein calories. For adult patients, 1.5 to 2.0 g protein per kilogram lean body mass per day is a reasonable goal and for children, 3 g protein per kilogram lean body mass.[139,140] A nonprotein calorie to nitrogen ratio of 100:1 provides the patient with sufficient calories to support protein synthesis in the face of ongoing protein breakdown and reduces net protein loss.[141,142] The provision of dietary protein at these levels has been shown to positively impact patient outcome.[143] An increasing blood urea nitrogen level must be evaluated in terms of nitrogen overfeeding and the protein load recalculated to avoid uremia and an associated diuresis. Measurements of visceral proteins such as serum transferrin and albumin can be used to monitor the impact of the nitrogen content of the diet on the patient's nutritional status. These proteins are simply markers that can be followed over time and are probably best utilized in a trend analysis based on weekly determinations because albumin has a half-life of 20 days and transferrin 8 days. Thyroid prealbumin with a half-life of 2 days and retinal binding protein with a 12-hour half-life can be used to track short-term responses in selected patients.

To prevent the development of essential fatty acid deficiencies, lipids must be included in the diet but should not exceed more than 40% of the total calorie load or more than 3 g/kg body weight per day. Most enteral diets will contain adequate fat to prevent the development of essential fatty acid deficiency, and parenteral diet formulations typically contain long-chain fatty acids. The serum triglyceride concentration and the triene/tetraene ratio should be measured weekly to assess fatty acid status. If this ratio is greater than 0.4, an essential fatty acid deficiency exists that necessitates adjustment of the dietary fat content.[144] Supplemental medium-chain triglycerides can be given enterally but are associated with increased ketone production and may cause diarrhea.[39]

Complications

Serum electrolytes must be monitored to make necessary adjustments in the amount of free water, sodium, chloride, potassium, phosphorus, calcium, and magnesium provided to the patient. Laboratory values should be obtained at initiation of the feedings and daily during the stabilization phase and with each change in the patient's clinical status. During the first several days after admission, and with the initiation of nutritional support, there can be dramatic shifts in serum and plasma values of electrolytes and minerals. As noted above, hypernatremia can develop if free water replacement is insufficient to account for insensible water loss through the burn wound, which can be 2.0 to 3.1 mL/kg body weight/% burn/day.[145] Hypernatremia can also develop with persistent febrile episodes if free water replacement does not match the patient's needs. Hyponatremia may represent underreplacement of sodium but typically is related to free water excess. Correction of hyponatremia should be attempted with restriction of free water intake. For adults an increase in body weight of more than 400 g per day reflects water loading and should prompt a review of fluid intake and output records and adjustment of fluid administration.[2] Potassium and phosphorus must be given to meet the patient's needs, which often exceed initial estimates particularly when large loads of glucose are being given along with exogenous insulin.

In the course of the patient's care as the open wound area decreases and the hypermetabolic state slowly resolves, the nutrient load should be adjusted so that balance is maintained between metabolic needs and substrates delivered and the patient is not overfed. Alternatively, if a patient is found to have lost more than 10% of his or her admission weight, it is likely that caloric estimates are not being achieved or were underestimated. Although most experienced clinicians possess the skill to assess patient needs accurately, the performance of bedside indirect calorimetry can provide objective information as to the patient's resting energy expenditure, respiratory quotient, oxygen consumption, and carbon dioxide production. The results may indicate the need to adjust the total calorie load if the resting energy expenditure has been underestimated or modify the fuel substrate load if the respiratory quotient is approaching or greater than 1.

The patient should receive increased amounts of vitamin C, at recommended doses of 1 g/day for adults and 500 mg/day for children, which will aid in wound healing.[146] For patients with burns of greater than 20% of the total body surface area, zinc at doses of 220 mg/day will support wound healing as well as white cell function.[147] The routine provision of these nutrients avoids complications related to insufficient delivery and obviates the need to measure their levels in the patient.

In patients with prior surgery or preexisting medical conditions, special attention may be required to monitor for feeding intolerance and to ensure that adequate amounts of iron, folate, and vitamin B_{12} are being effectively delivered. For patients who have received extended courses of broad-spectrum antibiotics, vitamin K replacement beyond standard recommendations may be required to avoid the development of nutritionally related coagulopathy. The preservation of lean body mass requires more than just the appropriate amounts and blend of nutrients. Physical activity is important in directing the nutrients to muscle and reducing truncal fat deposition and the risk of hepatic steatosis.

In addition to providing appropriate calorie, protein, and nutrient loads to burn patients, it is now possible to modulate the metabolic response. Administration of beta-antagonists to children has been shown to be safe and to have a significant positive effect on outcome.[148] The administration of growth hormone, which is depressed following burn injuries, has met with variable results. Herndon et al.[149] have reported a positive effect in burned children given growth hormone, but a recent multicenter trial from Europe including critically ill patients showed an increased mortality in treated patients.[150] An alternative strategy that seems not to be associated with problems for adults and is efficacious for children is the use of the drug oxandrolone, although a recent study reported that the agent was associated with prolonged need for mechanical ventilation in trauma patients.[151–154] Additional strategies that might be utilized are the provision of selected nutrients in increased amounts. Glutamine, arginine, nucleotides, and omega-3 fatty acids have all been used in attempts to improve immune function above that seen with the optimal use of standard nutritional formulations.[155–159] The routine use of these measures requires a full understanding of the therapeutic benefits and the potential adverse consequences of each. Additionally, some studies have found such supplements to be ineffective.[160]

For patients who have established chronic renal failure or develop renal insufficiency during their course of care, changes in the nutritional formulation will have to be made to accommodate their altered clinical status. For patients who require dialysis, the frequency of dialysis should be adjusted so that the protein intake needed to meet metabolic needs can be given. For patients with significant injuries who are receiving large amounts of feeding through the GI tract, the health of the GI tract itself must be continuously monitored. The development of major GI complications, although not common, can adversely impact the patient's outcome. Complications can include ischemic necrotic bowel disease, intestinal obstruction, the development of *Clostridium difficile* colitis, and noninfectious diarrhea.[161–165] The patient's clinical status should be continuously monitored, and any changes in abdominal findings on physical examination should be aggressively followed up with appropriate diagnostic radiographic studies, endoscopy, stool cultures, and abdominal exploration before the patient deteriorates and develops an irreversible condition.

Transportation and Transfer

Many important advances have been made in the care and management of burn-injured victims during the past 50 years. One of the more significant advances has been the recognition of the benefits of a team approach in the care of critically injured burn patients. The American

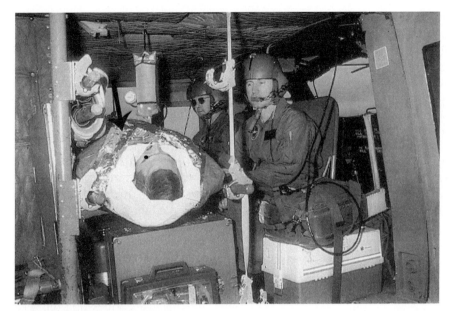

FIGURE 9.11. The transfer of patients to burn centers is often done by helicopter as shown here. Note the shiny metallic inner surface (black arrow) of the "space blanket" in which the patient has been wrapped to conserve heat and prevent excessive cooling during transport. The burn surgeon and burn nurse, sitting adjacent to the patient, monitor urinary output and, as needed, adjust the rate of infusion of the fluids suspended above the patient. The vibration, noise, poor light, and limited space that conspire to make monitoring and therapeutic intervention difficult mandate preflight physiologic stabilization of each patient who is to be transferred.

College of Surgeons and the American Burn Association have developed optimal standards for providing burn care and a burn center verification program that identifies those units that have undergone peer review of their performance and outcomes. Patients with burns and/or the associated injuries and conditions listed in Table 9.2 should be referred to a burn center.

Once the decision has been made to transfer a patient to a burn center, there should be physician-to-physician communication regarding the patient's status and need for transfer.[166] Institutions should have preexisting interhospital transfer policies in place to facilitate communication and patient transfers. It is critical that the patient be properly stabilized in preparation for the transfer. The flight transfer team should have the capability of providing the care required for a critically injured, severely burned patient throughout the entire transfer procedure. A surgeon, a respiratory therapist, and a licensed practical nurse, all experienced in burn care, comprise such a team for long-distance, fixed wing aircraft transfers. For short-distance transport by rotary wing aircraft, inclusion of a burn physician in the flight team optimizes the safety and quality of care of extensively burned patients, but patients with lesser burns may be adequately cared for by nonphysician helicopter flight team members (a flight nurse and/or an advanced paramedic) who are in ready contact with medical control. A flight team roster should be maintained and published so the surgeons and other members of the team will be available when needed. Physicians and other team members should be assigned to the flight (transfer) team only after 6 to 12 months experience at a burn center, which will enable them to become familiar with the complications that occur in burn patients during resuscitation and develop compe-

tence in the prevention, treatment, and resolution of these problems.

During transport the need to perform life-saving interventions such as endotracheal intubation or reestablishing vascular access may be very difficult to accomplish in the relatively unstable and limited space of a moving ambulance or a helicopter in flight (Figure 9.11). This difficulty makes it important to institute hemodynamic and pulmonary resuscitation and to achieve "stability" before undertaking transfer by either aeromedical or ground transport. A secure large-bore intravenous cannula must be in place to permit continuous fluid resuscitation. Patients should be placed on 100% oxygen if there is any suspicion of carbon monoxide exposure. If there is any question about airway adequacy an endotracheal tube should be placed and mechanical ventilation instituted before transfer begins. In-flight mechanical ventilatory support can be provided by a transport ventilator with oxygen supplied from a lightweight Kevlar tank transported in backpack fashion by the respiratory therapist. Patient safety during transport may necessitate chemical paralysis of the patient to prevent loss of the airway or vascular access.

In-transit monitoring for helicopter transfer includes pulse rate, blood pressure, electrocardiogram, pulse oximetry, end-tidal CO_2 levels, and respiratory rate. For long-distance transfer, the same physiologic indices should be monitored. In addition, the ultrasonic flowmeter should be used to assess the presence and quality of pulsatile flow in all four limbs on a scheduled basis, and excursion of the chest wall should be monitored to identify a need for limb or chest escharotomy, respectively. The hourly urinary output should also be monitored with fluid infusion adjusted as necessary. All patients should be placed on nothing-by-mouth status, and those with a greater than 20% body surface area burn require placement of a nasogastric tube. In essence, a mini intensive care unit should be established for the duration of the long-distance flight.

The burn wound should be covered with a clean and/or sterile dry sheet. The application of topical antimicrobial agents is not necessary before transfer, because they will have to be removed on admission to the burn center. Maintenance of the patient's body temperature is vital. Wet dressings, which can lead to hypothermia, particularly in small adults and children, should be avoided. The patient should be covered with a heat-reflective space blanket to minimize heat loss. Pain medication is given in sufficient dosage to control the patient's pain during transport while avoiding respiratory depression, airway comprise, or hypotension. Burn wounds, as tetanus-prone wounds, mandate immunization in accordance with the recommendations of the American College of Surgeons. As in the case of the transfer of any trauma victim, documentation must be thorough, flow sheets should be clearly marked, and a listing of all medications, including intravenous fluids that have been given, must be provided to the receiving physician. In the case of a patient suffering from significant multisystem trauma and burn injuries, it may be necessary to treat the patient's life-threatening mechanical injury before transfer if the transport time will be of long duration or the patient is unstable.[98]

Survival Data

During the course of the past half century, early postburn renal failure as a consequence of delayed and/or inadequate resuscitation has been eliminated, and inhalation injury as a comorbid factor has been tamed. Invasive burn wound sepsis has been controlled, and early excision with prompt skin grafting and general improvements in critical care have reduced the incidence of infection, eliminated many previously life-threatening complications, and accelerated the convalescence of burn patients.[167] All of these improvements have significantly reduced the mortality rate for burn patients of all ages. At the midpoint of the past century, a burn of 43% of the total body surface would have caused the death of 50 of 100 young adult patients (15 to 40 years) with such burns. Since that time, the extent of burn causing such 50% mortality (the LA_{50}) in 21-year-old patients has increased to 82% of the total body surface and in 40-year-old patients to 72% of the total body surface. In children (0 to 14 years) the LA_{50} has increased from 51% of the total body surface in the 1950s to 72% today, and in the elderly (>40 years) the LA_{50} has increased from 23% of the total body surface area to 46% (Table 9.5). Not only has survival

TABLE 9.5. Changes in burn patient mortality at U.S. Army Burn Center, 1945–1991.

Age group	Percentage of body surface burn causing 50% mortality (LA_{50})	
	1945–1957	1987–1991
Children (0–14 years)	51	72*
Young adults (15–40 years)	43	82†
		73‡
Older adults	23	46§

*Age 5 years.
†Age 21 years.
‡Age 40 years.
§Age 60 years.

improved, but the elimination of many life-threatening complications and advances in wound care have improved the quality of life of even those patients who have survived extensive severe thermal injuries.

Critique

It is well known that the Parkland formula is merely a *guideline* for fluid resuscitation and not a strict rule. The formula is particularly inaccurate for deep partial- and full-thickness burns greater than 60% total body surface area. However, volume resuscitation, which substantially exceeds the estimated amount, often reflects the extent of an associated inhalation injury.

Answer (B)

References

1. Brigham PA, McLaughlin E. Burn incidence and medical care use in the United States: estimates, trends, and data sources. J Burn Care Rehabil 1996; 17:95–107.
2. Pruitt BA Jr, Goodwin CW, Cioffi WG Jr. Thermal injuries. In Davis JH, Sheldon GF, eds. Surgery: A Problem-Solving Approach, 2nd ed. St. Louis: Mosby, 1995: 642–720.
3. Forjuoh SN. The mechanisms, intensity of treatment, and outcomes of hospitalized burns: Issues for prevention. J Burn Care Rehabil 1988; 19:456–460.
4. Stabilization, transfer, and transport. In Gamelli RL, ed. Advanced Life Burn Support Course Instructors Manual. Chicago: American Burn Association, 2001: 73–78.
5. Sheridan RL, ed. Burn Care Resources in North America. Chicago: American Burn Association, 2004.
6. Graitcer PL, Sniezek JE. Hospitalizations due to tap water scalds, 1978–1985. MMWR Morbid Mortal Wkly Rep 1988; 37:35–38.
7. Burn Injury Fact Sheet. Washington, DC: National Safe Kids Campaign, 1301 Pennsylvania Avenue NW, Suite 1000, 20004–1707, Dec 98.

8. Cadier MA, Shakespeare PG. Burns in octogenarians. Burns 1995; 21:200–204.

9. Acute Chemical Hazards to Children and Adults. Washington, DC: Directorate for Epidemiology, U.S. Consumer Product Safety Commission, NEISS Data Highlights, Vol. 12, 1988,

10. Baker SP, O'Neill B, Karpf RS. The Injury Fact Book. Lexington, MA: Lexington Books, 1984: 139–154.

11. Lopez RE, Holle RL. Demographics of lightning casualties. Semin Neurol 1995; 15:286–295.

12. Pruitt BA Jr, Goodwin CW, Mason AB Jr. Epidemiological, demographic, and outcome characteristics of burn injury. In Herndon DN, ed. Total Burn Care. Philadelphia: WB Saunders, 2002: 16–30.

13. Arturson G, Mellander S. Acute changes in capillary filtration and diffusion in experimental burn injury. Acta Physiol Scand 1964; 62:457–463.

14. Lund T, Bert JL, Onarheim H, Bowen BD, Reed RK. Microvascular exchange during burn injury I: a review. Circ Shock 1989; 28:179–197.

15. Lund T, Wiig H, Reed RK, Aukland K. A new mechanism for oedema generation: strongly negative interstitial fluid pressure causes rapid fluid flow into thermally injured skin. Acta Physiol Scand 1987; 129:433–436.

16. Arturson G, Soed AS. Changes in transcapillary leakage during healing of experimental burns. Acta Chir Scand 1967; 133:609–614.

17. Arturson G. Capillary permeability in burned and non-burned areas in dogs. Acta Chir Scand (Suppl) 1961; 274:55.

18. Brown WL, Bowler EG, Mason AD Jr. Studies of disturbances of protein turnover in burned troops: use of an animal model. In Pruitt BA Jr, ed. Annual Research Progress Report. Fort Sam Houston, TX: U.S. Army Institute of Surgical Research, 1981: 233–259.

19. Demling RH, Kramer GC, Gunther R, Nerlich M. Affect of nonprotein colloid on postburn edema formation in soft tissues and lungs. Surgery 1984; 95:593–602.

20. Mason AD Jr. The mathematics of resuscitation: 1980 presidential address, American Burn Association. J Trauma 1980; 20:1015–1020.

21. Nissen NN, Gamelli RL, Polverini PJ, DiPietro LA. Differential angiogenic and proliferative activity of surgical and burn wound fluids. J Trauma, 2003; 54(6):1205–1211.

22. DeMeules JE, Pigula FA, Mueller M, Raymond SJ, Gamelli RL. Tumor necrosis factor and cardiac function. J Trauma 1992; 32:686–692.

23. Cioffi WG, DeMeules JE, Gamelli RL. The effects of burn injury and fluid resuscitation on cardiac function in-vitro. J Trauma 1986; 26:638–642.

24. Ayala A, Chaudry IH. Platelet activating factor and its role in trauma, shock, and sepsis. New Horiz 1996; 4(2):265–275.

25. Asch MJ, Fellman RJ, Walker HL, Foley FD, Popp RL, Mason AD Jr, Pruitt BA Jr. Systemic and pulmonary hemodynamic changes accompanying thermal injury. Ann Surg 1973; 178:218–221.

26. Demling RH, Wong C, Jin LJ, Hechtman H, Lalonde C, West K. Early lung dysfunction after major burns: role of edema and vasoactive mediators. J Trauma 1985; 25:959–966.

27. Choudrhry MA, Fazal N, Goto M, Gamelli RL, Sayeed MM. Gut-associated lymphoid T-cell suppression enhances bacterial translocation in alcohol and burn injury. Am J Physiol Gastrointest Liver Physiol 2002; 282(6):G937–G947.

28. Kowal-Vern A, McGill V, Gamelli RL. Necrotic bowel is a complication in the thermally injured population. Arch Surg 1997; 132(4):440–443.

29. Murton SA, Tan ST, Prickett PC, Frampton C, Donald RA. Hormone response to stress in patients with major burns. Br J Plast Surg 1998; 51:388–392.

30. Loebel DC, Baxter CR, Curreri PW. The mechanism of erythrocyte dysfunction in the early postburn period. Ann Surg 1973; 178:681–686.

31. Deitch EA, Sittig KM. A Serial study of the erythropoietic response to thermal injury. Ann Surg 1993; 217:293–299.

32. Gamelli RL, Hebert JC, Foster RS Jr. Effect of burn injury on granulocyte and macrophage production. J Trauma 1985; 25(7):615–619.

33. McEuen DD, Ogawa M, Eurenius K. Myelopoiesis in the infected burn. J Lab Clin Med 1997; 89:540–543.

34. Gamelli RL, He LK, Liu H. Marrow granulocyte-macrophage progenitor response to burn injury as modified by endotoxin and endomethycin. J Trauma 1994; 37(3):339–346.

35. Santangello S, Gamelli RL, Shankar R. Myeloid commitment shifts toward monocytopoiesis after thermal injury and sepsis. Ann Surg 2001; 233(1):97–106.

36. Rico RM, Ripamonti R, Burns AL, Gamelli RL, DiPietro LA. The effect of sepsis on wound healing. J Surg Res 2002; 102(2):193–197.

37. Hahn EL, Tai HH, He L-K, Gamelli RL. Burn injury with infection alters prostaglandin E_2 synthesis and metabolism. J Trauma 1999; 47:1051–1057.

38. Sen S, Muthu K, Jones S, He L-K, Shankar R, Gamelli RL. Thermal injury and sepsis deplete precursor dendritic cells and alter their function. J Am Coll Surg 2003; 197:539–540.

39. Pruitt BA Jr, Goodwin CW Jr. Critical care management of the severely burned patient. In Parrillo JE, Dellinger RP, eds. Critical Care Medicine, 2nd ed. St. Louis: CV Mosby, 2001: 1475–1500.

40. Shock and fluid resuscitation. In Sheridan RL, ed. Advanced Burn Life Support Course Instructors Manual. Chicago: American Burn Association, 2001: 33–40.

41. Salisbury RE, Loveless S, Silverstein P, Wilmore DW, Moylan JA Jr, Pruitt BA Jr. Postburn edema of the upper extremity: evaluation of present treatment. J Trauma 1973; 13:857–862.

42. Warden GB, Wilmore DW, Rogers PW, Mason AD Jr, Pruitt BA Jr. Hypernatremic state in hypermetabolic burn patients. Arch Surg 1973; 106:420–427.

43. Klein GL, Langman CV, Herndon DN. Persistent hypoparathyroidism following magnesium repletion in burn-injured children. Pediatr Nephrol 2000; 14:301–304.

44. Pruitt BA Jr. The development of the International Society for Burn Injuries and progress in burn care: the whole is greater than the sum of its parts. Burns 1999; 25:683–696.

45. Cullinane DC, Jenkins JM, Reddy S, Van Natta T, Eddy VA, Bass JG, Chen A, Schwartz M, Lavin P, Morris JA Jr. Anterior ischemic optic neuropathy: a complication after systemic inflammatory response syndrome. J Trauma 2000; 48:381–387.

46. Ivy ME, Atweh NA, Palmer J, Possenti PP, Pineau M, D'Aiuto M. Intra-abdominal hypertension and abdominal compartment syndrome in burn patients. J Trauma 2000; 49:387–391.

47. Tasaki O, Goodwin CW, Saitoh D, Mozingo DW, Ishihara S, Brinkley WW, Cioffi WG Jr, Pruitt BA Jr. Effects of burns on inhalation injury. J Trauma 1997; 43:603–607.

48. Balakrishnan C, Tijunelis AD, Gordon DM, Prasad JK. Burns and inhalation injury caused by steam. Burns 1996; 22:313–315.

49. Rabinowitz PM, Siegel MB. Acute inhalation injury. Clin Chest Med 2002; 23:707–715.

50. Robinson M, Miller RH. Smoke inhalation injuries. Am J Otolaryngol 1986; 7:375–380.

51. Soejima K, Schmalstieg FC, Sakura H, Traber LD, Traber DL. Pathophysiological analysis of combined burn and smoke inhalation injuries in sheep. Am J Physiol Lung Cell Mol Physiol 2001; 280:L1233–L1241.

52. Abraham E. Neutrophils in acute lung injury. Crit Care Med 2003; 31:S195–S199.

53. Chen CM, Fan CL, Chang CH. Surfactant in corticosteroid effects on lung function in a rat model of acute lung injury. Crit Care Med 2001; 29:2169–2175.

54. Suchner U, Katz DP, Furst P, Beck K, Felbinger T, Thiel M, Senftleben U, Goetz AE, Peter K. Impact of sepsis lung injury and the role of lipid infusion on circulating prostacyclin and thromboxane A$_2$. Intensive Care Med 2002; 28:122–129.

55. Willey-Courand DB, Harris RS, Galletti GG, Hales CA, Fischman A, Venegas JG. Alterations in regional ventilation, perfusion, and shunt after smoke inhalation measured by PET. J Appl Physiol 2002; 93:1115–1122.

56. Ernst A, Zibrak JD. Carbon monoxide poisoning. N Engl J Med 1998; 339:1603–1608.

57. Weaver LK. Carbon monoxide poisoning. Crit Care Clin 1999; 15:297–317.

58. Weaver LK, Hopkins RO, Chan KJ, Churchill S, Elliott CG, Clemmer TP, Orme JF Jr, Thomas FO, Morris AH. Hyperbaric oxygen for acute carbon monoxide poisoning. N Engl J Med 2002; 347:1057–1067.

59. Vogel SN, Sultan TR, Ten Eyck RP. Cyanide poisoning. Clin Toxicol 1981; 18:367–383.

60. Mokhlesi B, Leikin JB, Murray P, Corbridge TC: Adult toxicology in critical care: part II: specific poisoning. Chest 2003; 123:897–922.

61. Nakae H, Tanaka H, Inaba H. Failure to clear casts and secretions following inhalation injury can be dangerous: report of a case. Burns 2001; 27:189–191.

62. Combes A, Figliolini C, Trouillet JL, Kassis N, Dombret MC, Wolf PM, Gilbert C, Chastre J. Factors predicting ventilator-associated pneumonia recurrence. Crit Care Med 2003; 31:1102–1107.

63. Levine BA, Petroff PA, Slade CL, Pruitt BA Jr. Prospective trials of dexamethasone and aerosolized gentamicin in the treatment of inhalation injury in the burned patient. J Trauma 1978; 18:188–193.

64. Brower RG, Fessler HE. Mechanical ventilation and acute lung injury and acute respiratory distress syndrome. Clin Chest Med 2000; 21:491–510.

65. Amshel CE, Fealk MH, Phillips BJ, Caroso DM. Anhydrous ammonia burn case report and review of the literature. Burns 2000; 26:493–497.

66. Gattinoni L, D'Andrea L, Pelosi P, Vitale G, Presenti A, Fumagalli R. Regional effects and mechanism of positive end-expiratory pressure in early adult respiratory distress syndrome. JAMA 1993; 269:2122–2127.

67. Rouby JJ, Lu Q, Goldstein I. Selecting the right level of positive end-expiratory pressure in patients with acute expiratory distress syndrome. Am J Respir Crit Care Med 2002; 165:1182–1186.

68. Esteban A, Alia I, Gordo F, dePablo R, Suarez J, Gonzalez G, Blanco J. Prospective randomized trial comparing pressure-controlled ventilation and volume-controlled ventilation in ARDS for the Spanish Lung Failure Collaborative Group. Chest 2000; 117:1690–1696.

69. Johnson B, Richard JC, Strauss C, Mancebo J, Lemaire F, Brochard L. Pressure-volume curves and compliance in acute lung injury: evidence of recruitment above the lower inflection point. Am J Respir Crit Care Med 1999; 159: 1172–1178.

70. Tripathi M, Pandy RK, Dwivedi S. Pressure controlled inverse ratio ventilation in acute respiratory distress syndrome patients. J Postgrad Med 2002; 48:34–36.

71. Wang SH, Wei TS. The outcome of early pressure-controlled inverse ratio ventilation on patients with severe acute respiratory distress syndrome in surgical intensive care unit. Am J Surg 2002; 183:151–155.

72. Yoder BA, Siler-Khodr T, Winter VT, Coalson JJ. High frequency ossitory ventilation: effects on lung function, mechanics, and airway cytokines in the immature baboon models with neonatal chronic lung disease. Am J Respir Crit Care Med 2000; 162:1867–1876.

73. Kornberger E, Mair P, Oswald E, Hormann C, Ohler K, Balogh D. Inhalation injury treated with extracorporeal CO$_2$ elimination. Burns 1997; 23:354–359.

74. Lyons B, Casey W, Doherty P, McHugh M, Moore KP. Pain relief with low dosage intravenous clonidine in a child with severe burns. Intens Care Med 1996;22:249–251.

75. Jellish WS, Gamelli RL, Flurry P, McGill VL, Fluder EM. Effect of topical local anesthetic application to skin graft harvest site for pain management in burn patients undergoing skin grafting procedures. Ann Surg 1999; 229:115–120.

76. McGill V, Kowal-Vern A, Gisher SG, Kahn S, Gamell RL. The impact of substance use on mortality and morbidity from thermal injury. J Trauma 1995; 38:931–934.

77. Bennett B, Gamelli RL. Profile of an abused child. J Burn Care Rehabil 1998; 19:88–94.

78. Czaja AJ, McAlhany JC, Pruitt BA Jr. Acute gastro-duodenal disease following thermal injury: an endoscopic evaluation of incidence and natural history. N Engl J Med 1974; 291:925.

79. Cioffi WG, McManus AT, Rue LW III, Mason AD, McManus WF, Pruitt BA Jr. Comparison of acid

neutralizing and non-acid neutralizing stress ulcer prophylaxis in thermally injured patients. J Trauma 1994; 36:541–547.

80. Swain AH, Azadian BS, Wakeley CJ, Shakespeare PG. Management of blisters in minor burns. Br Med J (Clin Res Ed) 1987; 295:181.

81. Rockwell WB, Ehrlich HP. Should burn blister fluid be evacuated? J Burn Care Rehabil 1990; 11:93–95.

82. Demling RH, Lalonde C. Burn trauma. In Blaisdell FW, Trunkey DD, eds. Trauma Management, vol. IV. New York: Thieme Medical, 1989: 55–56.

83. Hartford CE. The bequests of Moncrief and Moyer: an appraisal of topical therapy of burns B 1981 American Burn Association presidential address. J Trauma 1981; 21:827–834.

84. Hunter GR, Chang FC. Outpatient burns: a prospective study. J Trauma 1976; 16:191–195.

85. Miller SF. Outpatient management of minor burns. Am Fam Physician 1977; 16:167–172.

86. Nance FC, Lewis VL Jr, Hines JL, Barnett DP, O'Neill JA. Aggressive outpatient care of burns. J Trauma 1972; 12:144–146.

87. Heinrich JJ, Brand DA, Cuono CB. The role of topical treatment as a determinant of an infection in outpatient burns. J Burn Care Rehabil 1988; 9:253–257.

88. Smith-Choban P, Marshall WJ. Leukopenia secondary to silver sulfadiazine: frequency, characteristics and clinical consequences. Am Surg 1987; 53:515–517.

89. Gamelli RL, Paxton TO, O'Reilly M. Bone marrow toxicity by silver sulfadiazine. Surg Gynecol Obstet 1993; 177: 115–120.

90. Lindberg RB, Moncrief JA, Mason AD. Control of experimental and clinical burn wound sepsis by topical application of Sulfamylon compounds. Ann NY Acad Sci 1968; 150:950–972.

91. Yin HQ, Langford R, Burrell RE. Comparative evaluation of the antimicrobial activity of Acticoat antimicrobial barrier dressing. J Burn Care Rehabil 1999; 20:195–200.

92. Strock LL, Lee MM, Rutan RL, Desai MH, Robson MC, Herndon DN, Heggers JP. Topical Bactroban (mupirocin) efficacy in treating burn wounds infected with methicillin-resistant staphylococci. J Burn Care Rehabil 1990; 11:454–460.

93. Pruitt BA Jr. Burn wound. In Cameron JL, ed. Current Surgical Therapy, 5th ed. St. Louis: CV Mosby, 1995: 872–879.

94. Pruitt BA Jr, McManus AT, Kim JH, Goodwin CW. Burn wound infections: current status. World J Surg 1998; 22: 135–145.

95. Jackson D, Topley E, Caso JS, Lowbury EJ. Primary excision and grafting of large burns. Ann Sur 1960; 152: 167–189.

96. Tompkins RG, Remensynder JP, Burke JF, Tompkins DM, Hilton JF, Schoenfield DA, Behringer GE, Bondoc CC, Briggs SE, Quinby WC. Significant reductions in mortality for children with burn injuries through the use of prompt eschar excision. Ann Surg 1988; 208(5):577–585.

97. Burke JF, Bondoc CC, Quinby WC. Primary burn excision and immediate grafting: a method of shortening illness. J Trauma 1974; 14:389–395.

98. Santaniello JM, Luchette FA, Esposito TJ, Gunawan H, Davis KA, Gamell RL. Ten years experience of burn, trauma and combined burn/trauma injuries comparing outcomes. J Trauma 2004; 57:696–700.

99. McManus WF, Mason AD Jr, Pruitt BA Jr. Excision of the burn wound in patients with large burns. Arch Surg 1989; 124:718–720.

100. Janzekovic Z. A new concept in the early excision and immediate grafting of burns. J Trauma 1970; 10:1103–1108.

101. Desai MH, Herndon DN, Broemeling L, Barrow RE, Nichols RJ, Rutan RL. Early burn wound excision significantly reduces blood loss. Ann Surg 1990; 211:753–759.

102. Herndon DN. Perspectives in the use of allograft. J Burn Care Rehabil 1997; 18:S6.

103. Chatterjee DS. A controlled comparative study of the use of porcine xenograft in the treatment of partial thickness skin loss in an occupational health center. Curr Med Res Opin 1978; 5:726–733.

104. Demling RH. Burns. N Engl J Med 1985; 313:1389–1398.

105. Supple K, Halerz M, Aleem R, Gamelli RL. Transcyte as an alternative dressing for use in the pediatric burn patient. J Burn Care Rehabil 2003; 24(2):S129.

106. Sheridan RL, Choucair RJ. Acellular allodermis in burn surgery: 1 year results of a pilot trial. J Burn Care Rehabil 1998; 19:528–530.

107. Rue LW III, Cioffi WG, McManus WF, Pruitt BA Jr. Wound closure and outcome in extensively burned patients treated with cultured autologous keratinocytes. J Trauma 1993; 34:662–667.

108. Mozingo DW, Smith AA, McManus WF, Pruitt BA, Mason AD. Chemical burns. J Trauma 1988; 28:642–647.

109. Kohnlein HE, Merkle P, Springorum HW. Hydrogen fluoride burns: experiments in treatment. Surg Forum 1973; 24:50.

110. Pardoe R, Minami RT, Sato RM, Schlesinger SL. Phenol burns. Burns 1976; 3:29–41.

111. Pruitt BA Jr. Management of burns in the multiple injury patient. Surg Clin North Am 1970; 50:1283–1299.

112. Bangs CC. Hypothermia and frostbite. Emerg Med Clin North Am 1984; 2:475–487.

113. Miller BJ, Chasmar LR. Frostbite in Saskatoon: a review of 10 winters. Can J Surg 1980; 23:423–426.

114. Britt LD, Dascombe WH, Rodriguez A. New horizons in management of hypothermia and frostbite injury. Surg Clin North Am 1991; 71:345–370.

115. IAEA, June 1996, The Radiological Accident at the Irradiation facility in Nesvizh, IAEA (vienna, Austria), on line at IAEA http://www-pub-iaea.org/MTCD/publications/PDF/Pub1010_web.pdf.

116. Tsujii H, Akashi M, eds. The Criticality Accident in Tokaimura: Medical Aspects. Proceedings of an International Conference, December 14 and 15. Chiba, Japan: National Institute of Radiological Sciences, 2000. (NIRS-M-146).

117. Mettler, FA, Voelz, GL. Major radiation exposure—what to expect and how to respond. N Engl J Med 2002; 346:1554–1561.

118. Roujeau JC, Kelly JP, Naldi L, Rzany B, Stern RS, Anderson T, Auquier A, Basliju-Garin S, Corlea O, Locate F. Medication use and the risk of Stevens Johnson syndrome

or toxic epidermal necrolysis syndrome. N Engl J Med 1995; 333:1600–1607.

119. Viard I, Wehrli P, Bullani R, Schneider P, Holler N, Salomon D, Hunziker T, Saurat J, Tschopp J, French L. Inhibition of toxic epidermal necrolysis by blockade of CD95 with human intravenous immunoglobulin. Science 1998; 282:490–493.

120. Becker DS: Toxic epidermal necrolysis. Lancet 1998; 351:1417–1420.

121. Rasmussen JE, et al. Erythema multiforme, Stevens-Johnson syndrome and toxic epidermal necrolysis. Dermatol Nuc Dermatol Nurs 1995; 7:37–43.

122. Heimbach DM, Engrav LH, Marvin JA, Harnar TJ, Grube BJ. Toxic epidermal necrolysis: a step forward in treatment. JAMA 1987; 257:2171–2175.

123. Speron S, Gamelli RL. Toxic epidermal necrolysis syndrome versus mycosis fungoides. J Burn Care Rehabil 1997; 18:421–423.

124. Brown KM, Silver GM, Halerz M, Walaszek P, Sandroni A, Gamelli RL. Toxic epidermal necrolysis: does immunoglobulin make a difference? J Burn Care Rehabil 2004; 25:81–88.

125. Dougherty W, Waxman K. The complexities of managing severe burns with associated trauma. Surg Clin North Am 1996; 76:923–958.

126. Purdue GF, Hunt JL. Multiple trauma and the burn patient. Am J Surg 1989; 158:536–539.

127. Wilmore DW, Orcutt TW, Mason AD Jr, Pruitt BA Jr. Alterations in hypothalamic function following thermal injury. J Trauma 1975; 15:697–703.

128. Carlson DE, Cioffi WG Jr, Mason AD Jr, McManus WF, Pruitt BA Jr. Resting energy expenditure in patients with thermal injuries. Surg Gynecol Obstet 1992; 174:270–276.

129. Alverdy J, Aoys E, Moss GS. Total parenteral nutrition promotes bacterial translocation from the gut. Surgery 1988; 104:185–190.

130. Wilmore D, Long J, Mason A, Skreen RW, Pruitt BA Jr. Catecholamines: mediators of the hypermetabolic response to thermal injury. Ann Surg 1974; 180:653–669.

131. Kudsk K, Brown R. Nutritional support. In Mattox K, Feliciano D, Moore E, eds. Trauma. New York: McGraw-Hill, 2000: 1369–1405.

132. Demling RH, Seigne P. Metabolic management of patients with severe burns. World J Surg 2000; 24:673–680.

133. Bessey PQ, Jiang ZM, Johnson DT, Smith RJ, Wilmore DW. Posttraumatic skeletal muscle proteolysis: the role of the hormonal environment. World J Surg 1989; 13:465–470.

134. Mochizuki H, Trocki O, Dominion L, Brackett KA, Joffe SN, Alexander JW. Mechanism of prevention of postburn hypermetabolism and catabolism by early enteral feeding. Ann Surg 1984 ;200:297–300.

135. Wood RH, Caldwell F Jr, Bowser-Wallace BH. The effect of early feeding on postburn hypermetabolism. J Trauma 1988: 28:177–183.

136. Chiarelli A, Enzi G, Casadei A, Baggio B, Valerio A, Mazzoleni F. Very early nutrition supplementation in burned patients. Am J Clin Nutr 1990; 51:1035–1039.

137. Van Den Berghe G, Wouters P, Weekers F, Verwaest C, Bruyninckx F, Schetz M, Vlasselaers D, Ferdinande P, Lauwers P, Bouillon R: Intensive insulin therapy in critically ill patients. N Engl J Med 2001; 345:1359–1367.

138. Askanazai J, Rosenbaum S, Hyman A, Silverberg PA, Milic-Emili J, Kinney JM. Respiratory changes induced by the large glucose loads of total parenteral nutrition. JAMA 1980; 243:1444–1447.

139. Peck M. Practice guidelines for burn care: nutritional support. J Burn Care Rehabil 2001; 12:59S–66S.

140. Waymack J, Herndon D. Nutritional support of the burned patient. World J Surg 1992; 16: 80–86.

141. Wolf R, Goodenough R, Burke J, Wolfe M. Response of proteins and urea kinetics in burn patients to different levels of protein intake. Ann Surg 1983; 197:163–171.

142. Matsuda T, Kagan R, Hanumadass M, Jonasson O. The importance of burn wound size in determining the optimal calorie: nitrogen ratio. Surgery 1983; 94:562–568.

143. Alexander J, MacMillan B, Stinnet J, Ogle CK. Beneficial effects of aggressive protein feeding in severely burned children. Ann Surg 1980: 192:505–517.

144. O'Neill JA, Caldwell MD, Meng HC: Essential fatty acid deficiency in surgical patients. Ann Surg 1977; 185:535–542.

145. Harrison HN, Moncrief JA, Duckett JW Jr, Mason AD Jr. The relationship between energy metabolism and water loss from vaporization in severely burned patients. Surgery 1964; 56:203–211.

146. Mayes T, Gottschlich M, Warden G. Clinical nutrition protocols for continuous quality improvement in the outcomes of patients with burns. J Burn Care Rehabil 1997; 18:365–368.

147. Selmanpakoglu ACC, Sayal A, Isimer A. Trace element (Al, Se, Zn, Cu) levels in serum, urine, and tissues of burn patients. Burns 1994; 20:99–103.

148. Herndon DN, Hart DW, Wolf SE, Chinkes DL, Wolfe RR. Reversal of catabolism by beta-blockade after severe burns. N Engl J Med 2001; 345(17):1223–1229.

149. Herndon D, Barrow R, Kunkel K, Broemling L, Rutan R. Effects of recombinant human growth hormone on donor site healing in severely burned children. Ann Surg 1990; 212:424–429.

150. Talala J, Ruokonen E, Webster N, Nielsen MS, Zandsta DF, Vurdelinckx G, Hinds CJ. Increased mortality associated with growth hormone treatment in critically ill adults. N Engl J Med 1999; 341:785–792.

151. Demling R. Comparison of the anabolic effects and complications of human growth hormone and the testosterone analog, oxandrolone, after severe burn injury. Burns 1999; 25:215–221.

152. Demling R, Orgill D. The anticabolic and wound healing effects of the testosterone analog oxandrolone after severe burn injury. J Crit Care 2000; 15:12–17.

153. Demling R, DeSanti L. Oxandrolone, an anabolic steroid, significantly increases the rate of weight gain in the recovery phase after major burns. J Trauma 1997; 43:47–51.

154. Bulger EM, Jurkovich GJ, Farver CL, Klotz P, Maier RV. Oxandrolone does not improve outcome of ventilator-dependent surgical patients. Ann Surg 2004; 240:472–480.

154. Saito H, Trocki O, Wang S, Gonce SJ, Joffe SN, Alexander JW. Metabolic and immune effects of dietary arginine supplementation after burn. Arch Surg 1987; 122:784–789.

156. Souba W. Glutamine: a key substrate for the splanchnic bed. Annu Rev Nutr 1991; 11:285–308.

157. Alverdy JC. Effects of glutamine-supplemented diets on immunology of the gut. J Parenteral Enteral Nutr 1990; 14:109S–113S.

158. Ziegler T, Young L, Benfell K, Scheltinga M, Hortos K. Clinical and metabolic efficacy of glutamine supplemented parenteral nutrition after bone marrow transplantation: a randomized, double-blind controlled trial. Ann Intern Med 1992; 116:821–830.

159. Alexander J, Saito H, Trocki O, Ogle C. The importance of lipid type in the diet after burn injury. Ann Surg 1986; 204:1–8.

160. Saffle JR, Wiebke G, Jennings K, Morris SE, Bartor RG. Randomized trial of immune-enhancing enteral nutrition in burn patients. J Trauma 1997; 42:793–802.

161. Kowal-Vern A, McGill V, Gamelli R. Ischemic necrotic bowel disease in thermal injury. Arch Surg 1997; 132:440–443.

162. Scaife C, Saffle J, Morris S. Intestinal obstruction secondary to enteral feedings in burn trauma patients. Proceedings of the Western Trauma Association, Crested Butte, CO, February 1999. J Trauma 1991; 47:859–863.

163. Marvin R, McKinley B, McQuiggan M, Cocanour C, Moore F. Nonocclusive bowel necrosis occurring in critically ill trauma patients receiving enteral nutrition manifests no reliable clinical signs for early detection. Am J Surg 2000; 179:7–12.

164. Grube B, Heimbach C, Marvin J. *Clostridium difficile* diarrhea in critically ill burned patients. Arch Surg 1987; 122:655–661.

165. Gottschlich M, Warden G, Michel M, Havens P, Kofcha R, Jenkings M, Alexander JW. Diarrhea in tube-fed burn patients: incidence, etiology, nutritional impact and prevention. J Parenteral Enteral Nutr 1988; 12:338–345.

166. Cioffi WG, Pruitt BA Jr. Aeromedical transport of the thermally injured patient. Med Corp Int 1989; 4(3):23–27.

167. Pruitt BA Jr. Centennial changes in surgical care and research. Ann Surg 2000; 233:287–301.

10
Electrical and Lightning Injuries

Raphael C. Lee

Case Scenario

A 23-year-old industrial mechanic sustains a high-voltage electrical injury. He has a circumferential full-thickness injury of the right upper extremity. The patient develops hand paraesthesia and then numbness. Which of the following is the management of choice at this time?

(A) Decrease fluid resuscitation and elevate the involved extremity
(B) Increase fluid resuscitation and administer mannitol
(C) Continue to monitor the extremity
(D) Perform escharotomy and monitor the extremity
(E) Perform escharotomy and fasciotomy of the involved extremity

---

Pathophysiology and Manifestations

Because of the multiple modes of electrical force action on biologic tissues, electrical injury can produce a very complex pattern of injury and resulting clinical manifestations.[1,2] Electrical forces cause tissue injury primarily by permeabilization of cell membranes and thermal denaturation of tissue proteins. When high-energy arc-mediated contacts occur, there is often a strong thermoacoustic blast force generated, which adds blunt mechanical trauma. Associated falls and skin burns are frequent, adding to victim injury.

Electrical current passing through the body imposes electrical forces acting on cell membranes. The longer the cell projects in the direction of current flow, the stronger the force. Large cells, such as skeletal muscle and nerve, experience strong enough forces during electrical shock to disrupt their membranes. This produces the increased permeability to electrolytes in solution that subsequently

leads to metabolic energy depletion, free radical generation, and cellular necrosis. The resistance to current passage is highest at the skin contact points, which explains the occurrence of deep burns at the contact point, as shown in Figure 10.1.

Similarly, victims of direct lightning strikes experience a multimodal injury. The current passes in the air *between* the cloud, and the lightning strikes the victim. Although very little of the lightning current penetrates the body, the current pulse sets up a large magnetic field pulse that readily penetrates the body. The magnitude of this pulse is sufficient to induce large internal currents that cause neuromuscular, cardiac, and central nervous system damage. The thermoacoustic blast (i.e., thunder)–related barotrauma can be significant.

Peripheral nerve and skeletal muscle tissues are the most vulnerable to membrane permeabilization by electrical force. The rapidity of this process is such that only millisecond duration contacts are required to generate significant damage accumulation. With more prolonged contacts, on the range of seconds, thermal damage in the subcutaneous tissues occurs. Because the vulnerability to supraphysiologic temperature exposure is similar across different tissue types, victims of prolonged contact suffer direct thermal damage to all tissues in the current path.[3] The rate of tissue heating scales with the square of the tissue current density. As a consequence of the variation in current density with extremity cross-sectional area, the anatomic distribution of tissue injury varies considerably. Both heat and electrical forces lead to disruption of cellular membranes, extensive swelling, and compartment syndromes (Figure 10.2).[4]

The extremities are nearly always involved because most victims that require inpatient hospital care are young industrial or construction workers using their hands. In industrial high-voltage shocks, conduction of electrical current through the body takes place before mechanical contact is made. Electrical contact can occur through the electrical arc. Exposure to the expanding arc

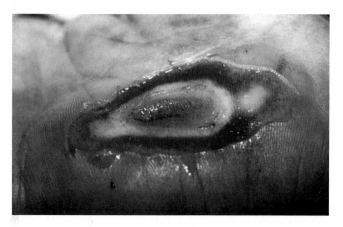

FIGURE 10.1. Characteristic appearance of an electrical contact wound. The central area has experienced very high temperatures, resulting in tissue coagulation. It can be expected that this injury extends along the current path beneath the skin. The same pattern results regardless of the direction of the current. The depression of the wound is caused by coagulation, not by the momentum of ionic current passage.

TABLE 10.1. Basic management of electrical injuries.

- **Resuscitation and assessment**
  - Evaluate and support vital organ function
  - Manage cardiac injury if present
  - If myoglobinuria present, increase urine output to 2 cc/kg
  - Perform fasciotomies as needed within 6 hours of injury
  - Use diagnostic imaging (MRI) to assess extent of injury
  - Provide tetanus prophylaxis
- **Initial debridement**
  - Remove grossly devitalized tissue
  - Provide temporary wound coverage
  - Provide antibiotic coverage
  - Release tense muscle compartments
- **Wound closure**
- **Provide nutrition support**
  - Repeat debridement at 24–48 hours
  - Close the wound
- **Neurologic and psychiatric assessment**
  - Provide pain control
  - Perform baseline psychiatric assessment and follow-up
  - Perform neuropsychological evaluation at 6 months postinjury
- **Rehabilitation**
  - Muscle strengthening and endurance enhancement
  - Scar management
  - Occupational therapy

or flash brings the victim in the circuit. The involuntary muscle spasm that results may lead to joint dislocations and spine fractures. When currents of more than 100 mA are passed hand-to-hand or hand-to-foot, there is enough electrical force generated in the heart to cause cardiac arrhythmias.

Approach to Management

Electrical injury patients can present complex medical management challenges. In severe cases, the widespread destruction of tissue causes tremendous life-threatening physiologic stress unlike any other form of trauma. On the other extreme are the apparently minor cases, wherein insidious injury to the nervous system presents substantial diagnostic and management challenges. Many electrical shock survivors present with delayed-onset neurologic and neuropsychological problems. In general, medical providers must be aware that electrical shock patients can require involvement of every medical and

surgical specialty. A basic management strategy is listed in Table 10.1.[5]

Acute Care

In the field, the first priority is to disconnect the patient from the electrical power source. When high-capacity circuits are involved, this must not be attempted before the circuit is deenergized. If the circuit is a commercial power distribution line, great care has to be exercised. High-voltage, high-current-capacity lines can generate enough electrical field in the ground around a victim to cause injury to anyone approaching to aide. In addition, these commercial power circuits have automatic shut-off and automatic power return breakers. These high-voltage circuits can turn on while emergency crews are attempting to extract the victim. Therefore, it is strongly recommended that the emergency crews contact the electrical utility to shut down the line before extracting.

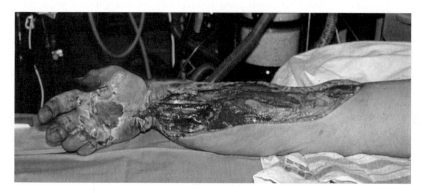

FIGURE 10.2. The incredibly destructive nature of just a brief contact with high-voltage electrical power is shown. The muscle contraction has ripped the muscle away from the tendons, and there is massive swelling requiring full fasciotomies. Both thermal and nonthermal injuries are evident, resulting in extensive tissue destruction.

While extracting the victim, it is safest to assume spine injury until proven otherwise. Although this manifestation is unusual, it is well established that fractures and joint dislocations can follow the muscle spasm that occurs during electrical shock. Prolonged cardiopulmonary resuscitation may be necessary before the stunned myocardium regains the ability to sustain a coordinated rhythm. This is particularly true following lightning injury. Large-bore peripheral intravenous lines delivering a balanced salt solution at a rate sufficient to generate a 30 to 50 cc/hr urine output, supplemental oxygen, and a Foley catheter are essential. If the urine is visibly pigmented with hemochromogens, the urine output should be doubled and alkalinized to a pH > 6.

As soon as the patient arrives in the emergency care department, clothing and debris on wounds should be removed and the wounds cleaned. Large skin burn wounds are often present because of arc-mediated contacts and clothing ignition. Care should be taken to prevent rapid loss of body heat through open wounds. When skin contact wounds are present or the contact voltage is in excess of 200 volts, transfer to a burn center for definitive evaluation and care should occur. The immediate goal is to support vital organ function to achieve patient stabilization. Begin initial resuscitation with potassium-free solutions such as normal saline, which is preferred until serum chemistries are known. In the absence of significant skin burns the initial fluid administration rate is based on clinical signs such as blood pressure, pulse rate, and clinical intuition. Subsequently the fluid is adjusted as needed to maintain 30 to 50 cc of urine output per hour. If the urine is visibly pigmented, intravenous fluid should be increased to double the hourly urine output until it clears. It is recommended that the urine pH is alkalinized to above 6.0 by adding bicarbonate to the intravenous solutions. Providing adequate nutritional support, especially though enteral tube feedings, is very important. Supplemental oxygen may be helpful to edematous tissues.

Cardiac arrhythmia must be immediately controlled by appropriate antiarrhythmic agents and correction of pH and electrolyte abnormalities. Brain injury can manifest with seizures, which may need to be controlled with antiepileptic agents and with correction of serum chemistries.[6] Patients who have lost central nervous system control or respiration or airway should be intubated and mechanically ventilated. A feeding tube should be passed to begin gastrointestinal alimentation within 6 hours of injury. Clearly, enteral feeding is contraindicated if abdominal viscera are injured by current. Substantial intraabdominal injuries are known to occur in electrical trauma. Ruptures of colon, gallbladder, and other organs have been reported. Fortunately, these severe intraabdominal injuries are unusual. A paralyzed ventilated patient may need electroencephalographic monitoring to assess the quality of seizure control.

Diagnostic Evaluation

Cardiac arrhythmias must be rapidly detected by examination of the pulses and measurement of blood pressure and then diagnosed by electrocardiogram. The major initial diagnostic challenge is to determine the location and extent of all tissue damage, particularly that which is beneath undamaged skin. Lateral spine x-rays are needed to rule out unstable spine fracture patterns. X-ray images of the extremities involved are also important to rule out skeletal fractures or joint dislocations. Blood chemistries should be immediately evaluated and monitored. Metabolic acidosis and elevated serum potassium level may occur as a consequence of extensive skeletal muscle injury. Over several hours creatine phosphokinase level will rise if there is significant skeletal muscle cell lysis.

Thermally damaged tissue is recognizable on gross inspection, whereas tissues damaged by electropermeabilization usually simply appear edematous. Within minutes after injury, tissue edema begins to increase due to increased vascular permeability and release of intracellular contents into the extravascular space. Compartment syndrome and compression neuropathies are common manifestations of an electrically traumatized extremity. Injured skeletal muscle and nerve frequently underlie uninjured skin (see Figure 10.1). If a fast magnetic resonance imaging (MRI) scanner is available, T_2-weighted images can localize muscle and nerve edema, and gadolinium enhanced T_1-weighted images can demonstrate tissues with cell membrane permeabilization.[7] It is important to remember that edema cannot form in the absence of tissue perfusion. Thus, where severe heating has left coagulated vessels, tissue injury may exist in the absence of edema.

The presence of edema on MRI should guide attention to potential problem areas. Compartment pressures should be measured where edema is present. Tense muscle compartments are not reliably diagnosed by manual palpation. Muscle compartment fluid pressures should be measured and documented. If MRI is not available, then the muscle compartments within the current path between contact points should be monitored for elevated interstitial fluid pressure. Elevated compartment pressures may not manifest until the patient has been resuscitated. It may be necessary to check the pressures every 8 hours for 24 hours. Radionucleotide scanning with Tc^{99m}-pyrophosphate may be useful to localize hidden tissue injury, especially in cases of less extensive injury.[7] However, these scans take 4 to 6 hours to complete and are mostly useful in the less severe injuries.

Neurologic complaints are almost invariably present. When symptoms exist, neurodiagnostic studies are required to determine the extent of neuromuscular dysfunction. Compound nerve conduction velocity and electromyography are standard studies that are widely available. Unfortunately, they lack sensitivity and specificity. Our protocol is to use refractory period spectral analysis, which permits separately measuring the responses of the different nerve fiber types present in compound nerves. Major peripheral nerves contain thousands of fibers that exist in several different types. The large myelinated fast fibers are most susceptible to electrical forces generated by passage of current through the extremity while small-diameter unmyelinated fibers are the least susceptible. Thus, peripheral nerve injury is mixed in pattern. Diagnostic evaluation by refractory period spectral analysis of nerve function is most useful because of its capability to discriminate each axon type separately.[8]

Unless the victim was water submerged, at least two skin contact wounds are present. Because 60-Hz commercial power frequency current reverses direction every 8 msec, nearly always all wounds serve as both entry and exit points into the body. Therefore, the commonly used terminology of "entrance" or "exit" wounds is basically incorrect. Differences in wound area, depth, and topography are determined by the size and shape of the object with which the victim was in contact. Ophthalmologic examination with emphasis on signs of corneal burns or abrasions should be performed. The ignition of a high-energy arc generates a loud noise or blast, which can lead to tympanic membrane rupture and/or closed head trauma. If there is a history of loss of consciousness, a computerized tomogram of the head is indicated.

Early Management

Perfusion to edematous tissue must be restored as soon as possible. Diminished pulses or decreased tissue oxygen detected by transcutaneous pulse oximetry are indications for escharotomy releases. Assessing the need for fasciotomy is an important consideration. The classic clinical signs of pain in acute compartment syndrome cannot be relied on because of the nerve injury that frequently accompanies electrical shock. When there are circumferential (or near-circumferential) extremity skin burns, muscle compartment pressures can be elevated because of eschar compression.

If the muscle, abdominal, chest, or other compartment pressures remain elevated after escharotomy, then fasciotomy is indicated in the operative theater under adequate lighting. Because the compartment pressure needs to exceed only 30 mm Hg to reduce gas exchange in the muscle, measurement for a distal arterial pressure drop is not an early indicator of the risk of ischemic muscle injury. A muscle compartment fluid pressure of greater than 30 cm H_2O is the indication for fasciotomy. When a muscle compartment requires release in an electrical shock victim, the adjacent ones should also be decompressed. It must be remembered that permanent muscle

damage can be appreciated after only 2 hours of warm ischemia, and a no-reflow state can occur after 6 hours of warm ischemia time. To be effective, the epimyesium must also be released under full view. Release of skeletal muscle compartments is often followed by massive bulging of muscle and a readily observed increase in tissue perfusion. Care to avoid tissue drying or desiccation is important. In addition to topical antimicrobial coverage, the wound should be covered using an evaporative barrier.

In addition to decompression of extremity muscle compartments, decompression of nerve within edematous fibroosseus conduits (e.g., carpal tunnel, Guyon's canal, and tarsal tunnel) should be carried out to help prevent compression neuropathy. Unless thermally burned, nerve and tendons should not be debrided at the initial visit to the operating room. Well-fashioned splints are essential to maintain joints in a position of function and to protect vascular perfusion during hospitalization. With modern surgical reconstruction techniques, amputations are required less often now.

The risk of infection must be kept in mind. Tetanus prophylaxis should be administered as established by the World Health Organization guidelines. Anaerobic bacterial infection of devascularized skeletal muscle is a commonly expressed concern and intravenous penicillin G and/or hyperbaric oxygen as prophylactic antibiotics are utilized by some but has unproven value. Radiographs taken to rule out fractures may reveal air bubbles in the subcutaneous tissues. This probably results from boiling from Joule heating and may indicate irreversible heat damage. Most importantly, in the triage and acute care setting, soft tissue air bubbles should not be interpreted as a sign of anaerobic sepsis.

Debridement of nonviable tissue should be performed in the operating theater as soon as the patient has been stabilized and the evaluations completed. Quinby et al.[9] proposed early muscle debridement under histologic control. Although accurate, this method prolongs general anesthesia and may result in increased morbidity. Arteries and veins that are burned should be replaced with healthy vein grafts as soon as possible. A second-look procedure 48 hours later is often needed to be certain of a complete debridement. The most widely practiced approach is to reinspect and debride the wounds in the operating theater within 48 to 72 hours so that systemic toxicity and local infection risk are minimized.

Wound closure should wait until the wound is free of all dead and/or marginal tissue and quantitative bacteriologic counts rule out invasive wound sepsis. In most cases, the major vessels have not been heat damaged and can be used to support microvascular free flaps. Wound closure can also be accomplished by local fasciocutaneous flaps or skin grafts. The choice of procedure should be made with the view toward optimizing rehabilitation potential. Local skin and fascial flaps in an injured extremity have been shown to be reliable. Doppler presurgical assessment of the vascular pedicles is desirable. Tendons and nerves should be kept physiologically moistened and protected with vascularized tissue as soon as possible. Effective wound closure should be accomplished whenever possible within the first week.

Rehabilitation

Rehabilitation into society and gainful employment is the ultimate objective and often the biggest challenge. Survivors of industrial accidents are often young and proud of their capabilities. After injury, they are often limited by pain and worried about their ability to return to gainful employment. For severely injured victims this requires functional muscle and nerve reconstruction as well as correction of scar contractures. Psychological problems are the rule and require involvement of serial neuropsychological assessment and protracted support.[10] Persistent neurologic problems are also common and often require therapeutic intervention from a pain management specialist.[11] Work force reentry should be guided by consultation with employer, patient, co-workers, and an experienced rehabilitation team.[12] Under investigation are therapeutic surfactant copolymers that mimic the effects of natural cellular chaperones that promise to reduce tissue loss after electrical injuries.[13]

Critique

The development of paraesthesia in an extremity with a circumferential full-thickness burn is a compartment syndrome until proven otherwise. In addition to this patient requiring an escharotomy, a fasciotomy is also needed given the mechanism of injury—a high-voltage electrical injury. Muscle damage with subsequent swelling should be suspected.

Answer (E)

References

1. Lee RC. Tissue injury from exposure to power frequency electrical fields. In Lin J, ed. Advances in Electromagnetic Fields in Living Systems, New York: Plenum Press, 1994; 81–127.
2. Capelli-Schellpfeffer M, Lee RC, Toner M, Diller KR. Correlation Between Electrical Accident Parameters and Sustained Injury. IEEE /PCIC Transactions, September 1996.
3. Remensnyder JP. Acute electrical injuries. In Martyn JAJ, ed. Acute Management of the Burned Patient. Philadelphia: WB Saunders, 1990; 66–86.
4. Lee RC, Cravalho EG, Burke JF, eds. Electrical Trauma: The Pathophysiology, Manifestations and Clinical Management. Cambridge: Cambridge University Press, 1992; 133–152.
5. Lee RC, Capelli-Schellpfeffer M, Kelley KM, eds. Electrical injury: a multidisciplinary approach to therapy, prevention and rehabilitation. Ann NY Acad Sci 1994; 720.
6. Dasgupta RA, Schulz JT, Lee RC, Ryan CM. Severe hypokalemia as a cause of acute transient para plegia following electrical shock. Burns 2002; 28:609–611.
7. Fleckenstein JL, Chason DP, Bonte FJ, et al. High-voltage electric injury: assessment of muscle viability with MR imaging and Tc-99 m pyrophosphate scintigraphy. Radiology 1995; 195(1):205–210.
8. Abramov G, Bier M, Capelli-Schellpfeffer M, Lee RC. Alteration in sensory nerve function following electrical shock. Burns J 1996; 22(8):602–606.
9. Quinby WC Jr, Burke JF, Trelstad RL, Caulfield J. The use of microscopy as a guide to primary excision of high-tension electrical burns. J Trauma 1978; 18:423–429.
10. Pliskin NH, Ammar AM, Fink JM, Hill SK, Malina AC, Kelley KM, Meiner BA, Lee RC. Neuropsychological effects of electrical injury. J Int Neuropsychol Soc 2006; 12:17–23.
11. Wilbourn AJ. Peripheral nerve disorders in electrical and lightning injuries. Semin Neurol 1995; 15(3):241–256.
12. Chico M, Capelli-Schellpfeffer M, Kelley KM, Lee RC. Management and coordination of post-acute medical care for electrical trauma survivors. Ann NY Acad Sci 1999; 888:334–342.
13. Lee RC, River P, Pan FS, Ji L, Wollmann RL. Surfactant-induced sealing of electropermeabilized skeletal muscle membranes in vivo. Proc Natl Acad Sci USA 1992; 89:4524–4528.

11
Soft Tissue Infections

Anthony A. Meyer, Jeffrey E. Abrams, Thomas L. Bosshardt, and Claude H. Organ, Jr.

Case Scenario

A 57-year-old renal transplantation patient develops a necrotizing soft tissue infection in the perineum. She is febrile, tachycardic, and hemodynamically labile with deterioration of renal function. Which of the following is *not* essential to the management of the patient?

(A) Fluid resuscitation
(B) Antimicrobial therapy
(C) Nutritional support
(D) Debridement of necrotic tissue
(E) Hyperbaric oxygen therapy

Necrotizing soft tissue infections are infections that cause tissue necrosis by both direct cell destruction and ischemia secondary to thrombosis of blood vessels that pass through the fascial and subcutaneous fat to the skin. Infections can occasionally involve muscle as well. Necrotizing soft tissue infections represent a spectrum of infection that may be localized to a relatively small area, take days to progress, and have minimal systemic effects or spread rapidly to involve more than 25% of the body's surface, with profound hemodynamic instability and death within 12 to 24 hours. Such soft tissue infections mandate acute surgical intervention.

These infections have been known by many names, including "hospitalism," "hemolytic streptococcal gangrene," "necrotizing erysipelas," "necrotizing cellulitis," and "necrotizing fasciitis." Recently, the name "necrotizing soft tissue infection" (NSTI) has become the accepted name. However, the terminology of NSTI is of secondary concern when physicians are challenged by a pattern with this aggressive illness. Distinguishing the specific category of necrotizing infection serves little purpose. The primary emphasis must be focused on rapid recognition and prompt treatment. To limit severe morbidity and to reduce mortality, early treatment with aggressive surgical intervention and appropriate antimicrobial therapy is essential. The NSTIs must be considered a surgical emergency. In an excellent clinical account of NSTI in Civil War medicine, over 60% mortality for serious infections was reported.[1–3] Mortality rates reported for this disease process have varied dramatically, depending on the patient population and treatment available. Meleney,[4] in a review of cases from China in 1920, reported lower mortality (20%), but described a less aggressive spectrum of disease because patients with more virulent infections would not survive to reach care. Recent series in the United States have also varied in the type of disease process that is seen, the patient population, and outcomes. In general, the mortality rate for NSTI generally remains in the 20% to 40% range.[2,5,6]

Increased attention has been focused on NSTIs in recent years. This may have to do with studies coming out documenting potentially new and more virulent types of the disease. Other reasons for greater attention may be the sensational accounts of individual cases in the tabloid press, including descriptions of "flesh-eating bacteria" and "flesh-eating viruses." Clearly, there is evidence that the actual incidence of these infections is increasing.[7–9]

Hospitals that treat a large number of critically ill patients, such as teaching and public hospitals, have described an increase in the number of NSTI patients. The rise in the incidence of the disease may also be explained by the increasing numbers of immunosuppressed or chronically ill patients, who appear to be more susceptible to these infections, the increased obesity in the population, and a better recognition and diagnosis of the process.[10–12] The magnitude by which correct diagnosis is contributing to an increased perceived incidence is yet to be determined.

The etiology of the disease remains poorly understood, but it is clear that NSTIs remain a major clinical problem.

The pathophysiology will be reviewed to understand why the disease is so morbid and to provide an understanding of how to diagnose and treat this challenging spectrum of soft tissue infections.

Pathophysiology

The potential causes of NSTIs include tissue injury, bacterial inoculation, superficial skin infection, and any of the many possible mechanisms for initiating cutaneous infections. There is often tissue damage or injury, including the injury of a surgical incision. Wounds combine a means for introduction of bacteria with a potential medium in which the bacteria can multiply. By whatever mechanism, a bacterial inoculum gets into dermal or subcutaneous tissue and, rather than create a simple abscess or cellulitis, initiates a cascade of cell destruction, inflammation, and ischemia. This creates a means by which the infection moves into normal tissue and causes necrosis and secondary ischemia of more superficial tissue by thrombosis of vessels that pass through the infected tissue.[5,13,14]

Patients who are at increased risk for NSTIs include diabetics, immunosuppressed patients, and intravenous drug users.[15,16] Whether the continued inoculation of contaminated material or the debilitating lifestyle that is associated with intravenous drug use is the principle cause of the infection is unclear.[13,17,18] There are many other medical problems that are associated with increased incidence of NSTIs. Diabetics have impaired blood flow to skin and other soft tissue, decreased ability to fight bacterial infection, and other metabolic changes that make them more susceptible to any infection. Patients who undergo immunosuppression to limit transplant rejection or for treatment of cancer are also at increased risk for these severe soft tissue infections. Furthermore, these immunosuppressed patients are more likely to develop infections from atypical organisms than the most common types, which are discussed later.[19] There are patients, however, in whom there is no obvious cause who present with a clinical picture suspicious for NSTI. It is important to understand that the lack of an obvious associated medical condition or injury should not preclude a potential diagnosis of NSTI. There is ample evidence that early identification and treatment are important to improving outcome and ultimately decreasing the morbidity of this rapidly progressing infection. It is important also to remember that the management of NSTI in patient groups at increased risk is no different from management in patients without these risks. The presence of risk factors should only make the physician more aggressive at pursuing early diagnosis.

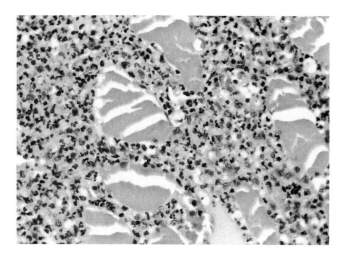

FIGURE 11.1. Histology of NSTI, demonstrating acute inflammation within muscle bundles.

Microbiology

The microbiologies of the organisms cultured from NSTIs in different studies vary widely and are dependent not only on the disease and patient population but also surgical and laboratory techniques as well. The bacteriology of NSTI is well recognized, and the infectious process is independent of specific bacteria.[17,20–23] Although NSTIs can be monomicrobial, most are polymicrobial and involve aerobic and anaerobic organisms behaving synergistically. These bacteria can invade the subcutaneous tissue, fascia, and even muscle to result in necrosis and destruction (Figures 11.1 and 11.2). In our series of patients treated at an urban hospital, 78% of cases were polymicrobial and 2.8 organisms were recovered per patient.[17] Anaerobes, skin flora, and Gram-negative rods were commonly encountered (Table 11.1). Elliott et al.[21]

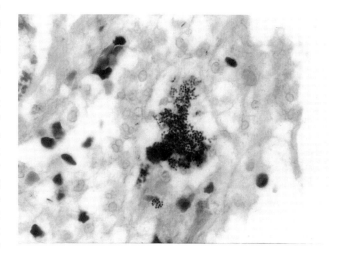

FIGURE 11.2. Bacterial invasion of the soft tissues by Gram-positive cocci.

TABLE 11.1. Bacteriologic findings in patients with necrotizing soft tissue infections.

Organism	No. of patients
Anaerobes	
Mixed anaerobes	16
Clostridium sp.*	8
Diphtheroids	3
Bacteroides fragilis	2
Bacteroides buccae	2
Peptostreptococcus sp.	1
Total	32
Gram-positive cocci	
Streptococcus viridans	8
Hemolytic group A streptococci	7
Enterococcus faecalis	6
Total	21
Gram-negative rods	
Mixed gram-negative rods	6
Proteus mirabilis	4
Escherichia coli	3
Eikenella corrodens	3
Enterobacter sp.	1
Serratia marcescens	1
Total	18
Skin flora	
Staphylococcus coagulase negative	14
Staphylococcus aureus	14
Mixed skin flora	4
Total	32

*Includes *C. perfringens, C. septicum, C. sordellii, C. tetani,* and *C. botulinum.*
Source: Reprinted with permission from Bosshardt et al.[17]

analyzed 182 patients with NSTI over an 8-year period, focusing on the microbiology of the infectious process, and found 154 polymicrobial infections out of 182 total cases, with an average of 4.4 microbes per NSTI (based on original wound cultures). The most common organisms, in order, were *Bacteroides* species, aerobic *Streptococcus*, staphylococci, enterococci, *Escherichia coli*, and other Gram-negative rods.

Monomicrobial infections are usually caused by hemolytic group A *Streptococcus*, *Staphylococcus aureus*, or clostridial species. Group A streptococcal NSTIs not uncommonly involve younger patients and the extremities and are associated with a streptococcal toxic shock-like syndrome. These infections may appear suddenly in previously healthy patients and are often exceedingly rapid in progression. Organ system dysfunction can be out of proportion to the extent of local signs and symptoms.[8,24,25] Recent reports indicate that NSTIs can be caused by group B *Streptococcus*[26] and group G *Streptococcus*,[27] demonstrating that serious invasive streptococcal infections may be on the rise.

Clostridial infections are classically associated with myonecrosis (gas gangrene), severe toxicity, and higher mortality. *Clostridium perfringens c. novyi* and *c. septicum* are often cultured, and clinical signs include intense pain, swelling, crepitus, and a thin watery discharge.[21,28,29] On exploration necrotic, sometimes blackened muscle is encountered.

There are many other monomicrobial NSTI pathogens that are less frequently encountered, including *Vibrio vulnificus*[30] and *Cryptococcus neoformans.*[31] Table 11.2 summarizes some of the organisms seen with NSTI, their characteristics, and some general recommendations.

It must be remembered, however, that the microbiology of soft tissue infections is not usually known until days after treatment has been initialed, at which time the patient is improving or deteriorating or has died. The identification of the NSTI is not done by the microbiology but by clinical evaluation and surgical exploration of the infected tissue. It is the clinical evidence of tissue destruction by the advancing soft tissue infection causing necrosis rather than infection of necrotic tissue that defines NSTI.

The mechanisms that determine whether organisms will only colonize or will cause rapidly progressing tissue destruction and potential death in hours or a few days remain unclear. It is probably a combination of the virulent organism, the local milieu of the infection, the general condition of the patient, and other unknown factors during the early spread of the infection that are most important. Once the organisms start to grow in the tissue, the infection appears to progress on the basis of two principle areas: The first is the destruction and breakdown of normal tissue components by proteolytic and lipolytic enzymes. This causes a breakdown of tissue and provides more nutrients for bacteria that allow the infection to progress. Furthermore, tissue breakdown helps eliminate barriers that would allow normal septations to limit progression of infection to normal healthy tissue.

TABLE 11.2. Organisms seen with necrotizing soft tissue infection, their characteristics, and general recommendations.

Organism group	Relative prevalences	Clinical problems
Group A *Streptococcus*	Common	Often spreads rapidly
Staphylococcus	More common with cutaneous origin of infection	May have multiple sites
Bacteroides sp.	Most common anaerobe	Need tissue to process for culture
Gram-negative organisms	Common in mixed infection	More often seen in postoperative wound infections
Candida and other fungi	Most associated with immunosuppressed patients	May require microscopic tissue evaluation for diagnosis
Clostridia	Relatively uncommon	Often leads to profound sepsis and rapid death

The second component of tissue destruction is the cytokine release secondary to initiation of these infections. There is evidence that the cascade of cytokines that can be released by these infections impacts the patient both locally and systemically. The massive release of tumor necrosis factor and other tissue destruction cytokines contribute to the necrosis seen in infected tissue. This provides additional nutrients for bacterial growth. Furthermore, the cytokines, lymphokines, and other mediators, including leukotrienes and products of the coagulation and complement cascades, cause vasodilatation, hypotension, and sepsis syndrome, leading to altered organ function and potentially multisystem organ failure.[32–34] The eventual outcome of these processes is a rapidly progressing systemic sepsis, triggered by the advancing soft tissue infection. Understanding these physiologic changes is essential to rapidly diagnosing the problem and rationally treating the unique differences in each patient.

Presentation and Diagnosis

The presentation of NSTI is highly variable and can range from early sepsis with obvious skin involvement to minimal cutaneous manifestations with a disproportionate (even alarming) underlying necrotizing fasciitis. The infections often develop in deep tissue planes, resulting in the epidermis appearing relatively uninvolved until late in the course of the disease. This may lead to difficulty differentiating serious NSTI from cellulitis or non-necrotizing infections.

The clinical presentation of NSTI usually begins with localized pain and a deceptively benign appearance. Clinical clues (summarized in Table 11.3) that may assist in establishing an early diagnosis are pain out of proportion to physical appearance, edema beyond the area of erythema, small skin vesicles, crepitus, and the absence of lymphangitis. Additional local signs suggesting deep infection include skin induration, dermal thrombosis, epidermolysis, or dermal gangrene. Bullae formation and a thin, gray, foul-smelling discharge from the skin and subcutaneous tissue develop late in the process and are typically associated with systemic manifestations of sepsis, including shock and multiple organ failure.[2,17,29,35–38] Figure 11.3 illustrates an advanced case of NSTI secondary to intravenous drug use. The extremities are the predominant location of NSTIs in most large series of patients. The perineum, trunk, and gluteal region are other common anatomic sites. Although no area of the body is safe from NSTI, infections of the chest and head and neck region are less common.[6,17,38–42]

Early recognition is the sine qua non for the assessment of risk factors. Multiple risk factors increase the

TABLE 11.3. Signs and symptoms of necrotizing soft tissue infections.

Physical examination
  Erythema
  Edema
  Inflammation
  Induration
  Bronzing of skin
  Vesicles or bullae
  Crepitance
  Local anesthesia
  Pain out of proportion to physical findings
  Loss of function
  Foul odor
  Discolored thin drainage
  Necrosis

Systemic signs
  Fever
  Tachycardia
  Confusion or obtundation
  Shock
  Systemic inflammatory response syndrome
  Multiple-organ dysfunction or failure

probability of a life-threatening infection.[43] Those comorbid conditions include diabetes mellitus, peripheral vascular disease, malnutrition, malignancy, obesity, advanced age, immunocompromised states (AIDS, steroid therapy), and chronic alcohol or intravenous drug abuse (Table 11.4). These factors are associated with underlying defects in immune function, and they all affect patient outcome. In the urban setting, intravenous and subcutaneous injections of illicit substances have become a more prevalent risk factor and should raise one's suspicion. Our experience with NSTIs treated at an urban medical center revealed that 67% of patients were actively

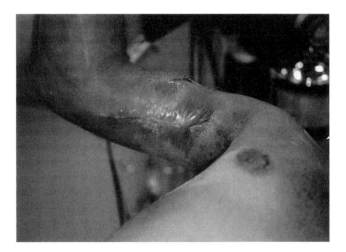

FIGURE 11.3. Advanced necrotizing soft tissue infection of the upper extremity secondary to intravenous drug abuse. Large bullae, bronzing and induration, and weeping of thin gray fluid signify severe underlying infection and necrosis.

TABLE 11.4. Risk factors for necrotizing soft tissue infections.

Diabetes mellitus
Intravenous drug abuse
Obesity
Malnutrition
Chronic alcoholism
Peripheral vascular disease
Age greater than 60 years
Immunocompromised state
   Steroid therapy
   HIV/AIDS
   Malignancy

practicing parenteral drug use.[17] Additional studies demonstrated similar results.[38,44–46]

The etiology of an NSTI is not always obvious and usually involves some form of tissue damage. The most common etiologies include trauma (blunt and penetrating), postoperative wound complications, cutaneous infections, intravenous or subcutaneous illicit substance injection, perirectal abscesses, strangulated hernias, perforated viscous (i.e., diverticulitis), and idiopathic causes.[6,17,35,37,38,47] Necrotizing soft tissue infections have also been linked to nonsteroidal antiinflammatory drugs (NSAIDs). However, this association remains unclear, as other comorbidities and risk factors are frequently found.[48–50]

Necrotizing soft tissue infections must be diagnosed clinically. There has been some investigation of the use of frozen section or other techniques to diagnose NSTI, but, other than with fungi such as *Aspergillus*, invasive infection is not diagnosed microscopically. The defining characteristic of NSTI is tissue destruction caused by advancing infection, which can be best and quickest determined by clinical assessment, usually in the operating room.

Initially when presented with a patient with extensive soft tissue manifestations of infection as evidenced by any one or all five of the classic components of inflammation (pain, swelling, redness, and increased temperature and loss of function), a clinician should consider NSTI. If there are questions as to whether this is indeed an NSTI or a simple soft tissue infection, a reasonable approach is to start treating the patient for a simple soft tissue infection by standard treatments—intravenous antibiotics, elevation and immobilization of the area—and frequently reexamine the area every 4 to 6 hours. The limits of erythema should be marked on the skin with a pen, with attention to determine if the border of infection appears to progress beyond this mark in subsequent examinations. If infection progresses beyond the previous delineated areas of infection, then NSTI should be strongly considered and surgical intervention should be planned immediately. Even failure to improve over a period of 8

to 24 hours with appropriate treatment should be a reason for surgical exploration or very close attention.[13] Wong et al.[51] have described a diagnostic tool to distinguish what they describe as necrotizing fasciitis from other soft tissue infections. They developed the Laboratory Risk Indicator for Necrotizing Fasciitis (LRINEC) score that includes white cell count, hemoglobin, sodium, glucose, creatinine, and C-reactive protein as variables. However, these are all measures of physiologic derangement and inflammation and are not specific enough for infection. Furthermore, there is no comparison of LRINEC to clinical judgment by an experienced surgeon.[51]

The use of imaging studies to determine the presence of NSTI is limited by the relatively low percentage of patients who have soft tissue gas or other means of diagnosis. Inflammatory changes in soft tissue may be very clear on computed tomography or magnetic resonance imaging but are very nonspecific and not as useful as an examination by a clinician experienced with NSTIs.

Clinical aspiration of fluid to look for bacteria also is insufficient. Cultures often take too long to make a timely diagnosis and the Gram stains are not able to make a diagnosis of necrotizing infection.

Operative exploration for diagnosis should be an incision down to the muscular fascia (and through it to fully evaluate the fascia and muscle). The area should be examined for gray-brown fluid ("dishwater pus"), change of the fascia from glistening white to gray, and easy separation of the subcutaneous fat from the fascia. If any of these are found, a presumptive diagnosis of NTSI is made. Ultimately the diagnosis is made with a high index of suspicion and confirmed at the time of surgical exploration of the area involved.[44]

Clinical Management

The clinical management of NSTIs requires rapid and simultaneous resuscitation, antibiotics (and possible other antimicrobial agents), aggressive surgical debridement, and supportive care. It is important to understand that all aspects of treatment must be initiated promptly to limit tissue damage, morbidity, and mortality.

Resuscitation should begin immediately for patients who are suspected of having any type of soft tissue infection, even if the diagnosis is unclear and the patient is being closely monitored. The magnitude of resuscitation will depend on the patient's physiologic status and response to initial treatment. Intravenous fluid resuscitation is essential because these patients are often intravascularly depleted, despite having localized and sometimes even generalized edema. Adequate intravascular volume is important to maintain good tissue oxygen delivery as well as limit the adverse effects of multiple organ failure.

Intravenous lactated Ringer's solution given in large volumes is the appropriate way to resuscitate these patients. The use of colloid resuscitation is generally not of benefit and may lead to other potential problems, including coagulopathy, if synthetic colloid is used. The amount of fluid resuscitation should be targeted to provide adequate perfusion of organ systems. Urine output remains the best single measure of determining adequacy of resuscitation. The use of pulmonary artery catheters or other means to look at cardiac index can increase risk to the patient given the potential systemic nature of the infection. Furthermore, many patients will have high cardiac output states, and invasive monitoring will be of limited benefit.

Patients who have profound cardiac or cardiopulmonary dysfunction may require a pulmonary arterial catheter to monitor and guide treatment when the benefit exceeds the risk. Patients who have evidence of multiple organ dysfunction or failure need support of the affected system(s). This may include intubation and mechanical ventilation for acute respiratory failure, use of vasoactive drugs for profound hypotension, hemofiltration or dialysis for acute renal failure, and other organ-system support as needed. Hyperglycemia should be closely managed to best treat the infection. It is important to integrate the surgical management of the infection with the critical care management of the patient. However, critical care management is an adjunct, not the primary treatment of NSTIs. Delaying surgical management until the patient is "stable" or "improved" by resuscitation in the intensive care unit will fail. Appropriate and aggressive surgical debridement and appropriate antibiotics must be included in the immediate resuscitation plan.

Critical Care Management

Hemodynamic support from vasoactive drugs such as dopamine or alpha agents may be useful. Beta-adrenergic agents such as dopamine or alpha-adrenergic agents should be used if the patient is unable to maintain a blood pressure sufficient for renal autoregulation. Systolic blood pressures of only 75 to 80 in septic patients are often sufficient, and use of alpha agents to raise the blood pressure even higher may be deleterious to the heart. Patient care should be focused on treating the disease process more than treating the organ-system consequences of the infection.

Mechanical ventilation, when needed, should be initiated quickly to prevent complications of respiratory failure and/or aspiration. Good pulmonary toilet will need to be part of this supportive care. Treatment of other organ-system dysfunction, such as coagulopathy, should be initiated immediately as well. Nutritional support should be considered as soon as the infection is improving.[52,53]

Attention is often focused on what antibiotics to use for these patients. Given the sometimes complex nature of the infections, broad-spectrum antibiotics should be started first, with narrowing of the spectrum once the causative organisms are known. Intravenous penicillin G remains the other treatment of choice for group A streptococcal infections, although there is some evidence that clindamycin may provide equal benefit. However, no comparative study has demonstrated a superior response to clindamycin in NSTI. Penicillin G, if chosen, should be given at a high dose, such as 20 to 24 million units a day for adults, to have as rapid an impact as possible. One million units hour of penicillin G in continuous infusion avoids some of the low levels associated with bolus dosing cited by the proponents of clindamycin.

Until Gram-negative organisms can be ruled out, coverage for them is important. This can be done with an aminoglycoside or other agent effective against the common Gram-negative organisms in individual hospitals. If previously hospital-acquired organisms such as resistant *Staphylococcus* are suspected, vancomycin would be recommended for use in the initial antibiotic treatment for these infections. If there is suspicion of *Candida* or fungi such as *Aspergillus*, based on either wound inspection or pathology, antifungal agents should be included.

The specific antibiotics chosen should be based on the patient's acute infection, underlying pathology, medical history (including allergies), and the bacteria and other organisms seen in the respective hospitals. Consideration of the antimicrobial sensitivities of different organisms in a specific hospital should also be used when selecting which agents to use. These antibiotics should be adjusted when cultures and sensitivities are complete.

Some physicians have recommended the use of intravenous immunoglobulins (IVIG) for NSTI.[54,55] It is unclear whether IVIG works as a nonspecific opsonin or by specific binding to a bacterial antigen and activation of specific and nonspecific inflammatory mechanisms. Intravenous IG may also have an effect on the circulating cytokines to control the systemic inflammatory response. There are no comparative trials yet to assess the efficacy of IVIG for NSTIs.

The fundamental approach to NSTI still remains aggressive surgical debridement in the acute or initial setting. Operative exploration of the wound not only permits definitive diagnosis of the NSTI but also puts the surgeon in position to provide the most crucial part of the treatment.[19,56] Some research suggests that surgery can be delayed or potentially avoided.[57] However, most thorough studies conclude that the most important part of the treatment of NSTIs is surgical debridement, and the earlier it is done, the better the outcome.[5,58] True NSTIs will not be successfully treated without aggressive surgical debridement.

For patients who are hemodynamically unstable or who have not yet responded to rapid resuscitation, delay in surgery until "normalization" has been achieved may limit the patient's chance of survival. Often, patients will respond to resuscitation only after the infected tissue is debrided and the area drained.

Surgical Debridement

Surgical debridement of an NSTI has many different techniques; however, wide excision of all inflamed or infected tissue is the most accepted therapeutic approach. Initial debridement should involve an incision in the most inflamed, tender, or indurated area or in a central area of soft mass if one is present. This should be carried down to the fascia. If the fascia is a gray, dull, or a stringy type of tissue as opposed to the normal pearly, tough fascia, a diagnosis of NSTI can be made. Whether or not the fascia is abnormal, it should be incised to examine the muscle underneath. If the fascia is abnormal as described, then the skin and soft tissue above the abnormal fascia should be lifted away to see how far the abnormality extends in the fascia. The necrotic fascia should be excised, and the overlying skin and subcutaneous fascia should be excised with it. This avoids the possibility of leaving large flaps of heavily infected skin, allowing continued spread of the infection and drainage of the inflammatory mediators into the lymphatics and veins. The skin and subcutaneous fascia should be cut back to viable bleeding tissue that appears normal in color and texture. The viable tissue will likely be edematous but it will be otherwise normal.

It is uncommon to see classic thick, creamy purulence in NSTIs. The classic description has been "dishwater pus," which is a brownish-tan fluid that weeps from the infected site.

The debridement should be done expeditiously either with a curved Mayo scissors or cautery. The difficulty with cautery is that it is hard to assess the quality of the tissue once it has been cut with the Bovie. If cautery is to be used, cutting current is more likely to be effective with specific attention either to tie off or to coagulate isolated vessels. If the infection is in the extremity and has caused considerable muscle necrosis and/or destruction of neurovascular components, consideration should be given to guillotine amputation.[59]

No attempt should be made to close any wounds such as extremity stumps in the face of such NSTIs. If the patient is profoundly unstable with an extremity infection, guillotine amputation may be the fastest way to attempt to salvage the patient's life.

It is important that the patient be brought to the operating room as soon as possible. If it is unclear that the patient has an NSTI and the patient is being closely monitored, observation examinations are important. However, once the diagnosis is made and the suspicion is high, rapid transfer to the operating room for exploration should be done. Attempts to try to do this in unstable patients outside the operating room should be very limited. Once the diagnosis is made, transport the patient to the operating room because the magnitude of debridement, fluid resuscitation, and potential blood loss that could occur are best managed there.

Preoperative preparation should include type and cross with at least four units of blood and warming the operating room. The wound exploration and debridement should be considered similar to excision of a large burn area, because the fluid and potential bone losses are similar and the need for maintenance of body temperature is important.

After aggressive debridement, it is likely that the patient will actually improve hemodynamically and clinically. It is important, however, that the patient be reexamined in the operating room within 24 hours to assess whether or not the advance of the infection has been stopped.[2,6,13] If there is additional necrotic tissue, then it should be again debrided aggressively. Necrotic tissue should not be left for subsequent debridement, hoping that more tissue will not have to be taken. If the tissue has a reasonable chance of being viable, then it should be noted where this is so it can be considered for further debridement if necessary on subsequent exploration. Repeated operative debridements are often necessary; one study reported an average of 3.3 debridements per patient.[6] Once a wound appears to be stable and there is no evidence of advancing infection, dressing may occur in an appropriate facility, not necessarily in the operating room.

Necrotizing soft tissue infections are often treated in a burn center. Burn centers are often experienced with the massive fluid resuscitation and management of very critically ill and unstable patients required not only in burns but in NSTIs as well. Furthermore, the wound care and wound coverage teams needed for these patients has considerable overlap between burns and NSTIs.[12,60,61]

Wound Care

Dressing the wounds between debridements is best done by using a moist dressing, such as saline or lactated Ringer's. In general, it is best to avoid topical antimicrobial agents such as Silvadene, which cause discoloration in the tissue and make it difficult to determine whether tissue is viable or nonviable. Other soluble topical antimicrobials that do not stain tissue can be used, but they are not a substitute for adequate excision and debridement from the NSTI. Antimicrobial solutions that cause cellular damage such as betadine solution should be avoided.

Hyperbaric oxygen (HBO) has been proposed as an integral part of treatment of NSTIs.[62,63] Although it is used in some centers, there is no prospective evidence that outcomes are superior with HBO compared with standard care approaches. A recent study by Riseman et al.[64] compared 12 patients treated before HBO with 17 patients treated after HBO, with an improvement in mortality from 67% to 23%. However, it was not a prospective, randomized, or case-controlled study.[64] Some studies examining the use of HBO have described patients who have slow-healing soft tissue wounds with positive surface cultures rather than NSTIs. When HBO can be compared in a comprehensive prospective randomized trial, the appropriateness of this technique for NSTIs can be determined.

Once the patient is stable, the subsequent wound coverage should be planned. This is often done using a simple skin graft, but sometimes complex reconstruction such as for perineal wounds may be needed. Perineal infections resulting in large debridement of perianal tissue occasionally requires colostomy but often can be managed without it. If the scrotal skin has to be resected during debridement of the NSTI, the testicles are almost always viable and can be left behind. If they retract into the inguinal canal, they can be mobilized, brought down, and sutured together with absorbable sutures beneath the penis and then skin grafted over to form a new scrotal area.

More complex wound coverage can be done in conjunction with plastic surgery when necessary. However, early closure with skin graft is usually advantageous with subsequent reconstruction once the patient is well and recovering not only from the infection but also the other complicated medical problems.

Supportive care of the patient during this process is important. Nutritional support is important, especially as the patient is recovering and becomes anabolic again.[52] Tube feedings may be necessary for adequate caloric and protein intake because patients may be intubated or unable to take in sufficient calories and protein just by eating. Appropriate vitamins and minerals such as zinc are essential. These patients will have increased caloric and protein demands because of the loss of fluid through the open wounds as well as the hypermetabolism associated with this infection.

Patients often need rehabilitation. When amputation is required, contact with a prosthetist to determine how best to eventually shape the stump will be important. Rehabilitation should begin as early as the patient is stable and able to participate and not put off until discharge. It may take months for patients to regain strength even after relatively straightforward management of the NSTI.

Burn centers again are often useful places to treat these patients because burn centers have many of the elements and the experienced staff necessary to treat this problem. However, treatment could be effectively done in other units that have the surgical expertise, nursing and hospital support, and experience in management of these problems.

In summary, an NSTI is a surgical disease that needs to be quickly recognized and aggressively treated. The time required to treat the patients is considerable, and the temptation is often to look for someone else to manage this life-threatening but uncommon problem. However, a well-trained general surgeon with comprehensive skills should be able to manage most of the patients.

The pattern of these infections will continue to change as the microbial flora, antibiotic use, and patient population evolves. This disease process will continue to require rapid evaluation and treatment based on clinical experience and a high index of suspicion. New techniques for diagnosis and treatment are still being evaluated. Diagnosis and management of NSTIs will still require the attention and skill of a committed general surgeon.

Critique

The mainstay of management of any necrotizing soft tissue infection is early and aggressive surgical debridement. Antibiotics, fluid resuscitation (particularly for a hemodynamically labile, septic patient), and nutritional support are required adjuncts. However, without surgical debridement, the adjuncts will not provide definitive management. Also, there have been no phase III blinded, prospective, randomized trials demonstrating the efficacy of hyperbaric oxygen therapy.

Answer (E)

References

1. Dellinger FL. Severe necrotizing soft-tissue infections. Multiple disease entities requiring a common approach. JAMA 1981; 246(15):1717–1721.
2. Malangoni MA. Necrotizing soft tissue infections: are we making any progress? Surg Infect (Larchmt) 2001; 2(2): 145–152.
3. Quirk WF Jr, Sternbach G. Joseph Jones: infection with flesh eating bacteria. J Emerg Med 1996; 14(6):747–753.
4. Meleney. Hemolytic *Streptococcus* gangrene. Arch Surg 1924; 9:317–364.
5. Ahrenholz DH. Necrotizing soft-tissue infections. Surg Clin North Am 1988; 68(1):199–214.
6. McHenry CR, et al. Determinants of mortality for necrotizing soft-tissue infections. Ann Surg 1995; 221(5):558–565.

7. Bisno AL, Stevens DL. Streptococcal infections of skin and soft tissues. N Engl J Med 1996; 334(4):240–245.

8. Chelsom J, et al. Necrotising fasciitis due to group A streptococci in western Norway: incidence and clinical features. Lancet 1994; 344(8930):1111–1115.

9. Demers B, et al. Severe invasive group A streptococcal infections in Ontario, Canada: 1987–1991. Clin Infect Dis 1993; 16(6):792–802.

10. Chao CS, et al. Necrotizing soft tissue infection in heart transplantation recipients: two case reports. Transplant Proc 1998; 30(7):3347–3349.

11. Cheung AH, Wong LM. Surgical infections in patients with chronic renal failure. Infect Dis Clin North Am 2001; 15(3):775–796.

12. Kuncir EJ, et al. Necrotizing soft-tissue infections. Emerg Med Clin North Am 2003; 21(4):1075–1087.

13. Schecter WP, Schecter G. Necrotizing fasciitis of the upper extremity. J Hand Surg 1982; 7:15–20.

14. Lewis RT. Soft tissue infections. World J Surg 1998; 22(2): 146–151.

15. Huang JW, et al. Necrotizing fasciitis caused by *Serratia marcescens* in two patients receiving corticosteroid therapy. J Formos Med Assoc 1999; 98(12):851–854.

16. Wai PH, et al. *Candida* fasciitis following renal transplantation. Transplantation 2001; 72(3):477–479.

17. Bosshardt TL, Henderson VJ, Organ CH Jr. Necrotizing soft-tissue infections. Arch Surg 1996; 131(8):846–854.

18. Ebright JR, Pieper B. Skin and soft tissue infections in injection drug users. Infect Dis Clin North Am 2002; 16(3):697–712.

19. Hill MK, Sanders CV. Skin and soft tissue infections in critical care. Crit Care Clin 1998 14(2):251–262.

20. Childers BJ, et al. Necrotizing fasciitis: a fourteen-year retrospective study of 163 consecutive patients. Am Surg 2002; 68:109–116.

21. Elliott DC, Kufera JA, Myers RAM. The microbiology of necrotizing soft tissue infections. Am J Surg 2000; 179:361–366.

22. Giuliano A, et al. Bacteriology of necrotizing fasciitis. Am J Surg 1977; 134:52–56.

23. Sudarsky LA, et al. Improved results from a standardized approach in treating patients with necrotizing fasciitis. Ann Surg 1987; 206:661–665.

24. Wood TF, Pooter MA, Jonasson O. Streptococcal toxic shock-like syndrome: the importance of surgical intervention. Ann Surg 1993; 217:209–214.

25. Wolf JE, Rabinowitz LG. Streptococcal toxic shock-like syndrome. Arch Dermatol 1995; 131:73–77.

26. Gardam MA, et al. Group B streptococcal necrotizing fasciitis and streptococcal toxic shock-like syndrome in adults. Arch Intern Med 1998; 158:1704–1708.

27. Humar D, et al. Streptolysin S and necrotising infections produced by group G streptococcus. Lancet 2002; 359:124–129.

28. Lewis RT. Soft tissue infections. World J Surg 1998; 22:146–151.

29. File TM. Necrotizing soft tissue infections. Curr Infect Dis Rep 2003; 5:407–415.

30. Holow KD, Harner RC, Fontenelle LJ. Primary skin infections secondary to *Vibrio vulnificus*: the role of operative intervention. J Am Coll Surg 1996; 183:329–334.

31. Marcus JR, et al. Risk factors in necrotizing fasciitis: a case involving *Cryptococcus neoformans*. Ann Plast Surg 1998; 40:80–83.

32. Fast DJ, Schlievert PM, Nelson RD. Toxic shock syndrome–associated staphylococcal and streptococcal pyrogenic toxins are potent inducers of tumor necrosis factor production. Infect Immun 1989; 57(1):291–294.

33. Muller-Alouf H, et al. Cytokine production by murine cells activated by erythrogenic toxin type A superantigen of *Streptococcus pyogenes*. Immunobiology 1992; 186(5):435–448.

34. Muller-Alouf H, et al. Comparative study of cytokine release by human peripheral blood mononuclear cells stimulated with *Streptococcus pyogenes* superantigenic erythrogenic toxins, heat-killed streptococci, and lipopolysaccharide. Infect Immun 1994; 62(11):4915–4921.

35. Elliott DC, Kufera JA, Myers RAM. Necrotizing soft tissue infections: risk factors for mortality and strategies for management. Ann Surg 1996; 224:672–683.

36. Majeski JA, John JF Jr. Necrotizing soft tissue infections: a guide to early diagnosis and initial therapy. South Med J 2003; 96:900–905.

37. Chapnick EK, Abter EI. Necrotizing soft tissue infections. Infect Dis Clin North Am 1996; 10:835–855.

38. Lille ST, et al. Necrotizing soft tissue infections: obstacles in diagnosis. J Am Coll Surg 1996; 182:7–11.

39. Singh G, et al. Necrotising infections of soft tissues—a clinical profile. Eur J Surg 2002; 168:366–371.

40. Callahan TE, Schecter WP, Horn JK. Necrotizing soft tissue infections masquerading as cutaneous abscess following illicit drug injection. Arch Surg 1998; 133:812–818.

41. Urschel JD, Takita H, Antkowiak JG. Necrotizing soft tissue infections of the chest wall. Ann Thorac Surg 1997; 64:276–279.

42. McMahon J, Lowe T, Koppel DA. Necrotizing soft tissue infections of the head and neck: case report and literature review. Oral Surg Oral Med Oral Pathol Oral Radiol Endod 2003; 95:30–37.

43. Francis KR, et al. Implications of risk factors in necrotizing fasciitis. Am Surg 1993; 59:304–308.

44. Wall DB, et al. A simple model to help distinguish necrotizing fasciitis from nonnecrotizing soft tissue infection. J Am Coll Surg 2000; 191:227–231.

45. Bangsberg DR, et al. Clostridial myonecrosis cluster among injection drug users. Arch Intern Med 2002; 162:517–522.

46. McGuigan CC, et al. Lethal outbreak of infection with *Clostridium novyi* type A and other spore-forming organisms in Scottish injecting drug users. J Med Microbiol 2002; 51:971–977.

47. McHenry CR, et al. Idiopathic necrotizing fasciitis: recognition, incidence, and outcome of therapy. Am Surg 1994; 60:490–494.

48. Kahn LH, Styrt BA. Necrotizing soft tissue infections reported with nonsteroidal antiinflammatory drugs. Ann Pharmacother 1997; 31:1034–1039.

49. Forbes N, Rankin APN. Necrotizing fasciitis and non steroidal anti-inflammatory drugs: a case series and review of the literature. NZ Med J 2001; 114:3–6.

50. Lesko SM, et al. Invasive group A streptococcal infection and nonsteroidal antiinflammatory drug use among children with primary varicella. Pediatrics 2001; 107:1108–1115.

51. Wong CH, et al. The LRINEC (Laboratory Risk Indicator for Necrotizing Fasciitis) score: a tool for distinguishing necrotizing fasciitis from other soft tissue infections. Crit Care Med 2004; 32(7):1535–1541.

52. Graves C, et al. Caloric requirements in patients with necrotizing fasciitis. Burns 2005; 31(1):55–59.

53. Green RJ, Dafoe DC, Raffin TA. Necrotizing fasciitis. Chest 1996; 110(1):219–229.

54. Stevens DL. Streptococcal toxic shock syndrome associated with necrotizing fasciitis. Annu Rev Med 2000; 51:271–288.

55. Laupland KB, et al. Intravenous immunoglobulin for severe infections: a survey of Canadian specialists. J Crit Care 2004; 19(2):75–81.

56. Voros D, et al. Role of early and extensive surgery in the treatment of severe necrotizing soft tissue infection. Br J Surg 1993; 80(9):1190–1191.

57. Hsiao GH, et al. Necrotizing soft tissue infections. Surgical or conservative treatment? Dermatol Surg 1998; 24(2):243–248.

58. Bilton BD, et al. Aggressive surgical management of necrotizing fasciitis serves to decrease mortality: a retrospective study. Am Surg 1998; 64(5):397–401.

59. Anaya DA, et al. Predictors of mortality and limb loss in necrotizing soft tissue infections. Arch Surg 2005; 140(2):151–158.

60. Barillo DJ, et al. Burn center management of necrotizing fasciitis. J Burn Care Rehabil 2003; 24(3):127–132.

61. Edlich RF, et al. Massive soft tissue infections: necrotizing fasciitis and purpura fulminans. J Long Term Eff Med Implants 2005; 15(1):57–65.

62. Clark LA, Moon RE. Hyperbaric oxygen in the treatment of life-threatening soft-tissue infections. Respir Care Clin North Am 1999; 5(2):203–219.

63. Wilkinson D, Doolette D. Hyperbaric oxygen treatment and survival from necrotizing soft tissue infection. Arch Surg 2004; 139(12):1339–1345.

64. Riseman JA, et al. Hyperbaric oxygen therapy for necrotizing fasciitis reduces mortality and the need for debridements. Surgery 1990; 108(5):847–850.

12
The Open Abdomen: Management from Initial Laparotomy to Definitive Closure

Fred A. Luchette, Stathis J. Poulakidas, and Thomas J. Esposito

Case Scenario

A 67-year-old patient has undergone a prolonged and complicated operation for mesenteric ischemic (embolic etiology). Circulation has just been restored to the ischemic bowel; however, the patient is hypothermic (34°C), acidotic, and coagulopathic. Which of the following is the appropriate management at this time?

(A) Wood's lamp assessment of bowel viability
(B) Repeated on-table angiography after 45 minutes
(C) Administration of mannitol
(D) Immediate fascial closure of the abdomen
(E) Creative abdominal closure

The establishment and management of the open abdomen is now a main component of the armamentarium in acute care surgery. Pringle was the first to report use of the open abdomen for management of soldiers sustaining catastrophic abdominal injuries during World War II. It was abandoned because of the poor results encountered with recurrent bleeding at the time of pack removal and late infections. Lucas and Ledgerwood[1] reintroduced the technique with a prospective study conducted from 1968 to 1973. Subsequent patient series reports by Calne et al.,[2] Feliciano et al.,[3] Svoboda et al.,[4] and Carmona et al.[5] demonstrated the utility of packing for devastating abdominal injuries with subsequent patient survival.

Today, the concept of "damage control" has been well accepted in the management of critically ill and injured patients. Promulgated by Rotondo and colleagues,[6] this operative management strategy has become the mainstay in major trauma centers throughout the United States. The strategy has been utilized to avoid and treat the complications of primary and secondary abdominal compartment syndrome (ACS) related to intraabdominal hypertension. The acute care surgeon will also encounter ACS in patients presenting with other nontraumatic abdominal catastrophes.[7–14]

Additionally, the damage-control technique has applications in general surgery, vascular surgery, urology, gynecology, and even thoracic surgery.[8,9] Surgeons treating intraabdominal infection at the end of the nineteenth century respected the "enormous increases of intraabdominal tension."[10] Effective treatment for both primary and secondary ACS became available with the introduction of the open abdominal technique,[11,12–14] which allowed practitioners to realize the benefits of this new strategy on impaired physiology that resulted from abdominal hypertension.[15–17] This has been used adjunctively with open peritoneal lavage for the management of severe feculent peritonitis. With the evolution of the open abdomen for trauma and peritonitis, the challenge of dealing with the temporarily open abdomen and its eventual closure has grown. This chapter details the complex care of such patients and the decision processes culminating in the definitive closure of the abdomen.

Indications for Leaving the Abdomen Open

Utilizing the strategy of damage control, physicians have increasingly incorporated truncated operations into routine practice. For trauma patients, the initial procedure of abdominal exploration is designed to control hemorrhage and contamination. For nontrauma indications, these basic principles are also applied most commonly for control of an infectious source. The decision to terminate the initial operation is determined by the patient's overall capacity to withstand the physiologic stress posed by the extended operative time needed to complete the operation (Table 12.1).

The complex decisions dealing with choice of temporary closure, timing of return to the operating room for

TABLE 12.1. Indications for the damage-control approach.

1. Inability to achieve hemostasis because of coagulopathy
2. Inaccessible major venous injury
3. Time-consuming procedure in a patient with suboptimal response to resuscitation
4. Management of extraabdominal life-threatening injury
5. Reassessment of intraabdominal contents
6. Inability to reapproximate abdominal fascia because of visceral edema

Source: Reprinted with permission from Shapiro et al.[47]

reconstruction, and definitive closure of the abdomen are dictated by individual patient variables, including the constellation of injuries or other conditions, physiologic reserve, response to resuscitation, and available resources. A critical factor at the first operation is the preservation of the abdominal wall fascia for use at the time of eventual closure. All available synthetic materials can be temporarily secured directly to the skin, recognizing that this may lead to minor skin loss and potential compromise of an ideal cosmetic result. A choice of temporary closure should be based on anticipated needs, including repeated access to the peritoneal cavity, porosity, durability, pliability, interaction with adjacent structures, and cost.

The temporary coverage of the exposed viscera allows a bridge to resuscitation and thereby the reversal of shock and other physiologic derangements such as fluid and heat loss and dessication. The most common goal during resuscitation in the intensive care unit is correction of hypothermia and underlying coagulopathy. Aggressive cardiovascular resuscitation with both crystalloid and blood products should also occur in order to optimize oxygen delivery and consumption. One should anticipate progressive pulmonary failure requiring manipulation of ventilatory modes to maintain oxygenation and ventilation.

Return to the operating room will be dictated by the time required to achieve restoration of physiologic reserve defined as correction of hypothermia, coagulopathy, and acidosis. This typically requires 24 to 96 hours. The patient's response to treatment or onset of further problems will determine the time and location of additional operative intervention. Ongoing hemorrhage (transfusion requirement of more than 10 units of packed red blood cells), persistent or worsening acidosis, or the development of ACS will necessitate an early unplanned return to the operating room for intervention. When ACS develops as a result of ongoing resuscitation, the surgeon may decide to proceed with decompression of the peritoneal cavity in the intensive care unit. If there is a concern that the ACS is a result of ongoing hemorrhage, the operating room offers the optimal setting for controlling the hemorrhage in contrast to the intensive care unit.

Definitive closure of the open abdomen often requires complex planning and the involvement of other surgical disciplines with expertise in wound management. A particularly vexing complication of the open abdomen is an enteral fistula, which is now open to the air without interposing tissue. Management of the open abdominal wound while controlling the fistula output is challenging. The incidence ranges between 2% and 25% of injured patients undergoing damage control management. With this in mind, most acute care surgeons make efforts to close the open abdomen as soon a physiologically possible. This can be performed as early as several days after the original operation or electively at weeks or months after the initial procedure. Delayed operations allow time for catabolism to abate and for the patient's physiologic reserve to return as signaled by wound contracture and granulation, improving nutritional parameters (nitrogen balance, prealbumen, transferrin) reflected by weight gain, and return of general well being. The choice of procedure or prothesis will vary based on the constellation of injuries and tissue available for reconstruction. Because each patient's wound is unique, no single technique or prosthesis is ideal for every patient's situation. Frequently, a combination of techniques must be utilized with some degree of creativity and flexibility because of the complex nature of these wounds and the attendant complications that can be associated with them. Cipolla et al.[18] have proposed an algorithm linking the clinical situation with specific techniques used for management of the open abdomen.

Temporary Wound Management Techniques for the Open Abdomen

Temporary closures can be categorized into two types: those involving closure of the skin and those that do not. When the skin can be approximated, coaptation can be achieved with a running suture or towel clips. In contrast, there are multiple techniques for temporary closure that leave the skin as well as fascia separated. All include some type of protective barrier applied over the peritoneal contents (Table 12.2).

Towel clip closure of the skin is the most rapid of the temporary techniques. The clips are placed at 1-cm intervals. Some surgeons advocate orienting the handles of the towel clip toward the center of the incision. This facilitates dressing coverage of the towel clips and reduces artifact on subsequent radiographs. A surgical cloth is then applied as a wound drape over the towel clips. The entire assembly is held in place with an adhesive plastic drape, thereby reducing ascitic fluid irritation of the abdominal skin. Advantages of a towel clip closure are its rapid technique, low cost, maintenance of core

TABLE 12.2. Various techniques for temporary bridging of an open abdomen.

Method	Material	Expense
Skin closure (running monofilament suture or towel clips)	The most rapid technique and most effective at reducing heat and fluid loss	Low
Nonadherent materials (Bogotá bag, bowel bag, silicone sheet)	Biologically inert, maintains heat and reduces fluid loss, reexploration is easy; evisceration occurs when material tears at suture sites	Low
Polyglactin 910 (Knitted Vicryl Mesh, Ethicon, Somerville, NJ)	Absorbable, noninfectious, partially incorporated into granulation tissue; complications include tearing at suture line with evisceration and/or enteric fistulae	Moderate
Polyglycolic acid (Dexon Mesh, Davis & Geck, Danbury, CT)	Absorbable, noninfectious, rapidly incorporated into granulation; complications include enteric fistulae	Moderate
Removable prosthesis (Wittman patch, Starsurgical, Inc., Burlington, WI)	Extended time of open abdomen with repeated reexploration in the intensive care unit; limitation is requirement for suturing to fascia	High
Vacuum-assisted closure KCI USA, Inc., San Antonio, TX)	Reduced incidence of abdominal compartment syndrome while prolonging time of temporary closure before fascial closure; requires manufacturer's equipment	High

Modified with permission from: Rutherford EJ, Skeete DA, Brasel KJ. Management of the patient with an open abdomen: Techniques in temporary and definitive closure. Cur Prob Surg 2004;41:824.

temperature, and minimization of fluid losses. Despite close application of the clips, as intraabdominal pressure increases, there may be development of secondary ACS, evisceration of bowel between the towel clips, and pressure necrosis of the skin.

The Bogotá bag utilizes a large sterile intravenous (IV) bag, which is usually split open, to cover the abdominal viscera.[19–22] The bag can be secured to either the skin or fascia, but preferentially one should use the skin to minimize trauma to the fascia. When securing the bag to the skin, it is preferable to use a tapered needle, which minimizes the tearing of the bag at the suture sites. In comparison, the IV bag may tear when secured to the skin with a cutting needle. Other materials that can be employed in a similar fashion include intestinal bag, steri drape, parachute sheeting,[23] silicone sheeting,[24] PTFE (polytetrafluoroethylene; Gortex®) patch, or rayon cloth.[25] All of these materials minimize fluid loss and are easy to remove, relatively inexpensive, and biologically inert, thus minimizing adhesions. The downside of using these materials is that they all easily tear, creating the potential for subsequent intestinal evisceration.

Mesh materials include nonabsorbable and absorbable types. The nonabsorbable have fallen out of favor because of high cost and increased association with fistulae. The absorbable mesh, if left in place, eventually will be incorporated into the granulating wound. There are two commercially available absorbable meshes, polyglactin[11,12] and polyglycolic acid.[26–30] Both can be secured to either the skin or fascia. Again, it is preferable to utilize the skin and preserve the fascia for later definitive closure. Both types of meshes are resistant to infection,[28,29] improve early wound strength,[25] and, if used for definitive closure, result in a planned ventral hernia (Figure 12.1). A noteworthy problem with polyglactin[11,12] is that the smaller interstices can impair fluid drainage.

Additionally, when secured with a tapered needle, the mesh tends to tear at the suture site. In contrast, polyglycolic acid has large interstices, which more easily allows egress of peritoneal fluid and also less tearing during needle placement.

The major disadvantage of all mesh closures is the association with enteric open-air fistulae if the wound is allowed to desiccate. The fistulae can be minimized if the mesh is covered with a moist dressing. With the mesh in place, no further procedures may be required for wound care in the critically ill patient. However, if the patient's physiologic state permits, the mesh can be reefed (tightened) at the bedside. This gradually draws the fascial edges closer together and may allow early definitive primary closure of the abdomen. If this is not possible, the wound is allowed to granulate through the mesh and contract. This can be covered with a skin graft at a later date or be allowed to naturally epithelialize over time.

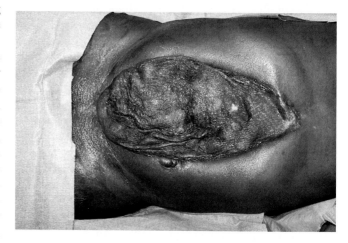

FIGURE 12.1. Ventral hernia after closure of abdomen by secondary intent with skin graft.

Mortality rate has been reduced with use of the "open" abdominal technique in the management of patients with intraabdominal sepsis.[31] Several techniques have been described to maintain abdominal integrity and yet allow frequent reexploration and lavage in the critically ill septic patient. These include slide fasteners, zippers, and the Wittman patch.[32–36] All were designed to eventually be removed with delayed primary closure. The Wittman patch has been extensively studied and is made of two adherent leaves of polyamiden and polypropylene with a Velcro-type closure (Figure 12.2). The leaves are sutured to the fascia and then secured to each other via the Velcro fastener. At the time of each reexploration, the leaves are trimmed to allow staged closure of the incision. In the final operation, the patch is removed and a definitive closure performed. Advantages of this device include easy reexploration at the bedside, maintenance of abdominal domain, and little need for chemical paralysis. The disadvantages

are the expense and multiple manipulations of the fascia.

The vacuum-assisted closure (VAC) for large chronic wounds is used in an effort to promote healing by constant application of negative pressure. It has subsequently been adapted for use in acutely managing the open abdomen.[37–41] This is a component dressing beginning with a nonadherent plastic drape placed beneath the anterior abdominal wall peritoneum to protect the abdominal viscera (Figure 12.3).[37–41] Multiple perforations are placed in the drape to allow for fluid drainage (Figure 12.4A). Moist surgical wound towels are then placed over the drape and Jackson Pratt drains positioned over the wound towels (Figure 12.4B). The dressing is then secured to the skin with an adhesive plastic drape (Figure 12.4C,D). It is critical to have a good seal to the skin to maintain negative pressure.

An alternative is a commercially available dressing (VAC dressing, KCI). In this system, a polyurethane

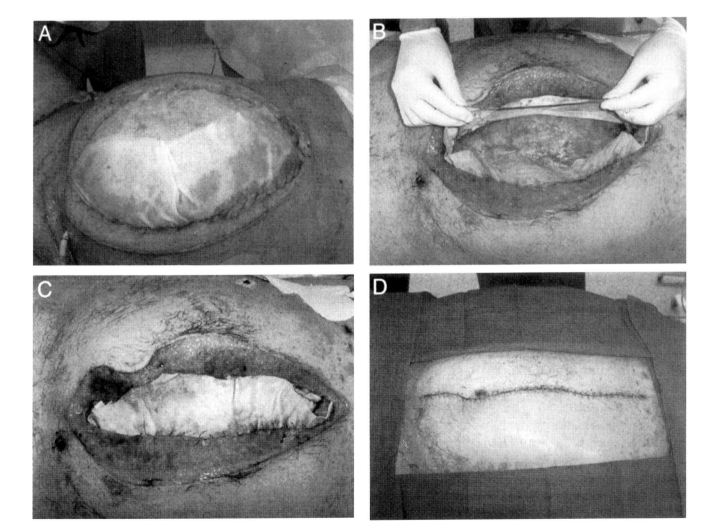

FIGURE 12.2. (A) Insertion of Wittman patch for open abdomen on postoperative day 8 after damage-control surgery for trauma. (B) Advancement of Velcro leaflets. (C) Approximation of fascial edges. (D) Primary closure of abdomen on postoperative day 18. (A–D, reprinted with permission from Cipolla et al.[18])

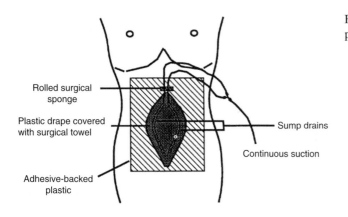

FIGURE 12.3. Schematic illustration of application of vacuum pack. (Reprinted with permission from Brock et al.[38])

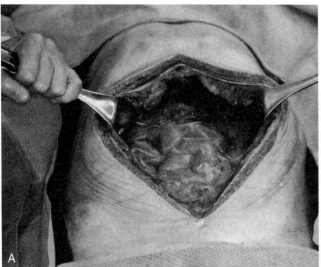

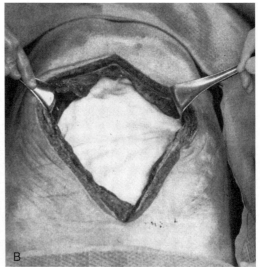

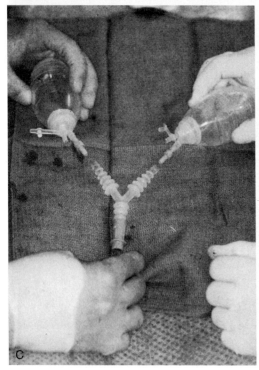

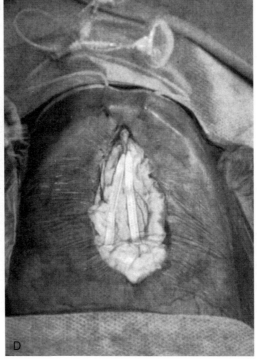

FIGURE 12.4. Barker vacuum dressing. (A) Polyethylene sheet placed over the peritoneal viscera and beneath the parietal peritoneum. (B) A moist surgical towel(s) folded to fit the fascial defect, on top of the polyethylene sheet, but below the skin edges. (C) Bulb suction devices connected to each drain using a Y-adapter. Alternatively, each drain may be attached to an individual bulb suction. (D) Final vacuum dressing after application of occlusive barrier and suction to drains. (A–D, reprinted with permission from Barker et al.[37])

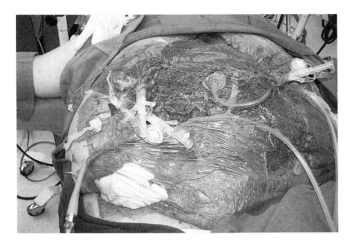

Figure 12.5. Vacuum-assisted closure dressing applied to the abdominal wound.

sponge is cut to the appropriate size of the open abdominal wound and placed over a sterile drape. An 18-F suction tube is inserted into the sponge, and then the sponge, tubing, and skin are covered with an adherent occlusive drape. Suction is applied to the sponge continuously from a portable pump. The dressing is changed every 2 to 3 days to allow inspection of the wound and viscera (Figure 12.5).

Advantages with either VAC dressing include decreased incidence of ACS, maintenance of abdominal domain, avoidance of chemical paralysis, elimination of temporary fascial suturing, and early fascial closure. Utilization of a nonadherent bowel bag with both the VAC-assisted dressing and the Wittman patch extend the time interval between dressing changes. Disadvantages of the commercial VAC system include the need for special equipment, expense, and minimal long-term follow-up data. Recent studies have reported use of the VAC device in patients for 21 to 49 days after injury with a primary closure rate of 40% to 92%.[46,50]

The temporary closure techniques necessitate further operative intervention. Although no single technique is ideal for every patient, priorities should include minimizing loss of abdominal domain while preserving the fascia, expense, minimization of heat and fluid losses, and expeditious closure. Thus, a common sequence in clinical practice is as follows: initial temporary coverage of the viscera followed by mesh or VAC dressing and then possible split-thickness skin graft or natural epithelialization.

Timing of Reconstruction and Subsequent Laparotomies

Patients undergoing a damage-control laparotomy with gastrointestinal discontinuity should be returned to the operating room as soon as possible for reconstruction.

This should be based on adequacy of cardiovascular resuscitation and restoration of oxygen delivery and consumption as well as correction of hypothermia and coagulopathy. Clearly if the patient has ongoing hemorrhage or develops a secondary ACS, they should have these problems immediately addressed either in the operating room or at the bedside in the intensive care unit. In the absence of pressing indications for early reexploration,[9,42,43] the reoperation should be scheduled when the probability of achieving complete fascial closure is greatest. This occurs usually 3 to 4 days after the initial celiotomy. Generally, by this time, diuresis and negative fluid balance have occurred. Decreasing abdominal girth and decreasing peripheral edema are evident and represent a reduction in visceral edema and abdominal wall edema. Despite this, often the abdomen cannot be closed, resulting in the acceptance of a subsequent ventral hernia that generally requires planned repair at a later date.[44]

When packing has been utilized in an effort to control solid organ bleeding, every effort should be made to remove the packing as soon as possible to minimize infectious risk (Figure 12.6). The rate of abdominal abscess formation in association with packing has been recorded as high as 24%.[9] This high incidence of infection in these immunocompromised patients may cause physicians to continue prophylactic antibiotics for a protracted course. However, this strategy has been shown to offer no reduction in infectious complications even in the face of intestinal injuries.[9,45–47] This may also predispose patients to the risk of superinfection with resistant organisms.[9] Thus there is no good evidence to support extended use of antibiotics in solid organ injuries that require packing for control of hemorrhage.

For patients requiring open abdomen management for secondary and tertiary peritonitis, many authors report bedside "washout" or peritoneal lavage in an effort to

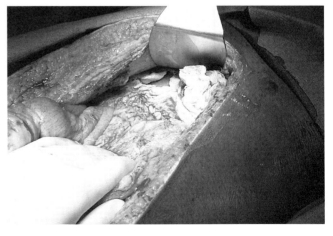

Figure 12.6. Perihepatic packing with laparotomy pads at the time of reexploration.

minimize septic complications. Repeated laparotomy can be performed safely in the intensive care unit, but it may not affect the incidence of subphrenic or pelvic abscess.

Techniques for Delayed Primary Closure

Ideally, all open abdomens should undergo definitive closure in a timely fashion. Every effort must be made to avoid unnecessary tension on the closure to avoid necrosis, dehiscence, and subsequent incisional hernia. The patient must also not be placed at risk for resultant incidence of secondary ACS. If primary closure can be achieved, there is minimal risk of the infection, enteric fistula, and wound problems that are typically seen with an open abdomen. This delayed primary closure of the original celiotomy wound can be performed days to weeks after the original operation.

If delayed primary closure is not possible in a timely fashion, options for wound management include closure with a permanent prosthetic material, closure with autologous tissue, or closure with temporary prosthetic material with an anticipated ventral hernia. The latter approach requires definitive closure months to years after the original wound closure. Most acute care surgeons avoid the use of a permanent wound prosthetic particularly with an open contaminated wound for obvious concerns with infection. Most open abdomens will thus be managed with one of several commercially available biologic materials. Use of an extracellular matrix from animal or human tissue, cadaveric fascia, or autologous tissue in the form of flaps avoids or reduces the frequency of wound infections and/or enterocutaneous fistulae.

Small Intestinal Submucosa

Porcine small intestine submucosa (SIS®) is an extracellular matrix composed primarily of type I collagen. It is prepared by removal of the mucosa's muscularis externa, leaving an acellular submucosa that is preserved by freeze-drying and then sterilized with ethylene oxide. Before full implantation, it is reconstituted in warm saline for 10 minutes. It is available as 1-, 2-, 4-, and 8-ply sheets. This has been studied in both animal models and clinical practice for repair of hernia defects using the 4-ply preparation. Unfortunately, only short-term follow-up data are available.[48–50] When histologic analysis was performed after use in repairing animal abdominal wall hernia defects, at 12 and 20 weeks postimplantation, the SIS had been well organized into the host tissue. The SIS was shown to be superior when compared with wounds closed with Marlex mesh or Dexon mesh. Furthermore, the occurrence of intraabdominal adhesions was minimal.[48,49] Because of the early vascular ingrowth and subsequent resistance to infection, SIS has been successfully utilized in contaminated or potentially contaminated ventral and/or inguinal hernias.[50] Unfortunately, there has been limited use of this material as a prosthetic for closure of open abdomens.

Human Acellular Dermis

Human acellular dermis (AlloDerm®) has similar biologic properties to porcine SIS. AlloDerm is prepared from cadaveric skin using a unique proprietary method. Once processed, all cellular components are removed, leaving the intact basement membrane and dermal collagen matrix. Thus, this acellular human dermis lacks the ability to induce an antigenic response.

AlloDerm functions as a biologic scaffold for ingrowth of autogenous tissue, with many of the same advantages as SIS. It is available in two sizes: $2 \times 4\,cm$ and $3 \times 7\,cm$. Before implantation, it must be rehydrated for 10 minutes in warm saline. An additional advantage over SIS is that several pieces of AlloDerm may be sutured together to cover larger defects (Figure 12.7). When compared with PTFE (Gortex®) in an animal model, there was no difference in mechanical wound strength.[51] Unfortunately, long-term follow-up data are not yet available.[52] However, more acute care surgeons are gaining experience with this new biologic prosthesis for wound closure and find it clinically superior to SIS.

Additional Techniques

Tissue expander devices can be useful in facilitating wound closure utilizing native tissue without creation of

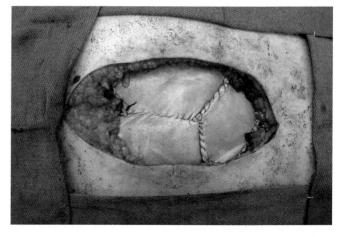

FIGURE 12.7. AlloDerm® placement for reconstruction of abdominal wall.

flaps and/or grafts. Large abdominal wall defects may be covered with native tissue after use of tissue expanders. The earliest report of soft tissue expansion described the use of pneumoperitoneum in 1931.[53] Current use of this strategy primarily involves soft tissue enhancement, using balloon devices strategically placed in surrounding tissues to increase their capacity to accommodate reconstruction, and closure is used to repair the fascial hernia. Small series have reported good results with short follow-up periods.[54] A recent series of 31 patients, which included seven trauma patients, claimed a success rate of 71%.[55]

Local advancement flaps in combination with absorbable mesh is another option for abdominal closure. This approach avoids split-thickness skin grafting and minimizes the risk of intestinal fistula.[56] It is generally employed when fascial closure is either not possible or would predispose to ACS. This method of closure should only be used when there are no further planned surgical interventions.

The flaps are created by separating the skin and subcutaneous tissue from the rectus sheath and external oblique fascia. The dissection is carried to the anterior axillary line from both sides of the open fascia. The fascial opening is then bridged with absorbable mesh, and the skin flaps are sutured in the midline. When there is unnecessary tension on the midline closure, a relaxing counterincision is made at the level of the anterior axillary line. Once the soft tissue edema resolves, these incisions will contract and close by secondary intention without the need for skin grafts. Depending on the size of the resultant ventral hernia, this may require repair of the ventral hernia at a later date. Most commonly this is performed using fascial component separation or standard mesh repair.

Autologous flap techniques include rectus femoris flap for the suprapubic area, component separation, free myocutaneous flaps, and tensor fascia lata flaps. Tensor fascia lata is an ideal autologous tissue for management of large infected wounds or a contaminated field. The fascia lata is harvested from the thigh; the thigh wound is closed over suction drains. The fascial graft is oriented so that the deep surfaces are in contact with the peritoneal cavity. Experimental models have demonstrated that the rate of collagen synthesis and deposition is increased fivefold after implantation of this autologous tissue graft. Within 2 weeks, revascularization from the surrounding abdominal wall occurs.[57–59] Unfortunately, recurrent hernia rates are rather high and reportedly range from 9% to 29%.[57,60,61] Other disadvantages of tensor fascia lata flaps grafts include the creation of an additional wound on the thigh and the requirement for epidermolysis and potential for necrosis of the skin closed over the fascial flap.

Component Separation

Ramirez et al.[62] first described component separation in 1990. This technique allows closure of the midline defect with an innovative advancement flap of muscle and fascia. First, a subcutaneous flap of adipose tissue is created by separating the subcutaneous adipose tissue from the fascia of the anterior rectus sheath and continuing laterally onto the external oblique aponeurosis to the level of the midaxillary line. The external oblique is then divided in a longitudinal fashion approximately 2 cm lateral to its insertion into the rectus sheet and separated from the internal oblique (Figure 12.8). This incision should be continued up onto the lower chest and no higher than the origin of the rectus abdominus muscle. With adequate release of the external oblique and internal oblique, the rectus muscles can be closed without significant tension. When additional mobility is required, a second longitudinal incision is placed in the posterior rectus sheath separating the rectus muscle. Bilateral component separation will allow enough mobility to close defects as large as 10 cm in the epigastrium, 20 cm at the level of the umbilicus, and 6 cm at the suprapubic level. The subcutaneous flaps are closed over suction drains to minimize seroma or hematoma formation. Multiple modifications of this technique have been described.[43,63,64] Component separation avoids the complications associated with mesh implantation and has a more established profile of reliability than do biologic scaffolds. However, as with tensor fascia lata, the reported rate of recurrent hernia formation is significant, ranging from 22% to 32%.[61,65]

Appropriate utilization of the open abdomen and strategies for its subsequent closure have been increasingly associated with improved patient outcome. Management of these patients is a complex and challenging endeavor that should be an essential component of the acute care surgeon's repertoire of skills.

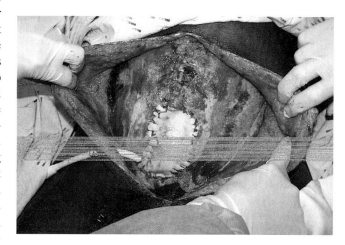

FIGURE 12.8. Component separation with placement of AlloDerm® to bridge fascial defect.

After the initial decision to leave the abdomen open, varying intervals of maintaining it temporarily open or transiently closed ensue. Definitive closure can be accomplished at the appropriate juncture either primarily or secondarily in a staged fashion, accepting a planned ventral hernia for some period of time. Noteworthy complications include secondary compartment syndrome; fistulae; intraabdominal and wound infections; tissue necrosis; evisceration; and dehiscence and incisional hernia.

Clinical acumen and knowledge of the indications for early termination of the initial operation are imperative and based on guidelines that are well described. Subsequent decisions for timing and number of returns to the operating room are rooted in a sound knowledge of patient physiology; options for staged closure; and the advantages, disadvantages, and potential complications of each as well as their management. This often requires the combination of a number of methods and some degree of flexibility and creativity. The use of native tissue, prosthetics, and general nutritional, pulmonary, immunologic, and psychological support, individually or in combination, are all integral to success.

Critique

This is a critical point in the case where continued operative management, even when definitive management has yet to be achieved, is deleterious. The "three dark angels of death" (hypothermia, acidosis, and coagulopathy) are absolute indicators for ending the operation as expeditiously as possible and establishing some type of creative closure (which includes simply packing the abdomen). Several options are usually available, including the creation of a "silo" by cutting a large panel from an irrigation bag. Further management of the patient needs to be done in an intensive care unit setting before any attempt at definitive intervention.

Answer (E)

References

1. Lucas CE, Ledgerwood AM. Prospective evaluation of hemostatic techniques for liver injuries. J Trauma 1976; 16:442–451.
2. Calne RY, McMaster P, Pentlow BD. The treatment of major liver trauma by primary packing with transfer of the patient for definitive treatment. Br J Surg 1979; 66:338–339.
3. Feliciano DV, Mattox KL, Jordan GL Jr. Intra-abdominal packing for control of hepatic hemorrhage: a reappraisal. J Trauma 1981; 21:285–290.
4. Svodoba JA, Peter ET, Dang DV, et al. Severe liver trauma in the face of coagulopathy: a case for temporary packing and early reexploration. Am J Surg 1982; 144:717–721.
5. Carmona RC, Peck DZ, Lim RC. The role of packing and planned reoperation in severe hepatic trauma. J Trauma 1984; 24:779–784.
6. Rotondo MF, Schwab CW, McGonigal MD, et al. "Damage control": an approach for improved survival in exsanguinating penetrating abdominal injury. J Trauma 1993; 35:375–383.
7. Wittman DH, Bansal N, Bergstein JM, et al. Staged abdominal repair compares favorably with conventional operative therapy for intra-abdominal infections when adjusting for prognostic factors with a logistic model. Theor Surg [now Eur J Surg] 1994; 25:273.
8. Berger RL, Dunton RF, Leonardi HK, Karlson KJ. Pack and close approach to persistent postcardiopulmonary bypass bleeding. J Am Coll Surg 1994; 178:353–356.
9. Rotondo MR, Zonies DH. The damage control sequence and underlying logic [review]. Surg Clin North Am 1997; 77:761.
10. Noetzel W. Die operativer Behandlung der diffusen eitrigen Peritonitis. Verh Dtsch Ges Chir 1908; 34:638.
11. Wittman DH, Schein M, Condon RE. Management of secondary peritonitis. Ann Surg 1996; 224:10.
12. Wittman DH, Wallace JR, Schein M. Open abdomen, planned relaparotomy, or staged abdominal repair: is there a difference? World J Surg 1994; 268:S49.
13. Wittman DH, Goris RJA, Ranga bashyam N, et al. Laparostomy, open abdomen, etappenlavage, planned relaparotomy and staged abdominal repair: too many names for a new operative method. In Ruedi TM, ed. State of the Art of Surgery. Reinach, Switzerland: International Society of Surgery, 1994:23.
14. Wittman DH. Staged abdominal repair: development and current practice of an advanced operative technique for diffuse suppurative peritonitis. Acta Chir Austriaca [Eur Surg] 2000; 32:171.
15. Neidehardt JH, Kraft F, Morin A, et al. Le traitement "La ventre ouvert" de certaines peritonites et infections parietals abdmoninales graves: etudes et technique. Chirurgie 1979; 105:272.
16. Maetani S, Tobe T. Open peritoneal drainage as effective treatment of advanced peritonitis. Surgery 1981; 90:804.
17. Porter JM, Ivatury RR, Nassoura ZE. Extending the horizons of "damage control" in unstable trauma patients beyond the abdomen and gastrointestinal tract. J Trauma 1997; 42:559–561.
18. Cipolla J, Stawicki SP, Hoff WS, et al. A proposed algorithm for managing the open abdomen. Am Surg 2005; 71:202–207.
19. Myers JA, Latenser BA. Nonoperative progressive "Bogotá bag" closure after abdominal decompression. Am Surg 2002; 68:1029–1030.
20. Feliciano DV, Burch JM. Towel clips, silos, and heroic forms of wound closure. Adv Trauma Crit Care 1991; 6:231–250.
21. Frenandez L, Norwood S, Roettger R, Wilkins HE 3rd. Temporary intravenous bag silo closure in severe abdominal trauma. J Trauma 1996; 40:258–260.

22. Ghimenton F, Thomson SR, Muckart DJ, Burrows R. Abdominal content containment: practicalities and outcome. Br J Surg 2000; 87:106–109.

23. Howdieshell TR, Yeh KA, Hawkins ML, Cue JL. Temporary abdominal wall closure in trauma patients: indications, technique, and results. World J Surg 1995; 19:154–158.

24. Howdieshell TR, Proctor CD, Sternberg E, et al. Temporary abdominal closure followed by definitive abdominal wall reconstruction of the open abdomen. Am J Surg 2004; 188:301–306.

25. Bender JS, Bailey CE, Saxe JM, et al. The technique of visceral packing: recommended management of difficult fascial closure in trauma patients. J Trauma 1994; 36:182–185.

26. Lamb JP, Vitale T, Kaminski DL. Comparative evaluation of synthetic meshes used for abdominal wall replacement. Surgery 1983; 93:643–648.

27. Marmon LM, Vinocur CD, Standiford SB, et al. Evaluation of absorbable polyglycolic acid mesh as a wound support. J Pediatr Surg 1985; 20:737–742.

28. Dayton MT, Buchele BA, Shirazi SS, Hunt LB. Use of an absorbable mesh to repair contaminated abdominal-wall defects. Arch Surg 1986; 121:954–960.

29. Lopez Villata GC, Furio-Bacete V, Ortiz Oshiro E, et al. Experimentally contaminated reabsorbable meshes: their evolution in abdominal wall defects. Int Surg 1995; 80:223–226.

30. Morris JA Jr, Eddy VA, Rutherford EJ. The trauma celiotomy: the evolving concepts of damage control. Curr Probl Surg 1996; 33:609–708.

31. Bradley SJ, Jurkovich GJ, Pearlman NM, Stiegmann GV. Controlled open drainage of severe intra-abdominal sepsis. Arch Surg 1985; 120:629–631.

32. Heddirch GS, Wexler MJ, McLean AP, Meakins JL. The septic abdomen: open management with Marlex mesh with a zipper. Surgery 1986; 99:399–408.

33. Walsh GL, Chiasson P, Hedderich G, et al. The open abdomen: a Marlex mesh and zipper technique. Surg Clin North Am 1988; 1:25–40.

34. Wittman DH, Aprahamian C, Bergstein JM. Etappenlavage: advanced diffuse peritonitis managed by planned multiple laparotomies utilizing zippers, slide fastener, and Velcro analogue for temporary abdominal closure. World J Surg 1990; 14:218–226.

35. Aprahamian C, Wittman DH, Bergstein JM, Quebbeman EJ. Temporary abdominal closure (TAC) for planned relaparotomy (etappenlavage) in trauma. J Trauma 1990; 30:719–723.

36. Wittman DH, Aprahamian C, Bergstein JM, et al. A burr-like device to facilitate temporary abdominal closure in planned multiple laparotomies. Eur J Surg 1993; 159:75–79.

37. Barker DE, Kaufman HJ, Smith LA, et al. Vacuum pack technique of temporary abdominal closure: a 7-year experience with 112 patients. J Trauma 2000; 48:201–207.

38. Brock WB, Barker DE, Burns RP. Temporary closure of open abdominal wounds: the vacuum pack. Am Surg 1995; 61:30–35.

39. Smith LA, Barker DE, Chase CW, et al. Vacuum pack technique of temporary abdominal closure: a four year experience. Am Surg 1997; 63:1002–1008.

40. Garner GB, Ware DN, Cocanour CS, et al. Vacuum assisted wound closure provides early fascial reapproximation in trauma patients with open abdomen. Am J Surg 2001; 182:630–638.

41. Stone PA, Hass SM, Flaherty SK, et al. Vacuum-assisted fascial closure for patients with abdominal trauma. J Trauma 2004; 57:1082–1086.

42. Hirschberg A, Mattox KL. "Damage control" in trauma surgery. Br J Surg 1993; 80:1501.

43. Hirschberg A, Mattox KL. Planned reoperation for severe trauma. Ann Surg 1995; 222:3.

44. Fabian TC, Croce MA, Pritchard FE, et al. Planned ventral hernia: staged management for acute abdominal wall defects. Ann Surg 1994; 219:643.

45. Bloomfield G, Saggi B, Blocher C, Sugerman H. Physiologic effects of externally applied continuous negative abdominal pressure for intra-abdominal hypertension. J Trauma 1999; 46:1009–1016.

46. De Waele JJ, Benoit D, Hoste E, Colardyn F. A role for muscle relaxation in patients with abdominal compartment syndrome. Intensive Care Med 2003; 29:332.

47. Shapiro MB, Jenkins DH, Schwab CW, Rotondo MF. Damage control: collective review. J Trauma 2000; 49:969–978.

48. Dejardin LM, Arnoczky SP, Clarke RB. Use of small intestinal submucosal implants for regeneration of large fascial defects: an experimental study in dogs. J Biomed Mater Res 1999; 46:203–211.

49. Badylak S, Kokini K, Tullius B, et al. Morphologic study of small intestinal submucosa as a body wall repair device. J Surg Res 2002; 103:190–202.

50. Franklin JJ Jr, Gonzalez ME Jr, Michaelson RP, et al. Preliminary experience with new bioactive prosthetic material for repair of hernias in infected fields. Hernia 2002; 6:171–174.

51. Menon NG, Rodriguez ED, Byrnes CK, et al. Revascularization of human acellular dermis in full-thickness abdominal wall reconstruction in the rabbit model. Ann Plast Surg 2003; 50:523–527.

52. Dalla Vecchia L, Engrum S, Kogon B, et al. Evaluation of small intestine submucosa and acellular dermis as diaphragmatic prostheses. J Pediatr Surg 1999; 34:167–171.

53. Cady B, Brooke-Cowden GL. Repair of massive abdominal wall defects: combined use of pneumoperitoneum and Marlex mesh. Surg Clin North Am 1976; 56:559–570.

54. Paletta CE, Huang DB, Dehghan K, Kelly C. The use of tissue expanders in staged abdominal wall reconstruction. Ann Plast Surg 1999; 42:259–265.

55. Tran NV, Petty PM, Clay RP, et al. Tissue expansion–assisted closure of massive ventral hernias. J Am Coll Surg 2003; 196:484–488.

56. Fansler RF, Taheri P, Cullinane C, et al. Polypropylene mesh closure of the complicated abdominal wound. Am J Surg 1995; 170:15–18.

57. Disa JJ, Goldberg NH, Carlton JM, et al. Restoring abdominal wall integrity in contaminated tissue-deficient wounds using autologous fascia grafts. Plast Reconstr Surg 1998; 101:979–986.

58. Disa JJ, Chiaramonte MF, Girotta JA, et al. Advantages of autologous fascia versus synthetic patch abdominal

reconstruction in experimental animal defects. Plast Reconstr Surg 2001; 108:2086–2087.

59. Das SK, Davidson SF, Walker BL, Talbot PJ. The fate of free autogenous fascial grafts in the rabbit. Br J Plast Surg 1990; 43:315–317.

60. Feldt-Rasmussen K, Jensen OA. Large ventral herniae treated with free fascial grafts; a follow-up study. Acta Chir Scand 1956; 111:403–408.

61. Girotto JA, Chiaramonte M, Menon NG, et al. Recalcitrant abdominal wall hernias: long-term superiority of autologous tissue repair. Plast Reconstr Surg 2003; 112:106–114.

62. Ramirez OM, Uras E, Dellon AL. "Components separation" method for closure of abdominal-wall defects: an anatomic and clinical study. Plast Reconstr Surg 1990; 86:519–526.

63. Jernigan TW, Fabian TC, Croce MA, et al. Staged management of giant abdominal wall defects: acute and long-term results. Ann Surg 2003; 238:349–357.

64. Ennis LS, Young JS, Gampper TJ, Drake DB. The "open book" variation of component separation for repair of massive midline abdominal wall hernia. Am Surg 2003; 69:733–743.

65. de Vries Reilingh TS, van Goor H, Rosman C, Bemelmans MH, et al. "Components separation technique" for the repair of large abdominal wall hernias. J Am Coll Surg 2003; 196:32–37.

13
Acute Care Surgery and the Elderly

Patrick K. Kim, Donald R. Kauder, and C. William Schwab

Case Scenario

You are asked to evaluate an 80-year-old retired railroad porter who stumbled and fell while walking his dog. He has left upper extremity and forehead abrasions. According to his family, he lives alone and is completely independent. The patient denies any medical problems with the exception of diabetes mellitus and benign prostate hypertrophy. He has a normal mental status and is hemodynamically stable. Outside of the abrasion, patient's physical examination is unremarkable. Which of the following should be the management plan for this patient?

(A) Overnight observation in the hospital
(B) Outpatient management
(C) Refer patient to a rehabilitation center
(D) Obtain plain radiography of the head
(E) Obtain head computed tomography scan

Performing acute care surgery in the elderly poses a wide spectrum of challenging problems for the surgeon. The geriatric population is possessed of unique physiology, risk factors, anatomic considerations, and preexisting conditions that significantly impact outcome. Many of these issues arise simply as a result of the "normal" aging process. Those who suffer from conditions that require acute care surgical interventions and are subsequently exposed to the physiologic stress that accompanies them suffer high rates of complications and mortality.[1] As the cohort of elders increases, it is increasingly vital for the surgeon to understand how age affects their surgical evaluation and treatment.

No broad consensus exists regarding the age at which a person becomes "elderly," but generally this appellation has been applied to those variably between 55 and 75 years of age. Regardless of when elder years begin, this group continues to comprise a greater proportion of the American population. In 2000, 35 million Americans were 65 years or older (12.4% of the population). In 2001, the overall life expectancy in the United States was 77.2 years (74.4 years for men and 79.8 years for women).[2] By 2030, this number is expected to increase to 71 million (19.6% of the population).[3]

Acute care surgery in the elderly is associated with strikingly high rates of complications and mortality, carrying a 7- to 10-fold increase in mortality compared with the same procedures performed electively.[4,5] Those older than 74 years fare even worse than those between the ages of 64 and 74 years.[5] Interestingly, it appears that age contributes less to morbidity and mortality in acute care operations than the emergency nature of the process itself. One study suggests that the differences in mortality between octogenarians and septuagenarians are due to American Society of Anesthesiologists (ASA) grade and delays in surgical treatment, not to age.[6] It might be inferred, then, that variations in the physiologic reserve of persons of similar ages, as well as different rates of senescence among an individual's organ systems, are critical factors that influence outcome. Because age cannot be controlled, it becomes imperative to optimize the other factors during evaluation and definitive treatment.

Normal Physiologic Changes Associated with Aging

The physiologic changes associated with aging are well studied. Every organ system has age-related changes that have significance for the surgeon. Collectively, the normal physiologic changes associated with aging and the changes associated with chronic diseases result in diminished physiologic reserve available to handle the stress of acute surgical disease and surgical intervention.[7]

The cardiovascular system undergoes many changes.[7] Aging is associated with decreased responsiveness to beta-adrenergic stimulus, limiting both inotropy and chronotropy and, ultimately, cardiac output. The maximum achievable heart rate is decreased. Left ventricular reserve is diminished, resulting in less ability to increase ejection fraction under stress. Left ventricular hypertrophy results in decreased compliance. Ventricle filling is more dependent on atrial contraction, and cardiac output becomes more dependent on end-diastolic volume. Alterations in the arterial vascular system also affect myocardial function. Arterial intimal hyperplasia leads to increased stiffness of arterial walls, occurring independently of atherosclerosis. Diastolic pressure decreases, which worsens perfusion pressure of the myocardium.

Progressive aging has a significant effect on pulmonary physiology.[7] Alterations in chest wall mechanics and intrinsic changes in the lung parenchyma have an additive effect. As costal cartilage becomes calcified, the chest wall becomes more rigid. Respiratory muscle strength is decreased, and intercostal muscles atrophy and become weaker. All of these factors contribute to decreases in both forced expiratory volume and forced vital capacity. Breathing becomes more dependent on the diaphragm and abdominal muscles. Regarding the lungs themselves, the alveolar–arterial oxygenation gradient is increased, the shunt fraction is increased, ventilation–perfusion mismatch is increased, and diffusion capacity is decreased. All of these factors contribute to decreased arterial oxygenation. Addition of a large abdominal surgical incision in this setting, especially in the emergency situation when there is no opportunity to optimize pulmonary mechanics preoperatively, can have disastrous consequences on pulmonary physiology.

The renal system is relatively impaired in the elderly.[7] Anatomic changes include glomerulosclerosis, which decreases effective renal cortex mass. Functional changes include decreased glomerular filtration rate, decreased glomerular filtration reserve, decreased reabsorption and secretion by renal tubules, and blunted response to aldosterone and antidiuretic hormone. Intraabdominal surgical conditions are frequently associated with insensible and third-space fluid losses or hemorrhage. The resultant hypovolemia and hypoperfusion of the renal cortex puts the patient at high risk for developing clinically significant renal dysfunction.

Gastrointestinal function is relatively preserved in the elderly.[7] Most age-related changes involve the esophagus and the colon. Esophageal neuromuscular degeneration contributes to diffuse esophageal spasm, achalasia, and reflux. Dysfunction of the upper esophageal sphincter predisposes patients to aspiration, dysphagia, and pharyngoesophageal diverticula. Lower esophageal sphincter dysfunction contributes to gastroesophageal reflux. The stomach and small bowel structure and function remain relatively unaffected by aging. In the colon, thickening of the colonic muscular wall occurs.

Endocrinologic changes are numerous.[7] Even among nondiabetic patients, the elderly demonstrate some degree of insulin resistance, resulting in decreased glucose tolerance. Studies in surgical patients have demonstrated that intensive glycemic control is associated with a decrease in morbidity and mortality compared with more liberal glycemic control,[8] but the optimal glycemic range among the elderly who undergo acute care surgery is unknown. An important age-related change in the endocrine system is the decreased sympathetic response to stress, clinically manifested by a decreased vasoconstriction response to cold environments. This makes the elderly patient particularly susceptible to hypothermia in the perioperative period. Finally, regarding the thyroid gland, subclinical hypothyroidism is prevalent in the elderly population.[9] Subclinical hypothyroidism in the elderly has been shown to be independently associated with depression, dementia, and coronary disease.[10,11]

Neurologic and cognitive changes are numerous.[7] Physiologic and anatomic changes include cortical atrophy, decreased cerebral blood flow, and decreased cerebral oxygen consumption. Clinically the elderly are more likely to have blunted visual, auditory, and tactile sensation and increased pain threshold. The clinical significance is the increased prevalence of anxiety, agitation, and delirium in the perioperative period. The inappropriate use of narcotic analgesics and sedative/hypnotics can exacerbate underlying deficits. Decreased capacity to follow postoperative instructions related to pulmonary toilet, ambulation, and analgesic management can lead to unfavorable outcomes. Alterations in cerebellar function, as well as balance and gait disturbances, can predispose the patient to falls.

Clinical Presentation of Elderly Patients

Initial evaluation of the elderly patient with a suspected surgical emergency may be difficult. For both medical and surgical conditions, the elderly may present atypically or with nonspecific complaints.[12] The elderly patient may delay seeking medical attention because of a higher pain threshold, or an atypical or falsely benign presentation, or denial.[13–15] Preexisting alterations in mental status or neurologic status (i.e., dementia, delirium, prior stroke, and diabetic neuropathy) may also contribute to delayed presentation by the patient or referral by primary providers. The chief complaint may thus not immediately suggest the correct differential diagnosis. Furthermore, the history of present illness may be difficult to elicit, and the medical history may be complex, incomplete, or frankly inaccurate. Physical examination similarly may be deceptively benign. This may be particularly true of diseases that normally cause peritonitis, such as diverticulitis and appendicitis.[16–18] Among patients hospitalized in medical intensive care, altered mental status, absence of peritoneal signs, analgesics, antibiotics, and mechanical ventilation all contributed to delays in surgical evaluation and treatment.[19] Predictably, delays in presentation, referral, diagnosis, and treatment all contribute to dismal rates of morbidity and mortality among the elderly with acute surgical problems.

Preoperative Assessment

By its nature, acute care surgery precludes complete preoperative evaluation and risk stratification. Ideally, a complete medical history is obtained, and this information can be helpful in stratifying risk and optimizing the patient in the perioperative period. Eighty percent of the elderly have at least one chronic medical condition, and fifty percent have two or more.[20] In decreasing order, the most common chronic conditions are arthritis, hypertension, heart disease, cancer, diabetes, and stroke.[20] Of these, heart disease, hypertension, and diabetes have the greatest impact on outcomes following surgery and are the focus of active investigations.

The American College of Cardiology/American Heart Association (ACC/AHA) perioperative executive summary provides guidelines for cardiac risk stratification for patients undergoing noncardiac surgery.[21] Although the guidelines are primarily focused on patients who undergo *elective* noncardiac surgery, the same algorithm is used for postoperative risk stratification among patients who undergo acute care procedures. The ACC/AHA paradigm stratifies risk using three components: clinical markers, functional capacity, and surgery-specific risk. Clinical markers are classified as major, intermediate, and minor. Major predictors include acute or recent myocardial infarction (MI), unstable or severe angina, decompensated heart failure, "large ischemic burden" (clinically or by noninvasive testing), significant arrhythmias, and significant valvular disease. Intermediate predictors include mild angina, remote MI, compensated heart failure, diabetes, and serum creatinine level ≥2.0 mg/dL. Advanced age is classified as a minor predictor, along with abnormal electrocardiogram, nonsinus rhythm, history of stroke, uncontrolled hypertension, and low functional capacity. Functional capacity can be measured by metabolic equivalent (MET) levels, in which 1 MET is defined as the oxygen uptake at rest (approximately 3.5 mL/kg/min oxygen uptake).[22] Patients who cannot routinely tolerate a demand of 4 METs have increased perioperative cardiac and long-term risks. Four-MET activities include light work around the house, such as dusting or washing dishes, climbing a flight of stairs, or walking at a rate of 4 miles per hour.

Regarding surgery-specific risk of sustaining a cardiac event, major acute care surgery in the elderly is a priori considered high-risk surgery (>5% risk of cardiac event) and is grouped with aortic and other major vascular surgery, peripheral vascular surgery, and prolonged procedures associated with large fluid shifts and/or blood loss.[21] Intermediate-risk procedures (<5% risk of cardiac event) include intraperitoneal and intrathoracic surgery, carotid endarterectomy, head and neck surgery, orthopedic surgery, and prostate surgery. Low-risk procedures (<1% cardiac risk) include endoscopic and superficial procedures, cataract surgery, and breast surgery.

Pulmonary complications following surgery are common, and, similar to cardiac issues, pulmonary risks are classified as surgery related and patient related. High-risk surgical procedures are generally the same as those identified by the ACC/AHA, with the addition of upper abdominal surgery, which compromises pulmonary function.[23] Patient-related risk factors for pulmonary complications include chronic obstructive pulmonary disease, recent cigarette use, dependent functional status, an abnormal chest radiograph, renal insufficiency, and hypoalbuminemia.[23] Pulmonary risk stratification is not particularly improved by routine preoperative spirometry.

Diabetes mellitus at any age increases the risk of complications and death after surgery.[24] In a variety of medical conditions, hyperglycemia is associated with an increased length of stay in the intensive care unit and the hospital, as well as increased hospital and long-term mortality.[25] The presence of diabetes similarly worsens outcomes in elderly patients after cardiac or gastrointestinal surgery or trauma.[26] Recent clinical investigation revealed that intensive glycemic control in a general population of critically ill surgical patients improved mortality, regardless of whether or not the patients had a history of diabetes.[8] The optimal target of serum glucose in elderly surgical patients is yet to be determined.

Perioperative Management of the Elderly

Preoperative optimization of the elderly patient with surgical emergency is limited, because lifestyle modifications (e.g., smoking cessation, exercise, nutritional supplementation, and weight loss) obviously cannot be performed. Among pharmacologic interventions in the perioperative period, beta-blockade has been clearly demonstrated to decrease morbidity and mortality in select populations. For patients undergoing elective vascular surgery, a population with high cardiac risk, beta-blockade decreases rates of MI and improves survival.[27] Beta-blockade also seems to benefit patients at cardiac risk undergoing noncardiac surgery. In the perioperative period, beta-blockade improves hemodynamics and postoperative analgesia.[28] On long-term follow-up, perioperative beta-blockade was found to improve long-term survival.[29] In this study,[29] patients were defined at risk if two of the following conditions were met: age ≥65 years, hypertension, current smoker, serum cholesterol level ≥240 mg/dL, and diabetes mellitus. These criteria are similar to those of the ACC/AHA, and most elderly patients satisfy these criteria. On the basis of these and other studies, perioperative beta-blockade has been recommended for all patients with a history of angina, myocardial infarction, heart failure, and diabetes, especially if the planned procedure is vascular, thoracic, or major abdominal.[30] Although there are no studies that specifically address beta-blockade for elderly patients undergoing noncardiac *acute care* surgery, the fact that a procedure is an emergency puts the patients into the high-risk category for a cardiac event. It is reasonable then to consider the use of beta-blockade in this setting. Despite good evidence, beta-blockers are probably underutilized in clinical practice, although beta-blockade has been shown to be safe and effective for patients with heart failure and pulmonary disease.[31]

It had been dogma that high-risk surgical patients benefit from invasive hemodynamic monitoring during the perioperative period. However, routine pulmonary artery catheterization in this group of patients is now controversial. Studies with high-risk surgical patients have variably demonstrated benefit, equivalence, and harm; a recent prospective study of high-risk elderly (≥60 years of age) patients undergoing predominantly elective surgery suggests that the use of pulmonary artery catheters neither worsened nor improved survival.[32] At present it is unclear whether the elderly who undergo acute care surgery uniformly benefit from pulmonary artery catheterization. Pulmonary artery catheters are likely to provide the most benefit to patients selected by factors besides age.

From a respiratory standpoint, several interventions may prove beneficial in the perioperative period. For patients who undergo elective surgery and have a history of significant pulmonary disease, optimization of chronic obstructive pulmonary disease and asthma, deep breathing exercises, incentive spirometry, and epidural local anesthetics reduce the risk of postoperative pulmonary complications in elderly surgical patients.[23] Epidural anesthesia may provide equal or superior analgesia compared with parenteral opioids in certain elective procedures,[33] but the benefit of epidural anesthesia when initiated after acute care operations is not known.

Acute Care Surgery: Specific Considerations

Although there are innumerable circumstances and a variety of body regions in which acute care surgery is warranted, surgical disease of the abdominal contents and the abdominal wall is commonly encountered. Gastrointestinal operations performed emergently in the elderly carry

higher rates of complication or mortality than their elective counterparts. Surgery for peptic ulcer disease is performed less commonly in the era of effective medical therapies. However, the spectrum of the disease has shifted to higher acuity caused by complications of perforation or intractable bleeding. Perforated gastric or duodenal ulcer is associated with high morbidity and mortality in elderly patients.[34] Case series suggest that for duodenal perforation, closure without vagotomy is associated with higher mortality than closure with vagotomy. For gastric perforation, gastrectomy is associated with higher mortality than simple closure. Paraesophageal hernia repair has higher mortality when performed emergently,[35] especially with associated gastric volvulus.[36]

Cholelithiasis is common among the elderly. Among patients who undergo expectant management of symptomatic gallstone disease, the mortality is high, suggesting that elderly patients with symptomatic gallstone disease should not have operative intervention withheld strictly because of age.[37] With elective cholecystectomy and common bile duct exploration, elderly patients have comparable outcomes to nonelderly patients.[38] In the acutely ill, percutaneous cholecystostomy with interval laparoscopic cholecystectomy is relatively safe and effective,[39] and one may be able to avoid cholecystectomy altogether in poor operative candidates. In patients older than 70 years, acute care cholecystectomy (particularly for suppurative cholecystitis) carries a high mortality compared with elective cholecystectomy, with much of the mortality attributable to concomitant cardiovascular and respiratory causes.[40]

Acute care colorectal procedures also demonstrate a pattern of generally higher morbidity and mortality in the elderly. Among patients 75 years or older, acute care operation for colorectal carcinoma is a statistically significant predictor of mortality. Similarly, octogenarians fare poorly after acute care colon surgery compared with elective colon surgery, with increased mortality and morbidity rates.[41] However, some series have suggested that emergent operative management of colorectal cancer, even among the most elderly (age >90 years), carries acceptable perioperative morbidity and mortality rates.[42] As expected, comorbidities negatively influence outcome after acute care colon operations.[43] Among the frailest patients, staged resection is probably indicated.[44] Several studies have suggested that elderly patients present with later stages or greater severity of peritonitis from appendicitis or diverticulitis than younger patients.[17,18,45,46] Dismal outcomes in elderly patients who have perforated appendicitis or diverticulitis are likely caused by the combination of a virulent disease process, delay in diagnosis, compromised host, and physiologic derangement.

Repair of abdominal or groin hernias is one of the most common procedures in general surgery and carries minimal morbidity and extremely low mortality when performed electively. The combination of advanced age and need for acute care operation for hernia drastically increases morbidity and mortality compared with elective repair.[47-49] Again, contributing factors include delay in presentation, atypical presentation, presence of comorbidities, and bowel obstruction, incarceration, or strangulation. Thus, for elderly patients with known abdominal or groin hernia, elective repair is strongly recommended.[48-51] Finally, among patients who undergo laparotomy urgently or electively, the incidence of late incisional hernia is higher following acute care laparotomy than elective laparotomy,[52] underscoring the importance of elective operation when possible.

The elderly injured patient is at higher risk for morbidity and mortality than younger injured patients.[53-56] Compared with younger patients, elderly patients have higher mortality rates for a given injury severity score[53] or mechanism of injury, are more likely to fail nonoperative management of solid organ injury,[57] have worse recovery after head injury,[58] and are more likely to require assistance after discharge from acute care. From a physiologic standpoint, mortality rate for the elderly trauma patient is prohibitive in the presence of hypotension,[55] significant base deficit,[59] and low respiratory rate (<10).[55] However, among injured patients, chronologic age itself is not uniformly predictive of outcome. Rather, it is the presence of preexisting diseases,[53] especially heart failure, obstructive pulmonary disease, hepatic disease, renal disease, and malignancy, that greatly increases the likelihood of poor outcome after trauma.[60] As a result, advanced age per se should not be used to justify withholding of care from the injured patient.[61] In fact, a low threshold is suggested for triage of the elderly injured patient to a trauma center.[61] (61). Not surprisingly, the multiply-injured elderly trauma patient requires significant use of health care resources,[54] which will only increase with the growing ranks of this cohort.

Ethical and End-of-Life Issues

The central component of the physician–patient relationship is patient autonomy.[62] The patient with decision-making capacity has the right to determine level of care or specific treatments as long as he or she retains that capacity. Advance directives may aid decision making by physicians and next of kin when the elderly patient cannot participate in the decision-making process. Advance directives are not invoked unless the patient is incapacitated, as deemed by the treating physician.[63] Furthermore, advance directives are not legally binding, serving only to outline patient preferences. Unfortunately, many patients presenting with acute surgical processes have no advance directive. In the absence of such a document, health care providers may give more aggressive care than the patient desired.[64] For the elderly patient who presents with a life-threatening acute surgical process, the physician should communicate to the patient or surrogate in understandable terms the diagnoses, management options, and expected outcomes and in turn ascertain the aggressiveness of care desired by the patient or surrogate, because it can be argued that patient suffering can result from either deficiency or excess of care.

In summary, caring for the elderly patient with an acute surgical process is particularly challenging because of unique presentation, diminution or absence of physiologic reserve, and comorbid conditions. The number of acute care procedures for elders will grow as the size of this group increases. Morbidity and mortality rates of emergent surgery for the elderly are consistently higher than those of procedures performed for the nonelderly or procedures performed electively. Options for optimizing preoperative conditions are limited by the nature of surgical emergencies. Prospective studies, largely composed of elderly elective surgery patients, suggest that perioperative therapies such as beta-blockade and intense glycemic control can improve outcomes. The benefits may extend to emergently operated elders. Good communication between physician and patient or surrogate is crucial to providing the appropriate level of care for patients who suffer acute surgical processes or injury.

Critique

There should be no apologies for liberal use of computed tomography scanning of the head in this situation, for what appears to be an unremarkable or normal neurologic status still could be an evolving intracranial injury in the elderly population. Age-related cerebral atrophy can allow for injury/hemorrhage to become more extensive before there is any clinical manifestation. Therefore, this subset of patients should have a computed tomography evaluation of the head.

Answer (E)

References

1. Pedersen T, Eliasen K, Henriksen E. A prospective study of mortality associated with anaesthesia and surgery: risk indicators of mortality in hospital. Acta Anaesthesiol Scand 1990; 34:176–182.
2. Arias E. United States Life Tables, 2001. National Vital Statistics Reports, vol 52, no 14. Hyattsville, MD: National Center for Health Statistics, 2004.
3. U.S. Census Bureau. International Database. Table 094. Midyear Population, by Age and Sex. Available at

http://www.census.gov/population/www/projections/natdet-D1A.html.

4. Keller SM, Markovitz LJ, Wilder JR, et al. Emergency and elective surgery in patients over age 70. Am Surg 1987; 53:636–640.

5. Barlow AP, Zarifa Z, Shillito RG, et al. Surgery in a geriatric population. Ann R Coll Surg Engl 1989; 71:110–114.

6. Arenal JJ, Bengoechea-Beeby M. Mortality associated with emergency abdominal surgery in the elderly. Can J Surg 2003; 46:111–116.

7. Aalami OO, Fang TD, Song HM, et al. Physiological features of aging persons. Arch Surg 2003; 138:1068–1076.

8. Van den Berghe G, Wouters P, Weekers F, et al. Intensive insulin therapy in critically ill patients. N Engl J Med 2001; 345:1359–1367.

9. Levy EG. Thyroid disease in the elderly. Med Clin North Am 1991; 75:151–167.

10. Davis JD, Stern RA, Flashman LA. Cognitive and neuropsychiatric aspects of subclinical hypothyroidism: significance in the elderly. Curr Psychiatry Rep 2003; 5:384–390.

11. Biondi B, Palmieri EA, Lombardi G, et al. Effects of subclinical thyroid dysfunction on the heart. Ann Intern Med 2002; 137:904–914.

12. Emmett KR. Nonspecific and atypical presentation of disease in the older patient. Geriatrics 1998; 53:50–52.

13. Morrow DJ, Thompson J, Wilson SE. Acute cholecystitis in the elderly: a surgical emergency. Arch Surg 1978; 113:1149–1152.

14. Smithy WB, Wexner SD, Dailey TH. The diagnosis and treatment of acute appendicitis in the aged. Dis Colon Rectum 1986; 29:170–173.

15. Levkoff SE, Cleary PD, Wetle T, et al. Illness behavior in the aged. Implications for clinicians. J Am Geriatr Soc 1988; 36:622–629.

16. Horattas MC, Guyton DP, Wu D. A reappraisal of appendicitis in the elderly. Am J Surg 1990; 160:291–293.

17. Franz MG, Norman JG. Delay in presentation accounts for the majority of inflamed appendices. Ann Surg 1996; 223:105–106.

18. Watters JM, Blakslee JM, March RJ, et al. The influence of age on the severity of peritonitis. Can J Surg 1996; 39:142–146.

19. Gajic O, Urrutia LE, Sewani H, et al. Acute abdomen in the medical intensive care unit. Crit Care Med 2002; 30:1187–1190.

20. Centers for Disease Control and Prevention. National Center for Health Statistics Supplement on Aging Study and Second Supplement on Aging Study. Atlanta, GA: CDC, 1995.

21. Eagle KA, Berger PB, Calkins J, et al. ACC/AHA guideline update for perioperative cardiovascular evaluation for noncardiac surgery—executive summary. Circulation 2002; 105:1257–1267.

22. Fletcher GF, Balady G, Froelicher VF, et al. Exercise standards: a statement for healthcare professionals from the American Heart Association. Circulation 1995; 91:580–615.

23. Smetana GW. Preoperative pulmonary assessment of the older adult. Clin Geriatr Med 2003; 19:35–55.

24. Hoogwerf BJ. Postoperative management of the diabetic patient. Med Clin North Am 2001; 85:1213–1228.

25. Khoury W, Klausner JM, Ben-Abraham R, et al. Glucose control by insulin for critically ill surgical patients. J Trauma 2004; 57:1132–1138.

26. Watters JM, Moulton SB, Clancey SM, et al. Aging exaggerates glucose intolerance following injury. J Trauma 1994; 37:786–791.

27. Poldermans D, Boersma E, Bax JJ, et al. The effect of bisoprolol on perioperative mortality and myocardial infarction in high-risk patients undergoing vascular surgery. N Engl J Med 1999; 341:1789–1794.

28. Zaugg M, Tagliente T, Lucchinetti E, et al. Beneficial effects from beta-adrenergic blockade in elderly patients undergoing noncardiac surgery. Anesthesiology 1999; 91:1674–1686.

29. Mangano DT, Layug EL, Wallace A, et al. Effect of atenolol on mortality and cardiovascular morbidity after noncardiac surgery. N Engl J Med 1996; 335:1713–1720.

30. Fleisher LA, Eagle KA. Lowering cardiac risk in noncardiac surgery. N Engl J Med 2001; 345:1677–1682.

31. Gottlieb SS, McCarter RJ, Vogel RA. Effect of beta-blockade on mortality among high-risk and low-risk patients after myocardial infarction. N Engl J Med 1998; 339:489–497.

32. Sandham JD, Hull RD, Brant RF, et al. A randomized, controlled trial of the use of pulmonary-artery catheters in high-risk surgical patients. N Engl J Med 2003; 348:5–14.

33. Park WY, Thompson JS, Lee KK. Effect of epidural anesthesia and analgesia on perioperative outcome: a randomized, controlled Veterans Affairs cooperative study. Ann Surg 2001; 234:560–571.

34. Duggan JM, Zinsmeister AR, Kelly KA, et al. Long-term survival among patients operated upon for peptic ulcer disease. J Gastroenterol Hepatol 1999; 14:1074–1082.

35. Hallissey MT, Ratliff DA, Temple JG. Paraoesophageal hiatus hernia: surgery for all ages. Ann R Coll Surg Engl 1992; 74:23–25.

36. Haas O, Rat P, Christophe M, et al. Surgical results of intrathoracic gastric volvulus complicating hiatal hernia. Br J Surg 1990; 77:1379–1381.

37. Arthur JD, Edwards PR, Chagla LS. Management of gallstone disease in the elderly. Ann R Coll Surg Engl 2003; 85:91–96.

38. Paganini AM, Feliciotti F, Guerrieri M, et al. Laparoscopic cholecystectomy and common bile duct exploration are safe for older patients. Surg Endosc 2002; 16:1302–1308.

39. Patterson EJ, McLoughlin RF, Mathieson JR, et al. An alternative approach to acute cholecystitis. Percutaneous cholecystostomy and interval laparoscopic cholecystectomy. Surg Endosc 1996; 10:1185–1188.

40. Burdiles P, Csendes A, Diaz JC, et al. Factors affecting mortality in patients over 70 years of age submitted to surgery for gallbladder or common bile duct stones. Hepatogastroenterology 1989; 36:136–139.

41. Bender JS, Magnuson TH, Zenilman ME, et al. Outcome following colon surgery in the octogenarian. Am Surg 1996; 62:276–279.

42. Catena F, Pasqualini E, Tonini V, Avanzolini A, Campione O. Emergency surgery for patients with colorectal cancer

over 90 years of age. Hepatogastroenterology 2002; 49:1538–1539.

43. Tsugawa K, Koyanagi N, Hashizume M, et al. Therapeutic strategy of emergency surgery for colon cancer in 71 patients over 70 years of age in Japan. Hepatogastroenterology 2002; 49:393–398.

44. Koperna T, Kisser M, Schulz F. Emergency surgery for colon cancer in the aged. Arch Surg 1997; 132:1032–1037.

45. Temple CL, Huchcroft SA, Temple WJ. The natural history of appendicitis in adults: a prospective study. Ann Surg 1995; 221:278–281.

46. Franz MG, Norman J, Fabri PJ. Increased morbidity of appendicitis with advancing age. Am Surg 1995; 61:40–44.

47. Primatesta P, Goldacre MJ. Inguinal hernia repair: incidence of elective and emergency surgery, readmission and mortality. Int J Epidemiol 1996; 26:835–839.

48. Arenal JJ, Rodriguez-Vielba P, Gallo E, et al. Hernias of the abdominal wall in patients over the age of 70 years. Eur J Surg 2002; 168:460–463.

49. Alvarez Perez JA, Baldonedo RF, Bear IG, et al. Emergency hernia repairs in elderly patients. Int Surg 2003; 88:231–237.

50. Brittenden J, Heys SD, Eremin O. Femoral hernia: mortality and morbidity following elective and emergency surgery. J R Coll Surg Edinb 1991; 36:86–88.

51. Ohana G, Manevwitch I, Weil R, et al. Inguinal hernia: challenging the traditional indication for surgery in asymptomatic patients. Hernia 2004; 8:117–120.

52. Mingoli A, Puggioni A, Sgarzini G, et al. Incidence of incisional hernia following emergency abdominal surgery. Ital J Gastroenterol Hepatol 1999; 31:449–453.

53. Morris JA Jr, MacKenzie EJ, Damiano AM, et al. Mortality in trauma patients: the interaction between host factors and severity. J Trauma 1990; 30:1476–1482.

54. Schwab CW, Kauder DR. Trauma in the geriatric patient. Arch Surg 1992; 127:701–706.

55. Knudson MM, Lieberman J, Morris JA Jr, et al. Mortality factors in geriatric blunt trauma patients. Arch Surg 1994; 129:448–453.

56. McMahon DJ, Shapiro MB, Kauder DR. The injured elderly in the trauma intensive care unit. Surg Clin North Am 2000; 80:1005–1019.

57. Harbrecht BG, Peitzman AB, Rivera L, et al. Contribution of age and gender to outcome of blunt splenic injury in adults: multicenter study of the eastern association for the surgery of trauma. J Trauma 2001; 51:887–895.

58. Vollmer DG. Age and outcome following traumatic coma: why do older patients fare worse? J Neurosurg 1991; 75:S37–S49.

59. Davis JW, Kaups KL. Base deficit in the elderly: a marker of severe injury and death. J Trauma 1998; 45:873–877.

60. Grossman MD, Miller D, Scaff DW, et al. When is an elder old? Effect of preexisting conditions on mortality in geriatric trauma. J Trauma 2002; 52:242–246.

61. Jacobs DG, Plaisier BR, Barie PS, et al. Practice management guidelines for geriatric trauma: the EAST practice management guidelines work group. J Trauma 2003; 54:391–416.

62. Angelos P. Ethical guidelines in surgical patient care. J Am Coll Surg 1999; 188:55–58.

63. Baluss ME, Lee KF. Legal considerations for palliative care in surgical practice. J Am Coll Surg 2003; 197:323–330.

64. Darzins P, Molloy DW, Harrison C. Treatment for life-threatening illness. N Engl J Med 1993; 329:736.

14
Acute Care Surgery in the Rural Setting

Dana Christian Lynge, Nicholas W. Morris, and John G. Hunter

Case Scenario

A 25-year-old pregnant patient is brought to the trauma bay after sustaining devastating injuries in a motor vehicle crash. The patient was intubated in the field. She is in the third trimester (34 weeks) and has what is thought to be a lethal closed head injury (Glasgow Coma Scale of 3). While in the trauma bay, she has a precipitous and sustained drop in blood pressure, refractory to body positioning and fluid resuscitation. Which of the following should emergency management do at this time?

(A) Emergency cesarean section
(B) Computed tomography evaluation of the abdomen
(C) Initiation of pressors
(D) Immediate transfer to a tertiary facility (20 miles)
(E) Initiation of do not resuscitate order

Almost one fourth of the American populace lives in rural areas. A large proportion of these more than 55 million people are elderly and/or impoverished. Despite improvements in transportation, travel to urban medical centers is not an option for many of these patients. For surgical emergencies of a traumatic and nontraumatic nature, most rural residents in this country still rely on the presence, skill, and commitment of the local general surgeon.

General surgeons working in the rural setting perform a wide variety of acute care operations. Some of these operations are similar to those performed by their urban counterparts (e.g., appendectomy, splenectomy secondary to blunt trauma), whereas others are more specific to rural areas (e.g., farming- and mining-related injuries) (Figure 14.1). The mechanism of injury and the condition of the patient are different in rural surgery. The surgical

principles are the same. The central difference between urban and rural surgical practice is not one of training or skill, but rather of resources and case mix. Rural surgeons have fewer resources at their disposal while dealing with a wide variety of cases of varying complexity. The disparity in resources varies from situation to situation and from day to day. It can include the lack of crucial colleagues (pathologists, anesthesiologists, radiologists, gastroenterologists, and/or even a lack of a competent first assistant for major operations) and lack of technology (imaging studies such as computed tomography [CT] and magnetic resonance imaging [MRI], on-site blood banks, adequate intensive care facility).[1] Because of this reality, rural surgeons often find innovative ways to deal with surgical problems and must be constantly evaluating when and what kind of patients to transfer and what kind of patient to operate on locally. Rural surgeons must master the logistics of transfer and referral from what can be very isolated situations. When weather or other factors prevent an appropriate transfer, rural surgeons can be called on to undertake major surgical procedures outside their normal "comfort zone" in order to save lives.

Defining Rurality and the Rural Surgeon

Any discussion of acute care surgery in the rural setting must first define its terms. There have been many proffered definitions of rural.[2] Some define rural based on whether the economic base is centered around agriculture or the extraction industries. Others use numerical indices such as number of persons per square mile or, in the case of the historically accepted Metropolitan Statistical Index system, the population of largest town in a given area. One of the more accurate and increasingly accepted systems is the rural–urban commuting area (RUCA) designation developed in collaboration

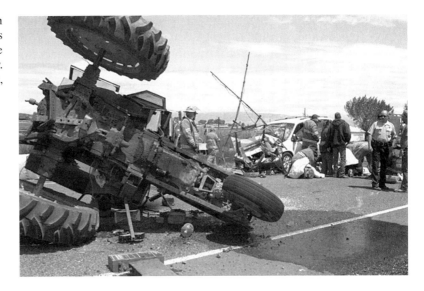

FIGURE 14.1. The collision of slow moving farm equipment with automobiles on rural roadways creates unique challenges for rural trauma care delivery. (Photograph by Steve Moseley. Reprinted with permission of the *Powell Tribune*, Powell, Wyoming.)

between the Department of Agriculture's Economic Research Service and the WWAMI Rural Health Research Center at the University of Washington.[3] This system takes into account commuter flow and actual proximity to urban services and can be used to break populations down into three categories: "urban" (metropolitan core with population greater than 50,000), "large rural" (large town core with a population between 10,000 and 50,000) and "small or isolated rural" (towns with populations of 2,500 to 10,000 or areas without an urban core population of at least 2,500). The principal advantage of using this system is the differentiation between "large rural" and "small or isolated rural"—as opposed to lumping them both together under the designation of "rural." Previous data have suggested that the surgeon-to-population ratios and individual surgeon case lists of "urban" and "large rural" surgeons are, in general, more similar than those of "large rural" and "small or isolated rural" surgeons. Because surgeons in "small or isolated" areas appear to form a group distinct from their "urban" and "large rural" counterparts—often working with fewer resources, colleagues, and subspecialists—this chapter focuses on surgery as performed by this group as being in a truly rural setting.

Finally, any examination of the practice of general surgery in the "small or isolated" rural areas of this country will reveal innumerable permutations of practice: general surgeons in solo practice as the "only surgeon in town"; general surgeons in group practice that cover several towns; general surgeons who practice in a community where there are gastroenterologists, orthopedic surgeons, and obstetrician/gynecologists; those who practice where there are no gastroenterologists or surgical subspecialists at all, and so forth. In this chapter, the practice model/template is that of a general surgeon in

solo practice in a "small or isolated rural" area of the western states with no resident gastroenterologist and limited surgical subspecialist services (e.g., orthopedics and obstetrician/gynecologist). This situation is that of the second author (N.M.), and the variety of situations contained herein reflect his experience.

An emergency is defined by *Webster's Ninth New Collegiate Dictionary* as "an unforeseen combination of circumstances or the resulting state that calls for immediate action." For this chapter, "immediate" is defined as within 24 hours.

Prehospital Care, Stabilization, and Transportation

Prehospital care in the rural setting is less standardized than in urban settings. It is carried out by a wide variety of "first responders," including volunteer medics, search and rescue organizations, and local volunteer fire departments. The qualifications and training of these personnel vary widely and are usually less extensive and standardized than the professional ambulance corps and fire departments of urban areas. Often their training is at a Basic Life Support level.[4] They are less apt to be trained in establishing airways, intravenous (IV) access, and resuscitation. There is evidence to suggest that improving training of prehospital care personnel to advanced life support (ALS) status improves outcomes.[5] The state of Vermont chose to focus on improving their prehospital care system and personnel, studies based on that indicated that the prehospital phase of care for rural patients was associated with the highest morbidity and mortality rates.[6]

In some cases, the local prehospital care system is completely bypassed and the rural patient evacuated from the roadside or domicile by air to a tertiary care facility. Some studies done in urban area trauma systems have made a case for superior outcomes with this approach.[7] However, studies of rural hospitals in trauma systems have failed to consistently show a downside to stabilization at the rural hospital before transport.[8,9] This is probably because of the frequent delays in discovery and distances involved in rural trauma that make immediate transfer to a Level I trauma center impossible and mandate stabilization at the rural hospital before transport. One type of injury where the "scoop and run" approach may be superior to local stabilization before transport is penetrating vascular injury with exsanguinating hemorrhage. However, in rural trauma, distance and weather may make this unfeasible, necessitating a "damage-control" procedure by the general surgeon at the rural hospital followed by transfer to a tertiary center with a larger blood bank, more intensive care resources, and relevant surgical specialists.

Modern transportation technology has revolutionized rural surgical emergency care. Patients who would have previously expired because of lack of resources and manpower in small, rural hospitals now routinely are evacuated to regional centers. "Med-evac" helicopters and fixed-wing aircraft are a common resource in many rural parts of the country at present. The use of air evacuation was developed by the military during the Korean and Vietnam wars and led to a reduction in deaths caused by penetrating injury.[10] Some studies of surgical trauma have shown increased mortality rates in areas where previously extant rotor-wing medical evacuation services were withdrawn.[11] Studies indicate that the advantage of emergency air transport is not necessarily a reduction in transport time but rather that the on-board personnel are highly trained in resuscitation, intubation, chest tube placement, and so forth, and function as a direct extension of the receiving trauma center physicians.[12,13] It should be noted, however, that, despite the evidence of utility of air transport in severely injured patients, not all rural states/areas can afford this expensive technology, and there is evidence to suggest that more lives would be saved by focusing efforts on earlier discovery and response and improving the training of rural volunteer medics and rural emergency department staff (who often lack advanced trauma life support [ATLS] training and are not always MDs).[6]

Early Management of the Surgical Emergency

The initial patient management by the general surgeon is to resuscitate, stabilize, diagnose, and treat. This approach is clearly outlined in ATLS protocols. Preparedness in the emergency department is crucial. Most rural hospitals have a trauma team and liberal activation criteria. Because of distances to the scene and the prevalence of radio communication between "first responders" and the rural hospital, the emergency room team and the surgeon have some time to activate the trauma team and prepare. During this time the surgeon ensures that all the members of the trauma team (there are rarely any backup members) are present and know their assignments. The surgeon should also check for med-evac and operating room availability. Frequently the need to transport to a referral center can be determined by on-scene emergency medical technician [EMT] reports before the patient arrives at the hospital. Unique to rural surgery, the surgeon must not only captain patient care but also rapidly formulate a decision plan based on the response of the patient to resuscitation, the patient's diagnoses, and available resources. Figure 14.2 outlines a rural surgeon's algorithm for emergency management.

Resources fall into three categories: hospital, personnel, and external. In small rural hospitals, there is often only one operating room team. If this team is not available, the surgeon must activate a backup plan. He or she

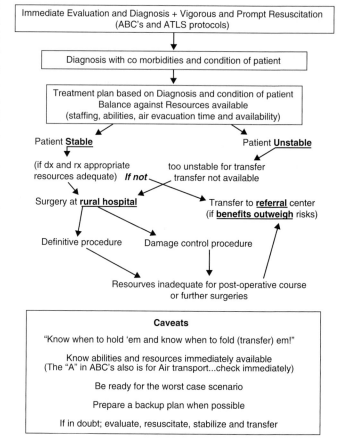

FIGURE 14.2. Management of emergency surgery in the rural setting: triage and flow scheme.

must assess blood availability and expected needs immediately. If massive transfusion is anticipated, other local hospitals must be notified so that they can send blood by ambulance or state police. Expected ongoing blood loss is a compelling reason to transfer a patient. Most rural hospitals have approximately 20 units of blood and fresh-frozen plasma, but no platelets. Radiology resources vary from rural hospital to hospital. Many have CT scanners. All have equipment for basic studies such as C-spine, chest, pelvis, and long bone. Interventional radiologic capabilities are uncommon in the true rural environment. The availability of an intensive care unit and ventilator care varies from place to place. Prolonged care in the intensive care unite—especially for the ventilated patient—is a tremendous effort in most rural settings and a drain of thin resources. In the interests of both the patient and the rural hospital, transfer should be carried out, if possible, for these patients.

Trauma Systems, ATLS, and Referral

There are good data that suggest that mortality rates for rural trauma are significantly higher than those in urban trauma.[14] This difference is ascribed to various factors, including length of time to discovery, length of time until arrival of medics, lack of professional medics, transport time (either to the local hospital or to a Level I trauma center), and lack of staffing or expertise at the rural hospital. The preponderance of available evidence in the literature suggests that the crucial factors are length of time to discovery, severity of injuries, age of patient, and, in the case of rural motor vehicle accidents, a higher vehicular velocity, likelihood of unrestrained driving, and alcohol ingestion.[15]

Trauma systems have been instituted in many states and regions, and overall the evidence suggests that they improve trauma management in rural areas through education of personnel and streamlining of the referral process.[16] As alluded to above, there is much debate about whether rural trauma patients have better outcomes when transferred to a Level I trauma center from the scene of the accident versus getting transferred from the rural hospital after stabilization. The available literature does not consistently reveal any increased mortality or morbidity with stabilization at the rural hospital, although, as mentioned above, there may be some cases (e.g., penetrating vascular trauma) when, if circumstance and proximity permit, the patient may be better off if transferred directly to a Level I hospital for definitive treatment.

Rural surgeons play a vital role in trauma systems both as educators (they are usually the local ATLS organizers and instructors) and as practitioners.[17] Studies indicate

TABLE 14.1. Errors in stabilization and transport of surgical patients.

1. Failure to document neurologic status
2. Inadequate cervical-spine immobilization when indicated
3. Failure to intubate patient when indicated
4. Failure to place tubes (chest tubes, nasogastric tubes, and Foley catheters) when indicated
5. Inadequate fluid resuscitation with crystalloid and/or blood
6. Failure to recognize problems that need urgent surgical attention
7. Delaying transport to obtain unnecessary x-rays (e.g., plain films of long bones and skull)

that there are fewer errors made in trauma management in small hospitals with ATLS-trained staff than in institutions where staff do not have the benefit of ATLS training.[16] A number of papers have retrospectively analyzed trauma deaths and elucidated the errors that contribute to patient demise during the prehospital and emergency department phases.[18] Table 14.1 lists some of the more common mistakes. All of these are largely avoidable if ATLS guidelines are followed.

Finally, rural surgeons should have their own non-trauma system referral network for surgical emergencies (e.g., abdominal aortic aneurysms [AAAs], necrotizing pancreatitis, necrotizing fasciitis) that require more personnel, resources, and facilities than they have available locally. Many rural surgeons will have trained in the state or area where they work and have a "ready-made" referral network for such cases. For rural surgeons not familiar with the surgical staff of their regional tertiary centers state, American College of Surgeons chapter meetings are an invaluable for finding regional experts and consultants with the resources to take on such cases. Good communication and mutual respect among rural and referral surgeons will improve outcomes and patient care.[19]

Crucial Colleagues

Urban surgeons, in addition to having well-staffed intensive care units and replete blood banks at their disposal, are able to take on complex patients with major physiologic impairment because of the support of specialist colleagues and the sophisticated and expensive technologies these colleagues can bring to bear upon a problem (not to mention the extra personnel in the form of house staff at academic institutions). A complete radiology service will have ultrasound, CT, and MRI available immediately. Those with interventional capabilities provide therapeutic (e.g., percutaneous drainage of abscesses) and diagnostic capability (e.g., fine-needle aspirates to diagnose infection or malignancy). The presence of these specialists enables the surgeon to handle more complex cases.

Data from Colorado revealed that only 40% of rural hospitals had radiologists on staff.[1] Rural general surgeons should develop expertise in reading plain films and CT scans and performing ultrasounds such as the focused abdominal sonography for trauma (FAST) examination.

A study of rural hospitals in Washington and Montana revealed that remote rural hospitals were significantly less likely to have anesthesiologists on staff and more likely to have their needs met by visiting certified registered nurse anesthetists (CRNAs).[20] There is evidence in the literature that anesthesiologist presence is associated with decreased mortality rate and decreased failure to rescue.[21] Anesthesia is needed both for airway management and ventilation as well as for any surgery. The CRNAs play a critical role at many rural hospitals and perform superbly. In some cases neither CRNAs nor anesthesiologists are available, leaving the general surgeon alone to manage intubation and ventilation. Practice intubating in the elective case is most useful.

General and Vascular Emergencies

The operative aspects of general and vascular emergencies are the same in the urban and rural settings. The central issue on what the rural surgeon does with traumatic or nontraumatic injury has to do with what resources they have available and how sick the patient is. These two realities dictate what the solo, rural surgeon should take on, whether they should stabilize with a "damage-control" procedure (when a definitive repair is not possible or ill advised for a patient who is unstable because of acidosis, hypothermia, and coagulopathy) followed by possible transfer and when the only procedure should be a transfer.[9]

For patients with massive hepatic trauma, limited blood bank and intensive care unit resources mandate packing and transferring to a larger facility.[22] An analogous nontraumatic case would be necrotizing pancreatitis, where transfer to a tertiary facility with more extensive intensive care unit capacity and personnel (including surgical residents) would be indicated before necrosectomy. Surgeons in solo rural practice with limited anesthesia, blood bank, and intensive care unit resources would probably be best advised to air transport a patient with a symptomatic AAA to a tertiary facility, because, even if they were able to perform the operation successfully and get the patient off the table, the personnel and resources required for resuscitation and monitoring in the immediate postoperative period might be

prohibitive in the rural practice situation. In brief, most operations performed infrequently (less than one a year) with high complexity, transfusion requirements, or intensive care unit care are better treated in a center with greater resources to care for these patients.

Surgical Subspecialty Emergencies

As described mentioned earlier, surgical subspecialty presence in rural communities can vary widely. General surgeons must assess the subspecialty needs in their communities and meet the need as best as possible. This need can be met by further training, such as taking a mini-fellowships or spending time with the relevant specialists at referral centers.

Neurosurgeons are seldom present in rural communities, yet neurotrauma is present in a significant proportion of rural motor vehicle accidents. This reality often leads to a patient with multiple injuries, including head trauma, being stabilized (i.e., this could entail anything from simple intubation to laparotomy) and transferred with ongoing bleeding and elevated intracranial pressure. A group of general surgeons from Montana sought to remedy this less than ideal situation by obtaining additional training and developing a treatment protocol with their regional trauma center and consultant neurosurgeon.[23] This collaboration has resulted in excellent patient outcomes.

Obstetrician/gynecologists are the third most common "surgical" specialists in rural America, after general and orthopedic surgeons. Many family practitioners are trained and credentialed to perform cesarean sections. However, there are still many parts of the country where general surgeons are called upon to perform cesarean sections and even hysterectomies.[24] Given the fact that few, if any, currently graduating general surgery residents receive any training in performing cesarean sections and other obstetric- and gynecologic-related surgery, a general surgeon in this situation would want to consider additional training in this procedure.[24] Other emergent subspecialty cases in which rural general surgeons might be called upon to address—depending on their training, the patient's acuity, and the availability of a subspecialist and/or transport—include bladder and urethra trauma, fractures of the extremities and even hips, and hand injuries.[24]

Endoscopy

The largest single difference in case content between urban and rural (including both large rural and small rural/isolated) surgeons submitting their previous year's case list prior to their 10-year recertifying examination was that rural surgeons performed significantly more endoscopies as part of their elective and emergency practice than their urban counterparts.[25] The ability of rural surgeons to endoscopically diagnose and even treat (by injection, cautery, etc.) the various causes of upper and lower gastrointestinal bleeding can save many needless transfers and "blind" emergency operations.

Telemedicine

Telemedicine is already in use in rural America, despite ongoing issues surrounding malpractice litigation and remuneration. It has proved useful in areas of medicine that rely on photographic or electronic interpretation (e.g., dermatology, cardiology, pathology, and orthopedics).[26] In Vermont, preliminary results have shown a positive impact on trauma patient care at the rural hospital.[27] The Vermont group is exploring ways to use wireless video technology to enable the trauma surgeon at the tertiary hospital to be virtually present in the ambulance with the volunteer medics and participate in the resuscitation from the outset. Ultimately, telemedicine has the potential to significantly reduce over-triage and under-triage rates, thus significantly improving emergency surgical care.

Surgical Education

The proper training and preparation for the practice of rural general surgery is currently under debate. What is clear is that current graduating chief residents in general surgery get very little, if any, true operative experience in obstetrics/gynecology or orthopedics and almost none in urology, otolaryngology, and neurosurgery.[28] The 10-year recertification case data cited by Ritchie et al.[25] revealed a profound difference in the amount of endoscopy that rural surgeons were doing compared with their urban counterparts, but did not reveal major differences in cases done outside the realm of "general surgery." However, the recertification data in this paper do not separate out the surgeons practicing in "small rural or isolated" areas, whose surgeon-to-population ratio, resources, and probable case distribution type differ from those of their "large rural" colleagues.[29]

A needs assessment study performed by Hunter and Deveney[30] in rural Oregon revealed that many surgeons in towns less than 10,000 there were performing orthopedic and obstetric/gynecologic procedures. Data from other parts of the country reveal that, although modern transportation and litigation concerns make subspecialty cases less common for rural general surgeons than in

years past, there are many parts of the country where general surgeons may be called on to perform cesarean sections, as well as basic orthopedic and urologic procedures.[28] It seems evident that trainees going into rural practice need something beyond the usual general surgical residency to equip them—at the very least, additional endoscopic skills and possibly some surgical subspecialty skills, depending on where they end up.

Several remedies to this educational conundrum have been put into effect. Oregon Health & Science University has designed and implemented a fourth-year rotation that takes place in a large rural hospital where the trainees can learn relevant subspecialty skills and includes several months working in a more isolated practice where they will have to use these skills.[30] At Basset Hospital in Cooperstown, NY, a 3- to 6-month rural fellowship is offered where graduated or practicing general surgeons can go to acquire the specific skills they need for their rural surgical practices. In Tennessee, surgical residents are offered a 3-month rural rotation as part of their training during which they do a lot of endoscopy and some gynecology, and, perhaps most importantly, they get to experience first hand what practicing in a small town is like and see if it is for them.

Conclusion

As mentioned earlier, the central difference between urban and rural surgeons when it comes to dealing with surgical emergencies is one of resources. Rural surgeons frequently have to deal with a wider variety of surgical emergencies with fewer resources in terms of both colleagues and technology. Accordingly, they need to be broadly educated in general surgical principles and techniques, including vascular and thoracic surgery. Depending on their individual practice situations, they may need to seek out additional training in acute care procedures in the areas of neurosurgery, orthopedic surgery, obstetrics/gynecology, and urology. This can be done as part of residency training or during their career as the situation demands. If they practice in a true remote/small rural area, they will want to obtain good training in diagnostic and therapeutic endoscopy, as this will form a large part of their elective and acute care practice. They will want to be part of a trauma or acute care system (either formal or informal), be active in teaching ATLS to other rural health care practitioners, and take part in the organization and training of their local prehospital care personnel. Their success will, in part, depend on developing a good referral network with regional centers and consultants for both trauma and nontrauma cases. They will need to have mastered the local resources and logistics of transferring patients at all times of the day and night and under a variety of weather conditions.

Finally, rural surgeons will need to develop—through education and experience—excellent "on the spot" judgment. It is this judgment that they most summon, not only to decide when to transfer and when not to, but also determine what to do when transfer of a very sick patient proves impossible due to lack of available vehicle (uncommon) or weather (more common). It is here that rural surgeons face challenges unique to their calling and bring all their training and experience to the saving of their patient's life.

Critique

This lethal injury to the mother will, inevitably, result in the demise of the near-term fetus. Therefore, the intervention that could make a difference is an emergency cesarean section. The rural setting should not preclude the acute care surgeon from performing such a life-saving intervention if the scenario is as described here.

Answer (A)

References

1. Majure J, Abernathy C. Rural surgeons of Colorado: the scope of their practice. Bull Am Coll Surg 1981; 66(2):11–16.
2. Ricketts T, Johnson-Webb K, Taylor P. Definitions of Rural: A Handbook for Health Policy Makers and Researchers. Rockville, MD: Office of Rural Health Policy, 1998.
3. Larson E, Johnson K, Norris T, et al. State of The Health Workforce in Rural America: Profiles and Comparisons. Seattle, WA: WWAMI Rural Health Research Center, 2002.
4. Grossman D, Hart L, Rivara F. From the Roadside to the Bedside: The Regionalization of Motor Vehicle Trauma Care in a Remote Rural County. Seattle, WA: WWAMI Rural Health Working Paper Series, Working Paper 24, 1993.
5. Rutledge R, Fakhry S, Meyer A. An analysis of the association of trauma center with per capita hospitalizations and death rates from injury. Ann Surg 1993; 218(4):512–524.
6. Rogers F, Osler T, Shackford S, et al. Population-based study of hospital trauma care in a rural state without a formal trauma system. J Trauma 2001; 50(3):409–413.
7. Sampalis J, Denis R, Frechette P, et al. Direct transport to tertiary trauma centers versus transfer from lower level facilities: impact on mortality and morbidity among patients with major trauma. J Trauma 1997; 43(2):288–295.
8. Rogers F, Osler T, Shackford S, et al. Study of the outcome of patients transferred to a Level I hospital after stabiliza-

9. tion at an outlying hospital in a rural setting. J Trauma 1999; 46(2):328–334.
10. Weinberg J, McKinley K, Petersen S, et al. Trauma laparotomy in a rural setting before transfer to a regional center: does it save lives? J Trauma 2003; 54(5):823–826.
11. Urdaneta L, Miller B, Ringenberg B, et al. Role of an emergency helicopter transport service in Rural trauma. Arch Surg. 1987; Sept. 122:992–996.
12. Mann N, Pinkney K, Price D, et al. Injury following the loss of air medical support for rural interhospital transport. Acad Emerg Med 2002; 9(7):694–698.
13. Sharar S, Luna G, Rice C, et al. Air transport following surgical stabilization: an extension of regionalized trauma care. J Trauma 1998; 28(6):794–798.
14. Moylan J, Fitzpatrick K, Beyer J, et al. Factors improving survival in multi-system trauma patients. Ann Surg 1988; 207(6):679–685.
15. Baker S, Whitfield R, O'Neill B. Geographic variations in mortality from motor vehicle crashes. N Engl J Med 1987; 316:1384–1387.
16. Rogers F, Shackford S, Hoyt D, et al. Trauma deaths in a mature urban vs rural trauma system. Arch Surg 1997; 132:376–381.
17. Olson C, Arthur M, Mullins R, et al. Influence of trauma system implementation on process of care delivered to seriously injured patients in rural trauma centers. Surgery 2001; 130(2):273–279.
18. Bintz M, Cogbill T, Bacon J, et al. Rural trauma care: role of the general surgeon. J Trauma 1996; 41(3):462–464.
19. Esposito T, Sanddal N, Hansen J, et al. Analysis of preventable trauma deaths and inappropriate trauma care in a rural state. J Trauma 1995; 39(5):955–962.
20. Rinker C, Sabo R. Operative management of rural trauma over a 10-year period. Am J Surg 1989; 158:548–552.
21. Dunbar P, Mayer J, Fordyce M, et al. Availability of anesthesia personnel in rural Washington and Montana. Anesthesiology 1998; 88(3):800–808.
22. Silber J, Kennedy S, Even-Shoshan O, et al. Anesthesiologist direction and patient outcomes. Anesthesiology 2000; 93(1):152–163.
23. Wemyss-Holden S, Bruening M, Launois B, et al. Management of liver trauma with implications for the rural surgeon. Aust N Z J Surg 2002; 72:400–404.
24. Rinker C, McMurry F, Groeneweg V, et al. Emergency craniotomy in a rural Level III trauma center. J Trauma 1998; 44(6):984–988.
25. Callaghan J. A twenty-five year survey of a solo practice in rural surgical care. J Am Coll Surg 1998; 44(6):984–990.
26. Ritchie W, Rhodes R, Biester T. Work loads and practice patterns of general surgeons in the United States, 1995–1997: a report from the American Board of Surgery. Ann Surg 1999; 230(4):533–543.
27. Reid J, McGowan J, Ricci M, et al. Desktop teleradiology in support of rural orthopedic care. Proc AMIA Ann Fall Symp 1997; 4:403–407.
28. Rogers F, Ricci M, Caputo M, et al. The use of telemedicine for real-time video consultation between trauma center

and community hospital in a rural setting improves early trauma care: preliminary results. J Trauma 2001;51(6):1037–1041.

28. Landercasper J, Bintz M, Cogbill T, et al. Spectrum of general surgery in rural America. Arch Surg 1997;132(5):494–497.

29. Thompson M, Lynge D, Larson E, et al. Characterizing the General Surgery Workforce in Rural America. Seattle, WA: WWAMI Rural Health Working Paper Series, Working Paper 77, 2004:1–11.

30. Hunter J, Deveney K. Training the rural surgeon: a proposal. Bull Am Coll Surg 2003;88(5):14–17.

15
Prehospital Care in the Acute Setting

Norman E. McSwain, Jr.

Case Scenario

A 16-year-old gang leader sustains a stab wound to the midchest (precordial area). He is found by the paramedics collapsed on the street with a thready pulse rate. With a Level I trauma center 11 miles away and a Level II facility four blocks away, which of the following should be the prehospital management decision?

(A) Perform endotracheal intubation and establish intravenous access
(B) Arrange air evacuation to the Level I facility
(C) Transport directly to the Level II facility
(D) Fully stabilize the patient in the field before any transport
(E) Pronounce the patient dead at the scene

For the acute care surgeon to be involved in the field care does not mean that the surgeon must be present in the field physically. However, the surgeon must be present philosophically in the field by being involved in the education of the prehospital provider, understanding what happens in the field, engaging in quality assurance, and having the confidence in the emergency medical technicians' (EMTs') ability and skill. The EMTs must "feel" this presence. This is achieved by (1) spending time with them, providing education both in the emergency room and in their classroom experiences; (2) riding with them on the street and understanding the conditions under which they carry out their responsibilities in the field; and (3) working with the emergency medical services (EMS) committee of the medical society or the acute care center.

An understanding of prehospital care is divided into two components: (1) understanding the EMS system and (2) understanding the physiology, pathophysiology, and management of the patient requiring acute care in the field just as they understand those same components in the hospital environment. The emergency training service (ETS) must understand and be conversant with both components of care in the field, just as the ETS in the hospital, to be effective, must understand the hospital system and the physiology, pathophysiology, and management of patient care to function effectively and provide proper care for those patients that the physician serves.

Emergency Medical Services Systems

An EMS system is to EMS and the EMT as the hospital is to medicine and the individual physician. It is the EMS system that provides a "home" for the EMTs, supervision of their function, quality assurance of their practice, delineation of their privileges, definition of their scope of practice, and financial support of the organization to provide patient care. *The key to running an effective EMS system that provides good care is strong physician oversight and quality control with attention to the details of patient outcome, skill utilization, and report analysis.*

Personnel

When J.D. "Deke" Farrington and Sam Banks, MD, FACS, started developing an educational program for the Chicago Fire Department in the late 1950s and when Walter Holt, MD, wrote the EMT textbook for the American Association of Orthopaedic Surgery in 1968, there was only one level of prehospital providers.[1] Most of their care was devoted to the management of trauma resulting from vehicular collisions, although rudimentary maintenance of some medical conditions was included. The medical component of this rapidly expanded, and, with the initiation of a mobile coronary care unit by Dr. J.F. Pantridge in Ireland[2] and its adaptation in the United States by physicians who were mostly anesthesiologists and cardiologists, an advanced level of medical and cardiac care was developed.

In the early 1970s, the U.S. Department of Transportation codified the EMT into three levels, which, with some small exceptions, are the national standard of the 21st century. These are the Emergency Medical Technician-Basic, Emergency Medical Technician-Intermediate, and Emergency Medical Technician-Paramedic. These have been abbreviated into EMT-B, EMT-I, and EMT-P. Many discussants further abbreviate this to use the term "EMT," meaning the basic emergency medical technician, and "paramedic," meaning the EMT paramedic. To follow the national standard, this chapter uses the terms EMT-B, EMT-I, and EMT-P for the individual levels and EMT as a generic term indicating all three levels.

Emergency Medical Technician-Basic

The EMT-B has completed a minimum of 110 contact hours of training following the objectives as outlined in the U.S. Department of Transportation's National Standard Curriculum and tested either by the National Registry for EMTs or by the individual state licensing agency or both. Depending on the state, re-registration is required every 2, 3, or 4 years to maintain that license. Each state has varying criteria for re-registration. Emergency medical service runs can generally be divided into three groups. Approximately one-third are trauma, one-third are medical, and one-third are cardiac. The EMT-B training program is divided essentially along these lines, with emphasis on life- or limb-threatening injuries such as cardiac arrest, airway problems, childbirth, hemorrhage control, fracture immobilization, and seizures. Additional training includes defensive driving, utilization of communication systems, ethics, laws, and report writing.

Emergency Medical Technician-Intermediate

The EMT-I has been trained to the level of an EMT-B, frequently has 1 or 2 years' experience on the streets functioning as an EMT-B, and takes approximately 200 hours of additional education, which includes intravenous fluid administration, advanced airway management, and, in some states, limited use of drugs.

Emergency Medical Technician-Paramedic

The EMT-P is trained with an increased emphasis on utilization of drugs for pain control, airway assistance (rapid sequence intubation [RSI], in some systems), seizure and cardiac management, and additional drug usage in specific situations, usually not trauma. The drugs on the unit usually consist of advanced blood pressure cardiac medications, glucose and insulin for the management of diabetic patients, and pain and seizure medication. The

training program to reach the EMT-P level varies from state to state, but it is traditionally in the range of 1,000 to 1,200 hours in addition to the EMT-I. This includes not only didactic lectures but also time in various patient care areas in the hospital, such as the operating room, emergency room, and intensive care unit, and a supervised field internship. At the completion of the training program, the student takes the state examination, the examination of the National Registry of EMTs, or both to obtain a license to function at the Advanced Life Support (ALS) level. Re-registration to maintain this license is required every 2, 3, or 4 years depending on the state. The re-registration depends on sustainment education in trauma cardiac and medical conditions, as well as skill demonstration and practice, such as with intravenous and endotracheal intubation.

A growing number of EMS services throughout the United States are utilizing RSI with drug control for airway management. Research results of the use of RSI in the field have been mixed. Some studies demonstrate effectiveness, some not. Many of those that do not demonstrate effectiveness in the use of an endotracheal tube seem to have problems associated with the actual skill of postintubation management and not the EMT's skill of placing the tube.

Emergency Medical Technician-Paramedic

There is a fourth level of care that is used by some systems in the United States and Canada. A physician responds to almost all ALS runs. The physicians assume control of the situation as soon as they arrive, and the EMS personnel on the scene are the assistants. The physicians provide decision making, primary care, and total control of the scene. This arrangement has not been proven as effective as EMT-Ps working alone in the field in those EMS systems that have been studied.[3–7]

Other systems have a physician riding the streets with a supervisor. This physician provides radio medical control, medical supervision, and education on the scene and adds to the quality assurance process. This type of arrangement has been thought to be effective, especially in the immediate and retrospective medical control. An emergency medicine resident usually responds to scenes on an ad lib basis, and some systems, usually not in the United States, have a physician assigned full time in the ambulance.

Communications

Prehospital communication systems are divided into two major categories. Each has its own purpose, and in most instances the two work on different frequencies. These are (1) dispatch/administrative communications with the

EMS system control and (2) medical communications with the hospital or physician.

In the United States, most of the EMS dispatch is done by an emergency citizen access arrangement using the 9-1-1 phone number. The communication arrangement may be separated into police, fire, and EMS, but some communities combine fire and EMS. Other communities combine law enforcement and EMS. In some communities, especially in rural areas, it is all done with one unit. Other countries have a similar communication system but a different phone number. Regardless of the system used, the function is to receive a phone call from a patient, family member, or a bystander; identify the type of call; dispatch the appropriate vehicle; and provide assistance by telephone to the caller while the ambulance is en route. The ambulance attendants, once on the scene, must survey the scene, identify if additional resources or backup are required, notify the dispatch of such needs, and begin to address patient care.

A medical communication system can be set up utilizing a cell phone or radio connection to a hospital and the medical control physician. Both systems are used by some services. Medical communication has three components: (1) notification of the hospital of the patient's condition and the expected time of arrival; (2) transmission of electronic data that may be beneficial to the hospital either to prepare for the arrival of the patient or to enhance the care of the patient while en route (electrocardiograms are commonly used, but photos have their supporters); and (3) use of a physician or a trained nurse to alter the protocols that have been developed for the EMS system and to provide specific care for a specific patient.

Transmitted electronic data, such as electrocardiograms, have limited usefulness. Training EMTs to read the electrocardiograms and to provide care according to previously developed protocols by the EMS system has been found to be much more effective. This is another example of providing the EMT with knowledge and allowing appropriate decisions to be made in the field.

Most systems now have fairly in-depth guidelines that direct EMT care without the need to contact the hospital for initial orders. Further orders and advanced medical direction can be utilized and are especially helpful with long transport times such as in rural areas or with the use of arrow medical transportation systems.

Protocols Versus Standing Orders

Distinguishing between protocols and standing orders has been difficult because early on these terms where not properly defined. Currently, protocols are defined as guidelines approved by the medical authority overseeing the EMS system, and standing orders are a specific set of care to be provided in specific circumstances.

Medical Control

Emergency medical technicians at all levels work as surrogates of physicians. In most states, they work on the license of the medical director of the EMS service. They are not independent practitioners. The various state licenses do not allow independent nonphysician practitioners to exist within the EMS. Several of the larger EMS systems have tried to make them independent practitioners so that they could carry out a nursing home practice and bill for this care. This has been fought successfully to this point and should be in the future.

Medical control is important for the health and welfare of both the patients and the EMS system. Medical control occurs at three different times[8,9]:

Prospective: initial development of the EMS system and needed modifications as the system matures and medical knowledge improves

Immediate (while the EMTs are in the field caring for the patients): direct (on-line) medical control

Retrospective: quality assurance, discipline, education, or indirect (off-line) medical control

Direct Medical Control (On Line)

Direct medical control is a function of a physician or designee answering the radio and talking directly to the EMTs in the field. The EMTs explain the situation, the scene, the condition of the patient, the scene care provided, and the care to be provided en route and ask for further direction in the management of the patient if required. Further direction can range from bringing the patient to the hospital as quickly as possible to administering specific drugs or procedures that should be administered for the health of the patient either before transport or while the patient is being transported.

Indirect Medical Control (Off Line)

Indirect medical control is retrospective analysis of the individual's run reports and analysis of statistics gained from compiling various data points from the field (which may include response times, time on the scene, skills, attempted skills completed successfully, time to complete the skills, drugs used, and, the most difficult of all, assessment of the judgment used by the EMTs in the management of the patient). Such data can be used to change protocols, add or subtract personnel or vehicles, change the ambulance placement strategy, and redesign protocols, sustainment education, and skills practiced. These are examples of things that can be analyzed and changed to improve the outcome of the patient.

Quality Assurance

Detailed quality assurance became a standard in EMS long before it came into universal use in the hospital. In the early 1970s, in many EMS systems each run was reviewed manually by the physician, the training officer, or a nurse in the hospital. The goals were to check the ambulance placement strategy, the skill deterioration of the individual EMT, the need for re-education in assessment and management, and even the attention to detail. One EMS service used it to detect the EMTs' abilities to function with long duty hours. (This was something started in EMS long before it became a consideration in the work week of the physician resident in training.) As EMS services became busier and computer technology became available, analyses were done by scanning the run reports and watching for trends as well as the response of the individual EMT.

Kinematics (Mechanism of Injury)

Critical in understanding the potential of injury in a patient is the mechanism of injury. Upwards of 95% of injuries can be anticipated before even examining the patient by understanding the energy exchange on the human body at the time of impact. These are based on some very simple laws of energy and motion:

1. Body at rest or body in motion will remain in that state until acted on by some outside force.
2. Energy can be neither created nor destroyed, but it can be changed in form.
3. Mass × acceleration = force = mass × deceleration.
4. Kinetic energy = mass/2 × velocity^2

Cavitation

Many games that we play are based on the physics principle of energy exchange from one object to a cluster of other objects. The cluster is broken apart. The game of bowling is a classic example. The bowling ball is rolled down the hardwood floor aimed at a rack of pins in the middle of the lane. The energy given to the ball by the bowler breaks the rack apart. Pool is a similar game in which a force of muscle motion of the arm is applied through the cue stick to the cue ball. The ball goes down the table to the rack of balls at the other end and exchanges the energy into the rack of balls, which is broken apart. A similar force on the human body occurs when the energy from the explosion that occurred inside the barrel of a gun drives the bullet al.ong the length of the muzzle and into tissue of the human body. The energy of the explosion is transmitted into the bullet, which in turn transmits the energy into the tissues of the body and

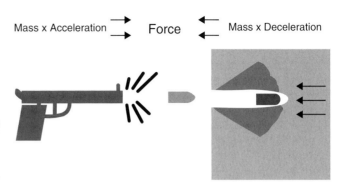

FIGURE 15.1. The energy created by the explosion of the gunpowder in the muzzle of the weapon drives the bullet outward. When the bullet impacts another object, the entire amount of energy of the original explosion must be absorbed for the bullet to stop. This is Newton's First Law of Motion.

"blows them apart." This creates a cavity. One is temporary, depending on the elastic tissue and is unseen by the examiner, but must be imagined as the patient is assessed. The other is permanent and can be seen or partially seen when the injured patient is assessed.

Energy is neither created nor destroyed, but it can change in form. The energy of the explosion in the weapon was exchanged for motion of the bullet. This was changed to motion of the tissue particles being knocked from their position in an organ or being damaged by the force of the energy exchange. Mass × acceleration = force = mass ×deceleration (Figure 15.1).

The same force occurs when an automobile hits a pedestrian or an occupant of the vehicle hits the inside of the vehicle. The energy of the force is exchanged onto the energy tissue of motion to produce tissue destruction.

The elasticity of the tissues of the human body frequently makes this energy exchange/cavitation/tissue damage difficult to detect on initial examination of the patient.

An analogy is to visualize the side of a steel drum hit with a baseball bat. Examine the dent made in the steel drum by the baseball bat. Take the same baseball bat and swing it with the same force into a roll of foam rubber and examine the foam rubber. There is no cavitation or dent visible, although the hitter knows that such a cavitation was produced at the time of impact. Such are the changes that occur within the human body, particularly when the force is spread out over an area too wide to penetrate the skin (blunt trauma). The cavity is directly away from the movement of the baseball bat (or automobile). The elastic tissue of the body reforms the cavity quickly but not the damage created by the energy exchange.

Because energy can be neither created nor destroyed, but can be changed in form, the exchange of energy from the impacting object to the tissue cells forces these cells away from their usual position or moves anatomic structures away from their attachments. One can appreciate the overall changes produced by the exchange onto the human body and injury to the organs and other structures that are in the direct pathway of the forces. For simplicity's sake and ease of understanding, the forces are divided into blunt and penetrating trauma. The readers should realize, however, that the only difference in these two forces is the penetration of the object into the tissue and the direction of the cavitation. The cavitation is at 90° from the pathway of the bullet but 0° from the pathway of the blunt object.

Blunt Trauma

The energy exchange in blunt trauma has four components: shear, compression (crush), overpressure (paper bag effect), and cavitation. Each, to a greater or lesser extent, is involved in every crash. These are the results of deceleration if the body suddenly stops or acceleration if the body is suddenly put into motion away from the point of impact.

To better understand the forces of blunt trauma, these are divided into motor vehicle crashes (subdivided into automobiles, motorcycles and pedestrians), falls, and blasts.

Vehicular Collisions

Vehicular impacts are further subdivided according to the direction of the forces and the vehicle in which the patient was riding. There are five separate types of collision each of which has its own individual patterns: frontal, lateral, rear, rotational, and rollover.

Frontal

The occupant riding in the vehicle is traveling at a speed produced by the energy created in the engine from the burning of gasoline. When this vehicle strikes an immovable object directly in the front, the vehicle rapidly slows as the bending metal absorbs the energy of the momentum of this speed. If the car stops and the occupant inside the vehicle stops, then all of the energy of the momentum was absorbed by the vehicle or the patient. Figures 15.2 and 15.3 show two types of energy absorption: one locally at the front and the other as energy is absorbed by the frame.

The energy of the motion of the occupant is only absorbed when the energy is dissipated into the stretching of the seatbelt, the impact into the air bag, or, if neither safety device is available, such energy is dissipated into the tissues of the body as the passenger impacts the dashboard or steering column. Generally, the unstrained occupant can follow two pathways: forward into the dash or steering column as the energy of the vehicle is absorbed and stops (1) with the head as the lead point of the human missile, the "up and over" pathway;

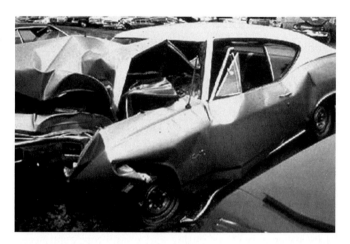

FIGURE 15.2. The energy of the collision is absorbed at the point of impact, but the rest of the vehicle continues to move forward until the remaining energy is absorbed by the ending of the metal in other parts of the car.

or (2) where the knee is the lead point of the human missile into the dash or the floor, the "down and under."

Down and Under. The vehicle stops its forward motion against some immovable object, and the frame or front is bent as it absorbs the energy. The continued forward motion of the occupant's lower torso impacts the knees into the dash (Figure 15.4). The dash stops the forward motion of the knees, but the continued energy of the torso pushes into the upper portion of the lower extremity. This energy is absorbed by dislocation of the knee, fracture along the shaft of the femur, or, if the femur remains intact, the pelvis continues to travel forward with the acetabulum overriding the head of the femur (Figure 15.5). The result is a posterior dislocation at the hip. As the lower half of the torso comes to rest, the upper half of the torso continues forward, bending at the hips

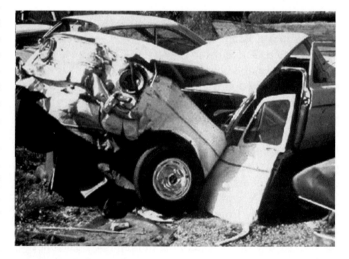

FIGURE 15.3. The entire front of the car is involved in the impact, but the energy of the continued motion of the rear of the car is not absorbed until the body parts bend.

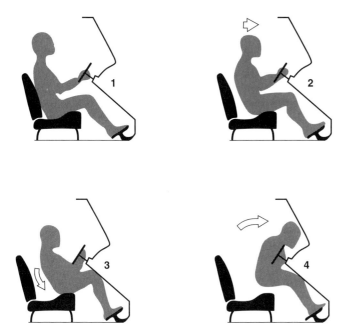

FIGURE 15.4. (1) The occupant and the vehicle are moving forward at the same speed. (2) The vehicle stops, but the occupant continues to move forward. (3) The occupant impacts the front of the passenger compartment first with knees. (4) Then the second rotation occurs: the impact of the torso and head into the steering wheel or windshield.

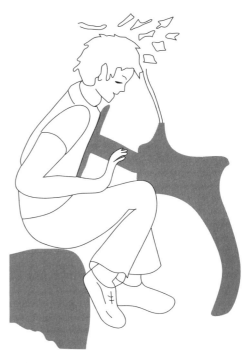

FIGURE 15.6. The movement of external body parts onto the passenger compartment at the time of impact. (Adapted with permission of Elsevier from McSwain et al.[9])

and impacts the dash or the steering column with the patient's head or chest (Figure 15.6).

Up and Over. The chest is the lead point of the human missile. The sternum stops its forward motion against the

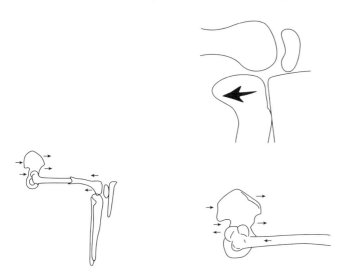

FIGURE 15.5. The energy of the forward motion of the lower extremity is absorbed on the tibia (if that is the only point of impact). The femur overrides and produces a dislocation of the knee. Similarly, if the femur is the point of impact, the energy must be distributed along the shaft of the femur, which either breaks the femur or causes a dislocation at the acetabular pelvic junction. (Adapted with permission of Elsevier from McSwain et al.[9])

steering column, but the continued motion of the posterior thoracic wall from behind bends and eventually fractures the ribs, crushes the lungs between the forward motion of the posterior thoracic wall and the anterior components of the ribs and/or sternum, or compresses the heart between the vertebral column and the sternum. Refer to Figure 15.2 as an illustration of energy absorption to the chest and rib cage (see also Figure 15.7).

If the energy forces are such that the head becomes the lead point of the human missile impacting into the "A" pillow, the wind screen, or the roof of the car, the anterior part of the skull stops its forward motion, but the continued motion of the skull fractures the area of the impact. The continued energy forces produce compression, crush, or lacerations of the brain matter itself.

The brain is not attached to the inside of the skull, but floats in the cerebral spinal fluid. Once the skull stops, the brain continues to move forward until the energy is absorbed by compression and laceration of the brain. This tears the vessels loose posteriorly and pulls the brain away from the spinal cord at the brain stem (Figure 15.8). Parts of the fractured skull may stick into the brain tissue itself.

Once the head has stopped its forward motion, the continued force of the torso from behind distributes energy onto the unprotected cervical vertebrae, producing compression, hyperextension, or hyperflexion injuries (Figure 15.9). Such injuries to the cervical spine can lead to spinal cord damage at the time of impact or are

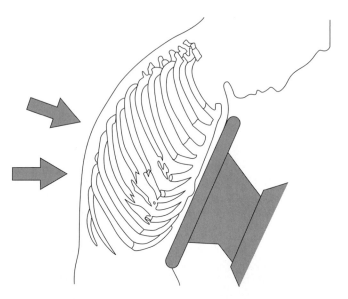

FIGURE 15.7. The impact of the sternum into the steering column stops the sternum, but the posterior thoracic wall continues in forward motion until the energy is absorbed by breaking of the ribs, cardiac compression, or pulmonary compression. (Adapted with permission of Elsevier from McSwain et al.[9])

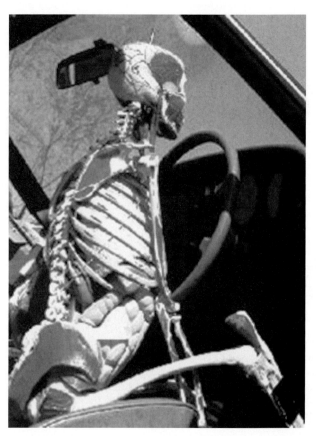

FIGURE 15.9. The head stops its forward motion against the windshield, but the continued forward motion of the torso is absorbed onto the relatively unprotected cervical spine.

unstable, which can lead to further injury to the patient en route to the hospital or in the hospital. Therefore, the entire spine must be appropriately protected on a backboard and in a cervical collar.

Concomitant energy exchange can occur in the chest and abdomen. The anterior chest stops abruptly against the steering column. The posterior chest wall only stops when its energy of forward motion has been absorbed. This energy absorption is onto the ribs, resulting in lateral fractures, compression of the lung (pulmonary contusion), or compression of the heart. Rapid reduction of the intrathoracic volume and increase in intrathoracic pressure (overpressure; Boyles law) can rupture the lung (like a paper bag hit with the hand) (Figure 15.10), tearing the parenchyma and producing a pneumothorax. Although a

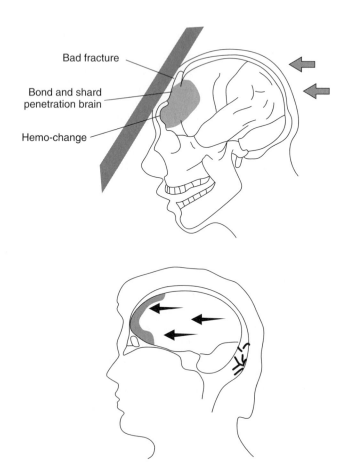

FIGURE 15.8. The brain and skull move forward at the same time. If the skull stops its forward motion, the brain continues its forward motion until the front of the brain is contused and the back of the brain is separated from the skull, resulting in hemorrhage. (Adapted with permission of Elsevier from National Association of Emergency Medical Technicians. KITES: Basic and Advanced Prehospital Trauma Life Support, 5th ed. Philadelphia: Mosby, 2003.)

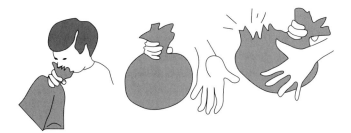

FIGURE 15.10. Impact of the thoracic cavity and lung with compression on the posterior thoracic wall is similar to blowing up a paper bag and hitting it with a hand. The paper bag pops. The lung does the same. (Adapted with permission of Elsevier from McSwain et al.[9])

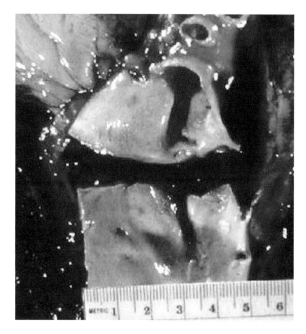

FIGURE 15.12. A tear of the thoracic aorta secondary to sheer injury and blunt trauma. (Reprinted with permission of Elsevier from McSwain et al.[9])

sharp edge of the fractured rib can lacerate the lung, the paper bag effect is more common.

The heart and arch of the aorta are not firmly attached to the chest wall, but the descending aorta is. The heart and arch can decelerate at a different rate from the descending aorta (Figure 15.11). This produces shear forces at the junction of the arch and the descending aorta. The shear results in tears of the aorta at that point. If the rupture extends in to the thoracic cavity, immediate exsanguination results (Figure 15.12). However, in 20% or so of the situations, the blood is contained within the adventitia surrounding the aorta as a pseudoaneurysm (Figure 15.13).

The abdomen is an organ cavity similar to the thorax. The organs can be subject to compression from the continued motion of the posterior abdominal wall (crush of the liver, spleen, pancreas, or kidney), shear to the vascular attachments of the solid organs during deceleration (spleen and kidney), shear of the liver around the ligamentum teres (especially in the down and under pathway), or overpressure to the abdominal cavity (diaphragmatic rupture into either the left or the right pleural cavity).

As a starting point to estimate the energy potential of the crash, a description of the damage to the vehicle by the EMTs to the emergency department personnel gives the ETS a visual picture of what happened to the patient as the initial energy exchange happened. The same type of damage happens to the patient as happens to the vehicle. Examination of the vehicle reveals the direction of impact into it and the amount of force involved in a crash. This information can be translated as the amount and direction of the energy that is exchanged between the reduced speed of the vehicle and the continued motion of the occupant.

Lateral

Lateral impact collisions are frequently the result of an intersection (T-bone) crash (Figure 15.14). This actually

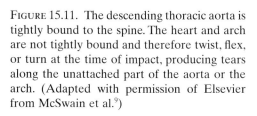

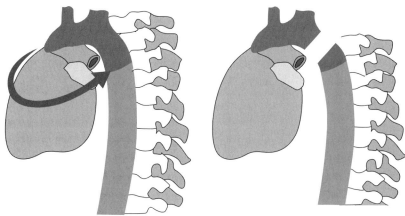

FIGURE 15.11. The descending thoracic aorta is tightly bound to the spine. The heart and arch are not tightly bound and therefore twist, flex, or turn at the time of impact, producing tears along the unattached part of the aorta or the arch. (Adapted with permission of Elsevier from McSwain et al.[9])

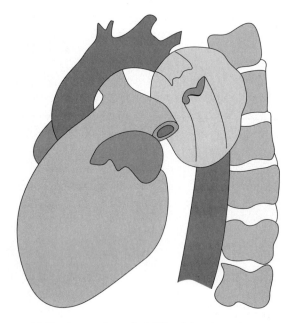

Figure 15.13. Approximately 80% of the thoracic aorta tears result in immediate exsanguination. Approximately 20% produce a pseudoaneurysm, which may remain intact for up to 3 days. (Adapted with permission of Elsevier from McSwain et al.[9])

and pulmonary contusions. The acceleration, in the lateral direction, affects the internal organs by moving those rapidly attached to the torso, particularly the aorta, away from the site of the impact while those unattached organs (the heart and arch) begin motion as they are pulled along by the aorta. The same segment of the aorta is sheared as described above (frontal). Approximately 25% of aortic sheer injuries occur in lateral impact collisions. Approximately 75% occur as a result of frontal collisions.

- The shoulder can be involved in this part of the lateral impact as well. A clavicle fracture can result.

Although there is not direct contact between the head and the vehicle itself, the acceleration of the torso laterally happens first, with the head being pulled along afterwards. The center of gravity of the head is anterior and superior to the cervical spine; therefore, this motion causes rotation of the head toward the impact and lateral flexion of the neck in the same direction. The effect is opening of the facets on the contralateral side of the spine and rotation of the upper vertebra as the head turns. Dislocations, lateral compressing fractures, and jumped facets result.

results in two types of collision patterns. One vehicle is involved in a lateral impact collision, the other in a frontal collision. A careful history obtained from the EMS personnel will allow the examining physician to identify which vehicles were involved and which impact and therefore be able to appropriately assess the individual patients.

At the time of the collision, the occupants in the target vehicle are usually traveling in a forward direction. The bullet vehicle impacts the target vehicle from the side. This energy exchange accelerates the target vehicle in the direction of the impact and away from the bullet vehicle. The unrestrained occupants remain in the forward motion until impacted by the interior of their own vehicle. This initially crushes the side of the patient at the impact point, then rapidly accelerates the patient away from the point of the impact. The occupant on the near side receives more energy than the far side as the door and "B" pillows come into direct contact with the occupant. This contact and acceleration to lateral motion initially affects three parts of the body:

- Impact on the femur tends to push the femoral head into and through the acetabulum. As the force continues, the door contacts the pelvis proper.
- The second point of impact is the lateral chest wall or the shoulder or both. This compression fractures ribs (flail chest), contuses the lung in the chest, and crushes the liver or spleen, depending on the site of the impact

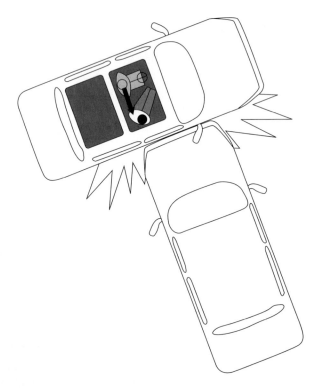

Figure 15.14. A lateral impact collision moves the target car away from the point of impact. The occupants inside the passenger compartment move only when they are impacted by the side of the compartment. (Adapted with permission of Elsevier from McSwain et al.[9])

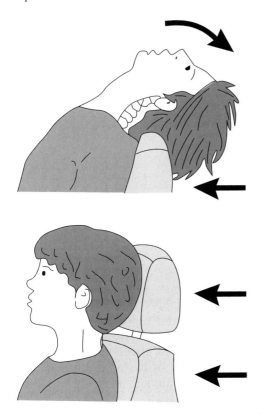

FIGURE 15.15. Hyperextension of the head is prevented in rear impact collisions if the head restraint is in its proper position to contact the occiput at the time of impact. Improperly positioned head restraints allow hyperextension and muscular injury to the neck. (Adapted with permission of Elsevier from McSwain et al.[9])

Because the acceleration forces are in line with the body posterior to anterior, except as noted above with spinal injuries, the injuries to the occupant at the initial impact are minimal. Much force is absorbed by the springs. Additional injuries can occur if there is a second collision with the target vehicle being pushed forward into another target vehicle, and the collision suddenly becomes frontal.

Rotational

If the initial impact is off center, that part of the vehicle stops forward motion while the rest of the vehicle continues in forward motion. This puts the current rotation around this pivot point, and therefore the occupants can receive collisions of frontal or lateral or both.

Rollover

In a rollover collision, the unbelted occupant flies freely throughout the passenger compartment and impacts all aspects of the vehicle. The patterns associated with these injuries are extremely difficult to predict.

Falls

The "g" force on earth is 32 feet per second per second. Speed significantly increases over time and distance. The greater the distance, the more energy the potential patient has when suddenly stopped at the bottom of the fall. The initial impact is on that part of the body that makes contact first, but there is continued energy/motion of those other components that have not stopped their fall. The old adage of "in a fall one breaks his S" is very true. The energy compresses the concavity of the S and stretches the convexity. The neck of the femur, posterior lumbar spine, anterior thoracic spine, and posterior cervical spines are all aligned to encounter this energy exchange. Compression fractures such as the talus into the tibia, the calcaneus itself, the shaft of the femur, and tibia are vulnerable. Deceleration/sheer injuries will occur to the kidneys, spleen, liver, and arch of the aorta.

These are all the kinds of injuries that one would expect if the patient lands on his or her feet. The multiple other directions and the energy exchange in them can be figured out.

Motorcycle Collisions

Three different types of collisions are associated with motorcycle crashes: ejection or partial ejection of the biker and hitting another object or the road (Figure 15.16); body pinned between the motorcycle tank/engine and the another object (Figure 15.17) (legs, pelvis, chest, and unprotected skull and underlying brain); and "lying the bike down" (Figure 15.18) to prevent impact with

Rear

The target vehicle is stopped or moving at a significantly slower rate than the bullet vehicle as the contact between the two vehicles transpires. The bullet vehicle imparts a significant amount of its energy differential to the target vehicle. This accelerates the target vehicle and all components inside the car that are attached to the car. Those components not tied to the car (which includes the occupants) start to move forward only as the parts of the vehicle such as the seats add force to them. Some of the energy is absorbed in the springs of the seat. Those portions of the occupant that touch the seat are accelerated almost simultaneously with the vehicle (Figure 15.15).

Those body parts not touching the seat (for example, the head when the head rest is in the down position) are only accelerated as they are pulled along by their attachments to the body. Only if the acceleration force reaches or exceeds 15 g's is the energy exchange at a high enough level to cause significant damage to the occupant. When the energy exchange is below 15 g's, the acceleration of the thorax out from under the head produces only ligaments or muscle strain and spasm.

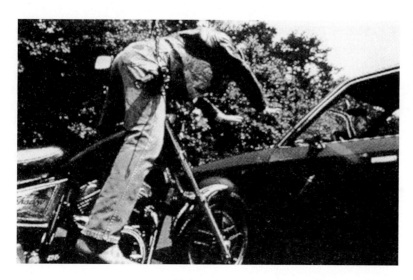

FIGURE 15.16. In a bicycle impact, the bike stops its forward motion, and, on impact, the occupant continues forward, impacting the legs into the handlebar or ejecting the occupant completely from the vehicle. (Reprinted with permission of Elsevier from McSwain et al.[9])

another object, but sliding on the road and losing skin and other tissue during the slide.

Blast Force

Blast injuries are a result of three separate mechanisms: The primary zone, overpressure injuries; secondary zone, flying particles and debris; tertiary zone, the victim becomes a missile (Figure 15.19).

Penetrating Trauma

Energy

Penetrating trauma is a result of the energy exchange onto the human body covering a small enough surface area that the skin itself is penetrated. The deeper the penetration, the more damage will occur.

In blunt trauma, the energy exchange to the body produces compression forces from the initial impact and organ sheer at their point of attachments from the acceleration or deceleration of the tissue. In penetrating trauma, only the compression forces are involved, these from the direct impact to the missile and from the cavitation that surrounds it. How much energy exchange occurs onto the human body to produce injury is a result of the direct impact of the penetrating object onto the human tissue. The amount of energy varies according to the number of tissue particles hit. The *size of the frontal area* of the penetrating object and the *density* of the tissue impacted determines the number of tissue particles hit and therefore the amount of energy exchange that occurs.

Density of body tissue is a continuum but can simplistically be divided into three categories: air density, soft (water) tissue density, and bone density. The least amount of energy exchange would occur when the bullet impacts an object with a lot of air, such as the lung. The most amount of energy exchange would occur when the bullet impacts a very dense tissue, such as bone. Soft tissue density (water density) is in between.

The size of the frontal area of impact depends on three variables of the bullet itself. The spin imparted to the

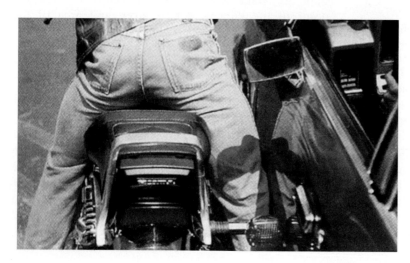

FIGURE 15.17. Off-center impacts tend to center the motorcycle into the vehicle, and the leg is trapped between the two, producing injuries. (Reprinted with permission of Elsevier from McSwain et al.[9])

FIGURE 15.18. To protect themselves from hitting the car, motorcyclists will frequently lay the bike down. (Reprinted with permission of Elsevier from McSwain et al.[9])

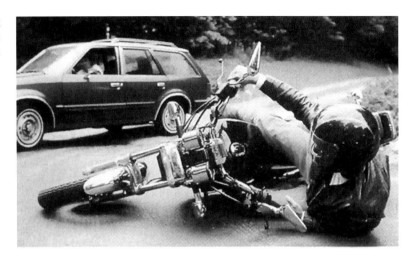

bullet as it comes out of the barrel and the shape of the bullet are constructed in such a manner so that the bullet flies aerodynamically as straight as possible passing through the air. The least amount of air resistance during travel to the target is beneficial. To get the greatest crush effect, a rapid increase in resistance (therefore large exchange of energy) immediately on impacting the target is desired.

These variables are used to increase the frontal surface area of the bullet:

1. *Profile modification* can occur, such as a hollow point bullet that expands and spreads (mushrooms) on impact.
2. *Tumbling* of the bullet rotates to present a broad side. At the 90° point of this rotation there is the greatest exchange of energy.
3. *Fragmentation* can occur either as the missile is leaving the muzzle, such as a shotgun, or after impact. Some bullets are made to actually explode after the bullet enters the tissue.

The two factors that influence the severity of the injury from a penetrating object are the amount of energy exchange that occurs and the organs on which that energy exchange is a result. The amount of energy exchange can be grossly estimated before the patient is examined in the operating room by dividing penetrating objects into three groups based on energy:

1. Low energy would be a knife that creates no temporary cavity and only lacerates tissue.
2. A medium-energy weapon is generally a handgun with a muzzle velocity of approximately less than 1,000 feet per second, which creates a temporary cavity approximately five to seven times the diameter of the missile.
3. A high-energy weapon is one of high velocity, which is greater than 2,000 feet per second, and can create a temporary cavity as much as 20 times the diameter of the missile.

Anatomy

In attempting to identify those organs that are injured, determining the probable pathway through the body is helpful. This can be established if one can identify the wound of entrance and the wound of exit. In most cases (but not all), this is fairly straightforward and follows an easy diagnostic trail. In some cases, it is more difficult. A wound of entry will be oval or round in shape as it punches through the skin against a firm back support of muscle and fat, like pushing a biscuit cutter through biscuit dough. Additionally, the spinning of the bullet as it goes into the tissue will abrade the outside of the skin

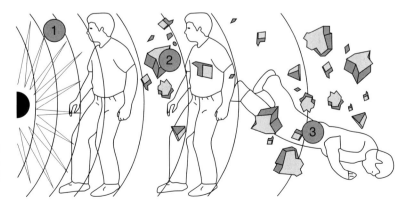

FIGURE 15.19. There are three components to the blast injury: pressure and heat; debris; and projection of the victim. (Adapted with permission of Elsevier from McSwain et al.[9])

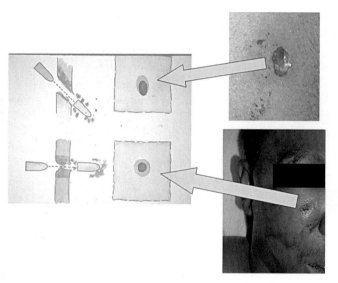

FIGURE 15.20. Angle versus direct impact.

that it has pushed in front of it. This will create a round hole with a pink rim.

If the bullet enters at an angle and produces an ovoid wound, then the side of the wound with the most abrasion will be the entry. The side with the least abrasion (or none) will be the travel side through the body (Figure 15.20).

The wound of exit, because it has no backing, will be blown apart. The wound has no discrete shape. It may well be stellate with several fragments. There will be no abraded rim, because this is under the skin, not on the surface (Figure 15.21).*

---

*For more detailed information, please see National Association of Emergency Medical Technicians. PHTLS: Basic and Advanced Prehospital Trauma. Life Support Revised Reprint, 5th ed. Philadelphia: CV Mosby, 2003.

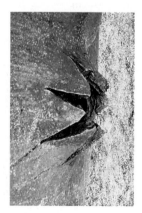
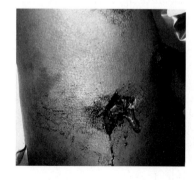

FIGURE 15.21. Exit wound.

Assessment and Management in the Field

Assessment in the field is composed of two separate steps: assessment of the scene (safety and situation) and assessment of the patient. Safety comes first.

Safety

A rescuer provides no benefit to the patient if he or she gets injured. In fact, this complicates the state of affairs by adding to the number of people needed to be cared for and reducing the number of caregivers at the scene. Therefore, selfish though it may seem, the safety of the rescuers is paramount.

The next component of safety is that of the patients. Identify hazards in the area: chemical, weather, perpetrator of the incident, unruly bystanders, fire, and so forth. Questions always to be asked by the EMS team of themselves, other professionals on the scene, and bystanders include the following: Are there any biological or chemical hazards in the area? Is there an unknown liquid on the ground? Is there an unusual cloud or smell in the air? Is there gasoline on the ground? Is there a fire risk? Is the patient's car in a precarious situation? Is the scene secure from the perpetrators of the incident? Is law enforcement needed?

Situation

Assessing the situation includes evaluating the condition of the patients and asking the following questions: What is the mechanism of injury? How many patients are there? Does the number of patients or the conditions exceed the resources available? What is the situation? What is the cause of the collision? What are the potential injuries that can be anticipated from the mechanism of injury? Is there anyone on the scene who can provide information about the situation, about any of the patients, or about additional patients who are not visible?

Initial Patient Assessment

There are many similarities between the initial assessment on the scene and the initial assessment in the emergency department. In fact, the ATLS pattern of the initial assessment was based on a similar system used by EMS. The basic goal on the scene is also similar to the basic goal of the initial assessment in the emergency department. What is wrong with the patient, and what steps are necessary to be able to transport the patient to the next level of care? In the emergency department, the next level of patient care is generally the operating room, the intensive care unit, or advanced diagnostic methods.

On the scene, the next level care is the emergency department.

Just as wasting time in the emergency department delays moving the patient rapidly to that next level is important, so it is on the scene, except perhaps more so. Almost never is the field the best place to assess or to care for the trauma patient. The patient should be moved into the ambulance as quickly and as safely as possible, and the ambulance should be en route to the emergency department quickly, while following the dictum of "*do no further harm.*"

"Do no further harm" includes sins of *omission* as well as sins of *commission*. To move the patient quickly without ensuring that the airway is open, that the patient is breathing, and that the patient has cardiac output or without stabilizing the fractures is a sin of omission. Starting unnecessary intravenous lines; doing the secondary survey in the field when the patient is crashing; and performing unnecessary diagnostic tests such as otoscopic evaluations, osculation of the abdomen, cervical spine clearance, and ultrasound are examples of sins of commission. These do further harm to the patient and should not be a part of field care. It is the ETS' responsibility through education and quality assurance to make certain that these sins are not committed.

The components of the initial assessment (primary survey, resuscitation, secondary survey, definitive care) are present in the field just as they are in the emergency department. The methods and the extent to which they are used are different, however, in two major respects:

1. For the severely injured patient with hemodynamic instability, the secondary survey may never be completed. The intent of the prehospital provider should be devoted to managing life- and limb-threatening conditions while transporting the patient to the hospital. Other, less severe conditions can wait.

2. The equipment used, the skills, and the process of patient care are extremely different when carried on outside in the rain, snow, with a large crowd of people around, when a patient is trapped in the vehicle, or when the perpetrator of the crime may still be in the area than when in the warm, dry, controlled environment of the emergency room or the operating room.

Primary Survey

As part of the scene size-up and the primary survey, the general impression of the patient is obtained immediately upon acquiring visual contact with him or her. The first few seconds when the EMT sees the patient lying in a ditch, lying in the street with a motorcycle 30 feet away, leaning over the steering wheel without the deployed air bag, or lying in the street with blood coming from the chest and clothes soaked with blood provides a general impression of what is going on and aims the prehospital care provider in a general direction toward what needs to be quickly accomplished before initiation of transport.

Efficiency in the field is critically important if the patient is to be moved to the hospital safely and rapidly. That initial general impression must identify what is wrong with the patients, what it will take to get them stabilized before loading them in the ambulance, and what care would need to be provided en route to the hospital. Also important is the assessment of which patients are the most severely injured and which will require attention first. The rate of the patients' ventilations, whether they are talking, how intact the mental process is when they are asked to describe "what happened," and what the patient says when asked "where are you hurt" solidify the general impression as to whether this is an immediately critical condition that requires rapid evacuation or whether attention be placed on other components of the scene.

The objective of the field primary survey is to identify the severity of the patients' injuries so that they can be delivered to the correct hospital and so that the injuries that will not continue to do harm to the patient (such as a fractured femur) are appropriately managed in the field and during transportation.

The general impression of the patient includes those important medical factors that must also be gathered in the emergency room; the prehospital provider must make an early decision of the condition of the patient and the need to transport to a trauma center. Will a helicopter be required? Is extrication going to be a problem? Is a patient in extremis so that the rapid extrication maneuver should be utilized to get the patient out of the car quickly without taking time for backboard stabilization of the cervical spine? Can this patient be handled with basic life support alone or will ALS be required? How far away is ALS? Should there be an ALS intercept en route to the hospital? What are the impediments to keeping prehospital scene time as short as possible?

The same ABCs that are addressed in the emergency room are also addressed in the primary assessment in the field. Airway management must take into consideration the possibility of a cervical spine fracture. However, when the EMT arrives on the scene, the initial decision as to the possibility of a cervical spine injury must be made. The patient is not in a cervical collar or on a long board (like when they arrive in the emergency room) to alert the EMT that there is a possibility of a cervical spine fracture. This must be ferreted out by looking at the mechanism of injury, the injuries of the patient, the condition of the patient, and other factors. The second question that needs to be answered is what kind of cervical spine immobilization is required immediately? Is this one hand on each side of the head with the forearms on the clavicles to provide stabilization while someone secures the airway? Is this a situation where a cervical spine injury is likely?

A: Airway

Airway management is different when the patient is trapped in a car versus on a stretcher in the emergency room. For patients lying on the ground, there is not enough time to move the patient to the stretcher; therefore, intubation must be accomplished "where they lie."

The airway can be managed in the field as in the hospital by manual, mechanical, or transtracheal methods. These are discussed in the special skills section. As an example of how the management is different in the field than in the emergency department, the problems intubating a patient while lying on the ground are discussed later. Add to this, cold, rain, dark, and gawking bystanders.

There are several positions for the EMT to achieve this intubation. The two preferred by the author are described here. Both are accomplished while one EMT kneels beside the patient's chest with the palms of his or her hands over the patient's ears, forearms resting on the patient's clavicle so that the head and neck are stabilized in line, while the operator doing the intubation elevates the mandible alone with the laryngoscope (Figure 15.22). The EMT can position himself or herself lying flat on the ground with the elbow of the left hand planted on the ground beside the patient's left ear and elevating the mandible to visualize the larynx using wrist action alone.

In the second technique position, the operator positions himself or herself with the patient's head (and the hand and palms of the EMT supporting the cervical spine) between his or her legs. The operator clamps the inner thighs around the head of the patient, and the feet are placed on either side of the chest so that the knees are bent over the shoulders. After placing the laryngo-

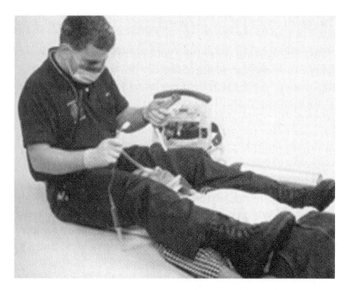

FIGURE 15.23. Sitting intubation. (Reprinted with permission of Elsevier from McSwain et al.[9])

scope in the patient's mouth, the operator leans back at approximately a 45° angle. This gives him or her direct vision into the larynx. The endotracheal tube can be quickly inserted (Figure 15.23).

Once the endotracheal tube is in place, the correct placement is assessed. Techniques available to verify intubation are divided into two groups: clinical assessment and adjunctive devices.[10]

Clinical assessment includes

1. Direct visualization of the tube passing through the cords
2. Presence of bilateral breast sounds and absence of air sounds over the epigastrium
3. Visualization of chest rising or falling during ventilation
4. Fogging (vapor condensation in the endotracheal tube)

Adjunctive devices include

1. Esophageal detector device
2. Carbon dioxide monitoring
3. Color-metric carbon dioxide detector
4. Endotracheal carbon dioxide monitoring (capnography)
5. Pulse oximetry

None of these methods is 100% accurate. Therefore, all of the clinical assessment methods should be used unless impractical. In addition, at least one (preferably two) of the adjunctive techniques should be added.[11,12]

Once the tube is in place and secured, then the attention of the operator should be directed at immobilizing the cervical spine with a long backboard and hard collar

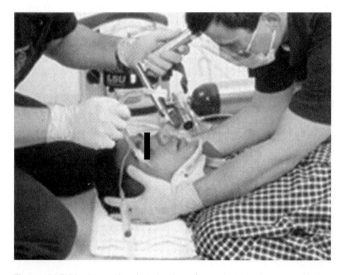

FIGURE 15.22. Kneeling intubation. (Reprinted with permission of Elsevier from McSwain et al.[9])

while the spinal immobilization is being maintained by the other EMT. It has been fairly well documented that lateral rotation of the head and anterior/posterior extension and flexion of the head can move the tip of the endotracheal tube 1 to 2 cm. One to two tip movements can easily pull the endotracheal tube out of the trachea and allow it to reposition itself into the esophagus. Any time the patient is moved, verification of the position of the endotracheal tube must be repeated. These movements are placing the patient on the backboard, placing the backboard on the stretcher, placing the stretcher in the ambulance, removing the patient from the ambulance at the hospital, and moving the patient from the stretcher to the emergency room resuscitation gurney.

Various studies have indicated that the successful field intubation rate was between 80% and 90%. Therefore, the EMT must be skilled in backup techniques for airway management. These include retrograde intubation, digital intubation, laryngeal mask airway, intubating laryngeal mask airway, percutaneous transtracheal ventilation, or a surgical airway. The skills learned to perform any of these and other techniques tend to deteriorate rapidly. A well-accepted study[13] has indicated that skills can deteriorate in as little as 6 months. Close monitoring of the EMT's success rate, field observation of the EMT, and sustainment skill retraining are mandatory to preserve the efficiency and quality of patient care in the field. This is especially true for skills that are not required on a frequent basis. Even in a busy urban EMS system, EMTs may use surgical airway techniques only once or twice every 5 to 10 years. Maintaining these skills can be time consuming and laborious for the training division of the EMS service.

B: Breathing and Ventilation

The first step in ensuring that red cells are adequately oxygenated to deliver the oxygen to the tissue cells is an open airway. The second step it to ensure adequate volume expansion of the lungs. Traumatic conditions that interfere would be physical limitation of expansion (pneumothorax), reduced expansion of the chest cavity (rib pain), or reduced neurologic drive (high spinal fracture, brain injury, or alcohol or drug excess).

Bag valve mask (BVM) ventilation is the standby for the severely injured immediately and if the patient cannot be intubated. Some studies have shown that the outcome using BVM ventilation and endotracheal intubation is the same. Unfortunately, none of these studies has been done in a randomized fashion. Most are retrospective or prospective with historical controls.

The ventilation rate tends to be much faster than required in the urgency of an emergency situation when the EMT must multitask to get the patient packaged, properly placed in the ambulance, and moved to the hospital in the back of a bumpy ambulance that swerves around curves. It has been recognized for some time by anecdotal reports, personal experience, isolated observation, and recent reports that intubated patients are ventilated at a much higher frequency than is required. There are implications that such hyperventilation was the cause of an increased mortality following head injury when drug-assisted intubation was used.

While en route to the hospital, the lone EMT in the patient compartment—the other EMT is driving—must maintain proper position of the mandible and tongue in order to achieve BVM ventilation, reassess vital signs, monitor intravenous administration rate, observe for hemorrhage, and attempt secondary survey while strapped in the seat at the head of the patient. For all of the above reasons, many of the EMTs do not use restraint systems while in the back of an ambulance, therefore increasing their own hazard during violent motions and increasing the chance of moving the endotracheal tube or even pulling it out.

Another difficulty associated with ventilation in the field is maintaining an open airway and holding the mask on with one hand while squeezing the bag with the other while on the scene, in the back of an ambulance, or in the emergency department. Studies have shown that use of both hands on the bag and someone else holding the mask in place is the ideal. Unfortunately, most EMS services operating in the United States do not have the luxury of more than two trained EMS individuals in an ambulance.

Assessment of correct ventilation is best achieved by pulse oximetry and capnography in the field as well as in the emergency department. However, such devices are expensive and difficult to maintain in the environment of an ambulance: heat, cold, rain, snow, dust, dirt, and rough handling are all factors. Most EMS services in the United States are underfunded, and therefore expensive adjunctive devices are not in use. The major factor that the EMT must depend on is clinical observation. The ideals of someone holding a pulse oximeter on the patient's finger during the rough ride to the hospital or applying a sticky pulse oximeter of operating quality are expensive, difficult to achieve in the rain or snow or blood of an emergency scene situation, and require time and additional hands. These oximeters are generally not available in the back of an ambulance. The same is true for capnography, which requires an additional device that must be secured to the stretcher or to the patient during transportation, loading and unloading from the ambulance, and moving into the emergency department.

Thoracic injury adds to the potential ventilation difficulty. The major problems encountered that will affect patient ventilation management include pneumothorax, pulmonary contusion, flail chest (multiple rib fractures), and hemothorax.

Hemothorax includes the additional complication of vascular volume redaction while limiting the expansion of the lungs to properly oxygenate the patient. This is not an easily identified or easily treated condition in the prehospital period. It is only mentioned to acknowledge its existence and not to recommend a method of treatment.

Generally, the EMT has only two clinical skills to assist in the assessment of adequate pulmonary excursion: stethoscope and pulmonary compliance. In the field and during transportation, the high noise level may make the stethoscope a difficult instrument to use accurately. Similarly, pulmonary compliance is extremely subjective and requires frequent experience with abnormal conditions to maintain this assessment skill.

C: Cardiac Evaluation

From the perspective of a prehospital care provider, cardiac arrest in the trauma patient usually indicates a nonsurvivable trauma condition secondary to exsanguination. The American College of Surgeons/Committee on Trauma (ACS/COT) and the National Association of EMS Physicians (NAEMSP) have developed a position paper outlining when and when not to initiate cardiopulmonary resuscitation (CPR) in the field on a trauma patient 4.[14,15]

The C in the primary resuscitation does not indicate that CPR should be started, but it does recognize the importance of hemodynamic instability as an indication to package and move as rapidly as possible to the trauma center if available. Cardiac evaluation includes pulse slow or fast, delay in capillary refill, and location of pulse. Other factors can be better determined in the secondary assessment or at least during resuscitation.

The more important factors are recognizing the shock-like state, taking steps to address this issue, addressing its etiology (controlling hemorrhage if present), and rapidly transporting the patient to the trauma center so that operative hemorrhage control and blood product replacement can be carried out quickly in the operating room if required. An understanding of the use of the pneumatic antishock garment (PASG) for hemorrhage control, whether intraabdominal or retroperitoneal or pelvic, is important (for long transportation times).[16] The associated benefits in severe shock (pressure less than 60) have been demonstrated in the literature for this device as well.

D: Disability

Although technically disability indicates the need to assess the mental status, the major factor is assessment of the brain as an end-organ for perfusion and oxygenation. A mental status examination at this point is for gross assessment for signs of a head injury, such as unequal pupils and appropriate staging with the Glasgow Coma Score.

Resuscitation

At the completion of the primary survey, the EMS personnel should have decided whether this patient requires immediate transport to the emergency department of a Level I trauma center, if available, or whether the secondary assessment can continue, intravenous lines get started, and each fracture immobilized individually before extrication and revised after extrication.

If extrication is a factor, the decision must be made regarding rapid extrication with only manual protection of the spine or whether the scene situation and patient conditions are such that total immobilization of the patient before extrication should be accomplished. In the latter situation, the general principle of removal of the car from the patient is much more appropriate than removal of the patient from the car. In the former situation, rapid extrication requires removal of the patient from the car.

In the mid-1980s, the process of rapid extrication was developed and taught. This is best done with a minimum of four individuals to immobilize the spine and with team lifting move the patient onto a long backboard where other methods of stabilization of fractures can be accomplished (Figure 15.24). By 2003, however, it had become apparent that, because most EMS systems in the United States did not respond with three or four trained responders, but only with two, a mechanism for two-person rapid extrication needed to be developed. This is demonstrated in Figure 15.25.

This extrication technique has risks and limitations. The cervical spine is not completely and safely immobilized on a short board before being turned and moved to a long board. If the patient is in critical condition, the delay to apply the short board is a risk in itself. The EMTs on the scene must make the decision in the best interest of the patient. Is the risk of extrication with only manual cervical spine immobilization less than the risk of leaving the patient in the vehicle to be a victim of fire, inappropriate airway management, or additional injuries from other sources? The long-held maxim from Hippocrates of "do no further harm" is followed. The EMS personnel should be well trained and experienced in various extrication techniques, as well as adequate methods of assessment of the patient so that appropriate decisions as to type of extrication can be made.

The resuscitation phase of prehospital care is also different from the resuscitation phase in the emergency room. Intravenous fluid administration, for example, is carried out en route to the hospital and not in the field, as this would delay transportation. It is more difficult to start an intravenous line in a crowded moving ambulance

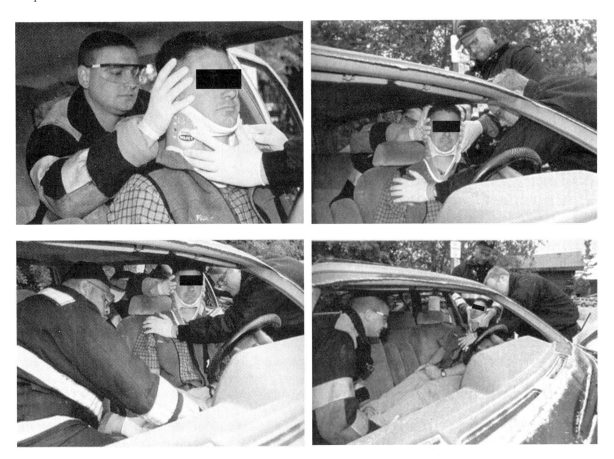

FIGURE 15.24. Rapid extrication. (Reprinted with permission of Elsevier from McSwain et al.[9])

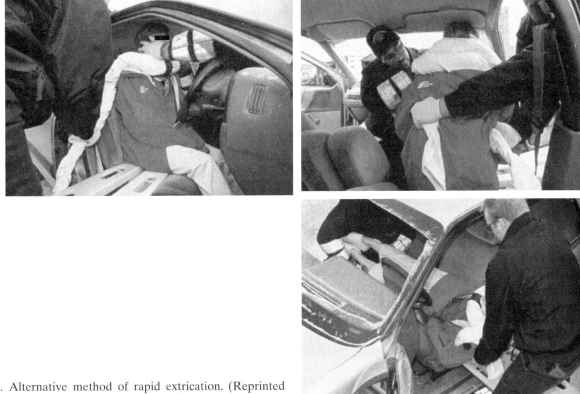

FIGURE 15.25. Alternative method of rapid extrication. (Reprinted with permission of Elsevier from McSwain et al.[9])

compared with in the open emergency room with the stable platform on which the patient is lying.

Based on the individual situation, the road surface and curves in the road, the confines of the back of the ambulance, and the condition of the patient, the EMT must again assess the entire situation and make decisions as to what of the many things that the patient needs has priority. Certainly of significance in these situations is the length of travel time to the hospital. If the scene of the emergency is 4, 5, or 6 minutes away from the hospital, then only certain things can or should be done. On the other hand, if the incident has occurred 30 to 45 minutes away from the hospital, when there is a far greater chance of the patient's deterioration en route, then a different set of priorities will be required.

Secondary Survey

Another difference between the back of an ambulance and the emergency department is removal of all of the patient's clothes to do an adequate secondary survey. Environment, bystanders, and other conditions dictate that the patient's clothes should not be removed before he or she is loaded into the ambulance. While en route the patient must remain stabilized to the backboard and to the roller; therefore, removing the straps to cut the cloths free is difficult and in general not productive to the long-term outcome of the patient (unless severe hemorrhage is present), again preventing a complete secondary assessment. The EMT's assessment is limited to those parts of the body that are freely visible while immobilized.

In most situations, therefore, the secondary survey is not completed before arrival at the hospital. The general principle of mobilization as a unit on the long backboard is frequently the best method of transporting the patient and stabilizing all of the fractures or potential fractures. The EMT, therefore, is not to be criticized for missed injuries, particularly during the short transport. All injuries have been immobilized by the long backboard and managed in the time available. It is just that they have not been individually identified as time, space, and personnel allow to be achieved in the emergency department. This does not imply in any way that life-threatening injuries such as external hemorrhage, airway problems, pneumothorax, and flail chest should not be addressed while providing rapid access to the trauma center or local hospital.

Early ultrasound examinations in the hands of many experienced people in the hospital have an early 30% false-negative rate. The EMS personnel have little imaging experience. Adding such a device would only delay transportation with minimal or even confusing diagnostic information.

Definitive Field Care

Like other steps in the assessment and management of the patient, definitive field care is different from definitive care in the emergency department. Definitive care by the prehospital personnel is appropriate packaging and safe and quick delivery to the emergency department.

Shock and Fluid Resuscitation

Of all the physiologic principles that the prehospital provider needs to grasp, shock is first. The EMS personnel have to make decisions regarding transporting patients to the trauma center (rapid vs. timely), requesting aeromedical scene pick-up, bypassing a local hospital to travel to a more distant trauma center, need for fluid replacement, and managing the patient during long transportation in rural and wilderness areas.

Depending on the educational program used by the individual/local EMS program, there is significant information provided to the EMTs or minimal information provided for the understanding of shock. Much of the inequality comes from trying to make shock a more complex subject than it needs to be for EMS personnel, the instructors themselves not understanding shock, having minimal physician input to the education, or physicians lecturing at a complex rather than a simple level. Additionally, some educational programs are so protocol driven that understanding of this process has no place in their educational scheme. It is incumbent on the ETS who works with EMTs to ensure that their basic foundation in shock is strong.

The primary emphasis should be on the following:

- Interruption of energy production at the cellular level when anaerobic metabolism replaces aerobic metabolism
- Decreased oxygenation of the cells secondary to either lack of oxygenation of the red cells in the lungs or lack of delivery of the red cells to the tissue cells (Fick principle)
- Understanding of the physiology of fluid replacement
- The Bernoulli principle
- Resuscitation of controlled versus uncontrolled hemorrhage

Energy Production

Metabolism produces injury-utilizing oxygen and glucose as fuel with byproducts of carbon dioxide and water. There are two pathways to achieve this: one with and one without oxygen. Aerobic metabolism is the most efficient and produces a larger amount of adenosine triphosphate (ATP) than anaerobic metabolism (38 vs. 2).

Additionally, anaerobic metabolism increases the production of lactic and anaerobic acids with resultant total body acidosis. The increased acid will result in an increased ventilatory rate, which may be the first sign of the beginning of shock. Increasing ventilation frequently precedes an increasing pulse rate and certainly precedes a decreasing blood pressure.

The heart and other components of the cardiovascular system *compensate* for the loss of blood volume and loss of oxygenation (decreased oxygen delivered to the cells) by an increased peripheral vascular resistance, thereby improving blood pressure, and by a rapid heart rate to increase the frequency of red cell passage through the tissue cells. This isolates some body organs from oxygen delivery. As the blood loss continues (uncontrolled hemorrhage), the physiologic systems cannot keep up and blood pressure can no longer be sustained (*uncompensated* shock).

The outcome of a prolonged hypoperfusion will result in impairment of organ function up to and including organ death. Many of the complications that occur result from hypoperfusion and hypo-oxygenation during the first hour that EMS is with the patient. These may not manifest themselves for several hours or days. Examples of this would be cardiac failure, lung failure (adult respiratory distress syndrome), acute renal failure, acute hepatic failure, and immune system failure (sepsis). The more short-term complications are myocardial ischemia and cerebral ischemia (brain edema and brain death). It is the responsibility of the EMT to understand the process of shock, assess these potentials, and provide appropriate management.

Oxygen Delivery

The cardiovascular system has three components: the pump (heart), a container and delivery system (vascular system), and the circulating fluid (blood). Failure of any component of this system can lead to failure of perfusion and therefore decreased oxygen delivery.

In trauma, failure of the heart to pump blood is the result of (1) hypoxia/ischemia of the myocardium secondary to severe blood loss; (2) interference with the pumping system (pericardial tamponade); or (3) rhythm disturbance. Failure of the vascular system occurs when the vessels are maximally constricted to maintain as much of the blood as possible in this initial onset of acute blood loss (hemorrhage) or vasodilatation from neurogenic or sepsis reasons. Sepsis is not generally a component of shock from trauma within the first hour; therefore, this should not be a concern on most EMS runs.

Acute volume loss affects both the red cell mass and the volume needed for delivery. Loss of either the fluid itself (dehydration) or blood cell mass and fluid (hemorrhage) or decreased red cells alone (anemia) can all affect oxygen delivery to the cells. In most emergency and trauma situations, hemorrhage is the etiology. Components of the

Fick principle include (1) oxygenation of the RBCs in the lung, (2) delivery of the oxygenated RBCs to the tissue cells, and (3) off loading of the oxygen to the tissue cells.

Physiology of Fluid Replacement

When determining how and what fluids to use for resuscitation, the ETS must know if the hemorrhage is *controlled* or *uncontrolled*. With controlled hemorrhage, the patient can be resuscitated back to normal hemodynamics without concern. Conversely, with uncontrolled hemorrhage, increasing the blood pressure and flow back to normal can increase the blood loss. With controlled hemorrhage, either large-volume fluid resuscitation or hypertonic saline fluid resuscitation works well.

Resuscitation of the blood volume using fluids alone (such as Ringer's lactate) has two potential negative outcomes:

1. Resuscitation with large volumes of Ringer's lactate when there is little blood dilutes the red cell mass. This reduces the delivery of oxygen to the tissue cells.
2. The return of blood pressure to the normal range may "pop the clot" short term.

In the face of *uncontrolled* hemorrhage, resuscitation should be back to a level of oxygen delivery that hemorrhage is not increased but oxygenation of the tissue is maintained. As of 2004, this "set point" has not been determined.

The short-term use of volume-restricted resuscitation method in one study demonstrated that there was increased mortality rate associated with hemorrhage from the thoracic cavity but no clinically significant changes in hemorrhages from other parts of the body.[17] This study has not been repeated in other EMS systems, so the research has not been substantiated. The ideal setting for restricted fluid protocols is with uncontrolled hemorrhage. However, it is logical to believe that, based on the Bernoulli principle, increasing blood pressure without increasing the tissue pressure will cause greater blood loss, which will lead to decreased perfusion.

Bernoulli Principle

According to the Bernoulli principle:

Rate of leakage ~ Size of the hole × transmural pressure

Transmural pressure = intraluminal pressure/extramural pressure

A decrease in the intramural pressure will decrease the transmural pressure and therefore reduce the rate of leakage out of the hole in the vessel. Conversely, an increase in the intramural pressure will increase the transmural pressure and thereby increase the rate of blood flow out of the hole. This is the theory behind the restricted fluid resuscitation technique.

Compression dressings for hemorrhage control work on the bottom side of the equation. By increasing the extraluminal pressure, the transmural pressure is decreased and the rate of leakage is decreased. Compression dressings of all sorts have been shown to work well, from elastic bandages to pneumatic dressings. (Blood pressure cuffs, pneumatic splints, and PASG are examples.) The damage-control laparotomy and the PASG work in a similar manner for intraabdominal and retroperitoneal hemorrhage. The new pelvic sling mid the PASG work in the same manner on the pelvis.

Assessment

There are a variety of techniques that have been successfully used to quickly assess the level of shock in a trauma patient:

1. Pulse: Three components of the pulse need to be evaluated on initial arrival of EMS personnel:
    a. Rate: Rate will give some initial ideas for patient care. On first contact, determining merely fast or slow is all that is needed. Tachycardia indicates at the very least compensated shock. A very slow pulse (less than 50) would indicate in most people the onset of the bradycardia associated with myocardial ischemia;
    b. Strength: Is it strong or thready?
    c. Location: A radial pulse indicates that there is decent perfusion with the systolic pressure somewhere above 80 to 90 mm Hg; absence of a similar pulse indicates that the pressure is probably below 70 systolic, and absence of carotid pulse indicates that blood pressure is 50 to 60 or below systolic.
2. Skin color: Pink versus cyanotic versus pale.
3. Skin temperature: Cool and clammy versus warm and dry.
4. Capillary refilling time: Less than 2 seconds or greater than 2 seconds.

All of these signs are in themselves not a test of shock but a test of perfusion of that portion of the body wherein they are detected. Perfusion can be a function of interruption of the blood supply proximal to the point of assessment. Hypothermia, vascular trauma, dehydration, or a variety of conditions can reduce the perfusion to the point that all of the above changes.

Blood Pressure

An important sign of shock, however, is that its change is frequently not noted until 30% to 40% of the blood volume has been lost. This is because of strong compensatory systems, described early, that maintain the pres-

sure. Blood pressure can then be divided into three general groups:

1. Normal blood pressure with normal pulse and respiration, skin color capillary refilling, and so forth
2. Normal *compensated* blood pressure but with other signs of decreased perfusion such as tachycardia and decreased capillary refilling time
3. *Uncompensated* shock, in which the body is no longer able to maintain blood pressure using these various compensatory mechanisms and the pressure itself actually starts to drop

Field Special Skills

Airway

Skills of the airway are divided into three groups: manual, mechanical, and transtracheal.

Manual

Manual skills include jaw thrust and jaw lift. These are effective because the tongue is the most common obstruction of the posterior pharynx (particularly when the patient is in the supine position or unconscious) and can be managed simply by moving the mandible forward. Unobstructing the airway can be achieved without moving the cervical spine, thereby protecting this structure from further injury in the airway-compromised patient.

The *jaw thrust* is done standing in front of the patient while the thumbs are placed on the maxilla, the long finger on the angle of the mandible, and scissors closed so that the mandible is thrust forward. When standing behind the head of the patient, the thumbs are similarly placed on the zygoma and the long finger on the angle of the mandible, but the mandible is thrust forward by the long finger.

When using the *jaw lift* on a conscious patient facing the rescuer, the mandible can be grasped with the thumb and index finger in front of and behind the symphysis and pulled forward, or, if the patient is totally unconscious, the thumb can be placed behind the lower incisors and lifted forward.

Mechanical

Four types of mechanical devices are used to sustain the airway once it has been pulled open with either the jaw lift or the jaw thrust. The *nasal airway* can be placed through the nose into the posterior pharynx, or the *oral airway* can be placed in the patient without a gag reflex posterior to the tongue in the posterior pharynx holding the airway open. Both of these techniques are very effec-

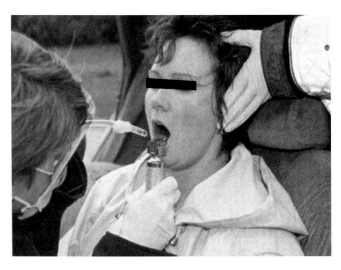

FIGURE 15.26. Face-to-face intubation. (Reprinted with permission of Elsevier from McSwain et al.[9])

tive but do not isolate the esophagus from the trachea. Aspiration may result.

To isolate the trachea from the esophagus, the first choice of airway would be the *endotracheal tube* placed orally. Certain situations occur when the EMT cannot get above the patient's head to place the endotracheal tube. An example is the patient upright in the seat of a car who cannot be moved. The EMT faces the patient, reverses the position of the laryngoscope (blade down, not up), places the blade behind the tongue, pulls the mandible out, visualizes the cords, and places the tube in the trachea. This is face-to-face oral intubation (Figure 15.26).

Spinal immobilization is the first step. The patient's head cannot be put in the sniffing position, which hyperextends the head at C1 and C2 and hyperflexes at C5 and C6, the two most common areas of cervical spine fracture (Figure 15.27). Rather, one rescuer positions himself

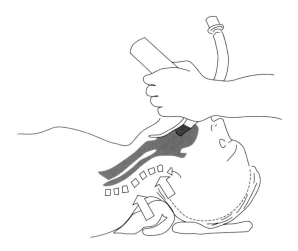

FIGURE 15.27. Intubation in sniffing position.

below the patient placing the palms of the hands directly over the ears with the fingers spread out. This puts the little finger in the occiput and the thumb along the zygoma. The forearms are then braced against the patient's clavicle and chest, which secures the neck into a single unit, preventing movement of any of the seven cervical vertebrae and the first couple of thoracic vertebrae.

Transtracheal

Although there are three methods of transtracheal airway management, the *tracheostomy* is not an emergency procedure either in the hospital or outside of the hospital; therefore, EMTs are not taught this technique. They are taught either percutaneous transtracheal ventilation or surgical cricothyroidotomy.

There is no question that a *percutaneous transtracheal* placement of a large 14- or 12-gauge needle is simpler because the operator does not have to place the device through the cricothyroid membrane but can place it anywhere along the length of the trachea in the neck. One easy method to do this is for the operator to stand on the left side of the patient, stabilizing the trachea and larynx with the thumb and index finger of the left hand. The needle is then placed in the midline, angled down at approximately 45°, and inserted sharply into the trachea. Aspiration through the needle ensures presence in the air passage (Figure 15.28).

Ventilation can be accomplished by connecting an oxygenation administration catheter, which has two female ends, one around the hub of the needle and the other into a 15 L/min oxygen source cutting a hole in the tube of the size to be totally occluded by the thumb. The thumb can occlude the hole for 1 second and open the hole for 4 seconds. This allows ventilation at 12 times per minute, promptly expands the lungs with 100% oxygen, but allows deflation when the catheter is opened. Oxygenation without compromising CO_2 buildup has been accomplished for 45 minutes without difficulty.

A *surgical cricothyrotomy* is accomplished by the operator standing on the right side of the patient, stabilizing the larynx with the left hand, incising the skin and cricothyroid membrane with the right hand, and then using a curve motion, inserting the tracheostomy tube directly into the trachea.

Double Lumen Airway

There are several types of double-lumen tube airways available. Initially the *esophageal obturator airway* (EOA) was used successfully for airway management by prehospital providers in the late 1960s. The EOA was actually a single-lumen tube that was inserted directly into the esophagus and a balloon blown up to occlude in the esophagus. This prevents regurgitation of material

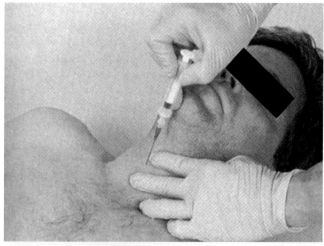

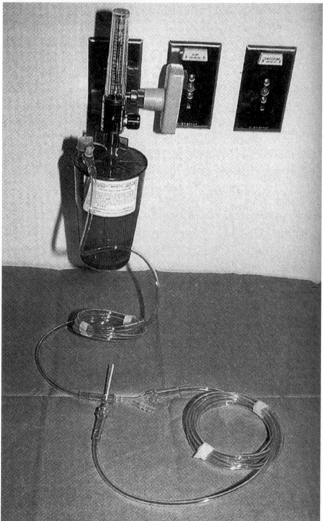

FIGURE 15.28. Percutaneous transtracheal ventilation. (Reprinted with of Elsevier permission from McSwain et al.[9])

into the trachea and allows ventilation to be accomplished with a mask seal in a standard BVM type of ventilation. Other more recent tubes have utilized a double-lumen airway, one of which is inserted blindly into the oropharynx and posterior pharynx. One tube will go into the esophagus and the other will go into the trachea or into the vicinity of the trachea so that whichever tube has the best access to the trachea is used as a ventilation port. The *combitube* and the *pharyngeal tracheal laryngeal* (PTL) airway are examples.

Laryngeal Mask Airways

A more recent tube is the *laryngeal mask airway* (LMA), which is a minimask surrounding the hypopharynx and sealing it off effectively when the balloon around the mask is blown up, again effectively separating the trachea from the esophagus but allowing good positive ventilation. Although this device was developed in Europe, it has rapidly been adopted by anesthesiologists in the United States and is commonly used in the operating room for ventilation.

A modification of this is the *intubating laryngeal mask airway* (ILMA), which allows for the insertion of an endotracheal tube down through the ventilating tube. Because of the positioning of the laryngeal mask, the endotracheal tube is guided directly into the trachea. This mask requires minimal skills compared with the endotracheal tube. Recently, on the international space station and the shuttle, the ILMA has taken precedence over the orally inserted endotracheal tube.

Spinal Immobilization

Field Clearance of the Cervical Spine

Clearing the cervical spine in the field is an extremely controversial subject. In many discussions, both pro and con, field cervical spine clearance is not well defined, and all such "clearances" are too often lumped together. The components should be divided into several groups for ease of understanding. The most obvious of the confounding variables is the setting:

1. The emergency department, with well-trained personnel available (this discussion is left to the many articles and book chapters available in the literature).

2. The field, with a very ill patient or with critical situations existing, such as a fire or precarious extrications: immobilization of the patient to the backboard; in this situation, take care of any possible fractures.

3. A calm field situation in which there are no severely injured patients and all patients are walking around when

the EMTs arrived: patients walking around can be easily assessed if the EMT is well trained and experienced.

4. Prolonged time to access to medical care with difficult transportation of an injured patient such as exists in a wilderness area several miles from a trailhead: carrying a patient on a litter over rugged terrain long distances with few personnel and inadequate equipment is perhaps more dangerous to the patient than walking out if the condition seems stable.

5. The scene is dangerous to the caregivers and the patients because of fire, heavy smoke, biological weapons or toxic chemicals, or military combat: in a combat or other situation in which the caregiver is at risk as well as the patient and the patient needs to be rapidly removed from the environment, then the potential of a cervical spine fracture is overridden by the potential danger of leaving the patient on the scene long enough to assess before movement.

Immobilization of every patient in the field with mechanism of injury or potential injuries to the cervical spine versus selective immobilization has been controversial for several years. On one side of the controversy is the emergency physician who has learned to clear cervical spines by clinical methods in the emergency room and becomes frustrated when most of the trauma patients are brought in with cervical spine immobilization. The responsibility to clear the cervical spine then falls to the physician. These physicians (in order to lighten their own work load) insist that EMS personnel clear the cervical spine in the field, while at the same time they insist that field time be kept very short and the patient be brought rapidly to the hospital. These two situations are mutually exclusive. The EMT makes a rapid decision either to immobilize the patient and go directly to the hospital or to take 5, 10, or 15 minutes to perform a total neurologic examination on the patient to "clear the cervical spine."

It is obvious that the EMT is not as well educated as the physician and therefore does not understand anatomy, physiology, and pathophysiology nearly as well. Forcing EMTs to accept this responsibility when they do not have adequate knowledge, background, or training is incorrect. Additionally, EMTs do not see cervical spine injuries frequently enough to be able to appreciate the subtleties of such injuries.

There is a middle ground, however. This is demonstrated well in immobilization algorithms. These are indications for immobilization, not reasons to "clear" the cervical spine—a very different philosophy. It indicates, as many have believed for a long time, that for penetrating trauma without a neurologic defect there is no indication for immobilizing the cervical spine. The patient should be rapidly transported to the hospital without

immobilization. The long backboard can be used as a device for moving the patient; unless necessary, the cervical collar does not need to be added.

With blunt trauma, the decision is a little more convoluted:

- When there is an altered level of consciousness secondary to injury, hypoxia, drugs, or alcohol, then the patient should be immobilized.
- If there is tenderness to the cervical spine and neurologic defect, or deformity of the cervical spine, the patient should be immobilized.
- If the mechanism of injury is such that there is a potential cervical spine injury or if there are distracting injuries, the patient should be immobilized.
- If none of these conditions is present, then immobilization is not indicated, and transportation to the hospital for evaluation is acceptable and a position of comfort.

For cervical spine immobilization, EMTs must have the skills to perform front, supine, and rear positioning of the head to maintain spine stability while accomplishing a jaw thrust or chin lift maneuver, BVM ventilation, insertion of nasal airways, oral airways, endotracheal tubes, or adjunctive devices.

Cervical Collars

Even the best of cervical collars provides only about 50% to 60% restriction in motion in the three standard positions of anterior/posterior, lateral flexion, and rotation. Therefore, the hard cervical collar cannot be relied on alone for such immobilization. The soft cervical collar does not immobilize the neck in any way whatsoever and is certainly not indicated for acute care and trauma patients, if it is ever indicated for any patient. It is referred to by many EMS services as a "neck warmer" as distain for its clinical function. When combined, however, with a long or short backboard, the hard collar does become an effective device (a belt and suspenders approach) in case the backboard for one reason or another slips or an unruly patient gets out of it.

Backboard

Properly placing a patient on either a long or a short board immobilizes the spine from the pelvis to the head, fulfilling the admonition of immobilization of the joint above and joint below the possible fracture. The proper management for cervical immobilization is to keep the patient's head in the neutral position as closely as

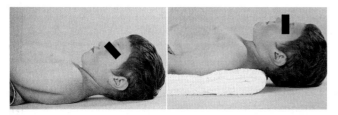

FIGURE 15.29. Small child with large head size requires padding beneath the shoulders. (Reprinted with permission of Elsevier from McSwain et al.[9])

possible. The thoracic structure, curvature of the thoracic vertebra, and head size are all factors in placing a patient properly on a backboard. If a child is to be immobilized, the smaller the child, the larger the head in contrast to the size and position of the thoracic spine makes it important to pad beneath the torso of the child (Figure 15.29). For the older adult and particularly for the kyphotic elderly adult, padding must be placed beneath the head to preserve the patient in the neutral position (Figure 15.30).

When a patient is placed on the backboard, the torso should be immobilized first while the head is maintained manually; the head is mobilized second. The reason for this is obvious. If the head is mobilized first and the

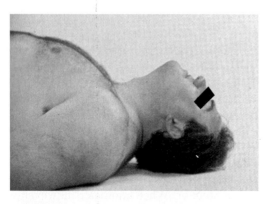

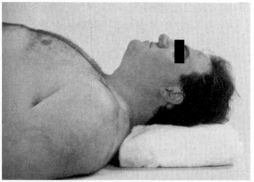

FIGURE 15.30. Kyphotic adult patient requires padding beneath the head. (Reprinted with permission of Elsevier from McSwain et al.[9])

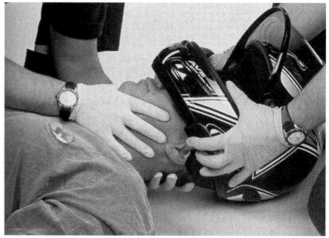

FIGURE 15.31. Helmet removal with spinal precautions.

patient becomes unruly and twists the torso or for some reason falls off of the board, then severe angulation of the cervical spine can occur.

Field Helmet Removal

Removal of motorcycle, bicycle, and football helmets is taught and practiced by every EMT in training and is taught again in the prehospital trauma life support courses. Physicians are almost never taught how to remove a helmet and almost none have practiced it on a consistent basis; therefore, it is appropriate for EMS personnel to remove helmets in the field to better immobilize the patient for transport. The key to removal of a motorcycle helmet is lateral expansion to clear the ears and rotation to clear the nose while the head is immobilize with the hand position in the occiput and on the chin by the second EMT from below. This is demonstrated in Figure 15.31.

For removing a football helmet, it is important to know (1) that the liner is best removed with a screwdriver and (2) when the shoulder pads are left in place, the head must be heavily padded to prevent hyperextension of the neck when placed on the backboard.

Musculoskeletal Trauma

Patients with severe musculoskeletal trauma are in the hands of the EMT 30 minutes or more before they arrive in the hospital. Therefore, an understanding of proper immobilization techniques is critical. Extremity trauma is probably the most common trauma seen and dealt with by EMTs.

First and most serious is severe hemorrhage. As in the operating room or the emergency department, *direct pressure* on the bleeding site is the most effective method of achieving control. This can be done with direct pressure with the hand pushing gauze into the wound, with a tight bandage such as an elastic bandage, or with an air splint. There are some situations in which this will not work. For years, pressure points have been taught in both first aid courses and in EMT courses, but most likely are not effective.

Tourniquets, both in the operating room and on the battle field, have been demonstrated to be effective to not cause the severe harm once thought to occur. It is certainly not true that application of a tourniquet mandates amputation at that level. Tourniquets have their place in both civilian and military situations.

Immobilization of fractures can be achieved by immobilizing the injured extremity to a board, wire lateral splint, the opposite extremity, or the torso for transportation. The diagnosis in the field does not have to be made as to whether the extremity is fractured, sprained, or strained. The diagnosis is only that one of these types of injury is possible; therefore, immobilization is utilized.

For a fractured femur or potentially fractured femur, the traction splint is an excellent device. Early literature from World War I reports that the use of the Thomas Whole Ring or the Thomas Half Ring Splint on soldiers receiving femur injuries reduces the mortality rate by 80%. More recent analysis of these reports indicates that the reduction of mortality may well have been closer to 40%, but nonetheless this is a significant change by the use of such a device.[18] They work by applying traction between the pelvis and the ankle, stretching the leg, pulling the fracture back into position, and relieving the muscle spasm and the hazard of open bones continuing to tear and lacerate the surrounding muscle. Such traction was actually described initially by Hippocrates, later expanded on by Galen, perfected by Oliver Thomas, and polished into the Hare® and Sigar® devices. Figure 15.32

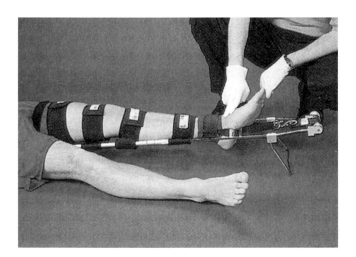

FIGURE 15.32. Traction splint. (Reprinted with permission of Elsevier from McSwain et al.[9])

demonstrates the correct method to apply such immobilization.

In summary, there is little difference in the overall principles of the prehospital management of the trauma victim or the person requiring acute surgical intervention for a nontraumatic problem. The general sequence in which the various steps are taken and the procedures to accomplish these steps are similar. An optimal prehospital environment is an essential component in acute care surgery.

Critique

It is well documented that arrest at the scene from any mechanism of injury significantly decreases the likelihood of survival. Also, several studies have demonstrated the futility of aggressive resuscitation and an emergency thoracostomy if a patient has had a prehospital blunt traumatic arrest. However, there is no indication that this patient has arrested. What could possibly save this patient's life is the intervention that can only occur at the trauma center. With a Level II trauma center being just a few blocks away, this patient should be immediately and directly taken to this facility. This is a situation where the paramedics should "scoop and run."

Answer (C)

References

1. McSwain NE. 71st Scudder Oration, Prehospital Care from Napoleon to Mars: The Surgeon's Role. Fracture Oration presented before the Clinical Congress of the American College of Surgeons, Chicago, IL, October 21, 2003.
2. Barkley, KT. The Ambulance. Hicksville, NY: Exposition Press, 1978; 148.
3. Liberman M, Mulder D, Sainpalis J. Advanced or basic life support for trauma: meta-analysis and critical review of the literature. J Trauma 2000; 49(4):584–599.
4. Sampalis JS, Tamim H, Denis R, et al. Ineffectiveness of on-site intravenous lines: is prehospital time the culprit? J Trauma 1997; 43(4):608–616.
5. Sampalis JS, Boukas S, Lavoie A, et al. Preventable death evaluation of the appropriateness of the on-site trauma care provided by urgences-sante physicians [see comments]. J Trauma 1995; 39(6):1029–1035.
6. Sampalis JS, Lavoie A, Williams JT, et al. Impact of on-site care, prehospital time, and level of in-hospital care on survival in severely injured patients. J Trauma 1993; 34(2):252–261.
7. Samplis JS, Lavoie A, Williams JT, et al. Standardized mortality ratio analysis on a sample of severely injured patients from a large Canadian city without regionalized trauma care. J Trauma 1992; 33(2):205–212.

8. McSwain NE Jr. Medical control—what is it? JACEP 1978; 7(3):114–116.

9. McSwain NE Jr, Frame S, Salomone JP, eds. Prehospital Trauma Life Support: Basic and Advanced Prehospital Trauma Life Support, 5th ed. St. Louis: Mosby, 2003.

10. Bigeleisen PB. An unusual presentation of end-tidal carbon dioxide after esophageal intubation. Anesth Analg 2002; 94(6):1534–1534.

11. Shankar KB, Posner M. A normal capnogram despite esophageal intubation. Can J Anaesth 2002; 49(4): 439–440.

12. Asai T, Shingu K. Case report: a normal capnogram despite esophageal intubation. Can J Anaesth 2001; 48(10):1025–1028.

13. Skelton MB, McSwain NE Jr. A study of cognitive and technical skill deterioration among trained paramedics. JACEP 1977; 6(11):436–438.

14. Hopson LR, Hirsh E, Delgado J, Domeier RM, McSwain NE Jr, Krohmer J. Joint position statement: guidelines for withholding or termination of resuscitation in prehospital traumatic cardiopulmonary arrest: joint position statement of the National Association of EMS Physicians and the American College of Surgeons Committee on Trauma. J Am Coll Surg 2003; 196(1):106–112.

15. Stockinger ZT, McSwain NE Jr. Additional evidence in support of withholding or terminating cardiopulmonary resuscitation for trauma patients in the field. J Am Coll Surg 2004; 198:227–231.

16. McSwain NE Jr. Pneumatic anti-shock garment (PASG): state of the art 1988. Ann Emerg Med 1988; 17(5):506–525.

17. McSwain NE Jr. Assessment and management In McSwain NE Jr, Frame S, Salomone JP, eds. Prehospital Trauma Life Support: Basic and Advanced Prehospital Trauma Life Support, 5th ed. St. Louis: Mosby, 2003: 62–89.

18. Henry BJ, Vrahas MS. The Thomas splint. Questionable boast of an indispensable tool. Am J Orthop 1996; 25(9): 602–604.

16
Disaster and Mass Casualty Management

Eric R. Frykberg

Case Scenario

You are the field medical director of the emergency system for your region. While patrolling an area being prepared for the upcoming state fair, a bolt of lightning strikes a concentrated area of workers who were hovering around one of the main tents. You arrive on the scene immediately and place a dispatch call for medical backup. Several fragments of the frame of the tent have impaled some of the victims. You see the following persons down:

(A) Two workers with metal frames impaled in lower extremities who are calling out for help
(B) One worker decapitated
(C) One worker with no vital signs of life and no obvious injuries
(D) One worker with abdominal evisceration who is moaning in pain
(E) One worker who is entrapped by a large metal plate with no vital signs of life

Which victim(s) require your immediate attention?

A sudden flash, a blast and then a cataclysmic earthquake—fire, lightning, earthquake—all the representatives of disaster and death, each following the other

Hiroshima Diary[1]

Health care providers have been confronted by an increasing number and frequency of major hazardous events throughout the world in recent decades, prompting an awareness of how challenging and different are the approaches to medical care in these settings. A *disaster* is generally defined as an event involving major damage and injury to people and property of sufficient magnitude to create a temporary imbalance between the large scale needs of a community or hospital and the availability of resources to address these needs.[2–4] Most basically, a dis-

aster represents a major departure from the normal experiences of daily life and requires a major change in thinking and approach to successfully manage. From a medical perspective, it is the large number of casualties in these events that most commonly overwhelms medical resources, requiring some degree of external assistance. This is what constitutes a true mass casualty event. The goal of the medical response is to optimize the survival and health of the casualties.

Disasters tend to be viewed as "acts of God" in terms of their unpredictability and randomness, leading to the perception that they cannot be prevented or that preparation for dealing with their consequences is futile. The very term *disaster* is derived from the Latin words for "evil star," implying an uncontrollable fate. Further strengthening this misguided idea is that the problems encountered in specific forms of disasters, such as fires, shootings, explosions, floods, tornadoes, earthquakes, airline crashes, or chemical spills, are all very different in many aspects (Figure 16.1). Even disasters of one specific mechanism may greatly vary in different locations and at different times.[5–11] However, certain patterns and common sets of problems can be anticipated in most disasters, allowing some general principles to be derived from which rational preparation and planning can be developed.

Surgeons and other acute care providers should always be at the forefront of disaster planning and casualty management because of the overwhelming predominance of bodily injury that occurs in most forms of disaster. However, most physicians, including surgeons, are quite unprepared for the unique requirements of disaster and mass casualty management. It is not a routine part of any medical training. The rarity of these events does not allow a widespread body of knowledge or experience to develop among medical professionals, and complacency and apathy are consequently common, especially in the historically safe but increasingly threatened haven of the United States.[12–14] This chapter reviews the classification,

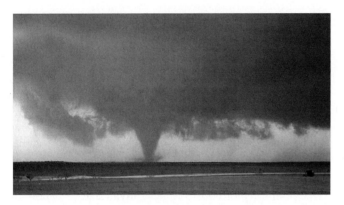

Figure 16.1. Tornadoes are an ongoing cause of natural weather-related disasters responsible for extensive property damage and injuries in the American Midwest every year.

medical consequences, and epidemiology of disasters and the basic concepts of mass casualty planning and management in order to emphasize and justify the importance of surgical involvement in these settings.

Classification of Disasters

There are several characteristics that can be used to stratify disasters into useful categories for study and comparison (Table 16.1). This should allow us to better understand and prepare for these events and ultimately to improve outcomes.[15]

Level of Response

Classification of disasters based only on numbers of casualties is difficult because of the variable impact that location, mechanism, and available resources have at any specific time. Very few disasters in world history have resulted in more than 1,000 casualties, and only 10 to 15

Table 16.1. Disaster classification schemes.

Level of response
  Local (I)
  Regional (II)
  State/national/international (III)
Mechanism
  Natural
    Weather-related
    Geophysical
  Man-made
    Intentional
    Unintentional
Nature of injuries
Extent and timing
  Closed
  Open
  Finite
  Ongoing

disasters each year result in more than 40 casualties.[4] Regardless of number, only about 10% to 20% of casualties are typically seriously injured or impaired.[16,17] Rather than absolute numbers, disaster severity is best classified according to the level of response and resources required to manage the casualty load and damage to property and infrastructure.[15] The level of response is determined by such factors as the size of the area involved, the size of the affected community, the extent of damage to people and property, and the extent to which local resources are overwhelmed and require outside help.

A Level I incident can be handled by local resources alone. It generally involves an escalated response by the local emergency medical services and cooperation with local community agencies, such as the office of emergency preparedness, public health department, police, and community hospitals.[7,18]

A Level II incident requires a regional response beyond the local community. It must involve outside resources from surrounding communities and counties, such as major urban medical centers, other police and fire departments, and regional mobilization of necessary personnel, transportation, and equipment.[9–11]

A Level III incident requires the involvement of state and federal government assets to manage the most extensive and severe forms of disaster. The widespread destruction and large casualty loads following major hurricanes, tornadoes, and earthquakes are examples of this level of disaster severity.[5,19,20]

Mechanism

Perhaps the simplest classification is based on the specific mechanism of the event. Examples include earthquakes, floods, explosions, contaminations (biological, chemical, or radiation), and industrial accidents. Each mechanism involves unique aspects of casualty numbers and injury patterns, logistical and resource requirements, and community impact. These mechanisms may be grouped within a variety of larger categories, such as natural (geophysical, weather related) or man made (intentional, such as terrorist attacks, or unintentional, such as industrial accidents).

Nature of Injuries

A number of different types of disasters may result in very similar patterns of injuries and injury severity, providing a level of predictability that allows for future planning and preparedness. On the other hand, the specific nature of injuries encountered may require very different resources and personnel to manage. Examples include hypothermia and frostbite, burns, chemical and radiation effects, drowning, infectious diseases and epidemics, blast injuries, physical trauma, and mental health issues.[19] Explosions result in well-established patterns of blast injuries and standard forms of trauma.[12,20,21]

Extent and Timing

Some disasters occur at a single site as a single occurrence. These are called *closed* disasters, usually involving technological failures such as industrial explosions, structural collapse, and transportation accidents. They tend to occur in populated areas with an abundance of medical resources. They may actually create a paradoxical set of problems involving too many first responders and onlookers in a small area. Societal infrastructure and resource availability generally remain intact in these events, but prompt and appropriate disposition of assets may be difficult because of overcrowding. Traffic gridlock is often found.[16,23] Hospitals near to the disaster scene tend to be swamped with a disproportionate share of casualties unless there is a rapid establishment of leadership and organization (the *geographic effect*). Although closed disasters may result in large casualty loads and extensive property damage, the logistical considerations are quite different and less complex than those that typify *open* disasters (i.e., tornadoes, earthquakes, floods, hurricanes), which occur over more extensive areas or many discrete sites.[5,9,10] In these, it is important that the incident management system keeps a proper perspective on the "big picture."

Another implication of disaster location is the level of isolation, such as rural areas having less availability of resources and longer transport times to care than urban locations. This factor could impact casualty outcomes.[12,18,20,22]

Finite disasters are those with a definite beginning and predictable and obvious end, usually over short periods of time, such as hurricanes and tornadoes. Most victims will be rescued and receive medical care within a few hours, and efforts may be concentrated on casualty welfare rather than avoidance of continued injury and damage and conservation of resources. *Ongoing* disasters are more problematic, with causative factors that may continue over indefinite periods, perhaps days to weeks, requiring a longer range plan for containment and resource allocation. The multiple aftershocks following an earthquake, infectious disease pandemics, and sustained armed conflicts are examples of such incidents.

Phases of Disaster Response

It is important to recognize several key elements and chronologic events that commonly occur in every disaster so as to optimize planning and casualty care and to avoid past mistakes. A disaster response tends to evolve

TABLE 16.2. Phases of disaster response.

Chaotic
Initial response/reorganization
Site clearing
Search and rescue
Recovery
Medical care
    Initial
    Definitive

in identifiable patterns that, once understood, can be controlled and exploited to the best advantage.[15,24] Many of these response phases occur simultaneously, others occur sequentially, and some are deliberately instituted to ensure proper scene management, casualty distribution, and medical care (Table 16.2).

Chaotic Phase

The chaotic phase is the period of disorganized confusion in the initial minutes to hours after a disaster strikes and is characterized by panic, fear, and lack of leadership or direction over those at the immediate scene and in the general population. This is most prominent in disasters involving unexpected major disruptions, such as bombings, airplane crashes, and earthquakes. In urban settings, it generally lasts less than 1 hour,[24] but in more isolated areas it may last several hours because of a paucity of resources and personnel to organize rescue efforts. The most critically injured casualties are at greatest risk of death during this phase. The least severely injured casualties generally walk themselves to the nearest hospital, causing a rapid inundation of large numbers of people who do not require urgent care, which could unnecessarily overwhelm scarce medical resources. This influx may be the first indication to health care providers that a disaster has occurred and may cause early confusion among them. Thus, chaos may extend from the disaster scene to the hospital. Many well-meaning volunteers may converge on the disaster scene in this phase in a misguided attempt to help, adding to the gridlock of arriving emergency service personnel, police, fire services, and victims. The earlier that firm leadership and command authority is instituted at the scene and in hospitals to end this phase, the less risk there is that further injury and damage will occur.[25]

Initial Response and Reorganization

The second phase begins when professional first responders arrive at the disaster scene to assume command and control, including those personnel who are trained to secure the area to prevent further damage, evaluate the medical needs of casualties, and establish a command center that interacts with the central command authority.

These personnel typically include firemen, police, and prehospital emergency medical services. The initial chaos should be supplanted by organized efforts and progress during this phase. A leader should be designated to take control of the scene at this time, to assess the nature of the event, to determine whether available resources are adequate to manage the logistical and medical needs, and to decide whether the disaster plan should be activated and a command post established.[15] The possible presence of biological, chemical, or radiation exposure must be determined and decontamination procedures initiated.

Several elements of the disaster response are initiated during this phase. A central emergency operations center must be established to coordinate communications and resource distribution with the scene command post. Search and rescue efforts are begun by mobilizing and transporting the appropriate equipment. Security at the scene is usually established by police and other law enforcement personnel in order to restrict access, maintain order among the large numbers of first responders, casualties, and volunteers, and ensure the safety of victims and first responders to prevent further injury. Traffic lanes must be kept open to ensure adequate flow of resources and casualties.[15,26]

Site Clearing

Once organization of the chaotic response is established, a thorough examination of the damage at the disaster scene must proceed, and the plan for clearing debris, rescuing casualties, and transporting casualties to medical care is executed. Generally the fire department has the responsibility to clear the area of dangers that could impede the rescue and clearing operations and further jeopardize both casualties and responders. These immediate dangers include active fires, downed power lines, gas leaks, and leaks or spills of toxic chemicals. Damaged buildings must be inspected by engineers to ensure stability, and personnel must be kept clear if there is danger of collapse. It is during this phase that attention must be focused on the management of any biological, chemical, or radiation contamination of the disaster scene that may have been detected. Specialized response teams may be necessary to rapidly identify these hazardous materials in order to minimize the duration and extent of exposure and initiate decontamination procedures.[27]

Another specific danger that exists in terrorist bombing disasters is the possibility of a second bomb that may be detonated later, with the intent of killing first-line responders arriving at the scene to help. This emphasizes the importance of strict control of access to any disaster scene by the command authority, allowing only those personnel who are trained to address these dangers to enter the area. It is critical to avoid the added injury and death of this "second hit" phenomenon, especially among health care providers, who typically want to help in these areas but who have essential duties elsewhere in casualty management. This could unnecessarily magnify the casualty load and adversely affect casualty outcome.[12,24,28,29]

Search And Rescue

Once the disaster scene is reasonably secure, a search for casualties is undertaken. Those who have died should be transported to a prespecified area for identification and examination by forensic personnel. This area must be separate from areas designated for surviving casualties and should be protected from public view.[15,30]

Surviving casualties should be immediately assessed for the nature of their injuries and the urgency of treatment needs after being rescued from the disaster site. In many disaster scenes, extensive extrication must be carried out to safely free these victims from collapsed rubble. This requires special equipment that must be transported to the scene and specialized expertise to provide any needed medical care in confined spaces while extrication proceeds. Care providers should be prepared for prolonged entrapment of victims in collapsed structures and rubble and for the prolonged field life support that may have to occur remotely. Respiratory impairment, hypothermia, hypovolemia, dehydration, crush syndrome, and skeletal injuries are examples of major problems that entrapped victims may suffer, which must be supported during this period.[31]

Once again, the safety of the rescuers must be of paramount importance, as their death or injury compounds the danger to surviving victims. Rescue personnel should be restricted to those with training and experience in this field, and proper protection gear must be worn. This should be the responsibility of a safety officer who oversees all rescue efforts at the scene and who answers to the central command authority. Dangers include not only secondary structural collapse, falling debris, and airborne dust, toxins, and biological, chemical or radiologic agents but also deliberate "second hit" booby traps designed to kill first responders, such as delayed bomb blasts.[24]

Search and rescue workers are the most common *secondary victims* of disasters due to the significant psychoemotional stress they undergo from both acute stress reactions and fatigue, as well as more chronic forms of post-traumatic stress disorder.[32] Critical incident stress management (CISM) is a mechanism involving the recognition and defusing of traumatic psychological effects that major disasters can inflict on rescue workers. Impaired workers are removed from the scene to undergo short interventions of debriefing and rest. This essential component of any disaster response should provide regular relief for rescue workers, with multiple shifts of personnel as a means of preventing adverse emotional consequences.[33]

In most disasters, it is rare to find live victims after 24 to 48 hours. At this point, search and rescue efforts convert to simple recovery efforts, which are focused on clearance of mechanical debris and identification and transportation of dead bodies.[24] A definitive recovery phase of disaster response has been recognized that involves restoring the community and society to a new state of "normal," which is never quite the same as the predisaster condition. It evolves over a long period of time, during which damaged property and infrastructure are rebuilt, economic losses are recouped, and long-term emotional stabilization of all involved people occurs.

Medical Care of Casualties

The medical care of disaster victims begins at the first moment of rescue and extends for hours, days, weeks, or longer through all phases of definitive care and rehabilitation. The more quickly care is instituted, the better the outcome. This requires early and rapid rescue, evaluation, and evacuation of casualties to hospital facilities (Table 16.3). It is within the first minutes and hours following a true mass casualty disaster that the major differences in medical management from our normal everyday care of injured patients become evident. There are two major phases of medical care following mass casualty disasters.

Initial Phase

The large numbers of casualties caused by most disasters require rapid assessment, with no time for detailed examinations, laboratory work, or imaging studies. Typically only a minority of surviving victims have life-threatening problems that require immediate care, and these must be identified quickly and, through the process of *triage*, separated from those with less severe problems requiring less urgent attention.[12,34] Although there are five widely recognized triage categories in mass casualty management (Table 16.4), the first triage performed at the disaster scene should be highly abbreviated to determine only those who need immediate treatment and those who do not.[24]

TABLE 16.3. Casualty flow following disasters.

Search and rescue/extrication
   proceeds to
Sorting and life support (triage)
   proceeds to
Decontamination
   proceeds to
Evacuation
   proceeds to
Definitive treatment

TABLE 16.4. Triage categories.

Immediate
Delayed
Minimal (walking wounded)
Expectant
Dead

It is essential to properly distribute the casualty load at the scene to as many different hospitals as possible, in accordance with the resources available at each hospital or in the area as a whole. This principle of sequential casualty distribution, also known as "leap frogging," prevents any one facility from being overwhelmed with such numbers that patient care capabilities are paralyzed.[24,28,35] In fact, this is typically what happens to the hospital that is nearest to any disaster scene if prompt organization is not established. The orderly casualty distribution process can only be effective if all hospitals in any community are equally prepared for the unique demands of a mass casualty event.[36]

An important concept in disaster management is that of *surge capacity*. This is the ability of a hospital to expand its resources to accommodate the large number of casualties in this setting that would otherwise overwhelm its capabilities under normal conditions. This involves increasing the number of available beds and patient care staff acutely, which generally requires discharge and transfer of existing patients elsewhere. *Surge capability* is a related concept that refers to the provision of special needs to disaster victims with unique injuries or conditions, such as burn care, pediatric care, crush injuries, biological, chemical, or radiation injuries, geriatric demands, specialty surgical care in such areas as orthopedics, plastics, neurosurgery, or ophthalmology, and mental health support.

The initial care provided in a mass casualty scenario must be as little as necessary to evaluate and stabilize a patient in a matter of seconds so as to be able to quickly recognize that small minority who may require urgent attention. This principle of *minimal acceptable care* represents a major departure from the normal evaluation and care rendered to individual patients in everyday practice in which the goal is optimal care for all, with essentially unlimited time and resources. In a true mass casualty disaster, medical resources are limited and must be carefully allocated on the basis of not only need but also the potential salvageability of the victim. Such rationing of care is quite contrary to the training and experience of all health care providers. In this setting, the goal of treatment must change from the greatest good for each victim to the greatest good for the greatest number, or maximizing the salvage of as many casualties as possible. The focus of medical care must change from the individual to the population as a whole in order to apply the limited resources where the most chance of success lies. There is no place in this setting for heroic time-consuming measures, such as cardiopulmonary resuscitation or emergent thoracotomy, which waste resources and may prevent the salvage of many more victims.[12,19,21,24,34,37]

Triage at the disaster site is best supplemented by a second level of triage and urgent stabilizing care that is located between the scene and the hospital in a safe area, known as a *casualty collection point*.[15] Those casualties with nonurgent injuries should be assigned to an area that is supervised by nonsurgical physicians who can monitor them for any deterioration and assess and document the nature of injuries and what care is needed. This allows the areas of the hospital best suited to emergent interventions to be free for the most urgent casualties, such as the emergency department, operating rooms, or intensive care units. The receiving area of the hospital, most commonly the emergency department, should rapidly be cleared of all existing patients, who should be transported to other spaces and overseen by designated health care providers for the duration of the mass casualty event.

The principles of advanced trauma life support (ATLS) should be applied to urgent casualties, assessing for the most critical injuries and intervening when found.[38] Radiologic imaging should be minimized, as clinical management decisions must be based only on a rapid physical examination if all casualties are to be assessed. Focused abdominal sonography for trauma (FAST) is among the few acceptable diagnostic tools in this setting consistent with minimal acceptable care, in view of its simplicity and rapidity.[24,34,39,40] The operating rooms should be utilized only for immediate life-saving procedures, such as laparotomy for liver or spleen hemorrhage or burr holes for intracranial hematoma. Damage-control principles should be applied in the operating room to maintain a rapid turnover to accommodate incoming casualties.[34,41] Bedside laparotomies or other surgical interventions may have to be carried out in the intensive care unit if operating rooms are not available. Blood transfusions should be strictly limited and are often not necessary in this setting.[42] A forward traffic flow must be maintained from the emergency department onward, consistently moving casualties as quickly as possible to other areas as determined by their needs, and never backward (see Table 16.3), again so as to ensure room for incoming casualties and to avoid chaotic backlogs and bottlenecks.[12,39]

This initial phase of disaster medical care lasts as long as the influx of casualties persists. The length of time of this influx and the ultimate number of casualties that will be brought to the hospital typically are not known and are largely unpredictable during the event.[34] This is due to the almost universal breakdown of communications between the scene and the hospital in these events.[10,42] This phase may last from hours to days, emphasizing the importance of strict and rapid triage, minimal acceptable care, damage-control surgery, and regular relief of medical workers in order to conserve essential hospital and personnel resources. Computer modeling studies have shown that the quality of medical care inevitably declines as the casualty load increases, although this decline can be mitigated by planning and preparedness.[43]

Definitive Phase

Once the casualty flow into the hospital has stopped, more time can be devoted to casualty care and distribution as order is restored to the situation. All casualties can be more thoroughly reevaluated. Available hospital resources can be inventoried and applied as necessary to casualty needs without the worry that they may be depleted by more incoming victims. Casualties initially denied care due to the prohibitive nature of their conditions, who are still alive, can be reassessed for the possibility of initiating care based on their needs and available resources. Hemodynamically stable victims requiring surgery for less urgent injuries (i.e., hollow viscus rupture, open fractures, soft tissue wounds, peripheral vascular injuries) should now undergo operation and more definitive treatment. Specialty care can now be initiated by plastic surgeons, otolaryngologists, ophthalmologists, vascular surgeons, neurosurgeons, orthopedic surgeons, and surgical intensivists for such common injuries as blast lung, ruptured eardrums, ocular disruption, and skeletal fractures. A more liberal use of imaging is now permissible to facilitate detailed evaluation, with such modalities as contrast studies, computed tomography (CT) scans, magnetic resonance imaging (MRI), and angiography.

Most nonurgent casualties can tolerate several hours delay before undergoing surgery or other interventions, allowing those with urgent and severe injuries to first be fully evaluated and treated. These delays can be shortened by transferring some of these less injured victims to other area hospitals for definitive care, where casualty loads may be less and there is greater capacity for care. This *secondary distribution* of casualties helps to equalize the burden among different facilities. Although this principle is rarely practiced in mass casualty events, it should be considered and included in the disaster plans of hospitals and communities.[10,24,36]

Record Keeping

An essential factor in the medical care of mass casualties following disasters is accurate record keeping. Continuity of care can be easily lost as large numbers of casualties are rapidly transported through successive echelons of evaluation and management without any health care providers following them. Without a written record that follows the patient, missed injuries and redundant triage are likely, wasting time and increasing the possibility of adverse outcomes. These records should be brief and concise, describing the injuries, treatment given, associated conditions, and what further care is necessary. They should be secured in a reliable way to the patient to avoid being lost. Plastic lamination is one suggested method to prevent tearing, moisture, and soiling, especially in austere environments. The forms should be those in routine use by caregivers so as to minimize the time required to become familiar with new forms.[12,21,22,42,44,45]

Another advantage to accurate medical records of each victim is the opportunity they provide to retrospectively assess injury patterns, outcomes, and problems encountered in medical care and administrative management of the disaster response, which can then be disseminated to enhance the education of others. They facilitate early postdisaster debriefings and critiques, which are recommended in order to determine the success of the disaster response and medical care and to revise disaster planning accordingly to improve the approach to future events. They provide the basis for a critical analysis of the event, from which comparison to other disasters can be made to determine patterns and improve understanding of disaster management.[12,42,46] Without such records, all these essential lessons can be lost.

It is important that the information on casualty injury patterns and outcomes be standardized and published for widespread dissemination.[12,18,20–22,28,34,35,44,45,47] An objective method for determining injury severity is essential for this purpose, as the most accurate assessment of the success of medical management is the outcome of the most severely injured. Many published reports of disasters have applied the injury severity score (ISS) to this end, with an ISS > 15 being widely accepted as an indication of critical injuries.[21,22,47] This allows the patterns of casualty injuries and severity to be identified and studied and objective and standardized comparisons to be made with similar disasters (Figure 16.2). A *critical mortality*

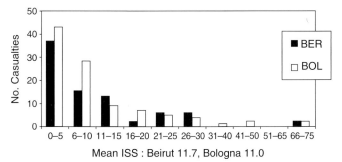

FIGURE 16.2. A graphic comparison of injury severity in survivors of the terrorist bombings of the Bologna, Italy (BOL), train terminal in 1980 and the U.S. Marine barracks in Beirut, Lebanon (BER) in 1983, demonstrating the consistent pattern of noncritical injuries (injury severity score [ISS] <16) among most casualties. (Data from Frykberg et al.[22] and Brismar and Bergenwald L.[47])

rate can be derived from these data, which are the percentages of deaths that occur only among the minority of critically injured casualties who are truly at risk of death. This outcome measure is considered a more accurate reflection of the quality of medical care than the overall mortality rate, which is falsely diluted by the great majority of casualties who are not severely injured and not at any real risk of death.[12,21]

The Role and Importance of Triage

As mentioned previously, the evaluation and distribution of patients according to severity of injury and urgency of required care is known as *triage*, from the French word meaning "to sort." This concept was popularized by Napoleon's battlefield surgeon Dominique Jean Larrey and has become a prominent part of military medical care.[48,49] Triage is practiced only occasionally, and on small scales, in ordinary medical care in developed countries because the abundance of resources makes any form of rationing unnecessary. However, triage assumes major importance in the care of mass casualties following major disasters in which setting resources are, by definition, limited, requiring institution of the principle of the *greatest good for the greatest number*.[15,45,50]

The process of triage normally depends on two factors—the severity of injury and the urgency of treatment needs, with those having the most critical life-threatening injuries typically being assigned to immediate care for rapid life-saving interventions. Additional factors that must be considered in mass casualty scenarios are the potential salvageability of the casualty and the extent of time, personnel, and resources that would have to be devoted to properly treat the injuries. The abandonment of some victims who normally would undergo heroic treatment measures goes firmly against our training and commitment to life, but must be applied in the setting of a disaster if salvage of the population is to be maximized. This principle translates into the paradoxical practice of actually denying care to the most severely injured casualties, who intuitively would seem to be the obvious candidates for immediate care.[12,15,34]

Triage Categories

Five major triage categories are generally applied in mass casualty response (Table 16.4). The *immediate category* includes those life-threatening injuries and conditions that require rapid but relatively simple intervention to save a life, such as hypotension, active external hemorrhage, burns of intermediate depth and extent, open chest wounds, tension pneumothorax, and airway compromise. The *delayed* category includes hemodynamically stable victims with injuries that will require some form of treatment but for whom delay of treatment will not significantly affect their outcome, such as open extremity fractures, pelvic fractures, extremity vascular injuries, soft tissue wounds, and penetrating torso wounds. The *minimal* category, sometimes referred to as "walking wounded," includes casualties with minor injuries and normal mental status who require no treatment beyond first aid (i.e., minor lacerations, abrasions) and who are typically identified by their ability to walk under their own power.

The *expectant* category includes casualties who show signs of life, but with such severe injuries and low likelihood of survival that necessary treatment would potentially jeopardize the salvage of many more victims by directing the limited resources away from them (i.e., severe head injury with unconsciousness, open skull fractures with extruding brain, extensive and deep burns, imminent cardiac arrest). These casualties should still be provided comfort care, and personnel should be assigned to monitor for any improvement that may warrant reconsideration for more immediate care, at least during the period of casualty influx when the adequacy of resources is uncertain.

The *dead* category is important to recognize so as to separate these bodies from live casualties for identification and autopsy, as well as to properly inform families as to their outcome. Any victim who is unresponsive and without signs of life (i.e., no pulse, spontaneous respirations, or cranial nerve reflexes) should be considered dead, especially with evidence of major physical trauma. There should be no efforts made to resuscitate these victims.[17,25,35,51]

Triage Accuracy

The accuracy of triage may certainly affect casualty outcome in the setting of a mass casualty disaster. *Undertriage* refers to the inappropriate assignment of casualties with severe injuries who need immediate care to a delayed, nonurgent category, with the obvious potential for preventable death. In all settings, undertriage is considered a medical problem that must be minimized. *Overtriage* is the assignment of noncritical casualties to the most urgent category of immediate care[52]; it is generally accepted as a necessary economic, logistical, and administrative burden in the routine practice of trauma and emergency care that helps to minimize undertriage,[53] although it has been suggested to potentially threaten lives in some emergency room settings.[54] Devoting resources to noncritical patients who present in small numbers over long periods of time and who in retrospect did not need such care certainly strains finances, personnel, and hospital bed availability, but it is not believed to

TABLE 16.5. Relation of overtriage to critical mortality in terrorist bombing survivors.

Event (Ref)	Year	No. survivors	No. critically injured (%)*	No. overtriage (%)†	No. critical mortality (%)‡
Cu Chi[61]	1969	34	3 (9)	9 (75)	1 (33)
Craigavon[59]	1970s	339	113 (33)	29 (20)	5 (4)
Old Bailey[56]	1973	160	4 (2.5)	15 (79)	1 (25)
Guildford[60]	1974	64	22 (34)	2 (8.3)	0
Birmingham[58]	1974	119	9 (8)	12 (57)	2 (22)
Tower of London[57]	1974	37	10 (27)	9 (47)	1 (10)
Bologna[47]	1980	218	48 (22)	133 (73.5)	11 (23)
Beirut[22]	1983	112	19 (17)	77 (80)	7 (37)
AMIA[62]	1994	200	14 (7)	47 (56)	4 (29)
Oklahoma City[20]	1995	597	52 (9)	31 (37)	5 (10)
Total		1,880	294 (16)	364 (53)	37 (12.6)

*Percentage of total survivors.
†Number of noncritical survivors triaged to immediate care, as a percentage of all casualties triaged to immediate care.
‡Number and percentage of all critically injured survivors who died.
Source: Reprinted with permission from Frykberg.[12]

represent a medical problem that impacts patient outcomes.

However, it is reasonable to postulate that in the setting of mass casualties, when large numbers inundate a hospital all at once, overtriage could be just as much a threat to casualty survival as undertriage because of the barrier it creates to the rapid detection of that small minority of critically injured victims who require immediate intervention.[12,21,25,55] In fact, a review of the published results of 10 major mass casualty terrorist bombings in which data on overtriage and critical mortality were provided[20,22,47,56-62] (Table 16.5) confirms a direct linear relationship between the degree of overtriage and the critical mortality rate of severely injured surviving casualties in this unique setting (Figure 16.3). This shows that triage decisions must not only be rapid but also highly accurate and discriminating in a mass casualty event to minimize *both* overtriage and undertriage in order to maximize casualty survival.

The triage officer must be experienced in handling the types of injuries that each specific disaster is likely to cause and must also be trained in the unique principles of mass casualty management. This person must also have absolute authority to make decisions as to casualty disposition if smooth and rapid flow is to be achieved. This triage officer need not necessarily be a physician. In some settings, experienced emergency or critical care nurses, or prehospital personnel, may serve in this role. In some unconventional disasters, other specialists may best direct triage, such as radiation biologists for radiologic events,

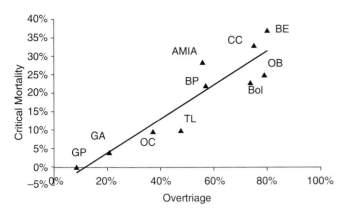

FIGURE 16.3. Graphic demonstration of the direct linear relationship between overtriage and critical mortality following major terrorist bombings. GP, Guildford pubs bombings, UK; CA, Craigavon bombings, Northern Ireland; TL, Tower of London bombing; BP, Birmingham pubs bombings, UK; AMIA, Buenos Aires bombing; OB, Old Bailey bombing, UK; OC, Oklahoma City bombing; Bol, Bologna, Italy, bombing; Be, Beirut bombing; CC, Cu Chi, Vietnam bombing. (Reprinted with permission from Frykberg.[12])

toxicologists for chemical disasters, or infectious disease or public health physicians in biological disasters. In the most common and most likely mass casualty events that involve bodily injury, surgeons and emergency medicine physicians are generally the best candidates to serve as triage officers because of their experience with the acute care of trauma victims.[63]

It has been shown that the use of physicians in triage roles in the routine transport, evaluation, and care of trauma victims improves triage accuracy, especially by reducing overtriage, when compared with nonphysician providers.[64] A computer simulation of a mass casualty scenario demonstrated that reducing overtriage from 50% to 25% did not significantly alter casualty outcomes, suggesting that the triage officer need not necessarily be the most experienced surgeon available and that triage accuracy need not be perfect.[39] However, a more recent computer modeling scenario that more realistically simulates constant casualty influx demonstrated a substantial degradation in the quality of casualty care when overtriage rates are increased up to 75%.[43]

Generally, a fine line must be established in the effort to maximize triage accuracy, because the more selective is the triage process, in order to reduce overtriage, the more likely will undertriage be increased. Cook and co-workers[65] showed that physiologic indicators and anatomic criteria are superior to mechanism in reducing overtriage in a standard trauma system. They further showed that reduction of overtriage can be accomplished without compromising undertriage as long as proper controls on triage accuracy are maintained. In recent terrorist events in Israel, some potentially lethal injuries in

victims with multiple penetrating wounds from firearms and bomb shrapnel initially presented with little symptomatology and were often triaged to the walking wounded category, only to later deteriorate and require urgent surgery.[66] Such undertriage is best avoided by learning to recognize and act on certain mechanisms and injury patterns despite the subtle clinical presentation. Assignment of medical personnel to the areas where delayed or minimal casualties are kept, in order to closely monitor any worsening, also serves to minimize the consequences of such undertriage.

The most severely injured casualties are those most prone to mistriage, especially on the side of overtriage. Expectant casualties who should be denied care, due to the extent of resources required for their level of expected salvageability, or dead casualties may be triaged to immediate care by inexperienced triage officers. This should be recorded as overtriage in the postevent analysis and could result in unnecessary loss of life among more salvageable casualties. Deaths among expectant casualties should similarly *not* be included among survivor deaths but should be included among immediate deaths, as they never were provided medical care. If they are improperly included in critical mortality among survivors, this would falsely skew the critical mortality rate toward a worse outcome and falsely impact the results of medical care. All cases of undertriage must be analyzed to learn how they could be avoided in the future. One marker of undertriage that should also require audit is any death that occurs among noncritically injured casualties.[12,21]

Triage Decisions

What exactly constitutes an expectant casualty will necessarily differ with each specific disaster according to the disaster mechanism, the casualty numbers, and the resources available. This determination cannot be strictly defined in advance planning but should be made only in the earliest phases of a disaster response by a consensus of those in charge of the medical operations. It is only at this time that a realistic assessment of the casualty load is possible. For instance, the need for mechanical ventilation may be limited by the number of ventilators, auxiliary equipment, and personnel available to provide this support. A lack of electrical power will significantly alter available resources for treatment. The need for major surgery must be adjusted according to the number of operating rooms and surgeons available. These considerations will determine which casualties will receive immediate treatment, with their potential salvageability a major factor in the decision.

Triage must be a dynamic process, with constant reevaluation of all casualties by those health care providers assigned to their care. This requires that no casualty be forgotten, but constantly monitored. Once casualty influx has abated, or once all those assigned to immediate care have been treated, and the remaining resources have been ascertained, expectant casualties who are still alive may be reconsidered for treatment. Victims in the delayed category may also be assigned to immediate treatment at this point, according to the priority their injuries require. Any deterioration of delayed or minimal casualties should be noted and may require reassignment to a higher priority of care[67]

Important elements that should be analyzed in the postevent debriefing and critique of any disaster include the quality of the triage decisions that were made, the quality of monitoring and medical care provided, and their potential impact on casualty outcome.[43] This analysis provides essential lessons that should be used to further train triage officers so as to improve future outcomes. Disaster drills and regional exercises are necessary to implement these lessons for proficiency in disasters.[49,50]

Incident Command

As complex as most disasters are, an effective disaster response requires multiple organizations, agencies, and disciplines to achieve control and fulfill the goals of minimizing damage to people, property, and the societal infrastructure. These disparate elements include a wide range of expertise and capability but must function together smoothly in a strictly coordinated fashion in order to succeed. It is widely accepted that the earlier command and control is instituted over the chaos of a disaster scene, the faster and more effectively will the disaster response proceed.[25]

The Incident Command System (ICS) is generally considered the best organizational model for disaster response management and has been adopted by most local, state, and national agencies in the United States as the key element in their disaster planning and management. The ICS had its origins in California in 1970 in response to a failure of adequate command and control over a series of wildfires that required the coordination of firefighters from several jurisdictions. It has since proved quite successful at providing the structural framework for a rapid and coordinated response to virtually any emergency or major disaster, and it involves the appropriate allocation of people, services, and resources. The flexibility it allows in adapting to a variety of contingencies is its major asset.[68]

The ICS organizational hierarchy is based on functional requirements and revolves around five major management activities—Command, Operations, Planning, Logistics, and Finance/Administration (Figure 16.4). This structure can be scaled up or down to match the nature

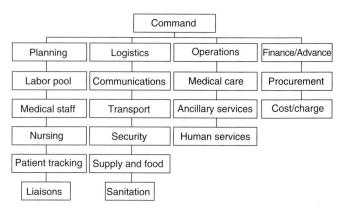

FIGURE 16.4. Structural organization of the functions of the Incident Command System.

and extent of the emergency. Individual hospitals in most communities can adopt this structure to their own internal disaster plan, as the Hospital Emergency Incident Command System (HEICS), and it can easily be expanded into a larger ICS function as needed for an entire community, region, or state. It can function only if all participants are willing to subjugate their functions under one command authority. An understanding of its functional components is important to its proper application to any disaster response.

Command

The incident commander is the one person tasked with overall responsibility for the management of a disaster response and for supervision, control, and decision making over each of the other components of the ICS. The command structure often includes a public information officer to manage the flow of information to the media and public, a liaison officer to coordinate efforts among all involved agencies and services, and a safety officer who is responsible for the safety of the responders and the public. In different forms of disasters, this structure does not change, only the skills of the individuals do (i.e., radiation biologists in radiologic events, toxicologists in chemical events, infection control specialists in biological events).

The ICS command structure demonstrates the concept of *unity of command* in bringing a variety of different services and jurisdictions under one authority for the purpose of achieving the common goal of disaster response and mitigation. When several disparate elements or incident command systems must integrate their functions under one overall command authority, such as several hospital HEICS systems functioning under a regional Emergency Operations Center for a widespread disaster (i.e., tornadoes, earthquake, or flood), a *unified command* is formed. The ICS also involves the concept of *chain of command* in which each part of the command structure, and every person in it, knows its responsibility and who it reports to within the hierarchy. When properly implemented, these concepts provide the organization and flexibility necessary for control of the most complex and extensive disasters.[68]

Operations

Operations is responsible for all efforts directly involved in controlling the disaster and minimizing its damage to people and property, and it is the only part of the ICS that directly interfaces with the public. All other ICS sections exist to support this one. It includes the activities of fire-fighting, law enforcement, scene search and rescue, crowd control, victim staging, decontamination, and medical management of casualties at all echelons from the scene through the hospital and evacuation to definitive care.

Planning

Planning is responsible for *situational awareness* and anticipation, including ongoing evaluation of the disaster and its aftermath, so as to keep the incident commander informed of progress and problems. It is responsible for the development of an incident plan to be carried out by Operations and for establishing documentation of the incident, which may be used by, among others, Logistics or Finance/Administration. Damage assessment, resource allocation, technical specialist provision, and demobilization plans are other functions of Planning. The goal of this activity is to stay ahead of problems, issues, and needs to facilitate smooth operations.

Logistics

Logistics implements the incident plan in support of Operations by providing the nuts and bolts of services and support as needed. It includes communications, transportation, security, medical personnel and supplies, food provision and distribution for workers and victims, inventory capabilities, sanitation, and facilities for shelter and care.

Finance/Administration

Finance/Administration is responsible for keeping track of costs and procurement of needed resources. Its major activities include a time unit to record all personnel and equipment time devoted to the incident, a procurement unit for equipment and supplies, and a compensation and claims unit to determine costs and develop cost-saving methods.

All of these ICS functions are directed toward management of the entire disaster scenario. The actual

location at which the key members of the ICS structure manage the overall operations is the Emergency Operations Center (EOC). The EOC may be supplemented by satellites, such as a forward command center near the disaster scene, a logistics center, and a triage staging center, depending on the size and extent of the incident.

Terrorism

. . . from a terrorist perspective, the true genius of this attack is that the objective and means of attack were beyond the imagination of those responsible for Marine security.

Report of the U.S. Department of Defense Commission
on Beirut Airport Terrorist Act, October 23, 1983

Terrorism is the unlawful exercise of random and ruthless violence against property or individuals, usually innocent civilians, in order to intimidate governments or societies for political or ideological purposes.[69] Terrorist attacks on civilian populations have become the most prominent and threatening cause of mass casualty disasters around the world in recent years, and they pose the most obvious reason why health care providers must be trained in the unique aspects of mass casualty management. In the United States, physicians have largely taken a back seat to other nonmedical organizations in disaster preparedness efforts. Surgeons in particular have not stepped up to their natural leadership role in this area, ceding this to other specialties,[13] although the looming threat of increased attacks in future years makes disaster planning and preparedness quite important.

The two major goals of terrorist attacks, maximal casualty generation and maximal lethality, are best achieved by the weapons of mass destruction of biological, nuclear or radiologic, incendiary, chemical, and explosive (BNICE) mechanisms. However, even the mere threat of these attacks may be sufficient in some settings to achieve the public chaos and societal disruption that terrorists seek. It is essential that the medical community be prepared to meet these threats through a study of their epidemiology, pathophysiology, and injury patterns so as to best organize and execute medical care.

Biological Agents

Bioterrorism refers to the use of microorganisms, or toxins derived from them, to intentionally inflict disease and death on large populations. The most unique feature that distinguishes biological weapons from all other weapons of mass destruction is the slower time course of its effects, and thus of the evolution of the disaster and its response, because of the incubation period required for disease to manifest after the initial exposure. A large number of casualties may occur before the medical community is first aware of an attack and able to institute containment measures. The number of potential victims depends on the type of agent, its virulence, the susceptibility of the population to its infectious or toxic effects, the mode of dissemination, and the concentration of the population exposed. Front-line health care providers must know the clinical manifestations of these agents and have a high index of suspicion for their deliberate use in order to contain an attack as early as possible.

Anthrax is considered by the U.S. Centers for Disease Control and Prevention as a Category A agent, being the most likely to be used in a biological attack.[70,71] Its spores can be easily produced in large quantities with little training, they can be stored for years without loss of potency, and they are easily spread in the air by delivery mechanisms such as sprayers, bombs, and missiles. When inhaled, anthrax has a high fatality rate. One report estimates that an aerosolized release of 100 kg of spores could result in up to 3 million deaths in the Washington, DC, area.[71] The incubation rate is between 2 and 60 days and has three clinical forms—cutaneous, gastrointestinal, and pulmonary. The cutaneous form occurs naturally, has a 20% fatality rate, and is the most common form in developed countries. The gastrointestinal form requires ingestion of contaminated meat and manifests with non-specific gastrointestinal symptoms that may progress to bleeding and peritonitis if untreated. The pulmonary form is 100% fatal if untreated and 80% fatal if treatment is initiated after the onset of symptoms; it is considered the most likely to result from a terrorist attack. Penicillin is the treatment of choice. Prophylaxis of personnel at high risk of exposure is done with a combination of antibiotics and vaccination.

Botulinum toxin is a neurotoxin and is one of the most poisonous substances known, causing neuromuscular blockade that leads to respiratory failure. Although most commonly caused by ingestion of contaminated food, the likely method of deliberate attack would be through an aerosolized form that can cause widespread disease very quickly as it is tasteless, colorless, and odorless. Treatment is supportive care and antitoxin.[72]

Bubonic plague and tularemia are bacterial infections, and smallpox is a virulent viral disease, and all have high infectious potential and lethality and an established history of causing millions of deaths. All can be transmitted by airborne contamination, all have actually been prepared, and in some instances used, as biological weapons intended to decimate large populations, and all are considered major threats as bioterrorist agents.[73]

The process of *syndromic surveillance* is a system of recognition of patterns of illness over a wide area that is essential to allow early determination of disease pandemic and terrorist-related attack.[74] Personal protection measures must be initiated among health care providers in these settings to protect against the further spread of infection through mucosal surfaces, respiratory system, and skin. Public health officials and infectious disease experts should be integrally involved in the response to bioterrorist disasters.

Chemical Agents

Toxic chemicals have a proven capability to cause severe and widespread morbidity and mortality among large populations as well as spread panic, which in itself could lead to societal disruption, and thus pose a major threat from their intentional use by terrorists. These agents can exert their deadly effects through inhalation of aerosolized or gaseous forms, ingestion of poisoned foods, and direct contact with the skin and eyes. Poison gases have been used extensively in warfare, especially in the twentieth century, with as many as 1 million casualties of these agents in World War I. The worst chemical disaster in history occurred in Bhopal, India, in 1984, when the accidental release of 40 tons of gaseous methyl isocyanate led to 6,000 deaths and 400,000 injuries, demonstrating the potential of these agents as effective terrorist weapons. The bomb that exploded in the World Trade Center in 1993 in New York City contained enough cyanide to contaminate the entire building, but it was destroyed by the blast.[75] In 1995, the first terrorist use of the nerve agent sarin on a civilian population occurred in Tokyo, Japan, leading to 12 deaths and 5,000 injuries.[76] The major categories of chemical poisons and their treatments are listed in Table 16.6.

The initial phase of management of chemical attacks requires early detection, which is often difficult without a high index of suspicion. Patterns must be recognized that involve large numbers of patients with similar symptom clusters, and this requires a knowledge of signs

TABLE 16.6. Potential chemical terrorism agents.

Category	Agents	Treatment
Vesicants (blistering)	Mustard	Decontamination
	Lewisite	Hypochlorite (bleach)
	Phosgene oxime	Dimercaprol
Pulmonary irritants	Phosgene	Decontamination
	Chlorine	Water cleansing
	Ammonia	Bronchodilators
	Mace	Mechanical ventilation
Blood agents	Cyanide	Decontamination
		100% oxygen
		Amyl nitrite
Incapacitating agents (anticholinergics)	BZ	Intravenous hydration
		Physostigmine
Nerve agents	Tabun, sarin	Atropine
	saman, VX	2-Pam
		Diazepam
		Airway management
		Decontamination

and symptoms associated with chemical toxicity. The source of contamination must be identified and neutralized, victims must be evacuated to prevent further contamination, and effective treatment must be initiated. The classic symptoms that should heighten awareness of chemical poisoning include coughing and choking, dry mouth and mucous membranes, seizures, eye irritation, and cholinergic symptoms as described by the DUMBELS mnemonic (diarrhea, urination, miosis, bronchospasm or bronchorrhea, emesis, lacrimation, salivation).

Health care workers must wear personal protective equipment to prevent inhalation of "off-gassing" exposure that may emanate from some victims, as well as skin and eye exposure. Triage and decontamination must be established outside the hospital to prevent disabling contamination that will prevent treatment of victims. All victims must undergo decontamination as early as possible. Simply removing clothing and showering with soap and water can remove up to 90% of all contaminating agents and is called *gross decontamination*. More intensive *technical decontamination* can then follow for specific forms of exposure, such as hypochlorite washing for mustard agents and copious eye irrigation with saline solutions. Poison control centers, public health officials, pharmacologists, local or regional poison control centers, and toxicologists are important resources and personnel who should be involved in the planning and management of chemical disasters.

Nuclear/Radiologic Agents

Dispersal of radioactive substances poses a major potential for a terrorist attack because of the theoretical damage that could be imparted on large populations, although a deliberate attack on civilian populations outside of war has never occurred. These agents also carry the potential of large-scale psychosocial effects and panic because of the mystique that is associated with radiation among the general population, which is far out of proportion to many of the actual dangers. Radiation exposure from a terrorist attack is generally easier to manage than biological and chemical attacks because of easy detection methods with various forms of dose-rate meters and Geiger counters, the large number of hospital and government personnel who regularly deal with radiation, and the well-known clinical effects that can be monitored with simple laboratory tests.[77,78]

Ionizing radiation damages living tissue, especially of the gastrointestinal tract and bone marrow, through its direct energy, as well as indirect effects from the creation of unstable, toxic hyperoxide molecules. The two major forms of ionizing radiation include electromagnetic (gamma rays and x-rays, which have high penetration and cause the most damage) and particle (alpha and beta par-

ticles, which have very low penetration and cause harm only if ingested; and neutrons, which have high penetration and destructive energy). The major factors that determine the severity of biological effects are time, distance, and shielding. The absorbed dose decreases rapidly with the square of the distance from the source so that doubling the distance reduces the dose rate to one-fourth of the original level.

The two major forms that a terrorist radiologic attack could take are the dispersal of common radioactive materials used in industry and medicine (cobalt-60, cesium-137, iridium-192), most likely through explosions (*dirty bombs*), and the atmospheric release of large amounts of intense ionizing radiation through the sabotage of nuclear power plants or the detonation of nuclear weapons. Dirty bombs are easy to construct with little training. They could spread contamination over a few city blocks at most and also cause bodily injuries from the blast, as well as fear and panic in the affected population. Actual damage to property and individuals are unlikely to be extensive, and the relatively small area of contamination should be easily monitored and contained for long-term cleanup. Terrorist nuclear events, on the other hand, are considered relatively low risk to occur, because they require significant technical expertise and money to carry out. However, these weapons pose the threat of substantial destruction to property and people over a range of hundreds of miles because of the physical effects of air blast, the thermal and blinding effects of the ensuing fireball, and the intense ionizing radiation thrown into the atmosphere that can spread lethal levels of radioactive fallout over large areas.

Medical treatment of radiologic casualties is largely supportive, consisting of symptomatic care and isolation for the gastrointestinal (nausea, vomiting, diarrhea, bleeding) and hematopoietic (bone marrow depression) manifestations that make up *acute radiation syndrome*. In acute doses of <1.0 gray (Gy) unit (equivalent to 10 rads), the only effects are possible long-term malignancies. Local effects from low-penetration alpha- and beta-particle contamination include thermal burns with erythema, desquamation, and blistering. The effects of whole-body exposure from highly penetrating gamma rays, x-rays, and neutrons are dose and duration dependent and do not cause contamination, and thus they do not require decontamination. Ten gray is considered the highest survivable dose exposure with maximal medical therapy and is marked by the severest gastrointestinal symptoms and blood cell count depression monitored by lymphocyte counts. With doses >10 Gy, symptoms develop within minutes, and in excess of 30 Gy cardiovascular and nervous system collapse cause death in 24 to 72 hours.

There is no "antiradiation" drug. Internal contamination through inhalation, ingestion, or skin absorption can be treated by dilution, blockage, displacement by nonradioactive materials, minimizing absorption, mobilization of renal and gastrointestinal elimination, and chelation. These measures have little overall effectiveness, including bone marrow and stem cell transplantation, or may have some effect only against specific radioisotopes. Potassium iodide does effectively block thyroid uptake of radioactive iodine, which is found after nuclear explosions or spills, but only if given within 4 hours of exposure, and it only has substantial clinical utility for children. External contamination is easily managed by removing clothing and showering with soap and water, which should remove close to 100% of the contamination. The clothing and runoff fluids should be bagged and properly disposed; open wounds that have been exposed to doses >1.0 Gy or contaminated should be scrubbed, debrided, and closed as soon as possible to prevent them from becoming portals for lethal internal contamination; and wound excision should be considered for contamination with long-lived radionuclides (i.e., alpha emitters). External radiologic contamination does not constitute the medical emergency for victims or medical personnel that chemical contamination does and should be considered much the same as dirt—something that is preferably cleaned off by decontamination prior to treatment but should not delay life-saving interventions or lead to suboptimal care in any way. Medical personnel should adhere to standard universal precautions and are not at risk of any significant radiation exposure even with the highest levels of contamination and exposure of casualties.[78–80]

Management of a radiologic disaster should involve proper planning and preparation through personnel training and education, accurate scene and hospital triage, and contact of national government resources for guidance in the recognition and management of radiation exposure[78] Severely injured victims with radiation exposure/contamination should be transported for definitive management to different facilities from those used for victims who are not seriously injured in order to facilitate containment of radiation spread. Procedures for dealing with the stress and psychosocial effects that are inevitable in victims, medical personnel, and the overall population should be established.

Explosive Disasters

Explosive devices have usually been categorized as conventional weapon threats, but the magnitude of force that terrorist bombings have achieved over the past three decades, and the thousands of resulting casualties, clearly demonstrate that these agents are as much weapons of mass destruction as those discussed earlier. Moreover, explosives have by far been the most common weapons used by terrorists historically and therefore remain the most prominent and most likely threat for which we must be prepared in the future. The technology is easily learned, and the cost-effectiveness in relation to the number of casualties and extent of societal disruption is unsurpassed. These considerations have led to an exponential increase in the worldwide frequency of these events over the past few decades.[12,13,24,81] Even within the relatively safe United States, over 30,000 instances of terrorist bombings have occurred over the past 30 years, resulting in thousands of deaths and extensive property damage and economic disruption, and these also continue to increase in frequency.[81–83]

Blast Physics and Pathophysiology

Low-energy explosives release energy slowly in a process called *deflagration*. However, terrorists typically employ high-energy explosives that create a pressure pulse traveling at supersonic speeds of 3,000 to 8,000 m/sec, called a *blast wave*. The edge of this radially propagating wave is called the *blast front*. Blasts begin with a *peak overpressure* phase lasting only a fraction of a second as the blast pressure rises far above ambient air pressure. This instantaneous rise in pressure gives the blast wave the unique characteristic of *brisance*, or shattering ability. This is followed by a more gradual ebbing of pressure that can last up to 10 times longer and ends in a negative pressure as a relative vacuum is created from the initial outward force, into which air and debris can be sucked before returning to atmospheric pressure. *Blast wind* refers to the rapid movements of air back and forth. This negative pressure phase accounts for the *implosion* of surrounding structures and for the creation of tidal waves in the vicinity of large bodies of water.[12,60,84–86]

The severity of injuries to casualties is determined by four factors—the magnitude of the explosive force, the distance from the blast, the location indoors or outdoors, and the surrounding medium of air or water. The magnitude of the explosion determines the destructive force of the peak overpressure. The blast magnitude also dissipates rapidly in proportion to the cube of the distance from it so that moving three times the distance away reduces the force 27-fold. Indoor detonations magnify rather than dissipate the blast wave as it reflects off walls, floors, and ceilings, causing much more damage than open-air blasts.[87,88] Underwater blasts propagate greater distances with longer duration of peak overpressure due to the increased density of water compared with air.

Although several forms of explosives have been used by terrorists, an especially popular one is the ammonium nitrate (simple fertilizer)–based device that is constructed as a fuel–air explosive to create a chain reaction of detonation that greatly magnifies the original blast to reach magnitudes of several tons of TNT equivalence. This is extremely easy to build and execute, which explains why it has been used in several major terrorist bombings (Beirut, 1983; Buenos Aires, 1994; Oklahoma City, 1995; U.N. Headquarters, Baghdad, 2003).[12,81]

There are three major categories of injury imparted by explosions. Primary blast injury is caused by the passage of the blast wave through the body, which results in turbulence, or *spalling*, at air–liquid interfaces, such as the lungs, bowels, eyes, and ears, and subsequent disruption of these tissues. Tympanic membrane rupture is a sensitive marker for primary blast injury.[89] The lung is the most common visceral organ damaged by primary blast effects in air blasts, whereas the bowel is damaged by this mechanism in only the most powerful explosions and most commonly in underwater blasts.[60,85,87] Most victims of primary blast lung injury following terrorist bombings die immediately, as this injury occurs only in those closest to the blast because of the rapid dissipation of the blast wave, thus suffering lethal bodily injury. Only 0.6% of survivors of terrorist bombings have been found to have blast lung, in which group this injury is a marker of severity and high risk of death.[21] A higher incidence of blast lung in bombing survivors tends to occur in urban locations as a result of rapid triage and transport to medical care, allowing those who would otherwise die very quickly to be saved by early ventilatory support.[90] Blast lung is characterized by progressive pulmonary insufficiency, with radiologic and pathologic findings similar to severe pulmonary contusion, and death is caused by massive cerebral and coronary air embolism.[91,92]

Secondary blast injury is caused by the impact of objects set in motion by the blast. Tertiary blast injury involves the displacement of the victim's body to crash into other objects. Both of these forms of blast injury cause the standard forms of blunt trauma that predominate among survivors of terrorist bombings.[21,47,60,87] Secondary blast injury has also increasingly included penetrating trauma in recent years from destructive shrapnel placed in the bombs[18,34,93] and from body parts of suicide bombers that become embedded in victims. A unique and bizarre implication of this latter form of injury to casualties and medical personnel is that these body parts may transmit chronic diseases to the victims, such as HIV, hepatitis, and other infectious diseases, that serve to magnify the level of injury and terror.[37]

Quaternary blast injuries, otherwise called *miscellaneous* blast injuries, are indirect consequences of bombings and include burns, crush injuries, inhalational injuries from dust and toxic chemicals, and ocular injuries.[24,37] Building collapse as a consequence of indoor detonations could be considered in this category.[86] The dissemination of biologic, chemical, or radiologic agents in dirty bombs, or shrapnel, would also fall in this category, and is also

called *combined* blast injury.[13,86] Some have labeled a new category of *quinary* blast injury, which is the pathologic dissemination of toxic chemicals that are incorporated into the explosive charge, which can poison victims through inhalation, ingestion, or skin exposure (Sorkin et al., Poster, unpublished data, Eastern Association for Surgery of Trauma Annual Scientific Assembly, Amelia Island, FL, January 2004).

Patterns of Injury, Mortality, and Severity

Major terrorist bombings result in very consistent patterns of injury and mortality in all published reports.[12,20–22,44,47,58,59,61,62,94–96] The incidence of immediate mortality is related to the magnitude of the explosion, its location (indoors vs. outdoors, urban vs. isolated), and the association with building collapse. Building collapse greatly magnifies the lethality and casualty generation of any explosion, which is why terrorists increasingly place bombs indoors, preferably in large buildings. In the AMIA bombing in Buenos Aires, Argentina, in 1994, involving the collapse of a seven-story building, the immediate death rate of all casualties was 29%, but it was 94% among those within the building.[62] In the terrorist suicide truck bombing of the U.S. Marine barracks in Beirut in 1983, involving the complete collapse of a four-story building housing over 350 men (Figure 16.5), 68% of all casualties were immediately killed.[22,44] In the Oklahoma City bombing of the Murrah Building in 1995, there was only a partial collapse of the building, with an overall immediate death rate of 29%, and 9.6% were critically injured.[20] However, those casualties within the collapsed portion of the building had significantly higher death and severe injury rates than did those not in the collapsed portion (Table 16.7). This was remarkably different from the 3.3% immediate death rate among 574 casualties of the Khobar Towers bombing in Saudi Arabia in 1996, in which there was no building collapse.[97]

Most survivors of terrorist bombings are not critically injured, for the most obvious reason that those with the most severe injuries are immediately killed.[12,21] Trauma to the head, chest, and abdomen, as well as blast lung and traumatic amputation, are the most common body system injuries found in immediate fatalities. The same injuries are found in only a small minority of survivors (10% to 20%), although they contribute significantly to all late deaths among survivors and should be considered important markers of severity that mandate rapid and comprehensive care. The great majority of survivors have noncritical skeletal and soft tissue injuries that are not life threatening and may be delayed in their care for hours to days if necessary in order to maximize casualty flow and immediate care of critical injuries (Table 16.8). The major implications of these patterns for overtriage, and its

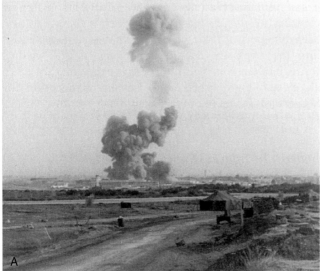

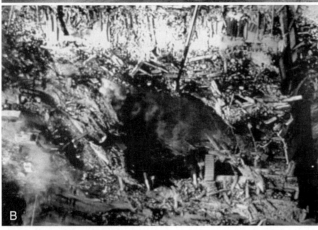

FIGURE 16.5. **(A)** Blast of the suicide truck bombing of the four-story U.S. Marine barracks at Beirut, Lebanon, international airport, October 23, 1983, using an ammonium nitrate–based bomb constructed as a fuel–air explosive, from 1 mile away. **(B)** The resulting complete building collapse with over 350 men inside.

TABLE 16.8. Patterns of injury and mortality in 3,357 victims of terrorist bombings.*

Specific injury	Incidence in immediate deaths (%)	Incidence in survivors (%)	Specific mortality*	% Survivor deaths with specific injury[†]
Head	71	31	1.5	52
Chest	25	2	15	21
Blast lung	47	0.6	11	4
Abdomen	30	1.4	19	21
Traumatic amputation	—	1.2	11	10
Skeletal	—	11	0	0
Soft tissue	—	55	0	0

*Number of survivor deaths with injury/total number of survivors with injury.
[†]Number of survivor deaths with injury/total number of survivor deaths.
Source: Data from Frykberg and Tepas.[21]

adverse impact on survival, were emphasized earlier in the section on triage (see Figure 16.3).

An important consideration for medical management of terrorist bombing casualties is the second hit phenomenon, mentioned earlier in this chapter, that is increasingly inflicted by terrorists to effectively magnify casualty generation. This commonly involves the delayed detonation of a second explosion to injure and kill the predictably large influx of first responders, volunteers, and unwitting onlookers who flock to the scene of the initial explosion. This threat should mandate that responders to a disaster scene be strictly limited and certainly that medical personnel not be allowed at the scene. The delayed collapse of the World Trade Center towers after the initial airline impacts, resulting in the loss of over 400 first responders drawn to the initial event, represents a new iteration of the classic second hit phenomenon that must be anticipated in all disasters to minimize unnecessary loss of life.[12,15,24,28]

Disaster Planning and Reporting

Advance preparations are essential for the success of any disaster response, because disasters occur randomly and unpredictably. Their magnitude additionally requires a response that is organized, rapid, and comprehensive, as well as far more extensive and different than the routine approach used in our daily practice of emergency care. The many disparate elements that comprise an effective disaster response could not possibly function properly without a detailed plan that is accepted by all and is rehearsed on a regular basis.[25,29] These rehearsals must include disaster drills not only within individual hospitals but also in community-wide disaster exercises that integrate regional resources.

TABLE 16.7. Effect of building collapse on morbidity and mortality in Oklahoma City terrorist bombing, 1995.*

Casualty location	No. casualties*	No. dead (%)	No. survivors	No. survivors hospitalized (%)
Collapsed	175	153 (87)	22	18 (82)
Uncollapsed	186	10 (5)	176	32 (18)
Total	361	163 (45)	198	50 (25)

*Includes only 361 casualties who were inside the Murrah Building, stratified by portion of building they were in at the time of the bombing.
Source: Data from Mallonee et al.[20]

All communities and all health care facilities should have plans in place for disaster and mass casualty events, as disasters tend to be local, and communities and hospitals must be prepared to function for several hours to days on their own with no help from outside.[25,36] However, many hospital disaster plans are not realistic or well conceived and are not rehearsed appropriately with frequent drills that are followed by after-action critiques that result in meaningful revisions of the plan.[98]

A realistic disaster plan must be based on the known patterns of behavior and injuries that are abundantly documented in the medical literature, as well as on the many barriers to an effective disaster response that are consistently identified in published reports of actual disasters. Because disasters are so rare, prior experience and mistakes provide the only way to learn how to best respond to future events. However, the fact that the most common critique typically made in the aftermath of most disasters is how useless the existing disaster plan was demonstrates that this planning process is typically not performed appropriately and is not based on valid assumptions derived from widely published reports.[16,42]

Klein and Weigelt[42] reported that the four major impediments to an effective disaster response in a series of three aircraft crashes in Dallas, Texas, were overwhelmed and ineffective communications, unclear lines of authority and responsibility, poor security of the disaster scene and of the hospital, and a disorganized system of medical care for surviving casualties. They found, as so many others have,[18] that there are usually too many physicians trying to help, resulting in paralyzing all care efforts, as well as misguided attempts to enlist the public to help, such as in calls for blood donation.[19,99] The same problems are reported in virtually every major disaster,[10,11] which by itself tends to confirm that we do not learn from the past, allowing the same mistakes to constantly be repeated. The authors emphasized the importance of early postdisaster critiques and debriefings that should result in revisions to the plan designed to avoid future mistakes.

Effective planning requires a large number of different entities to participate who do not normally work together yet whose cooperation is essential for a successful overall disaster response (Table 16.9). The planning process must include firm commitments from all the necessary resources and a firm leadership to guide all entities. The Incident Command System has become the most effective functional structure that allows large-scale disaster responses to work smoothly and effectively, as described earlier in this chapter. Disaster plans must have a built-in flexibility in order to adapt to the many aspects of every disaster that are unique and unpredictable and provide that "imagination" so necessary to anticipate the most unexpected forms of attack. They must incorporate a method for continuing to care for the everyday emergent medical problems that will continue to present while simultaneously dealing with the disaster victims.[99] They must also provide for effective *crisis management*, or the handling of the immediate problems during the initial phases of disaster response, as well as effective *consequence management* of the longer term effects that disasters create that allow recovery to normal conditions. Hirshberg and coworkers[43] have provided scientific evidence from computer modeling that disaster preparedness from effective planning improves casualty care in this setting.

Above all, it is essential that surgeons become integrally involved in disaster planning by participating in their local disaster committees and in hospital disaster drills and community disaster exercises. These activities promote an understanding of the surgeons' proper role in actual disasters and allow their valuable input into an appropriate disaster response. The most common mass casualty disasters that have historically occurred, and thus the most likely to occur in the future, involve casualties with physical trauma in large numbers over short periods of time. This, in fact, is what surgeons are trained to handle and what they actually do on a regular basis every day, albeit on smaller scales.[14,63] Trauma centers, and their complement of surgeons and other acute care providers who commonly manage injured patients, should serve as the ideal template for a regional and national disaster system, in view of their extensive resources and collective experience, as well as their already established liaisons with so many other personnel, agencies, and organizations essential to disaster management (i.e., prehospital assets, transportation, law enforcement, public health, local and state governments).[9,29,35,37] Statewide disaster systems based on regional trauma centers have already been developed for this purpose[100] and should serve as excellent models for larger national systems of disaster preparedness.

TABLE 16.9. Essential elements and participants in disaster planning.

Hospital assets	Community assets
Medical and nursing staffs	Emergency operations center
Administration	Public health department
Security	Prehospital EMS services
Food services	Law enforcement
Hospital incident command (HEICS)	Fire department
Volunteer pool	Search and rescue
Blood bank/laboratory	Media
Imaging services	Transportation/evacuation services
Operating room staff	Area blood banks/Red Cross
Intensive care unit staff	Area hospital representatives
Public information office	Mental health services
Chaplains	Local medical society
Rehabilitation assets	Civil engineers

Critique

With the exception of probably two people (B and E), all will require expeditious medical attention. However, the victim who requires the most immediate intervention is the one who has no vital signs of life and no obvious injuries. Cardiac dysrhythmia is the most common cause of arrest resulting from a lightning strike. Therefore, aggressive cardiopulmonary resuscitation should be done immediately on this person first.

Answer (C)

References

1. Hachiya M. Hiroshima Diary. Chapel Hill: University of North Carolina Press, 1955.
2. Shemer J, Shapiro SC. Terror and medicine—the challenge. In Shemer J, Shoenfeld Y, eds. Terror and Medicine: Medical Aspects of Biological, Chemical, and Radiological Terrorism. Lengerich, Germany: Pabst Science Publishers, 2003; 17–23.
3. American College of Surgeons Committee on Trauma. Disaster management. In Resources for Optimal Care of the Injured Patient. Chicago: American College of Surgeons, 1998; 87–91.
4. Hogan DE, Burstein JL. Basic physics of disasters. In Hogan DE, Burstein JL, eds. Disaster Medicine. Philadelphia: Lippincott Williams & Wilkins, 2002; 3–9.
5. Sheng, CY. Medical support in the Tangshan earthquake: a review of the management of mass casualties and certain major injuries. J Trauma 1987; 27:1130–1135.
6. Lillehei KO, Robinson MN. A critical analysis of the fatal injuries resulting from the Continental flight 1713 airline disaster: evidence in favor of improved passenger restraint systems. J Trauma 1994; 37:826–830.
7. Beyersdorf SR, Nania JN, Luna GK. Community medical response to the Fairchild mass casualty event. Am J Surg 1996; 171:467–470.
8. Vosswinkel JA, McCormack JE, Brathwaite CEM, et al. Critical analysis of injuries sustained in the TWA flight 800 midair disaster. J Trauma 1999; 46:617–621.
9. May AK, McGwin G, Lancaster LJ, et al. The April 8, 1998 tornado: assessment of the trauma system response and the resulting injuries. J Trauma 2000; 48:666–672.
10. Millie M, Senkowski C, Stuart L, et al. Tornado disaster in rural Georgia: triage response, injury patterns, lessons learned. Am Surg 2000; 66:223–228.
11. Cocanour CS, Allen SJ, Mazabob J, et al. Lessons learned from the evacuation of an urban teaching hospital. Arch Surg 2002; 137:1141–1145.
12. Frykberg ER. Medical management of disasters and mass casualties from terrorist bombings: how can we cope? J Trauma 2002; 53:201–212.
13. Ciraulo DL, Frykberg ER, Feliciano DV, et al. A survey assessment of preparedness for domestic terrorism and mass casualty incidents among Eastern Association for the Surgery of Trauma members. J Trauma 2004; 56:1033–1041.
14. Frykberg ER. Principles of mass casualty management following terrorist disasters. Ann Surg 2004; 239:319–321.
15. Waeckerle JF. Disaster planning and response. N Engl J Med 1991; 324:815–821.
16. Quarantelli EL. Delivery of Emergency Medical Services in Disasters: Assumptions and Realities. New York: Irvington, 1983.
17. Sklar DP. Casualty patterns in disasters. J World Assoc Emerg Disaster Med 1987; 3:49–51.
18. Feliciano DV, Anderson GV, Rozycki GS, et al. Management of casualties from the bombing at the Centennial Olympics. Am J Surg 1998; 176:538–543.
19. Mahoney LE, Reutershan TP. Catastrophic disasters and the design of disaster medical care systems. Ann Emerg Med 1987; 16:1085–1091.
20. Mallonee S, Shariat S, Stennies G, et al. Physical injuries and fatalities resulting from the Oklahoma City bombing. JAMA 1996; 276:382–387.
21. Frykberg ER, Tepas JJ. Terrorist bombings: lessons learned from Belfast to Beirut. Ann Surg 1988; 208:569–576.
22. Frykberg ER, Tepas JJ, Alexander RH. The 1983 Beirut Airport terrorist bombing: injury patterns and implications for disaster management. Am Surg 1989; 55:134–141.
23. Murphy MF. Emergency medical services in disaster. In Hogan DE, Burstein JL, eds. Disaster Medicine. Philadelphia: Lippincott Williams & Wilkins, 2002: 90–103.
24. Stein M, Hirshberg A. Medical consequences of terrorism: the conventional weapons threat. Surg Clin North Am 1999; 79:1537–1552.
25. Berry FB. The medical management of mass casualties: the oration on trauma. Bull Am Coll Surg 1956; 41:60–66.
26. Barrier G. Emergency medical services for treatment of mass casualties. Crit Care Med 1989; 17:1062–1067.
27. Plante DM, Walker JS. EMS response at a hazardous materials incident: some basic guidelines. J Emerg Med 1989; 7:55–64.
28. Jacobs LM, Ramp JM, Breay JM. An emergency medical system approach to disaster planning. J Trauma 1979; 19:157–162.
29. Jacobs LM, Goody MM, Sinclair A. The role of a trauma center in disaster management. J Trauma 1983; 23:697–701.
30. Hooft PJ, Noji EK, Van de Vorde HP. Fatality management in mass casualty incidents. Forensic Sci Int 1989; 40:3–14.
31. Goodman, CS, Hogan DE. Urban search and rescue. In Hogan DE, Burstein JL, ed. Disaster Medicine. Philadelphia: Lippincott Williams & Wilkins, 2002; 112–122.
32. Oster NS, Doyle CJ. Critical incident stress. In Hogan DE, Burstein JL, eds. Disaster Medicine. Philadelphia: Lippincott Williams & Wilkins, 2002; 41–46.
33. Hammond JS, Brooks J. Helping the helpers: the role of critical incident stress management. Crit Care 2001; 5:315–317.
34. Almogy G, Belzberg H, Rivkind AI. Suicide bombing attacks: updates and modifications to the protocol. Ann Surg 2004; 239:295–303.
35. Ammons MA, Moore EE, Pons PT, et al. The role of a regional trauma system in the management of a mass dis-

aster: an analysis of the Keystone, Colorado chairlift accident. J Trauma 1988; 28:1468–1471.

36. Einav S, Feigenberg Z, Weissman C, et al. Evacuation priorities in mass casualty terror-related events—implications for contingency planning. Ann Surg 2004; 239:304–310.

37. Stein M, Hirshberg A. Limited mass casualties due to conventional weapons—the daily reality of a Level I trauma center. In Shemer J, Shoenfeld Y, eds. Terror and Medicine: Medical Aspects of Biological, Chemical and Radiological Terrorism. Lengerich, Germany: Pabst Science Publishers, 2003; 378–393.

38. American College of Surgeons Committee on Trauma. Advanced Trauma Life Support, 6th ed. Chicago: American College of Surgeons, 1997.

39. Hirshberg A, Stein M, Walden R. Surgical resource utilization in urban terrorist bombing: a computer simulation. J Trauma 1999; 47:545–550.

40. Sarkisian AE, Khondkarian RA, Amirbekian NM, et al. Sonographic screening of mass casualties for abdominal and renal injuries following the 1988 Armenian earthquake. J Trauma 1991; 31:247–250.

41. Hirshberg A. Damage control for abdominal trauma. Surg Clin North Am 1997; 77:813–820.

42. Klein JS, Weigelt JA. Disaster management: lessons learned. Surg Clin North Am 1991; 71:257–266.

43. Hirshberg A, Scott BG, Granchi T, et al. How does casualty load affect trauma care in urban bombing incidents? A quantitative analysis. J Trauma 2004; 57:446.

44. Frykberg ER, Hutton PMJ, Balzer RH. Disaster in Beirut: an application of mass casualty principles. Milit Med 1987; 11:563–566.

45. Rignault DP. Recent progress in surgery for the victims of disaster, terrorism and war. World J Surg 1992; 16:885–887.

46. Caro D. Major disasters. Lancet 1974; 2:1309–1310.

47. Brismar B, Bergenwald L. The terrorist bomb explosion in Bologna, Italy, 1980: an analysis of the effects and injuries sustained. J Trauma 1982; 22:216–220.

48. Burris DG, Welling DR, Rich NM. Dominique Jean Larrey and the principles of humanity in warfare. J Am Coll Surg 2004; 198:831–835.

49. Llewellyn CH. Triage: in austere environment and echeloned medical systems. World J Surg 1992; 16:904–909.

50. Hogan DE, Lairet J. Triage. In Hogan DE, Burstein JL, eds. Disaster Medicine. Philadelphia: Lippincott Williams & Wilkins, 2002; 10–15.

51. U.S. Department of Defense. Emergency War Surgery. Washington, DC: U.S. Government Printing Office, 1975.

52. Kreis DJ, Fine EG, Gomez GA, et al. A prospective evaluation of field categorization of trauma patients. J Trauma 1988; 28:995–1000.

53. American College of Surgeons Committee on Trauma. Field categorization of trauma patients (field triage). Bull Am Coll Surg 1986; 71:17–21.

54. Boutros F, Redelmeier DA. Effects of trauma cases on the care of patients who have chest pain in an emergency department. J Trauma 2000; 48:649–653.

55. Rignault DP, Deligny MC. The 1986 terrorist bombing experience in Paris. Ann Surg 1989; 209:368–373.

56. Caro D, Irving M. The Old Bailey bomb explosion. Lancet 1973; 1:1433–1435.

57. Tucker K, Lettin A. The Tower of London bomb explosion. BMJ 1975; 3:287–290.

58. Waterworth TA, Carr MJT. Report on injuries sustained by patients treated at the Birmingham General Hospital following the recent bomb explosions. BMJ 1975; 2:25–27.

59. Pyper PC, Graham WJH. Analysis of terrorist injuries treated at Craigavon Area Hospital, Northern Ireland, 1972–1980. Injury 1982; 14:332–338.

60. Cooper GJ, Maynard RL, Cross NL, et al. Casualties from terrorist bombings. J Trauma 1983; 23:955–967.

61. Henderson JV. Anatomy of a terrorist attack: the Cu Chi mess hall incident. J World Assoc Emerg Disaster Med 1986; 2:69–73.

62. Biancolini CA, Del Bosco CG, Jorge MA. Argentine Jewish Community Institution bomb explosion. J Trauma 1999; 47:728–732.

63. Frykberg ER. Disaster and mass casualty management: a commentary on the American College of Surgeons position statement. J Am Coll Surg 2003; 197:857–859.

64. Champion HR, Sacco WJ, Gainer PS, et al. The effect of medical direction on trauma triage. J Trauma 1988; 28:235–239.

65. Cook CH, Muscarella P, Praba AC, et al. Reducing overtriage without compromising outcomes in trauma patients. Arch Surg 2001; 136:752–756.

66. Peleg K, Aharonson DL, Stein M, et al. Terror-related injuries: gunshot and explosion—characteristics, outcomes, and implications for care. Ann Surg 2004; 293:311–318.

67. Briggs SM, Brinsfield KH. Advanced Disaster Medical Response. Boston: Harvard Medical International Trauma and Disaster Institute, 2003.

68. Irwin RL. The incident command system (ICS). In: Auf Der Heide E, editor. Disaster Response: Principles of Preparation and Coordination. St. Louis: Mosby, 1989: 133–163.

69. U.S. Department of State. International Terrorism. Selected documents, No. 24. Government Printing Office, 1986.

70. Inglesby TV, Henderson DA, Bartlett JG, et al. Anthrax as a biological weapon: medical and public health management. JAMA 1999; 281:1735–1745.

71. Eachampati SR, Flomenbaum N, Barie PS. Biological warfare: current concerns for the health care provider. J Trauma 2002; 52:179–186.

72. Arnon SS, Schecter R, Inglesby TV, et al. Botulinum toxin as a biological weapon: medical and public health management. JAMA 2001; 285:1059–1070.

73. Henderson DA. The looming threat of bioterrorism. Science 1999; 283:1279–1282.

74. Green MS, Kaufman Z. Syndromic surveillance for early detection and monitoring of infectious disease outbreaks associated with bioterrorism. In Shemer J, Shoenfield Y, eds. Terror and Medicine: Medical Aspects of Biological, Chemical and Radiological Terrorism. Lengerich, Germany: Pabst Science Publishers, 2003; 81–95.

75. Jenkins BM. Understanding the link between motives and methods. In Roberts B, ed. Terrorism with Chemical and

Biological Weapons: Calibrating Risks and Responses. Alexandria, VA: Chemical and Biological Arms Control Institute, 1997; 43–52.

76. Keim M. Intentional chemical disasters. In Hogan DE, Burstein JL, eds. Disaster Medicine. Philadelphia: Lippincott Williams & Wilkins, 2002; 340–349.

77. National Council on Radiation Protection and Measurement: Management of Terrorist Events Involving Radioactive Material. NCRP Report No. 138. Bethesda, MD: National Council on Radiation Protection and Measurement, 2001.

78. Mettler FA, Voelz GL. Major radiation exposure—what to expect and how to respond. N Engl J Med 2002; 346:1554–1560.

79. Fong FH. Medical management of radiation accidents. In Hogan DE, Burstein JL, eds. Disaster Medicine. Philadelphia: Lippincott Williams & Wilkins, 2002; 237–257.

80. Yehezkelli J, Lehavi O, Dushnitsky T, et al: Radiation terrorism—the medical challenge. In Shemer J, Shoenfield Y, eds. Terror and Medicine—Medical Aspects of Biological, Chemical and Radiological Terrorism. Lengerich, Germany: Pabst Science Publishers, 2003; 335–346.

81. Slater MS, Trunkey DD. Terrorism in America: an evolving threat. Arch Surg 1997; 132:1059–1066.

82. Karmy-Jones R, Kissinger D, Golocovsky M, et al. Bomb-related injuries. Milit Med 1994; 159:536–539.

83. Federal Bureau of Investigation. 1997 Bomb Summary. Bomb Data Center, Washington, DC: U.S. Department of Justice, 1997.

84. Clemedsson CJ. Blast injury. Physiol Rev 1956; 36:336–354.

85. Hill JF. Blast injury with particular reference to recent terrorist bombing incidents. Ann R Coll Surg Engl 1979; 61:4–11.

86. Dire DJ, Gatrell CB. Conventional terrorist bombings. In Hogan DE, Burstein JL, eds. Disaster Medicine. Philadelphia: Lippincott Williams & Wilkins, 2002; 301–316.

87. Candole CA. Blast injury. Can Med Assoc J 1967; 96:207–214.

88. Leibovici D, Gofrit ON, Stein M, et al. Blast injuries: bus versus open-air bombings—a comparative study of injuries in survivors of open-air versus confined-space explosions. J Trauma 1996; 41:1030–1035.

89. Phillips YY. Primary blast injuries. Ann Emerg Med 1986; 15:1446–1450.

90. Gutierrez de Ceballos P, Fuentes T, Diaz P, et al. The terrorist bomb explosions in Madrid, Spain. An analysis of the logistics, injuries sustained, and clinical management of casualties treated at the closest hospital. Crit Care 2005; 9:490–499.

91. Clemedsson CJ, Hultman HI. Air embolism and the cause of death in blast injury. Milit Surg 1954; 114:424–437.

92. Rawlins JSP. Physical and pathophysiological effects of blast. Injury 1977; 9:313–320.

93. Boffard KD, MacFarlane C. Urban bomb blast injuries: patterns of injury and treatment. Surg Ann 1993; 25:29–47.

94. Rutherford WH. Experience in the accident and emergency department of the Royal Victoria Hospital with patients from civil disturbances in Belfast, 1969–1972, with a review of disasters in the United Kingdom, 1951–1071. Injury 1972; 4:189–199.

95. Kennedy TL, Johnston GW. Civilian bomb injuries. BMJ 1975; 1:382–383.

96. Hadden WA, Rutherford WH, Merrett JD. The injuries of terrorist bombing: a study of 1,532 consecutive patients. Br J Surg 1978; 65:525–531.

97. Thompson D, Brown S, Mallonee S, et al. Fatal and nonfatal injuries among U.S. Air Force personnel resulting from the terrorist bombing of the Khobar Towers. J Trauma 2004; 57:208–215.

98. Auf Der Heide E. Disaster Response: Principles of Preparation and Coordination. St. Louis, MO: CV Mosby, 1989.

99. Shamir MY, Weiss YG, Willner D, et al. Multiple casualty terror events: the anesthesiologist's perspective. Anesth Analg 2004; 98:1746–1752.

100. Jacobs LM, Burns KJ, Gross RI. Terrorism: a public health threat with a trauma system response. J Trauma 2003; 55:1014–1021.

17
Principles of Injury Prevention and Control

M. Margaret Knudson and Larisa S. Speetzen

Case Scenario

Because of your leadership in the field of acute care surgery, you are asked to address a group of bicycle enthusiasts who support motorcycle helmets but feel that such a requirement should not be applied to the leisure bicyclist. Which of the following is accurate and should be the theme of your message with respect to use of bicycle helmets?

(A) The helmets can often be obtained at no cost
(B) There is no difference between the two regarding morbidity and mortality
(C) The helmet requirement should not be a legislated requirement but an individual's choice
(D) Helmet use has resulted in significant reduction of bicycle-related head injuries
(E) A task force should be established to investigate the efficacy of helmet protection with cycling

Injuries (both unintentional and intentional) are the leading cause of death among persons aged <35 years and the fourth leading cause of death among persons of all ages in the United States. In the year 2000, 16.3% of the U.S. population or 44.7 million people were treated for at least one injury. The causes of fatal injury are summarized in Figure 17.1. The cost of caring for these injuries comprised 10.3% of the total medical expenditures in the United States in 2000, an estimated $117.2 billion.[1] As staggering as this figure seems, however, the true economic burden of injury is much greater when one considers the value of life lost in premature mortality, loss of patient and caregiver time, nonmedical expenditures associated with disabilities, insurance costs, property damage, litigation, decreased quality of life, and diminished functional capacity.

In all, injuries are the number one public health problem in the United States and are emerging as a major health threat globally. Although organized trauma systems have resulted in a decrease in mortality among patients cared for after injury, more than half of the injury deaths occur before entry into a trauma system. Decreasing these scene deaths can only be accomplished by prevention. Taken together, these facts present a strong case for a national focus on programs that address injury prevention and control.

Basic Principles of Injury Prevention and Control

The field of injury control has been greatly advanced by standardized reporting of "E codes," which assign "intentionality" to the injury. For example, although firearm injuries are a major cause of deaths among adolescents, the approach to reducing youth violence and homicides is considerably different from that required to decrease gun-related teen suicides. The second major advance in this area is the realization that injuries are not "accidents" or random events but that they are, in fact, preventable.

Although medical professionals are most familiar with *tertiary* prevention, that is, acute medical care to improve the outcome of the injury, they should also be advocates for *primary* and *secondary* prevention efforts. Primary prevention aims at preventing the event from occurring at all (such as an automated breath-analyzer that prevents a drunk driver from starting his or her car). Secondary prevention lessens the degree of injury after the event occurs (e.g., deployment of an air bag). The public health approach to injury addresses these three phases of the injury (pre-event, event, and postevent) as well as focuses on the host, the agent, and the environment, as initially outlined by Haddon et al.[2] Additionally, injury control efforts must include the following four major areas:

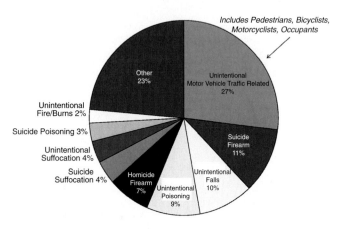

FIGURE 17.1. Top ten causes of fatal injury: all age groups in 2001. (Adapted from Centers for Disease Control and Prevention. Web-based Injury Statistics Query and Reporting System [WISQARS] [online], 2003. National Center for Injury Prevention and Control, Centers for Disease Control and Prevention (producer). Available at www.cdc.gov/ncipc/wisqars.)

- Engineering (examples: countdown lights for pedestrians, helmet designs)
- Enforcement (examples: video cameras to capture red-light runners; primary seatbelt laws)
- Economics (examples: taking cars away from drunk drivers; fines for guns not properly stored)
- Education (examples: public campaigns to promote the use of bicycle helmets, lowering the temperature of a water heater)

With these principles in mind, this chapter addresses the major causes of injury and includes information on what is known and what can be done to control each specific injury. The final section addresses education in injury control and evaluation of injury prevention efforts.

Motor Vehicle Crashes

In 1999, motor vehicle crashes (MVCs) were the cause of more than 42,000 deaths and resulted in more than 4 million emergency department visits.[3] In all age groups, MVCs are the leading cause of death from unintentional injuries and of years of potential life lost. Although major efforts have been made in the area of highway and automobile designs to address safety, the sad fact is that people continue to drive drunk and without restraint devices (Table 17.1).

According to the Centers for Disease Control and Prevention (CDC), more than half of the people involved in fatal crashes were not retrained, and 38% of fatal crashes involve alcohol.[3] Child safety-seat use reduces the likelihood of fatal injury by an estimated 71% for infants and 54% for toddlers, but car seats are frequently utilized improperly or children are riding in the incorrect location

in the car.[4] The addition of airbags as standard equipment in passenger cars has undoubtedly prevented many deaths and injuries, but a recent review has documented that 263 pediatric injuries were caused by the airbag deployment itself, and 159 were fatal.[5] Sadly, only 2% of the children who were injured or killed by airbags were properly secured, suggesting that the proper child restraint and seating position could have prevented the injury.

Seatbelts are the single most effective safety device in preventing serious injury and death in MVCs, but currently only 75% of motor vehicle occupants routinely use restraints. Increasing the national seatbelt use rate to 90% would prevent an estimated 5,536 fatalities and 132,670 injuries and save the nation $8.8 billion annually.[6] Currently, every state but New Hampshire has seatbelt legislation, but only 19 jurisdictions have primary seatbelt laws. "Primary" safety belt laws allow a citation to be issued whenever a law enforcement officer observes an unbelted driver or passenger. "Secondary" safety belt laws require the officer to stop a violator for another traffic infraction before being able to issue a citation for not using a safety belt. "Primary" seat belt laws have been shown to increase safety belt use by 24% in the year following implementation.[7] Thus, strong legislation and enforcement, which are crucially important to the success of safety belt laws, could significantly impact the rates of death and disability after an MVC.

Another area where prevention efforts should be focused is elderly drivers. Projections indicate that by 2050, for the first time in history, the world's population of elderly persons will exceed the population of children.[8] As they age, most Americans plan to remain in their own homes, and access to transportation is essential for the majority of seniors. Surveys indicate that the mode of transportation preferred by most seniors is automobiles. However, as people age, physical changes associated with aging and disease often affect the perceptual, motor, and cognitive abilities required for driving an automobile safely. It is not surprising, then, that older drivers are

TABLE 17.1. Motor vehicle crashes.

What we know	What can be done
• Leading cause of death/disability	• Implement alcohol screening and intervention
• 38% of traffic fatalities involve alcohol	• Enforce severe penalties for drunk driving
• Teens are at highest risk right after obtaining a full license	• Implement graduated licensing for teenage drivers
• 75% of people involved in fatal crashes were not restrained	• Enact primary seatbelt laws and enforce universal child safety/booster seat use
• Drivers 65 years and older have higher death rates per miles traveled than all age groups except teenage drivers	• Improve methods for evaluating elderly drivers

involved in a disproportionate number of traffic crashes. In fact, drivers 65 years and older have higher crash death rates per mile driven than all but teenage drivers, and rates for motor vehicle–related injury are twice as high for older men as for older women.[3] Strategies to address elderly driver safety might include on-road driving evaluations specifically to help older adults make more responsible decisions about continuing or stopping driving and to help them drive safely longer.[8] Another potential method of identifying older drivers at inflated risk of MVCs would be using an off-road simulator.[9] Finally, for drivers at risk, providing acceptable alternative means of transportation might enhance the quality of life for this growing population.

It is common knowledge that teenage drivers are at increased risk of crashing their cars, and recent research has demonstrated that although those driving with a learner's permit are at low risk of crashing, this risk rises dramatically upon initial licensure, with a more than sixfold increase in the risk of crash in the first month of driving without supervision (Figure 17.2).[10] Other high-risk driving situations for teenagers include late-night driving and transporting passengers. To address teenage driving safety, many states have implemented graduated licensing. Graduated licensing is a method of managing initial on-road driving experience, providing new drivers with the opportunity to gain driving experience under conditions that minimize the exposure to risk. As experience and competency are gained, exposure to more demanding situations is phased in. Research has demonstrated that graduated licensing has reduced the overall crash rate among 16-year-old drivers by 27%, with a reduction of injury and fatal crash involvement of 25% (Figure 17.3).[11] Clearly, this is compelling evidence for the adoption or strengthening of graduated driver licensing laws in each state.

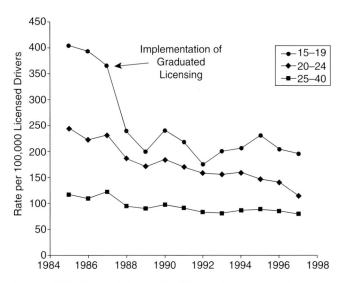

FIGURE 17.3. Rate of driver fatalities and hospitalizations per 100,000 licensed drivers, 1984–1998. (Reprinted with permission of Elsevier from Begg D, Stephenson S. Graduated driver licensing: the New Zealand experience. J Safety Res 2003; 34(1):99–105.)

Pedestrian Injuries

In 2001, nearly 5,000 pedestrians were killed in traffic crashes in the United States, and 78,000 were injured (one person every 7 minutes!).[12] Populations at greatest risk for pedestrian injuries are the very young and the very old (Table 17.2). Children are at particular risk because of their small size (making it difficult for drivers to see them), their lack of understanding of traffic signals, and their inability to judge distances and vehicle speeds accurately. Importantly, children are more likely to be struck outside of intersections as they dart out between cars or jay walk. In addition to improved supervision of children by parents and caregivers, prevention programs that have

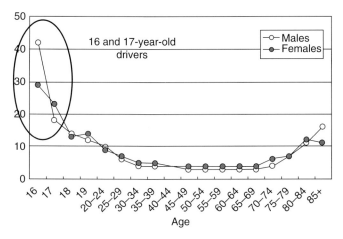

FIGURE 17.2. Driver crash involvement per million miles traveled, 1995. (Reprinted with permission of Elsevier from Williams.[10])

TABLE 17.2. Pedestrian injuries.

What we know	What can be done
• Pedestrians account for 11% of all motor vehicle–related deaths	• Use traffic calming and diversion tactics in high-risk areas
• The elderly are at highest risk of being struck and killed	• Improve signage, signal timing, and illumination at intersections
• Nearly 25% of children killed in traffic crashes are pedestrians	• Provide safe crossings near school zones
• Alcohol is a factor in 50% of adult pedestrian deaths	• Use interventions for problem drinkers
• Hospital charges for pedestrian injuries average $25,000 per victim	• Use surveillance to target interventions that will create maximal impact

had some success with teaching pedestrian safety to children include a desktop virtual reality program designed to educate and train children to safely cross intersections, games that identify risk-taking children most likely to make harmful crossing decisions, and practical roadside pedestrian training of children by volunteers.[13–15]

At the other end of the spectrum, older pedestrian (ages 70+) account for 18% of all pedestrian fatalities and 4% of all pedestrians injured in 2001.[12] In 2000, the death rate for this group was 3.17/100,000 population, higher than for any other age group. Interventions most likely to be successful in decreasing geriatric pedestrian injuries include traffic engineering changes such as traffic-calming measures (roundabouts and speed bumps), strategies to improve road sharing and to separate pedestrians from traffic, and enforcement strategies such as red-light cameras.[3] Identification of high-risk intersections using surveillance data and modifying these intersections with the installation of lights (including countdown timed lights) may also prove valuable.

Finally, although there is a tendency to blame the driver for all pedestrian crashes, the pedestrian is just as likely to be at fault. Although alcohol involvement, either for the driver or the pedestrian, has been reported in 47% of traffic crashes that resulted in pedestrian fatalities, the pedestrian is twice as likely to be drunk when struck.[12] Targeted prevention efforts for the alcohol-impaired driver and the inebriated pedestrian should focus on areas with greater bar densities, greater population and cross-street densities, and areas where low-income families reside.[16]

Nontraffic Injuries in Children

Until recently, national attention concerning motor vehicles and child safety has focused primarily on protecting children as occupants transported in traffic on public roads. However, recent studies suggest that young children are at greater risk in private driveways and parking lots than as occupants of motor vehicles (Table 17.3). The CDC reported that from July 1, 2000, through June 20, 2001, an estimated 9,160 children aged 14 years and younger were treated in U.S. hospital emergency departments for injuries caused by being left untended in or around motor vehicles.[17] By mechanism, these injuries include being left in a car in hot weather, being backed over by a car, being injured while putting the car in motion, being locked in a trunk, and being strangled by power accessories. Sadly, 85% of these deaths occur in children ages 4 years and younger. In another study that included 78 children injured in driveways, 75% were younger than 5 years of age, and 96% of the injuries occurred while the vehicle was being backed out of the

TABLE 17.3. Nontraffic injuries in children.

What we know	What can be done
• In 2002, over 100 children died in nontraffic-related incidents because they were left unattended in and around cars	• Penalize parents/ caregivers for leaving children unattended inside vehicles
• 27% of these deaths resulted from children overheating	• Distribute sensing devices that alarm when a child is left in a car seat and the key has been removed from the ignition
• 50% of the deaths were caused by a child being backed over by a motor vehicle	• Install "backover prevention technology" in trucks, minivans, and other large vehicles
• In rollover incidents, the driver is usually a parent	• Separate play areas from driveways
• The National Highway Traffic Safety Administration does not maintain a database for nontraffic vehicle-related incidents and fatalities	• Require the National Highway Traffic Safety Administration to maintain a database for nontraffic vehicle-related incidents and fatalities
• In 20% of driveway fatalities, a child puts the car in motion	• Educate parents on the dangers of leaving children unattended in and around cars

child's own driveway.[18] All but one of the drivers was related to the child, and 70% involved light trucks and vans as opposed to passenger cars. As might be expected, children run over by small trucks or vans had serious injuries, especially to the head, with 31% requiring admission to the intensive care unit and a 3% death rate. In a similar study of driveway crush injuries, there was a 10-fold higher mortality rate for children under 5 years of age when compared with similar aged children involved in other types of pedestrian crashes.[19] Most parents and caregivers are unaware of the fact that in many vehicles, especially popular sport utility vehicles and trucks, there is a large blind spot located behind the vehicle that cannot be visualized with a standard rearview mirror (Figure 17.4).

This area of pediatric trauma should be a prime target for prevention efforts, which might include data collection on injuries to children in driveways and parked cars, separation of play areas from driveways, improving vehicle designs to include sensing devices that alarm when children are left in car seats when the key is out of the ignition, and improved backup warning devices. The national organization KIDSANDCARS has done much to advocate for improved vehicle designs and to educate the public in this important area of preventable pediatric injuries.[20]

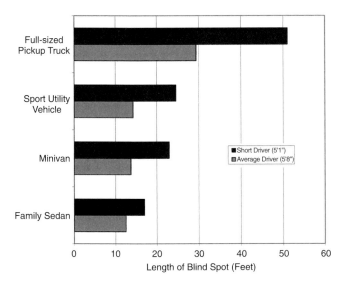

FIGURE 17.4. Lengths of blind spots behind vehicle types. The distance noted is how far behind the vehicle a 28-inch traffic cone had to be placed before the driver could see its top by looking through the rear window. (Data from Consumer Reports. The problem of blind spots: the area behind your vehicle can be a killing zone. March 2004. Available at www.consumerreports.org.)

Motorcycle and Bicycle Helmets

In 1999, 750 bicyclists died in crashes, and more than 25% of these were children.[3] Sadly, more than 95% of the bicyclists killed were not wearing helmets (Table 17.4). It has been clearly demonstrated that helmet use is associated with an 85% reduction in the risk of head injury and an 88% reduction in the risk of brain injury.[21] Armed with this information, investigators from the Harborview Injury Prevention and Research Center launched a mul-

TABLE 17.4. Motorcycle and bicycle helmets.

What we know	What can be done
• If every bicycle rider wore a helmet, 150 deaths and 100,000 nonfatal head injuries would be prevented each year	• Support local, state, and federal legislation regarding bicycle helmet use
• Bicycle helmets reduce the risk of serious head injury by 85%	• Conduct bicycle helmet campaigns
• Only 25% of children ages 5–14 wear helmets	• Provide discount coupons for the purchase of bicycle helmets
• Helmeted motorcycle riders have an 85% reduction in severe brain injuries	• Campaign for universal motorcycle helmet laws in all states
• Universal helmet laws result in near 100% compliance; repealed or partial helmet laws decrease helmet use and increase both injuries and health care costs.	• Educate legislators on the medical and societal costs associated with unhelmeted motorcyclists

tifaceted community-based campaign to increase the use of helmets in the Seattle area.[22] The campaign included information provided to parents and children about helmets in the newspapers, on the radio and the television, in their doctor's office, at school, and at youth groups. Additionally, discount coupons for the purchase of bicycle helmets were widely distributed. These efforts resulted in an increase in helmet use from 1% to 57% by children and to 70% by parents. Additionally, admissions to Seattle-area hospitals for bicycle-related head injuries dropped by two-thirds. Similar efforts are underway in other states, but a universal federally mandated approach to the use of bicycle helmets is clearly indicated.

In 2001, 3,181 motorcyclists died in the United States, and 60,000 more were injured in highway crashes.[23] Head injury is the leading cause of death in motorcycle crashes, and wearing a helmet is the single most important factor in surviving motorcycle crashes. Despite multiple studies demonstrating the reduction in fatalities, serious injuries, and costs associated with a *universal* motorcycle helmet law, many states have either repealed or weakened their helmet laws (e.g., enacted a *partial* helmet law applicable to only riders <18 years). Arguments against helmets are primarily those based on personal freedoms, but some argue that hearing and sight are impaired with the helmet, that they are uncomfortable to wear, or that they increase the incidence of spinal cord injuries. None of these arguments has any scientific backing. Although universal helmet laws result in nearly 100% compliance, partial or no laws decrease helmet use to 50% or less and correlate with higher death rates.[24] Sadly, the high cost of caring for brain-injured motorcycle riders is borne primarily by the public, and these costs underestimate the real impact on society of the productive years lost.[25,26] Enactment and preservation of full motorcycle helmet laws in all areas of the country should be the goal of all public health advocates.

Falls by the Elderly

One in three elderly Americans fall each year, and falls are a leading cause of death in this age group (Table 17.5).[27] Falls typically result in hip fractures or brain injuries, and many elderly patients who suffer nonfatal injuries never return to their preinjury level of function. Factors that may contribute to falls include hazards in the home or nursing facilities (including loose rugs, unsafe stairways, uneven floors, poor lighting, etc.); medications that affect balance; diseases such as stroke, arthritis, and Parkinson's disease; and visual and cognitive impairments.[28] The approach to preventing falls by the elderly must be multifaceted and might include a program of muscle strengthening and balance training, home hazard assessment and modifications, withdrawal of

TABLE 17.5. Falls by the elderly.

What we know	What can be done
• Leading cause of injury death among the elderly	• Carefully assess the home environment for hazards that increase fall risk
• Hip fractures are among the most serious fall-related injuries, and 50% of older people with hip fractures never regain their previous function	• Review medications for those causing hypotension or dizziness
• Falls represent the most common mechanism of traumatic brain injury in the elderly	• Encourage exercise programs to improve balance and strength
• Women are three times more likely to fall than men, but men are more likely to die after falling	• Improve lighting and vision and consider hip pads

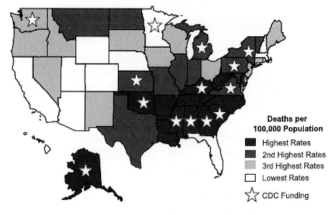

FIGURE 17.5. Unintentional fire and burn-related death rates, United States, 1995–1998. States marked with stars were funded by the Centers for Disease Control and Prevention for 3 years to install smoke alarms in high-risk homes and educate residents about fire safety and the importance of having and practicing an escape plan. (From National Center for Injury Prevention and Control.[3])

psychotropic medications, and nutritional counseling.[29] As the American population ages, fall prevention must take a higher priority among injury-control researchers.

Burns

The United States has the fourth highest fire death rate of all industrialized countries.[30] Approximately 85% of all U.S. fire deaths occur in homes, and smoking is the leading cause of fire-related deaths (Table 17.6).[31] Population-based surveillance studies have identified groups at highest risk for burn injuries and deaths, and these include the elderly, minority groups, low-income populations, and those living in buildings without smoke detectors (Figure 17.5).[32] Although distributing smoke detectors to the high-risk groups would seem a logical prevention strategy, studies have demonstrated that this approach alone has not achieved the desired reduction in fire-related injuries, mostly because few alarms were actually installed and/or maintained.[33] Clearly, educa-

TABLE 17.6. Burns.

What we know	What can be done
• Every 27 minutes someone is killed or injured in a home fire	• Research fire prevention technology, such as long-lasting smoke alarms and residential sprinkler systems
• In 1999, 383,000 residential fires killed 2,900 people and injured 16,050 in the United States	• Support development and distribution of a fire-safe cigarette
• Most fire deaths occur in the home, and 40% involve alcohol	• Promote awareness about residential fires and their prevention
• Residential fires result in $5 billion yearly in property damage	• Standardize water heater temperatures at 120°F
• For every $1 investment in smoke alarms, $69 is saved in fire-related costs	• Cook on back burners and cover electrical outlets when children are in the home

tional efforts promoting awareness about residential fires and their prevention must accompany smoke alarm distribution programs to increase their effectiveness in reducing burn injuries.[34] The value of working smoke alarms and sprinkler systems should also be investigated.

Although only 4% of all residential fires are reportedly caused by smoking materials, the fire fatality rate is nearly four times higher than the overall residential fire rates and injuries are more than twice as likely. Smoking fires typically occur in the early morning when victims are asleep and affect both smokers and nonsmokers alike, particularly children and the elderly. Traditional cigarettes burn continuously even when unattended. However, a fire-safe cigarette is designed to extinguish itself when not actively smoked. In June of 2004, New York State enacted the World's first law requiring hat cigarettes include design alternations to make them fire safe and similar laws are under consideration in other states. Mandating safer cigarettes can have an immediate impact on the morbidity and mortality from cigarette fires. (Additional information on burn prevention can be obtained from the Phoenix Society for Burn Survivors at www.phoenix-society.org.)

Children ages 4 and under are at greatest risk for burn and scald injuries, and preventing such injuries begins with ensuring that the home is child-proof. One simple primary prevention method to guard against scald injuries is to simply turn the water heater temperature down from 140°F (standard) to 120°F. A child exposed to hot tap water at 140°F for just 3 seconds will sustain a third-degree burn[36] Many communities have enacted local ordinances or building codes that require the installation of antiscald plumbing devices. Matches, gasoline, lighters, and all other flammable materials must be locked away and out of children's reach. Children should never be left alone in the kitchen, and, when someone is cooking, the back burners should be utilized and pot handles turned to the back. Additionally, hot foods and liquids should be kept away from the table and counters, especially those prepared in a microwave. Such simple measures can be effective in reducing the estimated 22,600 scald burns among children treated in the United States each year, with a price tag approximating $2.1 billion.

Water-Related Injuries

America is a water-oriented society, and many of our recreational and residential activities involve water. Most pediatric drownings occur in backyard pools, and children gain access through open doors to unfenced pools. According to information from the CDC, however, fencing would prevent only one-fifth of the drownings among children under age 5 years.[3] In addition to the need for constant adult supervision around residential and public pools, it appears that pool covers and alarms in combination with mandatory fencing and community education might be needed to address the 1,000 pediatric drownings that occur each year. African American males aged 5 to 14 years are another high-risk group for drowning, and it has been suggested that training in swimming and water safety in schools might be effective in decreasing drowning rates in this group.[37,38]

A study from Florida found that most drowning victims were engaged in a nonpool-related activity before the incident, most drowning victims could not swim, and most died at the scene.[39] Another investigation revealed that less than 10% of victims of watercraft-related drowning were wearing personal flotation devices, and elevated blood alcohol levels were detected in 44% of those who drowned.[37] Table 17.7 summarizes the prevention efforts

that should be considered to improve water safety and to decrease drowning rates.

Suicide

Suicide is a major public health problem and results in more deaths than homicides. Although females attempt suicide more often than males, males are more likely to succeed (Table 17.8).[40] The elderly are at highest risk for suicide, and factors that might contribute to the feelings of despair in the geriatric population include not only depression but also physical illness, alcohol use, impulsiveness, and help-seeking behavior.[41] Among youths, suicide rates have tripled since 1950, and suicide is now the third leading cause of death in the 15- to 24-year-old group, behind unintentional injury and homicide.[40]

Clearly, the approach to preventing suicide will be different among different populations and ages, but preventing access to guns would dramatically decrease the number of suicide attempts that are successful. Promising prevention strategies for youth suicide include school-based skills training for students, screening for at-risk youths, education of primary care physicians, media education, and lethal-means restriction.[42] Many elderly patients who commit suicide visit a nonmental health provider within the last month of their lives. This finding stresses the important role that primary care providers can play in identifying risk factors for suicide and referring patients with suicidal intentions for treatment.[43] Ongoing studies that will likely impact our understanding of suicide include investigations into the role of alcohol and other drugs in suicide, as well as the effect of prior psychiatric treatment on at-risk individuals. Finally, training for all health and human services professionals (including clergy, teachers, and other community leaders) concerning suicide risk assessment should be a high priority for our society.

TABLE 17.7. Water-related injuries.

What we know	What can be done
• Drowning kills 4,000 people each year; this is an average of 12 people per day	• Promote legislation to mandate pool fencing used together with pool alarms and covers
• Drowning is the second leading cause of death among children ages 1–14 years	• Include training in swimming and water safety in school curriculum
• Alcohol use is involved in 25%–50% of adolescent and adult drowning deaths	• Ban alcohol on boats
• 89% of people who drowned in boating-related episodes were not wearing flotation devices	• Mandate flotation devices for all boaters

TABLE 17.8. Suicide.

What we know	What can be done
• In 2000, suicide took the lives of 29,350 Americans	• Improve recognition and treatment of depression, substance abuse, and other mental illnesses associated with suicide risk
• Suicides outnumber homicides almost 2:1	• Eliminate barriers to the provision of quality mental health treatments
• The groups at highest risk for suicide are adolescents and people ages 65 and older	• Provide school-based screening programs to identify at-risk adolescents
• 57% of suicides involve a firearm	• Reduce gun availability for at-risk groups
• Females attempt suicide more often than males, but males are more likely to succeed	• Work with the media to ensure informed portrayal of suicide

Child Maltreatment

The Childhood Abuse Prevention and Treatment Act identifies four major types of maltreatment: physical abuse, neglect, sexual abuse, and emotional abuse (Figure 17.6).[3] These can be defined as follows:

- *Physical abuse:* infliction of physical injury as the result of punching, beating, kicking, biting, burning, or shaking
- *Child neglect:* failure to provide for the child's basic physical, educational, or emotional needs
- *Sexual abuse:* fondling a child's genitals, intercourse, incest, rape, sodomy, exhibitionism, and commercial exploitation
- *Emotional abuse:* acts of omission by the parents or other caregivers that have caused or could cause serious behavioral, cognitive, emotional, or mental disorders.

As can be seen from Table 17.9, childhood maltreatment is a significant cause of death and disability in the United States and can lead to long-term behavioral problems as the child matures. Although reporting suspected child abuse is mandated by law, physicians and other health care professionals must be trained to recognize signs of abuse because they will likely only be seeing those injuries severe enough to require medical attention. Interventions to promote improvements in parenting skills among high-risk mothers have shown some promise in addressing the issues associated with child maltreat-

TABLE 17.9. Child maltreatment.

What we know	What can be done
• 900,000 children in the United States are at risk for abuse	• Recognize and report suspected child maltreatment
• In 2000, 1,200 children died from maltreatment	• Support programs promoting positive parenting skills
• 25% of infant shaken-babies die	• Evaluate programs aimed at decreasing parental stress
• Abused children are at risk for suicide and adult violent behavior	• Encourage home visits for at-risk children

ment.[44] Another approach to the problem involves home visits during early childhood years for families considered "at risk."[45] Equally important is the development of data collection and tracking systems that will capture all children at risk for abuse, not just those severe enough to come to the attention of child protective services. Finally, strategies aimed at reducing child maltreatment need to be rigorously evaluated as to their effectiveness so that evidence-based best practices can be developed in this area where they are sorely needed.

Intimate Partner Violence

Intimate partner violence is actual or threatened physical or sexual violence or psychological and emotional abuse directed toward a spouse, ex-spouse, current or former boyfriend or girlfriend, or current or former dating partner (including heterosexual and same-sex partners).[3] As can be seen from Table 17.10, women are most often the victims of this type of violence, which may begin as relatively minor injuries but may also escalate into serious injuries and even death. Intimate partner violence may also escalate during pregnancy.

TABLE 17.10. Intimate partner violence.

What we know	What can be done
• 1.5 million women and 834,700 men experience intimate partner violence annually	• Institute staff training and emergency department protocols to increase recognition of intimate partner violence
• Health care costs for intimate partner violence exceed $5.8 billion annually	• Accompany mandatory reporting with the provision of a safe environment
• 32% of all female homicide victims were murdered by an intimate partner	• Emphasize early recognition and intervention before escalation occurs
• Alcohol is associated with violence between partners	• Implement interventions for alcohol abuse
• 324,000 pregnant women experience intimate partner violence each year	• Recognize patterns of abuse injuries in pregnancy

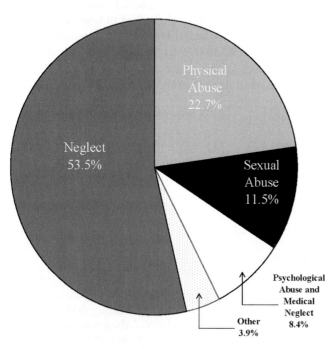

FIGURE 17.6. Types of child maltreatment. (From National Center for Injury Prevention and Control.[3])

Common types of injuries seen include contusions, abrasions, and minor lacerations, as well as fractures or sprains. Any implausible explanation for the injury or an unusual delay in seeking medical care should raise concerns about intimate partner violence. Presentations during pregnancy include injuries to the breasts, abdomen, and genital area; unexplained pain; substance abuse; poor nutrition; depression; late or sporadic accessing of prenatal care; and unexplained "spontaneous" abortions, miscarriages, and premature labor.

Increased awareness by health care providers is the first step in preventing intimate partner violence. A recent survey of internal medicine residents demonstrated that 37% did not screen for domestic violence and that 51% would not document this type of violence.[46] Clearly, educational interventions must be directed at remedying residents' gaps in knowledge and attitudes to improve screening for, documenting, and managing intimate partner violence. Similarly, baseline knowledge about domestic violence among surgeons and emergency physicians has been demonstrated to be poor.[47] On the other hand, after introducing a protocol for enhancing identification of battered women, one emergency department increased the identification of battered women from 5.6% to 30%.[48]

In another study, the Partner Violence Screen, consisting of the following three questions, has been tested recently in the acute care setting and found to detect 65% to 70% of domestic violence victims:

- Have you been kicked, hit, punched or otherwise hurt by someone within the past year? If so, by whom?
- Do you feel safe in your current relationship?
- Is there a partner from a previous relationship who is making you feel unsafe now?[49]

Finally, although detection of intimate partner violence may indeed be increased by education of health care providers, effective interventions must be linked to shelters and treatment programs that ensure the continued safety of the battered partner.[50]

Youth Violence

One of the first steps toward preventing violence, according to the public health approach, is to identify factors that place young people at risk for violent victimization and perpetration. According to the CDC, such factors include

- A history of early aggression
- Beliefs supportive of violence
- Poor monitoring or supervision of children
- Exposure to violence
- Parental drug/alcohol abuse

TABLE 17.11. Youth violence.

What we know	What can be done
- Homicide is the second leading cause of death among 15–19 year olds	- Promote involvement in community violence prevention programs
- Homicide is the leading cause of death among African Americans 15–24 years old	- Identify at-risk youth in emergency departments and trauma centers
- In a recent survey, 20% of high school students reported carrying a weapon	- Encourage school-based programs that include conflict resolution and problem-solving skills
- The recidivism rate in youth violence is at least 20%	- Link at-risk youth with community-based organizations that provide vocational training, drug counseling, and other needed services

- Peers engaged in high-risk behavior
- Academic failure
- Poverty and diminished economic opportunity[3]

Although a comprehensive approach to prevention of youth violence has yet to be developed, a few elementary steps have been made (Table 17.11). The first step is the commitment to participation by medical professionals. A recent survey of trauma surgeons revealed that although 71% of responding surgeons felt that violence prevention should be an integral part of trauma center activity, only 26% of them actually participated in such activities.[51] A position paper from the National Medical Association Surgical Section also challenged trauma surgeons caring for victims of violence to become actively involved in prevention efforts.[52] Intervention early in the cycle of violence will likely be most effective. One randomized control trial among elementary school children that utilized 30 specific lessons to teach social skills related to anger management, impulse control, and empathy demonstrated an increase in prosocial behavior in the intervention group that persisted for 6 months.[53]

Data from our trauma center document recidivism rates of between 16% and 50% among youths with violent injuries.[54,55] To address this problem, a new intervention program that targets patients at risk for repeated violent injuries has been initiated in the hospital. This program links patients with community-based organizations and social services that provide educational and vocational training, anger management skills, and other services once that patient is discharged.[55] Although it is too soon to evaluate the effects of the program in terms of reducing repeated violent injuries, it has been well received by the targeted youths and the targeted community.

Firearm Injuries

Although a comprehensive review of the complex issues of firearm injuries and deaths in American is far beyond the scope of this chapter, certain aspects such as gun safety should be mentioned. As can be seen in Table 17.12, firearms in general, and handguns in particular, are involved in the majority of homicides and suicides in the United States and contribute to a number of unintentional injuries and deaths each year as well. There is a marked and distressing disparity in homicides in the United States compared with other industrialized countries (Figure 17.7). In the United States, only motor vehicle crashes and cancer claim more lives among children than do firearms, and a disproportionately high number of 5 to 14 year olds die from suicide, homicide, and unintentional firearm injuries in states and regions where guns are more prevalent.[56]

It has been well documented that guns kept in the home are more likely to be involved in a fatal or nonfatal accidental shooting, criminal assault, or suicide attempt than to be used to injure or kill in self-defense.[57] Additionally, few handguns are currently equipped with safety devices that can prevent accidental firing, such as a loaded chamber indicator or a magazine safety, which could impact the rate of unintentional gun deaths.[58] Furthermore, many unintentional injuries could be prevented by promoting safe storage of guns in the home, particularly in homes where children and adolescents reside.[59]

As in other areas of injury prevention, changing the product design may be more effective in preventing injuries than trying to change personal behaviors. In that regard, emerging technologies that enable gun manufactures to "personalize" guns could prevent unauthorized users of any age from firing the weapon.[60] Other approaches that aim to reduce firearm violence include

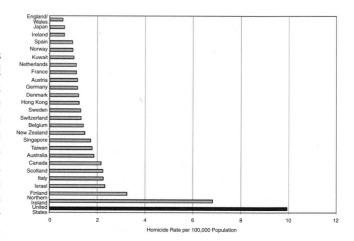

FIGURE 17.7. Homicide rates for 26 high-income countries: report years 1991–1995. (Reprinted with permission of Oxford University Press from Krug EG, Powell KE, Dahlberg LL. Firearm-related deaths in the United States and 35 other high- and upper-middle-income countries. Int J Epidemiol 1998; 27(2):214–221.)

stricter firearm regulations regarding purchasing, selling, and registration of all guns.[61] In certain areas of the country, comprehensive interventions to curb youth violence have significantly impacted the rate of gun injuries in children.[62] Recently, a National Violent Injury Surveillance System was initiated that will provide a true picture of the rate of both fatal and nonfatal firearm injuries in our country by location in order to better target prevention efforts.

Alcohol and Injury

The reader of this chapter will recognize that alcohol is involved to some extent in most injury areas described. Between 20% and 30% of patients seen in U.S. hospital emergency departments have alcohol problems, and nearly half of alcohol-related deaths are the result of injuries from motor vehicle crashes, falls, fires, drowning, homicides, and suicides.[3] Approximately 1.4 million drivers were arrested in 1998 for driving under the influence of alcohol or narcotics, and alcohol-related motor vehicle crashes cost the nation $26.9 billion that year. In one study of patients who fell, those who had consumed alcohol had a higher incidence of head injuries and severity correlated with the blood alcohol concentration.[63] It appears that intoxicated passengers involved in motor vehicle crashes are just as likely as the driver to be reinjured and have an increased mortality rate in the 5 years following the injury.[64] Thus, prevention efforts should be directed at both intoxicated passengers as well as drivers.

TABLE 17.12. Firearm injuries.

What we know in the year 2000	What can be done
• Firearms were used in 16,586 American suicides	• Reduce gun availability for at-risk groups
• Firearms were used in 10,801 American homicides	• Campaign for legislation to require personalized handguns
• Unintentional firearm injuries took the lives of 776 Americans	• Equip firearms with safety devices to prevent accidental discharge
• 75,685 people suffered nonfatal firearm injuries	• Promote legal purchasing and gun registration
• More than 2,200 Americans aged 18 and under died from bullet wounds; this is 6 young people daily	• Promote safe storage of firearms

Source: National Center for Injury Prevention and Control.[3]

In a recent evaluation of 756 consecutive deaths in a Texas trauma center, among unintentionally injured patients, 28% had a positive blood alcohol level; of the 206 patients with intentional injuries, 44% were intoxicated at the time of their death.[65] To date, community-based efforts have focused on alcohol-impaired driving, with random breath testing/sobriety checkpoints, reducing legal blood alcohol concentration of 0.08%, training the servers of alcohol, and enforcing "zero tolerance" laws for teenagers. However, to address all injured patients with alcohol problems, comprehensive screening programs are needed.

There is increasing support for screening programs by trauma surgeons nationwide, and most patients appear motivated to change their drinking habits after being injured.[66,67] A brief intervention that can be easily performed in the acute care setting involving feedback, responsibility, advice, empathy, and self-efficacy has been described and has been demonstrated in a randomized controlled study to reduce recurrent injuries by 47%.[68,69] Alcohol screening and interventions have the potential to significantly impact injury rates in many areas.

Education

A recent study of practicing surgeons and nurses, including those working in trauma centers, demonstrated that most were unaware of the basic concepts of injury prevention (Figure 17.8).[70] Currently, few surgeons receive any formal training in injury control and prevention. Indeed, without proper training, few physicians would volunteer prevention advice to their patients. In another study, pediatric residents who had received intensive training in the use and installation of child safety seats were found to be more likely to discuss their use with

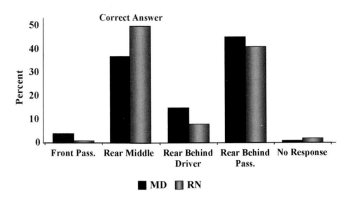

FIGURE 17.8. Physicians' (MD) and nurses' (RN) responses to identifying the safest place in a car for children. (Reprinted with permission of the American College of Surgeons from Knudson et al.[70])

parents than were those residents who had not received this training.[71] Despite this demonstration, only 50% to 60% of pediatric residency programs address injury prevention.[72] In a survey of emergency medicine residents, 97% of respondents believed that injury prevention was pertinent to emergency medicine, but only 44% had received lectures on this topic.[73] Indeed, we agree with Mucha,[74] who stated that trauma "prophylaxis" is the responsibility of every physician. To this end, we are developing a core curriculum for injury prevention and control for medical students, with advanced modules unique to each specialty to be added during residency training. Similar programs should be aimed at nurses, prehospital providers, and the public.

Program Evaluation

Prevention programs exist for nearly every type of unintentional and many intentional injuries. However, there has been a lack of rigorous research and evaluation of the effectiveness of most interventions. Important aspects to consider in an injury prevention program include the following[75,76]:

- Choice of focus area: Are local data being used to determine the type of program appropriate for the region?
- Budget and personnel: Is there a dedicated budget for the prevention program? Are the personnel adequately trained and of sufficient number to carry out the program?
- Has a formative evaluation process been conducted? Included in this evaluation would be a review of materials, an evaluation of how the target population gets information, and an identification of a spokesperson respected by the targeted population.
- Has a process evaluation been conducted? A process evaluation will reveal how well the program is working and problems that occur in reaching target populations; evaluate plans, procedures, and activities; and consider areas that need modification.
- Has an impact evaluation been conducted? An impact evaluation measures changes in the target population's knowledge, attitudes, and beliefs.
- Has an outcome evaluation been conducted? This is an evaluation of the degree to which the program met its ultimate goals, such as reduction of injuries in the targeted area and population.

We have tools to significantly improve the health of the American public by decreasing the burden of injuries. We need now only the commitment and the recognition that injury prevention and control should be in the scope of practice of every health care provider.

Critique

As a health care professional in the acute care setting, you have a responsibility to provide accurate information and counseling to the public, particularly regarding prevention of illnesses and injuries. Significant reduction of bicycle-related head injuries has been documented.

Answer (D)

References

1. Centers for Disease Control and Prevention. Medical expenditures attributable to injures—United States, 2000. MMWR Morbid Mortal Wkly Rep 2004; 53:104.
2. Haddon W, Vailen P, McCarroll JR, Umberger CJ. A controlled investigation of the characteristics of adult pedestrians fatally injured by motor vehicles in Manhattan. J Chronic Dis 1961; 14:655–678.
3. National Center for Injury Prevention and Control. Injury Fact Book 2001–2002. Atlanta, GA: Center for Disease Control and Prevention, 2001.
4. Department of Transportation, National Highway Traffic Safety Administration. Traffic Safety Facts: 1999 Occupant Protection, publication No. DOT HS 809090, 2000. Washington, DC: Department of Transportation.
5. Quinones-Hinojosa A, Jun P, Manley GT, Knudson MM, Gupta N. Childhood injuries to the central nervous system associated with automobile airbag deployment and improper restraints. J Trauma 2005; 59:729–733.
6. Department of Transportation, National Highway Traffic Safety Administration. The Presidential initiative for increasing seatbelt use nationwide, publication No. DOT HS 349. Washington, DC: Department of Transportation, 2001. Available at http://www.nhtsa.dot.gov/people/injury/airbags/bua4thresport/satus.html.
7. Kostyniuk LP, Shope JT. Driving and alternatives: older drivers in Michigan. J Safety Res 2003; 34:407–414.
8. Stutts JC, Wilkings JW. On-road driving evaluation: a potential tool for helping older adults drive safely longer. J Safety Res 2003; 34:431–439.
9. Lee HC, Lee A, Cameron D, Li-Tsang C. Using a driving simulator to identify older drivers at inflated risk of motor vehicle crashes. J Safety Res 2003; 34:453–459.
10. Williams AF. Teenage drivers: patterns of risk. J Safety Res 2003; 34:5–15.
11. Shope JT, Molnar L. Graduated driver licensing in the United States: evaluation of results from early programs. J Safety Res 2003; 34:63–69.
12. Department of Transportation, National Traffic Safety Administration. Traffic Safety Facts, publication No. DOT HS 809 478. Washington, DC: Department of Transportation, 2001.
13. McComas J, Mackay M, Pivik J. Effectiveness of virtual reality for teaching pedestrian safety. Cyperpsychol Behav 2003; 5:185–190.
14. Hoffrage U, Weber A, Hertwig R, Chase VM. How to keep children safe in traffic: find the daredevils early. J Exp Psychol Appl 2003; 9:249–260.
15. Thomson J, Whelan K. A Community Approach to Road Safety Education Using Practical Training Methods: The Drumchapel Project. Road safety research report No. 3. London: Department of Transport, 1997.
16. LaScala EA, Johnson FW, Gruenewald PJ. Neighborhood characteristics of alcohol-related pedestrian injury collisions: a geostatistical analysis. Prev Sci 2001; 2:123–134.
17. Centers for Disease Control and Prevention: Injuries and deaths among children left unattended in or around motor vehicles, United States, July 2000–Jun 2001. MMWR Morbid Mortal Wkly Rep 2002; 52:570–572.
18. Nadler ER, Courcoulas AP, Gardner MJ, Ford HR. Driveway injuries in children: risk factors, morbidity and mortality. Pediatrics 2001; 108:326–328.
19. Patrick DA, Bensard KK, Moore EE et al. Driveway crush injuries in young children: a highly lethal devastating and potentially preventable error. J Pediatr Surg 1998; 33:171–175.
20. www.KIDSANDCARS.org.
21. Thompson RS, Rivara FP, Thompson DC. A case–control study of the effectiveness of bicycle safety helmets. N Engl J Med 1989; 320:1361–1367.
22. Rivara FP, Thompson DC, Thompson RS. Bicycle helmet use: it's time to use them. BMJ 2000; 321:1035–1036.
23. NHTSA. Costs of injuries resulting from motorcycle crashes: a literature review. Available at http://www.nhtsa.dot.gove/people/injury/pedbimot/motorcycle/overview.html.
24. Branas CC, Knudson MM. Helmet laws and motorcycle death rates. Accid Anal Prev 2001; 33:641–648.
25. Max W, Stark B, Root S. Putting a lid on injury costs: the economic impact of the California motorcycle helmet law. J Trauma 1998; 45:550–556.
26. McSwain NE, Belles A. Motorcycle helmets—medical costs and the law. J Trauma 1990; 30:1189–1199.
27. Hornbrook MC, Stevens VT, Winfield DJ, et al. Preventing falls among community-dwelling older persons: results from a randomized trial. Gerontologist 1994; 34:16–23.
28. Nevitt MC, Cumming SR, Kidd S, Black D. Risk factors for recurrent nonsyncopal falls: a prospective study. JAMA 1989; 261:2663–2668.
29. Gillespie L, Gillespie W, Robertson M, et al. Interventions for preventing falls in elderly people. Cochrane Database Syst Rev 2003; 4:CD000340.
30. International Association for the Study of Insurance Economics. The World Fire Statistics: Annual Report to the UN Committee on Human Settlements. Geneva, Switzerland: The International Association, 2001.
31. Ahrens M. The U.S. Fire Problem Overview Report: Leading Causes and Other Patterns and Trends. Quincy, MA: National Fire Protection Association, 2001.
32. Istre GR, McCoy MA, Osborn L, et al. Deaths and injuries from house fires. N Engl J Med 2001; 344:1191–1196.
33. DiGuiseppi C, Roberts I, Wade A, et al. Incidence of fires and related injuries after giving out free smoke alarms: cluster randomized controlled trials. BMJ 2002; 325:995.

34. Mallonee S. Evaluating injury prevention programs: the Oklahoma City smoke alarm project. Future Child 2000; 10:164–174.

35. Barillo DJ, Brigham PA, Kayden DA, et al. The fire-safe cigarette: a burn prevention tool. Burn Care Rehabil 2000; 21:162–164.

36. The National SafeKids Campaign. Available at www.safekids.org.

37. Browne ML, Lewis-Michl EL, Stark D. Unintentional drownings among New York State residents; 1988–1994. Public Health Rep 2003; 118:448–458.

38. Asher KN, Rivara FP, Felix D, et al. Water safety training as a potential means of reducing risks of young children drowning. Inj Prev 1995; 1:228–233.

39. Rowe MI, Arango A, Allington G. Profile of pediatric drowning victims in a water-oriented society. J Trauma 1997; 17:587–591.

40. Starling SP, Boos S. Core content for residency training in child abuse and neglect. Child Maltreat 2003; 8:242–247.

41. Oslin DW, Zubritsky C, Brown G, et al. Managing suicide risk in late life: access to firearms as a public health risk. Am J Geriatr Psychiatry 2004; 12:30–36.

42. Gould MS, Greenberg T, Velting DM, Shaffer D. Youth suicide risk and preventive interactions: a review of the past 10 years. J Am Acad Child Adolesc Psychiatry 2003; 42:386–405.

43. The Institute of Medicine: Reducing Suicide: A National Imperative. Washington, DC: National Academy Press, 2002.

44. Peterson L, Tremblay G, Ewigman B, Saldana L. Multilevel selected primary prevention of child maltreatment. J Consult Clin Psychol 2003; 7:610–612.

45. Hahn RA, Bilukha O, Crosby A, et al. First reports evaluating the effectiveness for preventing violence: early childhood home visitation. MMWR Morbid Mortal Wkly Rep 2003; 52:1–9.

46. Varjavand N, Cohen DG, Gracely EJ, Novack DH. A survey of residents' attitudes and practices in screening for, managing and documenting domestic violence. J Am Med Women's Assoc 2004; 59:48–53.

47. Davis JW, Kaups KH, Campbell SD, Parks S. Domestic violence and the trauma surgeon: results of a study on knowledge and education. J Am Coll Surg 2000; 191:347–353.

48. McLeer SV, Answar R. A study of battered women presenting in an emergency department. AJPH 1989;79:65–66.

49. Feldhaus KM, Koziol-McLain J, Amsburg HL, et al. Accuracy of 3 brief screening questions for detecting partner violence in the emergency department. JAMA 1997; 277:1357–1361.

50. Sisley A, Jacobs LM, Poole G, et al. Violence in American: a public health crisis—domestic violence. J Trauma 1999; 46:1105–1113.

51. Tellez MG, Mackersie RC. Violence prevention involvement among trauma surgeons: descriptions and preliminary evaluation. J Trauma 1996; 40:602–608.

52. Cornwell EE, Jacobs L, Walker M, et al. National Medical Association surgical section position paper on violence prevention. JAMA 1995; 273:1788–1789.

53. Grossman DC, Nackerman HJ, Koepsell TE, et al. Effectiveness of a violence prevention curriculum among children in elementary school: a randomized controlled trial. JAMA 1997; 277:1605–1611.

54. Tellez MG, Mackersie RC, Morabito D, et al. Risks, costs and the expected complication of re-injury. Am J Surg 1995; 170:660–663.

55. Dicker R. The Wrap Around Project. Personal communication.

56. Miller M, Azrael D, Hemenway D. Firearm availability and deaths, suicide and homicide among 5–14 year olds. J Trauma 2002; 52:267–274.

57. Kellermann AL, Somes G, Rivara FP, et al. Injuries and deaths due to firearms in the home. J Trauma 1998; 45:263–267.

58. Vernick JS, Meisel ZF, Teret SP, et al. "I didn't know the gun was loaded"; an examination of two safety devices that can reduce the risk of unintentional firearm injuries. J Public Health Policy 1999; 20:427–440.

59. Ismarch RB, Reza A, Ary R, et al. Unintended shooting in a large metropolitan area: an incident-based analysis. Ann Emerg Med 2003; 41:10–17.

60. Teret SP, Culross PL. Product-oriented approaches to reducing youth gun violence. Future Child 2002; 12:118–131.

61. The Violence Prevention Task Force of the Eastern Association for the Surgery of Trauma. Violence in America: a public health crisis—the role of firearms. J Trauma 1995; 38:163–168.

62. Durkin MS, Kuhn L, Davidson LL, et al. Epidemiology and prevention of severe assault and gun injuries in children in an urban community. J Trauma 1996; 41:667–673.

63. Johnston JJ, McGovern SJ. Alcohol related falls: an interesting pattern of injuries. Emerg Med J 2004; 21:185–188.

64. Schermer CR, Qualls CR, Brown CL, Apodaca TR. Intoxicated motor vehicle passengers: an overlooked at-risk population. Arch Surg 2001; 136:1244–1248.

65. Stewart RM, Myers JE, Dent DL, et al. Seven hundred fifty-three consecutive deaths at a level 1 trauma center: the argument for injury prevention. J Trauma 2003; 54:66–70.

66. Schermer CR, Gentilello LM, Hoyt DB, et al. National survey of trauma surgeons' use of alcohol screening and brief interventions. J Trauma 2003; 55:849–856.

67. Apodaca TR, Schermer CR. Readiness to change alcohol use after trauma. J Trauma 2003; 54:990–994.

68. Dunn CW, Donovan DM, Gentilello LM. Practical guidelines for performing alcohol interventions in trauma centers. J Trauma 1997; 42:299–303.

69. Gentilello LM, Rivara FP, Donovan DM, et al. Alcohol interventions in a trauma center as a means of reducing the risk of injury recurrence. Ann Surg 1999; 230:478–483.

70. Knudson MM, Vassar MJ, Straus EM, et al. Surgeons and injury prevention: what you don't know can hurt you. J Am Coll Surg 2001; 193:119–124.

71. Tender J, Taft C, Mickalide A, Gitterman B. Pediatric residents' buckle up [abstract]. In Harris BH, ed. Progress in Pediatric Trauma, 4th ed. Colorado Springs, CO: Memorial Hospital Press, 2000: 187.

72. Zavoski IW, Burke GS, Lapidus GD, Banco LI. Injury prevention training in pediatric residency programs. Arch Pediatric Adolesc Med 1996; 150:1093–1096.

73. Anglin D, Hutson HR, Kyriacou DM. Emergency medicine residents' perspectives on injury prevention. Ann Emerg Med 1996; 28:31–33.

74. Mucha P. Trauma prophylaxis: every physician's responsibility. Mayo Clin Proc 1986; 61:388–391.

75. Thompson RS, Sacks JJ. Evaluating an injury intervention or program. In Rivara FR, Cummings P, Koepsell TD, Grossman DC, Maier RV, eds. Injury Control: A Guide to Research and Program Evaluation. Cambridge, UK: Cambridge University Press, 2001; 196–216.

76. Centers for Disease Control and Prevention. Demonstrating Your Program's Worth. Atlanta: NCIPC, 1998.

18
Education: Surgical Simulation in Acute Care Surgery

Lenworth M. Jacobs and Karyl J. Burns

Case Scenario

As a member of the Residency Review Committee, you are asked to consider mandating the incorporation of simulation training into the educational curriculum for all surgical programs, particularly acute care surgery training. Which of the following should likely guide your decision?

(A) The transference effect of simulation training is well established in surgery
(B) The high-tech simulators have been validated
(C) Low-tech simulation training should be required for all programs
(D) The utilization of simulation centers by residents is high
(E) Mandatory scheduled simulation training on site does not count when calculating the 80-hour duty limitation for resident trainees

This chapter describes simulation education with a focus on education for acute care surgery for trauma. It begins with a discussion of the advances made in the aviation industry and in anesthesiology. The various classifications of simulators used in surgical education are reviewed, as are the educational principles that guide education in general and those specific to simulation. Specific types of simulation in surgery are discussed. Finally, an exemplar of a simulation course for trauma surgery is presented. This example provides detail regarding the development and implementation of a simulation education program.

Simulators and various models are a means to deliver simulation education. Krummel[1] defines simulation as "a device or exercise that enables the participant to reproduce or represent, under test conditions, phenomena that are likely to occur in actual performance." Simulation education is education that uses some form of simulation or a simulator to achieve educational objectives. Typically the educational objectives are designed so that the student achieves a designated level of performance. This performance is usually specified to denote competence. Competence refers to safe and adequate action to achieve a goal. Perhaps the best known example of the use of simulation education is in the aviation industry where there is a long history of simulator use.

Aviators at the turn of the twentieth century realized that there was a need to standardize the education and training necessary to produce safe, competent pilots. In 1929, Link developed the early prototype simulation trainer. The purpose of this device was to educate prospective pilots on how an aircraft took off, maintained itself in flight, and landed. The initial concept was that of teaching novice pilots how to safely fly an aircraft. This concept progressed to teaching pilots how to fly different types of aircraft. The first concept was to take a novice pilot and develop competency in a simulated environment to the point that the novice could safely fly a real aircraft. The second concept was to take experienced pilots who had the necessary competence and skills to fly an aircraft and allow them to transition to a different type of aircraft or a different complexity of aircraft. This education was provided using simulators, and the experienced pilot progressed from competence in the initial aircraft to full competence in a new aircraft.

The next level of evolution was put in place once a pilot gained competence in basic flying skills. The simulated environment then produced numerous negative aviation problems and educated the pilot as to how to deal with these problems in a simulated environment. A number of examples of the kinds of situations the pilots experienced in a simulation environment were loss of an engine, a fire in the engine or in the cockpit, landing gear failure, an aileron failure, and tail assembly failure. These rare situations were presented to the pilot in a simulated environment, and the pilot had to develop a method to safely manage the negative event.

Simulation was further honed with a military aviation simulation model. Not only did pilots have to learn to fly the aircraft competently, but they also were required to gain competence in aerial combat. A simulation model evolved to include multiple operating systems such as guns, missiles, and bombs. The complexity of all of these systems was so great that different functions had to be assumed by different team members. This concept then developed to include a copilot, a bombardier, a weapons officer, and a navigator. All members of the team were integrated into a coordinated group. The simulated environment was an excellent one to teach all members of the team how to function effectively and harmoniously in all kinds of hostile environments. This concept has matured into the Cockpit Resource Management (CRM) model.

The CRM model emphasizes teamwork and communication among members of the cockpit.[2] This concept has been expanded to now include all team members that the pilot must interact with to manage a flight. These include ground and cabin personnel and traffic control. To reflect the new configuration, "CRM" now refers to Crew Resource Management. Helmreich and Schäfer[2] point out that anesthesiologists saw similarities between crew training and the practice of anesthesia and that the cockpit and operating room require a similar type of training. This prompted the development of Anesthesia Crisis Resource Management (ACRM).[3]

Anesthesiologists have effectively implemented an example of the evolution of simulated education. For example, they identified the anatomic and physiologic criteria that predict a difficult airway and required students to competently perform the task of intubation and avoid consequences of an incorrect intubation in a simulated environment. Management of other rare but fatal physiologic conditions such as malignant hyperthermia that need to be identified, diagnosed, and treated are taught using simulation education. Such experience helps to ensure that anesthesiologists successfully manage events that they may see only once in a career.

Several factors led surgical educators to implement simulation education. Reduced training hours for surgeons and the additional minimally invasive procedures that need to be learned have prompted surgical educators to incorporate simulation education into training programs. This ranges from the use of a simple simulator to teach intravenous insertion to complex procedures to performing an entire operation or managing a team during a trauma activation.

Classifications of Simulators/Simulations

Satava[4] proposed a taxonomy for simulators for surgical education. He classifies simulators according to four levels of skill to be practiced or taught using the simulator. The simplest type of simulators requires "precision placement" or a single motion. An example would be a latex arm for intravenous needle insertion. "Simple manipulation" simulators are more complex. They require basic skills but can offer a variety of situations in which manipulation of the instrument is required to achieve the goal of the task. An example is guiding a catheter, an endoscope, or some other instrument. "Complex manipulation" simulators require the performance of a single complex task. The models represent the visual and haptic presentation of tasks such as sewing an anastomosis or debriding a wound. Simulators for "integrated procedures" require the student to perform multiple tasks to accomplish a complete procedure. As described by Satava,[4] this might require the use of surgical skills such as cutting, dissecting, and sewing an anastomosis. He identifies three types of integrated simulators. These are virtual reality, mannequins, and hybrids of mannequins and virtual reality.

Another classification system has been proposed by Torkington et al.[5] This system bases simulation on the types of materials that are used in the simulation:

- Inanimate artificial tissues and organs
- Fresh tissue or animals
- Virtual reality and computers
- Moulage, where a situation is simulated and an actor plays the role of the patient in appropriate makeup

Helmreich and Schafer,[2] when comparing simulation in medicine and aviation, describe three levels of simulation training in medicine based on complexity of the task or tasks and the degree of coordination and integration of the medical team that is required. The first level is part-task simulation in which only a part of an "array of tasks" needs to be performed, such as intubating a patient. A second level of simulation recognized by these authors is Anesthesia Crisis Resource Management (ACRM),[3] which teaches critical events with a partial team. This level uses an instrumented mannequin as the patient and surgical personnel to act as the surgeon and operating room nurses. ACRM presents students with scenarios of crises situations that must be managed. The third level of simulation proposed by Helmreich and Schäfer[2] is Team-Oriented Medical Simulation (TOMS). This type of simulation is similar to ACRM except that the entire team of operating room personnel who are responsible for the care and disposition of the patient are involved in the simulation.

Goals of Simulations

The goals of simulation education exercises are to

- Increase competence in performing a skill or task
- Uncover errors during the performance of a task
- Allow the learner to discover the consequences of the error
- Allow the student to learn from his or her mistakes
- Correct the errors
- Practice the correct procedure
- Allow the learner to be exposed to uncommon complex difficult events that have the potential for disastrous consequences
- Develop confidence in performance of tasks and skills
- Develop multitasking teamwork skills

Educational Principles

Regardless of the type or class of simulation that is presented to the student, the principles of educational theory should guide the learning activity. Simulation education needs to be grounded in the entire curriculum. It cannot stand alone but must be fully integrated into the entire program of study.[4,6] This will allow for repetitive practice to promote the development of expertise over time. Issenberg et al.[6] point out that it is deliberate practice over a long period of time that separates elite performers from other less capable performers. Simulation offers opportunities for deliberate and repetitive practice.

Education Objectives

Simulation education should be used when it is the most appropriate method to achieve educational objectives.[7] In particular, simulators should not be used when other effective but less costly methods can be used. However, simulators should be used when harm to the patient is considered a possibility. Therefore, until a student has demonstrated a minimal level of competency, the student will need to receive instruction and practice with the simulator.

The educational objectives for a simulation must be explicitly stated. The exact behaviors that must be performed by the student must be identified. Murray and Henson[7] point out that educational activities using simulators are best for teaching the higher levels of cognitive knowledge. These are analysis, synthesis, and evaluation, as described by Bloom.[8] Therefore, the educational objectives of the simulation activity should reflect these levels of knowledge. This does not imply that technical skill or affective attributes are not involved. The practice of surgery requires the integration of cognitive, affective, and psychomotor skills.

Bloom[8] describes analysis as "the breakdown of the material into its constituent parts and detection of the relationships of the parts and of the way they are organized." Synthesis is defined as "the putting together of elements and parts to form a whole. This is a process of working with elements, parts, etc., and combining them in such a way as to constitute a pattern or structure not clearly there before."[8] Evaluation, the highest level of cognitive knowledge, is "the making of judgments about the value, for some purpose, of ideas, works, solutions, methods, material, etc. It involves the use of criteria as well as standards for appraising the extent to which particulars are accurate, effective, economical, or satisfying."[8] Educational objectives should be written to achieve learning at these levels. Similarly, evaluation methods must test these higher cognitive levels. Murray and Henson[7] suggest that these higher cognitive abilities are called upon when objectives use words such as "manage," "diagnose," "treat," and "adjust." Objectives that ask the student to merely "define," "recognize," "list," or "explain" are not suitable to simulation education and can be taught with less resource-intensive teaching methods.[7] Table 18.1 lists the higher level surgical skills.

TABLE 18.1. Examples of surgical skills at the higher cognitive levels.

Analysis: diagnosing an injury
  Must know what investigations to order
  Must recognize interruption of anatomy and physiology
  Requires ability to see the elements of the anatomy and physiology and their relationships

Synthesis: creating a repair
  Although repairs may be standard, some creativity may be involved to repair complex injuries
  Procedures may need to be combined and or modified

Evaluation: assessing the quality of the repair
  Determine the need for additional interventions
  Plan subsequent treatments.

Note: Analysis, synthesis, and evaluation are described further in Bloom.[8]

Teaching Strategies

Teaching strategies need to be designed to help the student achieve the educational objectives. In surgical education, objectives are usually aimed at the acquisition of certain cognitive, affective, and psychomotor skills and the integration of these three domains; students should know the proper application of certain techniques and procedures and adopt and perform these behaviors with confidence. Feeling confident promotes the adoption of new behaviors into one's repertoire.

A useful theory to frame the education and training of surgeons is Social Cognitive Theory.[9] A central construct of this theory is self-efficacy. Self-efficacy refers to "people's judgments of their capabilities to organize and execute courses of action required to attain designated types of performances."[9] People who have high levels of perceived self-efficacy readily and successfully accomplish tasks. Those with low levels avoid tasks or easily give up. Certainly surgeons must organize and execute complex actions to effect safe and adequate patient care. Therefore, teaching strategies should be directed at increasing students' perceived self-efficacy for the desired surgical skills. Bandura[9] describes four methods to increase self-efficacy. The most effective way is through "enactive attainment" or being successful at the task. A second way is through "vicarious experience" where a learner witnesses someone else being successful. Yet another way is through "verbal persuasion" where a learner is encouraged by another that success is achievable. Finally, people rely upon their "physiologic state" to provide perceptions of personal efficacy. Interpretation of somatic arousal in stressful situations can lead to debilitation and the inability to perform. Conversely, the maintenance of a calm state can reinforce capability and lead to success.

Teaching situations and activities should be structured so as to apply these four methods of increasing students' self-efficacy for the desired behaviors. Simulation education is particularly useful for providing opportunity for enactive attainment. With simulation, students can practice repeatedly until they are successful. Vicarious experience can be obtained by viewing media of someone else being successful, seeing fellow students achieve success during the simulation, or having the instructor demonstrate what needs to be done. Instructors can, and should, provide verbal persuasion by acting as cheerleaders. They need to offer their confidence that the students can be successful. Finally, instructors need to redirect any of the students' negative physiology. This means employing stress management techniques, breaking the task into smaller components to permit success, and pointing out previous successes. Qualified instructors are a requisite for any education activity.

Principles of Simulation Education

Simulation education activities need to adhere to the principles that guide this type of learning activity.[10] First, as with any educational endeavor, the objectives must be clearly specified, with identification of the exact behaviors that the students must perform successfully. Criteria for success must be determined. Next, students must be prepared for the simulation. They need to know what will happen, what is expected of them, what the role of the instructor is, what the roles of other students are, and what behaviors are acceptable during and after the simulation. The simulation must be designed to be plausible and true to life (Figure 18.1). Complexity should be based on the level of the learner. If scenarios are not preprogrammed, they must be developed to meet standard practice. The information for the development of the scenarios and the treatment methods should be derived from peer review and published documents to give credibility to the educational and therapeutic management protocols. The treatment algorithms must be correct, plausible, and have reproducible, reliable outcomes. A panel of experts can be helpful in determining that scenarios meet these criteria.

Finally, debriefing and feedback are critical components of the simulation exercise. Debriefing and feedback are necessary to help students assess their performance, identify strengths and weaknesses, and identify areas for further practice or future learning (Figure 18.2).

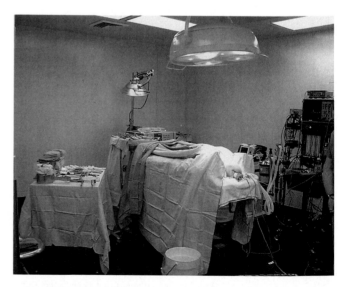

FIGURE 18.1. The simulation environment should be true to life as depicted in this operating room. (Reproduced with permission from Jacobs LM, Gross R, Luk S, eds. Advanced Trauma Operative Management: Surgical Strategies for Penetrating Trauma. Copyright © 2004 by Cine-Med, Inc., Woodbury, CT.)

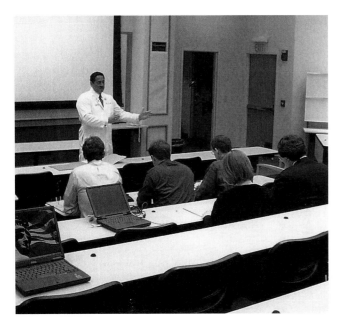

FIGURE 18.2. Debriefing and feedback are critical components of simulation education. (Reproduced with permission from Jacobs LM, Gross R, Luk S, eds. Advanced Trauma Operative Management: Surgical Strategies for Penetrating Trauma. Copyright © 2004 by Cine-Med, Inc., Woodbury, CT.)

Evaluation

Evaluation of learning should assess progress in the cognitive, affective, and psychomotor domains. Each educational objective needs to be evaluated to determine student achievement.

Knowledge can be assessed with multiple-choice tests, essay tests, or verbal responses. A multiple-choice test must be carefully prepared. Only one option should be correct. The stem and options must be grammatically correct. Questions that require the student to draw only on memory should be avoided. Essay and verbal responses are perhaps better suited to assessing the higher cognitive levels of analysis, synthesis, and evaluation. However, these can be time consuming to correct. For essay and verbal responses, the explicit criteria that must be met by the students need to be developed beforehand. Answer content must consider the correct sequence and timing of events. Content of examinations, in the form of multiple-choice essay, or verbal response, must reflect knowledge and practice that is current and standard.

For the affective domain, self-efficacy can be assessed. Self-efficacy provides the "most comprehensive understanding of the interplay of cognition, affect and behavior."[11] It can be assessed with instruments designed to quantify latent constructs.[11] Texts to develop such instruments should be consulted. However, the evaluator must keep in mind that self-efficacy judgments are best made for specific tasks and not global performances.[9]

The psychomotor domain is particularly important in surgical education. It is also difficult to assess, and no one method appears to be superior. However, attention to certain principles, some already mentioned, can help. Evaluation will typically take place in a laboratory environment where performance will be evaluated with a simulator or animal model. Again, the evaluation of psychomotor skill must coincide with the educational objectives. Here a set of critical behaviors that must be performed and the sequence of their performance must be available. A reference list can help. Students can be evaluated as to the degree of assistance that is required for them to complete a task. For instance, one point would be awarded if the student could not perform the task. Two points would be given if help was needed. Three points would indicate that the student performed the task independently. The score for all the tasks would then be summed to provide an overall score for the psychomotor portion of the simulation exercise.

Validity of Simulation

Simulation education must be documented to produce the expected outcomes of the educational process. Paisley et al.[12] state that surgical performance, with the use of a simulator, should

- Show a positive correlation with the experience of the trainee
- Improve with training
- Discriminate between groups who are expected to have low levels of surgical skill and those expected to have high levels of surgical skill

Assessing the validity of simulation as a teaching method requires that reliable and valid instruments be used to assess teaching outcomes. Validity of an instrument refers to its ability to accurately measure what it is suppose to measure.[13] Support for the validity of content should be sought from a panel of experts as to whether this is an instrument to assess the cognitive, affective, or psychomotor domains. For knowledge tests, correct responses should be documented with references from current or classic literature. In addition, support for validity of measurement instruments in all three domains can be obtained by using a procedure commonly referred to as "known groups." With this procedure, the examinations are given to groups of individuals who are known to possess low levels of the attribute of interest whether that is surgical knowledge or surgical self-efficacy and to those who are known to possess high levels of the attribute. Scores from the examinations are compared across the groups to determine if results are as expected. This would support the validity of the instrument. If the examination is given to individuals with various levels of

TABLE 18.2. Basis of simulation education.

Sound education principles
  Objectives
  Teaching strategies
  Evaluation methods
  Standardization
  Reliability and validity
  Qualified instructors

Essentials of simulation education
  Preparation of students
  True-to-life scenarios
  Debriefing and feedback
  Standardization
  Reliability and validity
  Qualified instructors

training, results should show a stepwise increase in the attribute as the level of training increases.

All instruments must be assessed for reliability. Reliability refers to the repeatability of results.[13] Assessment frequently is done by calculating internal consistency of the instrument or test–retest stability. Intra-rater and inter-rater reliability should be addressed for essays, verbal responses, and laboratory assessments for psychomotor skill.

Assessing reliability and validity of the instruments to document the effectiveness of simulation education is crucial. Without support for reliability and validity of the measurement instruments it cannot be determined if any lack of improvement is because of the ineffectiveness of the educational program or the inability of the measurement instruments to detect improvements. Similarly, without support for reliability and validity of the instruments, improvement in outcomes cannot be trusted. Indeed, attention to all aspect of the scientific method is critical in determining the benefits of simulation education. In a prospective randomized study, Lee et al.[14] demonstrated that students who trained using a patient simulator had higher mean trauma assessment test scores than students trained using a moulaged patient.

The validity of the educational and therapeutic protocols is critical. If the simulated education resulted in teaching students thought processes or technical skills that could harm patients, there would be serious negative clinical and medicolegal repercussions. Table 18.2 summarizes the components that form the basis of simulation education.

Simulations in Surgery and Traumatology

An example of the simplest simulator and what Satava[4] refers to as a precision placement simulation is an intravenous arm simulator or a Foley catheter simulator. The device is designed to be anatomically correct and allows the student to accurately identify the anatomy of a vein or a urethra. The student can use a real device such as an intravenous catheter or a Foley catheter and perform the task in exactly the same way that it would be performed in the human. With the addition of haptics, the anatomy and tactile feel and touch are so similar to the human that the student receives the same tactile feedback from the model as would be obtained from a human. This experience is so accurate and reproducible that the student is very well prepared to successfully perform the task on a human being. The experience is useful but fairly basic skill development model. However, practice on such devices before implementation on a human is required.

Another type of simulation utilizes computer programming to represent a disease process and sophisticated equipment to accurately diagnose the disease and employ the appropriate therapeutic intervention. These models have evolved considerably in the last five years and are now able to accurately reproduce the clinical disease process and use the correct equipment to generate therapeutic interventions.

Examples of this type of simulation are bronchoscopy and colonoscopy. The bronchoscopy model utilizes a flexible bronchoscope and an anatomically correct model of the tracheobronchial tree and the lungs. The student has to pass the bronchoscope through the anatomically correct model and not injure the patient in any way. The tip of the bronchoscope demonstrates the same anatomy that the student would see in the human. The mannequin can also respond to stimuli in the same way that a human would. For example, the mannequin can generate a cough and close the vocal cords if appropriate anesthesia has not been applied. Similarly, the number of times that the tip of the bronchoscope hits the side of the trachea or bronchus is identified and recorded. When the tip of the bronchoscope arrives at the carina, if a broncholithic antitussive agent has not been given, the mannequin will generate a cough. The appropriate intrapulmonary segment has to be identified and the tumor identified. A biopsy is then performed. All of these events are recorded and are available for interaction with both the student and the instructor. The time that all of these events takes is also recorded.

Because the anatomy is accurate and the physiologic responses are simulated to appear real, students are engaged in a very similar environment that they wound encounter with a human. At any time, students can switch to an educational mode, which will allow them to identify, with labels, the anatomic structures or segments of the endobronchial tree in which the tip of the bronchoscope is located. This concept is an interactive real education experience that effectively mimics the human experience.

A similar type of experience can be achieved with colonoscopy. Not only is the anatomy clearly demonstrated to be very similar to human anatomy but the positioning of the tip of the colonoscope exactly mimics the images seen when the colonoscope is in the lumen or in the side of the colon. It is, therefore, an interactive, accurate, real-time educational experience. Similarly, anatomically difficult areas of the examination, such as the splenic flexure and the hepatic flexure, have to be identified, and the appropriate maneuvers, such as pressing on the left upper quadrant, have to be performed by the student to facilitate passage of the scope. If the student is inept or rough in the manipulation of the colonoscope and elicits pain, the model reacts with appropriate moans. All of these events are recorded as is the time taken to perform the procedure. Even complex events such as rotating the tip of the colonoscope in the rectum to evaluate the anus are faithfully reproduced. Failure to do this procedure will also be recorded and would be a negative event for the student. The excellent anatomy and ability of the model to reproduce physiologic responses makes the entire experience very real. It has been demonstrated that as the student repeats these activities and gains confidence and competence, the number of errors, the elicitation of pain, and the time for completing the procedure dramatically decrease. This model is, therefore, a simulation with no disease and no human being, but an extremely accurate computer modeling of the event with a real colonoscope.

Another type of simulation used in surgical education involves a patient model with a disease or an injury-producing event that requires the student to take a history, generate a diagnosis, and formulate a treatment plan. The treatment plan is then implemented, and the clinical results of the interventions are integrated into the evolution of the management of the disease or injury. As in the human environment, if the treatment is successful, the patient improves and ultimately has a successful outcome. If the treatment plan is inappropriate or ineffective, the patient deteriorates. The plan then has to be modified to result in patient improvement; if the correct therapy is not implemented, the patient deteriorates and ultimately dies.

Again, the entire process is carefully recorded and monitored so that the instructor can review the interventions and the thought processes with the students. The students can then learn from their errors and redo the clinical interventions until a successful result is achieved. This level of simulation requires that each scenario be clinically correct. The clinical situation must closely mimic a real-life scenario so that the student understands that the situation that they are being presented with is a realistic one. This type of simulation requires either computer software programming or human programming from an instructor to fully engage and test the knowledge and skill level of the student.

Examples of the second type of simulation are the Advanced Cardiac Life Support (ACLS) course and the Advanced Trauma Life Support (ATLS) course. Both of these courses use real clinical situations to simulate and then evaluate the ability of a student to process information from a clinical event, develop a diagnosis, and then implement therapy.

The ACLS course utilizes a clinical heart attack scenario and allows the student to utilize physiologic parameters such as blood pressure and pulse rate as well as investigations such as electrocardiograms to diagnose the type and severity of the myocardial infarction. It then allows for drug and electrocardiographic interventions such as defibrillation, cardioversion, and pacemaker to return the patient to a stable hemodynamic state. The instructor can interact with the student by following the predetermined treatment plan or by creating a new scenario as the treatment and the disease process evolve.

The predetermined treatment plan has the advantage of a written consistent set of clinical events that require a fixed response. This method is completely reproducible and therefore has high intra-rater and inter-rater reliability between all instructors teaching the course.

The disadvantage of this type of simulation is that it becomes predictable and less interesting for both the instructor and eventually the student who has taken the course a number of times. The more complex, more sophisticated approach is to allow the instructor to dynamically change the scenario with each treatment intervention that the student employs. This method is interesting and engaging for the instructor but requires the instructor to be familiar with numerous correct treatment pathways. As the numbers of interactions and pathways increase, the chances of introducing bias and inappropriate or idiosyncratic treatment choices also increase. The learner can quickly become confused, and the fidelity, accuracy, and reproducibility of the model may decrease.

To standardize this process and develop a reproducible software application to interact with learners, an almost infinite number of scenarios and treatment plans need to be developed, validated, and programmed. In the human environment, where there are multiple variables of age, disease, changes in response of the disease to treatment, and numerous types of pharmacologic and other therapeutic treatment modalities, developing a sophisticated, accurate software model is a major challenge.

The ATLS model has been a useful interactive simulation model with clinical scenarios, radiographic and hematologic investigations, and moulaged models. The testing event again relies on an experienced, well-trained instructor guiding the student along a previously thought-out, safe pathway to a successful clinical outcome.

The American College of Surgeons has attempted to increase intra-rater and inter-rater reliability by requiring a potential instructor in ATLS to attend a day-long structured educational session taught by educators and surgeons to standardize the instructional process and to educate the instructor on the principles of providing a standardized, reproducible, sophisticated, interactive course. This process has dramatically increased inter-rater reliability. There have been criticisms that it has decreased the ability of instructors to introduce their own creative methods of dealing with the particular event. Although this is a reasonable criticism, the benefits of having a national and international trauma resuscitation method that is highly predictable and reproducible far outweighs the loss of creativity.

Another method to respond to the challenge of teaching technical operative surgery to surgeons in a simulated environment has been the use of virtual reality education. This methodology has been typified by laparoscopic simulators. The instruments used in laparoscopy are grasped by the surgeon as he or she looks at a screen that reproduces the movements of the tips of the instruments. The computer simulation accurately demonstrates appropriate three-dimensional movements generated by the handles of the instruments and is conveyed via the screen to display the tips of the instruments. In so doing, the surgeon can visualize exactly how his or her hands are functioning in a virtual operative environment. The simulations are sufficiently real enough that they accurately mimic an operation. The surgeon is able to develop surgical expertise in manipulating tissues, ligating vessels, and tying sutures.

A significant disadvantage of the early virtual reality models was that they did not accurately reproduce the tactile sensation of the tip of the instrument against tissues. Considerable effort has been spent in developing realistic tactile feedback impulses. This is known as haptics. The newer, more advanced models have resistances built into them that mimic putting a needle through different tissues such as skin, subcutaneous tissue, and fascia. Similarly, if a blood vessel is lacerated, the model can mimic blood being expressed into the operative field. The computer graphics have progressed, and they are now beginning to be realistic. There is still considerable room for growth and improvement in the development of these models.

The models have the advantage of being reproducible and having a grading system that measures the competence of the operator and also a timing system that measures the elapsed time to perform a given procedure. There is evidence that, with increased usage of these simulators, the operator increases surgical dexterity and decreases the time taken to successfully complete a given procedure. It is also clear that skills and competence learned in the virtual reality environment can be transferred to the human environment.

The next level of simulated experience used in surgical education provides a true to life environment with the exact same behavior of an injured patient in a single- or multiple-injury trauma event. The ideal environment would be for the learner to visualize the injury event and to appreciate and understand the kinetic injury forces that have produced this event. The most effective method of reproducing this event is to film a head-on, side impact, or rollover crash and visualize the patient sustaining this event. This can be provided by filming realistic dummies in the car. The "patient" can be unrestrained or restrained with a two-point or three-point seatbelt. The "patient" can have an airbag deployed or not. Cameras inside the car can demonstrate the effects of intrusion of the front, side, or top of the passenger compartment on the patient.

Similarly, films of investigations such as blood gas monitoring, ultrasound, x-rays, computed tomographic scans, angiograms, and magnetic resonance imaging can be archived and immediately retrieved by students. A computerized DVD retrieval system has the advantage of allowing students to order a test and immediately evaluate the results. The immediate availability of these studies allows students to generate a treatment plan based on the information that would be available in the clinical arena.

The clinical management process is conducted in the same environment in which a real patient would be treated. For example, an air medical resuscitation would occur in the helicopter with the same ambient noises that are present in a helicopter. Resuscitation in the trauma center is conducted in the same or similar room where the resuscitation team would perform an actual resuscitation. Here teamwork as describe by Helmreich and Schäfer[2] for ACRM or TOMS becomes an educational goal. The advantage of conducting education in the same environment is that the student has to function with the same audiovisual and environmental cues that would be present in the real scenario.

Many medical schools use a highly sophisticated simulation model and a human volunteer to educate medical students. The volunteer is either medically trained or has been specifically educated in the presenting symptoms and signs of a specific disease and can mimic the findings of that specific disease. An excellent example of this kind of simulated education is to use an adult female to simulate ovarian and gynecologic problems. The student elicits history from the patient, which may be specific to lower abdominal symptomatology. During the history taking process, the human volunteer gives the appropriate responses when asked. She does not help the student with her responses but gives clear and concise answers in response to appropriate questions. The student builds a differential diagnosis and on physical examination is able to perform all the appropriate evaluations, including a pelvic and rectal examination to confirm a diagnostic impression. The volunteer is well coached on how to present the appropriate physical findings of rebound tenderness and guarding. With appropriate coaching and significant experience, the human volunteer can become very effective in mimicking a given disease process.

An obvious advantage of this type of simulation is that, although the patient does not have the disease, he or she is able to appear to have the disease. The student is able to interact in a very sophisticated way with a thinking human being. Students also can be evaluated in a very precise manner on how they perform the physical examination and on how the patient perceives the examination. This educational experience has been reproducible and very beneficial in medical school education.

An important element of this type of simulation is that the volunteer has to understand all aspects of the disease process and be able to generate the appropriate responses on physical examination. The disadvantages are that it is invasive and requires humans who are prepared to subject themselves to multiple physical examinations from students. However, it fulfills the criteria of realism and sophisticated interaction, which are difficult to reproduce with a mannequin and even the most sophisticated algorithmic programming.

A final type of simulation useful in trauma is one where injuries that would occur in the human are presented to the student in a large animal model. The advantages of this type of presentation is that real injuries to the vena cava, heart, pancreas, and other organs can be created in a model that is alive and has all the cues of tactile stimuli, bleeding, deteriorating physiology, and accurate anatomy. The swine's organs are similar in size and consistency to the organs of a human.

The Advanced Trauma Operative Management (ATOM) course[15–17] utilizes this mechanism to produce penetrating injuries that are infrequently seen by the surgeon and allow the surgeon to identify the injury, develop an operative plan, and repair the injury in real time in a real operating room. This model represents penetrating trauma in a real environment with a nonhuman but live model. The ATOM course was developed by the authors and others at their institution and is described below to illustrate the development and implementation of an educational program using simulation.

ATOM: An Example of Simulation Education

The ATOM course was developed to provide surgeons-in-training and surgeons who infrequently encounter penetrating trauma an opportunity to develop or enhance surgical skill to repair such injuries. The course

was designed to give students a comprehensive learning experience.

The ATOM course begins by having the student review a CD-ROM of the management of penetrating injuries in the chest and abdomen. THE CD-ROM reviews the anatomic operative approaches to various structures in a cadaver. A number of case scenarios allow the learner to integrate the operative management strategies into clinical cases. Once the students have reviewed the cases, they attend six lectures that are confined to the operative management of injuries to the chest, major vascular structures, the solid organs within the abdomen, and the retroperitoneum and diaphragm.

This preliminary work prepares the student for the simulation experience. In addition to preparing students about the surgical procedures, the students are informed as to how the simulation will proceed and the behaviors that are appropriate. For instance, the students are told that they should act as though they are in an operating room operating on a human being. Therefore, all precautions such as gown, gloves, and protective eyewear that are taken for a human patient are taken for the simulated patient.

Students are then taken to the operating room where large 50-kg swine are used for operative experiences. Clinical scenarios are given to the students that reflect real-life trauma cases involving 14 penetrating injuries. Both the injuries and procedures are standardized and were evaluated by a panel of expert traumatologists as being important for course content.[16] The instructor creates a series of injuries while the student is out of the room. The student is then brought to the operating table to identify and manage these injuries. The student is asked to develop a competent treatment plan for each injury and then successfully demonstrate to the instructor one method of repairing the injury. The injuries become more severe and more difficult to repair as the operative experience continues. It is essential that the repairs are successfully completed and the animal is maintained in a stable state to the completion of all procedures. The animals are monitored in exactly the same way that the human would be monitored in the operating room (Figure 18.3). This realistic scenario creates the same visual, auditory, and mental cues that would alert the operating surgeon to a hemodynamically unstable situation in the human environment. The entire experience is designed to reproduce the tensions and stresses of managing a severely injured patient.

The teaching methods of the ATOM course are derived from Social Cognitive Theory[9] and provide the four methods to increase students' self-efficacy. The laboratory experience gives the students the opportunity to practice skills and successfully perform tasks. Along with the CD-ROM, the laboratory experience offers

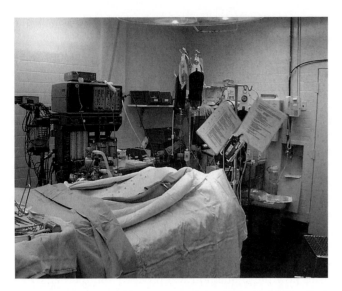

FIGURE 18.3. Monitoring equipment used in the ATOM course is the same as in a human operating room. (Reproduced with permission from Jacobs LM, Gross R, Luk S, eds. Advanced Trauma Operative Management: Surgical Strategies for Penetrating Trauma. Copyright © 2004 by Cine-Med, Inc., Woodbury, CT.)

observational learning in that the student can view the repair of injuries on the CD-ROM and also see faculty demonstrate techniques in the laboratory. The ATOM instructors act to champion the students' success by offering assurance that mastery of the task can be accomplished. Finally, ATOM instructors act to calm any debilitating physiology that the student may experience. Physiology can be managed by using stress reduction techniques, verbal encouragement, and having students initially perform smaller, more manageable tasks.

After the laboratory session, students have a debriefing session in which events of the simulation are reviewed. Instructors provide each student with information regarding strengths and weaknesses. Debriefing is necessary to help students reflect on their performance and integrate the experience. It also helps students and teachers identify areas for future learning.[10]

The ATOM participants are evaluated in cognitive, affective, and psychomotor domains.[16] A 25-item multiple-choice test assesses learning in the cognitive domain. The content of the test reflects the topics taught in the course, with each topic being equally represented. The answers to the questions were validated by a national panel of expert traumatologists and are supported with annotated references from the literature. To assess learning in the affective domain, a 25-item self-efficacy instrument asks participants to rate their level of confidence for performing the surgical procedures taught in ATOM using a 5-point Likert-type scale. A score of 1 on the self-efficacy instrument denotes very little confidence, and a score of 5 denotes quite a lot of confidence. The self-

efficacy instrument was administered to "known groups" to gather support for its validity. Anesthesiologists and acute care physicians were expected to score the lowest and attending surgeons and expert traumatologists were expected to score the highest. Surgical residents and trauma fellows were hypothesized to score according to their level of training.[16] All groups scored as expected, thereby supporting the validity of the self-efficacy instrument. The ATOM participants complete the knowledge test and the self-efficacy instrument on the World Wide Web prior to taking the ATOM course and immediately after completing it. Data from the first 50 participants have clearly shown substantial gains in both knowledge and self-efficacy after taking the ATOM course.[16]

In the laboratory, psychomotor skills are evaluated on a 3-point scale that indicates the degree of assistance needed by the student to perform the task. Students are required to accurately identify the injury, develop a treatment plan, and repair the injury. Critical behaviors necessary to accomplish these essential skills are posted in the laboratory for easy reference (Figure 18.4). These

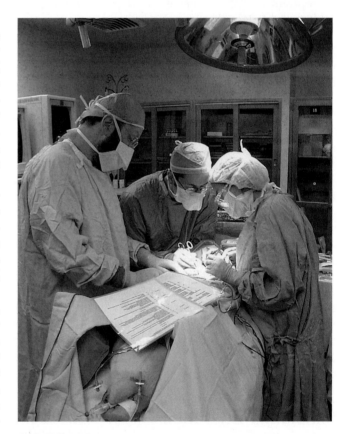

FIGURE 18.4. A list of critical behaviors for student performance and evaluation should be readily available. (Reproduced with permission from Jacobs LM, Gross R, Luk S, eds. Advanced Trauma Operative Management: Surgical Strategies for Penetrating Trauma. Copyright © 2004 by Cine-Med, Inc., Woodbury, CT.)

delineate precisely what must be done to identify each injury, develop a treatment plan, and competently repair the injury. On the 3-point scale, 1 indicates that the student could not perform the task. Two denotes that help was needed. Three indicates that the student independently performed the task. The items on the laboratory evaluation scale were evaluated and supported by a national panel of traumatologists. Inter-rater agreement was assessed when two instructors evaluated 12 students with 100% agreement.[16] In addition, ATOM participants are asked to complete course and instructor evaluations and a six-month follow-up assessment regarding the benefits of the ATOM course.[18]

All aspects of the ATOM course have been standardized to ensure accurate reproducibility.[16,17] Each lecture has been developed so that different instructors can deliver the same content. Similarly, in the operating room, the preparation of the animal, resuscitation, and monitoring are also standardized. The injuries to the swine are created using a systematic method. In this way each student is expected to repair an injury of the same severity. To achieve this standardization, a senior instructor demonstrates the injury to the junior instructor. The junior instructor must create the injury exactly as specified before being certified as an independent instructor. In addition, standardization is enhanced by having instructors view a film that was made of the injury creations. Requirements to become an ATOM instructor include board certification (or eligibility) in surgery and successful completion of the ATOM instructor-training course. The methods of standardizing the educational content, the delivery of the lectures, the education of the instructors, and the operating room instruments and procedures allow a uniform standard for the ATOM course no matter where it is offered.

In conclusion, surgical education for trauma requires methods that will produce unique educational outcomes. The nature of trauma requires surgeons to employ high cognitive and psychomotor skills in an environment where rapid diagnosis and treatment are crucial. This sets acute care surgery off from other specialties where time pressures are much less. Because of this, surgical education for trauma must also teach surgeons to deal with the crisis situations. Preparation must include team leadership in an arena that demands efficiency of diagnosis and treatment. The use of simulation in acute care surgery education is necessary. It can no longer be considered optional or an extra addition to an already complete curriculum. It is a vital component; without simulation education the curriculum is incomplete. Students must be able to practice and be successful at all essential skills, from the most basic intravenous or catheter insertion to the more complex situations of resuscitation and trauma surgery, including injury identification, development of a treatment plan, and repair of the injury. Ideally, students should confront and manage complex injuries in a simulated environment before such injuries are ever encountered in the emergency department or operating room.

Critique

The transference effect of simulation training has *not* been well studied in surgery. In addition, there are only three simulators that have been validated, to date: MIST-VR, TRAUMA MAN, and HUMAN MODEL. Unfortunately, even at institutions with elaborate simulation centers, the voluntary utilization by residents has been disappointing. Many institutions have to make this a *mandatory* requirement in order to increase resident participation. However, if simulation training is, indeed, mandatory and the residents are given times when they must attend, then the time spent must be included in the 80-hour limitation. The Residency Review Committee for Surgery (ACGME) has made low-tech simulation training a requirement for all surgical programs.

Answer (C)

References

1. Krummel TM. Surgical simulation and virtual reality: the coming revolution. Ann Surg 1998; 228:635–637.
2. Helmreich RL, Schäfer H-G. Turning silk purses into sows' ears: human factors in medicine. In Henson LC, Lee AC, eds. Simulators in Anesthesiology Education. New York: Plenum Press, 1998: 1–8.
3. Howard SK, Gaba DM, Fish KJ, et al. Anesthesia crisis resource management training: teaching anesthesiologists to handle critical incidents. Aviat Space Environ Med 1992; 63:763–770.
4. Satava RM. Surgical education and surgical simulation. World J Surg 2001; 25:1484–1489.
5. Torkington J, Smith SGT, Rees BI, et al. The role of simulation in surgical training. Ann R Coll Surg Engl 2000; 82:88–94.
6. Issenberg SB, McGaghie WC, Hart IR, et al. Simulation technology for health care professional skills training and assessment. JAMA 1999; 282:861–866.
7. Murray WB, Henson LC. Workshop on educational aspects: educational objectives and building scenarios. In: Henson LC, Lee AC, ed. Simulators in Anesthesiology Education. New York: Plenum Press, 1998: 57–64.
8. Bloom BS, ed. Taxonomy of Educational Objectives. The Classification of Educational Goals, Handbook I: Cognitive Domain. New York: David McKay Company, Inc., 1956.
9. Bandura A. Social Foundations of Thought and Action: A Social Cognitive Theory. Englewood Cliffs, NJ: Prentice Hall, 1986.

10. Hertel JP, Millis BJ. Using Simulations to Promote Learning in Higher Education. Sterling, VA: Stylus Publishing, LLC, 2002.

11. Gable RK, Wolf MB. Instrument Development in the Affective Domain: Measuring Attitudes and Values in Corporate and School Settings, 2nd ed. Norwell, MA: Kluwer Academic Publishers, 1993.

12. Paisley AM, Baldwin PJ, Paterson-Brown S. Validity of surgical simulation for the assessment of operative skill. Br J Surg 2001; 88:1525–1532.

13. Nunnally JC, Bernstein IH. Psychometric Theory, 3rd ed. New York: McGraw-Hill, Inc., 1994.

14. Lee SK, Pardo M, Gaba D, et al. Trauma assessment training with a patient simulator: a prospective, randomized study. J Trauma 2003; 55:651–657.

15. Jacobs LM, Lorenzo C, Brautigam RT. Definitive surgical trauma care live porcine session: a technique for training in trauma surgery. Conn Med 2001; 65:265–268.

16. Jacobs LM, Burns KJ, Kaban JM, et al. Development and evaluation of the advanced trauma operative management course. J Trauma 2003; 55:471–479.

17. Jacobs LM, Burns KJ, Luk S, et al. Implementation of the advanced trauma operative management course. Panam J Trauma 2004; 11:21–27.

18. Jacobs LM, Burns KJ, Luk S, Marshall WV III. Follow-up survey of participants attending the advanced trauma operative management course. J Trauma 2005; 58:1140–1143.

Part II
Organ-Based Approach

19
Pharynx and Larynx

Ernest M. Myers

Case Scenario

A 22-year-old hockey player sustains a forearm blow to the neck. He presents with expanding crepitus and some difficulty breathing. You are concerned that he has a laryngotracheal partial transection. The patient remains alert and is talking. Which of the following is the airway management of choice in this acute setting?

(A) Transnasal-translaryngeal endotracheal intubation
(B) Surgical cricothyroidotomy
(C) Needle cricothyroidotomy
(D) Tracheostomy
(E) Face mask

In a busy emergency room, nontraumatic ear, nose, and throat complaints are common in adult and pediatric patients. Most diagnoses are benign. However, hidden within the plethora of common complaints are potentially deadly conditions that present innocently. A heightened sense of suspicion by the alert physician thwarts the progression and rapid emergence of life-threatening conditions. Most veiled, hidden surgical emergencies of the pharynx and larynx present as airway obstruction, hemorrhage, infection/inflammation, caustic inhalation/ingestion, and foreign bodies (Figure 19.1).

Acknowledgments: Tanya Powell, Informatics and Manuscript Preparation; Jacqueline Sealey, Medical Illustrations; Patricia Randolph-Myers, PhD, Manuscript Review and Informatics. Dedication: Eustace Vanderpool, PhD, 1934–2003, microbiologist, teacher, scientist, father, husband, patient.

History and Physical Examination

When evaluating any medical or surgical problem, there is no substitute for a well-analyzed chief complaint, history, and a comprehensive, in-depth, physical examination.[1] The minimal factual requirements are onset, duration, and associated problems. In addition, past medical history, habits, occupation, and medications also are pertinent. The goals of the history and physical examination are preliminary diagnosis, disease assessment, and establishment of a doctor–patient relationship. To fulfill these goals, this section outlines basic data collection, describes the head and neck evaluation, and highlights fundamental analytical concepts.

History

Database

An accurate history, gleaned from open and directed questioning and attentive listening, is indispensable to define disease progression. Establishing the database is the beginning of the formal history. The essentials are name, sex, birth date, age, residence, telephone number, marital status, race or nationality, occupation, and closest relative or friend.

Chief Complaint

The *chief complaint* is the catalyst that prompts the patient to seek medical advice. As the history unfolds, head and neck complaints are assigned to one of five regions. The most common but not necessarily the only chief complaints for each region are

Region I (face): skin lesions (nonhealing ulcer or swelling)
Region II (sinonasal tract): rhinitis, sinusitis, nasal obstruction, rhinorrhea, epistaxis
Region III (orodigestive tract): sore throat, dysphagia

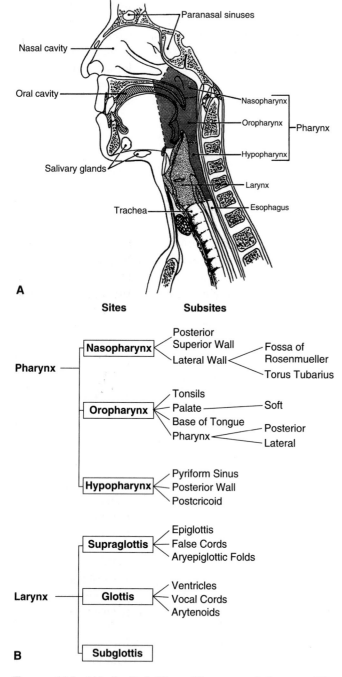

FIGURE 19.1. **(A)** Sagittal View: Pharynx and Larynx. **(B)** Pharynx and larynx: sites and subsites. (Reprinted with permission from Myers.[2])

Region IV (aerodigestive tract): upper, sore throat, dysphagia, otalgia; lower, hoarseness and airway obstruction

Region V (neck): neck mass or masses, pain

History of the Present Illness

The *history of present illness*, a succinct narrative of the disease process, includes time of onset, location, progres-

sion, severity, frequency of complaints, associated problems (weight loss, dyspnea, headache, visual changes), and pertinent negatives derived from the *review of systems*. In addition, as the history is gathered, the patient's general appearance, demeanor, expression, and emotions are observed keenly and recorded.

The history of the present illness fulfills three goals: (1) identification of the major region, (2) preliminary determination of the diagnosis and possible differential diagnoses, and (3) assessment of the patient's reaction and tolerance to the malady.

Past Medical History

The *past medical history* should include (1) medical illnesses and surgical conditions (current and past), (2) medications and homeopathic preparations, (3) allergies, (4) hospitalizations, (5) operations, (6) habits, (7) carcinogen exposure, (8) previous malignancy, (9) AIDS risk factors, (10) occupation, and (11) family history of illnesses.

Review of Systems

In the head and neck, the emphasis is: (1) eyes, (2) ears, (3) respiratory factors, (4) cardiac disease, (5) gastrointestinal factors, (6) neurologic factors, and (7) psychiatric factors.

Physical Examination

The physical examination begins with careful observation as the patient elaborates the chief complaint, review of systems, and history. The head and neck examination can be divided into *external* and *internal* evaluations whose methodologies encompass direct and indirect visualization, palpation, and auscultation (Table 19.1). The external examination includes inspection of the lips, facial skin, eyes, ears, and sinuses. The internal examination requires illumination and instrumentation.

External Examination

A wealth of information is obtained by careful observation and astute inspection of demeanor, level of discomfort, speech, airway, and evidence of medication, drug, alcohol, or heavy tobacco usage. The external examination, an assessment of facial symmetry, speech patterns, and airway, includes the following:

Symmetry

Observe for symmetry of the eyes (exophthalmos/enophthalmos, ptosis, proptosis), face (facial palsy, edema), and neck (mass).

TABLE 19.1. Physical examination of the head and neck.

Region	Inspection	Palpation	Auscultation	Special Techniques
I. Face				
Skin	+	+		Oto, In
Eyes	+	+	−	Oto, Fund, In
Ears	+	+		Oto, In, In
Lips	+	+		In
II. Sinonasal				Oto, Fund, In
Nasopharynx				In
Sinuses	+	+	−	Oto, Fund, In
Nose	+			In
III. Orodigestive				Oto, Fund, In
Oral cavity	+	+		In
Oropharynx	+	+	−	
IV. Aerodigestive		+		
Larynx	−	+	+	Oto, In
Hypopharynx				Oto, In
V. Neck	+	+	+	In

Oto (otoscopy); Fund (fundoscopy); In, (indirect laryngopharyngoscopy).
Source: Reprinted with permission from Ortiz.[1]

Speech

Characteristic, altered speech patterns are associated with *nasopharyngeal*, *oropharyngeal*, and *hypopharyngeal* maladies or lesions. Hyponasal voice is produced by nasopharyngeal, posterior nasal, and palatal problems (Region II). Muffled voice is associated with problems of the base of the tongue, epiglottis, and posterior pharyngeal wall (Region III). Wheezing and hoarseness are related closely to the hypopharynx and/or larynx (Region IV). Tongue-tied speech implicates the oral cavity, especially the anterior tongue and floor of the mouth.

Airway

Airway obstruction in head and neck patients often develops slowly and insidiously, producing low-pitched stridor, dysphonia, dysphagia, and mild dyspnea on exertion. Suprasternal retractions, accessory muscle usage, cyanosis, high-pitched stridor, tachycardia, and tachypnea are signs of severe airway obstruction. Despite severe airway compromise, many patients are asymptomatic at rest because of gradual metabolic compensation. Obviously, astute clinical suspicion and early airway assurance in compensated patients decreases mortality and morbidity.

Stridor, coarse inspiratory or expiratory breath sounds, is a cardinal sign of airway compromise. Inspiratory stridor is associated with supraglottic and glottic obstruction. High-pitched stridor implicates glottic pathology. Both inspiratory and expiratory stridor are found in subglottic and tracheal obstruction. Expiratory stridor, often confused with wheezing, characterizes intrathoracic or tracheal obstruction.

Skin

The examination of the skin consists of inspection (thickness, color, ulceration) and palpation (texture, fixation).

Ears

Careful otoscopy with emphasis on the appearance of the tympanic membrane is performed. Otalgia and/or serous otitis media may be associated with subtle complaints of head and neck maladies, inflammatory or neoplastic in nature.

Eyes

Proptosis, exophthalmos, enophthalmos, ptosis, and strabismus implicate sinonasal or orbital disease. Head and neck conditions may extend into the skull, temporal space or petrous apex and affect extraocular movements, visual acuity, and visual fields.

Nose and Sinuses

The examination of the nose and sinuses consists of both an *external* and *internal* examination. The *external examination* includes inspection and palpation. Inspect the upper and middle face for asymmetry and tenderness. Palpate the nasal dorsum and bony pyramids. Test with a cotton swab or pinprick for infraorbital hypesthesia. Absent sensation suggests a sinonasal tract lesion that may be inflammatory or neoplastic. The *internal examination* requires rhinoscopy with either an endoscope or a nasal speculum.

Lower Face, Mandible, and Salivary Glands

The lower face, mandible, and major salivary glands (parotid, submandibular, sublingual) are inspected and palpated. The complete examination includes bimanual palpation especially for pain, hypesthesia or induration of the mandible floor of the mouth and tongue. Mental nerve sensation is assessed routinely: anesthesia implies nerve injury or invasion. Dental occlusion or malocclusion may be apparent with external inspection.

Neck

A comprehensive evaluation includes assessment for tenderness, size, firmness, consistency, mobility, and

TABLE 19.2. Systems in the neck.

System	Structure
Integument	Scalp
	Neck skin
	Beard
Cardiovascular	Carotid artery
	Thyrocervical trunk
	Subclavian artery
	Innominate artery
	Internal jugular vein
	External jugular vein
Nervous	Sympathetics
	Nodose ganglia
	Parasympathetics
	Carotid body
	Lingual nerve (cranial nerve V)
	Facial nerve (cranial nerve VII)
	Glossopharyngeal nerve (cranial nerve IX)
	Spinal Accessory nerve (cranial nerve XI)
	Hypoglossal nerve (cranial nerve XII)
	Superior laryngeal nerve (cranial nerve X)
	Recurrent laryngeal nerve (cranial nerve X)
	Peripheral nerves
	Pharyngeal plexus
	Phrenic nerve
	Brachial plexus
Endocrine	Thyroid gland
	Parathyroids
Gastrointestinal	Salivary glands
	Tongue
	Hypopharynx
	Esophagus
Hematopoietic	Thymus
	Lymph nodes
	Thoracic duct
Musculoskeletal	Cervical spine
	Mandible
	Scapula
	Clavicle
	Sternum
	Cervical musculature
Respiratory	Larynx
	Trachea
	Lungs (apices)

Source: Reprinted with permission from Myers EM. Neck dissection. In: Myers EM, ed. Head and Neck Oncology: Diagnosis, Treatment, and Rehabilitation. Boston: Little, Brown & Company, 1991: 3–17.

auscultation (Table 19.2). Many neck masses are discovered by close observation, notably asymmetry, while obtaining the history. Palpation, invaluable but underutilized, can detect laryngeal fixation, abnormal position, or pain. Although rare, fixation is found with advanced neoplasms or extensive infection. The neck is palpated systematically and carefully in the submental, submandibular, carotid, and parotid regions. Preferably, the physician stands behind the patient and palpates, with both hands simultaneously, the anterior and posterior cervical triangles. The larynx is mobilized: absence of crepitance suggests fixation from either induration or neoplasm. Between the thumb, index, and middle fingers the thyroid gland is grasped. The sternocleidomastoid is relaxed as the carotid sheath is palpated gently. The head is flexed and rotated to decrease muscle tension and facilitate palpation. Finally, the suprasternal (thyroid) and carotid triangles are auscultated for murmurs or bruits.

Internal Examination

The basic requirements for the internal examination are illumination (headlight or head mirror), laryngeal mirrors (sizes 3–6), nasopharyngeal mirrors (sizes 0–2), and topical anesthesia, if needed. More sophisticated instruments such as the rod and fiberoptic laryngoscopes are invaluable when indicated. They can facilitate an excellent aerodigestive tract examination with minimal patient discomfort. After anesthetizing the nose with anesthetic gel or spray, the fiberoptic scope is passed through the nose, over the soft palate, to visualize the nasopharynx, oropharynx, hypopharynx, and larynx. The nasopharyngoscope is passed orally after topical anesthesia. A thorough, internal examination includes the oral cavity, nasopharynx, pharynx, hypopharynx, and larynx.

Nose

Aided by illumination and the nasal speculum, the nasal fossae are inspected for turbinate pathology, septal displacement with associated secondary nasal obstruction, mucosal ulceration, necrosis, hemorrhage, or purulence.

Oral Cavity/Oropharynx

With excellent illumination, the floor of the mouth, teeth, gingivae, tongue, tonsils, retromolar trigone, palate, buccal mucosa, and dentition are inspected. Possible significant findings are loose teeth, trismus, impaired tongue mobility or fixation, glossal palsy, tonsillar asymmetry, palatal palsy, and any leukoplakia or erythematous or ulcerative lesion. Occlusion or malocclusion is noted. Bimanual palpation is the final maneuver.

Nasopharynx

The nasopharynx is visualized either indirectly (by mirror) or directly (by the fiberoptic or rod laryngoscope). Indirect nasolaryngoscopy is performed by depressing the tongue and inserting the laryngeal mirror around the soft palate. After rotating the mirror *superiorly* 90°, the choanae, eustachian tubes (especially Rosenmuller's fossae), and posterior pharyngeal walls are inspected. Significant findings are edema, irregularity, nasal vault asymmetry, ulceration, and bleeding. For some

FIGURE 19.2. Laryngoscopy, indirect.

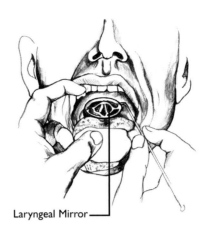

Laryngeal Mirror

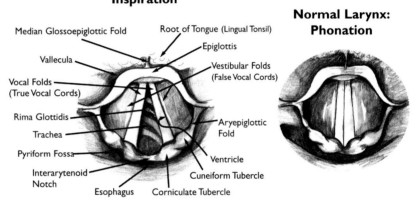

Normal Larynx: Inspiration

Normal Larynx: Phonation

Median Glossoepiglottic Fold

Root of Tongue (Lingual Tonsil)

Epiglottis

Vallecula

Vestibular Folds (False Vocal Cords)

Vocal Folds (True Vocal Cords)

Rima Glottidis

Trachea

Aryepiglottic Fold

Pyriform Fossa

Interarytenoid Notch

Ventricle

Cuneiform Tubercle

Esophagus

Corniculate Tubercle

patients, indirect nasopharyngoscopy is suboptimal; thus, rigid or fiberoptic instrumentation is necessary.

Hypopharynx and Larynx

The patient sits and faces the examiner. The tongue is grasped firmly and gently and pulled anteriorly and inferiorly. Anxious patients are topically anesthetized for a relaxed, systematic examination. The patient is instructed to breathe rhythmically as a warm mirror is placed in the oropharynx. With the mirror directed 90° *inferiorly*, the base of the tongue, epiglottis, lateral pharyngeal walls, pyriform sinuses, and endolarynx are visualized well (Figure 19.2). Erythema, ulcerations, swelling, pooling of saliva, and vocal cord irregularities or dysfunction are possible significant findings.

Diagnosis

Crafting a working diagnosis requires an in-depth history followed by a careful, general physical and thorough head and neck examination (Table 19.3).[2] As discussed in the previous section, the emphasis is on the ears, facies, oral cavity, oropharynx, hypopharynx/larynx, and neck. Aside from the otologic, nasopharyngeal, and hypopharyngeal/laryngeal examinations, no special instrumentation is required. As a basic dictum, a head and neck examination is incomplete without otoscopy and laryngoscopy (mirror or fiberoptic).

The data from the history and physical usually implicate a particular region. This in turn dictates the diagnostic modalities. Thus, laboratory screens, images, fine-needle aspiration and biopsy, when appropriate, are ordered (Table 19.4). In most instances, the diagnosis can be determined in minutes and rarely greater than 1 day. The simultaneous development of fiberoptic laryngoscopy, sophisticated imaging, and fine-needle aspiration/biopsy enhances early head and neck diagnosis. These exciting developments simplify and streamline diagnostic workups (Table 19.5). However, with emergencies, the diagnosis must be even more rapid and efficient. Critical surgical emergencies of the pharynx and larynx mandate responses that must be executed quickly without conclusive facts. This is especially true for decompensating, deteriorating patients.

TABLE 19.3. Basic workup.

Physical examination	Diagnostic radiology
Scalp and skin	Chest, anteroposterior and lateral views
Head and neck	Sinus series
Thorax and lungs	Soft tissue, anteroposterior and lateral neck
Breasts and axillae	Panorex
Abdomen*	Scans, CT/MRI
Pelvis and genitalia*	Barium swallow
Rectum*	
	Endoscopy
Laboratory	Indirect nasopharyngoscopy
CBC	Indirect laryngoscopy
Multiphasic screening	Flexible endoscopy
Urinalysis	
Human immunodeficiency virus[†] (HIV)	Empirical trial of antibiotics
Purified protein derivative[†] (PPD)	

*If neoplasm is suspected.
[†]Check if inflammation/infection is suspected.
Source: Reprinted with permission from Myers.[2]

TABLE 19.4. Head and neck diagnostic modalities.

Anatomic region	Special	CT	MRI	Other
Ear	Puretone Audiometry Tympanometry Brain stem evoked Audiometry/ENG	Temporal/bone Maxillofacial Sinuses	Head and neck	Magnetic resonance angiography
Nose	C&S, smear for eosinophilia, IgE Total eosinophil count	Maxillofacial	Head and neck	Plain sinus films Rhinoscopy
Sinuses	Transillumination	Maxillofacial	Head and neck	Nasopharyngoscopy
Pharynx	C&S	Neck maxillofacial	Neck	Barium swallow Laryngoscopy
Oral and cavity	C&S	Maxillofacial and neck	Neck	Plain sinus films Facial bone films Mandible series
Larynx	Pulmonary functions Flow loop studies	Neck	Neck	Barium swallow
Neck	Ultrasonography Fine-needle aspiration Thyroid function studies	Neck and chest	Neck and chest	Thyroid scans Laryngoscopy Nasopharyngoscopy Angiography Ultrasonography

C&S, culture and sensitivity; ENG, electronystagmography.

TABLE 19.5. Imaging modalities: hypopharynx and larynx.

Modality	Advantages	Disadvantages	Indications
Soft tissue films	Availability Inexpensive Speed	Soft tissue detail	Airway assessment Nasopharyngeal soft tissue assessment Retropharyngeal assessment
Computed Tomography	Soft-tissue detail Speed Reconstruction Multidimensional views	Cartilage invasion Mucosal detail Contrast allergy Expense Availability	Preepiglottic space Paraglottic space Subglottis Postcricoid area Lymphadenopathy
Magnetic Resonance Imaging	Soft-tissue detail Multidimensional views Allergy (contrast agents) Cartilage invasion	Availability Expensive Pacemaker malfunction Metal prostheses	Base of tongue Preepiglottic space Paraglottic space Pyriform sinus Parapharyngeal space

FIGURE 19.3. Pharynx (posterior view).

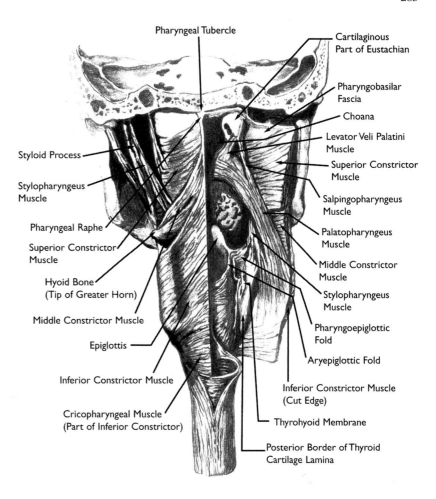

Pharynx

Anatomy

Posterior to the nasal/oral cavities and anterior to the prevertebral fascia, the pharynx continues lateral and posterior to the larynx (Figure 19.3).[3] It extends from the skull base to the inferior border of the cricoid cartilage anteriorly and the inferior border of C6 vertebra posteriorly. Widest opposite the hyoid bone and narrowest inferiorly, it merges with the cervical esophagus. Spanning the skull base and thoracic inlet, the pharynx can be divided into three areas.

The *nasopharynx* has ventilatory and respiratory functions as it begins posterior to the nose and choanae (Figure 19.4). Inferior to the sphenoid and occipital bones, the vaulted nasopharyngeal roof and posterior wall form a continuous surface.

Extending from the soft palate to the superior border of the epiglottis, the *oropharynx* has primarily a digestive function. It is delineated by the soft palate superiorly, the

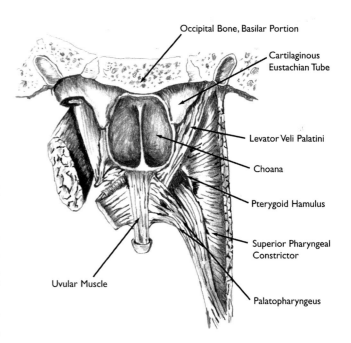

FIGURE 19.4. Posterior view of nasopharynx.

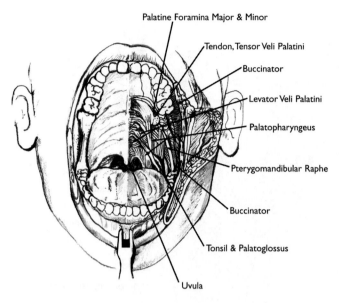

Palatine Foramina Major & Minor

Tendon, Tensor Veli Palatini

Buccinator

Levator Veli Palatini

Palatopharyngeus

Pterygomandibular Raphe

Buccinator

Tonsil & Palatoglossus

Uvula

FIGURE 19.5. Oropharyngeal muscles.

base of the tongue inferiorly, and the palatoglossal and palatopharyngeal arches laterally (Figure 19.5).

The *hypopharynx*, lying lateral and posterior to the larynx (C4 through C6), extends from the superior margin of the epiglottis and pharyngoepiglottic folds to the cricoid cartilage inferiorly, where it ends at the cervical esophagus. The hypopharynx merges with the endolaryngeal inlet anteriorly and the esophagus inferiorly.

The pyriform sinuses or fossae are small mucosal (lateral) troughs that flank the larynx, superior to the cer-

vical esophagus. These recesses are separated from the laryngeal inlet by the aryepiglottic folds. Medially, the pyriform recesses are bounded by the medial surfaces of the thyroid cartilage and the thyrohyoid membrane. Deep to the pyriform mucosa bilaterally are branches of the superior (sensory/autonomic) laryngeal and recurrent (motor/sensory) laryngeal nerves.

Physiology

Tympanomastoid Ventilation

The eustachian tube, linking the tympanomastoid air cell complex and nasopharynx, is composed of bone and cartilage covered by mucosa. The eustachian tube equalizes middle ear and atmospheric pressures to facilitate tympanic membrane compliance, thus contributing to hearing efficiency. Normally, it is closed and opened actively by levator veli palatini (pushing) and tensor veli palatini (pulling) contractions.

Swallowing

The complex process of swallowing, coordinated with laryngeal physiology, transports a bolus (food and saliva) from the mouth, through the pharynx and esophagus, into the stomach (Table 19.6; Figure 19.6). Deglutition, or swallowing, can be divided into three stages: (1) oral (voluntary), (2) pharyngeal (involuntary), and (3) esophageal (involuntary). Breathing ceases with swallowing to prevent aspiration. The larynx elevates superiorly and anteriorly. During the third stage of swallowing, the epiglottis and aryepiglottic folds involute and converge

TABLE 19.6. Pharyngeal muscles.

Layer	Muscle	Origin	Insertion	Innervation
External layer	Superior constrictor	Pterygoid hamulus, pterygomandibular raphe, posterior end of mylohyoid line of mandible, and side of tongue	Median raphe of pharynx and pharyngeal tubercle on basilar part of occipital bone	Cranial root of accessory nerve via pharyngeal branch of vagus and pharyngeal plexus
	Middle constrictor	Stylohyoid ligament and superior (greater) and inferior (lesser) horns of hyoid bone	Median raphe of pharynx	Cranial root of accessory nerve as above, plus branches of external and recurrent laryngeal nerves of vagus
	Inferior constrictor	Oblique line of thyroid cartilage and side of cricoid cartilage		
	Palatopharyngeus	Hard plate and palatine aponeurosis	Posterior border of lamina of thyroid cartilage and side of pharynx and esophagus	
	Salpingopharyngeus	Cartilaginous part of eustachian tube	Blends with palatopharyngeus	Cranial root of accessory nerve via pharyngeal branch of vagus and pharyngeal plexus
Internal layer (elevators)	Stylopharyngeus	Styloid process of temporal bone	Posterior and superior borders of thyroid cartilage with palatopharyngeus	Glossopharyngeal nerve

FIGURE 19.6. Pharyngeal muscles.

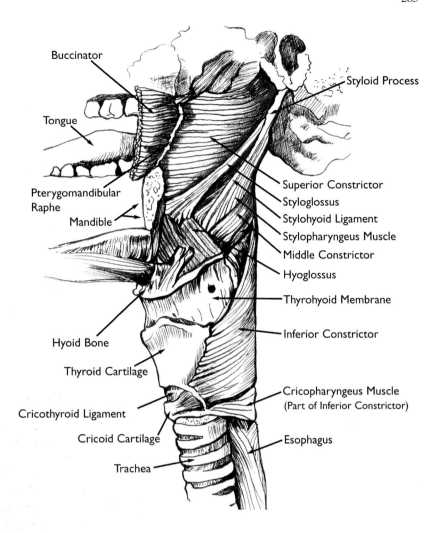

Buccinator

Styloid Process

Tongue

Pterygomandibular
Raphe

Mandible

Superior Constrictor
Styloglossus
Stylohyoid Ligament
Stylopharyngeus Muscle
Middle Constrictor
Hyoglossus
Thyrohyoid Membrane

Inferior Constrictor

Hyoid Bone

Thyroid Cartilage

Cricopharyngeus Muscle
(Part of Inferior Constrictor)

Cricothyroid Ligament

Esophagus

Cricoid Cartilage

Trachea

as the bolus flows and diverges around the larynx via the pyriform fossae. As the bolus passes into the esophagus, the vocal cords adduct to isolate the upper from the lower respiratory tract.

Taste

Taste, one of two chemical special visceral sensory afferents, is located in the oropharynx (base of tongue), oral cavity (anterior tongue), upper esophagus, and larynx. Taste buds are 50 to 100 chemoreceptors that synapse with primary afferent nerves. Most taste afferents are from glossopharyngeal and facial nerves, with minor contributors from the upper esophagus and larynx. Centrally, all taste afferents synapse in the nucleus of the solitary tract.

Complaints

Table 19.7 lists common general conditions of the pharynx.

TABLE 19.7. Pharynx: common general conditions.

Trauma	Head injury, complex facial fractures, mandibular fractures
Inflammation/allergy	Adenoiditis, tonsillitis, gastroesophageal reflux disease
Neoplasms	Benign (angiofibroma); malignant (squamous cell carcinoma, lymphoma)
Foreign bodies	Organic (bone, food); metallic; loose dentures
Caustic ingestion	Acids or bases
Autoimmune	Systemic lupus erythematosus, Wegener's granulomatosis
Infections	Peritonsillar abscess, retropharyngeal abscess, masseter space abscess, buccal space abscess, parapharyngeal space abscess, AIDS
Vascular	Hemangiomas, cystic hygroma, arteriovenous malformation
Congenital:	Cleft palate, trisomy disorders, head and neck syndromes
Degenerative	Cervical ankylosis/arthritis

Symptoms

Symptoms are sore throat, earache, hot potato voice, halitosis, nasal regurgitation, shortness of breath, difficulty swallowing, and fever.

Signs

Signs include hearing loss, hemoptysis, dysphagia, unilateral serous otitis media, epistaxis, obstruction (nasal), upper airway obstruction, trismus, neck mass, odynophagia, and weight loss.

Larynx

Anatomy

The larynx, located in the anterior neck between C3 through C6, has three primary functions: (1) *airway patency* between the upper and lower air passages, (2) *airway protection* or isolation of the upper and lower aerodigestive passages, and (3) *airway modulation* for voice production. The larynx is divided into the *supraglottis* (epiglottis, false cords), *glottis* (true vocal cords), and *subglottis* (inferior from the true vocal cords to the cricoid cartilage).[3,4]

The anterior border of the larynx is the epiglottis (laryngeal surface), thyrohyoid membrane, anterior wall of the subglottis, cricothyroid membrane, and the anterior arch of the cricoid cartilage. The posterior and lateral borders are aryepiglottic folds, arytenoids, interarytenoid space, and cricoid cartilage. The superior and lateral boundary is the tip and lateral border of the epiglottis. The inferior border is a plane passing through the inferior edge of the cricoid cartilage (Figure 19.7).

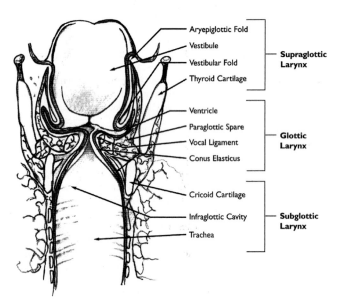

FIGURE 19.7. Larynx, coronal view.

Anterior View   **Posterior View**

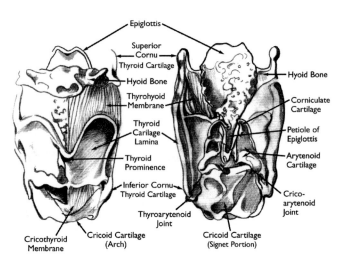

FIGURE 19.8. Laryngeal skeleton.

Laryngeal Skeleton

The laryngeal skeleton consists of nine cartilages linked together by ligaments and membranes (Figure 19.8). Three cartilages are single (thyroid, cricoid, and epiglottis), and three are paired (arytenoid, corniculate, cuneiform). The *thyroid* is the largest cartilage.

The *cricoid*, a complete ring of cartilage, has posterior signet and anterior arch components. Smaller than the thyroid cartilage, the cricoid cartilage is thick and strong. The *cricoarytenoid joints* slide, tilt, and rotate the arytenoid cartilages. These actions respectively approximate, tense, and relax the vocal folds.

Muscles

The *extrinsic* laryngeal or strap muscles suspend and move the larynx between the hyoid bone and sternum. The infrahyoid muscles depress, whereas the suprahyoid and stylopharyngeus muscles elevate the larynx.

The *intrinsic* muscles lengthen and tense the vocal folds, thus altering the size and shape of the rima glottidis (see Figure 19.2). With one exception, the intrinsic muscles are innervated by the recurrent laryngeal nerve, a branch of the vagus, cranial nerve X. This exception, the cricothyroid muscle, is supplied by the external branch of the superior laryngeal nerve, cranial nerve X.

Vasculature

Laryngeal branches of the superior laryngeal and inferior laryngeal arteries arise from the external carotid and the thyrocervical trunk, respectively. The superior laryngeal artery accompanies the internal branch of the superior laryngeal nerve through the thyrohyoid membrane. The inferior laryngeal artery is associated closely with the recurrent laryngeal nerve.

The superior laryngeal vein usually empties into the superior thyroid vein and drains into the internal jugular vein. The inferior laryngeal vein empties into the inferior thyroid vein or the venous plexus of thyroid veins on the anterior aspect of the trachea into the brachiocephalic veins.

Lymphatics

Laryngeal lymphatic vessels, superior to the vocal folds, accompany the superior laryngeal artery through the thyrohyoid membrane into the superior deep cervical lymph nodes. Inferior to the vocal cords, the lymphatics drain into the pretracheal or paratracheal lymph nodes and eventually into the inferior deep cervical lymph nodes.

Nerves

Arising from the inferior vagal ganglion, the superior laryngeal nerve divides into the internal laryngeal (sensory/autonomic) and the external laryngeal (motor) branches. The larger internal laryngeal nerve, with the superior laryngeal artery, pierces the thyrohyoid membrane. It supplies sensation to the endolarynx mucosa superior to the vocal folds. The smaller external laryngeal nerve, posterior to the sternothyroid muscle, aligned closely with the superior thyroid artery, supplies the inferior constrictor and cricothyroid muscles.

Physiology

Sphincteric action—isolation and protection of the upper and lower respiratory tracts—is the *primary* function of the larynx. A derivative of this primary function is valsalva, vital for lifting and bowel elimination. The *secondary* function is phonation, derived from vocal cord approximation, tensing, and relaxation. Speech and communication are its derivatives.[5]

The intrinsic laryngeal muscles are sphincters, adductors, abductors, tensors, and relaxers. The powerful sphincteric muscular activity adducts or closes the rima glottidis during swallowing and valsalva. Contraction of the lateral cricoarytenoids, transverse and oblique arytenoids, and aryepiglottic muscles adduct the aryepiglottic folds and pull the arytenoids toward the epiglottis. The lateral cricoarytenoid muscles are the principal abductors. They supplement the intrinsic thyroarytenoids that relax the larynx. Vital for effective respiration, the larynx is always active whether the patient is awake or asleep.

Complaints

Laryngeal complaints, head and neck lymphatics, and common general conditions of the larynx are listed in Tables 19.8, 19.9, and 19.10, respectively.

TABLE 19.8. Laryngeal complaints.

Site	Symptoms		Signs		Pathogenesis	Salient features
	Early	Late	Early	Late		
Supraglottis	"Lump in throat" Sore throat Earache	Hoarseness Hot potato voice Dysphagia Odynophagia	Exophytic or ulcerative lesion Neck mass	Vocal cord paralysis Hemoptysis Stridor Airway Obstruction	Preepiglottic space Base of tongue Vocal cord paralysis Early unilateral or bilateral cervical metastasis	Early: sore throat or vague complaints Intermediate: voice change Late: airway complaints, frequent early cervical metastasis
Glottis	Hoarseness	Shortness of breath Dyspnea on exertion	Vocal cord lesion/paralysis	Airway Obstruction Stridor Aphonia Vocal cord Paralysis Neck mass	Paraglottic space Thyrohyoid Membrane	Early: hoarseness
Subglottis	Shortness of breath Hoarseness	Shortness of breath Dyspnea on exertion	Subglottic lesion without cord paralysis	Cord paralysis Aphonia Neck mass Stridor Airway obstruction	Paraglottic space Cricoid membrane	Late: Airway complaints Neck mass

Source: Reprinted with permission from Hinton and Myers.[4]

Symptoms

Symptoms are hoarseness, shortness of breath, cough (croup vs. noncroup), wheezing, tachypnea, apnea, halitosis, and choking.

Signs

Signs include vocal cord paralysis, hemoptysis, stridor, cyanosis, neck mass, and dysphagia.

TABLE 19.9. Head and neck lymphatics.

Site	Origin	Group
Scalp	Frontal region	Preauricular/parotid
	Temporoparietal region	Postauricular/parotid
	Occipital region	Occipital
Pinna and external auditory canal	Anterior	Preauricular
	Posterior	Postauricular
	Inferior	Superior deep and superficial cervical
	Eyelids and conjuctiva	Parotid and submandibular
	Posterior neck	Parotid
	Anterior neck	Submandibular
	Ala	Submandibular
	Upper lip	Submandibular
	Lower lip (lateral)	Submandibular
	Central lower lip	Submandibular
	Temporal fossa	Deep facial
	Infratemporal fossa	Superior deep cervical
Nasopharynx	Skull base	Retropharyngeal
		Superior deep cervical
Nose	Anterior one half	Submandibular/submental
Paranasal sinuses	Posterior two thirds	Retropharyngeal
	Soft palate	Nose superior deep cervical
		Retropharyngeal
		Parotid
		Superior deep cervical
Oral cavity	Gingivae	Submandibular
	Hard palate	Parotid
	Anterior floor of mouth	Submental
	Lateral floor of mouth	Submandibular
	Tongue tip	Submental
	Lateral tongue	Superior deep cervical
Oropharynx	Hard palate	Submental/submandibular
	Lateral	Submandibular
	Base of tongue	Super deep cervical
	Tonsils	Ingodigastric
Hypopharynx/ larynx	Thyrohyoid membrane	Superior deep cervical
	Conus elasticus	Pretracheal and prelaryngeal
	Cricoid membrane and first tracheal ring	Inferior deep cervical

Source: Reprinted with permission from Myers EM. Neck dissection. In Myers EM, ed. Head and Neck Oncology: Diagnosis, Treatment, and Rehabilitation. Boston: Little, Brown & Company, 1991: 449–464.

TABLE 19.10. Larynx: common general conditions.

Trauma	Laryngeal fractures, cervical spine fractures, blunt trauma, penetrating wounds, subglottic stenosis, trauma (projectiles), intravenous drug injections, central venous catheter insertions, Iatiogenic (surgery)
Inflammation/ allergy	Fumes, prolonged intubation, smoke, noxious inhalations, gastroesophageal reflux disease
Neoplasms	Benign (nodes, polyps), malignant (squamous cell carcinoma, lymphoma), thyroid malignancies
Foreign bodies	Assorted foods, nonmetallic, metallic, dentures
Autoimmune	Sarcoidosis, rheumatoid arthritis
Infections	Croup, tuberculosis, diphtheria, epiglottitis
Vascular	Hemangiomas, arteriovenous malformations, cystic hygromas, vascular rings, cardiovascular accident sequela
Congenital	Laryngeal clefts, laryngomalacia, subglottic stenosis
Degenerative	Amyloidosis, laryngocele

Emergencies

Most head and neck surgical emergencies involve either the pharynx (Table 19.11) or larynx (Table 19.12). The common emergencies are airway obstruction, hemorrhage, infection/inflammation, caustic ingestion, and foreign bodies. First and foremost is airway obstruction, whose diagnosis and management is the key to safe treatment. More often than not, immediate or impending airway compromise is associated with the other emergencies (Figure 19.9). Whenever a patient presents with *any* head and neck emergency, the underlying question is, will it affect the airway?

Hemorrhage

Hemorrhage is common in the pharynx, notably the tonsils (oropharynx) and nasopharynx. Tonsillectomy bleeding, immediate or postoperative, is always vexing and, at times, life threatening. Nasopharyngeal bleeding may be confused with and associated with nasal sources. A less common site is bleeding from the larynx (subglottis) in the immediate/delayed post-tracheotomy patient or a patient with previous head and neck irradiation.

Infection/Inflammation

Again, the pharynx (oropharynx) is the principle site (i.e., tonsillitis or peritonsillar abscess). However, other areas such as the nasopharynx, hypopharynx, and supraglottic larynx may be involved. Examples respectively are peritonsillar parapharyngeal/retropharyngeal abscesses, epiglottis, and croup. Within the family of deep cervical abscesses, peritonsillar space abscesses are by far the most common. In the past, epiglottitis was a pediatric

TABLE 19.11. Pharynx: emergency conditions and treatment.

Initial Condition	Nasopharynx	Oropharynx	Hypopharynx	Treatment	Secondary Conditions

Obstruction	Neoplasm
	Adenoid hypertrophy
	Sinus pathology
		Tonsillar hypertophy
		Neoplasm
		  Tonsil
		  Base of tongue
		  Parapharynx
			Neoplasm	*Airway assurance*
				Treatment of primary
				  cause
					Airway obstruction
					Obstructive apnea
					Arrhythmia
					Respiratory arrest

Hemorrhage	Postadenoidectomy Epistaxis	Post-tonsillectomy Facial fractures Penetrating trauma	Rare	*Airway assurance* Packing Cauterization Ligation Embolization	*Airway obstruction* Aspiration Hemorrhagic shock

Inflammation/
infection
	Secondary to chronic
	  sinusitis
	Retropharyngeal
	  abscess
		Secondary to oral
		  cavity abscess
		Peritonsillar abscess
		Parapharyngeal abscess
			Parapharyngeal
			  Abscess
				Airway assurance
				Incision and drainage
					Airway obstruction
					Respiratory arrest

Foreign body	Vegetable matter	Fish bones
		Dentures
			Fish bones
			  loose teeth
			  Dentures
				Airway assurance
				Endoscopy and
				  extraction
					Airway obstruction
					Perforation
					Sepsis
					Septic shock

Caustic ingestion	Burns (rare)	Burns (common)	Burns (common)	*Airway assurance* Neutralization Lavage Endoscopy	*Airway obstruction* Perforation Sepsis Septic shock Stenosis

disease; however, today it is more common in adults. Croup, the quintessential pediatric airway inflammatory condition, must be differentiated from epiglottitis. Both may require emergency airway assurance.[6,7]

Caustic Ingestion

Caustic agents, whether basic or acidic, can affect the upper aerodigestive tract from the lips to the esophagus.[8–10] However, the most common sites are the pharynx (oro/hypopharynx) and esophagus. The gag reflex usually protects the larynx. Immediate measures include neu-

tralization, lavage, antibiotics, systemic steroids, and early bronchoscopy or esophagoscopy to assess damage. If no damage is evident, steroids are discontinued. However, for significant burns, steroids may be prescribed. Serial esophagoscopy every 10 days is performed until the injury stabilizes.

Foreign Body

Foreign body ingestion is more common in pediatric, mentally challenged, and elderly patients. The usual ingested objects are displaced dentures, bones, pins, coins,

TABLE 19.12. Larynx: emergency conditions and treatment.

Initial condition	Supraglottis	Glottis	Subglottis	Treatment	Secondary condition
Obstruction	Inflammation Allergic reaction Neoplasm	Inflammation Allergic reaction Neoplasm Vocal cord paralysis	Inflammation Allergic reaction Neoplasm Stenosis	*Airway assurance* Avoid tracheotomy	*Airway obstruction* Respiratory arrest
Hemorrhage	Foreign body	Blunt trauma	Hemangiomas Posttracheotomy	*Airway assurance* hemostatis	*Airway obstruction* Respiratory arrest Hemorrhage shock

Inflammation/
infection
	Epiglottis	Tuberculosis
		Gastroesophageal
		  reflux disease
			Croup	*Airway assurance*
				Treatment of underlying
				  condition
					Airway obstruction
					Respiratory arrest
					Sepsis
					Septic shock

Foreign body	Dentures	Food
		(beans, peas, corn)
			Tacks
			Pins
			Loose teeth
				Airway assurance
				Endoscopy and
				  extraction
					Airway obstruction
					Respiratory arrest
					Aspiration into lung
					  or esophagus

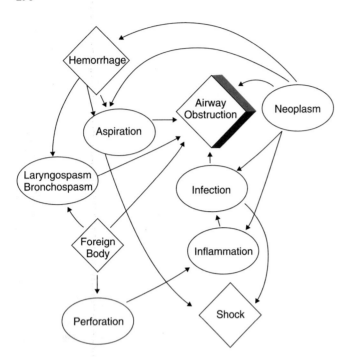

FIGURE 19.9. Web of complications. Diamond, start or finish; arrow, suggested pathway; oval, comment or variable (See also Figure 19.17.)

needles, toys, and food (corn, peanuts). Aspirated foreign bodies that obstruct the glottis, straddle the carina, or occlude a main stem bronchus, may be rapidly fatal. Foreign bodies lodged in the subglottis or trachea may perforate and initiate edema, segmental atelectasis, pneumonia, or abscess formation. Clinical suspicion must be heightened because the history may seem innocuous. Aspirated food may be asymptomatic initially, only to evolve (hours or days), into life-threatening obstruction, infection, inflammation, and edema. Following the physical examination, including auscultation, soft tissue lateral films of the neck, chest x-rays, and barium swallow are ordered as indicated.

Case Studies

Case 1 (Pharynx): "The Flickering Candle"

Indications

A 57-year-old diabetic woman presented with a 3- to 4-week history of decreasing vision in the left eye, leading rapidly to almost complete blindness. Soon thereafter she was hospitalized by her primary care physician for a mild stroke with transient left-sided paresis. After noting significant left proptosis, she was referred to an ophthalmologist who in turn referred her emergently to the otolaryngology service. Computed tomography (CT) of the sinuses revealed a large left sinonasal mass, (skull

base to the nose) that extended in an anteroposterior direction from the sphenoid sinus to the left maxillary sinus (Figure 19.10). The lamina papyracea was breached and the septum was bowed significantly to the right. Magnetic resonance imaging (MRI) of the head did not implicate skull base or intracranial involvement.

Operative Findings

Within 24 hours of the otolaryngologic evaluation, she was scheduled for emergent transendoscopic optic nerve decompression. Sinus endoscopy demonstrated inflammatory disease in the left nasal cavity associated with nasal polyps. Following polypectomy, a thick, green to brown substance with the consistency of peanut butter oozed from the left nasal cavity, the maxillary and sphenoid sinuses. Dramatically, 3 days after decompression, her vision returned completely. The final pathologic diagnosis was mucormycosis.

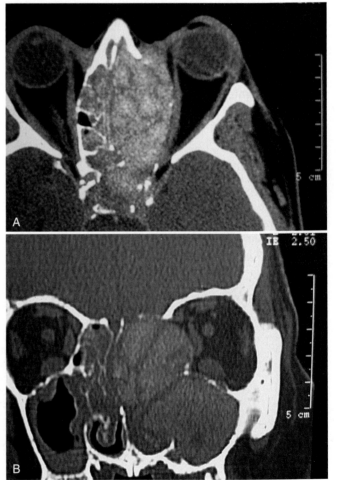

FIGURE 19.10. (A) Computed tomographic scan of the sinuses, axial view: extensive opacification of left sphenoid, ethmoid, and maxillary sinuses. (B) Computed tomographic scan of the sinuses, coronal view.

Discussion

Mucormyosis, an invasive fungal infection, is associated with permanent complications and high mortality.[11] These phycomycete fungi are three basic species: rhizopus, absidia, and mucor. They are especially aggressive in immune-compromised, poor-controlled diabetics and patients with bone marrow malignancies or renal failure. Early recognition and intervention are crucial for survival. These spores are ubiquitous but in the susceptible patient, they can invade blood vessels directly into the ethmoid sinuses, orbit, or skull base. If the skull base is violated, intracranial pathogenesis facilitated by intravascular thrombosis, is possible. This is a distinct possibility in the high-risk patient who complains of headache, orbital/facial pain, fever, visual changes with associated rhinorrhea or acute sinusitis. Grave clinical signs are periorbital/facial edema, altered mental status, ophthalmoplegia, and black, demarcated nasal or palatal mucosa (necrosis).

Mucosal biopsy specimens show nonseptated hyphae with 90° branching on Gomori methamine-silver stain. Images, CT or MRI, may demonstrate soft tissue and bony boundaries as well as skull base or intracranial extension. Surgical debridement may be targeted (endoscopy) or extensive (debilitating). If extensive, the prognosis is poor. Postoperative, long-term (months) therapy includes antifungals as well as correction of any predisposing underlying pathophysiology.

Conclusions

This case is a notable but important exception of common pharyngeal surgical emergencies. Some aggressive pharyngeal conditions may involve adjacent regions such as the skull base or thorax. However, dramatic reversal by aggressive, timely surgical intervention can preserve function and life.

Case 2 (Pharynx): "Routine Surgery"

Indications

A 2$\frac{1}{2}$-year-old girl, 2 months postadenoidectomy for documented obstructive sleep apnea that required a home apnea monitor. At the time of the original surgery the small tonsils seemed noncontributory to the obstructive process. Postadenoidectomy, initially, the patient did well, but a follow-up sleep study demonstrated persistent sleep apnea although less severe. Persistent apnea and significant hypoxia dictated a second procedure. Thus, she was reevaluated for tonsillectomy and possible uvulopharyngopalatoplasty rarely performed in a child.

Description of Procedure

Following intubation, the adenoid bed was reinspected and found free of any significant regrowth of adenoid tissue. The left tonsil, small to moderate in size, was dissected with the harmonic scalpel. Hemostasis was achieved with electrocautery. In a similar fashion the right tonsil was dissected and removed. Bleeding seemed to stop.

Momentarily, troublesome oozing in the inferior pole was observed. Again, hemostasis was attempted with electrocautery; however, suddenly, a major arterial bleeder erupted. The bleeding, very brisk and spectacular, required multiple hemostats for control. Several attempts were made to control three bleeding points in the deep inferior portion of the tonsillar bed, but suture ligatures were futile. Once the clamps were removed major arterial bleeding gushed profusely.

Within minutes, the patient lost approximately 1,000 cc of blood. The estimated circulating blood volume, based on weight, was approximately 1,400 cc. She was transfused with 3 units of whole blood, including one unit of type O nonspecific whole blood. Aggressive transfusions and 700 cc of crystalloid fluids maintained the blood pressure. Although the bleeding was controlled, more definitive efforts were necessary. At first large and then small titanium clips were applied, but these were inadequate. Medium-sized titanium clips were placed deep in the tonsillar bed around the major arterial bleeder. Approximately four clips were placed. Finally, the bleeding stopped, and the bed was oversewn with superior constrictor muscle. The vital signs were stable after definitive hemostasis and fluid resuscitation.

Discussion

An assessment of the events yielded the following analysis. The patient had a superficial left internal carotid artery in the inferior tonsillar fossa. Electrocauterization in this area disrupted the internal carotid artery, thus resulting in emergent hemorrhage. Stat consultations were requested from the pediatric and pediatric neurology services while the patient was in the operating room. The consultants recommended strongly that the patient have an immediate postoperative MRI of the head with contrast. While intubated, she was transported for the study. A long-term favorable prognosis was encouraged by intact bilateral cerebral circulation. A void in the area of the left internal carotid arteries was secondary to multiple titanium vascular clips (Figure 19.11).

Conclusions

Annually, thousands of tonsillectomies and adenoidectomies are performed safely. The possibility of life-

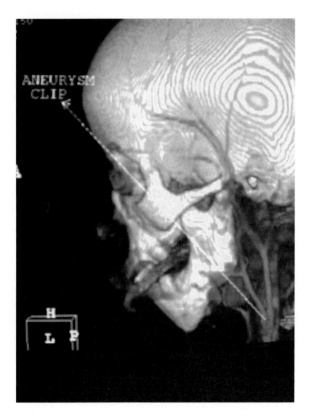

FIGURE 19.11. Magnetic resonance image of the head, showing left lateral reconstruction, vascularity, and post-titanium clipping of the internal carotid artery.

threatening complications is recognized but quite uncommon. Immediate or delayed life-threatening hemorrhage is always disconcerting, but fatalities are extremely rare. Nonetheless, this case illustrates dramatically that there is no such entity as *routine surgery*.

Case 3 (Pharynx): "Chokehold"

Indications

A 68-year-old man with an 8-to 10-month history of gradual dysphagia, difficulty breathing, and turning his neck sought medical care when he could only sleep propped up in a chair. He did not complain of hoarseness or of difficulty handling secretions. Fitful sleeping and progressive choking could no longer be ignored. Although the primary care physician did not detect any pathology on physical examination, he ordered a CT of the neck. The CT showed a large 4- to 6-cm mass in the right parapharyngeal space extending from the skull base to the carotid bifurcation (Figure 19.12). Indirect laryngoscopy by an otolaryngologist showed a right, posterior,

lateral, parapharyngeal mass that compressed extrinsically the airway.

Description of Procedure

An awake tracheostomy secured the airway. Following airway assurance, the patient was turned 180°, redraped, and reprepped. A cervical incision was performed from the right mastoid tip, approximately 2.5 finger breadths below the angle of the mandible to the submentum, in a natural skin crease. The carotid sheath was exposed after retracting the anterior border of the sternocleidomastoid muscle. The sheath was entered bluntly and the internal jugular vein and common carotid artery were identified and protected. For control, vessel loops were used. With retraction, the inferior portion of the firm mass was exposed. Aided by muscle relaxants, the mandible was dislocated anteriorly for increased exposure. At the skull base, the dissection proceeded cautiously. The vagus nerve, enveloped by the tumor at the skull base, was difficult to mobilize and dissect. Some bleeding was noted from the jugular vein as it emerged from the jugular fossa. This was controlled with vascular clips. The tumor was resected sharply and delivered. Postoperatively, he sustained a right vocal cord paralysis (cranial nerve X) and shoulder weakness (cranial nerve XI). The former responded to vocal Cora medialization and the latter to physical therapy.

Discussion

The parapharyngeal space boundaries are skull base (superior), mandible (lateral), pharyngeal wall (medial), cervical spine (posterior), and hyoid bone (inferior).

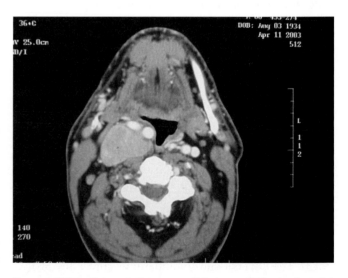

FIGURE 19.12. Computed tomographic scan of the neck, axial view, showing right poststyloid parapharyngeal mass displacing the carotid sheath anteriorly.

Carotid sheath contents, spinal accessory nerve, lymphatics, deep parotid lobe, and pterygoid muscles are crammed into this inverted cone-shaped space. Potentially, parapharyngeal space inflammation/infection or neoplasm can involve the retropharyngeal, peritonsillar, and submandibular spaces.[12]

The vast majority of parapharyngeal space neoplasms are benign (80%), notably mixed tumors of the deep parotid lobe, also called dumb-bell tumors. Lymphoma is the most common malignancy. The final pathologic diagnosis for this patient was glomus jugulare, a benign paraganglioma of the jugular baroreceptors. These slow-growing tumors present initially with airway compromise or as asymptomatic neck masses. When the tumor exceeds 2.5 to 3.0 cm, the patient may also complain of pain, dysphagia, trismus, or obstructive sleep apnea. Some present with vocal cord paralysis or Horner's syndrome, reflecting injury to the sympathetic trunk in the carotid sheath. Parapharyngeal masses are classified as pre- or poststyloid process. Unlike this case, the majority are prestyloid. There are a variety of surgical approaches: (1) transcervical, (2) transparotid, (3) combination transmandible/transcervical, (4) combination transmastoid/transcervical, and (5) preauricular fossa. Most surgeons advocate the transcervical approach, utilized in this patient, as the first option.

Conclusions

Although benign, potentially morbid consequences are associated with late diagnosis or inexpert excision. Many authors believe MRI is more accurate than CT. MRI classifies whether the lesions are pre- or poststyloid. This information helps to determine the surgical approach. Whatever the approach, the surgeon must secure the airway, isolate/protect the great vessels, preserve the facial nerve, and practice meticulous hemostasis.

Case 4 (Pharynx): "Cry Baby"

Indications

An irritable, crying, febrile 6-month-old infant seen in the early evening in the pediatric emergency room, had swelling in the right tail of the parotid and upper neck area. The oral cavity and oropharynx were clear. Computed tomography scans demonstrated findings compatible with an abscess in the tail of the parotid, upper neck area and possibly the parapharyngeal space (Figure 19.13). The parents and grandparents were advised and counseled extensively about emergent surgery. Reluctantly, they agreed. Surgery was performed early the next morning after overnight intravenous antibiotics.

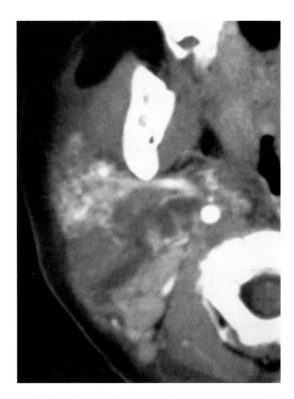

FIGURE 19.13. Computed tomographic scan of the neck, axial view, showing inflammatory changes in the right parotid gland and parapharyngeal space.

Description of Procedure

The baby had a large, fluctuant, indurated area involving the previously mentioned sites. A 2 centimeter incision one finger breadth below the angle of the incision was carried down through the skin/subcutaneous and platysmal layers to the sternocleidomastoid muscle. The carotid sheath was free of infection. However, 5 cm of pus was evacuated from the tail of the parotid gland. The right parapharyngeal space was explored and found free of involvement. The surgical site was irrigated copiously with normal saline and hydrogen peroxide after tissue samples were obtained. A small 1-inch Iodoform™ gauze pack was placed. The incision was approximated, and a pressure dressing was applied. Blood loss was minimal.

Discussion

Deep cervical inflammation or abscesses may be derived from multiple sites: 1, sublingual space (Ludwig's angina); 2, buccal space; 3, masseteric space; 4, peritonsillar space; 5, retropharyngeal space; and 6, parapharyngeal space. Sites 1 through 3 are oral or dental in origin. Sites 4 through 6 are oropharyngeal in origin. Rampant infections can progress to adjacent sites via interconnected fascial planes. Without timely treatment, airway obstruction or sepsis is the terminal event.

Conclusions

Early recognition and emergent surgery prevented this patient from developing morbid complications (see Figure 19.9). Precise surgery in inflammatory/infection emergency conditions is predicated on intimate knowledge of the fascial planes and potential spaces. Airway assurance, as always, is the prerequisite.

Case 5 (Larynx): "Wheezing"

Indications

The patient is a 19-year-old young man with a history of subglottic/tracheal stenosis following 16 days of intubation and mechanical ventilation for a closed head injury. Computed tomographic and MRI images of the neck and chest are normal. However, direct laryngoscopy and broncoscopy demonstrate a severe subglottal stenosis approximately 2.0 cm below the glottis that is dilated with a size 42 French filiform dilator. The patient is extubated and transferred to the Surgical Intensive Care Unit for overnight airway monitoring.

Description of Procedure

Initially, laser bronchoscopy and dilation are effective. However, within 3 months he presented to the emergency room, short of breath and wheezing, that began when he was playing basketball. He was admitted, reevaluated, and counseled for a more definitive procedure. Following bronchoscopy, end-to-end tracheoplasty, hyoid release, and blunt mediastinal dissection were performed (Figure 19.14).

Discussion

Subglottic stenosis, postintubation, a rare but debilitating complication, is often overlooked. Theoretically, cuff pressures exceeding 30 mm Hg impede mucosal capillary perfusion pressure, resulting in mucosal ischemia, ulceration, and chondritis. Secondary infection with granulation tissue proliferation and fibrosis creates a firm, stenotic scar. Postintubation stenosis may also involve the larynx and trachea.

Postdilation, the patient did well, but within 1 month the stridor evolved into dysphonia and impending airway obstruction. Tracheal stenosis is classified as grade I, <50% obstruction; grade II, 50% to <70% obstruction; grade III, 70% to 100%; and grade IV, no detectable lumen. Grades I and II are treated with dilation and/or with transendoscopic laser. However, grades III and IV require sophisticated open procedures. In this patient, the grade was underestimated. His persistent complaints prompted reevaluation.

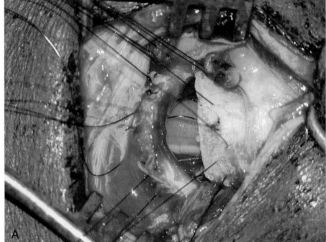

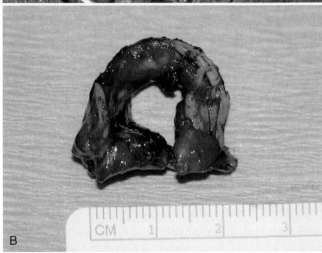

FIGURE 19.14. **(A)** Intraoperative view of trachea after stenosis resection before end-to-end anastomosis. **(B)** Resected stenotic segment.

Conclusions

A high index of suspicion was necessary to make this diagnosis. Definitive resection was executed after the stenosis was determined precisely by bronchoscopy. Unlike imaging, physical diagnosis and bronchoscopy were diagnostic. Tracheotomy was not performed because tracheoplasty after tracheotomy is much more difficult. Thus, if possible, it should be avoided if tracheoplasty is a surgical option.

Case 6 (Larynx and Bronchus): "The Cough"

Indications

Febrile (103°F) and coughing productively, a 5-year-old boy presented to the pediatric emergency room. The recent and past histories were negative. Centralized upper chest wheezing on auscultation prompted ordering

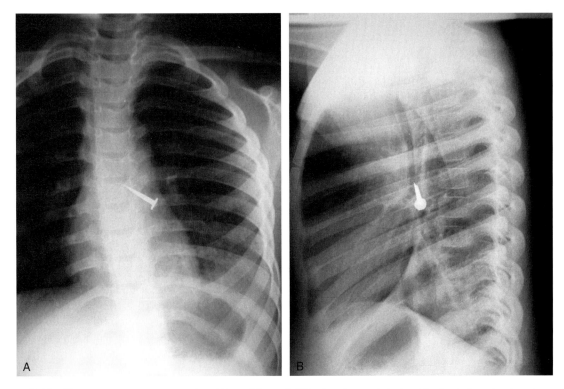

FIGURE 19.15. Chest x-rays, anteroposterior **(A)** and lateral **(B)**, showing tack lodged in the left main stem bronchus.

a chest x-ray. A tack was lodged in the left main stem bronchus (Figure 19.15). After hydration and intravenous antibiotics, it was removed the next morning.

Description of Procedure

Following laryngoscopy, a ventilating bronchoscope for general anesthesia was passed. A 2.7-mm telescope via the bronchoscope facilitated visualization. The right was clear, but the left main stem bronchus was obscured by profuse, purulent secretions that were aspirated to reveal the tack. With the point protected by the alligator forceps, it was extracted uneventfully.

Discussion

The diagnosis of a foreign body is made usually late after the emergence of respiratory signs and symptoms of inflammation or infection.[13] If the foreign body is large or the child is small, acute ingestion can fatally obstruct the glottis, subglottis or carina. An ingested foreign body can involve secondarily the gastrointestinal tract. The commonly involved sites in descending order are tonsil, base of tongue, pyriform sinus, and cervical esophagus (cricopharyngeus or the upper esophageal sphincter) (Figure 19.16). Sharp foreign bodies (bone, pins) have the potential to cause perforation. Perforation is a potentially morbid or mortal late complication, especially if the

foreign body lodges in the trachea or esophagus. Mediastinal perforation may evolve rapidly into mediastinitis, an infection that has a very high mortality rate.

Conclusions

For pediatric or mentally challenged patients, the physician must have a high index of suspicion and initiate

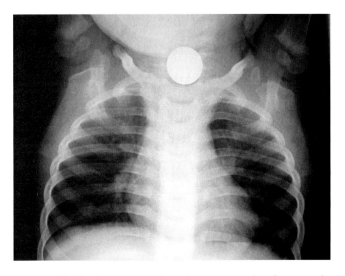

FIGURE 19.16. Anteroposterior chest x-ray, showing a coin (nickel) lodged superior to the cricopharyngeus in an infant.

timely surgical intervention. Unless a history of coughing paroxysms or ingestion is observed, the patient may be assumed to have an upper respiratory infection. Soft tissue lateral images of the neck and plain x-rays of the chest are usually sufficient for the diagnosis of a radiopaque foreign body. Radiotranslucent foreign bodies require endoscopy for diagnostic confirmation.

Case Study 7 (Pharynx and Larynx): "The Cobra"

The Arrival

1225 hours: The ambulance hurriedly drove the 57-year-old man to the Emergency Room. His wife had called frantically $1^1/_2$ hours after he began gasping and complaining of generalized tongue swelling.
He denied allergies (nuts or berries) but admitted to have been taking Zestril™ for 9 months.

1230 hours: Vital signs: pulse 112, respiration 22, blood pressure 148/102, oxygen saturation 100%

Physical Examination

Vital signs: temperature 97.9, pulse 102, respiration 24, blood pressure 138/85, oxygen saturation 100% (100% oxygen facemask). He was alert, oriented, dysphonic, and in mild distress secondary to gross tongue edema. The lungs were clear to auscultation.

Assessment

Angioedema secondary to angiotensin-converting enzyme (ACE) inhibitor

Treatment

IV heplock, CBC at *1227 hours*
Normal saline 1 L bolus at *1227 hours*
Solumedrol™ 125 mg IV at *1227 hours*
Benadryl™ 25 mg IV at *1229 hours*
Zantac™ 50 mg IV and epinephrine 0.3 mg (slowly) IV at *1230 hours*

1245 hours: Vital signs: 89, 20, 157/72 (100% O_2).
1300 hours: Airway patent, tongue swelling improving, normal sinus rhythm.
1310 hours: Vital signs: 92, 22, 149/67 (100% O_2).
1330 hours: Vital signs: 99, 22, 159/82; airway patent, angioedema unchanged, mild respiratory distress, normal sinus rhythm.
1400 hours: Vital signs: 88, 24, 138/77 99%; airway patent, mild distress, no change in angioedema, patient stated that he feels better.
1420 hours: No acute distress, SaO_2 99%, respirations unlabored, tongue swollen, awaiting bed in intensive care unit.

1445 hours: Vital signs: 81, 22, 153/67 (100% 0_2); nurse stated that "respirations were unlabored."
1500 hours: Patient sat on edge of stretcher talking with attending physician with oxygen mask in place. Pulse oximeter probe is in place. Suddenly he became anxious, breathing with extreme difficulty. The attending physician shouted for residents and nurses.
1505 hours: Cyanosis; resuscitation begun; attending physician requested racemic epinephrine. Resuscitative measures continued; patient was bagged with difficulty. Monitor showed bradycardia.
1520 hours: ACLS protocol initiated; for arrest and code, CPR is started. Atropine 1 mg started × 4; multiple oropharyngeal intubation attempts were unsuccessful.
1529 hours: Tracheostomy with No. 6 endotracheal tube placed by a surgeon after he was called frantically to the Emergency Room. After 5 minutes, a difficult tracheotomy was performed (fat, short neck, distorted anatomy secondary to grossly diffuse edema). Finally equal breath sounds are confirmed.
1530 hours: Asystole: epinephrine 1 mg started × 10.
1537 hours: Cardiac pacer placed.
1545 hours: Nasogastric tube placed.
1551 hours: $NaHCO_3$ 1 amp started × 5.
1555 hours: Dopamine 400 mg in 250 cc D5W IV wide open.
1600 hours: Calcium chloride started × 2.
1600 hours: Additional vascular access obtained.
1610 hours: Amiodarone 300 mg IV given.
1622 hours: Blood gases 7.17, 77 O_2, 49.5 pCO_2; rhythm remained asystolic.
1655 hours: Patient pronounced dead (total code time 1 hour and 35 minutes).

Discussion

The patient was evaluated, treated and monitored. However, the attending staff failed to recognize early intrinsic airway compromise that involved the entire upper respiratory tract from the oral cavity to the larynx. Consultations by airway specialists were not requested proactively. Deterioration was recognized immediately. Consultants with airway expertise were requested, and they responded when called.

Conclusions

In approximately $4^1/_2$ hours, an alert but acutely ill emergency room patient died. Although supportive measures were appropriate, the glaring error not to provide timely airway assurance cataclysmically triggered respiratory-cardiovascular arrest. In short, this case illustrates graphically untimely airway management. A proactive airway strategy could have saved this patient.

Discussion

Basic principles of diagnosis and treatment are illustrated by the Case Studies. A discussion of surgical emergencies of the pharynx and larynx focuses on timely airway assurance, hemostasis, and incision and drainage.

Airway

Patients suspected of having an immediate or impending airway emergency must be evaluated analytically and quickly (Tables 19.13 and 19.14).[14,15] An indirect (mirror) or direct (endoscope) method is fundamental to assess airway integrity. Cervical palpation and auscultation are also invaluable. Upper airway compromise may be triggered by loose dentures, tongue retrusion, edema, or inflammation. Simply clearing the oral cavity and oropharynx of blood, mucus, and vomitus may be sufficient to reestablish an airway. If the airway is assessed improperly, sedation and muscle relaxation may trigger acute respiratory and cardiovascular collapse (Tables 19.15 and 19.16). Moreover, in children, upper airway

TABLE 19.13. Symptoms and signs of airway obstruction.

Symptoms
  Psychological
    Apprehension
    Confusion
    Combativeness
  Visual
    Abnormal respirations (tachypnea)
    Retractions
    Sweating
    Anxiety
  Audible
    Dysphonia
    Aphonia
    Snoring
    Stridor
    Gagging
    Wheezing
    Grunting
    Hoarseness

Signs
  Integumental
    Cyanosis
    Sweating
  Respiratory
    Glottic edema
    Glottic obstruction (mass or inflammation)
    Vocal cord paralysis
    Rhonchi
  Cardiovascular
    Vital signs: tachycardia, hypertension, hypotension
    Electrocardiogram: ST segment elevation, prolonged QT interval, Q waves
  Musculoskeletal: use of accessory muscles of respiration

Source: Reprinted with permission from Myers.[14]

TABLE 19.14. The difficult airway: clinical assessment.

History
  Tracheal stenosis
  Maxillofacial trauma
  Previous difficult intubation
  Preoperative head and neck irradiation
  Previous head and neck surgery
  Cervical disc surgery fusion

Physical examination
  Congenital abnormalities
  Macroglossia
  Micrognathia
  Prognathia

Habitus
  Obese cervical anatomy
  Short or muscular neck
  Cervical arthritis or ankylosis

Dental assessment
  Loose teeth
  Protruding incisors
  Long, arched palate
  Temporomandibular joint ankylosis
  Trismus
  Dental implants

Head and neck infection/abscess
  Head and neck malignancy
  Large oral cavity neoplasm
  Large oropharyngeal neoplasm
  Marginal airway (associated with large laryngeal, hypopharyngeal, or thyroid malignancy)

Anticipated procedure
  Panendoscopy
  Laser endoscopy
  Interstitial implant
  Partial laryngectomy
  Jaw/neck dissection

Source: Reprinted with permission from Myers.[14]

TABLE 19.15. The difficult airway: objective assessment.

Physical examination
  Palpation
  Auscultation (neck and chest)
  Indirect or direct laryngoscopy

Diagnostic radiology
  Soft tissue films of the neck-AP and lateral
  Chest x-rays, anteroposterior and lateral
  Computed tomography scan of the neck*
  Computed tomography scan of the mediastinum*
  Computed tomography scan of the lungs*

Pulmonary function studies
  Arterial blood gases
  Flow-volume studies
  Spirometry

Fiberoptic laryngoscopy

Laboratory
  Complete blood count and differential
  Arterial blood gases

*When indicated.
Source: Reprinted with permission from Myers.[14]

TABLE 19.16. The difficult airway: anesthetic technique.

Premedication
    Mild sedative
    Anticholinergic

Induction: awake technique
    Nasoendotracheal intubation
    Shoulder roll (cervical hyperextension)
    Topical nasal and oral anesthesia
    Blind versus fiberoptic intubation

Oral-endotracheal intubation
    Shoulder roll (cervical hyperextension)
    Topical oral anesthesia
    Laryngeal mask
    Percutaneous retrograde catheterization

Backup
    Rigid bronchoscopy
    Cricothyrotomy
    Tracheotomy
    Jet ventilation

Source: Reprinted with permission from Myers.[14]

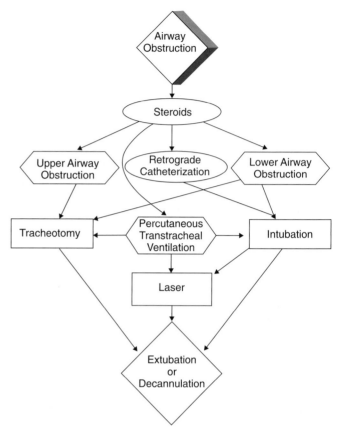

FIGURE 19.17. Airway strategy. Diamond, start or finish; arrow, suggested pathway; hexagon, question or decision; rectangle, instruction; oval, comment or variable. (See also Figure 19.9.)

manipulation may exacerbate a tenuous airway (i.e., epiglottis).

As the oral cavity is inspected, the patient is placed in a head upright or sitting position for maximum ventilation. Nasal or oral oxygen and pulse oximetry are vital adjuncts. Should the patient deteriorate, rapid, decisive action is necessary to avoid cerebral or myocardial hypoxia. The former may evolve quickly into irreversible anoxic encephalopathy and the latter into myocardial arrhythmia or ischemia. In short, a reliable airway is the first priority (Figure 19.17).

Intubation

Assessment

First, the head tilt, jaw thrust/jaw lift maneuvers with facial mask oxygen are initiated. If unsuccessful, then another airway option must be selected without hesitation. Endotracheal intubation is the preferred airway technique. An adequately inflated endotracheal tube cuff isolates and protects the lower from the upper respiratory tracts. For the difficult intubation, whether oral or nasal, the endotracheal tube may be passed under direct vision, utilizing the fiberoptic laryngoscope. Regardless of the route, nasal or oral, the optimal endotracheal tube position must be assessed by bilateral chest auscultation or chest x-ray and secured above the carina.

Nasal Intubation Nasotracheal intubation, blind or aided by fiberoptic laryngoscopy, is indicated for patients with cervical spine injury/ankylosis/immobilization, maxillofacial trauma, inflammation, or neoplasm. This technique is performed usually in an awake, semiconscious patient. It is the preferred route for unimpeded surgery in the oral cavity and oropharynx.

Oral Intubation Oral intubation is preferred for anticipated intubation problems, such as patients with short, muscular or fat necks, cervical arthritis, or anteriorly displaced larynges. Nasopharyngoscopy, nasal surgery and upper maxillofacial surgery are procedures that demand this technique. Endotracheal intubation requires minimal skill; however, it can be associated with complications.[16] It may also cause airway obstruction, especially in patients with upper airway lesions (i.e., neoplasms) (Tables 19.17 and 19.18).

TABLE 19.17. Intubation: disadvantages.

Requires constant tube position (assessment above the carina)
    23 cm from the teeth in men
    21 cm from the teeth in women

Altered respiratory physiology
    Diminished cough
    Increased secretions
    Mucous plugs

Increased airway resistance (notable with small-diameter tubes)
    Increases significantly in patients with respiratory insufficiency
    Increased work of breathing
    Predisposition for bronchospasm or laryngospasm

Source: Reprinted with permission from Myers.[14]

TABLE 19.18. Intubation: complications.

Site	Acute complications	Chronic complications
Oropharynx	Tooth avulsion	Pneumonitis secondary
	Tonsil laceration	to foreign body
	Tongue laceration	Cleft tongue
	Palate laceration	Cleft palate
Hypopharynx	Perforation	Cervical emphysema
		Pneumothorax
		Pneumomediastinum
		Mediastinitis
Supraglottis	Laceration	Supraglottic stenosis
and glottis	Cord edema	Polyps
	Cord abrasion	Granulomas
	Arytenoid dislocation	Cord fusion
Subglottis	Tracheoesophageal	Tracheoesophageal fistula
	perforation	Tracheoesophageal space
	Mucosal abrasion	abscess
		Mucositis, chondritis
		Subglottic stenosis
		Tracheitis
		Tracheomalacia
		Tracheal ring necrosis

Source: Reprinted with permission from Myers.[16]

Preparation

In an acute care situation, the most experienced physician or anesthetist intubates. The other members of the medical team stand by. If needed, they are prepared to assist or perform a tracheotomy. *Safe* intubation *requires* basic equipment: (1) suction, (2) shoulder roll, (3) oxygen source, (4) properly fitting face mask, (5) oral and flexible suction catheters, (6) nasal trumpet airway, (7) *fully* powered battery handle, and (9) straight (Miller) and curved (MacIntosh) laryngoscope blades (Figure 19.18). For most adults, 7- to 8-mm diameter tubes are sufficient. For children, an easy formula for tube size is internal diameter (millimeter) equals age divided by four plus 4.5. Flexible stylets are invaluable, especially for the difficult adult patient.

Anxious patients in the awake, tenuous state should be topically anesthetized and sedated intravenously. Laryngeal stimulation triggered by instrumentation may produce arrhythmias or hypotension. These physiologic reflexes are blocked by anticholinergics. Profound sedation or muscle relaxants are contraindicated for patients with impending upper airway obstruction. Such measures may precipitate complete airway obstruction.

Technique

All physicians, and especially surgeons, should be able to intubate; the potential for acute care airway obstruction exists for many patients. Ideally, intubation is performed in a controlled environment such as the Trauma Bay, Intensive Care Unit, or Operating Room. With the patient in the sniffing or neutral anatomic position, a shoulder roll is placed to facilitate cervical hyperextension. Any situation that compromises the oropharyngeal/laryngeal alignment undermines the technique. Dentures, mucus, blood, or vomitus is cleared for unobstructed visualization. The physician protects the upper dental arch, holds the laryngoscope with the nondominant hand, and inserts the endotracheal tube with the dominant hand. The straight or Miller blade, attached to a battery-operated laryngoscope, is recommended for patients with short, fat, or muscular necks.

Cricothyrotomy The cricothyrotomy technique is performed via a midline incision through the cricothyroid membrane. Cricothyrotomy, more straightforward than tracheotomy, is indicated for impending airway obstruction associated with either upper or lower airway obstruction. Once performed, cricothyrotomy is converted early to a standard tracheotomy. Contraindicated for pediatric patients, it has a high association with iatrogenic thyroid and cricoid cartilage fractures. These conditions predispose to chondritis and stenosis.

Tracheotomy In a tense acute care situation, tracheotomy can be a formidable procedure even for

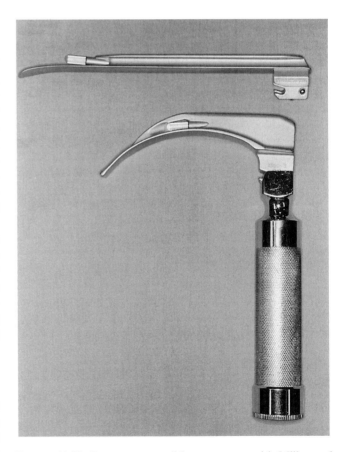

FIGURE 19.18. Battery-powered laryngoscope with Miller and MacIntosh (attached) blades. (Reprinted with permission from Myers.[4])

TABLE 19.19. Tracheotomy complications.

Immediate
  Hemorrhage
  Pneumothorax
  Pneumomediastinum
  Tracheoesophageal fistula
  Recurrent laryngeal nerve injury

Intermediate (<10 days)
  Hemorrhage
  Infection
  Aspiration
  Pneumonia

Late (>10 days)
  Hemorrhage
  Tracheal stenosis
  Stomal recurrence (laryngeal carcinomas)
  Tracheoesophageal fistula
  Tracheomalacia

Source: Reprinted with permission from Myers.[14]

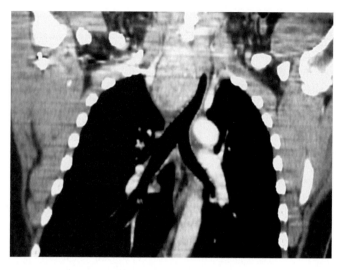

FIGURE 19.19. Computed tomographic scan of the neck, coronal view, showing a large substernal goiter.

experienced surgeons. Tracheotomy is performed preferably over an established airway (endotracheal tube or bronchoscope) in a controlled environment. Tracheotomy placement, of paramount importance, is usually between the second and third tracheal rings. Low placement is associated with immediate mediastinal emphysema, pneumothorax, and, later, possible innominate arterial or venous hemorrhage. At the end of the procedure, the surgery site must be thoroughly inspected for bleeding from anterior jugular or thyroid ima veins. Once the tracheotomy tube is placed, the patient must be monitored closely for intermediate and chronic potential complications (Tables 19.19 and 19.20).

Airway Strategy

The best airway team includes a surgeon comfortable with the difficult airway, a skilled anesthesiologist, and an experienced emergency room physician or neonatologist when appropriate (Figure 19.19). Assume the patient has a full stomach. Thus, if time permits, nasogastric decompression will prevent possible aspiration associated with airway placement. For the difficult airway, oral or nasal

TABLE 19.20. Tracheotomy general orders.

1. Give 40% oxygen via tracheotomy collar for humidification.
2. Deflate the cuff (if not on a respirator).
3. If the patient is on a respirator, inflate the cuff no greater than 5 cc of air.
4. Deflate the cuff 5 minutes each hour if the patient is on the respirator.
5. Do not change the tracheotomy ties for 72 hours.
6. Daily wound toilet; change the tracheotomy pad as needed.
7. Postoperative chest anteroposterior and lateral x-rays (optional).
8. Place the tracheotomy obturator at the bedside.
9. Inspect the tracheotomy site thoroughly if bleeding occurs.
10. Change the tracheotomy tube in 7–10 days.

Source: Reprinted with permission from Myers.[14]

intubation may be facilitated by fiberoptic intubation or laryngeal mask airway (LMA). The latter requires no special technique and may be a useful adjunct or bridge between masked ventilation and intubation. Should less invasive airway techniques fail, the airway team must proceed seamlessly to the next phase (Tables 19.21 and 19.22). The transition must be rapid and precise.[14,15]

Decannulation

Endotracheal Tube

Once ventilation is spontaneous and the underlying problem has been treated, the patient is a candidate for

TABLE 19.21. Etiology of airway compromise.

Blunt trauma
  Acceleration/deacceleration cervical injury
  Strangulation
  Soft tissue ecchymosis

Penetrating trauma (various sites)
  Maxillofacial trauma (LeFort fracture, midfacial or mandibular fractures)
  Laryngeal/tracheal fractures

Intrinsic obstruction
  Foreign body
  Caustic ingestion
  Inflammation (allergic reactions)
  Infection (croup, epiglottis)
  Granulomas (intubation, endoscopy)

Extrinsic obstruction
  Neoplasms (base of tongue, larynx, thyroid)
  Deep cervical fascial plane inflammation or infection
  Cervical spine injury

Iatrogenic (thyroid/parathyroid surgery, cervical spine surgery)
Thyromegaly

TABLE 19.22. Airway management: site versus technique (subtotally obstructive neoplasms).

Site	Intubation	Laser	Tracheotomy
Upper airway	2	3	1
Lower airway			
Hypoharynx	2	3	1
Larynx	2	3	1
Supraglottis	2	1	3
Glottis	2	1	3
Subglottis	2	1	3

1, First choice; 2, Second choice; 3, Third choice.
Reprinted with permission from Myers.[14]

decannulation. Immediately after decannulation, the patient is observed carefully and followed with sequential arterial blood gas monitoring. If there is any question of airway compromise, fiberoptic or indirect laryngoscopy is performed to assess the airway status.

Tracheotomy Tube

Tracheotomy is indicated for either temporary or permanent (long-term) airway management. However, the patient may be considered a decannulation candidate for the following: (1) reversal or elimination of the original indication for the airway, (2) decreased secretions, (3) reversal of coma, and (4) discontinuation of mechanical ventilation.

Options

If the attending or consulting physician is reticent, the patient is decannulated gradually. The usual protocol is tube downsizing every 24 hours (No. 6 Shiley™ to No. 4 Shiley™) and final decannulation. This conservative approach is preferable to immediate extubation, especially after normal duty hours or over the weekend.

Immediate decannulation is possible if the patient is (1) alert, (2) has an excellent cough, and (3) has fiberoptic or laryngoscopic documentation of clear upper or lower airways. As the tube is removed, the patient is suctioned sterilely. A clean gauze sponge is secured to the tracheotomy site with tape. The patient is instructed not to cough or talk without occluding the tracheotomy site. Tracheotomy site occlusion with a bandage enhances spontaneous closure by secondary intention. Peristomal infection is prevented with daily site cleansing with hydrogen peroxide or normal saline.

Ventilation

Following airway placement, some patients require mechanical ventilation. Ventilation is the movement of ambient air into the body and its distribution throughout the tracheobronchial system for effective alveolar gas exchange. Regardless of technique, vigilant nursing and monitoring is required for patients on mechanical ventilation. Tube displacement or mucous plugs is a constant potential risk. Pulmonary complications such as emphysema, effusion, and atelectasis must be monitored, preferably by sequential blood gases or pulse oximetry and frequent chest x-rays. Hypocarbia and hypercarbia are real risks. Nursing care must be superb. Thus, intubation and mechanical ventilation magnifies the complexity of airway assurance.

Hemostasis

Pharyngeal or laryngeal hemorrhage may be caused by epistaxis, tonsillectomy, maxillofacial cervical trauma, neoplasms, head and neck irradiation, and early or late complications of tracheotomy. After airway assurance, hemostasis is the next priority. Unique to the head and neck area, uncontrolled hemorrhage may precipitate airway compromise, as well as shock, in a rapidly spectacular and fatal fashion (see Figure 19.9).

Vascular Injury

Air Embolism

Poor control of the internal jugular vein during ligation or transection precedes air embolism. If suspected, the patient is ventilated vigorously by the anesthesiologist and placed in the left, lateral decubitus and Trendelenburg positions. This maneuver decreases the possibility of systemic and cerebral air emboli. Obviously, quick thinking and recognition are paramount. Surgery near the distal internal jugular vein must be precise to avoid brachial plexus, thoracic duct, or lung injury.

Carotid (Blow) Catastrophe

In the past, carotid (blow) catastrophe was more common especially in head and neck oncologic surgery or irradiation because the carotid artery was not protected routinely. Today, carotid coverage, closed-suction drains, and prophylactic antibiotics have decreased this complication markedly. However, it occasionally presents as a late complication of rampant, recurrent neck metastasis or head and neck irradiation.

If an impending carotid blow occurs or is suspected (sentinel bleed), quickly assume the following precautions:

1. Apply local pressure.
2. Consider early tracheotomy or intubation.
3. Resuscitate and maintain blood volume (adequate supplies of whole blood).
3. Transfer the patient to the Surgical Intensive Care Unit.
5. Plan for early great-vessel ligation.
6. Notify the family of the guarded prognosis.

As with most complications, cautious anticipation and good surgical technique decrease the morbidity and mortality from this dreaded complication.

Carotid Artery Injury

The most common causes of carotid artery injury are the removal of a tumor adherent to the internal jugular vein and common carotid artery, penetrating injury, and closed cervical injury. If practical, reconstructive angioplasty is performed but in the emergency situation the artery may have to be ligated. If ligation is anticipated, intraoperative electroencephalography is invaluable for monitoring cerebral function. Preoperative cerebral angiography and ophthalmoplethysmography are also helpful. Acute ligation has a high risk of secondary stroke especially in elderly patients.

Subclavian Artery

Fortunately rare, subclavian artery injury is caused by penetrating trauma, vigorous (distal) supraclavicular surgery, or a low tracheotomy. Primary repair is recommended because ligation or transection results in devastating upper extremity weakness. Intraoperatively, this diagnosis is considered if very brisk hemorrhage is encountered in the supraclavicular area. To facilitate exposure and control, sternotomy or removal of the medial portion of the clavicle may be necessary.

Transverse Cervical Artery

Transverse cervical artery injury may be associated with troublesome bleeding. Hemostasis by ligation has no long-term complication. However, the field must be well visualized to prevent injury to the phrenic nerve or brachial plexus.

Epistaxis

Nosebleeds, more common with nasal conditions or maxillofacial trauma, are uncommon with nasopharyngeal conditions.[17] Epistaxis may be either a nuisance or serious. Following a thorough history (Table 19.23), a complete head and neck examination is performed. Anterior rhinoscopy is facilitated after decongestion and topical anesthesia. If the source is still not apparent, fiberoptic nasopharyngoscopy is indicated. Diagnostic modalities such as CT or MRI scans may be required to ascertain inflammation, foreign bodies, or neoplasm as the ultimate etiology.

Contrary to popular misconception, a nose bleed may precipitate hemorrhagic shock and compromise the upper airway. Thus, regardless of the etiology, the physician must control the situation. All nose bleeds can be stopped; however, the means range from simple maneu-

TABLE 19.23. Etiology of epistaxis.

Local
  Trauma: self-induced, acute maxillofacial/nasal trauma/surgery, nasogastric tubes
  Mucosal irritation: topical nasal sprays, dessication
  Septal pathology: deviations, spurs, perforation, septoplasty

Inflammation
  Bacterial or viral diseases
  Allergic rhinosinusitis
  Sarcoidosis
  Wegener's granulomatosis

Neoplasms (benign or malignant)

Systemic
  Blood dyscrasias
  Coagulopathy: chemotherapy, anticoagulants, multiple transfusions
  Arteriosclerosis
  Hereditary hemorrhagic telangiectasia

vers to surgery. Hypertension and coagulopathies are common comorbid conditions.

Pressure

Pressure is the first maneuver. Simply pinching the nostrils together controls most minor (anterior) nosebleeds. Blunt or shearing midfacial force commonly involves the anterior nasal spine, nasal vestibule, and caudal septum. Kiesselbach's plexus, located in the caudal septum, is especially susceptible to injury even after vigorous nose blowing. A firm pinch collapses the mobile anterior nasal structures (lower lateral cartilages, ala, and membranous septum) onto the underlying caudal septum.

Vasoconstriction

Cold compresses constrict nasal vascularity, thus slowing bleeding in the anterior nose. In conjunction with local pressure, cold compresses can be very effective. If the bleeding persists, cotton pledgets impregnated with phenylephrine or dilute epinephrine are very useful. Careful blood pressure monitoring is necessary since vasoconstrictors can cause transient hypertension.

Packing

Cotton pledgets, impregnated (1/2 inch Vaseline)™ or special proprietary packs, are placed intranasally to control turbinate or midseptal bleeding. When preceded by topical anesthesia (Cetacaine™, Xylocaine™) and supplemented by vasoconstriction, packing is an effective control measure. A carefully layered (4- to 6-foot) bilateral or unilateral pack is sufficient for most anterior and some posterior nosebleeds.

Posterior nosebleeds are potentially more difficult to control. Hemorrhage from the posterior choanae, turbinate, nasopharynx, or skull base may not be controlled by even the most vigorous anterior pack.

Transnasal Foley catheter insertion (18 Fr, 30-cc bag) is the simplest means of controlling posterior epistaxis. If a Foley catheter is unavailable, rolled gauze sponges and vaginal tampons may be utilized. Posterior packs may require mild patient sedation and topical nasal anesthesia. Antibiotics usually are given after their insertion. All patients should receive low-flow humidified oxygen. Elderly patients and those with chronic obstructive lung disease must be monitored closely for transient hypoxia associated with acute posterior pack placement.

Embolization

On rare occasions, epistaxis may persist or recur despite all of the above measures. In centers staffed by skilled interventional radiologists, internal maxillary artery angiography and embolization are extremely effective. However, embolization (Gelfoam™ or Ivalon™) is contraindicated for high posterior or anterior ethmoid artery bleeds. Because both are endarteries of the internal carotid artery, embolization may cause blindness or cerebrovascular accident.[18,19]

Ligation

Surgery is reserved for patients with recurrent or severe epistaxis refractory to medical management.[20] Specific arterial ligation depends on the site of epistaxis (Table 19.24). Classically, vascular ligation is indicated for the internal maxillary and ethmoidal arteries. The former is accomplished transantrally (Caldwell-Luc) utilizing the operating microscope and the latter, hemoclips or with newer endoscopic techniques. However, in truly desperate situations, the ipsilateral external or common carotid arteries are ligated as illustrated earlier in Case 2.

Incision and Drainage

Incision and drainage, one of the oldest forms of surgery, probably predates written history. However, the foundation of modern precision surgery in the head and neck is well-understood anatomy and conceptualization of the

TABLE 19.24. Nasopharyngeal and nasal arterial vascularity.

External carotid artery
  Internal maxillary artery
    Sphenopalatine artery: posterior nasal septal artery, posterior
      lateral nasal artery, nasopalatine artery
    Descending palatine artery: greater and lesser palatine arteries
  External (facial) maxillary artery
    Superior labial artery: septal artery, alar artery
    Lateral nasal artery
    Angular artery
    Ascending palatine artery
Internal carotid artery
  Ophthalmic artery: anterior and posterior ethmoidal artery

cervical fascial planes. Fascial planes are a system of interconnected tissue envelopes that divide the neck into two compartments, *superficial* and *deep cervical* fascia. These compartments are potential spaces that may be expanded by abscesses, neoplasms, or surgery.[21,22] Superficial fascia, consisting of fat and connective tissue, envelopes the platysma muscle. The deep cervical fascia is divided into three layers: *superficial*, *middle*, and *deep*. These important concepts illuminate the potential complications of seemingly remote oral *pharyngeal* and *laryngeal* inflammatory/infectious conditions.

Superficial Layer

The *superficial layer*, extending from the skull base to the upper chest, invests the trapezius and sternocleidomastoid muscles and the submandibular and parotid glands. Superiorly, it splits into outer and inner layers near the lower mandibular border. The parotid gland and masseter muscle are covered by the outer layer. Attached to the mylohyoid ridge, the inner layer is superficial to the mylohyoid and anterior digastric muscles. Behind the angle of the mandible, these layers converge on the mastoid bone before encircling the entire neck. In summary, the superficial layer encloses two salivary glands (parotid and submandibular), two muscles (trapezius and sternocleidomastoid), and two anatomic triangles (suprasternal and posterior cervical).

Middle Layer

The *middle layer* of the deep cervical fascia encompasses the visceral neck structures. A portion invests the buccinator, tensor/levator palatine, and pharyngeal constrictors. Enveloping the larynx, trachea, esophagus, and thyroid gland, the middle layer stretches anteriorly behind the strap muscles and sternocleidomastoid. It is divided into two compartments: anterior (pretracheal space) and posterior (retropharyngeal space).

Deep Layer

The *deep layer* of the deep cervical fascia encircles the spine and paraspinous musculature, anterior to the cervical spine. The deep layer, originating from the spinous processes, extends to the trapezius muscles and covers the deep cervical musculature. It splits to form the anterior (alar fascia) and posterior (prevertebral) layers.

Carotid Sheath

The three layers of the deep cervical fascia converge to form the carotid sheath. Thus, the carotid sheath is a condensation of all layers of the deep cervical fascia. The sheath contains the internal jugular vein (anterolaterally), common carotid artery (medially), sympathetic trunk (posteriorly), and vagus nerve (laterally).

Final Comments

Surgical emergencies of the larynx and pharynx may present in a subtle fashion. "Colds," "flu," or "sinusitis:" the initial complaints seem innocent. However, any condition that progresses and fails to respond to symptomatic therapy is suspicious. Rapid deterioration can develop in seemingly healthy, pediatric, geriatric, and especially chronically ill patients. The common surgical emergencies of the pharynx and larynx are *airway obstruction, hemorrhage, inflammation/infection, foreign bodies*, and *caustic ingestion*.

Surgeons who treat these emergencies must be vigilant and astute. Their *diagnostic skills* must include (1) Well-developed history and physical examination, (2) rapid diagnosis, and (3) precise interpretation of appropriate images and laboratory screens. *Treatment* mandates: (1) thorough knowledge of anatomy and physiology, (2) airway assessment and strategy, (3) airway assurance (nonoperative and operative, (4) utilization of mechanical ventilation, (5) fluid resuscitation, (6) hemostasis including epistaxis management, (7) intimate understanding of the cervical fascial planes, and (8) endoscopy. Treatment begins as the workup proceeds.

A sense of urgency is embraced. Whatever the emergency, management of the airway is the key to patient survival. Finally, timely consultations with anesthesiologists, acute care physicians, pediatricians, neurosurgeons, and other professionals as indicated are sagacious.

Critique

The major management goal in laryngotracheal injuries is the establishment and maintenance of an airway. This particular injury is likely a partial transection at the laryngotracheal junction, that requires urgent airway management. In skilled hands, a transoral-translaryngeal approach for endotracheal intubation has been advocated. However, a tracheostomy is, the safest intervention.

Answer (D)

References

1. Ortiz JM. History and physical. In Myers EM, ed. Head and Neck Oncology: Diagnosis, Treatment, and Rehabilitation. Boston: Little, Brown & Company, 1991: 19–43.
2. Myers EM. Overview. In Myers EM, ed. Head and Neck Oncology: Diagnosis, Treatment, and Rehabilitation. Boston: Little, Brown & Company, 1991: 3–17.
3. Moore KL, Dalley AF. Clinically Oriented Anatomy. Philadelphia: Lippincott, William & Wilkins, 1999.
4. Hinton CD, Myers EM. Larynx. In: Myers EM, editor. Head and Neck Oncology: Diagnosis, Treatment, and Rehabilitation. Boston: Little, Brown & Company, 1991: 281–297.
5. Woodson GE. Laryngeal neurophysiology and its clinical uses. Head Neck 1996; Jan/Feb:78–86.
6. Friedman NR, Mitchell RB, Peira KD, et al. Peritonsillar abscess in early childhood. Arch Otolaryngol Head Neck Surg 1997; 123:630–632.
7. Hawkins DB, Miller AH, Sachs GB, et al. Acute epiglottitis in adults. Laryngoscope 1973; 83:1211–1220.
8. Tong MC, Woo JK, Sham CL, Vautlasselt CA. Ingested foreign bodies: a contemporary management approach. J Laryngol Otol 1995; 190:965–970.
9. Tucker J, Yarrington CT. Treatment of caustic ingestion. Otolaryngol Clin North Am 1979; 12:343–350.
10. Katzka DA. Caustic injury to the esophagus. Esophageal Dis 2001; 4(1):59–66.
11. Marple BF. Allergic fungal rhinosinusitis: current theories and management strategies. Laryngoscope 2001; 111:1006–1019.
12. Hughes KV, Olsen KD, McCaffrey TV. Parapharyngeal space neoplasms. Head Neck 1995; Mar/Apr:124–130.
13. Tucker J. Obstruction of the major pediatric airway. Otolaryngol Clin North Am 1979; 12:329–341.
14. Myers EM. Airway. In Myers EM, ed. Head and Neck Oncology: Diagnosis, Treatment, and Rehabilitation. Boston: Little, Brown & Company, 1991: 183–205.
15. Gonzalez RM, Herlich A, Krohner R, et al. Recent advances in airway management in anesthesiology: an update for otolaryngologists. Am J Otolaryngol 1996; 17(3): 145–160.
16. Myers EM. Hypopharyngeal perforation: a complication of endotracheal intubation. Laryngoscope 1982; 92(5):583–585.
17. Juselius H. Epistaxis: a clinical study of 1,724 patients. J Laryngol Otol 1974; 88:317–327.
18. Riche MC, Chiras J, Melki JP, Merland JJ. The role of embolization in the treatment of severe epistaxis. A review of 51 cases. J. Neuroradiol 1979; 6:207–220.
19. Chandler JR, Serrius AJ: Transantral ligation of the internal maxillary artery for epistaxis. Laryngoscope 1965; 75:1151–1159.
20. Siniluoto TM, Leinoneu AS, Karttunen AI, et al. Embolization for the treatment of posterior epistaxis. Otolaryngol Head Neck Surg 1993; 119(8):837–841.
21. Har-El G, Aroety JH, Shaha A, Lucente FE. Changing trends in deep neck abscess: a retrospective study of 110 patients. Oral Surg Oral Med Oral Pathol 1994; 77:446–450.
22. Myers EM, Kirkland LS, Mickey R. The head and neck sequelae of cervical intravenous drug abuse. Laryngoscope 1988; 98:213–218.

20
Head and Neck: Pediatrics

Reza Rahbar and Gerald B. Healy

Case Scenario

A child is discovered to have ingested a hearing aid battery. Radiographically, it is seen at the level of the distal esophagus. Which of the following represents the best management plan?

(A) No intervention; follow the patient clinically (inpatient)
(B) No intervention; follow the patient clinically (outpatient)
(C) Follow the progression of the foreign body radiographically
(D) Surgically remove the battery
(E) Remove the battery endoscopically

Emergencies of the head and neck region center around inflammatory disorders and trauma. Acute infections of the upper respiratory tract and neck constitute some of the most common causes of morbidity in children. Conditions such as supraglottitis, croup, and bacterial tracheitis are the most common acute inflammatory conditions affecting the pediatric airway. Infection in certain locations of the head and neck may lead to single or multiple space infections requiring urgent medical and surgical intervention. In the past two decades, there has been a rise in trauma in our society. Facial trauma and penetrating neck injury comprise some of the most commonly seen trauma in the pediatric population.

A thorough knowledge of the diagnostic and therapeutic modalities of acute inflammatory disease and trauma of the head and neck in the pediatric population is essential to ensure rapid resolution and avoidance of potentially life-threatening complications. The purpose of this chapter is to discuss the presentation of these disease processes, the role of radiographic studies, the value of endoscopic evaluation, the appropriate medical and surgical interventions, and the importance of cooperative effort among the pediatrician, anesthesiologist, and surgeon to ensure proper and timely treatment.

Inflammatory Disease of the Airway

Acute Supraglottitis

Historically, *Haemophilus influenzae* type B (HIB) was the most common cause of acute supraglottitis (Figures 20.1 and 20.2). With universal infant immunization with conjugate HIB vaccines, the incidence of supraglottitis caused by HIB has declined.[1,2] However, because of the severity of this condition and its occasional association with other organisms, it is essential that clinicians maintain an awareness and develop a protocol for its management.

Currently, the most common organisms associated with supraglottitis are pneumococci and beta-hemolytic streptococci. The usual presentation is a child with fever, odynophagia, and sonorous inspiratory stridor that may quickly progress to airway obstruction. The child often has a toxic appearance and sits in an upright position with the neck extended to maximize the size of the supraglottic airway. Drooling and muffled voice are commonly present. If the diagnosis of supraglottitis is suspected, any manipulation of the oral cavity and pharynx should be avoided as such action may result in complete airway obstruction. A chest and lateral neck x-ray should be done only if the diagnosis is uncertain and the patient is stable (Figure 20.3). A physician capable of intubating the patient should accompany the child to the radiology suite.

If one is suspicious of the diagnosis of supraglottitis in a child with respiratory distress, no radiographic studies should be obtained. Instead, the child should be taken to a setting where airway endoscopy, intubation, and possible tracheotomy can be performed. Depending on the institution's protocol and resources, this may take place in the operating room, intensive care unit, or emergency

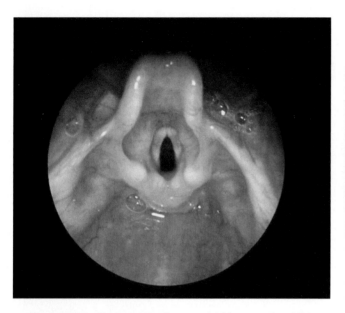

FIGURE 20.1. Endoscopic view: normal larynx of a child.

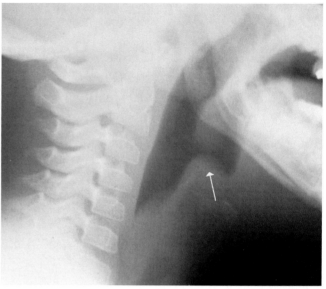

FIGURE 20.3. Lateral neck film: acute supraglottitis.

department. Regardless of the setting, it is essential that the anesthesia and surgical teams communicate in advance and discuss the protocol for airway evaluation and the provision of an artificial airway.

After airway endoscopy and confirmation of the diagnosis, the airway should be secured by oral or nasotracheal intubation. Cultures from the epiglottis and blood and routine blood sampling should be done only after the airway is secured. The patient should be monitored in an intensive care unit, and broad-spectrum intravenous antibiotics should be initiated. The first intravenous antibiotic should continue until the susceptibility of the

offending organism is known. The clinical status of the patient and direct visualization of the airway should determine when extubation should occur. Generally, extubation is possible after 48 hours.

Croup

Acute laryngotracheobronchitis (LTB), or croup, is a viral condition most commonly caused by parainfluenza virus types I and II. Other viruses causing croup are influenza virus types A and B, respiratory syncytial virus (RSV), and *Mycoplasma pneumoniae*. Croup most commonly presents between ages 6 months and 3 years and is seen primarily in the late fall and early winter.

The most common presentation is an upper respiratory infection with low-grade fever leading to biphasic stridor, barking cough, and increasing respiratory rate and respiratory distress. Stridor and respiratory symptoms are mainly caused by narrowing of the subglottis, which is the narrowest portion of the pediatric airway. One millimeter of subglottic edema in an 18-month-old child with an average subglottic diameter of 6.5 mm will decrease the cross-sectional airway area by approximately 50%[3] Children with croup usually have a normal white blood cell count and negative blood cultures. However, restlessness and tachycardia may be present because of hypoxia. Blood gases should be measured if there is any sign of respiratory failure. The diagnosis of croup is based on clinical presentation and radiographic findings. Chest and anteroposterior neck x-rays typically demonstrate the classic "pencil tip" or "steeple sign" of the subglottic region, a symmetric narrowing of subglottic space, as well

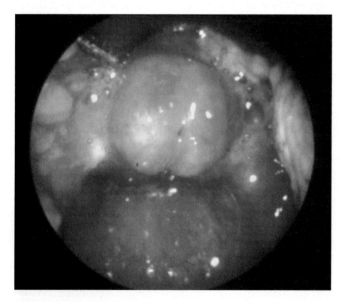

FIGURE 20.2. Endoscopic view: acute supraglottitis causing airway obstruction.

FIGURE 20.4. Neck film: normal subglottis on the left, and "steeple" sign in croup on the right.

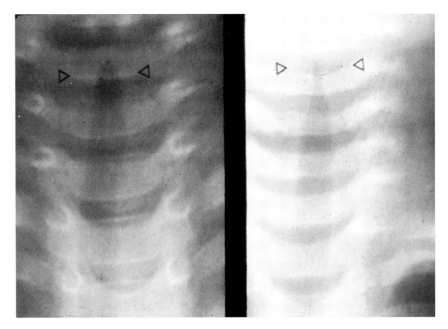

as hypopharyngeal distention, with normal configuration of the epiglottis (Figure 20.4).

Initial management consists of adequate hydration and cool humidification. At home, parents are instructed to take a child into the cool night air or into the bathroom with a running shower. The second component of therapy is racemic epinephrine inhalation therapy and systemic steroid administration. Racemic epinephrine is an alpha- and beta-agonist providing symptomatic relief by vaso-constriction and reduction of subglottic edema. Treatment with racemic epinephrine may not alter the natural history of the disease, but may postpone or eliminate the need for intubation. The rationale for systemic steroid use is to decrease mucosal edema and the inflammatory reaction in the subglottis.

Hospital admission and possible intubation may be required if there are retractions, restlessness, and an increased respiratory rate despite aggressive medical therapy. Intubation should be done in a controlled setting by experienced hands to prevent any secondary endotracheal tube trauma within the subglottis (Figure 20.5). There is a reported incidence of subglottic stenosis of less than 3% of children who undergo intubation for croup.[4] There is controversy with regard to the duration of intubation. As a general rule, extubation should not be attempted until the child is afebrile, an appropriate leak develops around the endotracheal tube, and there is a resolution of excessive secretions. Systemic steroids are beneficial prior to any attempt at extubation. Dexamethasone is particularly effective for this disease.

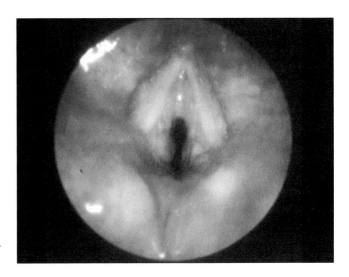

FIGURE 20.5. Endoscopic view: croup presenting with subglottic narrowing.

The drug has a long half life, and thus repeated small doses are not necessary. An initial dose of 1mg/kg may be used.

Bacterial Tracheitis

Bacterial tracheitis, also know as membranous laryngo-tracheobronchitis, is an acute airway infection presenting with subglottic edema and purulent tracheal secretions[5] The etiology is believed to be related to a bacterial super-infection of a preexisting viral upper respiratory tract infection. Patients often present with high fever, copious purulent secretions, respiratory distress, and a toxic appearance. Chest and lateral neck x-rays reveals irregular subglottic and tracheal narrowing.

The diagnosis is based on clinical suspicion and radiographic findings. Airway endoscopy in the operating room is essential to confirm the diagnosis, remove the dried and crusted tracheal secretions, and obtain appropriate cultures. Depending on the severity of the symptoms and findings at the time of endoscopy, the patient may require intubation and monitoring in an intensive care setting. The most common organisms are *Staphylococcus aureus*, HIB, beta-hemolytic streptococci, and *Moraxella catarrhalis* species. Broad-spectrum intravenous antimicrobial therapy should be immediately administered and modified based on the cultures and sensitivity. Currently, there are no standards with regard to the length of observation or antimicrobial therapy, but at least 14 days seems reasonable. Generally, fever and tracheal secretions decrease over 3 to 4 days, and extubation may be attempted in a controlled setting.

Inflammatory Diseases of the Neck

Peritonsillar Abscess

Peritonsillar abscess is the most common head and neck space infection. The "peritonsillar space" is located between the pharyngeal muscles and the capsule of the palatine tonsil. The anatomic boundaries of the peritonsillar space is the hard palate superiorly, piriform fossa inferiorly, and tonsillar pillars anteriorly and posteriorly. The patient with peritonsillar abscess presents with fever, dysphagia, trismus, and cervical adenopathy. The classic findings on the physical examination are medial displacement of the tonsil, displacement of the uvula to the contralateral side, and erythema and swelling of the peritonsillar region (Figure 20.6).

Historically, needle aspiration, incision and drainage, and immediate tonsillectomy "quinsy tonsillectomy" have all been advocated for the treatment of peritonsillar abscess.[6,7] Each of these treatment modalities has advantages and disadvantages in certain situations. Needle aspiration, when successful, is the least invasive

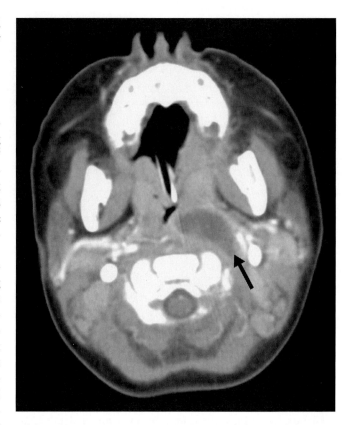

FIGURE 20.6. Computed tomography scan (axial view): peritonsillar abscess causing medial displacement of the tonsil. (Courtesy of Dr. Caroline D. Robson, Department of Radiology, Children's Hospital, Boston.)

and painful. In a cooperative child without any other associated complication, or in a child with bleeding diathesis, needle aspiration may be used as the initial treatment modality. Quinsy tonsillectomy is indicated if needle aspiration or incision and drainage fail to adequately drain the abscess or for a patient who presents with peritonsillar abscess causing airway obstruction. Appropriate cultures need to be obtained regardless of the method of drainage. Clindamycin should be started until the final culture and sensitivity measures are obtained because anaerobes may be present.

Retropharyngeal Abscess

Retropharyngeal abscess presents in the "retropharyngeal space," which is located between the posterior pharyngeal wall and the prevertebral fascia. The superior limit of the retropharyngeal space is the cranial base, and inferiorly it extends into the mediastinum to the level of the tracheal bifurcation. There are two groups of lymph nodes on either side of the midline of the retropharyngeal space that receive drainage from the nose, pharynx, and paranasal sinuses. Trauma to the pharynx may also provide a source of infection leading to abscess formation.

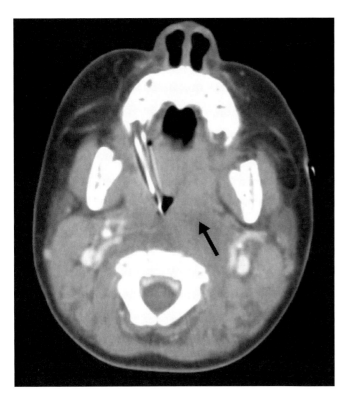

FIGURE 20.7. Computed tomography scan (axial view): retropharyngeal edema. (Courtesy of Dr. Caroline D. Robson, Department of Radiology, Children's Hospital, Boston.)

The most common presentation of retropharyngeal abscess in a child is fever, irritablility, dysphagia, muffled voice, neck adenopathy, and stiff neck.[8] In a cooperative child, one may see a posterior pharyngeal swelling. A lateral neck film may show an increased soft tissue density between the vertebrae and the pharynx. Inspiratory and expiratory films or airway fluoroscopy are more sensitive in detecting retropharyngeal abscess because a single lateral neck x-ray may give the impression of widening if taken in expiration. This is especially true with the young child. Computerized tomography (CT) reveals a rim-enhancing abscess in the retropharyngeal area that is often unilateral with surrounding edema (Figures 20.7 and 20.8).

A transoral approach is recommended for incision and drainage of the abscess. The patient must be intubated orally, and care must be taken to avoid puncture and sudden aspiration of the purulent material. The most common causative agents are beta-hemolytic streptococci, anaerobic streptococci, and *Staphylococcus aureus*. Clindamycin is the antibiotic of choice until the final results of the culture and sensitivity are obtained.

Lateral Pharyngeal Abscess

The lateral pharyngeal abscess forms in an "anatomic space" called the *parapharyngeal, pharyngomaxillary, pharyngomasticatory*, or, most commonly, the *lateral pha-*

ryngeal space. The lateral pharyngeal space is shaped like an inverted pyramid with superior extension to the cranial base and inferior extension to the hyoid bone. It lies medial to the pterygoid muscles and lateral to the buccopharyngeal fascia of the pharynx. The styloid process and attached fascia of the tensor veli palatine muscle divide the lateral pharyngeal space into an anterior "prestyloid" and posterior "poststyloid" compartments. The prestyloid compartment contains the internal maxillary artery, maxillary nerve, and the tail of the parotid gland. The poststyloid compartment contains the carotid artery, internal jugular vein, cranial nerves IX, X, XI, and XII, and the cervical sympathetic chain.

The most common source of infection in this space are the teeth, submandibular gland, tonsil, parotid gland, and retropharyngeal space. The usual presentation includes pain, fever, neck stiffness, and trismus. The patient may also present with shortness of breath and airway obstruction in cases of severe infection. In a cooperative patient, one may observe a fullness and medial displacement of the lateral pharyngeal wall. A CT scan is helpful in differentiating between an abscess and cellulitis and helps determine the extent of the infection (Figure 20.9). The treatment is surgical drainage in conjunction with intravenous antibiotic therapy. The approach for incision and drainage (intraoral, external, or combined) is based on the location and extension of the abscess.

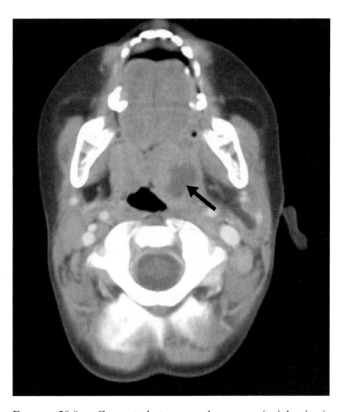

FIGURE 20.8. Computed tomography scan (axial view): retropharyngeal abscess. (Courtesy of Dr. Caroline D. Robson, Department of Radiology, Children's Hospital, Boston.)

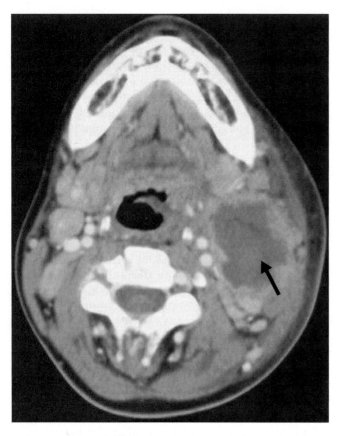

FIGURE 20.9. Computed tomography scan (axial view): lateral pharyngeal abscess. (Courtesy of Dr. Caroline D. Robson, Department of Radiology, Children's Hospital, Boston.)

Trauma

Many injuries that involve the head and neck are likely to compromise the airway. The primary tenet of all trauma management is to establish a safe and secure airway. Therefore, a rapid decision about airway management supersedes all other management decisions. The purpose of this section is to provide an overview of the presentation and management of the more common traumas impacting the head and neck region in children.

Facial Fracture

Historically, facial injuries were discussed and evaluated in terms of fractures of the upper, middle, and lower thirds of the facial skeleton. This resulted in a "segmentalized approach" in the management of these fractures.[9,10] In the past decade, because of the advances in diagnostic imaging and surgical techniques, there have been fundamental changes in the management of maxillofacial trauma. It has become evident that management of facial fractures based on arbitrary divisions of *upper,*

middle, and *lower* facial skeleton is illogical and may lead to suboptimal results.[9,10]

The proper management of a facial fracture should be done in coordination and consideration with other associated injuries such as oropharyngeal soft tissue, ocular, central nervous system, salivary glands, cranial nerves, and major vessels. Therefore, a team approach is essential to provide optimal care. It is of paramount importance to do a complete examination to rule out any other associated injury. The status of the airway and cervical spine should be addressed before any evaluation of the maxillofacial injury.[9] The patient should also be kept supine with the neck immobilized to protect the cervical spine until clearance of this area has been established.

Radiographic imaging has played an important role in the evaluation and management of these injuries. In the case of an isolated mandibular fracture, a panoramic radiograph is recommended to evaluate the mandible from condyle to condyle. It can adequately show fractures of the body, ramus, angle, and condyle. Axial and coronal CT scans have become an important and essential tool for the evaluation of more complex maxillofacial fractures. Areas that should be thoroughly inspected include the entire craniofacial horizontal and vertical buttress systems, frontal bone, and orbit. A three-dimensional reconstruction CT scan may help conceptualize the location and severity of the injury.[11]

The goal of modern facial fracture management is reconstruction of the bony and soft tissue injuries to provide the best functional and cosmetic outcome. Advances in metallic rigid internal fixation and bioresorbable implants have played a crucial role in the management of maxillofacial trauma. It is generally accepted that immediate reconstruction is less difficult and provides a better outcome. In the case of delayed reconstruction, the soft tissues surrounding the bony defect may contract and scar down, leading to a more difficult restoration of bone and soft tissue with suboptimal functional and cosmetic results.[9,10]

For the remainder of this section, we shall review the presentation and management of the nasal fracture, which is one of the most common facial fractures (Figure 20.10). Nasal fracture ranks third in incidence, behind fractures of the clavicle and wrist.[11] A history of significant trauma to the nose associated with epistaxis strongly suggests the possibility of a nasal fracture, and further evaluation is required. With proper assessment and management, most nasal fractures can be restored to proper alignment with good cosmetic and functional outcome.

Physical examination, including intranasal assessment, is the key to proper diagnosis and treatment. The nose must be inspected externally and internally to rule out deformity, septal deviation, laceration, and hematoma. Palpation should be performed systematically to assess tenderness, nasal bone depression, and displacement.

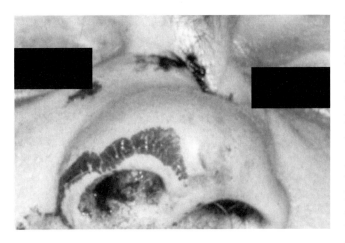

FIGURE 20.10. Nasal fracture: trauma.

Nasal and septal cartilages should be checked for possible fracture and displacement. Subcutaneous emphysema may be present secondary to attempts by the patient to blow clots from the nose. It is important to look for commonly associated injuries such as ocular trauma, dental fracture, and cerebral spinal fluid leak secondary to skull base fracture.

The usefulness and efficacy of radiographic studies in the evaluation of nasal fracture is controversial. The bony septum, dorsal pyramid, and lateral nasal walls can be evaluated on a Waters' and lateral view. Many surgeons have concluded that the time and expense of radiographic studies cannot be justified.[11,12] However, coronal and axial CT scans are recommended if there is any concern for associated facial injuries, orbital trauma, or cerebrospinal fluid leak.

Treatment options include closed or open reduction of the fractured nasal bone and septum. Significant swelling of the soft tissues of the nose and surrounding areas can preclude effective early management. Closed reduction has long been practiced as standard treatment for most nasal fractures. Most surgeons agree that closed reduction should be done within 3 to 7 days for children and within 5 to 10 days for adults.[13,14] Seven to 10 days after injury the nasal bones can become somewhat adherent and difficult to move. The success of closed nasal reduction is based on proper technique, adequate anesthesia, proper exposure, and splinting material.

Closed nasal reduction may not be possible in cases of complex nasal fracture or when other significant injuries exist. Open reduction can be done months later by an open septorhinoplasty technique. Traditionally, the septum is approached through a hemitransfixion incision on the side of dislocation. It is recommended to avoid a complete transfixion incision, which separates the septum

from the columella and may predispose to a lower tip height and introduce additional structural instability. Further access to the fracture lines is gained through bilateral intercartilaginous incisions. Regardless of the technique, it is essential to have a thorough discussion with the patient and his or her parent with regard to the potential for the injury or surgery to disturb the normal growth and development of the nasal complex.

Neck Trauma

Neck injuries can be divided into two basic groups depending on whether or not they are immediately life threatening. Urgent surgical exploration is mandatory in the case of a life-threatening neck injury presenting with airway obstruction, expanding hematoma, hemothorax, and/or hypovolemic shock. However, in case of a non-life-threatening injury, a thorough imaging investigation is recommended to determine the extent of the injury.

The initial care of patients with neck injuries should follow the basic rules of trauma care: (1) airway establishment, (2) blood perfusion maintenance, and (3) assessment and classification of the severity of the wound. Often a safe airway is established by intubation, cricothyroidotomy, or tracheotomy. In the case of extensive trauma, it may be difficult to completely evaluate the cervical spine until a safe airway is established. Intubation should be done by an experienced member of the trauma team to avoid the need for multiple attempts to establish the airway. Movement of the neck should be minimal until the status of the cervical spine is established. Large-bore intravenous lines should be placed immediately. Every patient with neck trauma should have routine anterior and lateral neck and chest radiographs.

Anatomically, the neck can be divided into three zones to help in the decision making for further diagnostic tests and management.[15] Zone I is the area below the cricoid and includes the vascular structures in the lower neck and thorax. The bony thorax and the clavicle act to protect the structures in zone I from injury. However, at the same time, they make it difficult to explore this area in case of an existing injury. In cases of suspected vascular injury, angiography is recommended to evaluate the status of the great vessels. If exploration is necessary, a low cervical incision may result in sufficient exposure, but a mediastinotomy extension or a formal lateral thoracotomy may be needed. Zone I injury has a mortality rate of approximately 10%.[16]

Zone II is the area between the angle of the mandible and the cricoid. This is the most commonly involved area in cases of neck trauma. There is controversy with regard to the use of mandatory exploration versus selective exploration in cases of injury to this area. In a stable patient with lack of physical signs of obvious major neck injury, a thorough diagnostic radiologic and endoscopic evaluation should be considered. Barium swallow, direct laryngoscopy, bronchoscopy, and esophagoscopy should be considered if there is associated drooling, dysphagia, hoarseness, subcutaneous emphysema, or hemoptysis.[15,16] Selective neck exploration is recommended if there is any clinical or radiographic indication of injury such as an expanding hematoma and hemodynamic or airway instability.

Zone III is located above the angle of the mandible. This area is protected by the mandible, facial bones, and skull base. It is recommended to consider angiography if there is any concern for injuries to the great vessels in this area.[16] It is difficult and treacherous to explore any high vascular injury in this area because of limited access caused by the skeletal structures and proximity of cranial nerves. A vascular injury can be temporized by pressure, and access may require a midline mandibulotomy. A temporary arterial bypass of the carotid artery and craniotomy may be required in the case of a high vascular injury in this area.

Laryngeal Trauma

Proper and timely management of laryngeal trauma is essential to preserve the patient's life, airway, and voice. Motor vehicle accident, sports injuries, and personal assaults are the most common causes of laryngeal trauma. Blunt trauma affects the larynx in the pediatric population different from in the adult patient. The pediatric larynx is located higher in the neck and is protected by the mandible. Also, laryngeal fracture is less common in children because of the elasticity of the pediatric larynx.

Regardless of the cause, the trauma may lead to mucosal laceration, fractures of the laryngeal cartilages, and airway obstruction. More severe trauma, such as a large amount of force to the neck, may lead to cricotracheal separation and bilateral recurrent laryngeal nerve injury. The classic symptoms of laryngeal trauma include hoarseness, laryngeal pain, dyspnea, and dysphagia. The most common signs of laryngeal trauma include stridor, hemoptysis, and subcutaneous emphysema.[17,18] Cervical subcutaneous emphysema indicates loss of the integrity of the mucosa of the upper aerodigestive tract.

Aphonia and airway obstruction may present in cases of severe trauma and require immediate establishment of an alternative airway. However, if the patient is stable, a complete examination to rule out any other injury should be performed. Care should be taken to avoid manipulation of the neck until the cervical spine has been cleared. Fiberoptic laryngoscopy should only be considered for a stable patient and performed by an experienced member of the team to assess the vocal cord mobility and the lack or presence of laryngeal laceration and hematoma.

In the past decades, CT scan has replaced the plain radiograph and laryngograms in the evaluation of laryngeal fracture.[18] Thin cut axial and coronal CT scans are

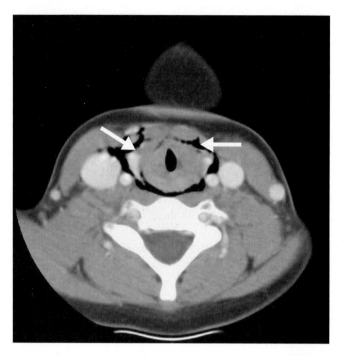

FIGURE 20.11. Computed tomography scan (axial view): laryngeal fracture. (Courtesy of Dr. Caroline D. Robson, Department of Radiology, Children's Hospital, Boston.)

not only helpful in identifying small fractures of the cricoid and thyroid cartilage but also help determine other associated injuries (Figure 20.11). Further evaluation of the upper aerodigestive tract by rigid endoscopy is based on the signs, symptoms, physical examination, and radiographic findings. A complete airway endoscopy under general anesthesia should be considered for any patient who presents with hoarseness, stridor, subcutaneous emphysema, vocal cord immobility, and laryngeal edema, laceration, or hematoma (Figure 20.12).

The medical or surgical management of laryngeal injury is based on the findings at the time of airway

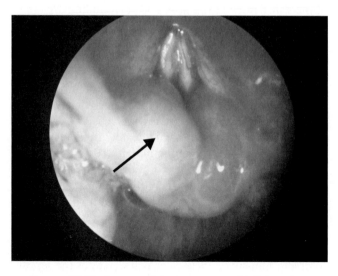

FIGURE 20.12. Laryngeal trauma: arytenoid dislocation.

endoscopy and on the radiographic findings. Conditions such as minimal mucosal edema, a small laryngeal laceration without exposed cartilage, or a small nondisplaced thyroid fracture may resolve spontaneously without any surgical intervention.[19] However, because of the uncertain course of laryngeal trauma, hospitalization for observation is recommended until the resolution or improvement of symptoms. The patient should have voice rest, cool humidification, and elevation of the head of the bed. We recommend the use of systemic corticosteroids and a broad-spectrum intravenous antibiotic to reduce laryngeal edema and decrease the risk of infection. Antireflux medication should also be utilized to reduce scarring potential.

Injuries that most likely require open laryngeal surgery and repair include laryngeal laceration with exposed cartilage, displaced laryngeal fracture, paralyzed vocal cord, and dislocated arytenoids.[19,20] The timing of surgical intervention remains controversial. Some authors advocate waiting a few days to allow the initial edema and swelling to resolve prior to any repair.[19] Other investigators recommend early exploration to allow for a complete assessment of the injury and possible repair with less risk of granulation tissue and scar formation.[17,20] Regardless of the timing of the surgery, all mucous membranes, muscle, and cartilage with a viable blood supply should be preserved and restored to their original position. Any laceration should be meticulously approximated and repaired, and any exposed cartilage should be covered to prevent granulation tissue and scar formation.

Care must be taken to approximate cartilaginous fractures with the help of wire, nonabsorbable suture, or miniplates. Even though the use of stents for laryngeal fractures remains controversial, clinical findings, such as extensive lacerations or multiple cartilaginous fractures that cannot be stabilized, may dictate their use. We recommend removal of the stent as soon as possible to prevent further mucosal damage. Long-term follow-up monitoring of these patients is essential to prevent delayed scar formation and airway stenosis.

Critique

Hearing aid batteries are the most common batteries swallowed. These alkaline batteries can cause severe corrosive injuries as a result of electrolyte leakage, pressure necrosis, and alkali seepage. Although still controversial, endoscopic removal of this foreign body should be done because the risks of leaving this object in the gastrointestinal tract outweigh the morbidity associated with endoscopy.

Answer (E)

References

1. Committee on Infectious Diseases. *Haemophilus influenzae* type B conjugate vaccines: recommendations for immunization with recently and previously licensed vaccine. Pediatrics 1993; 92:480–488.
2. American Academy of Pediatrics. Parainfluenza virus infections. In Peter G, ed. 1994 Red Book: Report of the Committee on Infectious Diseases, 23rd ed. Elk Grove Village, IL: American Academy of Pediatrics, 1994; 341–342.
3. Cressman WR, Myer CM III. Diagnosis and management of croup and epiglottitis. Pediatr Clin North Am 1994; 41:265–276.
4. McEniery J, Gillis J, Kilham H, Benjamin B. Review of intubation in severe laryngotracheobonchitis. Pediatrics 1991; 87:847–853.
5. Dennelly BW, McMillan JA, Weiner LB. Bacterial tracheitis: report of eight new cases and review. Rev Infect Dis 1990; 12:729–735.
6. Haeggstrom A, Gustafsson O, Engquist S, Engstrom CF. Intraoral ultrasonography in the diagnosis of peritonsillar abscess. Otolaryngol Head Neck Surg 1993; 108:243–247.
7. Holt GR, Timsley PP. Peritonsillar abscesses in children. Laryngoscope 1981; 91:1226–1230.
8. DiLorenzo RA, Singer JI, Matre WM. Retropharyngeal abscess in an afebrile child. Am J Emerg Med 1993; 11:151–154.
9. Stanley RB. The zygomatic arch as a guide to reconstruction of comminuted malar fractures. Arch Otolaryngol Head Neck Surg 1989; 115:1459–1462.
10. Stanley RB, Nowak GM. Midfacial fractures: importance of angle of impact to horizontal craniofacial buttresses. Otolaryngol Head Neck Surg 1985; 93:186–192.
11. Krause C. Nasal fractures: evaluation and repair. In Mathog RH, ed. Maxillofacial Trauma. Baltimore: Williams & Wilkins, 1984: 257–268.
12. Clayton MI, Lesser THJ. The role of radiography in the management of nasal fractures. J Laryngol Otol 1986; 100:797–801.
13. Altreuter RW. Nasal trauma. Emerg Med Clin North Am 1987; 5:293–300.
14. Waldron J, Mitchell DB, Ford G. Reduction of fractured nasal bones; local vs. general anesthesia. Clin Otolaryngol 1989; 14:357–359.
15. Brennan J, Meyers A, Jafek B. Penetrating neck trauma: a 5-year review of the literature, 1983–1988. Am J Otolaryngol 1990; 11:191–198.
16. Miller R, Duplechain J. Penetrating wounds of the neck. Otolaryngol Clin North Am 1991; 24:15–31.
17. Schaefer SD, Close LG. The acute management of laryngeal trauma: an update. Ann Otol Rhinol Laryngol 1989; 98: 98–104.
18. Schaefer SD, Brown OE. Selective application of CT in the management of laryngeal trauma. Laryngoscope 1983; 93:1473–1475.
19. Stanley RB, Cooper DS, Florman SH. Phonatory effects of thyroid cartilage fractures. Ann Otol Rhinol Laryngol 1987; 96:493–496.
20. Leopold DA. Laryngeal trauma. Arch Otolaryngol Head Neck Surg 1983; 109:106–112.

21
Esophagus

George C. Velmahos, Nahid Hamoui, Peter F. Crookes, and Demetrios Demetriades

Case Scenario

A college student presents to the emergency department after developing chest pain immediately after an episode of emesis. The patient is diaphoretic but hemodynamically stable chest. Chest x-ray demonstrates a pneumomediastinum. What would be the management plan at this point?

(A) Emergency thoracotomy
(B) Esophagogastroduodenoscopy
(C) Contrast swallow
(D) Chest tube insertion
(E) Celiotomy

General Considerations

The esophagus was once described as the surgical Tibet: a hostile region that is hard to reach, the location of frequent interspecialty turf wars, often visited by the ill-equipped person, and dangerous when once you get there. It is an unforgiving organ whose diseases have a high propensity to lead to serious complications, chiefly aspiration pneumonia, mediastinitis, empyema, cardiac arrhythmias, and multisystem organ failure. Aside from blunt and penetrating trauma to the esophagus, four major conditions dominate the acute care surgery of the esophagus, namely, perforation, caustic ingestion, foreign body impaction, and hemorrhage.

Traumatic and nontraumatic surgical esophageal emergencies share common principles of diagnosis and treatment but also differ in crucial details. For example, the diagnosis of a suspected injury to the esophagus consists of similar signs and tests regardless of the inflicting source, a bougie or a bullet. On the contrary, a perforation of an otherwise healthy esophagus from penetrating trauma may be managed quite differently from a perforation caused by cancer. For better clarity, we describe traumatic and nontraumatic diseases separately after some general considerations applicable to both.

Anatomic Considerations

The esophagus begins at the level of the sixth cervical vertebra immediately below the cricopharyngeal muscle and lies behind the trachea and slightly to the left of the midline. It passes to the mediastinum behind the great vessels and the left main stem bronchus. From this point it turns to the right and continues its course until it curves back to the left and crosses the diaphragm through the esophageal hiatus to join the stomach at the gastroesophageal junction.

The cervical portion of the esophagus measures 3 to 5 cm; the thoracic, 20 to 25 cm; and the abdominal, 3 to 5 cm; for a total length of 25 to 35 cm (40 to 50 cm if the distance from the incisors is taken into account by adding 15 cm for the mouth and pharynx). Blood supply is provided by numerous branches from the inferior thyroid, bronchial, intercostals arteries, and the aorta, forming a rich and tenuous plexus around the esophagus with relatively poor collateralization. This fact combined with the lack of serosa places anastomotic lines at risk and increases the likelihood of failure of surgical repair.

The neck is divided in three zones. Zone I extends from the sternal notch to the cricoid cartilage; zone II, from the cricoid cartilage to the angle of the mandible; and zone III, from the angle of the mandible to the base of the skull. Zone I and lower zone II penetrating injuries may involve the esophagus. Higher injuries usually place the pharynx—rather than the esophagus—at risk.

Because of the close association of the esophagus with major vessels, the trachea, and main bronchi, isolated esophageal injuries are unlikely. The presence of an esophageal injury should alert to the possibility of associated injuries. Vice versa, vascular or tracheal injuries of the neck and chest should prompt radiographic, endo-scopic, or surgical exploration of the esophagus.

Bacteriology

The esophagus is home to virulent Gram-positive and Gram-negative organisms, both aerobic and anaerobic, and frequently contains yeasts. Overgrowth occurs in several pathogenic conditions of the esophagus in which there is chronic stasis, such as achalasia and cancer. Recent studies of Chagas' disease have shed light on the spectrum of flora within the esophagus. Pajecki et al.[1] compared bacteria in esophageal aspirates from patients with Chagas' disease with those from patients with dys-peptic complaints. Both groups showed a predominance of aerobic Gram-positive and anaerobic bacteria; patients with Chagas' disease had a higher predominance of positive cultures overall and especially of certain anaerobic bacteria such as *Veillonella*. Another study[2] of pathogens in mediastinitis found the predominant aerobic organisms responsible for infection to be alpha-hemolytic *Streptococcus*, *Klebsiella pneumoniae*, and *Escherichia coli*, while the predominant anaerobic bacteria were *Prevotella* and *Porphyromonas* species, *Peptostreptococcus* species, *Fusobacterium* species, *Bacteroides fragilis*, and *Propionibacterium acnes*. Esophageal wall injury from whatever cause allows these organisms to spread within the soft tissue spaces of the neck and mediastinum, often with great rapidity. Knowl-edge of the likely organisms causing sepsis is important in choosing appropriate antimicrobial therapy at an early stage of the problem. Antimicrobial therapy for mixed aerobic and anaerobic bacterial infection should be administered. The Gram-negative anaerobic bacilli *Prevotella* and *Fusobacterium* species have increased their resistance to penicillins and other antimicrobials in the last decade, mainly through the production of beta-lactamase. Antimicrobial agents that can be used include cefoxitin sodium, clindamycin phosphate, imipenem-cilastatin sodium, and the combination of metronidazole hydrochloride and a beta-lactamase–resistant penicillin.

Traumatic Injuries

Frequency and Mechanism of Injury

Esophageal injury is uncommon. Penetrating trauma accounts for the overwhelming majority of cases, with blunt trauma being a very rare occurrence. Four mecha-nisms have been discussed following blunt trauma: (1) a sudden increase in the diameter of the esophagus from acute functional obstruction at the pharyngoesophageal junction, (2) a deceleration injury involving shearing of periesophageal vascular beds with resultant wall ischemia

and delayed perforation, (3) stretching over the spine (usually associated with major spinal injuries), and (4) direct laceration from fractured ribs. Crashes producing blunt esophageal injury are catastrophic and include major steering wheel damage, passenger space intrusion, or complete vehicle damage.[3] Blunt esophageal trauma in survivors is almost always in the neck and frequently involves the larynx or trachea.[4]

Following penetrating trauma, esophageal injuries are more common in the cervical region, with an incidence of 1.5% to 4% of all neck wounds.[5,6] Less than 0.5% of tho-racic gunshot wounds involve the esophagus.[7] This inci-dence is significantly lower for stabbings. Abdominal esophageal injury is equally uncommon.

Diagnosis

The diagnosis of esophageal injuries is notoriously diffi-cult. Delayed diagnosis leads to complications or death. A high index of suspicion is imperative.

Clinical Symptomatology

Clinical symptoms are subtle and revolve around the triad of odynophagia, subcutaneous emphysema, and hematemesis. Odynophagia is the most common symptom and occurs in almost all patients with penetrat-ing esophageal injury.[5] However, the specificity of the symptom is low, with less than 20% of the patients complaining of pain in swallowing found to have an esophageal injury. Subcutaneous emphysema is uncom-mon if the esophagus is the only injured organ. The amount of air contained in the esophagus may appear in radiographic studies but not clinically. However, because of associated laryngotracheal injuries, subcutaneous emphysema is not an infrequent finding. Hematemesis (or blood in the nasogastric tube) after a penetrating cer-vical or thoracic injury is a very specific symptom of esophageal perforation and should immediately prompt further workup. A clinical test has been used with occa-sional success for patients with suspected esophageal injury, particularly those who are clinically nonevaluable.[8] The tip of the nasogastric tube is placed in the cervical region, and air is inflated through it. The external wound is filled with saline. In the presence of an esophageal lac-eration, bubbles are observed coming through the wound. Alternatively, methylene blue can be injected through the nasogastric tube and visualized either through the neck skin wound or in the thoracostomy tube for thoracic esophageal injuries.

Plain Films

Air in the soft tissues of the neck or the mediastinum is a common radiographic finding but may be missed if not specifically suspected. In retrospective reviews the incidence of this finding is reported to be low.[9,10] Small quantities of air are invariably included in the esophagus and leak out through a perforation. Such small quantities may not be recognized in a superficial review of the film. Also, the interval between injury and radiologic examination plays a role. Plain films performed within 1 hour after the injury may not reveal air in up to 60% of the patients.[11] Additionally, the integrity of the pleura may confuse the picture. If the pleura is violated, the air may escape into the pleural cavity and show as pneumothorax rather than mediastinal or neck emphysema.[12]

Computed tomography (CT) identifies extraluminal air with higher sensitivity. Although air in the soft tissues should always alert for further workup, it is by no means pathognomonic of esophageal injury. Air can be present after tracheobronchial or lung injuries or just as part of the bullet trajectory without organ injury. The most common finding on chest radiograph is hemopneumothorax.[13]

Esophagography

Contrast esophagography localizes the site of perforation in the vast majority of patients with an esophageal injury. The sensitivity of the examination ranges from 89%[14] to 100%.[9, 15,16] Thoracic and abdominal esophageal injuries are easily discovered during esophagogram (Figure 21.1). However, cervical injuries particularly in the upper

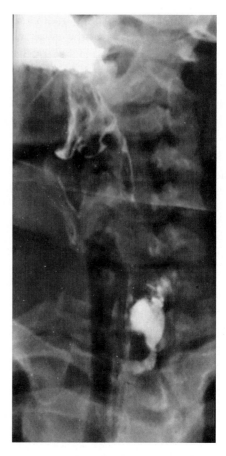

FIGURE 21.2. Contained contrast extravasation from perforation of the esophagus following a stab wound.

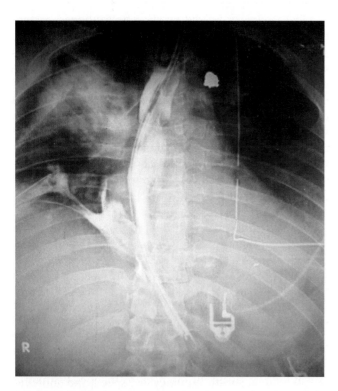

FIGURE 21.1. Contrast extravasation from perforation of the thoracic esophagus after a gunshot wound.

esophagus or pharynx may present a technical challenge in patients who are unable to cooperate by swallowing or in patients who are intubated. In these patients, the oral contrast is given through a nasogastric tube pulled to the level of the pharyngoesophageal junction (Figure 21.2). Proper positioning is important. Contrast progression may be too rapid if the patient is placed in the upright position. The study should be performed in the right or left lateral decubitus position, using multiple-plane radiographs.[11]

The preferred contrast agent is debated. Meglumine diatrizoate (Gastrografin, Squibb & Sons, Inc., Princeton, NJ) is water soluble and hyperosmolar. It does not produce soft tissue or mediastinal inflammation but causes severe pneumonitis if aspirated by an unconscious patient or in the presence of traumatic tracheoesophageal communication.[17] The balloon of the endotracheal tube should be maximally inflated in intubated patients undergoing esophagography to prevent aspiration. Barium is a better radiographic material and is isosmolar. Although it does not affect the lungs adversely like gastrografin, it may cause mediastinitis.[18] Probably thin barium is the ideal compromise between the two contrast agents, although the type and density of agent used should be tailored according to the suspected level of injury, suspected presence of associated tracheobronchial injuries, and status of the patient. Sometimes both agents are needed: the study starts with administration of gastrografin to be followed, if negative, by barium.[19]

Esophagoscopy

Direct visualization of the esophagus can be achieved by rigid or flexible endoscopy. Rigid esophagoscopy alone has a sensitivity of 70% to 89%[10,14,15] but in combination with esophagography increases to 100%.[10,14] Although many studies have cautioned against the use of flexible endoscopy,[4,14] newer evidence suggests that a sensitivity of 100% can be achieved.[20,21] The thoracic esophagus is easier to inspect through the endoscope than the upper cervical esophagus, and therefore an injury in this area is less likely to be missed. Direct evidence of a perforation may not always be apparent. On occasion, indirect evidence, such as mucosal abnormality or hematoma, should be used in conjunction with clinical findings to make a decision about the need for intervention. The specificity of flexible endoscopy is 83% to 96% because of occasional false-positive findings.[21,22]

An important point is brought forward by Cornwell et al.[23] in a study of 43 patients with aortic or esophageal injuries after transmediastinal gunshot wounds. The authors observed that, in the presence of hemodynamic stability, the likelihood of an aortic injury requiring immediate repair was almost nil. In contrast to this, esophageal perforations could occur in the face of hemodynamic stability. Diagnostic workup included first aortography and then esophagography, resulting in 11-hour delays on average from the time of injury to the time of esophageal surgery. The authors concluded that esophageal evaluation should precede aortography in the workup of stable patients with transmediastinal gunshot wounds.

Computed Tomography Scan

There are continuous technologic advancements in the field of CT. In a small series of only four patients with penetrating cervical esophageal injuries, Gonzalez et al.[24] reported that CT missed two injuries produced by stabbings, for a sensitivity of only 50%. The identical injuries were also missed by esophagography.

On the contrary, in a study of 24 patients with transmediastinal gunshot wounds, Hanpeter et al.[25] found CT to offer excellent specificity by defining bullet trajectories that were away from the esophagus and therefore tailoring the need for further esophageal studies to only 37.5% of a population that would have otherwise undergone in its entirety contrast esophagography or esophagoscopy. The sensitivity of CT cannot be determined from this

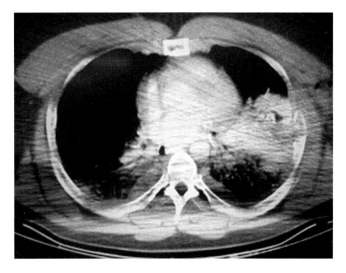

FIGURE 21.3. Computed tomographic scan of transmediastinal gunshot wound. The esophagus lies on the pathway of the bullet as it traverses the mediastinum, with an oblique left-anterior-to-right-posterior direction. Note the free air in the mediastinum. On esophagography, a perforation of the thoracic esophagus was found.

study because of the lack of esophageal injuries. However, it is expected that CT will gradually replace other diagnostic tests as the study of choice for penetrating injuries (and particularly gunshot wounds) of the neck and chest.

At this point, surgeons need to be cautioned against the exclusive reliance on CT, because convincing evidence of its diagnostic accuracy for esophageal trauma is lacking. However, the undisputable benefits of CT (convenience, noninvasiveness, additional information) will lead to its increasing use. If an injury trajectory is shown to be clearly away from the esophagus, no further specific workup is necessary. Patients who have suspicious or unclear trajectories on CT should be evaluated further with esophagography and/or esophagoscopy or simply explored based on the combination of clinical and radiographic findings (Figure 21.3).

Management

Selective Management or Routine Exploration of Penetrating Neck Injuries

The issue of selective management versus routine exploration of penetrating injuries to the neck or the mediastinum is only a debate of the past and mentioned here because of historic interest. Familiarity of surgeons with these injuries, development of expert trauma teams, advances in diagnostic accuracy and speed, and improvements in critical care have clearly shifted the balance toward selective management. There is overwhelming evidence that no patient should be routinely explored just for the mere presence of a cervical or mediastinal penetrating injury, even if this refers to a bullet traversing these regions from one side to the other.[25,26] It should be, rather, the clinical symptoms and radiographic or endoscopic findings that mandate the need for an operation.[26,27] Devastating complications from missed esophageal injuries in patients initially selected for nonoperative management attest to the failure of comprehensive clinical examination or adequate diagnostic workup rather than the failure of the method of selective management itself.[28]

Selective Operative Management of Documented Pharyngoesophageal Trauma

All thoracic and abdominal esophageal injuries should be operated on promptly because of the very real risk of mediastinitis, peritonitis, and death if left unrepaired. Although successful reports of nonoperative treatment exist for iatrogenic trauma or anastomotic leaks at the thoracic esophageal level, there is no evidence that traumatic perforation can be approached similarly, because the wounding agent has violated the tissue planes that may have contained the leak.[29] On the other hand, routine surgical repair is not mandatory for all pharyngeal and cervical esophageal perforations although the selection criteria for safe nonoperative management are not entirely clear cut. Three major factors should be taken into account: (1) location of injury, (2) size of injury, and (3) associated injuries.

The precise anatomic mapping of injury is important. The pharyngoesophageal complex could be divided into three areas for the purposes of making operative or nonoperative decisions.[30] The upper hypopharynx is defined as the space above a cross-sectional plane that crosses the tips of the arytenoid cartilages of the larynx. The lower hypopharynx lies below this plane and above the cricopharyngeus muscle. The esophagus lies immediately below this muscle. The upper hypopharynx is a low-pressure system, relatively open, and wrapped securely by the overlapping middle and inferior constrictor muscles. Perforations at this level are very likely to seal spontaneously. The lower hypopharyngeal region is narrower and enveloped only by the inferior constrictor muscle. Saliva and refluxed gastric contents pool in this area. Although the area is still well protected by muscles, perforations at this level are more likely to leak if left unrepaired. Below this level, the esophagus runs with little protection from surrounded muscles. Particularly the posterior wall is only separated by thin soft tissue layers from the spine. Perforations at this level can easily leak toward the mediastinum. As a general rule, it seems that upper hypopharyngeal injuries can be safely managed nonoperatively, esophageal injuries should be managed opera-

tively, and injuries in the region in between (lower hypopharynx) are managed on a case-by-case basis.

The size and mechanism of injury are other determinants of the decision to operate. There is little evidence that injuries more than 2 cm can be safely managed nonoperatively at any level.[30] Stab wounds are more likely than gunshot wounds to be managed without an operation. Associated injuries also significantly influence decision making. The presence of vascular or tracheal injuries that require surgical intervention makes repair of the pharyngeal or esophageal injury mandatory. The presence of a posterior esophageal wound that penetrates the spinal canal should most likely be repaired in order to avoid leakage and infection.

Four studies, two from South Africa, one from Colombia, and one from the United States, have described the results of nonoperative management of pharyngeal or esophageal wounds. Ngakane et al.[6] described four neck injuries (two stab wounds and two gunshot wounds) that showed gross oral contrast extravasation following oral contrast and were managed without an operation. The contrast examination was repeated 5 days later, and the leak had sealed spontaneously in all cases with no further sequelae. Information on the exact location and size of these injuries as well as associated injuries were not given for these four patients.

Yugueros et al.[31] reported on 14 patients with proven lesions of the hypopharynx produced by gunshot in 11, stabbing in 2, and shotgun in 1. The perforation was found on endoscopy in 9 patients and esophagography in 5. The size of the lesions ranged between 1 and 2 cm. Only 1 patient had an associated injury of the cervical spine. One patient developed a cervical abscess within the first week after injury. This patient had refused a nasogastric tube and initiated oral intake against medical advice. After surgical drainage of the abscess, his recovery was unremarkable. Five additional patients were subjected to follow-up esophagograms with no evidence of a leak. No complications were noted in 13 patients.

Stanley et al.[30] described 18 patients with upper hypopharyngeal injuries (11), lower hypopharyngeal injuries (6), and esophageal injury (1) who were initially managed without an operation. In 4 of them, the nonoperative management was unplanned because of a missed diagnosis. Five patients with lower hypopharyngeal injuries from a gunshot developed infections requiring drainage of the neck at intervals ranging from 32 hours to 11 days after injury. Four had associated vertebral fractures with spinal cord injuries. All five patients did well after drainage. The one patient with esophageal injury developed neck infection and mediastinitis, resulting in thoracotomy, cervical esophageal diversion, and distal esophageal exclusion. All 11 upper hypopharyngeal and one of five lower hypopharyngeal wounds were managed nonoperatively with success.

TABLE 21.1. Results of nonoperative management of proven pharyngeal and esophageal penetrating injuries.

Author, year	No.	Location	Complications
Ngakane et al.,[6] 1990	4	Unknown	None
Yugueros et al.,[31] 1996	14	Hypopharynx	1 cervical abscess
Stanley et al.,[30] 1997	18	11 upper pharynx, 6 lower pharynx, 1 esophagus	5 cervical abscesses, 1 mediastinitis
Madiba and Muckart,[32] 2003	17	Unknown	1 cervical abscess
Total	53		8 (15%)

Madiba and Muckart[32] reported recently on 17 patients with contained leaks on esophagogram following stab or firearm injuries. One of them required open drainage for local sepsis.

At this point, nonoperative management should be selected predominantly for small wounds that are at the higher rather than lower part of the pharyngoesophageal funnel and are not associated with other injuries requiring surgical repair. Careful mapping of the injury by endoscopy or contrast swallow is important, and a follow-up examination in 5 to 7 days, although not absolutely necessary, helps in the management. The duration of nasogastric suction, avoidance of oral feeds, and administration of antibiotics is tailored to the individual situation. The incidence of complications after nonoperative treatment is not negligible (Table 21.1) but is easy to manage. It primarily consists of local infection that is treated successfully by antibiotics and, if needed, percutaneous or surgical drainage. The feared complication of mediastinitis should always be kept in mind and ruled out in patients with signs of infection following a trial of nonoperative management.

Operative Therapy

The choice of repair is based primarily on the size and location of injury and the interval between injury and operation. In the majority of cases, primary closure of the perforation in one or two layers is all that is needed. Complex techniques are used rather infrequently and are described below. Sight should not be lost from the close association with injuries of the laryngotracheal system, which are far more emergent and life-threatening than the esophageal injuries. Airway compromise is a common problem following aerodigestive trauma and occurs in 29% of such patients.[33] Among those who are induced rapidly for intubation in the emergency room, 12% suffer loss of airway and require a cricothyroidotomy.[33]

Cervical esophageal injuries are approached through a lateral neck incision across the anterior border of the sternocleidomastoid muscle or a collar incision in the presence of bilateral neck injuries. A left lateral incision with medial retraction of the vessels allows the easiest exposure. Neither the number of suture layers nor the type of suture material used (absorbable or nonabsorbable) seems to influence the incidence of fistulization after repair.[17] We prefer two layers, a mucosal running layer with absorbable suture and a muscular interrupted layer with nonabsorbable suture. Muscle flaps are used in the presence of a combined tracheoesophageal or esophagovascular injury.[34] Usually, a vascularized flap of the sternocleidomastoid is inserted between the esophagus and the trachea or carotid artery repairs. Drains in the presence of vascular repairs should be placed anteriorly to avoid crossing over the site of vascular injury. Exteriorization of the esophagus is used by some authors for extensive combined injuries,[35] whereas others strive for repairing all injured structures in a one-stage intervention regardless of the complexity of repair.[36,37]

Insertion of a T-tube has been used for late traumatic esophageal perforations, when an environment of active inflammation precludes safe primary closure.[15,38] The short limbs of a 22 to 24 French T-tube are inserted through the perforation to lie above and below the level of the injury, and the long limb is exteriorized through the skin from a separate tract than the one created by the wounding agent. Near-total exclusion can be achieved by circumferential suture fixation of the lower arm of the T-tube.[39]

The value of drains is debated. Ten of 11 cervical injuries repaired surgically were not drained in a report of noniatrogenic esophageal injuries.[40] In our personal experience, we have used esophageal diversion only once for cervical esophageal injuries. Primary repair for cervical esophageal injuries was always feasible and safe. A drain was always left for a few days.

Thoracic esophageal injuries are challenging because they are frequently associated with long delays to diagnosis and surgical repair. The upper thoracic esophagus is approached through a right thoracotomy and the lower through a left thoracotomy. An average of 13 hours from admission to operation was reported in patients who were initially stable and underwent preoperative evaluation.[41] These patients had a higher complication rate than patients who were immediately taken to the operating room. In most cases, primary repair can be performed if the delay is less than 12 to 12 hours. Primary repair is usually done in two layers. Pleural, intercostal muscle, diaphragmatic, or pericardial wraps have been used to reinforce the esophageal repair, but their value is uncertain.[17,18,42,43] For injuries that are diagnosed after 24 hours, it is generally accepted that primary repair alone is at high risk of failure.[12,44] Principles of surgical therapy under such circumstances include any combination of the following procedures: double-layer closure, buttressing with flaps, cervical esophagostomy, exclusion of lower esophagus, gastrostomy, feeding jejunostomy, and wide drainage.[35] A second procedure may be needed following exclusion procedures, resulting in some occasions in the need for esophageal resection and colon interposition.

The abdominal esophagus is approached through a laparotomy. An increased index of suspicion must be maintained because other abdominal injuries and the absence of spillage or bleeding from the esophageal injury may detract the attention and risk overlooking this injury. Careful inspection of the gastroesophageal junction and exploration of existing hematomas should be part of the routine of a trauma laparotomy. Primary repair of esophageal perforations is usually adequate, although buttressing with stomach wall (Thal patch) or diaphragm has been suggested to improve results.[44,45] A formal gastric wrap has also been used in complex injuries.[40,46]

Complications of Operative Therapy

Overall, the range of major esophageal-specific complications following operations for esophageal injuries range from 0% to 74%.[34,35,40,47,48] This wide variation indicates the different populations that are treated in the various studies, including different parts of the esophagus, different types of injuries, and different types of operations.

The entire gamut of surgical techniques is directed toward preventing suture line dehiscence. As opposed to esophageal perforation leaks in nonoperatively managed patients, which are usually contained (Figure 21.4), leaks from suture lines of operated patients have the propensity of spreading to adjacent planes or cavities because the tissues surrounding the injury are already dissected during surgical exploration. Therefore, severe infections, such as mediastinitis, are possible. To avoid this, we recommend adequate drainage at the end of an esophageal operation, particularly at the thoracic level. In the presence of drains, a suture line leak is usually converted to an esophageal fistula, which can be managed usually with success by conservative methods.[47,48] The complexity of repair, severity of injury, and delay to operation are significantly associated with the likelihood for developing a leak.[41]

Stenosis at the site of repair is a complication that results from overzealous suturing in multiple layers, repair of complex injuries requiring extensive suture lines, or procedures for exclusion or diversion of the esophageal flow.[49] Most esophageal strictures resolve after esophageal dilatation, although resection and replacement may be required on occasion.

Other complications include tracheoesophageal fistula, blowout of carotid artery repair, osteomyelitis, meningitis, and pneumonia.[18,34,35] They usually occur because of a leak next to adjacent organ injuries (trachea, vessels, spine, spinal cord).

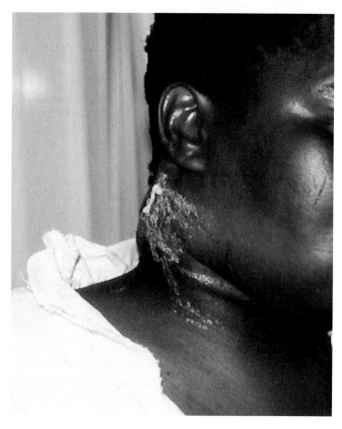

FIGURE 21.4. Neck abscess from a missed cervical esophageal injury.

Nontraumatic Emergencies

Esophageal Perforation

The single most common cause of esophageal perforation is iatrogenic: it is caused by esophageal instrumentation. Esophageal rupture can also occur spontaneously and is known as Boerhaave's syndrome. Other causes include foreign body ingestion and trauma and is considered separately.

Iatrogenic causes account for 43% of cases of esophageal perforation.[50] Diagnostic flexible endoscopy carries a very low risk of perforation (1:3,000); the use of the rigid endoscope carries three times this risk. Therapeutic interventions dramatically increase the risk of perforation. For this reason, most endoscopic perforations occur in patients who are undergoing therapeutic endoscopy and have underlying esophageal lesions. The incidence of perforation has been estimated at 0.4% after bougeinage and 0.3% after pneumatic dilation of stricture.[51] This incidence increases to 2% to 6% in achalasia because the balloon diameter is often twice as big as that used to dilate strictures.[52,53] Perforation has been reported in association with a variety of other forms of esophageal instrumentation, including nasogastric tube placement, overtube placement, sclerotherapy of esophageal varices, and endoscopic ultrasound. It has also been reported with placement of endotracheal tubes.[54–57] The site of perforation is typically at or just above the site of pathology, which in contemporary practice tends to be the distal esophagus. Cervical instrumental perforations are associated with the use of the rigid endoscope or maladroit attempts to insert an endotracheal tube.

Esophageal perforations can also occur as a result of a wide variety of surgical procedures, both esophageal (fundoplication, esophageal myotomy, and enucleation of a leiomyoma) and nonesophageal (vagotomy, pnemonectomy, thyroid resection, tracheostomy, thoracic aneurysm repair, thoracotomy tube placement, mediastinoscopy, and cervical spine surgery).[58,59] These are recognized either intraoperatively or in the early postoperative period and consequently rarely present to the emergency room. The most important to be aware of are those following Nissen fundoplication, where perforation can be caused by passage of the intraesophageal bougie used to size the fundoplication as well as by inexpert dissection behind the esophagus. Failure to recognize the injury is doubly serious because the patient may be sent home on the first or second postoperative day, only to return to the emergency room a day or two later with serious mediastinal or abdominal sepsis—the delay in diagnosis imposed by this interval worsens the prognosis.[60]

Spontaneous rupture of the esophagus is often termed Boerhaave's syndrome, named for the famous Dutch physician Hermann Boerhaave, who first described it in 1724. His report of the sudden tearing chest pain in a *bon viveur* attempting to vomit after a voluminous meal remains a classic description. This is still the most common presentation. Frequently the patient is attempting to resist vomiting, and the rupture is presumed to be secondary to a rapid increase in intraabdominal pressure, which in the presence of a closed upper esophageal sphincter is completely transmitted to the thoracic esophagus. The pain is typically of sudden onset, radiates to the back, and is associated with tachycardia and tachypnea, and diagnoses such as myocardial infarction and dissecting aneurysm are frequently considered first.

The classic presentation of any esophageal perforation is pain, fever, and the presence of subcutaneous or mediastinal air. Pain is the most common presenting symptom and is typically felt in the neck with cervical perforations and in the substernal area with thoracic perforations. Endoscopic perforations will typically present with chest pain after the patient has recovered from the sedation administered for the procedure, but, if the patient is discharged without suspicion of a problem, the pain may worsen and prompt a visit to the emergency room that night. Boerhaave's syndrome has been reported in a wide range of other situations causing raised intraabdominal pressure, for example, blunt trauma, straining, weight-lifting, severe coughing, and childbirth.[3,61] Mucosal disease that causes weakening of the esophageal wall is also associated with spontaneous perforation. The majority of these perforations develop in the distal esophagus on the left side.

Occasionally the general condition of a frail patient requiring intubation shortly after admission to the emergency department may conceal the underlying diagnosis of esophageal perforation. The patient is typically admitted to a medical intensive care unit with pleural effusion and presumed pneumonia—the diagnosis may only be made when the pleural effusion is subsequently tapped and found to contain gastric contents. Always consider the possibility of esophageal perforation for patients with unexplained pleural effusion. The basic message in all these situations is to have a high index of suspicion for the problem, because outcome depends on timely diagnosis and management.[62]

Assessment

Once the suspicion has been entertained, confirmation is important not just to make the diagnosis but for localization purposes. Many patients will require surgical exploration, and accurate identification of the site of leakage is helpful in planning the surgical repair.

Radiologic studies are the keystone of diagnosis. Chest radiographs may demonstrate subcutaneous emphysema, pneumomediastinum, mediastinal widening, pneumothorax, hydrothorax, pleural effusion, or pleural infiltrate. The earliest finding is a small linear streak of air just medial to the sternoclavicular joints (Figure 21.5). Suggestive abnormalities are found in 90% of patients, although in the first few hours after the injury the radiograph may be normal.[11] A contrast study is usually

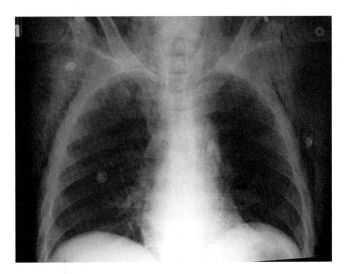

FIGURE 21.5. Chest radiograph after endoscopy showing mediastinal air, indicating esophageal perforation.

performed first with gastrografin, because it is much less harmful than barium if it leaks into the mediastinum. However, patients at high risk of aspiration should have a barium esophagogram as the first study because of the risk of pulmonary edema if the hypertonic water-soluble contrast medium is aspirated.[63] Gastrografin is less accurate than barium for diagnosing small perforations, so, if the gastrografin study is negative, a barium study should follow.[64] If a good-quality barium study is negative, the presence of esophageal perforation is very unlikely. Computed tomography scan can be used in equivocal cases or when an esophagogram is unavailable. Signs of esophageal perforation on CT scan include air in the mediastinum, abscess cavities adjacent to the esophagus, or a communication of an air-filled esophagus with an adjacent mediastinal air–fluid collection.

Treatment

Once the diagnosis is established, the earlier definitive treatment is begun, the better the outcome. In most large published series the mortality and morbidity are directly related to delay in initiating treatment. In addition to the time between the event and the onset of treatment, the other major factors that affect the choice of treatment are the presence of preexisting esophageal pathology (especially stricture, tumor, or achalasia) and the site of perforation. Not every patient needs operative repair. Some can be managed nonoperatively. The original report by Cameron et al.[65] listed several criteria for selecting nonoperative treatment. These include intramural perforation, perforations that are contained within the mediastinum and drain back into the esophagus, perforations that are not associated with esophageal obstruction or malignancy, and minimal evidence of clinical sepsis. These criteria are still broadly applicable today. There is a tendency to treat endoscopic perforations nonoperatively, because the patient was fasting and not vomiting or retching, and consequently the degree of mediastinal contamination is more limited. The principles of nonoperative treatment include restriction of oral intake, broad-spectrum antibiotics, and parenteral nutrition. If the patient develops no worsening sign of sepsis and the temperature, heart rate, and white blood cell count trend toward normal, the status of healing may be assessed by a barium swallow after 5 to 7 days. Oral intake may be resumed if the leak has healed.

Surgical treatment options include drainage alone, primary repair, diversion, or esophageal resection. In cervical perforations drainage may be sufficient. The cervical esophagus is exposed through the left side, making an incision along the border of the sternocleidomastoid. The right side may be used if the leak appears to track more on the right side. The recurrent laryngeal nerve has more variability on the right than on the left. The omohyoid is

divided, and the carotid sheath is retracted laterally and the trachea and larynx medially. It is critical to protect the recurrent laryngeal nerve, which lies posteriorly on the trachea and can be traumatized if a metal self-retaining retractor is used to hold the larynx medially. It is best if the assistant retracts gently using only a gauze sponge rather than a metal retractor. The esophagus is visible on top of the bodies of the cervical vertebrae. Circumferential mobilization is usually not necessary for drainage or repair. The laceration is usually posterior, and, if it is amenable to primary suture, it seems logical to close the defect. If it is a delayed perforation and the surrounding tissues are edematous and friable, then a soft drain should be positioned close to the perforation and the neck loosely closed.

For intrathoracic perforations, drainage is a less ideal option because of the propensity of the infection to spread throughout the mediastinum and pleural cavity. The best results are obtained when the perforation is accurately closed within 24 hours. A low (seventh or even eighth interspace), left-sided thoracotomy is made. All devitalized mediastinal and esophageal tissue should be removed, and the edges of the esophagus should be trimmed and closed. It is often not recognized that the esophageal mucosa is a tough and resilient layer, and every attempt should be made to close it precisely. It may even be necessary to elongate the muscular perforation to access the apex of the mucosal laceration. It should be repaired precisely and totally and then the muscle layer closed over it. A chest tube is positioned in the posterior mediastinum to act as a drain if the suture line should leak. Leakage of the suture line remains a serious problem and can be prevented to some extent by accurate suturing and by the use of an onlay patch. The easiest way is to dissect off a small flap of pleura and suture it over the closure. A perforation at the gastroesophageal junction, for example, after dilation for achalasia, may be reinforced with gastric fundus because partial fundoplication is part of the surgical strategy for achalasia. A centrally based tongue of diaphragm has also been advocated, but risks weakening diaphragmatic function and even diaphragmatic hernia later. The best method of patching the repair is to use a vascularized pedicle of intercostal muscle and pleura. This is best planned ahead of time, because it is difficult to harvest such a flap after a conventional thoracotomy has been made. The best method is to shingle out the seventh rib and divide the intercostal muscle very anteriorly, leaving the bulky intercostal muscle with its blood supply coming from the posterior. It is retracted out of the way during the repair and then sutured down over the esophagus, although not circumferentially encircling it.

Some authors have advocated approaching the perforation via the abdomen and even repairing it laparoscopically.[66] This approach may be adequate for very distal perforations when there is no stricture present; however, in the presence of a stricture, there is likely to be esophageal shortening, and access from the abdomen is likely to be very difficult.

Options for the Neglected Perforation or the Unstable Patient

There are situations when the patient is so unstable that thoracotomy with unilateral collapse of the lung may not be tolerated. Similarly, for perforations that have been unrecognized for days, primary closure may simply not be an option. The best solution to this problem is to divide the esophagus in the neck, leaving as long a proximal stump as possible to perform an esophagostomy, and to close the distal end, leaving retromanubrial sutures to aid subsequent reconstruction. Then staple off the cardia using a TA-55 stapler, insert a feeding jejunostomy, and insert a chest drain to drain the pleura and mediastinum. When the patient has recovered, it may be found that the staples in the distal esophagus have opened up, and it is possible to reconnect the esophagus in the neck. It often heals with a stricture, and the recurrent nerve is much more at risk after a second exploration of the neck, so the results of direct reversal of the esophagostomy are not always satisfactory. A substernal gastric pull-up or colon interposition may be better if the patient is otherwise in good health.[67]

Dealing with Associated Esophageal Disease

Free perforations associated with dilation for achalasia are usually treated with closure of the perforation with contralateral myotomy and a partial fundoplication. A stricture may be treated by fundoplication and the repair positioned below the diaphragm and the crura closed. If a perforated cancer is found, it is best to do an esophagectomy.[68] Because most cancers are now distal tumors arising in Barrett's esophagus, it may be possible to perform a transhiatal esophagectomy, excising a portion of the cardia and lesser curve, bring out a cervical esophagostomy, and insert a feeding jejunostomy. Subsequent reconstruction may be undertaken when the patient has recovered from the acute situation and will most likely be a substernal gastric pull up.

Caustic Ingestion

Caustic ingestions occur most commonly in two age groups: young children who accidentally ingest bleaches and other common household agents while exploring the domestic environment and young adults between 20 and 40 years of age in whom the ingestion is usually intentional. Injury tends to be more severe in the latter group because a larger volume is ingested. Before 1960, com-

mercial lye was produced in crystalline form. The immediate pain produced from burns to the mouth induced rapid expulsion of the crystals, preventing injury more distally in the gastrointestinal tract. The introduction of concentrated liquid forms of alkali has led to an increased incidence of injury to the esophagus and stomach.[69] Industrial changes sometimes lead to reduction of toxicity in one product only to find the emergence of a new source of caustics. The recent reports of ingestion of hair-relaxing preparations is one such example.[70]

The degree of injury depends on the concentration, duration, and quantity of the caustic agent. Alkaline agents cause liquefactive necrosis, resulting in a deep burn, whereas acids cause coagulative necrosis, forming an eschar that limits deeper tissue penetration. The sites of greatest injury in the esophagus are those of natural narrowing where liquid can pool: the cricopharyngeus muscle, the aortic arch, and the lower esophageal sphincter. Both alkali and acids can also cause reflex pylorospasm with pooling of the caustic agent in the antrum. Damage to adjacent structures, including colon and spleen, may occur when major ingestion has occurred.[71]

The typical patient presents with oral pain, constant drooling, and inability to swallow. Hoarseness and stridor are diagnostic of laryngeal injury and may indicate imminent loss of the airway. Retrosternal pain and acute epigastric pain are worrisome for full-thickness esophageal injury. Even patients with minimal symptoms may still have severe injury; however, a recent report of 85 pediatric patients showed that in the absence of symptoms serious caustic injuries did not occur.[72]

The immediate goals of therapy are airway assessment and fluid resuscitation. Evaluation should include direct visualization of the oropharynx. No attempt should be made to neutralize the agent, as this can cause the release of heat and further tissue damage. Giving syrup of ipecac is also dangerous, as emesis will reintroduce the upper esophagus to exposure with the corrosive agent. Plain films of the chest and abdomen should be performed to identify pneumoperitoneum, pneumomediastinum, or pleural effusions. Early endoscopy should be performed within the first 24 hours for all patients with stridor, all patients with intentional ingestions, and symptomatic children. Endoscopy is not necessary for asymptomatic children or patients with clear indications for operative exploration. Caustic injuries are classified endoscopically as first degree (hyperemia and edema), second degree (ulceration), and third degree (black discoloration or adherent slough, indicating full-thickness injury). Traditional teaching is to perform endoscopy and stop at the first sign of damage. However, in practice a skilled and gentle endoscopist can safely negotiate the esophagus and stomach and assess the extent of the injury more completely.

Treatment of first-degree injuries is observation for 24 to 48 hours. Patients with more severe injuries who do not require operative exploration should be placed in a monitored unit, kept on nothing-by-mouth (NPO) status, and given antibiotics such as penicillin, ampicillin, or clindamycin to provide coverage for oropharyngeal flora. Steroids were not shown to be effective in preventing strictures in a randomized controlled trial,[73] but retrospective data still suggest that they may be useful in severe injuries.[74] Gastric acid suppression is recommended to reduce gastroesophageal reflux and theoretically decrease the risk of stricture formation. Patients should be kept NPO until they can swallow their saliva and have no evidence of sepsis, after which their diet can be advanced as tolerated.

There are several treatment alternatives that have been used when recovery is delayed beyond 48 hours. A gastrostomy can be performed with passage of an orogastric string for retrograde dilation of strictures; this is commonly used for children.[75] A second alternative is intraluminal stent placement for prevention of strictures.[76] Nutrition can be provided using parenteral nutrition, or a feeding tube can be placed. The esophagus and stomach should be evaluated at 3 weeks, 3 months, and 6 months with a barium swallow for the development of stricture formation or gastric outlet obstruction.

Patients with full-thickness injuries require operative resection of devitalized organs. Signs of perforation include peritonitis, depressed mental status, shock, persistent acidemia, and the presence of free air on plain films. Delayed diagnosis is associated with increased morbidity and mortality rates. Some groups have recommended exploratory laparotomy for all patients with third-degree or circumferential second-degree burns,[77] but most surgeons determine the requirement for operative intervention on an individual basis, usually if there are signs of peritonitis or sepsis.

The esophagus is best approached through the abdomen, which allows evaluation of the stomach and adjacent organs. Esophagectomy can be performed using the transhiatal method, avoiding the need for a thoracotomy. A gastrectomy should also be performed if gastric necrosis is identified. A cervical esophagostomy should be performed and a feeding jejunostomy tube placed.

Delayed reconstruction is then performed when the patient is stable. Unlike many other inflammatory diseases, the scarring that follows caustic ingestion is dense, aggressive, and progressive. It continues for 1 year or more. It is common for the cervical esophagostomy to undergo stenosis, and the structuring may affect laryngeal function and even the tongue. Dense proximal scarring may eventually necessitate a laryngectomy as part of the reconstruction, because uncontrollable aspiration makes a conventional reconstruction useless. If one pyriform fossa is preserved, it may be possible to bring up a colon interposition to that location, and with the help of swallowing therapy the patient may learn to swallow safely. It is important not to perform reconstruction too early in the evolution of the stricture, as the anastomosis and pharynx are likely to undergo further dense structuring. Reconstruction can also be performed by a gastric pullup: this may not be possible if the stomach has been injured or resected at the time of the original injury.[78]

The longer term management of the deformities and disabilities as a consequence of scarring and structuring in the foregut is a complex subject and beyond the scope of this book. In general, the more distal the injury, the easier it is to treat. The stomach may become densely fibrotic and require resection. The distal esophagus when strictured may be repetitively dilated, but if patency cannot be maintained and the patient's social functioning and nutritional status continue to suffer, esophagectomy or esophageal bypass will be necessary. These reconstructions are complex and often require ingenuity and innovation when applied to individual patients. They should not be attempted by surgeons outside of a major esophageal center.

Foreign Body Impaction

Food

Impaction of a food bolus is a relatively common esophageal emergency. It presents with chest pain and abrupt, complete, dysphagia such that the attempt to clear the esophagus by drinking liquid promotes a spasm of coughing and the need to regurgitate the liquid. It is sometimes described as the steakhouse syndrome, and indeed meat is the offending food in 80% to 90% of cases. It is more common in the elderly and the edentulous. The impaction of a food bolus is unusual in an otherwise normal esophagus. Underlying esophageal pathology is often present, most commonly a stricture or a ring, but dysmotility and even tumors may present for the first time in this way. Consequently the management does not end with successful and atraumatic passage or extraction of the bolus: the underlying disease needs to be investigated subsequently.

Presentation

In most cases the history is obvious. In one particularly acute form the bolus lodges high in the esophagus, displacing or compressing the posterior trachea, and there is extreme stridor and shortness of breath in addition. This requires the Heimlich maneuver to treat. Sometimes the patient will feel that the bolus may have passed but will report residual discomfort. More commonly the esophagus is completely obstructed, and the patient arrives carrying a container for expectorated saliva. If the patient complains of pain in the throat and neck, the offending object is most likely a fish bone.

Assessment

The diagnosis is usually clear from the history. Pay particular attention to any evidence of preexisting esophageal dysfunction—a previous episode of impaction or a history of dysphagia, previous dilation, or esophageal surgery, such as Nissen fundoplication, stent insertion, or even gastric bypass surgery.

Physical examination is rarely helpful. It is typical to see a rather frightened patient holding a receptacle filled with tissues and expectorated saliva. The airway is rarely compromised.

Radiologic studies are not useful in cases of simple food impaction. Plain x-rays are useful when indigestible foreign objects or bony fragments have been ingested. Contrast studies are not indicated. They carry the risk of aspiration if hypertonic water-soluble contrast media such as Hypaque are used, and if barium is used it makes subsequent endoscopic extraction much more difficult.

Conservative Treatment

Several methods have been employed to avoid the need for urgent endoscopy. Glucagon was widely used because of its capacity to reduce lower esophageal sphincter pressure and, by inference, relax the distal esophagus. Success rates of about 50% were reported. However, more recent studies have shown that its effect on distal esophageal contractility is minimal, and in randomized controlled studies it has no advantage over placebo.[79,80] Others have reported success by attempting to digest a meat bolus by administering papain, usually in the form of Adolph's Meat Tenderizer. This material can also digest the esophageal mucosa and causes a particularly virulent form of pulmonary edema if aspirated.[81,82] It requires aspiration of saliva via a nasogastric tube before being administered. These disadvantages render it of little value in contemporary practice. Finally, carbonated beverages or administration of gas-forming agents, generally a combination of tartaric acid and sodium bicarbonate, have been given in the hope of inducing esophageal distension and allowing the bolus to pass more distally. Although there are some reports of success with these techniques, perforation has also been reported, and they are thus rarely employed.[83]

Endoscopic Treatment

Most patients with persistent food impaction can be managed by flexible endoscopy without much special equipment (Figure 21.6). Several different techniques can be employed, the choice of which depends on the coexisting esophageal pathology. The simplest is to push the

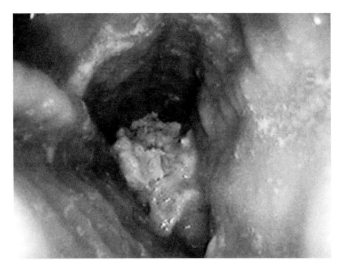

FIGURE 21.6. Esophagoscopy showing bolus of meat impacted in distal esophagus, causing complete occlusion.

bolus into the stomach.[84,85] This avoids the problem of fragmentation during extraction and the risk of accidentally dislodging the bolus into the airway during extraction. If the bolus cannot be advanced into the stomach, extraction is best performed using a polypectomy snare. The snare and scope are removed together, under direct vision, until the cricopharyngeal sphincter is reached; then the bolus and snare are pulled snugly against the endoscope and the whole assembly removed rapidly. If the bolus fragments, the triradiate grasping forceps can be used to retrieve individual pieces, and an overtube may be used if it is necessary to reintroduce the endoscope several times. An overtube can cause serious laceration of the esophagus if inserted incorrectly. Passing it over a loosely fitting scope can allow its sharp edge to catch on the esophageal mucosa and produce a long linear tear. It is safest if passed over a snugly fitting but lubricated Maloney bougie. The bougie is then removed and the endoscope passed through the overtube.

Identification of esophageal pathology is unlikely to be complete in the acute care setting, but it is important not to miss what information there is. Most often a localized stenosis in the distal esophagus will be found. This may be a Schatzki ring, a peptic or other fibrous stricture, or a cancer. Schatzki ring is a simple shelf or fibrous ring at the squamocolumnar junction that is readily dilated and generally associated with a hiatal hernia. Mild peptic strictures are similar in appearance (Figure 21.7). The recent presence of an impacted object and the trauma from attempts to remove it make it difficult to diagnose esophagitis with confidence. Barrett's esophagus may be seen, in which case the stricture is typically more proximal. The appearance of a cancer is usually obvious and presents as an ulcerating irregular mass. No attempt should be made to dilate a lesion resembling a cancer, but

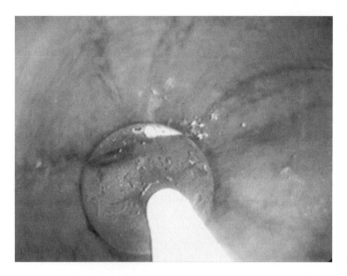

FIGURE 21.7. The underlying stricture of the same patient undergoing dilatation with a through-the-scope balloon.

a biopsy specimen should be taken and the patient referred for urgent evaluation to an esophageal center.

Indigestible Foreign Body

Humans have an amazing propensity to put objects in their mouths. The motivation ranges from exploration or mere inattentiveness for young children and the mentally impaired, to sexual gratification or suicide for adults, to protest or escapism for prisoners. When the objects are small enough to be swallowed but big enough or irregularly shaped to lodge in the esophagus, the consequences can be serious. Unlike food bolus impaction, the obstruction is rarely absolute: saliva and fluids can pass into the stomach. The risks are thus dominated by the threat of pressure necrosis with consequent mediastinitis or by the consequences of attempted removal rather than aspiration.

The variety of objects in clinical reports is enormous.[86] The leading contenders for children are coins, batteries, and parts of toys, but nails, safety pins, the small slotted plastic squares to close the plastic wrapping on loaves of bread, and aluminum rings on the tops of soda cans have all been frequently reported. For adults with suicidal intent, paper clips, razor blades, broken glass, and toothbrushes are added to the list, and the accidental swallowing of dental plates continues to be common.[87]

Presentation may be immediate or delayed. The patient, or more commonly the parent or caregiver, may report the event as soon as it occurs. If it is not witnessed, and the patient is too young or too incapacitated to give the history, there may be merely vague symptoms of chest or neck pain, which are easy to dismiss. The presence of fever or crepitus or an obvious radiopaque foreign body on the chest x-ray will prompt more detailed scrutiny.

Assessment

Once suspected, worry about sepsis. Fever and tachycardia may be present. Carefully examine the neck and chest for crepitus. A chest x-ray will show the impacted object if it is radiopaque, but many swallowed objects are not. It is worthwhile to x-ray the abdomen to detect other foreign bodies that may have passed, because the behavioral pattern is often repetitive. One area of controversy that remains is how extensively to investigate a child with a history, or mere suspicion, of foreign body ingestion. The logic is that many swallowed foreign objects are so small that most will have reached the stomach by the time of presentation. However, most physicians would agree that the presence of chest pain or the appearance of a radiopaque body on chest x-ray mandates endoscopic examination. Many small objects will indeed pass into the stomach, and the majority will be passed spontaneously in the stool. However, a sharp object, such as a pin, or a potentially dangerous one, such as a battery, should be removed endoscopically even if it has passed into the stomach.

The definitive treatment of these swallowed objects differs from that of food impaction in several important respects:

1. The esophagus is generally normal in caliber and function. There is no special tendency for these objects to impact at the distal end of the esophagus; if anything, they tend to be more proximal.

2. Much of the morbidity stems from damage inflicted by inexpert attempts to remove the object.

3. Flexible endoscopy is frequently unsuccessful, and rigid endoscopy may be required.

4. The problem may not end with successful removal of the object. Constant vigilance is necessary to ensure that there has been no perforation. Simple discharge from the emergency room is therefore rarely appropriate.

The development of safe techniques for removal of intraesophageal foreign bodies is always associated with the name of Chevalier Jackson, the famous ear, nose, and throat surgeon from Philadelphia a century or more ago. His invention and perfection of the rigid esophagoscope and a wide variety of grasping tools and his insistence on extreme gentleness in manipulating the objects continue to be the foundation of contemporary practice in this clinical situation.

Definitive Treatment

Most foreign bodies can be extracted endoscopically. It seems intuitive that what went down should also be capable of retracing its steps. The exception is when the object is especially angular or sharp and irregular. Several recent case reports have described the deliberate swallowing, by Bulgarian prisoners, of needles bent into a star shape. Attempts to remove these endoscopically will result in severe trauma to the esophagus, and a direct esophagotomy via thoracotomy is the safest option.[88]

For objects without sharp edges, such as coins and batteries, flexible endoscopy should be attempted first. It does not require general anesthesia and is more widely available in the emergency room. One major limitation is the size and strength of the grasping forceps that can be inserted down the biopsy channel. Use the biggest possible scope with the best suction channel. Sometimes it is necessary to remove accumulated secretions, food debris, or administered barium before the object can be clearly grasped. So-called rat-tooth forceps provide the best grip. Longer objects such as batteries or toothbrushes can be snared with polypectomy snare. As in the case of impacted food, the scope and object are removed slowly and gently under direct vision until the cricopharyngeal muscle is reached, and then the object is snugly brought up against the scope and the entire assembly removed rapidly. It helps to extend the neck during this maneuver. The critical thing to avoid is accidentally losing the grip of the object and allowing it to fall into the airway.

Unless the ingestion was recent and the extraction was simple and atraumatic, there is always the risk of perforation. Admitting the patient for observation and serial clinical examination to detect crepitus, fever, or tachycardia is the simplest option. Alternatively, a contrast swallow may be performed and permit earlier discharge. However, it is common for the condition to occur against the backdrop of serious psychosocial pathology, and overnight admission allows time for activation of social and psychiatric services to provide longer term support.

Esophageal Hemorrhage

The major source of esophageal hemorrhage is bleeding esophageal varices that are a consequence of portal hypertension. Similarly, Mallory Weiss syndrome, a linear tear at the gastroesophageal junction generally occurring after prolonged retching, can also be a source of hemorrhage. Nonvariceal esophageal hemorrhage is rarely as catastrophic as bleeding varices and typically presents with hematemesis without the serious hemodynamic instability associated with major or more rapid bleeds. The localization of the source of bleeding to the esophagus is usually only confirmed at endoscopy, but some clinical features may give a clue. Most esophageal bleeding comes from a diffuse alteration in the mucosa. The most common cause is still esophagitis due to gastroesophageal reflux disease (GERD).[89] Even though it is a rare complication, GERD is such a frequent condition in the population that in absolute terms it is still the most common source of esophageal hemorrhage. Infective esophagitis is relatively common in the immunosuppressed population, for example, in AIDS and after bone marrow transplantation.[90] Pill injuries, especially those caused by nonsteroidal antiinflammatory drugs (NSAIDs), are common in the elderly.[91]

In most of these cases, the diagnosis will be made by endoscopy. In GERD, there will be a history of longstanding heartburn and regurgitation, and it is likely that a hiatal hernia will be present. Infective esophagitis in AIDS is typically due to cytomegalovirus, herpes simplex, or *Candida*. All three types have characteristic endoscopic appearances.[92] The diffuse mucosal sloughing seen after chemotherapy or bone marrow transplantation is also easy to recognize. When endoscopy is carried out it is important to ensure that a more commonplace lesion in the stomach or duodenum has not been missed.

The treatment of diffuse esophageal bleeding is abolition of acid reflux, usually by proton pump inhibitors. Regular administration of mucosal protectants, such as Carafate suspension, has been shown to be beneficial.[93] It is given in the form of a slurry every 6 hours. The time-honored method of dripping a combination of milk and antacid via a nasogastric tube is still occasionally used but has only anecdotal support.

Major bleeding from an esophageal source initially presents like any severe upper gastrointestinal hemorrhage, and the acute care physician's initial approach is resuscitation while a diagnosis is being made. The airway is still the priority in this acute care situation, especially because major aspiration of blood and other gastric contents is a real risk. Any patient with a hemodynamically significant bleed and altered mental status is best intubated until the source can be determined and treated. The second priority is to obtain good venous access for administration of fluids and possibly blood products. Clinical clues to the site of bleeding may be sought pending definitive investigations—a history of alcoholism, or the presence of signs of portal hypertension (caput medusae, palpable spleen), or other signs of liver failure suggest bleeding esophageal varices. A history of peptic ulcers or heavy NSAID use suggests a bleeding peptic ulcer. A history of reflux disease, especially if Barrett's esophagus is known to be present, is a clue to an esophageal source.

Catastrophic nonvariceal esophageal bleeding may come from the rare condition of aortoesophageal fistula, which may occur when a thoracic aortic aneurysm erodes into the esophagus.[94,95] The pattern of hemorrhage is typically a massive hematemesis with circulatory collapse but with a history of smaller, self-limiting episodes of hematemesis in the preceding few days. The diagnosis of aortic pathology may be known or suspected from the mediastinal widening on chest x-ray, but it is difficult to confirm safely. This lesion has a high mortality rate, not just because definitive surgery is difficult and risky—it requires a high thoracotomy and operative replacement of a portion of the aortic arch—but also because during the investigations necessary to establish the diagnosis the patient may exsanguinate uncontrollably. Some reported successful outcomes have advocated the use of a Sengstaken-Blakemore tube with the esophageal balloon inflated while preparing the patient for the operating room.

Deep penetrating ulcers of the esophagus may occur in reflux disease and are usually associated with Barrett's esophagus. These resemble peptic ulcers in the stomach and duodenum in their tendency to penetrate deeply and occasionally cause massive bleeding. Modern endoscopic techniques of hemostasis—thermal coagulation and injection of epinephrine or saline—have been successfully used to arrest major hemorrhage caused by penetrating ulcers of the esophagus. Definitive treatment of the underlying condition is best performed at a specialist center, because this is not a straightforward case of reflux disease treatable by laparoscopic fundoplication: there is likely to be periesophageal scarring and esophageal shortening, and definitive surgery, if it is necessary, may be better carried out through the chest.

Acute Tracheoesophageal Fistula

Acute tracheoesophageal fistula (TEF) may occur when penetrating ulcers in the upper esophagus erode into the trachea. This condition may occur in patients with AIDS and ulcers associated with cytomegalovirus (CMV). A patient with a history of chest pain and dysphagia suddenly has uncontrollable cough superimposed on his or her former symptoms. Endoscopy typically shows one or more deep cavitating ulcers on the anterior esophageal wall. The fistula may be more easily identified at bronchoscopy and occurs on the membranous portion of the distal trachea or the left main bronchus. Esophageal carcinoma can also erode into the respiratory tract. In this situation, the patient may be from a social and ethnic group at high risk for squamous esophageal carcinoma (e.g., Asians and African Americans). It presents less dramatically, initially with refractory pneumonia. By definition, it represents advanced disease, and surgical cure is generally not possible. A very acute form of TEF can also occur in the process of dilating a high stricture. A proximal carcinoma that has been treated with definitive radiation will often have a very dense stricture that, if perforated, will open directly into the trachea or left main bronchus. The patient will immediately have a spasm of coughing as the respiratory tract becomes flooded with esophageal secretions. The diagnosis is obvious to the endoscopist.

The immediate treatment of acute TEF is the insertion of a covered esophageal stent. This can be done at the time it is discovered. It is frequently very successful in the short term. If the patient has an advanced malignancy,

this is often sufficient palliation. Cytomegalovirus ulcers in immunosuppressed patients will respond to antiviral treatment. For the patient with a radiation stricture, it may be best to bypass the esophagus by doing a substernal gastric pullup and drain the distal end of the esophagus into a Roux limb. Any attempt to resect the stricture will leave a large tracheal defect that may be extremely difficult to close.

Critique

The presentation is somewhat classic for Boerhaave's syndrome (retching-induced esophageal rupture). This patient is not in extremis and therefore should undergo diagnostic evaluation to confirm an esophageal perforation and the location. A contrast swallow would be the diagnostic modality of choice. A right thoracotomy will likely be required. However, if the rupture occurs at the gastroesophageal junction, there are some who advocate a transabdominal approach.

Answer (C)

References

1. Pajecki D, Zilberstein B, Azevedo dos Santos M, Ubriaco J, Quintanilha A, Cecconello I, Gama-Rodrigues J. Megaesophagus microbiota: a qualitative and quantitative analysis. J Gastrointest Surg 2002; 6:723–729.
2. Brook I, Fazier E. Microbiology of mediastinitis. Arch Intern Med 1996; 156:333–336.
3. Beal SL, Pottmeyer EW, Spisso JM. Esophageal perforation following external blunt trauma. J Trauma 1988; 28:1425–1432.
4. Pate JW. Tracheobronchial and esophageal injuries. Surg Clin North Am 1989; 69:111–123.
5. Demetriades D, Theodorou D, Cornwell EE, et al. Evaluation of penetrating injuries of the neck: prospective study of 223 patients. World J Surg 1997; 21:41–48.
6. Ngakane H, Muckart DJJ, Luvuno FM. Penetrating visceral injuries of the neck: results of a conservative management policy. Br J Surg 1990; 77:908–910.
7. Oparah RS, Maudal AK. Operative management of penetrating wounds of the chest in civilian practice. J Thorac Cardiovasc Surg 1979; 77:162–166.
8. Thal ER, Meyer DM. Penetrating neck trauma. Curr Probl Surg 1992; Jan:10–56.
9. Cheadle W, Richardson JD. Options in the management of trauma to the esophagus. Surg Gynecol Obstet 1982; 155:380–384.
10. Pass LJ, LeNarz LA, Schreiber JT, Estrera AS. Management of esophageal gunshot wounds. Ann Thorac Surg 1987; 44:253–256.
11. Parkin GJS. The radiology of perforated esophagus. Clin Radiol 1973; 24:324–332.

12. DeMeester TR. Perforation of the esophagus. Ann Thorac Surg 1986; 42:231–232.

13. Demetriades D, Theodorou D, Cornwell EE III, et al. Penetrating injuries of the neck in patients in stable condition. Physical examination, angiography, or color flow Doppler imaging. Arch Surg 1995; 130:971–975.

14. Weigelt JA, Thal ER, Snyder WH, et al. Diagnosis of penetrating cervical esophageal injuries. Am J Surg 1987; 154:619–622.

15. Hatzitheofilou C, Strahlendorf C, Kakoyanis S, Charalambides D, Demetriades D. Penetrating external injuries of the oesophagus and pharynx. Br J Surg 1993; 80:1147–1149.

16. Back MR, Baumgartner FJ, Klein SR. Detection and evaluation of aerodigestive tract injuries caused by cervical and transmediastinal gunshot wounds. J Trauma 1997; 42:680–686.

17. Sawyers JL, Greenfield LJ, Livingstone AS, et al. Esophageal perforation. Contemp Surg 1991; 39:91–110.

18. Hankins JR, Attar S. Esophageal injuries. In Turney SZ, Rodriguez A, Cowley A, eds. Management of Cardiothoracic Trauma. Baltimore: Williams & Wilkins, 1990: 197–218.

19. Ghahremani GG. Esophageal trauma. Semin Roentgenol 1994; 29:387–400.

20. Srinivasan R, Haywood T, Horwitz B, Buckman RF, Fisher RS, Krevsky B. Role of flexible endoscopy in the evaluation of possible esophageal trauma after penetrating injuries. Am J Gastroenterol 2000; 95:1725–1729.

21. Flowers JL, Graham SM, Ugarte MA, et al. Flexible endoscopy for the diagnosis of esophageal trauma. J Trauma 1996; 40:261–265.

22. Horwitz B, Krevsky B, Buckman RF Jr, Fisher RS, Dabezies MA. Endoscopic evaluation of penetrating esophageal injuries. Am J Gastroenterol 1993; 88:1249–1253.

23. Cornwell EE 3rd, Kennedy F, Ayad IA, et al. Transmediastinal gunshot wounds. A reconsideration of the role of angiography. Arch Surg 1996; 131:949–952.

24. Gonzalez RP, Falimirski M, Holevar MR, Turk B. Penetrating zone II neck injury: does dynamic computed tomographic scan contribute to the diagnostic sensitivity of physical examination for surgically significant injury? A prospective blinded study. J Trauma 2003; 54:61–64.

25. Hanpeter DE, Demetriades D, Asensio JA, Berne TV, Velmahos GC, Murray J. Helical computed tomographic scan in the evaluation of mediastinal gunshot wounds. J Trauma 2000; 49:689–695.

26. Velmahos GC, Souter I, Degiannis E, Mokoena T, Saadia R. Selective surgical management in penetrating neck injuries. Can J Surg 1994; 37:487–491.

27. Goudy SL, Miller FB, Bumpous JM. Neck crepitance: evaluation and management of suspected aerodigestive tract injury. Laryngoscope 2002; 223:791–795.

28. Nagy KK, Roberts RR, Smith RF, et al. Trans-mediastinal gunshot wounds: are "stable" patients really stable? World J Surg 2002; 26:1247–1250.

29. Flynn AE, Verrier ED, Way LW, et al. Esophageal perforation. Arch Surg 1989; 124:1211–1215.

30. Stanley RB Jr, Armstrong WB, Fetterman BL, Shindo ML. Management of external penetrating injuries into the hypopharyngeal-cervical esophageal funnel. J Trauma 1997; 42:675–679.

31. Yugueros P, Sarmiento JM, Garcia AF, Ferrada R. Conservative management of penetrating hypopharyngeal wounds. J Trauma 1996; 40:267–269.

32. Madiba TE, Muckart DJJ. Penetrating injuries to the cervical oesophagus: is routine exploration mandatory? Ann R Coll Surg Engl 2003; 85:162–166.

33. Vassiliu P, Baker J, Henderson S, Alo K, Velmahos GC, Demetriades D. Aerodigestive injuries of the neck. Am Surg 2001; 67:75–79.

34. Feliciano DV, Bitondo CG, Mattox KL, et al. Combined tracheoesophageal injuries. Am J Surg 1985; 150:710–715.

35. Ivatury RR, Rohman M, Simon RJ. Esophageal injury. Adv Trauma Crit Care 1994; 9:245–274.

36. Sokolov VV, Bagirov MM. Reconstructive surgery for combined tracheo-esophageal injuries and their sequelae. Eur J Cardiothorac Surg 2001; 20:1025–1029.

37. Weiman DS, Pate JW, Walker WA, Brossnan KM, Fabian TC. Combined gunshot injuries of the trachea and esophagus. World J Surg 1996; 20:1096–1099.

38. Andrade-Alegre R. T-tube insertion in the management of late traumatic esophageal perforations: case report. J Trauma 1994; 37:131–132.

39. Ozcelik C, Inci I, Ozgen G, Eren N. Near-total esophageal exclusion in the treatment of late-diagnosed esophageal perforation. Scand J Thorac Cardiovasc Surg 1994; 28:91–93.

40. Weiman DS, Walker WA, Brosnan KM, Pate JW, Fabian TC. Noniatrogenic esophageal trauma. Ann Thorac Surg 1995; 59:845–849.

41. Asensio JA, Chahwan S, Forno W, et al. Penetrating esophageal injuries: multicenter study of the American Association for the Surgery of Trauma. J Trauma 2001; 50:289–296.

42. Michel L, Grillo HC, Malt RA. Esophageal perforation. Ann Thorac Surg 1982; 33:203–210.

43. Nesbitt JC, Sawyers JL. Surgical management of the esophageal perforation. Am Surg 1987; 53:183–191.

44. Kelly JP, Webb WR, Moulder PV, Moustouakas NM, Lirtzman M. Management of airway trauma II: combined injuries of the trachea and esophagus. Ann Thorac Surg 1987; 43:160–163.

45. Goldstein GA, Thompson WR. Esophageal perforations: a 15 year experience. Am J Surg 1982; 143:495–503.

46. Defore WW Jr, Mattox KL, Hansen HA, Garcia-Rinaldi R, Beall AC Jr, DeBakey ME. Surgical management of penetrating injuries of the esophagus. Am J Surg 1977; 134:734–738.

47. Shama DM, Odell J. Penetrating neck trauma with tracheal and oesophageal injuries. Br J Surg 1984; 71:534–535.

48. Winter RP, Weigelt JA. Cervical esophageal trauma. Incidence and cause of esophageal fistulas. Arch Surg 1990; 125:849–852.

49. Armstrong WB, Detar TR, Stanley RB. Diagnosis and management of external penetrating cervical esophageal injuries. Ann Otol Rhinol Laryngol 1994; 103:863–871.

50. Jones WG 2nd and Ginsberg RJ. Esophageal perforation: a continuing challenge. Ann Thorac Surg 1992; 53(3):534–553.

51. Williamson WA, Ellis FH. Esophageal perforation. In Taylor MB, Gollan JL, Steer ML, Wolfe MM, eds.

Gastrointestinal Emergencies, 2nd ed. Baltimore: Williams & Wilkins, 1997: 31–35.

52. Reynolds JC, Parkman HP. Achalasia. Gastroenterol Clin North Am 1989; 18:223–255.

53. Kozarek RA. Hydrostatic balloon dilatation of gastrointestinal stenosis: a national survey. Gastrointest Endosc 1986; 23:15–19.

54. Ahmed A, Aggarwal M, Watson E. Esophageal perforation: a complication of nasogastric tube placement. Am J Emerg Med 1998; 16:64–66.

55. Lee J, Lieberman D. Complications related to endoscopic hemostasis techniques. Gastrointest Endosc Clin North Am 1996; 6:305–322.

56. Dinning JP, Jaffe PE. Delayed presentation of esophageal perforation as a result of overtube placement. J Clin Gastroenterol 1997; 24:250–252.

57. Ku PKM, Tong MCF, Ho KM, Kwan A, van Hasselt CA. Traumatic esophageal perforation resulting from endotracheal intubation. Anesth Analg 1998; 87:730–731.

58. Foster ED, Munro DD, Dobell AR. Mediastinoscopy. A review of anatomical relationships and complications. Ann Thorac Surg 1972; 13: 273–286.

59. Kelly MF, Rizzo KA, Spiegel J, Zwillenberg D. Delayed pharyngoesophageal perforation: a complication of anterior spine surgery. Ann Otol Rhinol Laryngol 1991; 100: 201–205.

60. Collet D, Cadiere GB. Conversions and complications of laparoscopic treatment of gastroesophageal reflux disease. Formation for the Development of Laparoscopic Surgery for Gastroesophageal Reflux Disease Group. Am J Surg 1995; 169:622–626.

61. Liang SG, Ooka F, Santo A, Kaibara M. Pneumomediastinum following esophageal rupture associated with hyperemesis gravidarum. J Obstet Gynaecol Res 2002; 28:172–175.

62. Muir AD, White J, McGuigan JA, McManus KG, Graham AN. Treatment and outcomes of oesophageal perforation in a tertiary referral centre. Eur J Cardiothorac Surg 2003; 23:799–804.

63. Trulzsch DV, Penmetsa A, Karim A, Evans DA. Gastrografin-induced aspiration pneumonia: a lethal complication of computed tomography. South Med J 1992; 85:1255–1256.

64. Tanomkiat W, Galassi W. Barium sulfate as contrast medium for evaluation of postoperative anastomotic leaks. Acta Radiol 2000; 41:482–485.

65. Cameron JL, Keffer RF, Hendrix TR, Mehigan DG, Baker RR. Selective non-operative management of contained intra-thoracic esophageal perforations. Ann Thorac Surg 1979; 27:404–408.

66. Bell RC. Laparoscopic closure of esophageal perforation following pneumatic dilatation for achalasia. Report of two cases. Surg Endosc 1997; 11:476–478.

67. Barkley C, Orringer MB, Iannettoni MD, Yee J. Challenges in reversing esophageal discontinuity operations. Ann Thorac Surg 2003; 76:989–994.

68. Gupta NM. Emergency transhiatal oesophagectomy for instrumental perforation of an obstructed thoracic oesophagus. Br J Surg 1996; 83:1007–1009.

69. Bautista Casasnovas A, Estevez Martinez E, Varela Cives R, Villanueva Jeremias A, Tojo Sierra R, Cadranel S. A retrospective analysis of ingestion of caustic substances by children. Ten-year statistics in Galicia. Eur J Pediatr 1997; 156:410–414.

70. Forsen JW, Muntz HR. Hair relaxer ingestion: a new trend. Ann Otol Rhinol Laryngol 1993; 102:781–784.

71. Cattan P, Munoz-Bongrand N, Berney T, Halimi B, Sarfati E, Celerier M. Extensive abdominal surgery after caustic ingestion. Ann Surg 2000; 231:519–523.

72. Lamireau T, Rebouissoux L, Denis D, Lancelin F, Vergnes P, Fayon M. Accidental caustic ingestion in children: is endoscopy always mandatory? J Pediatr Gastroenterol Nutr 2001; 33:81–84.

73. Anderson KD, Rouse TM, Randolph JG. A controlled trial of corticosteroids in children with corrosive injury of the esophagus. N Eng J Med 1990; 323:637–640.

74. Howell JM, Dalsey WC, Hartsell FW, Butzin CA. Steroids for the treatment of corrosive esophageal injury: a statistical analysis of past studies. Am J Emerg Med 1992; 10:421–425.

75. de Jong AL, Macdonald R, Ein S, Forte V, Turner A. Corrosive esophagitis in children: a 30-year review. Int J Pediatr Otorhinolaryngol 2001; 57:203–211.

76. Broto J, Asensio M, Jorro CS, et al. Conservative treatment of caustic esophageal injuries in children: 20 years of experience. Pediatr Surg Int 1999; 15:323–325.

77. Estera A, Taylor W, Mills LJ, Platt MR. Corrosive burns of the esophagus and stomach: a recommendation for an aggressive surgical approach. Ann Thorac Surg 1986; 41: 276–283.

78. Tran BA, Huy P, Celerier M. Management of severe caustic stenosis of the hypopharynx and esophagus by ileocolic transposition via suprahyoid or transepiglottic approach. Analysis of 18 cases. Ann Surg 1988; 207:439–445.

79. Trenkner SW, Maglinte DD, Lehman GA, Chernish SM, Miller RE, Johnson CW. Esophageal food impaction: treatment with glucagon. Radiology 1983; 149:401–403.

80. Tibbling L, Bjorkhoel A, Jansson E, Stenkvist M. Effect of spasmolytic drugs on esophageal foreign bodies. Dysphagia 1995; 10:126–127.

81. Goldner F, Danley D. Enzymatic digestion of esophageal meat impaction. A study of Adolph's Meat Tenderizer. Dig Dis Sci 1985; 30:456–459.

82. Hall ML, Huseby JS. Hemorrhagic pulmonary edema associated with meat tenderizer treatment for esophageal meat impaction. Chest 1988; 94:640–642.

83. Kaszar-Seibert DJ, Korn WT, Bindman DJ, Shortsleeve MJ. Treatment of acute esophageal food impaction with a combination of glucagon, effervescent agent, and water. AJR 1990; 154:533–534.

84. Longstreth GF, Longstreth KJ, Yao JF. Esophageal food impaction: epidemiology and therapy. A retrospective, observational study. Gastrointest Endosc 2001; 53:193–198.

85. Vicari JJ, Johanson JF, Frakes JT. Outcomes of acute esophageal food impaction: success of the push technique. Gastrointest Endosc 2001; 53:178–181.

86. Arana A, Hauser B, Hachimi-Idrissi S, Vandenplas Y. Management of ingested foreign bodies in childhood and review of the literature. Eur J Pediatr 2001; 160:468–472.

87. Kirk AD, Bowers BA, Moylan JA, Meyers WC. Toothbrush swallowing. Arch Surg 1988; 123:382–384.

88. Vassilev BN, Kazandziev PK, Losanoff JE, Kjossev KT, Yordanov DE. Esophageal "stars": a sinister foreign body ingestion. South Med J 1997; 90:211–214.

89. de Manzoni G, Catalano F, Festini M, et al. Esophageal non-variceal hemorrhage: a clinical and epidemiological study. G Chir 2002; 23:199–204.

90. Hashino S, Chiba K, Toyoshima N, et al. Exfoliative esophagitis early after autologous peripheral blood stem cell transplantation. Int J Hematol 2001; 74:461–463.

91. Ecker GA, Karsh J. Naproxen induced ulcerative esophagitis. J Rheumatol 1992; 19:646–647.

92. Mayeux GP, Smith JW. Massive esophageal bleeding from cytomegalovirus esophagitis. Am J Gastroenterol 1990; 85:626.

93. Yang WG, Hou MC, Lin HC, et al. Effect of sucralfate granules in suspension on endoscopic variceal sclerotherapy induced ulcer: analysis of the factors determining ulcer healing. J Gastroenterol Hepatol 1998; 13:225–231.

94. Snyder DM, Crawford ES. Successful treatment of primary aorta-esophageal fistula resulting from aortic aneurysm. J Thorac Cardiovasc Surg 1983; 85:457–463.

95. da Silva ES, Tozzi FL, Otochi JP, de Tolosa EM, Neves CR, Fortes F. Aortoesophageal fistula caused by aneurysm of the thoracic aorta: successful surgical treatment, case report, and literature review. J Vasc Surg 1999; 30:1150–1157.

22
Central Nervous System

Peter B. Letarte

Case Scenario

A construction worker falls from a scaffold that was positioned at the second-story level of a building. He has a severe closed heal injury with a Glasgow Coma Scale of 6. Admission computed tomography (CT) scan demonstrates diffuse axonal injury. No other injuries were found on secondary evaluation and CT evaluation of the cervical spine, chest, and abdomen. Which of the following is the preferred management for this patient?

(A) Forced diuresis
(B) Barbiturate administration
(C) Hyperventilation (72 hours)
(D) Craniotomy
(E) Intracranial pressure monitoring

Neurologic emergencies are among the most difficult and disconcerting emergencies facing providers of emergency care. These emergencies can result in high mortality and morbidity. Because neurologic emergencies are caused by a wide variety of pathologies, because the process of determining the pathologic process involved can often be complex or require special experience or expertise, and because, in the case of emergencies, the diagnosis must be arrived at quickly, these emergencies remain a challenge to most providers of emergency care.

The focus of the management of neurologic emergencies is the rapid determination of the nature of the pathology, its location, and the speed at which it is progressing. A decision must then be made as to whether surgical or nonsurgical intervention is the best option for the patient. Finally, the rapid planning and organization of the procedure must progress. In the chaos of the emergency department, the approach to neurologic emergencies can be focused by approaching each emergency seeking the answers to four questions: Where is it? What is it? How fast is it moving? What am I going to do about it?[1]

An Approach to Neurologic Emergencies

The Nature of the Pathology: What Is It?

To answer the question "what is it?" requires a general sense of the spectrum of neuropathology and of which conditions can lead to acute care presentations.

In the broadest terms, neurologic disease can be caused by congenital abnormalities, trauma, tumor, toxins, vascular disease, degenerative disease, infectious etiologies, and demyelinating syndromes. Usually, congenital abnormalities do not have acute presentations, although some sequelae of congenital conditions, such as seizures, can present in an acute care context.

Trauma, of course, is a common source of neurologic emergencies, both cranial and spinal pathology. Tumors often present as headache or progressive motor deficits. In the later case, the presentation can sometimes be similar to that of a stroke. Tumors can also present as new-onset seizures in an adult or as hemorrhage, both sources of acute care presentations. If intracranial tumors bleed, this more precipitous mass effect can lead to more acute and emergent intracranial pathology. Pituitary adenomas can create a unique emergency, pituitary apoplexy.

"Toxins" is a shorthand term for the wide variety of metabolic derangements that can disrupt the brain's delicate milieu and lead to neurologic dysfunction. A long list of conditions make up this list. Hypoxia, hypertension, alcohol and other drugs, endocrine disturbance, hypoglycemia, ketosis, sodium disturbance, hepatic failure, renal failure, hyperthermia, hypothermia, and sepsis can all lead to neurologic derangement.

Vascular diseases are among the most common neurologic emergencies. Most vascular neurologic emergencies present as cerebrovascular accidents. Strokes can be classified as hemorrhagic or ischemic. Hemorrhagic strokes involve some bleeding into the brain. The other form of stroke is ischemic or infarction from decreased blood flow to the brain. The most common cause of these strokes is emboli originating from the carotid arteries or heart.

"Degenerative diseases" refers to degenerative spine disease as well as certain brain conditions such as Alzheimer's disease. The intracranial degenerative processes rarely present as the direct cause of an acute care presentation, but, again, at times the sequelae of these diseases can result in acute care presentation.

Degenerative spine disease is also usually a chronic presentation. These conditions come to emergency attention usually when the condition progresses to a point where it becomes apparent that the condition is serious and the patient presents for emergent care. An example of this presentation is the patient with myelopathy from cervical stenosis whose myelopathy progresses to the point where the patient falls or cannot get out of bed and calls for help.

Degenerative disease combined with trauma can lead to an acute care presentation. Severe cervical stenosis combined with a relatively minor fall resulting in central cord syndrome can lead to acute care presentation.

Infections can be the cause of acute care presentation. Meningitis is an extreme emergency that requires immediate treatment. Subdural and epidural abscesses, both spinal and cranial, require acute care attention. Any opening of the dura, manifested as a cerebrospinal fluid leak, requires immediate attention. Demyelinating diseases rarely present as emergencies, although, like degenerative diseases, at times a chronic progression of multiple sclerosis will progress to a point where acute care attention is needed.

Identification of Pathology: The History

The best way to start defining what the presenting pathology is, as well as starting to determine how fast it is progressing, is through the presenting history. The standard for neuroscience is an exhaustive history that provides the details and background of the patient's presentation. In an acute care setting, however, the best approach is through a series of cycles of focused examinations and interventions. This approach has been made familiar by the Advanced Trauma Life Support course,[2] which emphasizes an initial examination focused on the identification of respiratory failure and shock. The more complete examination is only possible once these life-threatening conditions are addressed. Neurologic emergencies should be approached in the same fashion, with similar cycles of examinations and treatments, focused on the most immediate life-threatening conditions.

In an emergency the initial history may be limited to the prehospital provider's initial report, and subsequent history may have been obtained by emergency room personnel. Several features of the history can be particularly useful in an acute care setting.

Context of Presentation

The circumstance in which a patient presents may seem obvious but must not be ignored. The likely pathologies in a posttraumatic patient with neurologic decline are different from the pathologies likely to be present in patients found with a depressed mental status in their own bed. Patients who have been involved in high levels of physical exertion can present with hyperthermia or sodium derangement from sweating or excess free water intake. Hunters and others involved in cool or cold weather sports can present with hypothermia. In rural or industrial settings, toxic exposures are possible that can result in neurologic decline, organophosphate poisoning from pesticides being a common rural exposure resulting in altered mental status and other neurologic findings.

Past Illness

Certain past illnesses can be clues to the cause of a neurologic decline. Patients with previous neurologic disease, of course, may have experienced an exacerbation of their illness. If seizures have been a part of past neurologic disease or if there is a past history of seizures, then this may be the cause of the presentation, either as on-going status epilepticus or as a postictal state. Patients with seizures may also have experienced a rise in anticonvulsant levels from overdose, metabolic change, or change in other concurrently administered medications. Many patients with tumors or other conditions are treated with high-dose steroids. Inappropriate weaning or sudden discontinuation of steroids can lead to mental status changes. In a small percentage of cases, high or even normal doses of steroids can cause mania in the form of steroid psychosis. Similarly, patients taking endocrine replacement drugs who stop their medications can experience mental status decline.

Diabetics can present in ketosis or with hypoglycemia, and patients with renal or hepatic failure can present with uremia or elevated ammonia levels, respectively. Poorly controlled hypertension can lead to encephalopathy.

Age of Patient

The age of the patient is also an important contextual clue as to what pathologies may account for the neurologic decline. An adult who presents with focal weakness of the face and arm over hours is likely to be experiencing an intracerebral bleed or an ischemic stroke. A child who presents in this fashion is not likely to be suffering the consequences of advanced vascular disease but rather is likely to be suffering from an expanding hemorrhage from an ateriovenous malformation, aneurysm, tumor, coagulation disorder from leukemia, or thrombocytopenia from various causes.

Pattern of Presentation

The pattern of presentation is useful for determining how fast the pathlogy is moving, but also provides clues as to the nature of the pathology. For example, patients who present with the sudden onset of the worst headache of their lives are reporting the precipitous history characteristic of a subarachnoid hemorrhage from an aneursymal rupture. In contrast, a middle-aged individual who complains of the slower onset of face and arm weakness, over minutes to hours, is reporting the probable onset of a stroke, either hemorrhagic or ischemic. Repeated transient focal deficits such as transient focal weakness are more characteristic of emboli to the brain and trigger a search for the source of emboli in the carotid artery or perhaps the heart. The onset of focal weakness over weeks suggests a tumor or abscess, a slower, more progressive process.

Primary Survey: Immediate Actions

The primary survey is no less important in neurologic emergencies than in other acute care presentations. Limitation of hypoxia and hypotension is the key to limiting injury in most neurologic illnesses. The methods of assessment and early management of airway, breathing, and circulation are well-described elsewhere and are not repeated here.[2] In neurologic emergencies, there are additional considerations for the primary survey of the patient.

In many emergency departments, the approach to the patient has included an initial protocolized response to the treatable causes of metabolic depressed mental status. These protocols has been manifest as the so-called rally pack, a set of medications given on initial presentation. The medications given vary from institution to institution and are determined by local practice environment, custom, and training. One version of the rally pack includes dextrose, flumazenil, naloxone, and thiamine.[3]

Derangement of serum glucose levels is a common, serious, and treatable cause of depressed mental status, and it has been traditional to give 25 cc of D_{50} intravenous push (IVP) to patients presenting in coma. With the routine availability of point of care glucose obtained via a finger stick, immediate care of patients presenting in coma now includes a finger stick assessment of serum glucose before glucose administration. Of particular concern are levels below 70 mg/dL. Patients presenting with low levels should then receive at least 25 cc of D_{50} IVP. Patients who do receive glucose as a bolus or as a drip should also receive 50 to 100 mg of thiamine IVP as prophylaxis against Wernicke's encephalopathy.

Poisoning and overdose are common causes of neurologic emergencies. Over time, antidotes to common sources of overdose have become available and have, in some institutions, been routinely given. The two most common antidotes are naloxone and flumazenil.

Naloxone has also been a traditional part of the initial response to coma, because opioid overdose is a rapidly reversible cause of respiratory depression and depressed mental status. Care must be used when giving naloxone to chronic users of narcotics either as part of an abuse pattern or as part of a chronic pain management plan, and automatic administration before clinical assessment should be discouraged.

Flumazenil is a benzodiazepine antagonist. It is effective in reversing benzodiazepine overdose. Patients who chronically take benozodiazepines for seizure control and those who have taken other seizurgenic medications or alcohol are at high risk for seizures with flumazenil administration. Studies have shown high rates of inappropriate flumazenil use in acute care settings. Consultation with a poison center before administration of flumazinole is recommended.[3]

In certain rural and industrial settings, addressing poisoning as part of the primary survey is important because materials such as organophosphates can impact the ability to ventilate the patient. Successful resuscitation will hinge on management of the poisoning.

In a post 9/11 world, where the threat of chemical attack has unfortunately become a reality, the management of poisoning and other metabolic derangements as part of the primary survey of neurologically compromised patients has moved from the domain of an esoteric to a real consideration for all providers of emergency care.

Patients presenting with neurologic emergencies may have seizures, in particular status epilepticus, as a part of their presentation. Patients in status certainly require immediate attention to airway and breathing; at the same time, management of airway and breathing may be affected by the ongoing status.

Patients presenting in status epilepticus should be protected from self-injury and should have their airways assured. They should receive 4 mg or 0.1 mg/kg of lorazapam slowly over 2 minutes. This dose may be repeated every 5 minutes until the seizure is broken, up to a total dose of 9 mg. Valium 10 mg or 0.2 mg/kg repeated every 10 minutes up to 15 mg may also be used.

Simultaneously, the patient should be loaded with phenytoin or fosphenytoin. If the patient is not already receiving phenytoin, the patient should be loaded with

1,400 mg or 20 mg/kg given at rate of <50 mg/kg for phenytoin or <150 mg/kg for phosphenytoin.

If the patient is already receiving phenytoin and the serum level is known, 0.74 mg/kg may be given for each 1μm/mL increase desired. A serum level of 10 to 20μm/mL is therapeutic. A patient with a serum level of 5μm/mL would therefore receive 7.4 mg/kg to achieve a target level of 15μm/kg. If the patient is receiving phenytoin and the serum level is unknown, then a dose of 500 mg IV should be given. Additional 5-mg/kg IV doses can be given up to a total dose of 30 mg/kg until the seizures are broken.[4]

If phenytoin fails to stop the seizures, a phenobarbital drip at <100 mg/min may be started and continued to a total dose of 20 mg/kg. Care should be taken to monitor blood pressure during administration. Phenobarbital may take 20 minutes to work. Should the phenobarbital fail, the patient should then be placed under general anesthesia.[4]

Secondary Survey

The focus of the primary survey is to ensure that emergent life-threatening issues have been addressed. Once the patient's emergent resuscitation needs are addressed, the next critical goals are to more precisely identify the patient's pathology and then to localize it and finally to develop a plan and timeline for addressing it: Where is it? How fast is it moving? What am I going to do about it?

The computed tomography (CT) scan is a simple way to identify anatomic and therefore potentially surgical lesions. It is easy to understand how some providers may be tempted to progress to the CT scanner before any other evaluation. This should be avoided as much as the patient's condition will allow. The focused neurologic secondary survey, combined with the patient's history, provides an essential data base that allows for more intelligent analysis of the subsequent CT and appropriate monitoring of the patient in the CT scanner. Computed tomography scans interpreted in isolation from a focused, intelligent history and physical examination can lead to errors in management.

The Focused Neurologic Examination

A focused neurologic examination should include a rapid assessment of level of consciousness, cranial nerve function, motor examination and symmetry, and a brief directed sensory examination. The sensory examination should follow the guidelines of the American Spinal Injury Association,[5] which advocate rapid assessment of pinprick and light touch in each of the radiculotomes, an assessment that can be quickly accomplished. Reflexes can be checked, but drugs, alcohol, shock, and many other confounding factors present in the acute care setting make the assessment very difficult.

The key to this examination is to keep it focused on localizing the patient's pathology. The two key localizing determinations are to distinguish if the presentation is due to spinal or intracranial pathology and whether the lesion is focal or nonfocal, that is, localizable or generalized.

Patients with deficits in their extremities should be checked for deficits above the cervical spine, suggesting a possible intracranial pathology. Any cranial nerve deficits suggest supraspinal pathology. Examinations of pupils, extraocular motion, corneal reflex, facial symmetry, tongue deviation, and gag symmetry can be done quickly and establish the presence or absence of intracranial signs. Changes in cognition of course indicate intracranial pathology but are less specific.

A second goal of a focused neurologic examination is to search for asymmetry, such as a unilateral dilated pupil or weakness in one arm but not the other. An asymmetric examination finding is likely to be due to focal pathology, that is, pathology that is present on one side of the brain but not the other. although ischemic stroke can present in this fashion, pathologies such as bleeds, tumors, and impending herniation, that is, lesions that may require emergent surgical intervention, are also likely to present in this way. Identification of focal pathology increases the urgency of the workup and allows more critical evaluation of the CT scan.

Imaging

Once the focused neurologic examination is complete, most patients get a head or spine CT. A noncontrast head CT is the study of choice for identifying intracranial blood, the first priority in neurologic emergencies. Obtaining a contrasted head CT first confuses the search for blood, especially subarachnoid blood, and should be avoided. If contrast is administered as part of a later emergency room workup, it is important to document that fact for subsequent examiners.

The initial CT will identify intracranial bleeds, hemorrhagic stroke, and tumors. It can also identify subarachnoid hemorrhage from trauma or spontaneous aneurysm rupture. The CT will also often demonstrate mass effect from tumor, prompting appropriate follow-up magnetic resonance imaging (MRI) studies. Cerebral contusions and ischemic stroke will not appear for 12 to 24 hours, so patients with contused brains and early infarctions may have a relatively normal head CT initially.

For spinal trauma, CT can identify fractures and displacement of vertebrae. Computed tomography gives the best detail of the anatomy of most spinal fractures once they are identified.

Magnetic resonance imaging has little to no role in the acute management of head injury. In the case of spinal trauma, MRI has a distinct acute role. It is the best way to see the mass effect caused by hematomas, herniated disks, and other soft tissues in the spinal canal. In addition, the saggital images obtained with MRI offer the best overall image of canal compromise, spinal cord contusion, and edema and spinal alignment. Because plain films, CT, and MRI each have unique roles in the imaging of spine injury, all three are often obtained urgently as part of operative decision making and planning.[6] In the case of stroke, a noncontrast CT scan is essential to distinguish hemorrhagic from ischemic strokes.

Operative Decision Making

Once the resuscitation, focused neurologic examination, and imaging are complete, the last question must be answered: What are you going to do about it?

If surgical treatment is considered, the natural history of the pathology must be considered to determine how quickly surgery must occur or if there is time for another cycle of testing and examination. A patient with a ruptured arteriovenous malformation (AVM), for example, would ideally have an angiogram before proceeding to the operating room for evacuation of the clot and resection of the AVM. If the patient is rapidly progressing to herniation, however, the angiogram must be skipped, and the surgeon must proceed to the operating room with less than the desirable data base.

If pathology has been clearly identified, standardized grading scales are available to help with prognosis and decision making. Examples are the Glasgow Coma Scale[7] for grading comas caused by head injury, the Hunt-Hess scale[8] for grading ruptured aneurysms, the National Institutes of Health Scale for grading stroke, or the Karnofsky score[9] for assessing the functionality of patients with brain tumors. All of these scales have associated outcome data that offer information about the likelihood of survival and expected mortality and can be used as guides in deciding if and when to intervene.

Specific Disease Entities

Traumatic Emergencies

Glasgow Coma Score

The Glasgow Coma Score[7] is important in classifying the severity of head injury and determining its subsequent management. It is an important part of the primary survey. Patients with a Glasgow Coma Score of 14 to 5 are classified as having mild head injury; they have a 2% chance of elevated intracranial pressure (ICP), a 2% chance of any lesion on CT and <0.1% chance of that lesion being surgically significant. Moderate head injuries

have a score of 9 to 13, have a 20% chance of elevated ICP, and have an approximately 10% chance of having a lesion on CT scan. Severe head injuries have score of 3 to 8.[7,10,11] Patients with severe head injuries need to be intubated, have an approximately 50% chance of having elevated ICP, and, with the exception of low-risk patients with normal head CTs, need ICP monitoring.

Blunt Head Injuries

In blunt trauma, the rapid deceleration of impact can create rapid shifting of the brain within the intracranial space, causing contusions or vessel disruptions and bleeding, resulting in epidural, subdural, or intracerebral hematomas. In addition, metabolic sequelae of the injury, hypoxia, and hypotension can lead to loss of cell membrane integrity and cellular swelling, resulting in cerebral edema. Disruption of the vascular autoregulatory mechanisms in the brain can lead to vascular engorgement and vasogenic edema. All of these sources of mass effect can lead to herniation and subsequent increased morbidity and mortality.

Identifying and managing mass effect is therefore a primary goal in the management of head injury. Identification is usually via CT scan; management is accomplished by evacuation of hematomas, ventricular drainage, mannitol administration, and hyperventilation.[12]

Epidural Hematoma

Computed tomography will confirm the presence of significant space-occupying bleeds. Epidural hematomas will appear as lens-shaped hyperdensities along the inner table of the skull. They are usually the result of either skull fractures in the temporal bone, resulting in temporal hematomas, or disruptions of the transverse sinus, resulting in occipital hematomas. Epidural hematomas can form as late as 4 hours after an injury and thus early CT scans of the head can be obtained before hematoma formation.

Epidural hematomas exert mass effect on the brain with little associated underlying parenchymal injury. The mass effect will present as effacement of the cisterns and ventricles and midline shift.

Rapid removal of the hematoma and therefore the mass effect can result in excellent outcomes. Failure to remove the hematoma in a timely fashion can result in death or significant disability. The mortality rate of patients with epidural hematomas who are allowed to herniate from mass effect is estimated to jump from 2% to around 20%.[13]

Subdural Hematoma

Unlike epidural hematomas, subdural hematomas are often associated with underlying parenchymal injury and edema. Located under the dura, subdural hematomas present as crescent-shaped collections on the surface of the brain. Like epidural hematomas, subdural hematomas will present with the effacement of cisterns, ventricular effacement, and midline shift typical of mass effect. Unlike epidural hematomas, this mass effect can also be caused by the swelling of the brain beneath the subdural hematoma. This effect can be estimated by measuring the width of the subdural hematoma and the amount of midline shift. Any midline shift in excess of the width of the subdural is caused by cerebral swelling. This observation can often alert the surgeon to the fact that most of the mass effect is caused by cerebral edema and not by the subdural blood. Operative planning might then be changed to include a decompressive craniectomy to accommodate the swollen brain as well as removal of the hematoma.

Contusions

Cerebral contusions can also exert mass effect through cerebral edema and hemorrhage from injured smaller blood vessels. Contusions most commonly occur in the frontal and anterior temporal lobes.

Contusions are usually not apparent on the initial CT scan. Contusions progress for several days after the initial injury and do not start to appear on CT for 12 to 24 hours. Contusions are often hard to distinguish from intracerebral hematomas. Intracerebral hematomas are more likely to be visible on the initial CT.[14]

Because many patients who harbor contusions will initially present with normal or near-normal CT scans, it is easy to miss contusions in the early workup. The principle clue that patients are at increased risk for a contusion will be a Glasgow Coma Score less than 14. Many contusions present in moderately head-injured patients. Such patients should be admitted, observed, and reimaged at 24 hours to allow identification of contusions. Many moderately head-injured patients will require hospitalizations of several days to allow management of cerebral edema and its symptoms.[14]

Cerebral Edema

Cerebral edema, either cellular or vasogenic, can result in mass effect. Clues that edema is causing mass effect are similar to the clues available when hematomas are the cause of the mass effect. Swollen brain will cause effacement of basilar cisterns and ventricles and shift of the midline. Other CT clues will be loss of the distinction between gray and white matter on CT and loss of the normal gyral pattern, "gyral effacement."

Vascular Injury

Carotid Artery Trauma. Vascular injuries occur in less than 1% of all blunt head injuries. The incidence of carotid injury was 0.24% in a recent study.[15] Patients who present with potential arterial hemorrhage from mouth, nose, ears, or wounds, expanding cervical hematomas, cervical bruit in patients less than 50 years of age, or incongruous lateralizing neurologic deficit not explained by CT or other findings should have carotid dissection considered in their diagnosis. In addition, trauma patients who present with evidence of cerebral infarction should also have the diagnosis considered, although, like contusion, infarction does not present on CT scan for 12 to 24 hours after the infarction.

Patients suspected of harboring a carotid injury should undergo angiography on an emergent basis if they are otherwise stable. Recent aggressive protocols advocating angiography for asymptomatic patients have found carotid injuries in 0.86% of blunt trauma patients. The motivations for this more aggressive approach to diagnosis are the high rates of mortality and morbidity for the victims of blunt carotid injury, 23% and 48%, respectively. Criteria for angiography for asymptomatic patients include a history of severe hyperextension of the neck, soft tissue injury to the anterior neck, cervical spine fracture, fractures of face or mandible, and basilar skull fractures.[15]

Patients identified with vascular injury are thought to have a better prognosis with anticoagulation.[15] Repeated angiography at 7 to 10 days after injury and classification of identified injuries guide decision making about therapy.[16,17]

Vascular injuries range from disruption of the integrity of the vessel wall, to partial occlusion of the vessel lumen, to pseudoaneurysm or outpouching of the vessel wall, to complete occlusion, and finally to transection of the vessel.[18]

Vertebral Artery Trauma. Vertebral artery dissection is associated with trauma and cervical fractures. The symptoms used to screen symptomatic, as well as asymptomatic, patients for carotid artery injury also apply to vertebral artery injury. This means that patients suspected of posttraumatic vascular injury should receive a four-vessel angiogram to visualize both the carotid and vertebral arteries.[19]

The incidence of such injuries is relatively low, 0.53% in some series, and, traditionally, in asymptomatic patients, the outcomes were thought to be uniformly good without treatment. Recent literature has questioned this assumption of a benign course for this condition, quoting a 24% posterior circulation stroke rate and an 8% death rate from vertebral artery injuries. It has been suggested that early treatment with anticoagulation affects outcome.[19,20]

Management of Blunt Head Injuries

All victims of trauma require a primary and secondary survey. A CT scan of the head should then be obtained.

After prevention of hypoxia and hypotension, managing mass effect is the main priority. Based on the Glasgow Coma Score and the findings on CT, patients with a score less than 8 and findings on CT should have an ICP monitor placed. Patients with a score less than 8 and a normal head CT require ICP monitoring only if they have two of the following three conditions; age over 40 years, episode of hypoxia or hypotension, and lateralizing signs on examination. The ICP levels and the findings on CT will guide further therapy.[11]

Epidural and subdural hematomas greater than 1 cm in thickness require removal via craniotomy. Midline shift greater than 1 cm with association effacement of the basilar cisterns caused by cerebral edema, with or without associated subdural hematoma, should be considered for decompressive craniectomy. Patients without hematoma but with significant unilateral hemispheric or bifrontal edema may benefit from early decompressive craniectomy as part of their ICP management.[21]

For patients without a surgical lesion, cerebral spinal fluid drainage is the first therapy used to attempt further ICP control. For this reason, a ventriculostomy is the modality of choice for ICP monitoring. Should ICP not be controllable using cerebrospinal fluid drainage, mannitol given as a 1-g/kg bolus followed by 0.25-g/kg boluses is the next modality of choice. This therapy can be continued as long as the serum osmolality stays below 320 mOsm.

Serum pCO_2 should be kept at about 35 mm Hg. Should cerebrospinal fluid drainage and mannitol fail to control ICP, hyperventilation to a PCO_2 of 30 mm Hg can be used to try to reduce the pressure.

In desperate situations when hyperventilation is failing, further hyperventilation to a PCO_2 below 30 mm Hg can be attempted, and consideration can be given to pentobarbital coma. Pentobarbital coma can be induced by giving boluses of pentobarbital until a loading dose of 10 mg/kg over 30 minutes followed by 5-mg/kg boluses every hour ×3 has been given. Once the loading dose has been achieved, a pentobarbital drip can be started at 1 mg/kg/hr.[12,22]

Hypothermia has been used as a protective maneuver in trauma. Its efficacy and safety is the subject of ongoing studies.

Penetrating Head Injuries

Penetrating head injuries can be divided, somewhat artificially, into low-velocity and high-velocity injuries. Low-velocity penetrating injuries occur as a result of skull penetration with devices such as knives and nail guns. In this case the injury to brain tissue is the result of mechanical displacement and crushing by the object itself.

High-velocity injuries are caused by high-velocity projectiles that strike the head with significant energy. These projectiles also destroy tissue by actual displacement and crushing along their paths. These projectiles are preceded into the head by an impact shock wave or sonic wave that produces very little injury. As the projectile displaces tissue, however, it creates a wake whose size depends on the projectile's velocity. This wake displaces tissue away from the path of the projectile, creating a path that can be 10 to 20 times the size of the projectile. This wake then collapses, creating negative pressure behind the projectile, which sucks debris in after it. In a cyclical fashion the cavity then expands again and then contracts, often repeating this cycle several times and creating a sign wave–shaped wake behind the projectile. This enlarged path is not visible on CT but is manifest as a tract of contusion through the brain that is much wider than the projectile. Projectiles of this velocity and energy are almost exclusively bullets. This track width is also enhanced if the bullet tumbles as it passes through the brain.[23]

The energy with which the bullet strikes the brain is a function of the velocity that it leaves the barrel of the gun, the range at which it is shot, the bullet's aerodynamic properties, and the angle at which it strikes its target. Because the energy of impact is multifactorial, not all high-velocity weapons create high-velocity impacts.[23]

Unfortunately, many patients with gunshot wounds to the head present in very critical condition with, a mortality rate of 38% to 79% depending on the population studied.[24] Factors that appear to be correlated with outcome are Glasgow Coma Scale, papillary dilatation, coagulopathy, and bihemispheric penetration. Compilations of several reports on Glasgow Coma Scale and mortality from gunshot wounds to the head found an overall survival of only 8.1% for patients presenting with a Glasgow Coma Scale score of 3 to 5. The survival was 65.2% for a score of 6 to 8 and 93.3% for a score of 9 to 15.[25] Single, more-controlled sets of data show even grimmer odds of survival for patients with a score of 3 to 5.[25]

Bilaterally fixed and dilated pupils are also a grave prognostic sign, with a 79% mortality rate. Patients with unilaterally fixed and dilated pupils a 50% mortality rate, and those with bilaterally reactive pupils have a 5% mortality rate.[26] Bilaterally fixed and dilated pupils in patients with a Glasgow Coma Scale score of 3 to 5 are viewed by many as a marker of a very grave prognosis. Coagulopathy manifest as a single abnormal prothrombin time or partial thromboplastin time is also a poor prognostic marker, with patients with a coagulopathy having an 80% mortality rate versus a 7.4% mortality rate for those without coagulopathy.[27] Patients with disseminated intravascular coagulopathy have an 85% mortality rate.[25] Patients with bihemispheric involvement, ventricular involvement in the bullet path, and subarachnoid blood on CT have a worse prognosis.[26–28]

Each patient presenting with penetrating injuries to the head should be individually evaluated, and a thoughtful search for reversible factors such as space-occupying intracranial lesion or hypotension should be undertaken before accepting the verdict of poor prognostic indicators.[29] In most mortalities from penetrating injuries, death comes in the first 24 hours if multiple poor indicators are present.[24]

The principles of surgical management of gunshot wounds to the head for those who can benefit from treatment are debridement of the wound, removal of hematomas, control of vascular injury, and water-tight dural closure. Extensive exploration of the wound for removal of debris does not appear to reduce the risk of infection, and simple irrigation of the tract usually is sufficient. Any continuity with exposed sinus should be repaired.[30] Other management techniques for penetrating injury parallel those for blunt injury.[29]

Traumatic Spine Injury

Patients at risk for cervical spine injury should be immobilized in the field. Because excluding cervical spine injury in the field is a difficult task, the vast majority of trauma victims will have their cervical spines immobilized in the field. Immobilization should be accomplished with a combination of a rigid cervical collar and backboard immobilization, with the head secured to the backboard with head blocks and straps. The practice of immobilization with only sandbags and tape is not recommended.[2,31]

Spinal cord injuries should be defined in terms of neurologic deficit and not solely by radiographic criteria if possible. An excellent tool for performing a focused and efficient but thorough spinal cord injury evaluation is to use the American Spinal Injury Association (ASIA) international standards for neurologic and functional classification of spinal cord injury. This convenient examination is focused and grades injuries in ways that are very useful for further management decisions and for prognosis.[5]

After completion of the examination, patients who are awake, alert, not intoxicated, without neck pain or tenderness, able to focus, and have a high degree of reliability to cooperate with their examiner during examination of their spine may be clinically cleared and do no need radiographic examination.[2,32–34]

Distracting injuries, which often preclude clinical clearance of the spinal cord, can be thought of as any injury that prevents patients from giving their total attention to the examiner and to the process of clearing their spinal column. In addition to physical injuries, psychological and social circumstances may also distract trauma victims and prevent them from being able to adequately participate in the examination of their spine. Such patients should not be clinically cleared.[2,32,33–36]

Class I data have demonstrated that the vast majority of patients will require radiographic clearance of their cervical spine.[32] All major guidelines still recommend three-view cervical spine plain x-rays (anteroposterior, lateral, and odontoid views) for initial radiographic evaluation. For children younger than 9 years, anteroposterior and lateral views are sufficient. These x-rays are then supplemented by CT scans to better define suspicious areas or areas that are poorly visualized on plain films.[2,33,37,38]

The practice of using only CT to image the spine, without the use of plain films, is backed only by class II and III data. To date, this practice has not been condoned by any cervical spine clearance guideline.[33,37,38]

Patients who are awake and alert but have neck pain or tenderness and normal radiographic workup as described above can have their immobilization removed if normal dynamic flexion/extension radiographs can be obtained. These films should be obtained with the patient actively performing the flexion/extension. Passive flexion/extension of patients who cannot cooperate with the examination is to be absolutely avoided.[33,37] Immobilization can also be removed when a normal cervical MRI is obtained within 48 hours of the injury, although there is some disagreement among various guidelines on the efficacy of this approach.[33,37]

Patients who are obtunded and cannot cooperate with dynamic imaging may have immobilization removed after passive flexion/extension films are obtained under real-time fluoroscopic imaging by experienced and adequately trained personnel. Alternatively, the cervical collar can be removed if a normal MRI can be obtained within 48 hours of injury, although the qualifications on MRI mentioned above also apply here.[33,37]

Treatment of patients with neurologic deficits with intravenous methylprednisolone has become a standard of care. Patients are given a 30-mg/kg bolus in the first hour, followed by a 5.4-mg/kg/hr drip for the next 24 to 48 hours.[39] The data supporting this practice have been controversial, and recent neurologic surgery evidence-based guidelines have listed this treatment as an option with the statement that treatment of patients with acute spinal cord injuries "should be undertaken only with the knowledge that the evidence suggesting harmful side effects is more consistent than any suggestion of clinical benefit."[39]

Just as hypotension has been shown to be deleterious to the injured brain, it is also suspected of being harmful to the injured spinal cord. Maintaining victim's systolic blood pressure above 90 mm Hg as quickly as possible after injury and for the first 7 days after injury is thought to be beneficial to the injured patient.[34]

Management of Spinal Fractures

Patients with neurologic deficits but no radiographic abnormalities on screening x-rays should have CT scans of the suspected level obtained to look for occult injury. Magnetic resonance images should also be obtained. Imaging of the entire spinal column will at times reveal a deficit in another segment of the spine.[2]

Multiple fracture types are possible at the craniocervical junction. Some may be obvious on plain x-rays, such as a hangman's fracture with visible spondylolisthesis, odontoid fracture with significant displacement, or Jefferson fracture of C1. Others may be more subtle or not visible at all on plain x-rays, such as occipital condyle fractures, atlanto-occipital dislocation injuries, nondisplaced odontoid or hangman's fractures, or nondisplaced C2 body fractures.[33]

Patients with occipital tenderness, impaired range of motion in the neck, soft tissue swelling, or lower cranial nerve deficits as well as patients with soft tissue swelling in the upper cervical prevertebral area of a plain cervical spine x-ray should be suspected of upper cervical spine injury, should remain immobilized, and should receive a thin-cut CT through the occipital cervical junction and an MRI.[33] In addition, familiarity with specialized methods of plain film analysis to assess the relationship of the occiput to the cervical spine, such as the basion-axial internal-basion-dental interval method, can be useful in reviewing plain films of the cervical spine. Once upper cervical spine injury is identified or suspected, spine consultation for treatment is recommended.

Patients with identified fractures or dislocations of the subaxial spine should remain immobilized, with continuing cervical spine protection, and spine specialist consultation should be obtained.[2,33,41] Patients with subluxations or displaced subaxial cervical spinal fractures and patients with subaxial cervical facet dislocation injuries will require reduction and stabilization of their injuries. Although definitive realignment and stabilization will occur in the operating room, best evidence indicates that patients with fracture dislocation injuries should be urgently reduced using craniocervical traction. Early realignment is thought to offer the best possibility of recovery for these patients. There are reported cases of exacerbation of neurologic deficit by early reduction.[42] In order to prevent this complication, patients should be examined carefully before the placement of traction and monitored carefully during traction and realignment for signs of neurologic decline; if the examination declines, the traction should be discontinued. For obtunded patients who cannot cooperate with a neurologic examination, an MRI should be obtained to rule out an anterior disk herniation, the principle etiology of such neurologic injury from traction. The delay in reduction precipitated by MRI is controversial, and, although not warranted for awake patients, is thought by some to be appropriate for obtunded patients. For awake patients, MRI will usually be obtained subsequent to reduction, but is particularly indicated for patients who fail to reduce.[42] Patients with a second injury rostral to the fracture dislocation should not have closed reduction with craniocervical traction attempted.[42]

Patients with spinal cord injury without radiographic abnormality should remain in neck immobilization until the etiology of the deficit and/or spinal stability can be determined.[43]

Penetrating Spine Trauma

Penetrating spine trauma is managed similar to nonpenetrating trauma. In penetrating spine trauma, however, the efficacy of intravenous methylprednisolone has not been established, and its use is not recommended.[43–46]

Peripheral Nerve Injury

Peripheral nerve injuries can be difficult to diagnose early in the trauma resuscitation because of the need for a detailed neurologic examination in a cooperative patient. Initially, deficits may be attributed to cranial or spinal pathology, and only as the evaluation progresses does it become apparent that the pattern of deficit is consistent with peripheral nerve injury. At this point, or as soon as the patient is able to cooperate, repeated detailed examinations can better define the site of the injury, and a plan for managing the injury can be formulated.

Electromyography and nerve conduction velocity testing will ultimately be useful to further define peripheral nerve injuries. Because of the physiology of Wallerian degeneration and the tissue edema surrounding most peripheral nerve injuries, these studies are not useful for the first 14 to 21 days after the injury and should not be obtained.[47]

Most peripheral nerve injuries presenting in the context of trauma should be repaired in a delayed fashion. Only clean nerve lacerations that create a well-defined transection of the nerve, creating two nerve endings that can be easily reopposed, should be emergently repaired. Knife wounds or nerve lacerations from penetrating injuries with glass or other sharp objects are examples of such injuries. Bullet wounds do not require emergent repair because most peripheral nerve injuries from bullet wounds are concussive injuries from the shock wave and cavitation of the bullet and are not caused by direct transection of the nerve. When the nerve is transected by the bullet, the resulting nerve endings are badly macerated, disrupted, and inappropriate for early repair.[48,49]

Peripheral nerve injuries may be explored acutely in conjunction with the management of vascular or orthopedic injuries. Although early repair of the injury may not be indicated, early exploration in these settings allows exploration of the nature of the nerve injury and tagging of the damaged nerve endings, making subsequent repair easier.

Nontraumatic Emergencies

Outside of the context of trauma, neurologic emergencies present in a wide and often confusing array of presentations. Many neurologic emergencies have nonsurgical treatments, but surgeons will often become involved in the management of many of them.

Cerebrovascular Accidents

Patients with cerebral vascular accidents often present with the sudden onset of focal, usually unilateral, weakness, vision disturbance, or speech disturbance. Workup consists of a neurologic examination followed by a CT of the head. The initial goals of the workup are to define the location of the deficit and then to classify it as hemorrhagic or nonhemorrhagic. The later differentiation is accomplished with a noncontrasted CT scan of the head. Obtaining a contrasted CT scan of the head should be avoided because contrast will create a confusing picture where it is impossible to distinguish contrast from blood. The CT scan will distinguish between two patterns of bleeding, intraparenchymal and subarachnoid.

Hemorrhagic Cerebrovascular Accidents

Subarachnoid Hemorrhage. Blood only in the subarachnoid space, outside of the context of trauma, is usually caused by a ruptured cerebral aneurysm. This type of bleed will usually have been suspected from the history if the patient complained of the "sudden onset of the worst headache of my life." The apoplectic nature of this bleed is so severe that patients often think that they have been struck in the head as it occurs. No other stroke presents with this severity and rapidity of onset.

Once aneurysm is suspected, further management is dictated by the severity of the bleed and the patient's subsequent condition. Patients are classified using the Hunt-Hess scale. Patients who present asymptomatic or with only mild headache are classified Hunt-Hess I. Patients with significant headache and perhaps a cranial nerve deficit are classified Hunt-Hess II. Patients with mild deficits and lethargy or confusion are Hunt-Hess III, and patients with stupor and moderate to severe hemiparesis or decerebrate posturing are Hunt-Hess IV. Hunt-Hess V patients are in deep coma and have decerebrate posturing. Nuchal rigidity can be a common feature in all of these presentations.[8]

Patients who present with a Hunt-Hess score of V are considered to have little chance of good outcome and are often not treated, although some physicians have advocated surgery for this group. Grade IV patients are also very sick, and elderly grade IV patients or patients with preexisting conditions also might be patients for whom treatment might not be offered. Grades I to III patients are considered the best candidates for treatment and are those who often receive the most aggressive workup.

The immediate threats to the victim of subarachnoid hemorrhage are a rebleed of the aneurysm and hydrocephalus. A delayed complication is vasospasm.

Preventing rebleed is the first priority for the victims of a ruptured aneurysm. Patients who do rebleed have a dramatic jump in their mortality rate. To prevent rebleed, the aneurysm must be visualized and secured. Although many aneurysms can be seen on magnetic resonance angiography (MRA), the smallest, those <1 cm in diameter, cannot. For this reason, a cerebral angiogram is done as soon as possible. In institutions with interventional neuroradiology capability, coiling of the aneurysm is sometimes possible at the same time that the angiogram is obtained, thereby providing immediate protection from rebleed. Not all aneurysms are coilable, and sophisticated decision making and discussion are needed on the part of the neurosurgeon and the interventional neuroradiologist in these cases. If clipping is the best option for the patient, it is usually done within 72 hours of bleed.

Management of hydrocephalus is a concern in the early hours of a subarachnoid bleed. Subarachnoid blood is in the cerebrospinal fluid and can be transported to, among other places, the cerebral aqueduct, where it can interrupt cerebrospinal fluid flow. This interruption can lead to hydrocephalus, which can be a threat to the patient during the first hours after the bleed. Patients are carefully monitored for increasing lethargy, and CT scans are scrutinized for evidence of hydrocephalus and are repeated to monitor for expansion of the ventricles. The timing of placing an external ventricular drain to treat the hydrocephalus is problematic. Although the patient cannot be allowed to herniate from hydrocephalus, there is some concern on the part of neurosurgeons that drainage of cerebrospinal fluid may precipitate rebleed. An effort is made to place the external ventricular drain only if the patient has signs of hydrocephalus, ideally after the aneurysm is secured, although this is often not possible. It is often necessary to place the external ventricular drain before angiography to allow monitoring and treatment of ICP during angiography, a time when a neurologic examination is usually not available.

When patients develop hydrocephalus, their depressed mental status can be caused by this and not by the bleed. Some patients, after placement of a ventriculostomy, will have their Hunt-Hess grade improve with a resulting change in their management strategy. Similarly, large clots may exert mass effect that, if relieved, will improve the patient's mental status. In this way decisions about salvageability become intertwined with decisions about the timing of ventriculostomy placement and evacuation of large hematomas.

Vasospasm is the third complication of subarachnoid hemorrhage but occurs at 7 to 10 days after the bleed. It is not managed initially as part of the acute care. The risk of vasospasm can be estimated from the initial CT using the Fisher grading system[50]

Intraparenchymal Hematoma. Sometimes the bleeding pattern on CT scan reveals an intraparenchymal hematoma. These hematomas can be in a variety of locations, but many are located centrally, near the ventricles, or in the thalamus or basal ganglia.

Spontaneous intracerebral hematoma, also referred to as "hypertensive hemorrhage," present in this way. Such bleeds have an onset of focal symptoms over minutes to hours, with an intraparenchymal hematoma subsequently visualized on CT. "Hypertensive hemorrhage" can be a misnomer for this condition because 20% of patients have no history of hypertension. A process called "cerebral arteriosclerosis" is thought be responsible for these bleeds, causing the small branching vessels of the cerebral vasculature to become brittle and ultimately fracture and bleed, leading to dissection of other fragile vessels, vessel rupture, and further bleeding.[51]

There are multiple other causes of spontaneous intracerebral hematoma. Amyloid angiopathy is the result of amyloid deposits on the cortical vessel walls, making them brittle and more susceptible to fracture. These patients present with repeated subcortical bleeds often in the parietal and occipital lobes.[52]

Arteriovenous Malformations. Arteriovenous malformations are another source of intraparenchymal bleeds. These malformations result from aberrant vessels that shunt blood between the arteries and veins of the brain. These shunts create mass effect and at times bleed. Arteriovenous malformations can present as headache, seizures, or progressive neurologic deficit from mass effect or from a bleed. For the acute care surgeon, the bleed is the concerning scenario because in this case the onset of symptoms will be rapid, progressing over minutes to hours.

Management of Intraparenchymal Bleeds. No matter what the cause of the bleed, the approach to intraparenchymal clots is the same. Once the CT scan has identified an intraparenchymal clot, the next priority is to determine if surgery is required in its management. Many hypertensive hemorrhages have stopped expanding by the time of workup. For stable patients with both a clot and a deficit that are not progressing, it is not clear from the literature that surgery to remove the clot improves their outcome, and the role of surgery is still debated for these patients.[51] For patients who are herniating or who continue to progress as evidenced by expansion of the clot on repeated CT or declining neurologic examination, control of mass effect through removal of the clot is a lifesaving maneuver and should be undertaken if the clot can be removed without undue subsequent morbidity.

Removal of most intraparenchymal bleeds is a straightforward operation, but AVM surgery is complex and requires careful detailed planning to minimize the bleeding risk to the patient. The surgeon who operates on AVMs needs to know that they are present to properly prepare for the surgery. Because in many cases an AVM cannot be discerned from a hypertensive hemorrhage on routine CT or even MRI examination, many intraparenchymal bleeds require an angiogram for workup before surgery.[52]

If the patient is stable, that is, the bleed is not expanding, the patient's deficit is not progressing, and the patient is not herniating or is not in danger of herniation, then an angiogram can be obtained on an urgent basis. If, however, the patient has a progressing deficit or is herniating, there may not be time to obtain an angiogram. One of the important decisions in the management of these lesions is whether the patient is stable enough for an angiogram. Often, the patient must be taken to the operating room with less than ideal information available.

Ischemic Cerebrovascular Accidents

The management of ischemic stroke is largely nonsurgical. Once a CT scan has shown the absence of an intraparenchymal hematoma, various imaging modalities are used to attempt to identify the size of the infarction and to start decision making on treatments such as thrombolytic therapy.

Determining the etiology of the ischemic stroke is important. The majority of such strokes are caused by emboli usually from atherosclerotic plaque in the carotid artery, causing occlusion of midsized to large vessels in the brain. Thromblytic therapy works well for these patients if the infarction size is not large and the therapy can be started quickly, usually within 3 hours. Another cause of ischemic stroke is reduced cerebral blood flow from either carotid stenosis or reduced cardiac output.

Patients presenting with signs of stroke should receive a CT scan to differentiate hemorrhagic from ischemic stroke. Those with hemorrhage ruled out may have the size of their infarction assessed by CT, MRI, perfusion MRI, and/or diffusion MRI or by the presence of emboli confirmed by angiography, or they may undergo no further imaging, depending on local capabilities and protocols. Such protocols may also include the early administration of thrombolytics either intraarterial or catheter directed.[53,54] Further workup will include assessment of the carotid artery by carotid Doppler ultrasound, MRI/MRA or angiography, cardiac workup via electrocardiogram and echocardiography, and workup for hypercoagulable states.

Patients with progressing neurologic deficits or "stroke in progress" may require emergent carotid endarterectomy or carotid stenting, depending on institutional capabilities. Patients with complete occlusion of the involved carotid are often not candidates for emergent intervention. Angiography is often required to confirm complete occlusion because very low flow through the carotid ("string sign") is often not detectable by MRA. Patients with stable deficits will have such surgery delayed to allow the patient to be stabilized and to reduce the risk of reperfusion hemorrhage.

Surgeons can also become involved in the management of ischemic stroke if the patient experiences significant swelling and mass effect from the ischemia. For these patients, if the mass effect becomes life threatening, depending on the location of the edema, decompressive craniectomy or in some cases lobectomy can be considered as life-saving maneuvers. These issues, however, are usually addressed at the time of maximum swelling from the infarction, which is usually 3 to 5 days after to stroke when ICP management is becoming difficult.[55,56]

Brain Tumors

Brain tumors, either primary of metastatic, usually present with headache, seizure, or slow-onset neurologic deficit. These presentations are not emergent. At times, however, tumors that for various reasons have progressed undetected will present with patients on the edge of herniation. Decision making in this case involves deciding if medical management such as steroids or ICP control with ventricular drains or hyperventilation can stabilize the patient while the workup is completed or whether emergent debulking of the tumor is needed. Such decisions are particularly important with cerebellar tumors because compression of the posterior fossa contents can be rapidly lethal.

Many metastatic tumors and sometimes primary tumors will bleed and present similar to the spontaneous hemorrhages described above. The tumor will sometimes not be readily apparent on imaging, being masked by the bleed. Decision making for this presentation is similar to that for a spontaneous bleed, with life-threatening mass effect being treated by immediate evacuation and stable bleeds being temporized while further investigations to search for a primary tumor site are undertaken to determine if the tumor is metastatic or primary. Many tumors will require biopsy, either excisional or stereotactic.[57]

Pituitary Apoplexy

A rare but important neurologic emergency that will involve the surgeon is pituitary apoplexy. Pituitary apoplexy does not occur often and presents with a confusing array of symptoms that can cause it to be missed. These symptoms include headache, mental status changes, cranial nerve changes, vision changes, and systemic changes that are the result of endocrine derangements. Because much of the presentation involves

systemic illness, its intracranial source might not be considered, and a head CT might not be considered as part of initial workup. Recognizing this presentation is important in order to prevent unnecessary loss of vision or life.

The underlying pathology in pituitary apoplexy is hemorrhage in the pituitary fossa. This hemorrhage is usually caused by breakthrough bleeding from necrosis of an often large pituitary adenoma. This bleeding can cause compression of the optic nerves, leading to rapid visual loss, compression of the oculomotor nerve, leading to ophthalmoplegia, and sometimes cavernous sinus pressure leading to trigeminal nerve compression and dysfunction. Pressure on the hypothalamus can cause endocrine dysfunction, which can manifest as an addisonian crisis. In addition, compression on the hypothalamus and third ventricle can provoke coma via both hypothalamic dysfunction and hydrocephalous. Severe headache is an almost constant feature of the presentation and is often the first symptom. Computed tomography scanning will often show hemorrhage in the pituitary fossa. Occasionally, subarachnoid hemorrhage will also be present.

Immediate treatment should include stress dose steroids and external ventricular drainage if hydrocephalus is suspected from clinical presentation or CT. The differential diagnosis includes an anterior circulation ruptured aneurysm, migraine headaches, intracerebral hematoma, and brain stem infarction.

The operative treatment of choice is transsphenoidal removal of the clot; complete tumor removal is not mandatory. The goal of surgery is emergent decompression of the visual apparatus. Emergent decompression may also offer a better chance for endocrine function recovery. In the absence of acute visual loss, patients can have their clot removed on an urgent basis.[58]

Infection

Infection can establish itself in several ways in the intracranial space. Infection in the substance of the brain starts as a cerebritis that, as the brain becomes necrotic, progresses to an abscess. Infection in the ventricles and in their lining, or ependyma, is known as "ventriculitis." Infection on the surface of the brain, in the subarachnoid space, and involving the meninges is known as "meningitis." Infections in the subdural or epidural space form subdural or epidural abscesses.

Patients presenting with mental status change, nuchal rigidity, hemiparesis or hemiplegia, or seizures and fever should always have intracranial infection considered. The examination should always assess for nuchal rigidity.

The victims of trauma, especially open trauma, patients who have recently undergone an intracranial procedure, and patients with a foreign body in their head are all at high risk for cerebral infection. Intracerebral abscess occurs most frequently as spread from the paranasal sinuses. Patients commonly have a history of some form of trauma to the face or sinuses, recent otolaryngology procedure, or recent dental work. In addition, debilitated or immunocompromised patients have an increased propensity to intracerebral abscess. Debilitated patients with infections elsewhere in their bodies can develop abscesses. Interestingly, the organism grown from the abscess is often not the organism in the original infection.

Computed tomography scan in early cerebritis may show only mild hypodensity at the site of infection. At 2 to 4 weeks, abscess formation occurs as the cerebritis is walled off by a fibrotic rind. This fibrotic wall shows as an enhancing ring or "ring-enhancing lesion" on CT when contrast is given. The ring-enhancing lesion found with CT and MRI has a distinct differential diagnosis. Ring enhancement can occur in metastatic neoplasms of the brain, abscesses, gliomas, resolving cerebral infarctions, resolving contusions, rarely in demyelinating diseases, resolving hematomas, and lymphomas. The fact that resolving infarctions, contusions, and hematomas can, after a period of time, also appear as ring-enhancing lesions is important to remember. One high-risk group for cerebral infection is posttraumatic patients. When the victims of head injury who have sustained cerebral infarction, hematomas, or contusions develop fever several weeks into their recovery, these lesions will appear as ring enhancing lesions on CT and will be difficult to distinguish from an abscess. The surgeon will need to use clinical judgment to decide if the lesions represent abscess and whether surgery has a role in their management.

Subdural and epidural abscesses may be difficult to diagnose on CT because they may not be hyperdense but may appear as dark thickening of the epidural or subdural spaces on CT. The clinical examination will suggest the diagnosis.

Images of patients with meningitis will be normal in most cases. In more chronic meningitis, meningeal enhancement can sometimes be seen on MRI with contrast.

Patients suspected of meningitis should have an emergent lumbar puncture to confirm the diagnosis followed by initiation of antibiotics. For patients with space-occupying infections, such as abscess or epidural or subdural hematoma, the sensitivity of the lumbar puncture is low and there is some risk to lumbar puncture in the presence of a space-occupying lesion. Clinical judgment is needed to decide if the lumbar puncture is needed for clinical decision making.

Epidural and subdural abscesses should be emergently drained. Many epidural and subdural abscesses have an extensive fibrotic component. At surgery, instead of an easily drained pocket of liquid, a fibrotic mass is often encountered. This mass is often adherent to underlying dura or arachnoid. Although removal of the fibrosis from the dura poses no threat to the patient, extensive dissection of fibrosis from the arachnoid can lead to significant cortical injury. Surgical judgment is required in determining how much debridement is optimum.

For intraparenchymal abscesses less than 2 to 3 cm in diameter, antibiotic therapy alone has results comparable with surgical drainage. There is debate about the exact critical diameter that will respond to only antibiotics, but there is good agreement that smaller abscesses will respond without drainage. The operative goal for intraparenchymal abscess is to obtain material for organism identification and to reduce the size of the abscess to below 2 cm. Complete resection of the abscess and the capsule is not necessary. Often, these two operative goals can be achieved by simple aspiration of the abscess through a catheter or ventricular needle. Once the abscess is drained, further therapy for the cerebritis can be achieved with appropriate antibiotics and ICP control.[59,60]

Hydrocephalus

Patients with hydrocephalus can present with variety of signs and symptoms. The traditional presentation is headache, lethargy or somulence, nausea, vomiting, gait changes, and, occasionally, the traditional "sunset sign" or failure of upward gaze.

New-onset hydrocephalus can be caused by derangements of cerebrospinal fluid flow from tumors, hemorrhage, or infections. The diagnosis is confirmed by visualizing the enlarged ventricles on CT.

Shunt Malfunction

Patients with ventriculoperitoneal shunts in place may present with failure of the shunt. Shunt failure has the same pattern of presentation as hydrocephalus. Many patients in early failure have very mild symptoms and appear to have no more than an acute viral syndrome. Most importantly, most patients who have experienced hydrocephalus and shunt failure in the past can describe their unique pattern of presentation and can tell the practitioner if they suspect their shunt is failing. Careful attention to such history from parents or patients is critical to diagnosing shunt malfunction.

Workup includes a CT scan to assess ventricular size. This assessment is easier if a scan is available from when the patient was asymptomatic. In addition to a shunt series, plain x-rays of the head, chest, abdomen, and pelvis are obtained. This series is used to look for obvious disconnections in the shunt, which could account for the failure.

Subtle symptoms and small changes in ventricular size can make diagnosing shunt malfunction difficult. Ancillary testing such as a radionucleotide shunt series can sometimes be of use. Often open exploration of the shunt is required. Herniation from hydrocephalus is a real threat in these failures, and erring on the side of exploration is always prudent.[61,62]

Nontraumatic Spinal Emergencies

Patients with pathology of the spinal cord will present with deficits of the extremities and loss of bowel or bladder control but without deficits of cognition or of the cranial nerves. Out of the context of trauma, the majority of these deficits present over a protracted period of time and do not require emergent intervention. However, the sudden onset of numbness or weakness in the extremities or the acute loss of bowel or bladder control deserves emergent workup and, in some cases, emergent intervention.

The differential diagnosis for a patient with such a presentation includes pathologies that can cause acute spinal cord compression, such as spinal instability from tumors or infection, or spinal cord mass effect, again from tumors or infection, or large acute herniated disks or hematomas. Patients with apparently mild trauma and cervical stenosis can present with central cord syndrome. Patients with a previous history of spinal cord injury can present with a sudden progression of their deficit because of an expanding syrinx in their spinal cord. Patients can also suffer ischemic injury to the spinal cord from dissecting aortic aneurysms or from spinal AVMs, both of which can cause paraplegia. Finally, certain nonsurgical conditions, such as transverse myelitis, combined system disease, or radiation myelopathy must be part of the differential diagnosis if the imaging workup is negative.[63]

Patients presenting with nontraumatic progressive or sudden weakness should receive plain films of the suspected spinal segments. This should rapidly be followed by an MRI. If a compressive lesion is identified, plans should be made to decompress the spine. Depending on the location of the pathology, this may be done through a laminectomy or may require a more extensive anterior approach to the spine.

Practices for timing of surgery vary. In general, patients should be decompressed immediately. However, some surgeons believe that patients who have not progressed for 72 hours or more can be decompressed on a more routine basis.

Many spinal pathologies result in spinal instability. Tumors involving the vertebral bodies often destabilize the spine as well as cause spinal cord compression. Surgery to decompress the spine will often also involve instrumentation to stabilize the spine, further complicating operative planning. The key elements in surgical planning are the timing and approach for decompression and method of stabilization if required.

Patients presenting without neurologic deficits but with tumor or infection in the spinal column or canal may be candidates for nonoperative management, with either radiation or antibiotics. Nonoperative versus operative management is determined by ensuring that no deficit attributable to compression exists and that the spine is stable and likely to remain so and by estimating the natural progression of the presenting pathology.

Cauda Equina Syndrome

The most common acute syndrome associated with herniated disks occurs in the lumbar spine. From 80% to 90% of patients with lumbar disk disease never require surgery, responding instead to nonsurgical management. However, rarely, in 0.25% to 1% of cases, herniated lumbar disks present as the sudden onset of pain or weakness in the lower extremities, usually involving more than one nerve root with associated asymmetric sensory loss, which may include saddle anesthesia as the condition progresses and, importantly, often loss of bowel or bladder control, commonly urinary retention. Onset of weakness and loss of bladder control are sudden, but the patient may have had low back pain for several weeks. This syndrome is called "cauda equina syndrome." Without rapid decompression of the cauda eqina, permanent bladder dysfunction and weakness are likely.[64]

Critique

Intracranial pressure (ICP) monitoring is an essential component in the management of severe head injuries, because ICP can occur as a result of either primary or secondary brain injury. Intracranial pressure is normally 15 mm Hg or less. When intracranial pressure exceeds 20 mm Hg, the mortality rate increases exponentially. If rising intracranial pressure cannot be controlled, death is imminent. The patient in this scenario is comatose with a Glasgow Coma Scale of 6. He is clearly at risk for developing intracranial pressure elevation. Therefore, ICP monitoring is pivotal to the optimal management of this patient. Forced diuresis and administration of barbiturates would depend on the intracranial pressure. At this time, there is no indication for operative intervention. There have been no prospective, randomized studies that demonstrate the efficacy of hyperventilation for this period of time.

Answer (E)

References

1. Miller J. Lectures on the Approach to Neurotrauma. Unpublished work, 2005.
2. American College of Surgeons. Advanced Trauma Life Support. Chicago: American College of Surgeons, 2004.

3. Doyon S, Roberts JR. Reappraisal of the "coma cocktail." Dextrose, flumazenil, naloxone, and thiamine. Emerg Med Clin North Am 2005; 12(2):301–316.

4. Greenberg MS. Seizures. In Handbook of Neurosurgery. New York: Thieme, 2001: 254–284.

5. American Spinal Injury Association. International Standards for Neurological and Functional Classification of Spinal Cord Injury. Chicago: American Spinal Injury Association, 1996.

6. Holmes JF, Mirvis SE, Panacek EA, Hoffman JR, Mower WR, Velmahos GC, et al. Variability in computed tomography and magnetic resonance imaging in patients with cervical spine injuries. J Trauma 2002; 53(3):524–529.

7. Teasdale G, Jennett B. Assessment of coma and impaired consciousness: a practical scale. Lancet 1974; 2:81.

8. Hunt WE, Hess RM. Surgical risk as related to time of intervention in the repair of intracranial aneurysms. J Neurosurg 1968; 28:14–20.

9. Karnofsky DA, Burchenal JH. In: Macleod M, ed. Evaluation of Chemotherapy Agents. New York: Columbia University Press, 1949: 191–205.

10. Narayan RK, Greenberg RP, Miller JD. Improved confidence of outcome prediction in severe head injury: a comparative analysis of the clinical examination, multimodality evoked potentials, CT scanning, and intracranial pressure. J Neurosurg 1981; 54:751–762.

11. Narayan RK, Kishore PR, Becker DP. Intracranial pressure: to monitor or not to monitor? A review of our experience with severe head injury. J Neurosurg 1982; 56:650–659.

12. Brain Trauma Foundation. Management and Prognosis of Severe Traumatic Brain Injury, 2nd ed. New York: Brain Trauma Foundation, 2000.

13. Monroe D, Maltby GL. Extradural hemorrhage: a study of forty four cases. Ann Surg 1941; 113:192–203.

14. Stein SC, Ross SE. Moderate head injury: a guide to initial management. J Neurosurg 1992; 77:562–564.

15. Biffl WL, Moore EE, Ryu RK, Offner PJ, Novak Z, Coldwell DM, et al. The unrecognized epidemic of blunt carotid arterial injuries: early diagnosis improves neurologic outcome. Ann Surg 1998; 228(4):462–470.

16. Biffl WL, Moore EE, Offner PJ, Brega KE, Franciose RJ, Burch JM. Blunt carotid arterial injuries: implications of a new grading scale. J Trauma 1999; 47(5):845–853.

17. Biffl WL, Ray CE Jr, Moore EE, Franciose RJ, Aly S, Heyrosa MG, et al. Treatment-related outcomes from blunt cerebrovascular injuries: importance of routine follow-up arteriography. Ann Surg 2002; 235(5):699–706.

18. Biffle WL, Moore EE, Offner PJ, Brega KE, Francoise RJ, Burch JM. Blunt carotid arterial injuries: implications of a new grading scale. J Trauma Inj Infect Crit Care 1999; 47(5), 845.

19. Biffl WL, Moore EE, Elliott JP, Ray C, Offner PJ, Franciose RJ, et al. The devastating potential of blunt vertebral arterial injuries. Ann Surg 2000; 231(5):672–681.

20. Management of vertebral artery injuries after nonpenetrating cervical trauma. Neurosurgery 2002; 50(3 Suppl):S173–S178.

21. Schneider GH, Bardt T, Lanksch WR, Unterberg A. Decompressive craniectomy following traumatic brain injury: ICP, CPP and neurological outcome. Acta Neurochir Suppl 2002; 81:77–79.

22. Eisenberg HM, Frankowski RF, Contant CF. High-dose barbiturate control of elevated intracranial pressure in patients with severe head injury. J Neurosurg 1988; 69:15–23.

23. Part 1: Guidelines for the management of penetrating brain injury. Introduction and methodology. J Trauma 2001; 51(2 Suppl):S3–S6.

24. Part 2: Prognosis in penetrating brain injury. J Trauma 2001; 51(2 Suppl):S44–S86.

25. Kaufman HH, Levy ML, Stone JL, Masri LS, Lichtor T, Lavine SD, et al. Patients with Glasgow Coma Scale scores 3, 4, 5 after gunshot wounds to the brain. Neurosurg Clin North Am 1995; 6(4):701–714.

26. Shaffrey ME, Polin RS, Phillips CD, Germanson T, Shaffrey CI, Jane JA. Classification of civilian craniocerebral gunshot wounds: a multivariate analysis predictive of mortality. J Neurotrauma 1992; 9 Suppl 1:S279–S285.

27. Polin RS, Shaffrey ME, Phillips CD, Germanson T, Jane JA. Multivariate analysis and prediction of outcome following penetrating head injury. Neurosurg Clin North Am 1995; 6(4):689–699.

28. Levy ML, Rezai A, Masri LS, Litofsky SN, Giannotta SL, Apuzzo ML, et al. The significance of subarachnoid hemorrhage after penetrating craniocerebral injury: correlations with angiography and outcome in a civilian population. Neurosurgery 1993; 32(4):532–540.

29. Kaufman HH. Treatment of civilian gunshot wounds to the head. Neurosurg Clin North Am 1991; 2(2):387–397.

30. Surgical management of penetrating brain injury. J Trauma 2001; 51(2 Suppl):S16–S25.

31. Cervical spine immobilization before admission to the hospital. Neurosurgery 2002; 50(3 Suppl):S7–17.

32. Hoffman JR, Mower WR, Wolfson AB, Todd KH, Zucker MI. Validity of a set of clinical criteria to rule out injury to the cervical spine in patients with blunt trauma. National Emergency X-Radiography Utilization Study Group [see comment; erratum appears in N Engl J Med 2000; 344(6):464]. N Engl J Med 2000; 343(2):94–99.

33. Marion DW, Domeier R, Dunham CM, Luchette FA, Haid R, Erwood SC. EAST Practice Management Guidelines for Identifying Cervical Spine Injuries Following Trauma. East Northport, NY: Eastern Association for the Surgery of Trauma, 2000.

34. Radiographic assessment of the cervical spine in asymptomatic trauma patients. Neurosurgery 2002; 50(3 Suppl): S30–S35.

35. Hoffman JR, Wolfson AB, Todd K, Mower WR. Selective cervical spine radiography in blunt trauma: methodology of the National Emergency X-Radiography Utilization Study (NEXUS). Ann Emerg Med 1998; 32(4):461–469.

36. Velmahos GC, Theodorou D, Tatevossian R, Belzberg H, Cornwell EE, III, Berne TV, et al. Radiographic cervical spine evaluation in the alert asymptomatic blunt trauma victim: much ado about nothing. J Trauma 1996; 40(5):768–774.

37. Radiographic assessment of the cervical spine in symptomatic trauma patients. Neurosurgery 2002; 50(3 Suppl): S36–S43.

38. Daffner RH, Dalinka MK, Alazraki N, DeSmet AA, El-Khoury GY, Kneeland JB, et al. Suspected Cervical Spine Trauma. ACR Appropriateness Criteria. Reston, VA: American College of Radiology, 2002.

39. Pharmacological therapy after acute cervical spinal cord injury. Neurosurgery 2002; 50(3 Suppl):S63–S72.

40. Blood pressure management after acute spinal cord injury. Neurosurgery 2002; 50(3 Suppl):S58–S62.

41. Treatment of subaxial cervical spinal injuries. Neurosurgery 2002; 50(3 Suppl):S156–S165.

42. Initial closed reduction of cervical spine fracture-dislocation injuries. Neurosurgery 2002; 50(3 Suppl):S44–S50.

43. Spinal cord injury without radiographic abnormality. Neurosurgery 2002; 50(3 Suppl):S100–S104.

44. Heary RF, Vaccaro AR, Mesa JJ, Northrup BE, Albert TJ, Balderston RA, et al. Steroids and gunshot wounds to the spine. Neurosurgery 1997; 41(3):576–583.

45. Levy ML, Gans W, Wijesinghe HS, SooHoo WE, Adkins RH, Stillerman CB. Use of methylprednisolone as an adjunct in the management of patients with penetrating spinal cord injury: outcome analysis. Neurosurgery 1996; 39(6):1141–1148.

46. Prendergast MR, Saxe JM, Ledgerwood AM, Lucas CE, Lucas WF. Massive steroids do not reduce the zone of injury after penetrating spinal cord injury. J Trauma 1994; 37(4): 576–579.

47. Greenberg MS. Peripheral nerves. Handbook of Neurosurgery. New York: Thieme, 2001: 525–546.

48. Goodrich JT. Acute repair of penetrating nerve trauma. In Loftus CM, ed. Neurosurgical Emergencies. Rolling Meadows, IL: American Association of Neurological Surgeons, 1994: 299–312.

49. Robertson SC, Traynelis VC. Acute management of compressive peripheral nerve injuries. In Loftus CM, ed. Neurosurgical Emergencies. Rolling Meadows, IL: American Association of Neurological Surgeons, 1994: 313–326.

50. Greenberg MS. SAH and aneurysms. In Handbook of Neurosurgery. New York: Thieme, 2001: 754–803.

51. Greenberg MS. Intracerebral hemorrhage. In Handbook of Neurosurgery. New York: Thieme, 2001: 815–832.

52. Kaufman HH. Spontaneous intracerebral hematoma. In Loftus CM, ed. Neurosurgical Emergencies. Rolling Meadow, IL: American Association of Neurological Surgeons, 1994: 101–128.

53. Kothari RU, Hacke W, Brott T, et al. Cardiopulmonary resuscitation and emergency cardiovascular care. Stroke. Ann Emerg Med 2001; 37(4 Suppl):S137–S144.

54. Mielke O, Wardlaw J, Liu M. Thrombolysis (different doses, routes of administration and agents) for acute ischaemic stroke. [Update of Cochrane Database Syst Rev 2000; 2:CD000514; PMID: 10796381.] Cochrane Database Syst Rev 2004; 4:CD000514.

55. Greenberg MS. Occlusive cerebrovascular disease. In Handbook of Neurosurgery. New York: Thieme, 2001: 833–860.

56. Loftus CM. Emergency surgery for stroke. In Loftus CM, ed. Neurosurgical Emergencies. Rolling Meadow, IL: American Association of Neurological Surgeons, 1994: 151–164.

57. Mouw LJ, Vangilder JC. Emergency Treatment of Brain Tumors. In Loftus CM, ed. Neurosurgical Emergencies. Rolling Meadow, IL: American Association of Neurological Surgeons, 1994: 183–194.

58. Post KD, Shiau JSC. Pituitary apoplexy. In Loftus CM, ed. Neurosurgical Emergencies. Rolling Meadow, IL: American Association of Neurological Surgeons, 1994: 129–136.

59. Greenberg MS. Infections. In Handbook of Neurosurgery. New York: Thieme, 2001: 200–253.

60. Hall WA. Cerebral infectious processes. In Loftus CM, ed. Neurosurgical Emergencies. Rolling Meadows, IL: American Association of Neurological Surgeons, 1994: 165–182.

61. Greenberg MS. Hydrocephalous. In Handbook of Neurosurgery. New York: Thieme, 2001: 173–199.

62. McComb JG. Acute shunt malfunction. In Loftus CM, ed. Neurosurgical Emergencies. Rolling Meadows, IL: American Association of Neurological Surgeons, 1994.

63. Greenberg MS. Differential diagnosis by signs and symptoms. In Handbook of Neurosurgery. New York: Thieme, 2001: 864–901.

64. Greenberg MS. Spine and spinal cord. In Handbook of Neurosurgery. New York: Thieme, 2001: 285–351.

23
Chest Wall

John C. Mayberry and Donald D. Trunkey

Case Scenario

A 31-year-old man is involved in a single-car accident, which occurred when he lost control of his car and hit a tree. The airbag did not deploy, and it was reported that the steering wheel was bent. The evaluation of this patient reveals a sternal fracture. Chest x-ray demonstrates a normal cardiac silhouette, no hemothorax, and no pneumothorax. The patient has had no dysrhythmias, and the electrocardiogram is normal. However, the patient continues to complain of chest pain, located at the site of the fracture. Which of the following should be the management plan?

(A) Pain control and observation
(B) Admission to the intensive care unit
(C) Obtain an echocardiogram
(D) Sedate patient for cardiac catheterization
(E) Administer prophylactic antidysrhythmic drugs

Chest wall injuries are common, painful, and disabling. According to the National Center for Health Statistics, over 300,000 people with rib fractures were treated in emergency and ambulatory care departments in the United States in the year 2004, and this may actually be an underestimate because only three diagnoses were tracked per patient.[1] In addition, this survey of mostly nontrauma center emergency rooms and ambulatory care centers showed that 77% of patients with rib fractures were not admitted to the hospital. The Healthcare Cost and Utilization Project's Nationwide Inpatient Sample for the year 2003 indicates that 102,000 patients with rib fractures were admitted to U.S. hospitals, representing 7% of all injured patients.[2] The great majority of patients with chest wall trauma experience significant pain. Patients with rib fractures average pain levels on a 1- to 10-point scale of 5 at 1 week and 3.5 at 1 month, even while taking narcotics.[3] Rib fracture patients are significantly more disabled at 30 days postinjury than patients with chronic medical illness and lose an average of 70 days of work.[3] Patients with more severe chest wall injuries (e.g., flail chest) are at significant risk for permanent disability.[4,5]

The overwhelming majority (63% to 78%) of all chest wall trauma is caused by a motor vehicle crash (MVC), with the second most common cause, fall from a height, accounting for only 10% to 17%.[6-8] Although motor vehicle travel has become safer with each successive decade, 38% of the 101,000 deaths from unintentional injuries in the United States in 2001 were caused by an MVC.[9] A rough estimate of the risk of any injury in a significant MVC is 62% of which 14% will involve the chest.[10] However, half of these chest injuries are minor. During the last decade, an injury caused by an MVC occurred in the United States every 4 seconds and a death every 5 minutes.[11] Extrapolating these data, we can estimate that there are approximately 3,000 chest wall injuries caused by an MVC in the United States per day of which 1,500 are moderate to severe injuries. If 4% to 12% of patients with significant chest wall trauma will die, then we can estimate that 60 to 180 deaths caused by blunt thoracic trauma occur in the United States each day.[7,12]

Unfortunately, chest wall trauma comprises a higher percentage of thoracic injuries at the extremes of life. Blunt chest trauma accounts for 81% of thoracic injuries in children (12 years old and younger) and 78% in the elderly (60 years old and older).[6] Children are more likely to be injured as pedestrians (35%) than are the elderly (11%), whereas the primary mechanism of injury in the elderly is the MVC (69%).[6,13] Tragically, child abuse accounts for the majority of chest wall injury in children younger than 3 years of age.[14-16]

Injuries Associated with Chest Wall Trauma

Chest wall trauma is a marker for severe associated injury. Lee et al.[7] identified the presence of three or more rib fractures on radiograph as an indication of need for tertiary care. Patients with rib fractures are significantly more likely to require thoracotomy and laparotomy than are patients without rib fractures. The likelihoods of splenic and hepatic injuries are increased by 1.7 and 1.4 times, respectively. Interestingly, rib fractures do not influence the likelihood of aortic injury (see later discussion of biomechanics). Rib fractures are found in 52% of patients with documented blunt cardiac injury versus 27% without cardiac injury.[17] Mean lengths of stay in hospital and in the intensive care unit (ICU) are also significantly increased for patients with rib fractures, especially those who are older than 45 years of age.[7,18]

Mortality Rate

Excluding patients who are "dead on arrival," mortality rate doubles (1.8% vs. 3.9%) from those patients without rib fractures to those with three or more.[7] Gaillard et al.[12] studied all trauma patients requiring admission to a critical care unit at Hospital Henri-Mondor in France. The presence of chest trauma increased the risk of death from 27% to 33% overall ($p \leq 0.05$). Pneumothorax, hemothorax, pulmonary contusion, and flail chest were associated with 38%, 42%, 56%, and 69% risks of death, respectively. In the comprehensive study of Kemmerer et al.[19] of all traffic fatalities in New Orleans, rib fractures were the single most common injury (40%).

The elderly are especially at risk. Landercasper et al.[5] found a 13% in-hospital mortality rate for all patients with flail chest,[5] however, the risk of death for patients older than 65 years of age was 29% compared with 7% for those younger than 65 years. Each additional rib fracture increases the risk of death in the elderly by 19%.[20] Increased age was the strongest predictor of mortality when an artificial neural network was applied to a cohort of trauma patients with rib fractures.[21] Alexander et al.[22] stratified the risk of death for elderly patients with multiple rib fractures by whether they had preexisting cardiopulmonary disease. In their series, elderly patients with preexisting cardiopulmonary disease had a risk of death of 55%, whereas those without cardiopulmonary disease had a risk of death of only 13% ($p < 0.05$).

Rib fractures in children are an especially ominous finding. Because immature bone of children is more compliant than the mature bone of adults, pediatric rib fractures indicate that a high-energy transfer has occurred and that the patient is at significant risk of associated injuries. After accounting for head injury severity, there is a linear relationship between the probability of death and the number of ribs fractured.[14]

Biomechanics

The compression forces and impact velocities of trauma have been repeatedly studied with crash dummies, human cadavers, and anesthetized animals. A frontal chest impact equivalent to 17 mph has been shown to cause up to four rib fractures, and 18.5 mph causes extensive fractures.[23] Ribs subjected to either anteroposterior or lateral compression will frequently fracture in two places: laterally and posteriorly.[24,25] Force tolerance (kilonewtons [kN]) and stiffness (kN/cm) are lowest at 60° rotation from the sternum, the precise region where the ribs are thinner and less supported by the sternum or the spine (Figure 23.1).[24] This has important implications for automotive design, because 32% of passenger car fatalities

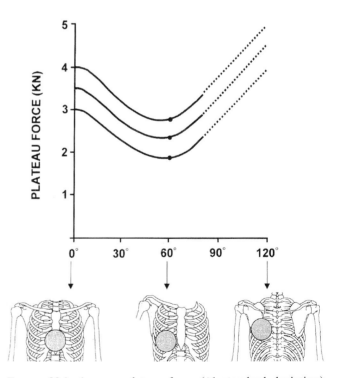

FIGURE 23.1. Average plateau force (±1 standard deviation) required for cadaver chest wall deflection at various locations on the chest wall. Solid lines indicate known data, and dotted lines indicate extrapolated data. (Reprinted from Viano DC, Lau IV, Asbury C, King AI, Begeman P. Biomechanics of the human chest, abdomen, and pelvis in lateral impact. Accid Anal Prev 1989; 21:553–574, with permission from Elsevier.)

occur in lateral impact crashes. Side-impact crashes more frequently involve the elderly, occur primarily at intersections, and usually involve driver error.[26] Better design of intersections and highway crossings would thus especially benefit the elderly (i.e., those least able to withstand a blunt thoracic force). The "round-about" intersection may be safer than the conventional "crossing" intersection.[26]

Although the primary determinant of chest wall injury (e.g., rib fractures) is the force compression of the chest wall, the primary determinant of intrathoracic injury is the *viscous criterion* (VC).[24,27,28] The VC is a time function derived from the velocity of deformation and the compression response of the body wall to a weighted, pneumatic pendulum device (Figure 23.2). In comparing the VC with both the force and the maximum compression in frontal and lateral impact, the VC had the strongest correlation with serious intrathoracic injury. In other words, soft tissue and organ injuries (except sustained crush injuries) occur at the time of peak *viscous response*, well before maximum compression. This explains how major intrathoracic injury (e.g., thoracic aorta rupture) may be found in the absence of rib fractures.[29] Blast or shock wave loading can cause appreciable intrathoracic trauma without chest wall deformation (Figure 23.3).[30] The chest wall transmits the shock wave through the lung parenchyma to concentrate at the hilum, heart, and great vessels.[31]

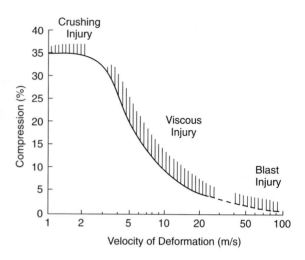

FIGURE 23.3. The various mechanisms of tissue injury can be differentiated by the percentage of compression of the chest wall in relation to velocity of deformation. (Reproduced with permission from Viano D. Live fire testing: assessing blunt impact and acceleration injury vulnerabilities. Milit Med 1991; 156:589.)

Injury Prevention

Lapbelts and shoulder harnesses (three-point restraints) prevent serious injury by minimizing the secondary impact of the victim with the interior elements of the vehicle.[32] Thus, rib fractures are common in unrestrained persons even at impacts less than 10 mph, but multiple rib fractures do not generally occur in restrained persons until frontal impacts of 30 mph are reached.[10] Torso seatbelt loading produces rib fractures generally located along the path of the belt.[33] Airbags, which are not designed to replace belt restraints, but rather to supplement them, provide further protection to the chest.[34] Side airbags provide an additional 68% to 75% risk reduction in head and chest injury.[35] Occupants who are too close to the steering wheel at the instant of inflation, however, may be injured by the force of the deployment. Lau et al.[36] laid anesthetized swine on airbag modules and studied postdeployment thoracic injuries.[36] Rib fractures were present in 52%, splenic laceration in 47%, cardiac contusion or perforation occurred in 41%, and liver laceration in 24%. In the one swine subjected to the highest inflation rating, no skeletal injury was found, but there was a cardiac contusion, inferior vena cava rupture, and a splenic tear. Interestingly, there was an overall lack of correlation of rib fractures with soft tissue trauma. Finally, four-point restraints (similar to those worn by flight attendants) plus airbags might give better protection.

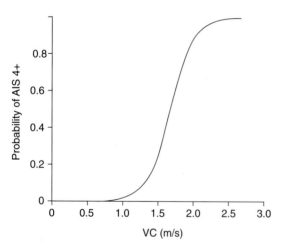

FIGURE 23.2. The probability of chest injury abbreviated injury scale (AIS) 4 or greater in relation to viscous response (VC). (Reprinted from Viano DC, Lau IV, Asbury C, King AI, Begeman P. Biomechanics of the human chest, abdomen, and pelvis in lateral impact. Accid Anal Prev 1989; 21:553–574, with permission from Elsevier.)

Acute Care Management: Initial Evaluation

The initial approach to chest wall trauma follows Advanced Trauma Life Support guidelines as published by the American College of Surgeons, with emphasis on evaluating the patient's airway, breathing, and maintenance of circulation.[37] The chest wall is examined for the presence of a flail segment and subcutaneous air. A tension pneumothorax is suspected when unilateral breath sounds are greatly diminished or absent and the patient presents with respiratory distress or shock. Placement of a 14-guage angiocatheter in the second intercostal space at the midclavicular line will emergently decompress a tension pneumothorax but needs to be followed by placement of an anterolateral chest tube thoracostomy. Open pneumothorax is emergently managed with a dressing occluded on three sides only. Inspired air will thus follow the path of least resistance through the patient's mouth instead of the open chest wall. Following completion of the primary survey, hemodynamically stable patients with no contraindications can be given intravenous narcotics for chest wall pain.

A supine chest radiograph is obtained immediately following the primary survey and is examined for evidence of pneumothorax, hemothorax, pulmonary contusion, or mediastinal hematoma. The extent of rib fractures and their location are documented, recognizing that plain radiographs underestimate the injury. Less than 40% of rib fractures are identified even by radiologists on the initial reading.[33] An urgent computed tomography (CT) scan of the chest with intravenous contrast is indicated for any patient injured in a high-speed MVC or a significant fall from height.[38–40]

Patients with significant chest wall trauma will often require ICU admission, although a minority will need mechanical ventilation. Any patient with known preexisting pulmonary insufficiency, cardiac disease, bleeding diathesis, or associated major injuries should be admitted to the ICU.[22] Many trauma centers, including our own, routinely admit thoracic trauma patients older than 65 years to the ICU. Aggressive pain control (see later), pulmonary toilet, and inhaled bronchodilators are cornerstones of treatment.

Categories of Chest Wall Injuries

Hematoma

The chest wall has a rich vascular network established by segmental intercostal arteries accompanying each rib and internal mammary (thoracic) arteries on either side of the sternum. The intercostal artery and vein are precariously located in the subcostal groove on the inferior and inner surface of the typical rib where the fracture could easily cause arteriovenous lacerations. Rib fractures also bleed from the raw surface of the bone and adjacent muscular tears. In addition, branches of the lateral thoracic artery supply the pectoral muscles and anastomose with the chest wall. Significant amounts of blood can be sequestered in the subcutaneous or extrapleural spaces of the chest. The elderly may especially be at risk because of skin and subcutaneous tissue laxity. Hematomas can require transfusion, correction of any coagulopathies, and evacuation.

Rib Fractures

The human thorax contains 12 pairs of semicircular ribs, more rigidly attached posteriorly to the spine than anteriorly to the sternum. Intervening anterior segments of cartilage provide essential flexibility. The second through seventh anterior ribs actually articulate with the sternum at synovial joints. Ribs 8 through 10 join the costal cartilage of rib 7 to form the acute angles of the costal margins. Ribs 11 and 12 are "floating," that is, attached only posteriorly. There are three layers of intercostal muscles running at right angles to each other, which at the least provide a dense barrier to penetration or pulmonary herniation. On inspiration, contraction of the intercostal muscles raises the ribs superiorly and laterally, thereby increasing both the anteroposterior and transverse diameters of the thoracic cage. The internal intercostal muscles are continuous with the internal oblique muscles of the abdominal wall. This symbiotic relationship inherent in the thoracic wall explains how just one rib fracture or muscle tear can affect all the muscles of respiration.

Because lateral rib fractures without displacement may be obscured by overlapping rib shadows, the chest radiograph grossly underestimates the presence and number of rib fractures.[33,41] Oblique films or special rib views would likely diagnose many that are missed, but the utility of additional films purely for documentation is questionable. Nuclear medicine scans, rib sonography, and three-dimensional (3-D) reconstruction of CT scan all approach 100% diagnostic accuracy.[42,43] These additional modalities, however, are usually unnecessary because treatment is based on clinical grounds. Injured patients with focal rib tenderness or crepitance may be presumed to have a rib fracture or intercostal muscle tear in the absence of radiographic findings.

Rib fractures secondary to sports-related injury have been well documented and occur in two unique types: first-rib fractures and floating rib fractures.[44] First-rib fractures are primarily caused by throwing and have been reported in tennis, baseball, surfing, windsurfing, football, dancing, rowing, and basketball. Most are located in a potential area of anatomic weakness—the shallow groove where the subclavian artery passes over the bone. The first rib is rigidly secured anteriorly and posteriorly; therefore, it has been suggested that sudden powerful contractions of the scalene muscles may cause a fracture at this thinnest part. Repetitive contractions may also result in bony fatigue and cause a "stress" fracture. Floating rib (numbers 11 and 12) fractures are avulsion fractures of the attachments of the external oblique musculature. Most athletic fractures heal spontaneously; however, rare significant complications have been described.[45] Athletic trainers often tape or splint these fractures for symptomatic relief, but, because of the concern for atelectasis, the use of compression for hospitalized patients with rib fractures is not advised. Cough fractures are another unusual cause of chest wall trauma and may be quite debilitating to these often frail patients.[46]

In 1975, a classic paper by Richardson et al.[47] established a trauma principle that, although challenged over the last three decades, is still widely believed: the presence of a first-rib fracture is an indication for a diagnostic thoracic angiogram. Of note, however, 78% of the patients in this series had other rib fractures, and 53% had a head injury. A similar study of multiply injured patients in 1978 led Wilson et al.[48] to recommend serious consideration to great vessel angiography in the setting of first- or second-rib fracture. However, Woodring et al.[49] have helped establish the principle that aortography is not indicated solely by the presence of first- or second-rib fracture on the radiograph but that other signs of mediastinal abnormality (e.g., widening, shift, obscuration of the aortic knob) are of greater significance. In their series of 105 thoracic angiograms, the incidence of abnormality was 14.5% in those *without* and only 8% *with* first- or second-rib fracture. Poole[50] reviewed all series of first- or second-rib fracture and found a 3% risk of aortic injury and a 4.5% incidence of injury to a brachiocephalic vessel. He found a possibly increased incidence of subclavian artery injury with first- or second-rib fracture but no association with thoracic aorta injury and no association between multiple rib fractures and aortic trauma.

Flail Chest

The strict definition of flail chest is the fracture of at least four consecutive ribs in two or more places (Figure 23.4); however, the functional definition is an incompetent segment of chest wall large enough to impair the patient's respiration. Paradoxical motion of the chest wall with inspiration hinders the creation of the expected ipsilateral negative inspiratory force. With expiration the affected segment lags behind and impedes the development of positive airway pressure. In large flail segments, mediastinal shift is possible with accompanying decreased venous return to the heart. The diagnosis of flail chest is ultimately determined by the physical exam-

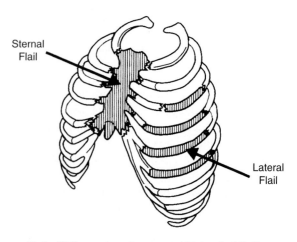

FIGURE 23.4. Oblique view demonstrating typical flail segments seen in blunt chest wall trauma. (Reproduced with permission of Elsevier from Wanek S, Mayberry JC. Blunt thoracic trauma: flail chest, pulmonary contusion, and blast injury. Crit Care Clin 2004; 20:71–81.)

ination of the chest wall during breathing, the appearance of the chest radiograph, and the physiologic impairment the patient is manifesting.

Flail chest is an independent marker of poor outcome among patients with chest wall trauma.[51] If significant associated injuries are present, intubation is unavoidable and should be accomplished early under controlled conditions.[51] Continuous positive airway pressure (CPAP) via mask with epidural pain control is an alternative for selected less-injured patients.[52] Positive pressure ventilation via mask or endotracheal tube provides "internal splinting" of the incompetent chest wall segment until fibrous stabilization develops. For intubated patients we use a combination of synchronized intermittent mandatory ventilation (SIMV) and pressure support (PS). Paralyzed patients are placed on pressure control (PC). The addition of positive end-expiratory pressure (PEEP) or CPAP has the theoretical advantage of atelectasis prevention by small airway "splinting."[53–55] The SIMV is usually weaned first followed by the level of PS. Tracheostomy should be reserved for cases of intubation longer than 5 days, failed extubation, persistent tracheal secretions, or severe head injury. Weaning from mechanical ventilation may take place in the face of a persistent flail defect as the overall physiologic status of the patient improves.

The majority of patients with flail chest who recover show evidence of long-term disability. Landercasper et al.[5] reviewed 62 consecutive patients with flail chest retrospectively from 1971 to 1982 and found that only 43% had returned to their previous full-time employment within 5 years. The most common long-term problem associated with flail chest is persistent chest wall pain exacerbated by physical exertion.[4] In contrast, the underlying pulmonary injury usually heals.[56]

Rib Fracture and Flail Chest Repair

The decision to surgically stabilize the chest wall in flail chest or to treat the acute pain and disability of rib fractures is currently based on the experience and judgment of the surgeon. Class III evidence, however, indicates that the surgical stabilization of rib fractures can reduce pain and decrease ventilator requirements for selected patients with flail chest.[57–60] For patients with flail chest, the goal would be to minimize the number of days of mechanical ventilation and to prevent long-term disability. Ahmed and Mohyuddin[57] compared patients with flail chest treated by Kirschner wire fixation with contemporary controls treated nonoperatively. Surgically treated patients had significantly less days of mechanical ventilation (1.3 vs. 15 days) and less tracheostomy, pneumonia, and mortality than a similar group treated nonoperatively. Voggenreiter et al.[58] also found significant improvements in early extubation with plate stabilization of flail chest, but only for patients without pulmonary contusions. Tanaka et al.[60] randomized 37 consecutive patients with flail chest requiring mechanical ventilation to rib fracture repair with Judet struts or no repair. They found less days of ventilation, less pneumonia, reduced costs, and a higher percentage of return to work at 6 months for patients with surgical stabilization with 2 weeks of injury compared with a similar cohort without stabilization. Granetzny et al.[60a] found similar beneficial results in a randomized trial of intramedullary wire fixation versus adhesive tape strapping for isolate flail chest.

For patients with rib fractures who have pain that is difficult to control with conventional nonoperative methods, the goal would be to relieve pain and shorten the time of disability. In the comparative trial of flail chest repair mentioned earlier, complaints of persistent chest tightness, chest wall pain, and dyspnea were less frequent in the surgically stabilized group at 12 months.[60] The resection of overlapping segments of rib fractures for the purpose of pain reduction has also been reported recently.[61] Our own experience indicates that selected patients with acute pain benefit from rib fracture repair.[62,63] Our experience with patients with chronic rib fracture pain associated with nonunion, however, has been mixed. Some patients have benefited dramatically.[64–66]

Our patient selection criteria for rib fracture stabilization are as follows. Patients with flail chest who are not weaning from mechanical ventilation after 5 to 7 days are offered repair with informed consent. The ideal candidate for flail chest repair is a patient with only moderate extrathoracic injuries whose weaning impediment clearly stems from his or her incompetent chest wall. After 5 to 7 days of weaning failure, the patient is placed on a T-tube or 5 cm of CPAP and the chest wall is viewed for the continued presence of the flail. If the flail segment continues to be prominent, then we conclude that weaning is likely to be facilitated by surgical stabilization. Patients with severe concomitant pathology that is preventing ventilator weaning (e.g., head injury, pulmonary contusion, or acute respiratory distress syndrome) are not considered for repair because their flail chest may not be the primary reason for their ventilator dependence. Patients with significant pain associated with fracture movement are offered surgical intervention with the understanding that the efficacy of the procedure for pain and disability reduction is not established. An ideal patient in this category has minimal or no extrathoracic injuries and has failed a 5- to 7-day trial of inpatient pain control (e.g., epidural analgesia or intravenous/oral narcotic regimens) or has already been discharged home and has failed oral narcotic pain control. A patient with multiple rib fractures or a flail chest who needs a thoracotomy for another indication (e.g., open pneumothorax or pulmonary laceration) is also a prime candidate for rib fracture repair.

Many techniques of rib fracture repair have been described, including using Kirschner wires and wire sutures, staples, and absorbable and steel plates.[57,63,67–69] Our preferred technique for rib fracture repair has evolved over the past two decades. Our initial approach was to reduce and fixate rib fractures with 3.5-mm Arbeitsgemeinschaft fur Osteosynthesefragen (AO) pelvic reconstruction plates (Synthes USA, Monument, CO) cerclaged with sternal wire. Standard thoracotomy incisions with muscle transection were the rule. In more recent years, smaller incisions, often multiple, have been employed to avoid unnecessary exposure, and muscle sparing has been attempted to decrease operative morbidity. Three-dimensional CT reconstructions are used to better define all rib fractures and the extent of their displacement and to help plan the surgical approach (Figure 23.5). Thorascopic assistance has also been added in order to facilitate a less invasive approach and to prevent injury to the lung during screw or wire fixation of the plates. Low profile titanium plates fixed with locking screws without wire cerclage and polylactide absorbable plates fixed with polylactide screws and absorbable suture cerclage have also been evaluated (Figure 23.6). When titanium locking plates and screws are chosen, wire cerclage is unnecessary. Polylactide plates are not made with locking screw capabilities. These less sturdy plates are not recommended for posterior rib repair and should always be cerclaged with absorbable suture for added strength.

Complications of rib fracture plating, both titanium and polylactide, have been very rare. Our most prominent complication, rib osteomyelitis, occurred when the surgical site was contaminated by the presence of a preoperative chest tube. We now recommend that all chest tubes be removed from the vicinity of the operative field at least 24 hours preoperative and that intravenous

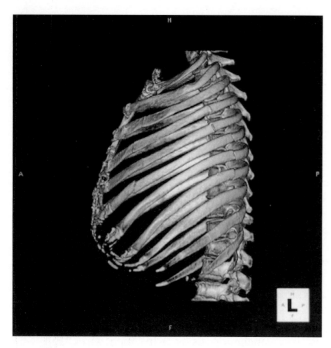

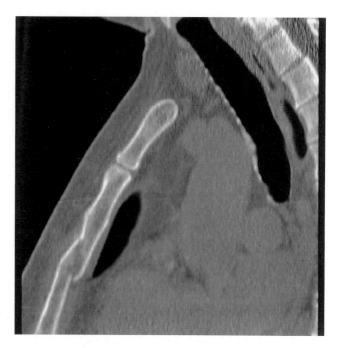

FIGURE 23.5. Three-dimensional (3-D) CT chest wall reconstruction of this patient struck in the chest by a boat trailer indicates multiple rib fractures of the left chest wall both anteriorly and posteriorly. This CT was used to plan a minimally invasive approach to her rib fracture stabilization.

Gram-positive–effective antibiotics be continued as long as the operative chest tube and subcutaneous drains are in place. Subcutaneous closed-suction drains are necessary to prevent significant postoperative seromas.

FIGURE 23.7. Sagittal CT reformation of sternal fracture sustained in fall from height.

Sternal Fractures

Sternal fractures are detected in less than 10% of all blunt chest trauma cases evaluated at trauma centers (Figure 23.7).[70,71] Most sternal fractures occur in the upper or midbody of the sternum, and an association with steering wheel impact has been established. Clinically sig-

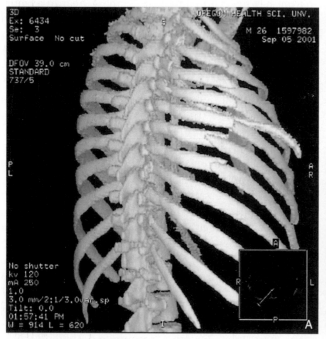

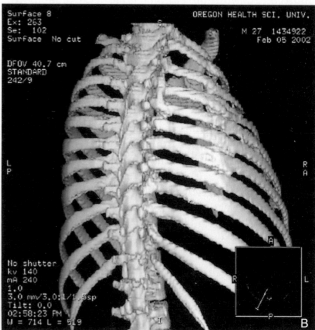

FIGURE 23.6. **(A)** Preoperative 3-D CT reconstruction of patient with multiple right posterior displaced rib fractures. **(B)** Same patient 5 months postoperative rib fracture stabilization with absorbable plates.

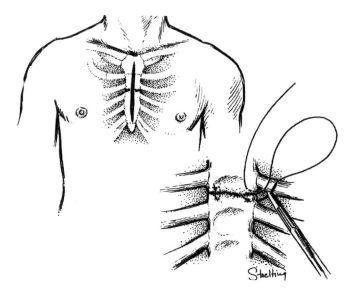

FIGURE 23.8. Sternal fractures can be repaired when indicated with sternal wire fixation (shown here) or plates and screws. (From Trunkey DD. Chest wall injuries. In Cervicothoracic Trauma, 2nd ed. New York: Thieme, 1994: 207. Reprinted with permission.)

nificant cardiac contusion occurs in approximately 6% of patients with sternal fractures and will be manifested by an abnormality on 12-lead electrocardiogram (ECG), a cardiac arrhythmia, or shock.[72] Isolated sternal fracture with no associated abnormality including a normal ECG and a normal chest radiograph is associated with an exceedingly low risk of intrathoracic injury.[70, 73] Any suspicion of mediastinal injury on radiograph, however, should be further evaluated with a thoracic CT. The vast majority of patients with sternal fracture will require no further evaluation or treatment. Rare complications reported include painful nonunion, persistent deformity, mediastinal abscess, and osteomyelitis.[71,74]

Indications for surgical reduction and fixation of a sternal fracture include severely displaced or overriding segments, significant instability with breathing, severe pain, or major deformity.[75] Proven techniques include the placement of a T-shaped titanium plate secured with screws or the use of sternal wire (Figure 23.8).[75,76] Early fixation is preferable to late (>10 days). External fixation has been successfully utilized in a case of manubrial-sternal dislocation associated with costosternal dissociation and rib fractures resulting in a flail chest.[77]

Fractures of the Clavicle and Shoulder

Clavicle fractures are common in injured patients but usually cause only moderate short-term morbidity and minimal long-term disability.[78–80] Frequently associated injuries are ipsilateral arm and hemithorax fractures. A cushioned figure-of-eight brace or a shoulder immobilizer can be fitted for the theoretical advantage of better alignment and cosmesis with bone union; however, in our

experience, many patients are noncompliant. Surgical management for both adults and children is normally reserved for nonunions or malunion deformities.[80–82] Patients with severely displaced clavicle fractures should be offered fixation early because they have a higher incidence of nonunion, and the fixation is less challenging before fibrous bridging occurs (Figure 23.9). Subclavian artery injuries have been reported with both operative and nonoperative treatment.[80–84]

Traumatic dislocation of the sternoclavicular joint is unusual because of the density of the ligamentous attachments. The diagnosis is usually made on physical examination where a prominent medial clavicular head indicates the presence of the more common anterior dislocation. Posterior dislocations may manifest a "hollowed" pocket or "step off" at the sternal edge. Relocation under sedation or general anesthesia is indicated especially for posterior dislocations.

Scapular fractures are rare and indicate a high-energy transfer.[85,86] Significant associated injuries include pulmonary contusion and rib fractures; however, the presence of a scapular fracture is not independently associated with an increased risk of mortality.[86] One study confirmed a higher incidence of ipsilateral subclavian, axillary, or brachial artery injury (11%) in patients with a scapular fracture than in those without a scapular fracture (0.4%).[85] Unfortunately, many scapular fractures are overlooked by the primary surgeon on the initial evaluation. Fortunately, the management of scapular fractures

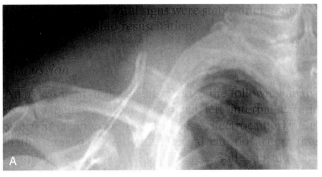
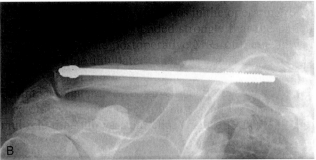

FIGURE 23.9. **(A)** Preoperative view of severely displaced clavicle fracture 9 days postinjury. **(B)** Clavicle fracture (same patient) stabilized on postinjury day 9 with an intramedullary pin.

is mainly nonoperative. Intraarticular and highly displaced fractures, however, may have a better outcome when stabilized surgically.[87]

"Floating shoulder" is an unstable injury caused by synchronous fractures of the scapular neck and ipsilateral clavicle.[88,89] Although surgical fixation of one or both fractures has historically been recommended, nonoperative immobilization with a sling or shoulder immobilizer has resulted in a 95% union rate.[88] Kirschner wire fixation of only the clavicular fracture is also an accepted minimally invasive operative treatment.[89]

Scapulothoracic dissociation is an extremely morbid injury caused by severe traction on the shoulder girdle that tears the ligamentous, muscular, and even neurovascular attachments of the scapula to the chest wall.[90] Significant chest wall hemorrhage can occur, and axillary artery and brachial plexus stretch injuries are common. The injury should be suspected when the patient presents with massive soft tissue swelling of the shoulder. Outcome is dependent on the severity of the neurologic deficit and not the arterial injury.[91] Subclavian or axillary artery occlusion is not necessarily an indication for vascular reconstruction because delayed lower arm amputation is often required for neurologic disability.[91,92]

Chest Wall Defects

Minimal to moderate-sized chest wall defects ($\leq 10 \times 10$ cm) can occur secondary to either penetrating missiles or impalement with surrounding objects during MVCs or falls (Figure 23.10).[93] Repair of both rib fractures and soft tissue is indicated to restore this incompetent segment of the chest wall even if the patient does not require mechanical ventilation. Unrepaired segments may lead to the development of chest wall herniation.[94] Comminuted rib fractures can be repaired with absorbable plates and absorbable suture cerclage.[63] Intercostal muscle defects may be closed by suturing the surrounding ribs together or by placing an intrathoracic patch of Alloderm® (Lifecell Corporation, Branchburg, NJ), an acellular dermal matrix derived from donated human skin tissue that can be used in a potentially contaminated field.[95] Larger chest wall defects such as those resulting from close-range shotgun blasts or explosions are a formidable therapeutic challenge.[96] A thorough debridement of devitalized muscle, bone, and skin and removal of foreign bodies will result in a large defect over which soft tissue coverage by rotation of myocutaneous flaps is necessary. Diaphragmatic transposition, detachment of the diaphragm peripherally and suturing it above the chest wall defect, has been described for lower chest wall defects.[97] This procedure converts the chest wall injury to an abdominal wall defect.

Intercostal pulmonary hernia is a rare complication of chest wall injury that can appear within several weeks or up to 40 years following injury.[94,98] The herniation of lung

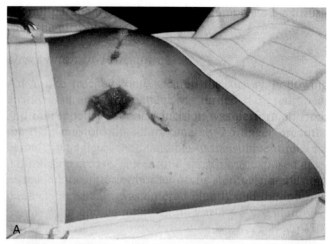

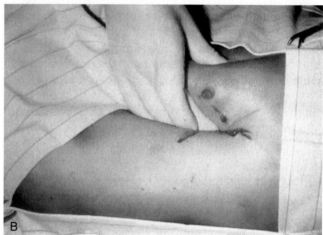

FIGURE 23.10. **(A)** Moderate-sized acute chest wall defect (with open pneumothorax) following steering wheel impact. **(B)** Palpation of the defect demonstrates incompetence of the chest wall secondary to comminuted rib fractures. Stabilization of the rib fractures with metal plates and closure of the skin and subcutaneous tissues was curative.

through an intercostal defect is presumed to be caused by damage or destruction of the muscle layers at the time of trauma. Spontaneous regression has been observed in children, but repair of the defect with a prosthetic patch or a local flap is curative.

Pain Management

Few nonsurgical conditions cause more pain than rib fractures. The pain may be more debilitating and potentially harmful than the injury itself. Fortunately, many pain control techniques and regimens have been devised and proven effective. The time-honored intercostal nerve block is no longer commonly used because of the inconvenience of repeated, multiple injections, but it can be of definite assistance for selected patients.[99] The placement of an intercostal catheter in the extrapleural space through which a long-acting local anesthetic is intermittently instilled is an attractive alternative to rib blocks. Both visual analogue scale pain level and incentive spirometry volume significantly ($p < 0.05$) improve 15 minutes after a 20-cc extrapleural bolus of 0.25% bupivacaine.[100] If the patient requires a chest tube, an accompanying long, thin catheter (e.g., an "epidural catheter") can be placed in the pleural space and similar boluses of long-acting local anesthetics intermittently instilled.[101,102] Mean duration of analgesia after 10 cc of 0.5% bupivacaine is about 4 hours. Care must be taken to avoid systemic local anesthetic overdose.

The use of chest wall taping and rib belts has not been well studied. Although patients often ask physicians whether taping the chest wall to externally stabilize fracture movement with respiration and thus decrease the pain of fracture movement is beneficial, surgeons are reluctant to recommend taping because of concerns about respiratory impairment. Norcross[103] reported subjective pain improvement in the majority of patients that he taped with zinc oxide straps secured to the chest wall with benzoin. Two small randomized trials have indicated that commercially available rib belts may be effective in decreasing rib fracture pain.[104,105] A rib belt should not, however, be used by patients with displaced rib fractures because of an increased risk of hemothorax.[105]

Continuous epidural analgesia for thoracic pain control has become more common in recent years as the expertise of anesthesia pain management services has spread. In many hospitals, it has become the pain management procedure of choice for postinjury and postoperative pain, especially given the convenience of continuous administration of the short-acting opioid fentanyl.[106] Fentanyl has the advantage of being lipophilic as opposed to morphine, which is relatively hydrophilic and therefore penetrates the spinal cord rather than migrating in the cerebrospinal fluid to the central nervous system where respiratory depression can result. Fentanyl has a rapid onset of action (5 to 10 minutes) and shorter duration of action than epidural morphine. Epidural fentanyl has proven effective in both pain relief and pulmonary function (maximum inspiratory pressure and vital capacity).[107] Epidural analgesia is an independent predictor of both decreased mortality ($p = 0.004$) and decreased pulmonary complications ($p = 0.009$) in thoracic trauma patients ≥60 years of age.[108] Local anesthetics, both short and long acting, can also be used alone or in combination with opioids in the epidural space, although hypotension can result.[109–111] Epidural analgesia with bupivacaine and morphine is superior to intravenous morphine patient-controlled analgesia in providing analgesia, improving pulmonary function, and decreasing the systemic inflammatory response.[112]

Other commonly utilized modalities for pain management include long-acting oral narcotics, transdermal patches, and nonsteroidal antiinflammatory drugs (NSAIDs). Transdermal fentanyl is not commonly used acutely but can be an important adjunct to oral pain medication chronically.[113] The smooth delivery of the opioid can provide an underlying level of pain relief to which oral narcotics or NSAIDs can be added. Transdermal lidocaine patches are a recent addition to our pain control regimen that may prove effective for chest wall pain.[114] Ketorolac, an intravenous/intramuscular NSAID commonly used to relieve inpatient acute pain, is quite effective but should be used cautiously to avoid renal damage or peptic ulcer sequelae.[115] It is typically used for only 2 or 3 days. Oral NSAIDs (e.g., ibuprofen or celecoxib) are a helpful adjunct to reduce the amount of narcotics required; however, ibuprofen may inhibit fracture healing.[116]

To summarize, chest wall injury is common and is a significant component of the morbidity resulting from thoracic trauma. Because these injuries are often very painful and potentially disabling, an in-depth knowledge of treatment options and the risk of associated injuries is essential for all clinicians who evaluate injured patients. Patients with multiple rib fractures not only are at high risk for associated injuries but also may experience respiratory deterioration that progresses to respiratory failure many hours or days after their initial presentation. The elderly are especially vulnerable to the deleterious effects that rib fractures have on pulmonary function. Rib fractures in children are an ominous indicator of high-energy transfer and should alert the clinician to look for serious intrathoracic associated injuries. Pain control is of paramount importance for all patients with rib fractures. Rib fracture repair is indicated for selected patients with acute pain caused by fracture instability and for selected patients with flail chest.

Critique

Sternal fractures constitute approximately 5% of all thoracic injuries. An isolated sternal fracture usually has no adverse sequelae except for pain. Although operative stabilization is advocated by some, such intervention is rarely needed. The possibility of myocardial contusion is always a concern with sternal fractures because of the energy kinetics and close proximity of the heart. However, with this patient *not* demonstrating hemodynamic instability and there being no associated dysrhythmias, a clinically significant myocardial contusion can be excluded. Also, patients with significant dysrhythmias usually present with electrocardiogram abnormalities. Therefore, a safe and appropriate management plan would be pain control and observation.

Answer (A)

References

1. National Center for Health Statistics, National Hospital Ambulatory Medical Care Survey. Available at http://www.cdc.gov/nchs/about/major/ahcd/nhamcsds.htm. 2004. Accessed May 2006.

2. Nationwide Inpatient Sample (NIS), Healthcare Cost and Utilization Project (HCUP), Agency for Healthcare Research and Quality. Available at www.hcupus.ahrq.gov/nisoverview.jsp. 2003. Accessed May 2006.

3. Kerr-Valentic MA, Arthur M, Mullins RJ, Pearson TE, Mayberry JC. Rib fracture pain and disability: can we do better? J Trauma 2003; 54:1058–1064.

4. Beal SL, Oreskovich MR. Long-term disability associated with flail chest injury. Am J Surg 1985; 150:324–326.

5. Landercasper J, Cogbill TH, Lindesmith LA. Long-term disability after flail chest injury. J Trauma 1984; 24:410–414.

6. Peterson RJ, Tepas JJ 3rd, Edwards FH, Kissoon N, Pieper P, Ceithaml EL. Pediatric and adult thoracic trauma: age-related impact on presentation and outcome. Ann Thorac Surg 1994; 58:14–18.

7. Lee RB, Bass SM, Morris JA Jr, MacKenzie EJ. Three or more rib fractures as an indicator for transfer to a Level I trauma center: a population-based study. J Trauma 1990; 30:689–694.

8. Shorr RM, Crittenden M, Indeck M, Hartunian SL, Rodriguez A. Blunt thoracic trauma. Analysis of 515 patients. Ann Surg 1987; 206:200–205.

9. Odds of Death Due to Injury, United States, 2001. Available at www.nsc.org/lrs/statinfo/odds.htm, 2004. Accessed April 2004.

10. Newman RJ, Jones IS. A prospective study of 413 consecutive car occupants with chest injuries. J Trauma 1984; 24:129–135.

11. Accident Facts, 1992 (National Safety Council). In Dorgan C, ed. Statistical Record of Health and Medicine. Farmington Hills, MI: Gale Research, Inc., 1995; 64.

12. Gaillard M, Herve C, Mandin L, Raynaud P. Mortality prognostic factors in chest injury. J Trauma 1990; 30:93–96.

13. Roux P, Fisher RM. Chest injuries in children: an analysis of 100 cases of blunt chest trauma from motor vehicle accidents. J Pediatr Surg 1992; 27:551–555.

14. Garcia VF, Gotschall CS, Eichelberger MR, Bowman LM. Rib fractures in children: a marker of severe trauma. J Trauma 1990; 30:695–700.

15. Bulloch B, Schubert CJ, Brophy PD, Johnson N, Reed MH, Shapiro RA. Cause and clinical characteristics of rib fractures in infants. Pediatrics 2000; 105:E48.

16. Cadzow SP, Armstrong KL. Rib fractures in infants: red alert! The clinical features, investigations and child protection outcomes. J Paediatr Child Health 2000; 36:322–326.

17. Healey MA, Brown R, Fleiszer D. Blunt cardiac injury: is this diagnosis necessary? J Trauma 1990; 30:137–146.

18. Holcomb JB, McMullin NR, Kozar RA, Lygas MH, Moore FA. Morbidity from rib fractures increases after age 45. J Am Coll Surg 2003; 196:549–555.

19. Kemmerer WT, Eckert WG, Gathright JB, Reemtsma K, Creech O. Patterns of thoracic injuries in fatal traffic accidents. J Trauma 1961; 1:595–599.

20. Bulger EM, Arneson MA, Mock CN, Jurkovich GJ. Rib fractures in the elderly. J Trauma 2000; 48:1040–1047.

21. Dombi GW, Nandi P, Saxe JM, Ledgerwood AM, Lucas CE. Prediction of rib fracture injury outcome by an artificial neural network. J Trauma 1995; 39:915–921.

22. Alexander JQ, Gutierrez CJ, Mariano MC, et al. Blunt chest trauma in the elderly patient: how cardiopulmonary disease affects outcome. Am Surg 2000; 66:855–857.

23. Patrick L, Mertz H, Kroel C. Cadaver knee, chest, and head impact wounds. Proceedings of the 11th Stapp Car Crash Conference, Warrendale, PA, 1967. Society of Automotive Engineers.

24. Viano DC, Lau IV, Asbury C, King AI, Begeman P. Biomechanics of the human chest, abdomen, and pelvis in lateral impact. Accid Anal Prev 1989; 21:553–574.

25. Kleinman PK, Schlesinger AE. Mechanical factors associated with posterior rib fractures: laboratory and case studies. Pediatr Radiol 1997; 27:87–91.

26. Viano DC, Culver CC, Evans L, Frick M, Scott R. Involvement of older drivers in multivehicle side-impact crashes. Accid Anal Prev 1990; 22:177–188.

27. Viano DC, Lau IV, Andrzejak DV, Asbury C. Biomechanics of injury in lateral impacts. Accid Anal Prev 1989; 21:535–551.

28. Sturdivan LM, Viano DC, Champion HR. Analysis of injury criteria to assess chest and abdominal injury risks in blunt and ballistic impacts. J Trauma 2004; 56:651–663.

29. Lee J, Harris JH Jr, Duke JH Jr, Williams JS. Noncorrelation between thoracic skeletal injuries and acute traumatic aortic tear. J Trauma 1997; 43:400–404.

30. Wightman JM, Gladish SL. Explosions and blast injuries. Ann Emerg Med 2001; 37:664–678.

31. Liu B, Wang Z, Leng H, Yang Z, Li X. Studies on the mechanisms of stress wave propagation in the chest subjected to impact and lung injuries. J Trauma 1996; 40:S53–S55.

32. Viano DC. Limits and challenges of crash protection. Accid Anal Prev 1988; 20:421–429.

33. Crandall J, Kent R, Patrie J, Fertile J, Martin P. Rib fracture patterns and radiologic detection—a restraint-based comparison. Annu Proc Assoc Adv Automot Med 2000; 44:235–259.

34. Groesch L, Katz E, Marwtiz H. New measurement methods to assess the improved injury protection of airbag systems. Proceedings of the 30th Annual Conference of the American Association for Automotive Medicine, Des Plains, IL, p. 235, 1986. Association for the Advancement of Automotive Medicine.

35. McGwin G Jr, Metzger J, Rue LW 3rd. The influence of side airbags on the risk of head and thoracic injury after motor vehicle collisions. J Trauma 2004; 56:512–517.

36. Lau IV, Horsch JD, Viano DC, Andrzejak DV. Mechanism of injury from air bag deployment loads. Accid Anal Prev 1993; 25:29–45.

37. American College of Surgeons. Advanced Trauma Life Support for Doctors. Chicago: American College of Surgeons, 7th edition, 2004.

38. Trupka A, Waydhas C, Hallfeldt KK, Nast-Kolb D, Pfeifer KJ, Schweiberer L. Value of thoracic computed tomography in the first assessment of severely injured patients with

blunt chest trauma: results of a prospective study. J Trauma 1997; 43:405–412.

39. Demetriades D, Gomez H, Velmahos GC, et al. Routine helical computed tomographic evaluation of the mediastinum in high-risk blunt trauma patients. Arch Surg 1998; 133:1084–1088.

40. Exadaktylos AK, Sclabas G, Schmid SW, Schaller B, Zimmermann H. Do we really need routine computed tomographic scanning in the primary evaluation of blunt chest trauma in patients with "normal" chest radiograph? J Trauma 2001; 51:1173–1176.

41. Thompson BM, Finger W, Tonsfeldt D, et al. Rib radiographs for trauma: useful or wasteful? Ann Emerg Med 1986; 15:261–265.

42. LaBan MM, Siegel CB, Schutz LK, Taylor RS. Occult radiographic fractures of the chest wall identified by nuclear scan imaging: report of seven cases. Arch Phys Med Rehabil 1994; 75:353–354.

43. Griffith JF, Rainer TH, Ching AS, Law KL, Cocks RA, Metreweli C. Sonography compared with radiography in revealing acute rib fracture. AJR Am J Roentgenol 1999; 173:1603–1609.

44. Miles JW, Barrett GR. Rib fractures in athletes. Sports Med 1991; 12:66–69.

45. Ochi M, Sasashige Y, Murakami T, Ikuta Y. Brachial plexus palsy secondary to stress fracture of the first rib: case report. J Trauma 1994; 36:128–130.

46. Sternfeld M, Hay E, Eliraz A. Postnasal drip causing multiple cough fractures. Ann Emerg Med 1992; 21:587.

47. Richardson JD, McElvein RB, Trinkle JK. First rib fracture: a hallmark of severe trauma. Ann Surg 1975; 181:251–254.

48. Wilson JM, Thomas AN, Goodman PC, Lewis FR. Severe chest trauma. Morbidity implication of first and second rib fracture in 120 patients. Arch Surg 1978; 113:846–849.

49. Woodring JH, Fried AM, Hatfield DR, Stevens RK, Todd EP. Fractures of first and second ribs: predictive value for arterial and bronchial injury. AJR Am J Roentgenol 1982; 138:211–215.

50. Poole GV. Fracture of the upper ribs and injury to the great vessels. Surg Gynecol Obstet 1989; 169:275–282.

51. Velmahos GC, Vassiliu P, Chan LS, Murray JA, Berne TV, Demetriades D. Influence of flail chest on outcome among patients with severe thoracic cage trauma. Int Surg 2002; 87:240–244.

52. Bolliger CT, Van Eeden SF. Treatment of multiple rib fractures. Randomized controlled trial comparing ventilatory with nonventilatory management. Chest 1990; 97:943–948.

53. Tzelepis GE, McCool FD, Hoppin FG Jr. Chest wall distortion in patients with flail chest. Am Rev Respir Dis 1989; 140:31–37.

54. Schweiger J, Downs J, Smith R. CPAP improves lung mechanics after flail chest injury. Crit Care Med 1996; 24:A110.

55. Schweiger J, Downs J, Smith R. Chest wall disruption with and without acute lung injury: effects of continuous positive airway pressure therapy on ventilation and perfusion relationships. Crit Care Med 2003; 31:2364–2370.

56. Livingston DH, Richardson JD. Pulmonary disability after severe blunt chest trauma. J Trauma 1990; 30:562–567.

57. Ahmed Z, Mohyuddin Z. Management of flail chest injury: internal fixation versus endotracheal intubation and ventilation. J Thorac Cardiovasc Surg 1995; 110:1676–1680.

58. Voggenreiter G, Neudeck F, Aufmkolk M, Obertacke U, Schmit-Neuerburg KP. Operative chest wall stabilization in flail chest—outcomes of patients with or without pulmonary contusion. J Am Coll Surg 1998; 187:130–138.

59. Lardinois D, Krueger T, Dusmet M, Ghisletta N, Gugger M, Ris HB. Pulmonary function testing after operative stabilisation of the chest wall for flail chest. Eur J Cardiothorac Surg 2001; 20:496–501.

60. Tanaka H, Yukioka T, Yamaguti Y, et al. Surgical stabilization of internal pneumatic stabilization? A prospective randomized study of management of severe flail chest patients. J Trauma 2002; 52:727–732.

60a. Granetzny A, El-Aal MA, Emam E, Shalaby A, Boseila A. Surgical versus conservative treatment of flail chest. Evaluation of the pulmonary status. Interact Cardiovasc Thorac Surg 2005; 4:583–587.

61. Sing RF, Mostafa G, Matthews BD, Kercher KW, Heniford BT. Thoracoscopic resection of painful multiple rib fractures: case report. J Trauma 2002; 52:391–392.

62. Mayberry JC, Terhes JM, Ellis TJ, Trunkey DD, Mullins RJ. Initial experience with rib fracture surgery: outcomes, complications, and recommendations. Pacific Coast Surgical Association Scientific Program, Las Vegas, NV, February 17, 2002.

63. Mayberry JC, Terhes JT, Ellis TJ, Wanek S, Mullins RJ. Absorbable plates for rib fracture repair: preliminary experience. J Trauma 2003; 55:835–839.

64. Cacchione RN, Richardson JD, Seligson D. Painful nonunion of multiple rib fractures managed by operative stabilization. J Trauma 2000; 48:319–321.

65. Slater MS, Mayberry JC, Trunkey DD. Operative stabilization of a flail chest six years after injury. Ann Thorac Surg 2001; 72:600–601.

66. Ng AB, Giannoudis PV, Bismil Q, Hinsche AF, Smith RM. Operative stabilisation of painful non-united multiple rib fractures. Injury 2001; 32:637–639.

67. Quell M, Vecsei V. Zur Operativen Stabilisierung von Thoraxwandbruchen. Unfallchirurg 1991; 94:129–133.

68. Reber P, Ris HB, Inderbitzi R, Stark B, Nachbur B. Osteosynthesis of the injured chest wall. Use of the AO (Arbeitsgemeinschaft fur Osteosynthese) technique. Scand J Thorac Cardiovasc Surg 1993; 27:137–142.

69. Actis Dato GM, Aidala E, Ruffini E. Surgical management of flail chest. Ann Thorac Surg 1999; 67:1826–1827.

70. Gouldman JW, Miller RS. Sternal fracture: a benign entity? Am Surg 1997; 63:17–19.

71. Velissaris T, Tang AT, Patel A, Khallifa K, Weeden DF. Traumatic sternal fracture: outcome following admission to a thoracic surgical unit. Injury 2003; 34:924–927.

72. Wiener Y, Achildiev B, Karni T, Halevi A. Echocardiogram in sternal fracture. Am J Emerg Med 2001; 19:403–405.

73. Jones A. Towards evidence based emergency medicine: best BETS from the Manchester Royal Infirmary. Admission of isolated sternal fracture for observation. J Accid Emerg Med 1998; 15:227–228.

74. Rehring TF, Winter CB, Chambers JA, Bourg PW, Wachtel TL. Osteomyelitis and mediastinitis complicating blunt sternal fracture. J Trauma 1999; 47:594–596.

75. Richardson JD, Grover FL, Trinkle JK. Early operative management of isolated sternal fractures. J Trauma 1975; 15:156–158.

76. Kitchens J, Richardson JD. Open fixation of sternal fracture. Surg Gynecol Obstet 1993; 177:423–424.

77. Henley MB, Peter RE, Benirschke SK, Ashbaugh D. External fixation of the sternum for thoracic trauma. J Orthop Trauma 1991; 5:493–497.

78. Jones GL, McCluskey GM 3rd, Curd DT. Nonunion of the fractured clavicle: evaluation, etiology, and treatment. J South Orthop Assoc 2000; 9:43–54.

79. Edwards SG, Wood GW 3rd, Whittle AP. Factors associated with Short Form-36 outcomes in nonoperative treatment for ipsilateral fractures of the clavicle and scapula. Orthopedics 2002; 25:733–738.

80. Kubiak R, Slongo T. Operative treatment of clavicle fractures in children: a review of 21 years. J Pediatr Orthop 2002; 22:736–739.

81. Marti RK, Nolte PA, Kerkhoffs GM, Besselaar PP, Schaap GR. Operative treatment of mid-shaft clavicular non-union. Int Orthop 2003; 27:131–135.

82. Jubel A, Andemahr J, Bergmann H, Prokop A, Rehm KE. Elastic stable intramedullary nailing of midclavicular fractures in athletes. Br J Sports Med 2003; 37:480–484.

83. Serrano JA, Rodriguez P, Castro L, Serrano P, Carpintero P. Acute subclavian artery pseudoaneurysm after closed fracture of the clavicle. Acta Orthop Belg 2003; 69:555–557.

84. Shackford SR, Connolly JF. Taming of the screw: a case report and literature review of limb-threatening complications after plate osteosynthesis of a clavicular nonunion. J Trauma 2003; 55:840–843.

85. Thompson DA, Flynn TC, Miller PW, Fischer RP. The significance of scapular fractures. J Trauma 1985; 25:974–977.

86. Veysi VT, Mittal R, Agarwal S, Dosani A, Giannoudis PV. Multiple trauma and scapula fractures: so what? J Trauma 2003; 55:1145–1147.

87. Cole PA. Scapula fractures. Orthop Clin North Am 2002; 33:1–18, vii.

88. Edwards SG, Whittle AP, Wood GW 2nd. Nonoperative treatment of ipsilateral fractures of the scapula and clavicle. J Bone Joint Surg Am 2000; 82:774–780.

89. Hashiguchi H, Ito H. Clinical outcome of the treatment of floating shoulder by osteosynthesis for clavicular fracture alone. J Shoulder Elbow Surg 2003; 12:589–591.

90. Witz M, Korzets Z, Lehmann J. Traumatic scapulothoracic dissociation. J Cardiovasc Surg (Torino) 2000; 41:927–929.

91. Zelle BA, Pape HC, Gerich TG, Garapati R, Ceylan B, Krettek C. Functional outcome following scapulothoracic dissociation. J Bone Joint Surg Am 2004; 86-A:2–8.

92. Sampson LN, Britton JC, Eldrup-Jorgensen J, Clark DE, Rosenberg JM, Bredenberg CE. The neurovascular outcome of scapulothoracic dissociation. J Vasc Surg 1993; 17:1083–1089.

93. Lang-Lazdunski L, Bonnet PM, Pons F, Brinquin L, Jancovici R. Traumatic extrathoracic lung herniation. Ann Thorac Surg 2002; 74:927–929.

94. Croce EJ, Mehta VA. Intercostal pleuroperitoneal hernia. J Thorac Cardiovasc Surg 1979; 77:856–857.

95. Tissue regeneration. Available at www.lifecell.com. Accessed August 2006.

96. Carrasquilla C, Watts J, Ledgerwood A, Lucas CE. Management of massive thoraco-abdominal wall defect from close-range shotgun blast. J Trauma 1971; 11:715–717.

97. Bender JS, Lucas CE. Management of close-range shotgun injuries to the chest by diaphragmatic transposition: case reports. J Trauma 1990; 30:1581–1584.

98. Forty J, Wells FC. Traumatic intercostal pulmonary hernia. Ann Thorac Surg 1990; 49:670–671.

99. Pedersen VM, Schulze S, Hoier-Madsen K, Halkier E. Airflow meter assessment of the effect of intercostal nerve blockade on respiratory function in rib fractures. Acta Chir Scand 1983; 149:119–120.

100. Haenel JB, Moore FA, Moore EE, Sauaia A, Read RA, Burch JM. Extrapleural bupivacaine for amelioration of multiple rib fracture pain. J Trauma 1995; 38:22–27.

101. Gabram SG, Schwartz RJ, Jacobs LM, et al. Clinical management of blunt trauma patients with unilateral rib fractures: a randomized trial. World J Surg 1995; 19:388–393.

102. Shinohara K, Iwama H, Akama Y, Tase C. Interpleural block for patients with multiple rib fractures: comparison with epidural block. J Emerg Med 1994; 12:441–446.

103. Norcross K. Strapping up the broken rib. Lancet 1980; 1:589–590.

104. Lazcano A, Dougherty JM, Kruger M. Use of rib belts in acute rib fractures. Am J Emerg Med 1989; 7:97–100.

105. Quick G. A randomized clinical trial of rib belts for simple fractures. Am J Emerg Med 1990; 8:277–281.

106. Ahuja BR, Strunin L. Respiratory effects of epidural fentanyl. Changes in end-tidal CO_2 and respiratory rate following single doses and continuous infusions of epidural fentanyl. Anaesthesia 1985; 40:949–955.

107. Mackersie RC, Karagianes TG, Hoyt DB, Davis JW. Prospective evaluation of epidural and intravenous administration of fentanyl for pain control and restoration of ventilatory function following multiple rib fractures. J Trauma 1991; 31:443–451.

108. Wisner DH. A stepwise logistic regression analysis of factors affecting morbidity and mortality after thoracic trauma: effect of epidural analgesia. J Trauma 1990; 30:799–805.

109. Worthley LI. Thoracic epidural in the management of chest trauma. A study of 161 cases. Intensive Care Med 1985; 11:312–315.

110. Cicala RS, Voeller GR, Fox T, Fabian TC, Kudsk K, Mangiante EC. Epidural analgesia in thoracic trauma: effects of lumbar morphine and thoracic bupivacaine on pulmonary function. Crit Care Med 1990; 18:229–231.

111. Wu CL, Jani ND, Perkins FM, Barquist E. Thoracic epidural analgesia versus intravenous patient-controlled analgesia for the treatment of rib fracture pain after motor vehicle crash. J Trauma 1999; 47:564–567.

112. Moon MR, Luchette FA, Gibson SW, et al. Prospective, randomized comparison of epidural versus parenteral opioid analgesia in thoracic trauma. Ann Surg 1999; 229:684–692.

113. Grond S, Radbruch L, Lehmann KA. Clinical pharmaco-kinetics of transdermal opioids: focus on transdermal fen-tanyl. Clin Pharmacokinet 2000; 38:59–89.

114. Gammaitoni AR, Alvarez NA, Galer BS. Safety and tol-erability of the lidocaine patch 5%, a targeted peripheral analgesic: a review of the literature. J Clin Pharmacol 2003; 43:111–117.

115. Forrest JB, Camu F, Greer IA, et al. Ketorolac, diclofenac, and ketoprofen are equally safe for pain relief after major surgery. Br J Anaesth 2002; 88:227–233.

116. Huo MH, Troiano NW, Pelker RR, Gundberg CM, Friedlaender GE. The influence of ibuprofen on fracture repair: biomechanical, biochemical, histologic, and histo-morphometric parameters in rats. J Orthop Res 1991; 9:383–390.

24
Lungs and Pleura

Riyad Karmy-Jones and J. Wayne Meredith

Case Scenario

A 59-year-old patient with end-stage renal disease required direct placement of a central line that resulted in a pneumothorax and a hemothorax. Even after insertion of two chest tubes over a 48-hour period, there was still radiographic documentation of a substantial amount of retained hematoma. The patient is hemodynamically stable with a normal coagulation profile. Which of the following should be the management option?

(A) Insertion of a third chest tube
(B) Urokinase administration (via chest tube)
(C) Video-assisted thoracic surgery
(D) Thoracotomy
(E) Continued observation

Although often discussed in isolation, acute care surgery of the lung parenchyma must take into account a number of issues, including cardiac status, airway management, and the pleural space. The basic principles include maximizing parenchymal expansion and fully draining the pleural space. Although lung resection can be relatively easy, in the setting of inflammation landmarks are often obscured, creating the possibility of catastrophic hemorrhage or injury to other chest structures. Planning requires flexibility, and a computed tomography (CT) scan can be invaluable in deciding the optimal approach. Although some problems are easy to sort out (e.g., a gunshot wound to the chest), others may require serial assessment of how the patient is doing clinically to decide if surgery should be done and what type of operation is required (e.g., lung necrosis).

Airway

With respect to surgery of the lung, airway management must take into account the advisability of providing lung isolation. The goals of isolation are twofold: to allow easier operative exposure and to prevent contaminating the nonoperative side (with blood and/or purulence). Whether or not this is possible depends on patient stability and associated conditions and may impact choice of operative approach. For stable patients who do not have contraindications (such as swollen airway, unstable cervical spine, or extremely high ventilator requirements) a double-lumen tube facilitates operation greatly. Usually a left-sided tube is easier to place, as difficulty in positioning a right-sided tube over the variable right upper lobe orifice may result in inadequate deflation or hypoxia.[1]

Double-lumen tubes are not ideal in the acute care setting, especially if major airway disruption is suspected, as they can be difficult to place and can exacerbate the injury. In addition, when placed in the setting of necrotic lung or hemoptysis, the smaller diameter of the lumens may obscure visualization, become plugged, and prevent adequate suctioning, and small-diameter lumens are often easily displaced at the most inopportune times. Newer endobronchial blocker systems (such as the Univent®) can be placed through a standard endotracheal tube and allow suctioning. These can be used in patients who are already intubated and again are easier to place in the left main stem bronchus. These are simpler to place and are often useful in an emergency when it becomes apparent that lung isolation is needed. The most basic method, a large uncut 8.0 or greater single lumen endotracheal tube, remains the mainstay.

If right lung isolation is need, this can be advanced into the left main stem. If left lung isolation is required, either a bronchial blocker can be placed or the tube can be advanced into the right main stem, again with the caveat that the right upper lobe orifice may be obstructed. Some patients may be anatomically suitable for lung isolation but physiologically unable to tolerate it. Options include brief periods of lung collapse and occasionally temporarily clamping the pulmonary artery to reduce shunt, but usually the surgeon must simply operate with the lung inflated.

Thoracotomy

Details regarding exposure of the trachea and main bronchi are discussed more fully in a later section. With regard to the lung itself, the best exposure is provided by a posterolateral thoracotomy, entering the chest at the fifth or sixth interspaces. While counting ribs, it is useful to remember that often the first rib cannot be palpated but the second rib can be identified by the strap muscles inserting on it. In addition, with a patient in the posterolateral position and the bed "broken," the tip of the scapula usually lies over the fifth intercostals space. A variety of muscle-sparing approaches are possible in elective cases, but in acute care cases exposure is usually a premium and these do not apply. If extensive pleural inflammation is suspected, performing a subperiostal resection of the chosen rib is a safer method of entering the pleural space. Usually resecting a tiny portion of the rib just deep to the longitudinal ligament ("shingling") allows easier rib spreading, although, if more exposure is required, there should be no hesitation in shingling adjacent ribs. Shingling under the ligament in malnourished or immune compromised patients reduces the risk of chest wall hernia.

Posterolateral approaches are often not possible. Reasons include instability, bilateral acute processes requiring simultaneous attention (such as a transmediastinal injury), or inability to achieve lung isolation in a patient at high risk of contralateral aspiration (massive hemoptysis or lung abscess). Although sternotomy offers ideal exposure of the heart and great vessels, as well as the medial aspects of the lung itself, the lateral, inferior, and posterior aspects are not well seen, particularly if bypass is not employed and/or lung isolation is not possible. A clam-shell approach is versatile, even if the area of concern is predominantly unilateral. The patient ideally should be positioned with both arms above the head, with a roll placed longitudinally along the spine and the bed flexed. In acute care situations, simply pulling the arms above the head in an exaggerated crucifix position will suffice. The incision should be made in the inframammary crease and extended upward to cross the sternum at the fourth or at most fifth intercostal space. The internal mammary arteries should be suture ligated.

Thoracoscopy

Thoracoscopy has been described for a variety of diagnostic and therapeutic indications. With respect to parenchymal conditions, the primary indications include treatment of air leaks and draining hemothorax/empyema. Although thoracoscopy can be performed on patients who require significant ventilator support, it should not be used in hemodynamically unstable patients where there is evidence of intrathoracic hemorrhage. "Rigid" thoracoscopy, utilizing a mediastinoscope, has advantages in that lung isolation is not required, blood and other debris can be evacuated through the larger port, pleural exploration is possible, and in many cases a single port can be used to complete the procedure.[2] Video-thoracoscopy (video-assisted thoracic surgery [VATS]) does require that the lung on the operative side be collapsed, but it offers a more panoramic view and is more flexible in terms of allowing advanced procedures such as repairing diaphragm or resecting injured lung parenchyma. Video-assisted thoracic surgery has been used acutely to treat ongoing bleeding and large air leak.[3] The management of empyema and retained hemothorax are discussed later in this chapter. Resolution of persistent air leak (>3 days) does appear to be shorter with VATS resection than with placing additional chest tubes.[4]

When entering the chest, it is important to avoid parenchymal injury by bluntly pushing a clamp through the intercostal space. Making the initial incision (if there is not a chest tube tract) in a manner that the intercostal muscle can be divided under direct vision reduces this risk. In addition, placing the ports as anteriorly as possible (where the rib spaces are wider) and minimizing the use of ports (which increase nerve trauma) can reduce the incidence of postoperative persistent pain, a complication that occurs in up to 7% of patients.

Trauma

Tracheobronchial Injury

Blunt tracheobronchial disruption occurs in only 1% to 3% of motor vehicle crashes, and >80% of victims die before reaching the hospital.[5,6] Kiser and colleagues,[6] in their review of the literature, found that the injury was within 2 cm of the carina in 76% of cases, within 1 cm in 58%, and specifically in the right main stem within 2 cm of the carina in 43%. Approximately half of the injuries are circumferential.[7] Right-sided injuries are more likely to be diagnosed within 24 hours (52%) than tracheal injuries (43%) or left main stem disruption (14%).[6] One reason may be that the left main stem is relatively more "buried" by mediastinal structures, including the arch of the aorta, and has significantly more peribronchial tissue that may maintain ventilation for a time.[8] Penetrating injuries involve the cervical trachea in >80% of cases.

Clinical evidence suggestive of tracheobronchial disruption includes subcutaneous emphysema, persistent air leak, and hemoptysis.[9] Chest radiography can demonstrate pneumothorax (60%), cervical emphysema and/or pneumomediastinum (70%), or occasionally the "fallen lung sign" in which the lung is seen to drop away from the hilum.[10] Spiral CT can also present important details, including demonstrating avulsion of the airway.[11] However, diagnosis can be difficult as many patients have underlying lung injury that could lead to air leak. In addition, one reason that the injury is not recognized is that mediastinal tissue, blood clot, or airway enfolding results in partial or complete occlusion preventing significant air leak. This can result in radiographic appearance of a persistent pneumothorax despite a well-placed chest tube (Figure 24.1).[10] Computed tomography bronchography may be more sensitive for evaluating airway anatomy and has been used both for diagnostic purposes and for planning surgery in the setting of congenital abnormalities and airway tumors, but it has not been used commonly following the trauma.[12,13] Penetrating cervical perforation may present with "bubbling" neck wound that stops after intubation. This is virtually diagnostic as it implies that the endotracheal tube has been passed distal to the injury site.

In the acute setting, the initial priority is airway control. Clearly simple oral intubation is the best option, but both flexible and rigid bronchoscopy can be diagnostic and possibly life saving. Flexible bronchoscopy can allow diagnosis, can be performed in a stable sedated patient or in

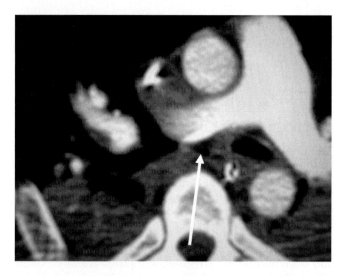

FIGURE 24.1. Computed tomography scan of a patient after blunt trauma with persistent pneumothorax but no air leak with chest tubes in place. Computed tomography demonstrates avulsion of the right main stem bronchus with infolding of mediastinal tissue (arrow).

a patient whose neck cannot be cleared, can act as an obdurator to pass an endotracheal tube, and can assess vocal cord function. The rigid bronchoscope can also maintain an airway and has a larger lumen to allow suctioning of blood or other debris.[14] If acute surgical airway is needed and there is a question of blunt laryngeal fracture, this is the one setting where tracheostomy as opposed to cricothyroidotomy is favored, as the latter can lead to complete upper airway separation. If there is a large slash wound in the neck, the distal trachea often retracts into the chest. It can be grabbed with clamps and elevated and the airway intubated directly.

Of those cases that are diagnosed late (>24 hours), most will manifest as obstructive pneumonitis develops with hemoptysis and/or signs of pulmonary sepsis. At least one fifth will present with late stricture formation and symptoms varying from "asthma" to dyspnea to recurrent pneumonia.[10] If parenchymal destruction has not occurred, airway reconstruction should be attempted, although stents may be possible as a temporizing or even definitive approach in some settings where the airway distal to the injury can be clearly seen at bronchoscopy.[7]

Intraoperative airway management depends on the acuity of the injury as well as its location. In elective situations, a double-lumen tube may be appropriate. In acute settings, especially if the diagnosis is not certain, an "uncut" endotracheal tube, preferably at least 8.0 Fr, should be used. This can allow bronchoscopy and adequate suctioning, can reduce the risk of aggravating the airway tear, is easier to place, can be passed across the injury site, and can be manipulated during surgery. On occasion, the distal airway must be intubated through the operative field to allow adequate exposure. Jet ventilation, with the tubes passed through the injury into one or both main stem bronchi, is also useful at times.

Operative exposure depends on site of injury and associated injuries. The proximal half of the trachea is best approached via a low-lying collar incision.[14] This also allows access to associated esophageal or vascular injuries in the neck. Extending this into a "T" over the manubrium will increase exposure of the middle one third of the trachea and allow proximal control of the innominate artery and vein. If there is a question of major great vessel, ascending aortic, and/or cardiac injury, sternotomy should be employed (Figure 24.2).[6] The distal one third of the trachea, carina, and right main stem bronchus are most easily approached via a right fourth intercostal space posterolateral thoracotomy (Figure 24.3). The left main stem bronchus can be approached via a left fourth or fifth intercostal incision, which also exposes the proximal left subclavian artery, the descending thoracic aorta, and lower esophagus. The very proximal left main stem is difficult to expose using this approach, requiring mobilization of the arch by dividing the ligamentum arteriosum.[14] Finally, a dedicated clam

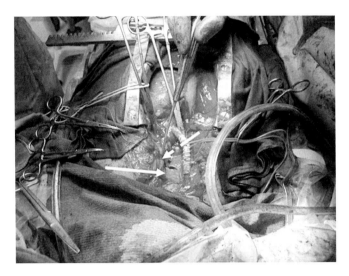

FIGURE 24.2. Sternotomy in a patient with torn innominate artery and tracheal laceration (viewed from the head). Pledgets mark the site of the innominate avulsion (broken arrow), and the tracheal disruption is indicated by the solid arrow.

shell can provide exposure of the distal trachea and carina.

Operative repair varies depending on timing of surgery and extent of injury. Distal airway injuries associated with lobar destruction (either acutely from trauma or chronically from infection) can be managed by simple lobectomy.[15] Small injuries, usually ones in which the membrane has torn away from the cartilage, can be primarily repaired. Simple lacerations can be closed with interrupted absorbable sutures of either monofilament or braided varieties. Dissection should be limited to the region to be resected to preserve blood supply. Muscle flaps can be used as an adjunct.[16] Where there has been complete disruption or significant airway injury, resection

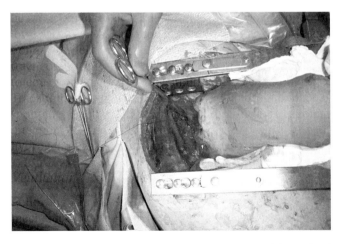

FIGURE 24.3. Right posterolateral thoracotomy with tracheal rupture extending into the right main stem bronchus.

and end-to-end anastamosis is required. Cervical resections should be buttressed with sternocleidomastoid muscle if there has been associated carotid or esophageal injury. End-to-end reconstructions in the chest should be buttressed with viable tissue, such as pericostal flap, thymic pedicle flap, or omentum.[10] Stricture and dehiscence occurs in 3% of patients following tracheobronchial reconstruction, the former presenting in many instances as new-onset wheezing.[10] If the stricture is limited, dilation and temporary stenting to allow remodeling can provide a permanently patent and functioning airway. In selected cases, endobronchial techniques or resuspension of the injured bronchus may be feasible.[17,18]

Parenchymal Injury

It has been estimated that 20% to 30% of patients who undergo thoracotomy following trauma will require some form of lung resection.[19,20] Considering all patients with chest trauma, as few as 2% of all blunt and 6% of penetrating traumas will require resection, although the need can vary widely.[21,22] Mortality rates as high as 3% to 50% following lobectomy and 70% to 100% following pneumonectomy reflect the severity of lung and overall injury in patients requiring extensive resection.[19,23,24] The use of nonanatomic and stapling techniques have been advocated as a method of both damage control and rapid definitive resection under appropriate circumstances, suggesting the potential for reduced operative time, blood loss, and increased parenchymal salvage.[20,25–28]

Most patients who present with penetrating injuries have peripheral injuries that are simple to manage, while extensive blast or blunt trauma often results in combinations of diffuse contusion, and lung maceration that is extremely difficult to salvage.[29] The most common procedures required are simple suture repair or wedge resection. Tractotomy (as discussed below) is used either to define deep injuries or to manage peripheral injuries that pass through the parenchyma (Figure 24.4). Lobectomy and pneumonectomy are rarely required and can be performed "nonanatomically" using staplers (so-called simultaneously stapled lobectomy or pneumonectomy) or anatomically. The latter is usually required in the setting of complete fissures, can take longer, and can be more difficult if there is diffuse edema and bleeding.

Minimal peripheral injuries are often encountered when operating for associated injuries.[29,30] Peripheral bullet tracts may spontaneously stop bleeding because of the relatively low pressure in the pulmonary circuit. To eliminate potential bleeding or air leaks, a wedge resection is performed. Standard stapling devices may be safely used without pledgets or oversewing of the edges.[28] The entire bullet tract must be contained within the excised specimen.

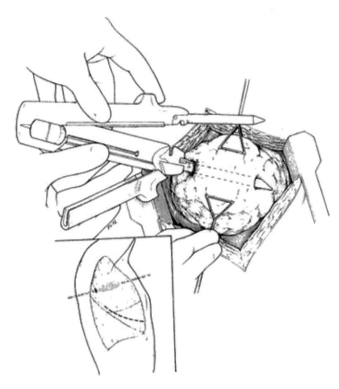

FIGURE 24.4. Tractotomy performed through a peripheral lung laceration. (Reprinted with permission from DiBardino DJ, Brundage SI. Abbreviated thoracotomy: the evolving role of damage control in thoracic trauma. In Karmy-Jones R, Nathens A, Stern E, eds. Thoracic Trauma and Critical Care. Boston: Kluwer Academic Publishers. With permission of Springer Science and Business Media.)

Whereas the management of the most severe and the most minor injuries is straightforward, the management of deep lobar injuries is more controversial. Simple oversewing of the entry and exit sites is insufficient, as there is invariably continued deep parenchymal hemorrhage that results in aspiration, pneumonia, and unremitting acute respiratory distress syndrome. In general, tractotomy should be performed.[20,26,28] It is common that, after tractotomy, there is such diffuse bleeding that simple suture ligation is inadequate. Placing large pledgeted mattress sutures, similar to liver stitches, from the depth of the wound to the edge provides excellent control. After completion of these initial maneuvers, a minority of patients will still have significant air leaks or long tracts of devitalized tissue. If these patients remain stable, they should be considered for resection up to and including lobectomy. Tractotomy was initially described as a damage-control technique. Although definitive for most cases, it may be associated with increased postoperative complications compared with lobectomy, but this is debated. Certainly if major blood loss continues, or there is obvious extensive lobar destruction, lobectomy must be performed as soon as possible. For patients with complete

fissures, a "stapled" lobectomy, similar to the pneumonectomy procedure described later, may be possible. Otherwise, anatomic lobectomy can be performed by skilled surgeons with almost the same rapidity.[30]

Patients with perihilar injuries or extensive lung maceration generally present with class III or IV hemorrhagic shock and are taken to the operating room quickly with minimal resuscitation. Survival correlates with the rapidity of control. If significant central bleeding is encountered, hilar control should be the first maneuver performed. The pulmonary ligament is taken down to the level of the inferior pulmonary vein. This allows torsion of the entire lung as a temporizing method. In addition, if the ligament is not taken down, the distance that a clamp or stapler is required to cover is tripled. Rarely, very proximal injuries may require intrapericardial control of the pulmonary artery.

For small injuries to a single structure, a noncrushing vascular clamp may be applied proximally and repair attempted. When both artery and vein are injured or when a significant length of vessel is damaged, the patient will benefit from an early decision to perform a pneumonectomy. A linear stapler is fired across the hilum and a "simultaneous stapled pneumonectomy" (SSP) performed. A TA-90 stapler with 3.5-mm staples (blue) is sufficient, although some medical centers use the 4.5-mm (green) staples. The stapler approach has the significant advantage over most vascular clamps in that the latter are often held slightly apart by the bronchial cartilages, and the thin-walled vessels can slip out of the clamp with fatal results when the lung is "amputated."[31] It must be emphasized that this represents a "damage-control" approach for the most extreme emergencies associated with central major hilar vascular trauma or the even rarer devastating complete parenchymal disruption.

Trauma pneumonectomy is generally associated with 50% to 100% mortality, and, although it should not be delayed, it should not be performed without at least quickly assessing whether lesser options are possible. One common cause for acute mortality is sudden right heart failure, a consequence of both volume of resuscitation and sudden halving of the pulmonary circuit. If this occurs immediately upon clamping, there is usually no hope. However, if it occurs hours or days later, supportive efforts can be tried with diuretics, vasodilators, and occasionally extracorporeal membrane oxygenation (ECMO). It is preferable fir patients with isolated hilar injuries to stop all fluid boluses when the hilum is controlled to avoid aggravating the right heart strain by excessive fluid administration. A second pitfall related to SSP is the potential for increased bronchial stump leak and/or empyema. In fact, animal models have shown that SSP stumps have similar bursting strengths when compared to individual ligation and oversewing of the artery, vein, and bronchus. Wagner and associates[31] noted a reduction in stump leak in survivors compared with individual stapling. Nevertheless, the bronchus is usually longer (particularly with right-sided pneumonectomies) than in elective cases, and this, in conjunction with the increased risk of empyema, has led to the suggestion that elective reexploration, washout, and stump reinforcement with viable tissue be performed as soon as the patient is stable enough to tolerate it.

A multicenter review identified 143 patients who underwent emergent lung resection following trauma (28 blunt)[29] Simple suture, tractotomy, and wedge resection were predominantly performed after penetrating injury. Relatively speaking, lobectomy and pneumonectomy were more often required after blunt trauma, which tended to be associated with significant diffuse parenchymal destruction. The choice of resection was determined by extent of lung injury, and each "increment" in resection was associated with an 80% relative risk of increased mortality, but the mortality was encouragingly low for this group of extremely unstable patients. Stapled lobectomy was associated with increased mortality, but this was predominantly because it was performed in more critically injured patients.[29]

Rarely, "elective" resection may be required. The role of thoracoscopy for persistent air leaks has been discussed previously. Lobectomy may be needed for persistent hemoptysis and/or progressive respiratory failure following high-velocity gunshot wounds or other focal devastating but relatively isolated injuries. During Vietnam, this was associated with a reduction in mortality.[32] Current indications are less clear, given the increased ventilator options available, but it may still be required if the patient cannot be transferred to a unit that can provide such support.

Whatever the reason for parenchymal resection, outcome will be significantly impacted by the degree of air leak at the time of closing and the residual space that is anticipated. For unstable patients, abbreviated closure must be employed with plans to reexplore and "wash out." For patients with extensive contamination or if it is anticipated that there will be significant residual clot, reexploration or placement of irrigation systems should be considered. The smaller the space, the sooner air leak will seal, and the lower the complication risk is.

Retained Parenchymal Missiles

Retained parenchymal foreign bodies may require resection, primarily because of infectious complications.[33] Irregularly shaped objects, those >1.5 cm in diameter, and/or those associated with severe contusion appear to pose the greatest risks of complications.[34] The University of Heidelberg reviewed the course of 55 patients who had retained bullets. Of the 55, 34 experienced recurrent bouts of hemoptysis (single episode in 8).[35] A Finnish

review of 502 patients managed over several years noted that 20% developed symptoms mandating surgery. These included chronic bronchitis (39), lung abscess (31), bronchiectasis (5), empyema (24), and bronchopleural fistula (10).[36]

The experience in World War II supported early removal. Early removal was associated with 0.9% mortality compared to 7.3% mortality associated with late removal of symptomatic foreign bodies.[35] However, waiting 2 to 6 weeks to allow parenchymal inflammation to diminish also appears to be associated with a lower incidence of complications.[37] Technique of removal varies. Peripheral small injuries can be managed by wedge resection. Deeper objects may be removed by tractotomy, although this may be associated with increased infectious complications. Deeper objects associated with significant destruction or necrosis may be better managed by lobectomy. It is ideal to wait 2 to 3 weeks if possible before removing the retained missiles or fragments to allow local inflammation to subside.

Foreign objects can migrate into more proximal bronchi, leading to obstructive pneumonitis and further risk of abscess formation. These may be removed by endoscopic techniques, and the lung abscess is treated by standard measures. Again, severe widespread destruction may mandate lobectomy. These objects can migrate peripherally or "fall" into the pleural space. Thoracoscopy offers a relatively minimally invasive way to both remove the object and allow irrigation to reduce any bacterial burden.

Retained Hemothorax

Tube thoracostomy fails to completely evacuate hemithorax in approximately 5% of cases.[38] Complications that may arise include empyema and/or fibrothorax. Conditions that predispose patients to both include prolonged ventilation, development of pneumonia, break in the pleura with residual blood (as is the case following tube thoracostomy), and/or other sites of infection.[39] On the other hand, stable, nonventilated patients with small effusions (less than one-fourth hemothorax) following blunt trauma with no obvious pleural disruption usually will resolve without sequelae. For these patients, the cornerstone of therapy should be observation.

Early evacuation of hemothorax has been shown to reduce the incidence of complications in military personnel, preferably within 7 days when loculations begin to complicate pleural debridement.[40] However, recognizing the extent of hemothorax can be difficult. Chest radiography can underestimate both the extent of parenchymal consolidation and the volume of retained blood, particularly in ventilated patients. Chest CT is much more accurate in this setting, but interpretation requires some individualization.[41] Briefly, nonintubated patients who are ambulating and have no infection risk whose hemothorax results in minor blunting of the costophrenic angle do not necessarily require further procedures.[2] On the other hand, even moderate effusions in ventilated patients or those with other risk factors should be aggressively drained when detected by CT.[39,42]

When recognized acutely following injury, the simplest and most expeditious treatment is to place a second chest tube. When recognized after 1 to 2 days, this may not be helpful in that it may simply increase pain, splinting, and the risk of pneumonia with subsequent seeding of the pleural space. Intrapleural streptokinase(250,000 units) or urokinase (40,000 units) has an efficacy of 65% to 90%.[43] Complications include fever and pain, but the risk of restarting bleeding is negligible. The down side of this approach is that it takes several days longer than more direct operative drainage and will not break down loculations. Thus, it may be more useful following debridement when it is suspected that the clot is relatively "soft."

Thoracoscopy offers the advantage of complete removal of all clot without the excess morbidity of a formal thoracotomy.[44] Meyer et al.[45] compared placement of a second chest tube versus thoracoscopy for treatment of retained traumatic hemothorax. Patients undergoing thoracoscopy had a shortened length of time requiring chest tube drainage, a shortened hospital stay (2.7 days less), and a decreased total hospital cost ($6000 less) compared with those patients treated with a second chest tube. There were no failures and no complications, and no patients required conversion to a formal thoracotomy in the group randomized to early thoracoscopy. In contrast, a second chest tube failed to completely evacuate the retained hemothorax requiring operative treatment in over 40% of the patients.

Thoracotomy through "mini" approaches is often sufficient to allow removal of soft gelatinous visceral and pleural rind, permitting full lung expansion. Irrigation with warm saline facilitates clot removal. The denser the adhesions, the greater the exposure must be, and if a formal decortication of a formed visceral peel is anticipated, a standard approach is required. This can be facilitated by excising a rib subperiosteally to allow safe identification of the pleura.

In summary, patients with retained hemothorax, at risk of empyema, should be managed aggressively, preferably by early thoracoscopic drainage.[39,44] There are occasional patients who present with delayed effusions, days after blunt injury, presumably partially because of missed small hemothorax and partially secondary to reactive fluid accumulation. If these patients have adequate pain control, have small effusions (less than one fourth of the hemithorax), and have no signs of infection, tube thoracostomy does not need to be performed as the risk of fibrothorax is negligible. Patients who present late (usually >3 months following injury) with an element of fibrothorax (but with no infection) should be managed nonoperatively because at 6 to 9 months in most cases there is some remodeling and adaptation, and if surgery is required there is no increased difficulty if it is undertaken at a later date.

Massive Pulmonary Embolism

Pulmonary embolus is usually a complication iliofemoral venous thrombosis (≥90%). However, the incidence of upper extremity deep venous thrombosis (DVT) has recently increased and is attributed to the use of central monitoring catheters. Regardless of the source, a DVT may be documented in as few as one third of patients suffering pulmonary emboli.[46] In addition, pulmonary embolism is often a subclinical event, with a higher incidence at autopsy than suspected during any given patient's clinical course.[47]

Presentation

Clinically acute massive pulmonary embolism is characterized by acute cor pulmonale and hypoxia. With shift of the septum to the left, compromising the "underfilled" left ventricle, progressive and rapid homodynamic deterioration occurs. The obstructive pathophysiology is further aggravated by ischemia–and blood component–mediated inflammatory response characterized by the release of cytokine agents with vasoconstrictive properties.[48,49] Dead space ventilation is subsequently combined with shunt pathophysiology, as high-flow pulmonary perfusion is directed to areas affected by bronchospasm and edema. The net effect is that acute massive pulmonary embolus has a dramatic presentation, which in severe cases includes sudden dyspnea, oppressive substernal chest pain, cyanosis, and hypotension.

Diagnosis

A variety of clinical tests have been recommended as initial screens to rule out other causes of sudden cardiorespiratory deterioration in patients at risk for pulmonary embolism (Table 24.1).[48,50] Once pulmonary embolism becomes the leading diagnosis, immediate therapy should begin with heparinization and inotropic support. A bolus (80 U/kg) should be followed by a continuous intravenous infusion (18 U/kg). Epinephrine is effective, as is dobutamine, which may help if systolic pressure can be supported by reducing pulmonary vascular resistance in the nonoccluded pulmonary arterial bed. Percutaneous cardiopulmonary bypass has been used to both resuscitate patients and allow a more orderly workup and plan for treatment. The next step depends, crudely speaking, on whether or not the patient

TABLE 24.1. Pulmonary embolism: initial diagnostic tests.

Test	Comment
Arterial blood gas	• ↑$PaCO_2$ consistent with >40% occlusion of pulmonary circuit • If preexisting hypercarbia, may see paradoxical ↓ in $PaCO_2$
Electrocardiogram	• Rule out myocardial infarction, pericarditis • $S_1Q_3T_3$ pattern, RBBB, right axis shift consistent with >35% occlusion
Chest x-ray	• Rule out other process • 40% of patients with pulmonary embolism have normal chest x-ray
D-dimer	• If negative, <5% incidence of pulmonary embolism
Duplex lower extremity	• Does not alter approach for unstable patients • Can be negative if upper extremity or ileofemoral clot
End-tidal CO_2	• Acute drop can reflect dead space ventilation due to pulmonary embolism • Differential includes pneumothorax and low CO

is in arrest or in shock but with a supportable pressure at least for the time being. For intubated patients, transesophageal echocardiography (TEE) usually reveals indirect evidence of pulmonary embolism with acute dilation of the right ventricle and elevated pulmonary artery (PA) pressures (if there is a tricuspid jet). Transthoracic echocardiography (TTE) and TEE can identify clot in the main PA and proximal right PA, but the proximal left PA is often obscured.[51,52] The primary benefit of TEE is to rule out segmental wall motion defects that might suggest acute infarction and tamponade and to define whether there is clot proximal enough to warrant an attempt at surgical removal.

If the pressure can be maintained, then there may be time for definitive tests. These include CT pulmonary angiography, echocardiography, and/or pulmonary angiogram.[53,54] Perfusion scan is useful but tends to be best used, in our opinion, in patients with hypoxia, without shock, and without associated underlying parenchymal conditions, and thus it is usually not considered in the setting of massive pulmonary embolism with instability. To a certain extent, the institutional preference with respect to treatment will determine the next "best" test.

Angiography remains the "gold standard" for diagnosing pulmonary embolism, but it too has its downfalls. The study is invasive, with a 0.3% to 4% mortality rate attributed to arrhythmias, acute right heart failure, and right ventricular perforation. Nephrotoxic contrast is necessary to define the pulmonary vasculature, and the study requires transporting a critically ill patient outside of the intensive care unit. However, angiography is both the most sensitive (63% to 100%) and specific (55% to 96%) study, and potential interventions can be undertaken in the angiography suite. Angiography should be the primary diagnostic test for patients who are unstable and for whom pulmonary embolism is the primary clinical diagnosis, as it can be both diagnostic and therapeutic. Institutions that favor percutaneous clot lysis and/or extraction favor this approach.

The dissatisfaction with ventilation perfusion scintigraphy and the morbidity and mortality of pulmonary angiogram have directed attention to CT as a useful diagnostic study for pulmonary embolus.[55–57] As with angiography, ionic contrast is required for this study. The scan can demonstrate emboli to the segmental level, and the sensitivity has been found to be better than with V/Q scanning. Although becoming more popular in the workup of pulmonary embolism, CT scan has not yet replaced angiography as the gold standard in all institutions. It appears to be particularly useful for intensive care unit patients who have decreased oxygenation with multiple potential causes that would be reasonably assessed by CT, such a pneumonia or empyema (Figure 24.5). A major issue with CT angiography is the "branch order resolution" of the CT angiogram. Better timing of contrast boluses and improved CT scanning have demonstrated that fourth order branches can be visualized. It remains to be seen whether a clot of nonocclusive type can be reliably excluded even in an optimized scan beyond third to fourth order branches with this technique. Recent improvements in contrast administration methods and findings with isosmolar contrast may also improve branch order resolving power, therefore improving sensitivity for clots in smaller pulmonary artery branches. This has yet to be universally accepted.

Treatment

Although still controversial for less severe embolic events, thrombolytic therapy (systemic or local) is

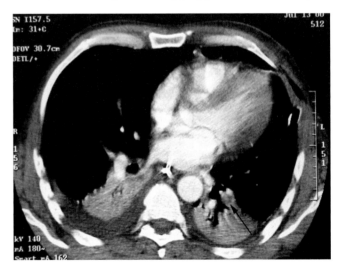

FIGURE 24.5. CTA in a patient with pneumonia and effusion. Pulmonary embolism noted in left lower lobe branch (arrow).

warranted for these patients if no contraindications are present. Either streptokinase or urokinase can be used. These agents lyse clot faster than heparin, and multivariate analysis suggests better outcomes when thrombolytic therapy is combined with anticoagulation compared with anticoagulation alone. Regardless, the hemorrhage risk associated with this therapeutic option is significant and must be considered. The dose has varied in the literature from 10 to 50mg intrapulmonary and/or an intravenous infusion. All clots can be laced with tissue plasminogen activator (tPA) and then the catheter removed, or tPA can be continually infused from the groin or other venous access. The need for catheter-directed therapy is unclear in this situation, because all intravenous tPA given goes via the right heart to the pulmonary circulation. Tissue plasminogen activator infusion has been shown effective in overnight thrombolysis.

Pulmonary artery embolectomy can be achieved percutaneously.[58–64] This technique is indicated for patients for whom thrombolytic therapy is not successful, and it can be carried out in the angiography suite. Basically there are two techniques, suction or fragmentation. Whichever of the two is used, postembolectomy tPA and anticoagulation result in a lower incidence of subsequent pulmonary hypertension.[65]

Some physicians believe that surgical approaches are better. According to this protocol, CT angiography or TEE is an acceptable initial tests with a plan to go to the operating suite immediately. Ideally, surgical removal is performed with cardiopulmonary bypass. On pump, with or without cardioplegic arrest, the main pulmonary artery can be opened and the clot extracted under more control. If needed, the right main pulmonary artery can be exposed between the superior vena cava and ascending aorta and a counterincision made to better expose distal clot.

If a patient arrests acutely, there are only two alternatives. One is to infuse systemic thrombolytics in the hope that this, combined with closed massage, may lyse the clot. There is significant bleeding, and, if cardiac massage has been performed for more than 10 minutes, thrombolytic therapy at that point is associated with massive pulmonary and mediastinal hemorrhage. The other option is to open the chest. If the arrest occurs in the operating room, this is preferred. Ideally, a sternotomy is performed, and if done promptly, open massage may break the clot enough to allow return of spontaneous circulation. Bypass can be used if immediately available to assist in both clot extraction and resuscitation. If the patient has distended right ventricle, but bypass is not immediately available, bicaval occlusion followed by opening the main PA can be performed, although salvage rates are extremely low. Outside of the operating room, open cardiopulmonary resuscitation (CPR) via left thoracotomy can also break up the PA clot and although

results in distal showering will at least relieve the acute cor pulmonale. This might be considered in the emergency room or on the ward for patients who have had a witnessed arrest, have been intubated early, and have undergone <10 minutes of CPR. Percutaneous bypass has been used to both resuscitate patients and support them through therapy, whether it be surgical or percutaneous embolectomy.[61,63] Interruption of the inferior vena cava is indicated for patients with recurrent embolus in the setting of therapeutic anticoagulation or for those who have life-threatening embolism requiring embolectomy by any approach.

Massive pulmonary embolus carries a significant morbidity and mortality. Immediate systemic anticoagulation is warranted after resuscitation has been instituted. All of the treatment options have themselves significant risks, which may add to the morbidity of the embolic event and clinical outcome. For those patients who survive, up to 6 months of anticoagulation with warfarin is required. This therapeutic period will be longer for patients found to have a hypercoagulopathy. For those patients with contraindications to anticoagulation, a caval filter must be placed.

Persistent Air Leak

Persistent air leak, either after trauma or in ventilated patients, can pose a significant dilemma depending on the severity of underlying lung pathology, whether the patient is ventilated, and how significant the respiratory support is. Air leak following traumatic injury in nonintubated patients is not an emergency. Management has tended to follow the management of persistent air leak in cases of spontaneous pneumothorax, and there is evidence, as mentioned earlier, that after 3 days surgical repair (by thoracoscopy or thoracotomy) can hasten resolution and shorten hospital stay.[4,66] for intubated patients, however, the indications and outcomes are not clear. There are two general situations that can be considered. The first is the medical patient with emphysema and air leak. These patients often have significant bullae, are taking steroids, and are developing pneumonia.[67] Resection of the dominant bulla requires thoracotomy, if only to be sure that the true site of the leak has been identified. Following the experience of lung volume reduction surgery, peristrips should be used, but this population already is a high-risk group, with an increased incidence of failure of the operation with the potential for even worse leak if the staple line falls apart.[68,69]

The second scenario may be the patient with diffuse parenchymal injury (acute respiratory distress syndrome), where, rather than fragile lung, dense parenchymal consolidation makes stapled resection difficult. In either case, primary therapy should be directed at minimizing airway pressure, including prone ventilation, permissive hypercapnia, and/or lung protective ventilation. Usually the air leak is in the setting of hypoxia rather than hypoventilation. One occasion, putting the chest tubes to water seal will reduce the transpleural gradient and diminish the volume of the leak, although careful watch for tension pneumothorax must be maintained.[70–72] If there is such a significant leak that hypoxia is impeded, or critical hypercarbia ensues, then repair should be considered. One temporizing approach is to isolate the offending lobe bronchoscopically and inject fibrin glue to temporarily occlude the airway. Some centers use ECMO to support patients through this period. If surgery is required, adjuncts include peristrips (as mentioned), topical fibrin glue, and/or muscle flaps to obliterate deep cavities.[69]

Surgical Management of Infections

Management of thoracic infections requires determining to what extent pleural space versus underlying parenchyma is involved. Although a variety of decisions are possible depending on this factor, ultimately the basic principles are simple: completely drain the pleural space; ideally the lung will expand to fill the space; if this is not possible, consider options for sterilizing the residual space.

Empyema

The diagnosis of empyema is based on documentation of an exudative effusion, characterized in particular by elevated pleural/serum lactate dehydrogenase ratio (>0.6).[73,74] In approximately 25% to 30% of cases, cultures will be "negative" because of suppression but not eradication of bacteria by antibiotics.[42] Many patients will present with indolent courses, often characterized by inability to wean, with radiographic evidence of persistent fluid after injury and despite tube drainage.[39] In many instances, once these "contaminated hemothoraces" are drained, the clinical picture rapidly improves.[42] Computed tomography scan with intravenous contrast can reveal a "rim sign" of enhancing pleura indicative of ongoing inflammation.

Surgical intervention for empyema most commonly occurs in one of three scenarios: parapneumonic empyema; empyema complicating traumatic hemothorax; or empyema occurring after lung resection and complicated by bronchopleural fistula (BPF).[75] In the first two conditions, the primary goal of therapy is directed at draining the pleural space and hopefully allowing full lung expansion. In the latter, although the infected pleural space must also be tackled, the approach must also take into account the persistent contamination via the airway into the empyema cavity and vice versa.

Empyema has been described as having three "stages." The first, usually within 1 to 7 days, is referred to as the "acute" or "serous" phase. This distinction is important as the thin, exudative fluid has a high likelihood of being successfully drained by tube thoracostomy. There have been regular attempts to treat this early stage by simple aspiration. Evidence of vigorous inflammation (pH < 7.0) almost universally predicts failure of this approach.[74] It is imperative that complete drainage be achieved or, failing that, that early operative drainage is performed before the progressive pleural obliteration characterizing the "subacute" and "chronic" phases occurs. Practically, palpation at the time of tube drainage, CT scans, or even chest radiographs can alert the surgeon to the presence of loculations that would indicate that simple tube thoracostomy will be unlikely to succeed.

One major reason for earlier intervention is that more minimally invasive approaches may succeed, while later, the combined impact of pleural space obliteration and lung trapping may make thoracotomy both mandatory and less effective. In this regard it is critical to note differences between empyema following traumatic injury as opposed to parapneumonic empyema (responsible for >85% of all empyema). Empyema following trauma is much more likely to require surgical intervention as the blood and inflammation create a vigorous inflammatory reaction.[75,76] Aggressive management of retained or "contaminated" hemothorax may reduce morbidity.[76,77] Patients with hemothoraces after chest tube placement that are detectable on chest x-ray (opacification or more than one-third hemithorax) should be considered for drainage. A number of other risk factors are listed in Table 24.2. On the other hand, asymptomatic patients who present with late effusions and who have not undergone tube thoracostomy do not necessarily require drainage.

The primary treatment goals of empyema are to drain the pleura and permit lung expansion. Thus, there are a number of "local" considerations when deciding which therapeutic approach is the most optimal in any given case (Table 24.3). Evidence of loculations suggests that simple tube drainage will be ineffective. Thrombolytic therapy has been used as an alternative to surgical intervention.[78] Current data suggest that compared with thoracoscopy as the primary intervention, thrombolytics are

TABLE 24.2. Risk of infection complicating residual hemothorax.

- Ventilated patient
- Splinting secondary to pain
- Onset of pneumonia
- Abdominal hollow viscous injury
- Chest tube in emergency room
- Extrathoracic infection

TABLE 24.3. Considerations when treating empyema.

- Residual space?
- Quality of lung parenchyma?
- Trapped lung?
- Density of loculations?
- Patient ventilated?
- Air leak?
- Lung abscess?

TABLE 24.4. Managing the residual space.

- Irrigation ± antibiotics
- Positive pressure ventilation: expands consolidated lung
- Bronchoscopy: rule out/treat obstruction
- Decortication: release trapped lung
- Open drainage: chronic treatment, particularly in debilitated patients
- Tissue flaps: fill space and close air leaks
- Combination, e.g., "Clagett" procedure

associated with greater failure rate, increased length of hospital stay, and greater cost.[79]

Thoracoscopy (VATS and rigid) approaches have been compared in an unselected manner to thoracotomy. Video-assisted thoracis surgery appears to be associated with decreased morbidity and length of stay, although it is usually attempted much earlier in the course, when loculations are less evident.[79] An alternative approach, when VATS is contraindicated, is rigid thoracoscopy. The major reasons intensive care unit patients are not VATS candidates are inability to use a double-lumen tube, inability to tolerate single lung ventilation, and pleural symphysis. One report documented results of rigid thoracoscopy combined with irrigation in the intensive care unit setting.[42] Fourteen procedures were successfully performed in 13 patients (one bilateral). Seven patients were ventilated, and in 11 cases a single lumen endotracheal tube was required. All were discharged alive from the hospital. Signs of sepsis abated within 48 hours of decortication.

The use of an irrigation system can be modified according to circumstances. We use a Jackson-Pratt® drain connected to intravenous tubing via a three-way stopcock. Postdecortication irrigation appears to be most beneficial in the immediate postoperative period, perhaps because the "new" blood is washed away. Usually antibiotics are not used, but in some instances (resistant bacteria, fungal infections) they can be added. The volume of irrigant varies. Often running 100cc/hr is sufficient, with care to ensure that pleurovac drainage does not "fall behind." It is important to close the deep tissue at all chest tube and port sites to avoid excessive leaking. When the irrigant is clear or 24-hour cultures are negative, it can be discontinued.[42] A potential disadvantage of irrigation is that it may inhibit postdecortication pleural symphysis, allowing residual spaces to be left. On the other hand, if a residual space is anticipated, irrigation appears to be particularly effective. If the irrigation is left in for more long-term management, repeated cultures from the chest tube, or serial lactate dehydrogenase evaluations may indicate whether pleural sepsis is controlled or not.

The residual pleural space remains a problem. A 3-year review of our experience with thoracoscopic drainage of empyema found that 4 of 21 early posttraumatic procedures failed due to "trapped" lung, whereas 15 of 81 non-traumatic and 3 of 7 late posttraumatic (developed after 1 month) procedures failed, 7 because of dense peel trapping the lung and the remainder because of residual space as a consequence of either lung resection or parenchymal consolidation. A variety of options are available, depending on the patient's overall condition and on whether a significant air leak is present (Table 24.4).

When performing thoracotomy for empyema, there are two technical variants that are helpful. First, avoid "counting ribs." This will reduce the chance of creating an extrathoracic infected space. Second, excise the rib rather than "shingling" it to provide a safer avenue for entering the thorax when the pleura is very inflamed and thick. When attempting visceral decortication, it is often necessary to maintain ventilation in the affected lung. This will allow both definition of the plane between visceral peel and underlying lung and confirmation that the lung will expand after the peel is removed. Significant peripheral lung leaks can be tolerated if the lung expands to obliterate the pleural space. If it is apparent, early on, that the lung parenchyma is too consolidated to expand, rather than the peel restricting expansion, it may be necessary to abandon pleurectomy in favor of a strategy aimed at the space.

Bronchopleural fistula and empyema following pneumonectomy are associated with a number of specific risk factors (Table 24.5). [80] Empyema following pneumonectomy can occur without BPF. Patients present with signs of sepsis and the diagnosis is almost confirmed if chest radiograph demonstrates fluid under pressure with the mediastinum shifted *away* from the operated side. Diagnosis can be confirmed by simple aspiration similar.

Bronchopleural fistula occurs in 3% of all lung resection and in 5% to 10% following pneumonectomy.

TABLE 24.5. Risk factors for bronchopleural fistula.

- Excessive stump length leading to pooling of secretions
- Devascularization of stump, possibly during radical lymph node dissection
- Poor tissue secondary to radiation
- Residual or recurrent cancer
- Closing stump in a manner that allows the mucosal membrane to buckle

Numerous factors have been implicated, but preoperative evaluation of the stump is important, as recognition that inflammation is present should prompt coverage with tissue, such as cardiac fat pad or onlay patch of intercostal muscle. Bronchopleural fistula usually manifests between 7 and 15 days after operation. A classic presentation is cough and, after pneumonectomy, a drop in the fluid level of two or more interspaces. In the acute setting, attention must first be given to prevent aspiration. The patient should be sat upright and a chest tube placed. The chest tube should be inserted above the thoracotomy scar to avoid injuring the diaphragm, which usually rises to the level of the incision.

Subsequent management depends on four features: how close to surgery did the BPF occur; was a pneumonectomy performed; how large is the BPF; and what is the patient's overall condition (how much sepsis or respiratory compromise exists). Bronchopleural fistula diagnosed within 7 to 10 days of operation can be considered for reoperation. Frank gangrene of the stump may require further resection. In the case of lower lobe stump leak, middle lobectomy (on the right side) may be an option. Upper lobe stump leaks may require completion pneumonectomy. Leaks after pneumonectomy can be debrided and closed via thoracotomy. All repairs should be buttressed with viable tissue, for which options include latissimus dorsi or serratus anterior if preserved, omentum, diaphragm, or intercostal muscle. Advantages of using bulkier chest wall skeletal muscle are that the potential space can be filled. Deschamps and associates[81] described managing postpneumonectomy BPF with an 80% success rate with transposition of skeletal muscles, open drainage, and repeated wet-to-dry dressings followed by delayed closure of the chest cavity. Regnard et al.[82] used a similar approach for BPF following a variety of resections. Initial treatment was open window drainage followed by flap closure of any large stump leak. Successful closure was achieved in 75% of cases. Gharagozloo and colleagues[83] modified the approach, using immediate stump reclosure and closed system irrigation with antibiotic solution. Of 22 patients, 20 were successfully treated by this approach. A further modification is repeated thoracoscopic debridement and drainage, which offers a chance to remove thicker purulent and necrotic debris. More recently, the use of betadine-soaked packs (1:100 solution) with serial repacking (up to three or four times) every 48 hours appears to be associated with good results, particularly if the omentum can be mobilized and placed over the open stump. Small BPF, not associated with gross air leak and not visible on bronchoscopy, may be temporized by instillation of fibrin glue.[84] Associated empyema should be drained and treated as noted above.

Bronchopleural fistula diagnosed weeks to months after pneumonectomy is technically challenging. Muscle flap closure or thoracoplasty can be tried, but in many instances the bronchus is rarely identifiable within the mediastinum, and adhesions to vascular hilar structures make dissection hazardous. In many instances a transsternal approach will be required. Incising the posterior pericardium between the superior vena cava and ascending aorta identifies the carina.[85] The right pulmonary artery can be redivided (in the case of right-sided BPF) or mobilized and the leaking mainstem re-resected. Dense adhesions will prevent removal of the stump, so the mucosa should be cauterized with silver nitrate. The new proximal resection line should be buttressed with omentum or another transposed portion of vascularized tissue. The risk is high, however, with perioperative mortality rates of approximately 25%.

In conclusion, the principles of treating empyema are to drain the space; debride the space; maximize lung expansion; if not possible, consider tissue flaps to fill the space; if this is not possible, consider chronic open drainage approaches; close significant BPF. Earlier intervention gives a greater chance of less invasive procedures (principally thoracoscopy) being successful. Thoracoscopy can still be considered in ventilated patients using "rigid" techniques. Patients who are malnourished and at high risk may be better managed by chronic open drainage.

Complex Parenchymal Infections

With the exception of cavitary lesions associated with hemoptysis, surgical intervention for parenchymal infection is rarely warranted. Rarely, persistent sepsis, hemoptysis, respiratory failure, and/or empyema may prompt considerations for intervention. The underlying condition is usually difficult to precisely define, as there is a spectrum of interrelated infections, necrotizing pneumonia, abscess, and/or lung gangrene that are often difficult to differentiate and yet the therapies for which can differ radically. Each, therefore, deserves to be discussed as a separate entity, but it must be remembered that in reality they usually coexist.

Necrotizing Pneumonia

Necrotizing pneumonia is characterized by consolidated lung with peripheral necrosis. Penicillin-resistant *Staphylococcus pneumoniae* has been an increasingly common offending agent.[86] Clinically, the picture is of rapid respiratory failure and onset of sepsis with diffuse parenchymal consolidation. On chest CT multiple small cavities less than 1 cm in diameter are noted (Figure 24.6). The parenchymal inflammation involves one or multiple lobes, and the reported 20% mortality rate depends on the extent of underlying disease. Complications of necrotizing pneumonia include abscess formation and frank gangrene. It is important to distinguish between abscess

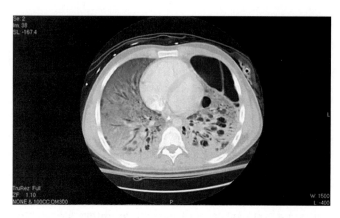

FIGURE 24.6. Computed tomography scan of a patient with diffuse necrotizing pneumonia demonstrating right-sided consolidation and multiple cystic changes in left lung.

and necrotizing pneumonia, and percutaneous drainage of pneumonia is associated with 100% failure and up to 70% incidence of BPF.[87] Because of the diffuse nature of the process, surgery has little to offer. One exception is drainage of empyema. Hemoptysis should be managed initially by endobronchial blockade and embolization, as surgery is associated with nearly 100% mortality. Typically, the lung heals from the periphery inward. Evidence of poor perfusion requires aggressive follow up to detect complications such as focal gangrene.[88]

Lung Abscess

Etiologies of abscess in the ICU population include aspiration, complications of necrotizing pneumonia, retained foreign body, septic emboli, and/or infected traumatic injury. For all patients, superinfection of a chronic cavity (e.g., aspergilloma) or cancer resulting in obstructing pneumonitis should also be considered. The management of lung abscess has remained relatively uniform over the past 20 years. In the three decades preceding this, there were some rapid advancements based on understanding the importance of antibiotics, recognizing the role of aspiration, and finally stressing the possibility of surgical intervention. Over this period, mortality has improved from nearly 50% to remain at approximately 10%. Initial therapy should be "medical," including aggressive drainage, bronchoscopy, and antibiotics.[89] Percutaneous drainage has allowed a reduction in the need for thoracotomy and can be performed in critically ill ventilated patients. Should empyema result, simple chest tube placement is sufficient in the majority of cases. The resultant BPF is rarely so significant as to impair oxygenation. A number of patients do not respond and require operative approaches (Table 24.6). When performing thoracotomy, key technical points include the following:

1. Prevent aspiration, preferably with double-lumen tube
2. Expose the proximal PA early because of risk of bleeding

TABLE 24.6. "Classic" indications for surgical intervention for lung abscess.

- >6 cm and not responding to medical therapy
- Persistent fever and signs of sepsis after 2 weeks of therapy
- Persistence after 6–8 weeks without reduction in size
- Recurrent or major hemoptysis
- Bronchopleural fistula
- Empyema
- Cannot exclude cancer

3. Place nasogastric tube or EGD in esophagus as anatomy may be obliterated
4. Small (<2 cm) abscess to do not need to be resected

Usually lobectomy will be the minimal resection possible as the parenchymal consolidation can prevent lesser approaches. In rare cases, the patient will not tolerate complete resection. Open drainage or closure with a muscle flap are reasonable alternatives. Air leak is not uncommon, and consideration should be given to placing an irrigation system for 24 to 48 hours to help clean the residual cavity.

Lung Gangrene

Pulmonary gangrene is an uncommon complication of bacterial pneumonia but one that has been reported in both seemingly immunocompetent as well as immunocompromised patients. It is often grouped with necrotizing pneumonia and lung abscess, but it has features that make it a distinct entity. Gangrene is distinguished by the development of central vascular obstruction, obstruction of the bronchus, and usually significant cavitation (Figure 24.7). These features, which are detected by chest CT,

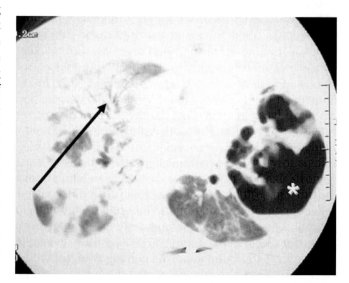

FIGURE 24.7. Patient with rapidly progressing necrotizing pneumonia over 36 hours. Computed tomography reveals right-sided consolidation and left upper lobe gangrene (*). Because of air trapping and inability to ventilate, she underwent successful left upper lobectomy.

TABLE 24.7. Pulmonary gangrene: radiographic findings and clinical significance.

- Lobar consolidation
- Cavitary changes → may be secondary to bronchopleural fistula and/or local hyperinflation
- "Mass within a mass" → necrotic lung
- Obstructed bronchus → inability to expectorate necrotic material
- Thrombosed vessels/no perfusion → inability of antibiotics to reach affected area

predict the failure of medical management (Table 24.7).[90,91] Computed tomography can also detect the development of peripheral BPF. As with necrotizing pneumonia, *S. pneumoniae* is increasingly reported as a cause of lung gangrene. Surgery is required in most cases, although the most important determinant is clinical progress (or lack thereof) rather than simply the radiographic findings. As previously noted, the loss of blood supply and obstruction of the bronchus prevent both the delivery of antibiotics and expectoration of necrotic material. Percutaneous drainage can be attempted but in the setting of necrotizing pneumonia appears to be associated with higher failure rates and increased complications. Surgical outcomes are determined by the extent of the underlying disease and the patient's overall condition. Lesnitski et al.[92] described a "diffuse" form with an overall mortality rate of nearly 40% and a "localized" form with a mortality rate of nearly 17%. Patients who are critically ill may be managed by procedures directed primarily at draining empyema (fenestration) followed by interval lung resection when they stabilize.[93] In most cases lobectomy or pneumonectomy is required. Although there are no data regarding the value of stump reinforcement in this specific setting, our bias is similar to that of other authors in providing some additional coverage. The risk of bronchial stump leak, especially for patients who have high airway pressures, may be increased because of either inflammatory change involving the stump or residual empyema eroding into the stump.[86] As with surgical management of empyema or abscess, one option might be to use muscle flaps and/or omentum both to fill the potential empyema cavity and to reinforce bronchial closure.

We reviewed our experience with 13 patients who underwent pulmonary resection for lung gangrene between April 1999 and June 2001.[86] Nine patients were ventilator dependent, 7 of whom could not tolerate independent lung ventilation. All had ongoing sepsis despite antibiotic therapy. Additional indications for resection included BPF (4), empyema (7), and hemoptysis (4). In 3 cases there was evidence of bilateral diffuse necrotizing pneumonia, whereas in 9 cases the process was localized to one side. Computed tomography scan revealed cavitation in 8 cases, absence of blood supply to the affected lung in 6 cases, and pulmonary artery psuedoaneurysm in 1. Surgical resection included wedge resection (2), bisegementectomy (1), lobectomy (7), bilobectomy (1), and pneumonectomy (2). In all cases the bronchial stump was reinforced with an intercostal flap. Postoperative empyema occurred in 2 cases, one treated by thoracoscopic decortication, the other by percutaneous drainage. There was one instance of stump leak, treated by open drainage. There were two deaths, one intraoperatively in a patient who was in septic shock and the other postoperatively of progressive cardiorespiratory failure in an elderly patient. All but one survivor have recovered and are at home. One patient (following pneumonectomy) remains chronically ventilated.

Despite the success of operative intervention, we reserve surgery for patients who are continuing to deteriorate clinically rather than based purely on the radiographic findings. It is not clear when surgery should be entertained for these high-risk patients. In some instances patients can be supported until respiratory status improves, with drainage of grossly necrotic areas. If the patient demonstrates continued improvement, surgery for BPF and/or abscess can be delayed until later (Figure 24.8).

In conclusion, parenchymal infections requiring resection or surgical drainage are uncommon. When the situation does arise, it is usually in nearly moribund patients with high ventilator requirements and persistent sepsis. Chest CT can identify pulmonary gangrene or other "focal" issues such as empyema, BPF, or PSA psuedoaneurysm that may be amenable to or indeed require surgery. Resection can be performed, even in the setting of high ventilator requirements, with acceptable results. Patients may not tolerate single lung ventilation, which does increase the technical difficulty. Bronchial stumps must be reinforced. Patients with residual spaces may benefit from routine irrigation of the cavity postoperatively. The residual space is at risk for development of postoperative empyema, and strategies, such as pleural irrigation, should be considered for preventing or treating this.

Descending Necrotizing Mediastinitis

Descending necrotizing mediastinitis (DNM) is a rare, often virulent, polymicrobial mediastinal infection originating as an oropharyngeal or a cervical level infection that makes its way into the mediastinum via the contiguous cervicomediastinal fascial planes and compartments. Less than 100 cases have been reported in the English literature since 1960. Mortality rates in most reported series are in the 30% to 40% range without much improvement in three decades or so despite modern antibiotic therapy. Surgeons can potentially have a huge impact on the outcome of this condition when the mortality rates are directly related to delays in posing the diagnosis and to a lack of aggressive surgical management.

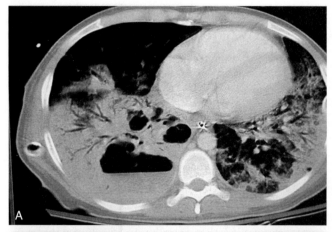

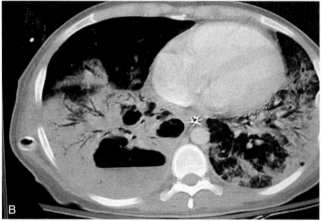

FIGURE 24.8. **(A)** Patient with sepsis requiring inotropic support and necrosis of right lower lobe. Because of diffuse parenchymal changes and hemodynamic instability, the abscess cavity was managed with percutaneous drainage. **(B)** Four weeks later, although still febrile, the patient was off inotropes. Because of persistent fever and elevated white count the right lower lobe was debrided and covered with latissimus flap. Following this, fever resolved and she was able to be extubated and ultimately discharged.

Estrera and colleagues[94] clearly defined DNM in 1983 as a severe necrotizing mediastinal infection as documented at surgery or autopsy associated with a primary oropharyngeal infection and by the recognition of a clear relationship between the two processes as well as the presence of the characteristic roentgenographic features. Acute mediastinitis secondary to esophageal perforations is not considered DNM and should be discussed as a different entity. In a collective review of the recent English literature, Freeman and colleagues[95] determined that the primary focus of infection was odontogenic in 64% of cases reported, peritonsillar abscesses in 20%, and retropharyngeal abscesses in 16%. As a result, DNM is most often a polymicrobial infection containing both aerobic and anaerobic organisms, many of which are gas-producing microbes.

The downward migration of the cervicopharyngeal infection into the mediastinum is promoted by the presence of anatomic fascial planes and spaces that communicate directly between the cervical and mediastinal compartments. The three resulting deep spaces are the pretracheal space, the retrovisceral space, and the prevertebral space. Gravity, respiratory movements, and the negative inspiratory intrathoracic pressure are also thought to facilitate such migration. As a result of these anatomic connections, DNM can potentially be complicated by infections involving the pleural spaces, the lung, the pericardial sac, and the subphrenic space.

Descending necrotizing mediastinitis affects mainly males in their fourth decade (8 to 1 male predominance). Symptoms on initial presentation may often be vague, characterizing the primary source of infection, without hints of DNM developing: facial and neck pain, otalgia, toothache, high cervical dysphagia, drooling, sore throat, fevers, odynophagia, dysphonia, hoarseness, stridor, and sensation of neck swelling usually associated with pain. On examination, poor dentition and the presence of carious teeth or a dental abscess may be noted. An established tonsillar abscess may be seen. Cervical tenderness and swelling and at times frank cervical cellulitis with subcutaneous emphysema imply progression of the primary process at least into the cervical soft tissues.

Diagnosis

Well-established DNM can easily be missed by plain chest radiography. Thus, one must have a high degree of suspicion for the occurrence of DNM in every patient presenting with a deep cervical infection, and some have recommended obtaining a contrast-enhanced CT of the neck and chest early in all such cases. Computed tomography findings of DNM can range from the subtle loss of normal mediastinal fat planes to the presence of mediastinal soft tissue infiltration with or without fluid collections and/or gas bubbles all the way to the identification of established mediastinal abscesses (Figure 24.9). Other thoracoabdominal spaces and compartments that are often involved in complicated DNM can also be evaluated by CT.

Management

The treatment of patients with DNM involves in most cases a multidisciplinary surgical team consisting of head and neck, oral, maxillofacial, and thoracic surgeons. After prompt initiation of empiric broad-spectrum intravenous antibiotics, early aggressive drainage and debridement at all levels involved is indicated. Considering the high mortality of DNM, it is probably prudent to err on the aggressive side upfront. One must treat the initiating focus of

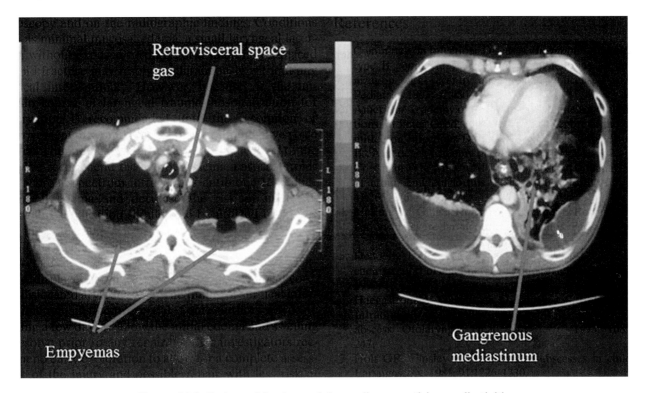

FIGURE 24.9. Patient with advanced descending necrotizing mediastinitis.

infection at the cervical level and establish wide-open drainage and debridement of all deep cervical spaces.

The routine use of tracheostomies in managing patients with DNM is somewhat a subject of debate. Although earlier series considered the mandatory establishment of a tracheostomy for every patient with DNM, a more selective use of tracheostomies has been advocated in more recent series.

Approaches to access the mediastinum are also a subject of controversy for these patients. Estrera and colleagues[94] concluded in 1983 that if the mediastinal process was limited to the mediastinum above the level of the T4 vertebra, a transcervical drainage of the superior mediastinum sufficed. However, others have estimated that transcervical mediastinal drainage is probably inadequate in 80% of the cases. In a literature review published in 1997, Corsten and colleagues[96] calculated a mortality rate of 47% in cases where transcervical drainage alone was used versus a mortality rate of 19% when, in addition, an open transthoracic approach was performed. The most recent reported series also conclude in favor of combining the cervical and the thoracic approaches to aggressively debride all fields affected.

Some have described the use of sternotomy, clamshell incisions, or VATS to tackle the mediastinal debridement and to permit access to both pleural spaces simultaneously. The fact remains, however, that the posterolateral thoracotomy gives optimal access to all mediastinal compartments, allowing evacuation, drainage, and debride-

ment. When treating a condition with a 30% to 40% rate of mortality, one should want the best access to achieve the best drainage and evacuation. A contralateral thoracotomy may at times be necessary to completely evacuate all of the compartments involved. Irrigation systems to allow further mechanical wash out of the mediastinum may possibly also be helpful in the management of DNM.

Second-Look Operations

In addition to being aggressive during the initial procedure in draining and debriding the neck and mediastinal compartments, there are definite merits in being aggressive in the follow up of these patients as well. A policy of routinely performing second-look exploration 48 to 72 hours after initial drainage follows such an aggressive plan of intervention. When the patient fails to improve or when there is clinical deterioration despite initial and/or repeat explorations, repeated contrast-enhanced Cervicothoracic–upper abdominal imaging by CT should be performed to look for undrained foci of mediastinal disease and/or the interval development of sepsis in adjacent compartments. In addition, Freeman and colleagues[95] recommend routine follow-up cervicothoracic CT imaging 48 to 72 hours after each exploration even when the condition appears stable or improved. In their series, 59% of such surveillance examinations identified findings leading to reexploration. An aggressive surgical approach favoring transthoracic evacuation in all cases of identified DNM combined with aggressive and repeated radiologic follow up are believed to explain their reported 0% mortality rate in their series of 10 consecutive patients with DNM.

In summary, DNM is an uncommon but highly lethal infection of the mediastinum complicating an oropharyngeal or cervical level primary infection. A high degree of suspicion for all patients at risk of developing DNM combined with a prompt evaluation by CT should allow a reasonably early diagnosis. Aggressive surgical drainage and debridement at all infected levels is necessary as soon as the radiologic diagnosis is made. An aggressive early follow-up policy including a planned second-look exploration at 48 hours for every patient and aggressive follow-up imaging with routine CT 48 hours after each reexploration, even when patients seem to be improving, possibly will allow DNM mortality rates to be reduced.

Lobar Torsion

Lobar torsion classically is said to occur following lung resection when the fissures are complete. The lobe most at risk is thought to be the right middle lobe. Torsion has also been described following trauma. The etiology may include mobility in conjunction with some "weight" on the affected lobe, such as focal hemorrhage following injury.[37] In practice, our belief is that the most common cause is not recognizing that the lobe has been torsed when putting the lung back into the chest at the end of the case. Prevention includes observing the lung expanding before closing the ribs and stapling the mobile middle lobe to the remaining upper or lower lobe. When it occurs, lobar torsion can present with a radiographic picture of lobar collapse, a clinical picture of fever and sputum production, and a bronchoscopic picture of "fish mouth" bronchus, although more commonly one sees simply purulence coming from the affected bronchus. The pathophysiology is one of torsion leading to gangrene, and in most cases when it is diagnosed because of symptoms a lobectomy must be performed.[37]

Massive Hemoptysis

Acute airway hemorrhage is a catastrophic event that is immediately life threatening. Survival is related to several factors, including volume of blood loss, underlying cardiopulmonary status, rapidity of recognition, and rapidity of control (Table 24.8).[97,98] The primary goals of intervention are to lateralize the source of bleeding and to directly protect the contralateral lung from drowning. Subsequent management may include simply antibiotics,

TABLE 24.8. Definitions of hemoptysis.

"Volume"
- "Massive": >600 mL/24 hr → 12%–50% mortality with medical management
- >600 mL/16 hr → 75% mortality with medical management
- "Exsanguinating": >1,000 mL at >150 mL/hr → 100% mortality with medical management

"Clinically significant" → one of the following:
- Causes death
- Requires hospitalization
- Associated with evidence of systemic blood loss, including ↓ hematocrit
- Requires transfusion
- Presents risk of aspiration and/or airway obstruction

embolization, and endobronchial ablation and/or resection, depending on etiology.

Etiology

Considering all forms of hemoptysis, approximately 85% are caused by inflammatory etiologies, with infection predominating.[99] The bronchial arteries are the major source of hemoptysis, making up 90% of cases.[97] Although tuberculosis continues to be the leading cause of hemoptysis worldwide, chronic inflammatory disease and bronchogenic carcinoma remain the most common causes in western societies.[100]

Uncommonly, massive hemoptysis may be a consequence of primary airway lesions or primary pulmonary malignancies. Inflammation or infection can result in erosion of adjacent great vessels into the bronchus. The propensity of anastomotic fistula arising after lung transplantation or sleeve resection (particularly of the right upper lobe) underlines the importance of wrapping the anastamosis with viable tissue (such as omentum or pericardium) or interposing intercostal flaps between the airway anastomosis and the pulmonary artery.[101] The "classic" airway-related procedure, however, does not involve resection but rather chronic intubation and pressure necrosis, namely, tracheoinnominate artery fistula. The underlying causes range from inappropriate low placement of the tracheostomy to anatomic variations. The published incidence of this potentially fatal complication ranges between 0.5% and 5%.

Diagnosis

Prior pneumonia, history of aspiration, smoking history, and prior surgery may all suggest the diagnosis. A travel history should always be sought when possible. Travelers to Asia, the Middle East, and South America may develop hemoptysis as a result of parasitic infection. Catamenial (endometriosis) hemoptysis may be suspected if recurrent episodes are associated with the patient's menstrual cycle. For children, bronchial adenoma, vascular anomalies, and foreign body aspiration are the most common cause. For adults, those over the age of 40 years and smokers are at risk for bronchogenic carcinoma. In addition, mitral stenosis and/or pulmonary infarction from embolism should be entertained when the clinical history is consistent.

The quality of the bleeding can suggest the source and thus the diagnosis. Brisk, bright red arterial bleeding usually implicates the bronchial circulation, most often secondary to inflammatory etiologies. Rarely, this can imply more major arterial sources, such as innominate artery or aorta, or, even more uncommonly, left atrium or pulmonary vein. Dark blood is more consistent with pulmonary artery bleeding, such as might be seen in the setting of a Rasmussen aneurysm.

"Occult" Massive Hemoptysis

Significant hemoptysis is rarely a diagnostic dilemma. However, it has been estimated that up to 30% of endobronchial clots, primarily in patients who have been ventilated for prolonged periods, with or without tracheostomy, occur without evidence of hemoptysis. In ventilated patients, the most notable manifestations are an acute rise in peak pressure accompanied by a decrease in tidal volume.[102] Multiple peripheral clots may result in transmission of elevated airway pressure to the rest of the thorax, resulting in decreased venous return and possibly hemodynamic compromise. More proximal clots, such as those at the end of the endotracheal tube, are usually associated with normal distal airway pressure and limited hemodynamic changes. A rare variation is a large clot that acts as a ball valve on the end of the endotracheal tube, allowing inspiration but preventing expiration. This may manifest as progressive lobar collapse in some areas while other areas are over distended, increasing difficulty in ventilation and recalcitrant hypoxemia. Recurrent pneumothoraces as a consequence of rapid hyperventilation have been reported. Diagnosis can be confirmed by flexible bronchoscopy, and for most cases this will be sufficient to break up the clot. Occasionally, rigid bronchoscopy with or without instillation of thrombolytics will be required.[99]

Initial Management

In the setting of massive hemoptysis, the initial concern should be to protect the airway and to stabilize the patient. Subsequently, lateralization, localization, and isolation to prevent drowning needs to proceed rapidly (Figure 24.10).[97] Bronchoscopy plays a central role in managing these patients. Bronchoscopy performed within 48 hours of the onset of hemoptysis is more likely

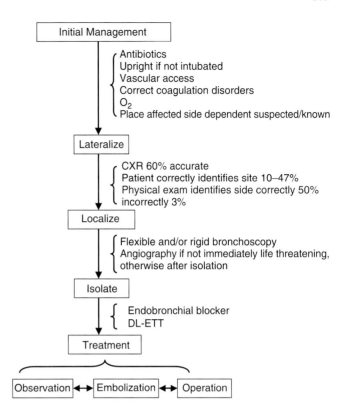

FIGURE 24.10. Rough schema for the initial management of massive hemoptysis.

to identify the site of bleeding than if performed later, for both rigid and flexible bronchoscopy. Rigid bronchoscopy has been able to identify the source of bleeding in up to 86% of cases when performed within 48 hours compared with 52% when performed later. Flexible bronchoscopy success rates range from 34% to 93% success rates with early intervention as opposed to 11% to 50% with later procedures.[101] Even when angioembolization control of the hemorrhage is being considered, bronchoscopic localization or even lateralization of the bleeding site may ultimately facilitate the angiographer's efforts to localize the feeding vessel(s). Rigid and flexible bronchoscopy are complimentary. Rigid scopes have better ability to suction large quantities of liquid and clotted blood, to maintain and secure an airway, to provide ventilation continuously, and to provide more technical options, including the use of large forceps to facilitate clot debridement and tumor debulking.[97] Flexible bronchoscopy has become more acceptable as an initial procedure, particularly for patients who are already intubated.[99] The flexible scope has a greater ability to evaluate the peripheral airways. Limitations include decreased suction capability and visualization through the smaller port in some settings. Also in some settings the endotracheal tube may obscure the source of hemorrhage.

When both techniques are available, a reasonable approach to bronchoscopy may be, for patients who are hemodynamically stable, already intubated, and in the intensive care unit, to perform flexible bronchoscopy first while arranging for surgical consultation, evaluating coagulation factors, and obtaining blood products. For unstable patients or patients with ongoing severe bleeding, the primary emphasis should be on transferring the patient to the operating room as soon as possible, where both flexible and rigid bronchoscopy can be performed. The desire to perform a flexible bronchoscopy should never impede transfer to the operating room.

In the presence of massive hemorrhage, flexible bronchoscopy is insufficient to adequately clear the airway of blood and blood clots. Rigid bronchoscopy will permit both aggressive bronchial toilet and ventilation. Initial control may be obtained by using ice-saline lavage or dilute epinephrine. If these initial maneuvers are successful, but no definite site of bleeding has been identified, flexible bronchoscopy can then be used through the rigid bronchoscope to further examine the bleeding side down to the lobar or segmental level. If significant bleeding continues, the bleeding side/site should be isolated using endobronchial techniques.

Strategies to Prevent Further Airway Contamination

A simple method to prevent further airway contamination is to advance the uncut endotracheal tube into the airway of the unaffected lung. This may be difficult if the site of bleeding arises from the left lung, as advancing the endotracheal tube into the right main stem bronchus often results in occlusion of the right upper lobe. However, in critical situations this can be tried as a temporizing measure. This will provide for unilateral ventilation while preventing further aspiration of blood. It does not, however, provide a means of control.

Double-lumen tubes may also be utilized. Well positioned, they allow excellent isolation of both lungs and prevent asphyxiation. These, however, may be at times difficult to place and require expertise, particularly in an acute care setting when time is of the essence. Even if successfully placed, technical difficulties such as displacement can lead to further aspiration and death. Garzon and colleagues[98] described a series of 62 patients, in which four of seven patients managed with a double-lumen tube ultimately died as a consequence of intraoperative tube dislodgment with subsequent continued aspiration of the unaffected lung during surgery. This was in contrast to six patients managed with left main stem intubation with a single-lumen tube and six further patients managed by single-lumen intubation coupled with balloon blockade of the left lung, none of whom died from aspiration.[98] Another drawback of double-lumen intubation relates to

the small caliber of each limb of the endotracheal tube which does not permit passage of bronchoscopes of adequate sizes to allow aspiration/toilet of the bleeding airway under direct vision. In this circumstance, one has to resort to "blind" catheter aspiration. The double-lumen tube is ideally utilized at the time of planned surgical resection.

Endobronchial blockers can be placed easily in the main bronchi or bronchus intermedius, although occasionally the individual anatomy of the patient will allow more precise control, such as into the orifice of the left lower, left upper, or right upper lobes. Not only will this approach prevent further aspiration of blood, but it also allows easier ventilation and further bronchoscopic assessment and toilet through the endotracheal tube. Inflation of the tracheal cuff helps secure the blocker in position against the tracheal wall, but additional fixation is obtained by tying the blocker to the secured endotracheal tube. A size 8 Fr Fogarty® blocker is usually needed to occlude the main airways. Smaller 4 Fr catheters are preferable for more selective occlusion at the lobar or segmental level. Recently, there have been bronchial blockers designed to be placed through an endotracheal tube, using a side port attachment and loop so that the blocker can be advanced and repositioned as needed. This form also has the ability to suction or irrigate through the blocker.

Endobronchial tamponade may by itself suffice to control bleeding.[103] The catheter is left inflated for 24 hours while coagulation parameters are corrected and the patient's condition is stabilized. The balloon is then deflated under bronchoscopic vision. If no further bleeding occurs, it is left in situ and deflated for an additional 24 hours. If there is no further bleeding, the catheter can be removed. Prolonged use of endobronchial blockers or double-lumen tubes may be associated with critical ischemia or obstructive pneumonitis. Antibiotic coverage should be provided.

Diffuse Parenchymal Bleeding

Rarely, the source of bleeding is diffuse, bilateral alveolar hemorrhage. In this setting, lung isolation is not sufficient. Bronchoscopy can confirm the bilateral nature of the hemorrhage and clear the airway of gross blood clots, which may allow some decrease in bleeding. Anecdotally applying increased positive end-expiratory pressure of 10 to 20 cm H_2O has resulted in diminishing bleeding until systemic therapy can be effective.

Subsequent Treatment

In the setting of massive hemoptysis, usually additional interventions are required after isolation. These can include topical or systemic agents (Table 24.9).[101,104] In

TABLE 24.9. Adjunctive pharmacological treatments of hemoptysis.

Topical
- Iced saline lavage → 50 mL aliquots at 4°C
- Topical epinephrine → 0.2 mL 1 : 1,000 in 500 mL normal saline
- Topical thrombin ± fibrinogen

Systemic
- Vasopressin → 0.2–0.4 U/min
- Tranexamic acid
- Steroids/cytotoxic agents/plasmapheresis → for autoimmune disorders
- Danazol → for catamenial hemoptysis

most cases the issue will be timing of angioembolization and whether or not surgical intervention, including resection, will be needed.

Angioembolization

Angiography can be used as both a diagnostic and a therapeutic tool.[105,106] Practically, it is much more efficient if the likely bleeding site has been localized before the study at bronchoscopy or by plain radiographs. A flush aortogram is first obtained to determine the number, location, and size of the bronchial arteries. There are a variety of bronchial artery anatomic variations. Most frequently, the bronchial arteries originate from the thoracic aorta between T3–T8, usually T5–T6. The three most common patterns are (1) a single left and right bronchial artery (30.5%), (2) a single right bronchial with an additional common trunk from which both a right and left bronchial arise (25%), and (3) two left bronchial arteries and a right intercostal origin to a right bronchial artery (12.5%).[99] If the bleeding site is from an upper lobe, the ipsilateral subclavian artery, internal thoracic, and at times intercostal arteries may also need to be studied because nonbronchial artery systemic collaterals exist in up to 45% of cases. This is particularly important when pleural thickening, indicating inflammation and a possible site of collateralization, is present.

Before embolization can be performed, digital subtraction angiography is used to determine whether or not a spinal arterial branch arises from the involved bronchial artery or arteries. If embolization can be carried out well distal to the spinal artery, embolization may still be feasible. Embolization can be performed using a variety of substances, but polyvinyl alcohol (350 to 590 μm) or gelfoam is preferred by most authors because these materials occlude neither the access vessel nor the smallest distal arterioles, which might lead to tissue infarction. Larger coils and detachable balloon, not only are associated with distal collateralization but, in the event that rebleeding occurs, appear to prevent reaccessing the target vessels. If a bleeding source cannot be iden-

tified or suspected, then a pulmonary angiogram will be required, especially if tuberculosis, other cavitary lesions, or a pulmonary arteriovenous malformation is suspected. The pulmonary artery is identified as the source of massive hemoptysis in only 8% of cases.

The initial success rates range from approximately 60% to 100%. Recurrent bleeding occurs in 20% to 30% of cases. Possible reasons for recurrence include the following:

1. Recanulization (usually between 2 and 7 months)
2. Increased blood flow via pulmonary artery–bronchial fistula
3. Diffuse systemic collaterals
4. Subsequent erosion of necrotizing inflammation into the pulmonary artery

Repeated procedures directed at the initial bronchial bleeding source or associated collaterals may increase the success rate in selected cases. Recurrent bleeding by 1 year occurs in 20% to 46% of patients, but usually is not massive. By 3 to 5 years, recurrent bleed rates are reported to be 23%.

Whether or not embolization should be accepted as definitive therapy depends on the underlying circumstances. Most critically ill patients have multiple problems, and embolization, with or without temporary airway control, may be the best therapy to allow improvement. However, patients with isolated lesions at high risk of rebleed (such as cavitary lesions or localized lung necrosis) may be better served with early resection when they have been stabilized.

Surgical Versus Medical Therapy for Massive Hemoptysis

Surgical intervention may be required to manage a specific large vessel bleed (such as tracheoinnominate artery fistula), or if there is a localized airway or parenchymal source that is resectable. Overall mortality rate in the setting of surgical resection (up to 50%) is somewhat lower than the maximum mortality described with medical management (up to 86%), but this probably reflects a degree of bias, as many of the medically managed patients were not considered surgical candidates because of extensive underlying disease processes.[107] If bleeding can be controlled and the patient stabilized, the mortality rate associated with surgery can be reduced to approximately 20%. In the acute setting, assuming that the patient is an operative candidate, surgery should be considered if there is ongoing bleeding despite airway control and embolization; if embolization is not technically possible; if bleeding recurs after embolization; and/or if a lesion is noted that has a high likelihood of rebleeding. Surgery is contraindicated if the underlying etiology is diffuse (such as bilateral necrotizing pneumonia) or if prebleed lung function is severely compromised ($FEV_1 < 1.0 L$).

In summary, airway hemorrhage is a potentially rapidly fatal condition. Death may occur within minutes from asphyxiation before control can be achieved. The primary prognostic factors are the rate of bleeding and the underlying cardiopulmonary status of the patient. Bronchoscopy is central to management, but the goals differ depending on circumstances. For stable patients with minimal hemoptysis, bronchoscopy can be used to diagnose the cause and to be the primary treatment modality. In the setting of massive and/or life-threatening bleeding, bronchoscopy is primarily performed to maintain ventilation and direct endobronchial blockade. Although flexible bronchoscopy is an acceptable mode initially, there should be no delay in performing rigid bronchoscopy when it becomes apparent that bleeding is too vigorous to permit successful airway exploration with the smaller flexible instrument. Once isolation of bleeding has been achieved, the choice needs to be made between embolization and surgical resection.

Tracheoinnominate Artery Fistula

Although not strictly a "parenchymal" problem, tracheoinnominate artery fistula (TIF) deserves to be included in the discussion of acute care lung surgery because it is as an important consideration for hemoptysis and because most patients requiring a tracheostomy do so because of underlying lung pathology. The seriousness of this feared complication of tracheostomy is the high mortality rate (87.6%) if it develops. Tracheoinnominate artery fistula arises as a consequence of proximity between the tube and the artery (below the fourth ring or high riding artery) or of pressure necrosis by the cuff. Tracheal capillary pressure ranges between 20 and 30 mm Hg, and tracheal wall circulation is impaired with cuff pressures at 22 mm Hg and totally obstructed at pressures of 37 mm Hg. High-volume low-pressure tracheal cuffs with cuff pressures <20 mm. Hg help reduce the risk. A useful adjunct to improve the tracheal blood supply is intermittent cuff deflation. However, despite these maneuvers to prevent tracheal wall necrosis, the ventilation pressures in some patients may necessitate a cuff pressure higher than that which is recommended simply to prevent cuff leak during the inspiratory phase.

Recognition and Initial Management

The only survivors (12.4%) are those with prompt diagnosis and treatment. Tracheoinnominate artery fistula has been reported as early as 30 hours to as late as 7 months, but 75% occur within 2 weeks of the tracheostomy. The two specific early warning signs are minimal tracheal

bleeding (herald bleeding) and pulsations of the tracheostomy tube. Approximately 50% of patients with TIF have a minor bleed that stops spontaneously; this is usually followed if untreated by exsanguinating tracheal bleeding within the next 2 days if left untreated. Tracheostomy tube pulsations occur in a minority of patients (5%) with TIF; furthermore, the sensitivity of this sign as a diagnostic criterion for TIF is likely very low.

Once the diagnosis is suspected immediate steps should be instituted to confirm or deny the diagnosis. If the hemorrhage is moderate to massive and the diagnosis is clinically suspected, then temporary control may be achieved by overdistension of the tracheostomy cuff. If this is unsuccessful, the tracheostomy tube should be replaced with an oral endotracheal tube whose cuff is below the site of the fistula. Removal of the tracheostomy tube and anterior digital compression of the innominate artery against the posterior surface of the sternum accomplish control of the hemorrhage. Once the airway and hemorrhage are controlled, the airway must be suctioned free of blood followed by immediate surgical exploration in the operating room.

In the more common scenario, tracheal bleeding is noticed that arouses the suspicion of TIF. However, there are many other causes of tracheal bleeding, ranging from stoma capillary erosions and inadequate posttracheostomy hemostasis (particularly in the presence of hemostasis disorders) to pulmonary or bronchial pathology as a cause of the bleeding. The dilemma here is that an accurate and prompt diagnosis of TIF is required before surgical exploration; clinical suspicion alone does not warrant a sternotomy, and delaying the diagnosis can be catastrophic. Investigation by angiography is both time consuming and ineffectual; the best test for TIF is intraoperative bronchoscopy, which should be performed in the operating room in order to institute immediate treatment, if the suspicion is confirmed. After general anesthesia is accomplished, orotracheal intubation is performed, leaving the endotracheal tube above the still indwelling tracheostomy tube. Flexible bronchoscopy is then performed through the tracheostomy tube, which is then gently removed, allowing for immediate bronchoscopic inspection of the anterior tracheal wall. If bleeding commences with removal of the tracheostomy tube or a fistula is visualized on bronchoscopy, the orotracheal tube is quickly advanced and a sternotomy is quickly performed.

Operative Repair

Surgical exploration is performed through a sternotomy, which provides immediate exposure for control of both the innominate artery and the trachea. Most authors do not recommend arterial grafting or repair because the risk of rebleed appears to outweigh the risk of neurologic damage among survivors of the initial operation. Most authors recommend excision of the area of the artery involved with the fistula and oversewing or stapling of the distal arterial ends, which should then be covered with healthy surrounding soft tissue. The tracheal fistula will usually heal by secondary intention, especially if also covered with healthy tissue. A low-lying stoma should quickly close with the assistance of an orotracheal tube; any subsequent tracheal surgery will depend on the recovery of the patient but should be deferred at least until adequate postoperative evaluation of the patient has been accomplished. Tracheoinnominate artery fistula is associated with a preoperative mortality rate of 32%, intraoperative exsanguination rate of 3%, and postoperative rebleeding leading to death in 19%. A further 19% of patients following successful surgical treatment of TIF will die of associated intensive care unit medical problems leading to an overall mortality rate of 73%.

In summary, TIF is an uncommon problem today because of recognition and prevention of the factors leading to the development of this life-threatening problem. Early diagnosis based on clinical suspicions with appropriate investigation and prompt and definitive surgical treatment is the only hope for a successful outcome for this problem.

Pulmonary Artery Catheter-Induced Hemoptysis

Pulmonary artery laceration is estimated to occur in 0.03% to 0.125% of all PA catheterizations. Most of the tears of the PA occur on the right side in the lower or middle lobe branches (93% of cases). Early mortality rates range from 41% to 70%. The tear is usually associated with an acute episode of massive hemoptysis or intrapleural hemorrhage. Late deaths have been reported from false aneurysms. These false aneurysms of the PA are clinically silent in 50% of cases; however 90% are visible on a plain chest x-rays.

Etiology

There are two situations leading to PA rupture from PA catheters: the operating room in preparation for or during cardiopulmonary bypass and in the intensive care unit during hemodynamic monitoring. In both scenarios the PA catheter is used for relatively sick patients, and the high mortality rate may in part stem from the compromised state of the patient on top of the pulmonary or circulatory consequences of the hemorrhage. The mechanism for PA rupture is the same in both situations: catheter perforation of the PA either by the tip of the catheter piercing the arterial wall or by balloon rupture

of the artery. Predisposing risk factors are old age and PA hypertension (both of which are associated with vessel wall fragility) and hypothermia, which can stiffen the catheter tips. Collapse of the lung, such as occurs with a pneumothorax in the ICU setting, or going on bypass in the operative setting have also been implicated.

Management

The management of a PA catheter tear in the operating room is often different from such an event occurring in the intensive care unit. Occasionally, minor hemoptysis occurs in preparation for cardiac surgery with positioning of the PA catheter. If possible the operation should be postponed and pulmonary angiography should be performed to determine if the bleeding is contained or if a false aneurysm has been created. The PA catheter should be deflated and retracted; further inflation of the balloon is thought to worsen the damage. If there is a critical need for bypass surgery to proceed or if the procedure has "gone past the point of no return" (e.g., the mammary has been harvested) then preparations for control of the PA should be anticipated with the understanding that there is a much higher mortality rate associated with this option. To some extent management is simplified, as bronchoscopy and lung isolation techniques can be performed while on bypass. The pleura should be opened to exclude free intrathoracic hemorrhage.

A PA catheter tear usually manifests itself during or shortly after weaning from bypass. Commonly there is only extensive parenchymal bleeding, which if controlled (visceral pleura intact) can permit nonoperative management.

If there is intrapleural rupture, the surgical options for the pulmonary artery are repair, resection of a proximal occluding vascular loop, or use of extracorporeal life support in the intensive care unit. As the arterial injury commonly occurs in the distal arterial branches, it is unlikely that the site can be found amid the parenchymal hematoma, precluding repair. Lung resection for these critically ill patients is best avoided. Central arterial injuries, which are uncommon, can be dealt with by repair on bypass. Surgical assessment of PA catheter tears on bypass is important, as recurrent pulmonary hemorrhage occurs in 45% of patients in the intensive care unit; this is massive in 89% and fatal in 78%.

Patients with PA catheter tears occurring in the intensive care unit need to be immediately assessed for a hemothorax. There have been occasional reports of pulling the PA catheter back and reinflating the balloon to obtain temporary proximal control, but this should be done only if the situation is extreme as the location of the catheter cannot be reliably ascertained and the tear may be aggravated. There is no survival without a thoracotomy in patients with PA catheter tears and a hemothorax. In the absence of a hemothorax, and for a stable patient, ventilation and positive end-expiratory pressure can be used to control bleeding. For all patients with suspected or documented PA catheter injuries, a follow-up angiogram should be performed as false aneurysms can occur, and some are effectively treated by embolization.

In conclusion, PA catheter-induced trauma carries a significant immediate mortality and, in the presence of a false aneurysm, a potential for delayed mortality. Hemoptysis induced by PA catheter insertion before commencement of a cardiac operation mandates postponement of the operation when possible. Hemoptysis presenting during surgery should be assessed for intrapleural bleeding; in the absence of hemothorax positive pressure ventilation and lung isolation may help to avoid lung resection.

Superior Vena Cava Syndrome

Depending upon the acuity, and thus on the development of collaterals, occlusion of the superior vena cava can lead to upper extremity and neck edema, loss of the airway, and cerebral edema. There are roughly four clinical scenarios to consider: malignancy, chronic mediastinal fibrosis, thrombosis (often related to dialysis), and traumatic asphyxia. The primary management is supportive, but interventions can include thrombolysis, stent grafting, bypass, or resection, depending on the setting.

Presentation

Classic findings include upper extremity and facial plethora and swelling, often with a demarcation line across the mid to upper chest. Marked superficial venous engorgement can also be prominent. In cases where there has not be time to develop collaterals, patients may present with stridor, eye edema, and headaches or dizziness suggesting increased intracranial pressure. Usually symptoms are worse when supine.

Initial Management

Patients should be positioned upright. If there is evidence of airway compromise and/or cerebral edema, steroids should be administered. Signs of impending airway loss require intubation, which may be safer in the operating room in case surgical airway or rigid bronchoscopy is required.

Computed tomography angiography or venogram can both confirm the diagnosis and identify the level of occlusion. Patients in whom the azygous vein is patent often decompress the superior vena cava, leading to less significant symptoms.

Treatment

The most common etiology is cancer, primarily non-Hodgkin's lymphoma and small cell lung cancer.[108] Most patients are not operative candidates, and the mainstay of treatment, once the diagnosis has been established, is radiation therapy, with/or without concurrent chemotherapy.[109] An uncommon etiology that can be confused with small cell cancer in particular is a substernal goiter.[110,111] A small subset of patients may have evidence of local invasion of the superior vena cava without evidence of mediastinal lymph node metastases or extrathoracic spread. These patients may, if they respond to induction therapy, be considered for lung resection in conjunction with partial or complete resection of the adherent superior vena cava.[112,113] Stent grafting can also be an option.[114-116]

Chronic fibrosing mediastinitis usually does not present with acute superior vena cava syndrome unless there has been acute thrombosis affecting the venous collaterals. Because chronic fibrosing mediastinitis is predominantly caused by fungal infection, surgery has little role as it is usually impossible to "debulk" the mediastinum. Occasionally mediastinal lymphoma can present in a similar fashion, and the primary role of surgery is to obtain a tissue diagnosis. Options include anticoagulation and possibly superior caval stenting.[114] Superior vena caval thrombosis for patients with dialysis catheters can be treated in a similar fashion.

The management of traumatic asphyxia is supportive, including elevation of the head, steroid administration, and intubation if there is airway compromise. Associated injuries such as cardiac rupture and contusion need to be ruled out.

If surgery is contemplated, bypass grafts from the innominate vein or jugular to the right atrium can be performed with an externally supported graft, femoral vein graft, a saphenous vein graft or a spiral vein graft.[117] A vein has the advantage of possibly a lower thrombosis rate but, more importantly, a higher recanulization rate than artificial material.

In conclusion, acute care surgery of the lung requires a comprehensive consideration of the state of the entire parenchyma, the pleural space, and the overall physiology of the patient. There must be a plan for the airway both acutely and postoperatively. The surgeon must be prepared for repeated explorations and anticipate postoperative complications. Ultimately, whatever the indications for surgery, the ideal goal is to achieve a fully expanded lung and completely drained pleural space. Although this is somewhat trite, in practice it can be difficult to achieve unless proper planning is employed.

Critique

Retained hemothorax, detectable on plain chest radiograph, despite tube thoracostomy, is at increased risk of developing empyema. Video-assisted thoracic surgery (VATS) is an accepted method of draining and washing out the chest, although there is a direct correlation between the timing of intervention and success. This should not be performed in patients with evidence of massive bleeding or instability. The main limitation of VATS is that endobronchial separation of the lungs is required as well and extensive pleural symphysis can prevent adequate visualization. Using "rigid pleuroscopy" (e.g., with a mediastinoscope) or miniaccess thoracotomy ports can overcome these limitations, but if there is evidence of dense loculations with early infection, there should be no hesitation to convert to thoracotomy if required.

Answer (C)

References

1. Slinger PD. Fiberoptic bronchoscopic positioning of double-lumen tubes. J Cardiothorac Anesth 1989; 3:486–496.
2. Karmy-Jones R, Vallieres E, Kralovich K, et al. A comparison of rigid -v- video thoracoscopy in the management of chest trauma. Injury 1998; 29:655–659.
3. Brusov PG, Kuritsyn AN, Urazovsky NY, Tariverdiev ML. Operative videothoracoscopy in the surgical treatment of penetrating firearms wounds of the chest. Mil Med 1998; 163:603–607.
4. Schermer CR, Matteson BD, Demarest GB 3rd, Albrecht RM, Davis VH. A prospective evaluation of video-assisted thoracic surgery for persistent air leak due to trauma. Am J Surg 1999; 177:480–484.
5. Kirsh MM, Orringer MB, Behrendt DM, Sloan H. Management of tracheobronchial disruption secondary to nonpenetrating trauma. Ann Thorac Surg 1976; 22:93–101.
6. Kiser AC, O'Brien SM, Detterbeck FC. Blunt tracheobronchial injuries: treatment and outcomes. Ann Thorac Surg 2001; 71:2059–2065.
7. Velly JF, Martigne C, Moreau JM, Dubrez J, Kerdi S, Couraud L. Post traumatic tracheobronchial lesions. A follow-up study of 47 cases. Eur J Cardiothorac Surg 1991; 5:352–355.
8. Taskinen SO, Salo JA, Halttunen PE, Sovijarvi AR. Tracheobronchial rupture due to blunt chest trauma: a follow-up study. Ann Thorac Surg 1989; 48:846–849.
9. Jones WS, Mavroudis C, Richardson JD, Gray LA Jr, Howe WR. Management of tracheobronchial disruption resulting from blunt trauma. Surgery 1984; 95:319–323.
10. Sattler S, Canty TG Jr, Mulligan MS, et al. Chronic traumatic and congenital diaphragmatic hernias: presentation and surgical management. Can Respir J 2002; 9:135–139.
11. Wintermark M, Schnyder P, Wicky S. Blunt traumatic rupture of a mainstem bronchus: spiral CT demonstration of the "fallen lung" sign. Eur Radiol 2001; 11:409–411.
12. Ferretti GR, Thony F, Bosson JL, Pison C, Arbib F, Coulomb M. Benign abnormalities and carcinoid tumors of the central airways: diagnostic impact of CT bronchography. AJR Am J Roentgenol 2000; 174:1307–1313.
13. Kawamoto S, Yuasa M, Tsukuda S, Heshiki A. Bronchial atresia: three-dimensional CT bronchography using volume rendering technique. Radiat Med 2001; 19:107–110.
14. Wood D. Tracheobronchial trauma. In Karmy-Joes R, Nathens A, Stern E, eds. Thoracic Trauma and Critical Care. Boston: Kluwer Academic Publishers, 2002: 109–122.
15. Rossbach MM, Johnson SB, Gomez MA, Sako EY, Miller OL, Calhoon JH. Management of major tracheobronchial injuries: a 28-year experience. Ann Thorac Surg 1998; 65:182–186.
16. Crouch RD, Nelson LE, Hawley PC, Frank DA, Williams TE Jr. Onlay patch repair of tracheobronchial rupture. Ann Thorac Surg 1997; 64:1158–1160.
17. Hira HS, Kumar D, Sondhi V, Kumar J, Jain SK. Bronchial stenosis after blunt chest trauma. J Assoc Physicians India 2002; 50:1189–1191.
18. Pilcher JA Jr, Ishitani MB, Rodgers BM. Left upper lobe bronchus reimplantation for nonpenetrating thoracic trauma. Ann Thorac Surg 2000; 69:273–275.
19. Carrillo EH, Block EF, Zeppa R, Sosa JL. Urgent lobectomy and pneumonectomy. Eur J Emerg Med 1994; 1:126–130.
20. Asensio JA, Demetriades D, Berne JD, et al. Stapled pulmonary tractotomy: a rapid way to control hemorrhage in penetrating pulmonary injuries. J Am Coll Surg 1997; 185:486–487.
21. Zakharia AT. Cardiovascular and thoracic battle injuries in the Lebanon War. Analysis of 3,000 personal cases. J Thorac Cardiovasc Surg 1985; 89:723–733.
22. Biocina B, Sutlic Z, Husedzinovic I, et al. Penetrating cardiothoracic war wounds. Eur J Cardiothorac Surg 1997; 11:399–405.
23. Robison PD, Harman PK, Trinkle JK, Grover FL. Management of penetrating lung injuries in civilian practice. J Thorac Cardiovasc Surg 1988; 95:184–190.
24. Stewart KC, Urschel JD, Nakai SS, Gelfand ET, Hamilton SM. Pulmonary resection for lung trauma. Ann Thorac Surg 1997; 63:1587–1588.
25. Stanic V. The advantages of limited resection vs. suture in the primary management of penetrating lung war wounds. Vojnosanit Pregl 1998; 55:583–590.
26. Cothren C, Moore EE, Biffl WL, Franciose RJ, Offner PJ, Burch JM. Lung-sparing techniques are associated with improved outcome compared with anatomic resection for severe lung injuries. J Trauma 2002; 53:483–487.
27. Wall MJ Jr, Soltero E. Damage control for thoracic injuries. Surg Clin North Am 1997; 77:863–878.
28. Wall MJ Jr, Villavicencio RT, Miller CC 3rd, et al. Pulmonary tractotomy as an abbreviated thoracotomy technique. J Trauma 1998; 45:1015–1023.
29. Karmy-Jones R, Jurkovich GJ, Shatz DV, et al. Management of traumatic lung injury: a Western Trauma

Association Multicenter review. J Trauma 2001; 51:1049–1053.

30. Gasparri M, Karmy-Jones R, Kralovich KA, Patton JH Jr, Arbabi S. Pulmonary tractotomy versus lung resection: viable options in penetrating lung injury. J Trauma 2001; 51:1092–1097.

31. Wagner JW, Obeid FN, Karmy-Jones RC, Casey GD, Sorensen VJ, Horst HM. Trauma pneumonectomy revisited: the role of simultaneously stapled pneumonectomy. J Trauma 1996; 40:590–594.

32. Geiger JP, Fischer RP, Guernsey JM, Thomas DE. Pulmonary resection: the treatment of choice for pulmonary contusion due to high velocity thoracic wounds. US Army Vietnam Med Bull 1971.

33. Kortbeek JB, Clark JA, Carraway RC. Conservative management of a pulmonary artery bullet embolism: case report and review of the literature. J Trauma 1992; 33:906–908.

34. Kortbeek JB, Kappor D, Karmy-Jones R. Thoracic missile emboli and retained bullets. In Karmy-Jones R, Nathens AB, Stern E, eds. Thoracic Trauma and Critical Care. Boston: Kluwer Medical Publishers, 2002: 151–158.

35. Vogt-Moykopf I, Krumhaar D. Treatment of intrapulmonary shell fragments. Surg Gynecol Obstet 1966; 123:1233–1236.

36. Laustela E. Thorax traumatology. Acta Chir Scand 1964; 332(Suppl):17.

37. Boyd AD, Glassman LR. Trauma to the lung. Chest Surg Clin North Am 1997; 7:263–284.

38. Eddy AC, Luna GK, Copass M. Empyema thoracis in patients undergoing emergent closed tube thoracostomy for thoracic trauma. Am J Surg 1989; 157:494–497.

39. Coselli JS, Mattox KL, Beall AC Jr. Reevaluation of early evacuation of clotted hemothorax. Am J Surg 1984; 148: 786–790.

40. Rosenblatt M, Lemer J, Best LA, Peleg H. Thoracic wounds in Israeli battle casualties during the 1982 evacuation of wounded from Lebanon. J Trauma 1985; 25:350–354.

41. Velmahos GC, Demetriades D, Chan L, et al. Predicting the need for thoracoscopic evacuation of residual traumatic hemothorax: chest radiograph is insufficient. J Trauma 1999; 46:65–70.

42. Karmy-Jones R, Sorenson V, Horst HM, Lewis JW Jr, Rubinfeld I. Rigid thorascopic debridement and continuous pleural irrigation in the management of empyema. Chest 1997; 111:272–274.

43. Inci I, Ozcelik C, Ulku R, Tuna A, Eren N. Intrapleural fibrinolytic treatment of traumatic clotted hemothorax. Chest 1998; 114:160–165.

44. Vassiliu P, Velmahos GC, Toutouzas KG. Timing, safety, and efficacy of thoracoscopic evacuation of undrained post-traumatic hemothorax. Am Surg 2001; 67:1165–1169.

45. Meyer DM, Jessen ME, Wait MA, Estrera AS. Early evacuation of traumatic retained hemothoraces using thoracoscopy: a prospective, randomized trial. Ann Thorac Surg 1997; 64:1396–1401.

46. The urokinase pulmonary embolism trial. A national cooperative study. Circulation 1973; 47:II1–108.

47. Goldhaber SZ. Pulmonary embolism. N Engl J Med 1998; 339:93–104.

48. Karmy-Jones R, Wilson M, Cornejo C, Gibson K, Engrav L, Meissner M. Surgical management of cardiac arrest caused by massive pulmonary embolism in trauma patients. J Trauma 2000; 48:519–520.

49. McIntyre KM, Sasahara AA. The hemodynamic response to pulmonary embolism in patients without prior cardiopulmonary disease. Am J Cardiol 1971; 28:288–294.

50. Worsley DF, Alavi A, Aronchick JM, Chen JT, Greenspan RH, Ravin CE. Chest radiographic findings in patients with acute pulmonary embolism: observations from the PIOPED study. Radiology 1993; 189:133–136.

51. Pruszczyk P, Torbicki A, Kuch-Wocial A, Szulc M, Pacho R. Diagnostic value of transoesophageal echocardiography in suspected haemodynamically significant pulmonary embolism. Heart 2001; 85:628–634.

52. Vieillard-Baron A, Qanadli SD, Antakly Y, et al. Transesophageal echocardiography for the diagnosis of pulmonary embolism with acute cor pulmonale: a comparison with radiological procedures. Intensive Care Med 1998; 24:429–433.

53. Qanadli SD, El Hajjam M, Vieillard-Baron A, et al. New CT index to quantify arterial obstruction in pulmonary embolism: comparison with angiographic index and echocardiography. AJR Am J Roentgenol 2001; 176:1415–1420.

54. Greenspan RH. Pulmonary angiography and the diagnosis of pulmonary embolism. Prog Cardiovasc Dis 1994; 37:93–105.

55. Blachere H, Latrabe V, Montaudon M, et al. Pulmonary embolism revealed on helical CT angiography: comparison with ventilation-perfusion radionuclide lung scanning. AJR Am J Roentgenol 2000; 174:1041–1047.

56. Harvey RT, Gefter WB, Hrung JM, Langlotz CP. Accuracy of CT angiography versus pulmonary angiography in the diagnosis of acute pulmonary embolism: evaluation of the literature with summary ROC curve analysis. Acad Radiol 2000; 7:786–797.

57. Remy-Jardin M, Tillie-Leblond I, Szapiro D, et al. CT angiography of pulmonary embolism in patients with underlying respiratory disease: impact of multislice CT on image quality and negative predictive value. Eur Radiol 2002; 12:1971–1978.

58. Hedegaard M, Lund O, Nielsen TT, Hansen HH, Albrechtsen O. [Aggressive treatment of acute pulmonary embolism. 132 consecutive patients treated with heparin, streptokinase or embolectomy, 1975–1987.] Ugeskr Laeger 1992; 154:2025–2030.

59. Glieca F, Santarelli P, Luciani N, et al. [What is the best treatment in massive pulmonary embolism: anticoagulants, thrombolytics or surgical embolectomy?] Minerva Cardioangiol 1990; 38:135–140.

60. Gamillscheg A, Nurnberg JH, Alexi-Meskishvili V, et al. Surgical emergency embolectomy for the treatment of fulminant pulmonary embolism in a preterm infant. J Pediatr Surg 1997; 32:1516–1518.

61. Sudo K, Ide H, Fujiki T, Tonari K, Nasu Y, Ikeda K. Pulmonary embolectomy for acute massive pulmonary

embolism under percutaneous cardiopulmonary support. J Cardiovasc Surg (Torino) 1999; 40:165–167.

62. Matis N, Groger A, Mayer N, Mohl W, Vecsei V. [Surgical embolectomy after reanimation in central pulmonary embolism.] Unfallchirurg 1999; 102:287–291.

63. Hsieh PC, Wang SS, Ko WJ, Han YY, Chu SH. Successful resuscitation of acute massive pulmonary embolism with extracorporeal membrane oxygenation and open embolectomy. Ann Thorac Surg 2001; 72:266–267.

64. Hirnle T, Oczko J, Wolan I, Muskala G, Michalak M. [Acute, massive pulmonary embolism treated with surgical embolectomy without cardio-pulmonary by-pass—a case report.] Kardiol Pol 2003; 58:481–483.

65. Meyer G, Diehl JL, Philippe B, Reynaud P, Sors H. [Pulmonary embolectomy in pulmonary embolism: surgery and endoluminal techniques.] Arch Mal Coeur Vaiss 1995; 88:1777–1780.

66. Carrillo EH, Schmacht DC, Gable DR, Spain DA, Richardson JD. Thoracoscopy in the management of post-traumatic persistent pneumothorax. J Am Coll Surg 1998; 186:636–640.

67. Cerfolio RJ, Bass CS, Pask AH, Katholi CR. Predictors and treatment of persistent air leaks. Ann Thorac Surg 2002; 73:1727–1731.

68. Hansson B, Jorens PG, van Schil P, van Kerckhoven W, van den Brande F, Eyskens E. Lung volume reduction surgery as an emergency and life-saving procedure. Eur Respir J 1997; 10:2650–2652.

69. Rice TW, Okereke IC, Blackstone EH. Persistent air-leak following pulmonary resection. Chest Surg Clin North Am 2002; 12:529–539.

70. Cerfolio RJ, Bass C, Katholi CR. Prospective randomized trial compares suction versus water seal for air leaks. Ann Thorac Surg 2001; 71:1613–1617.

71. Ayed AK. Suction versus water seal after thoracoscopy for primary spontaneous pneumothorax: prospective randomized study. Ann Thorac Surg 2003; 75:1593–1596.

72. Marshall MB, Deeb ME, Bleier JI, et al. Suction vs water seal after pulmonary resection: a randomized prospective study. Chest 2002; 121:831–835.

73. Aguilar MM, Battistella FD, Owings JT, Su T. Posttraumatic empyema. Risk factor analysis. Arch Surg 1997; 132:647–651.

74. Lemmer JH, Botham MJ, Orringer MB. Modern management of adult thoracic empyema. J Thorac Cardiovasc Surg 1985; 90:849–855.

75. Richardson JD, Carrillo E. Thoracic infection after trauma. Chest Surg Clin North Am 1997; 7:401–427.

76. Romanoff H. Prevention of infection in war chest injuries. Ann Surg 1975; 182:144–149.

77. Weissberg D, Refaely Y. Pleural empyema: 24-year experience. Ann Thorac Surg 1996; 62:1026–1029.

78. Robinson LA, Moulton AL, Fleming WH, Alonso A, Galbraith TA. Intrapleural fibrinolytic treatment of multiloculated thoracic empyemas. Ann Thorac Surg 1994; 57:803–814.

79. Wait MA, Sharma S, Hohn J, Dal Nogare A. A randomized trial of empyema therapy. Chest 1997; 111:1548–1551.

80. Deschamps C, Bernard A, Nichols FC 3rd, et al. Empyema and bronchopleural fistula after pneumonectomy: factors affecting incidence. Ann Thorac Surg 2001; 72:243–248.

81. Deschamps C, Allen MS, Miller DL, Nichols FC 3rd, Pairolero PC. Management of postpneumonectomy empyema and bronchopleural fistula. Semin Thorac Cardiovasc Surg 2001; 13:13–19.

82. Regnard JF, Alifano M, Puyo P, Fares E, Magdeleinat P, Levasseur P. Open window thoracostomy followed by intrathoracic flap transposition in the treatment of empyema complicating pulmonary resection. J Thorac Cardiovasc Surg 2000; 120:270–275.

83. Gharagozloo F, Trachiotis G, Wolfe A, DuBree KJ, Cox JL. Pleural space irrigation and modified Clagett procedure for the treatment of early postpneumonectomy empyema. J Thorac Cardiovasc Surg 1998; 116:943–948.

84. Regel G, Sturm JA, Neumann C, Schueler S, Tscherne H. Occlusion of bronchopleural fistula after lung injury—a new treatment by bronchoscopy. J Trauma 1989; 29:223–226.

85. de la Riviere AB, Defauw JJ, Knaepen PJ, van Swieten HA, Vanderschueren RC, van den Bosch JM. Transsternal closure of bronchopleural fistula after pneumonectomy. Ann Thorac Surg 1997; 64:954–959.

86. Karmy-Jones R, Vallieres E, Harrington R. Surgical management of necrotizing pneumonia. Clin Pulm Med 2003; 10:17–25.

87. Hoffer FA, Bloom DA, Colin AA, Fishman SJ. Lung abscess versus necrotizing pneumonia: implications for interventional therapy. Pediatr Radiol 1999; 29:87–91.

88. Reich JM. Pulmonary gangrene and the air crescent sign. Thorax 1993; 48:70–74.

89. Delarue NC, Pearson FG, Nelems JM, Cooper JD. Lung abscess: surgical implications. Can J Surg 1980; 23:297–302.

90. Curry CA, Fishman EK, Buckley JA. Pulmonary gangrene: radiological and pathologic correlation. South Med J 1998; 91:957–960.

91. Phillips LG, Rao KV. Gangrene of the lung. J Thorac Cardiovasc Surg 1989; 97:114–118.

92. Lesnitskii LS, Kostiuchenko AL, Tulupov AN. [Several problems of pathogenesis and treatment of pulmonary gangrene.] Grudn Khir 1989:39–44.

93. Refaely Y, Weissberg D. Gangrene of the lung: treatment in two stages. Ann Thorac Surg 1997; 64:970–974.

94. Estrera AS, Landay MJ, Grisham JM, Sinn DP, Platt MR. Descending necrotizing mediastinitis. Surg Gynecol Obstet 1983; 157:545–552.

95. Freeman RK, Vallieres E, Verrier ED, Karmy-Jones R, Wood DE. Descending necrotizing mediastinitis: an analysis of the effects of serial surgical debridement on patient mortality. J Thorac Cardiovasc Surg 2000; 119:260–267.

96. Corsten MJ, Shamji FM, Odell PF, et al. Optimal treatment of descending necrotising mediastinitis. Thorax 1997; 52:702–708.

97. Shamji FM, Vallieres E. Airway hemorrhage. Chest Surg Clin North Am 1991; 1:255–289.

98. Garzon AA, Cerruti MM, Golding ME. Exsanguinating hemoptysis. J Thorac Cardiovasc Surg 1982; 84:829–833.

99. Dweik RA, Stoller JK. Role of bronchoscopy in massive hemoptysis. Clin Chest Med 1999; 20:89–105.

100. Thompson AB, Teschler H, Rennard SI. Pathogenesis, evaluation, and therapy for massive hemoptysis. Clin Chest Med 1992; 13:69–82.

101. Karmy-Jones R, Cuschieri J, Vallieres E. Role of bronchoscopy in massive hemoptysis. Chest Surg Clin North Am 2001; 11:873–906.

102. Thomashow BM, Felton CP, Navarro C. Diffuse intrapulmonary hemorrhage, renal failure and a systemic vasculitis. A case report and review of the literature. Am J Med 1980; 68:299–304.

103. Swersky RB, Chang JB, Wisoff BG, Gorvoy J. Endobronchial balloon tamponade of hemoptysis in patients with cystic fibrosis. Ann Thorac Surg 1979; 27:262–264.

104. Tsukamoto T, Sasaki H, Nakamura H. Treatment of hemoptysis patients by thrombin and fibrinogen-thrombin infusion therapy using a fiberoptic bronchoscope. Chest 1989; 96:473–476.

105. White RI Jr. Bronchial artery embolotherapy for control of acute hemoptysis: analysis of outcome. Chest 1999; 115: 912–915.

106. Sundset A, Haanaes OC, Enge I. [Embolization of bronchial arteries in severe and recurrent hemoptysis.] Tidsskr Nor Laegeforen 1992; 112:2958–2962.

107. Garzon AA, Gourin A. Surgical management of massive hemoptysis. A ten-year experience. Ann Surg 1978; 187: 267–271.

108. Porte H, Metois D, Finzi L, et al. Superior vena cava syndrome of malignant origin. Which surgical procedure for which diagnosis? Eur J Cardiothorac Surg 2000; 17:384–388.

109. Varricchio C. Clinical management of superior vena cava syndrome. Heart Lung 1985; 14:411–416.

110. Dave ST, Kamath SK, Shetty AN, Naik LD. Anaesthesia management for subtotal thyroidectomy in a case of multinodular goitre with retrosternal extension and superior vena caval syndrome. J Postgrad Med 2001; 47:219.

111. Wesseling GJ, van den Berg BW, Kortlandt JG, Greve LH, Ten Velde GP. Superior vena caval syndrome due to substernal goitre. Eur Respir J 1988; 1:666–669.

112. Spaggiari L, Thomas P, Magdeleinat P, et al. Superior vena cava resection with prosthetic replacement for non-small cell lung cancer: long-term results of a multicentric study. Eur J Cardiothorac Surg 2002; 21:1080–1086.

113. Tagawa T, Uchiyama Y, Yamaoka N, Yamamoto S, Taguchi T. [Surgical treatment of lung cancer with combined resection of the aorta or superior vena cava.] Kyobu Geka 1999; 52:35–40.

114. de Gregorio Ariza MA, Gamboa P, Gimeno MJ, et al. Percutaneous treatment of superior vena cava syndrome using metallic stents. Eur Radiol 2003; 13:853–862.

115. Oudkerk M, Kuijpers TJ, Schmitz PI, Loosveld O, de Wit R. Self-expanding metal stents for palliative treatment of superior vena caval syndrome. Cardiovasc Intervent Radiol 1996; 19:146–151.

116. Wilkinson P, MacMahon J, Johnston L. Stenting and superior vena caval syndrome. Ir J Med Sci 1995; 164:128–131.

117. Gladstone DJ, Pillai R, Paneth M, Lincoln JC. Relief of superior vena caval syndrome with autologous femoral vein used as a bypass graft. J Thorac Cardiovasc Surg 1985; 89:750–752.

25
Heart

Matthew S. Slater

Case Scenario

Seven days after undergoing a thoracotomy and repair of a cardiac laceration, a 22-year-old patient develops tachycardia, substernal chest pain (worse on inspiration) and fatigue. He is afebrile and hemodynamically stable. On auscultation, a pericardial friction rub is discovered. Electrocardiography demonstrates ST segment elevation throughout the pericardium. Helical computed tomography scan shows no evidence of a pulmonary embolism. Chest x-ray reveals expanded bilateral lungs and a normal cardiac silhouette. Which of the following would be the most appropriate management approach?

(A) Administration of a nonsteroidal antiinflammatory agent
(B) Pericardiocentesis
(C) Reexploration
(D) Insertion of a pulmonary artery catheter
(E) Cardiac catheterization

Cardiac trauma, particularly penetrating cardiac trauma, represents an opportunity for salvage of critically injured patients. Achieving good outcomes in this patient group requires accurate diagnosis and effective interventions, all in a timely fashion. This was recognized as early as 1896 when Ludwig Van Rehn first repaired a cardiac injury. This chapter provides an overview of cardiac trauma, both blunt and penetrating. Although the epidemiology and pathophysiology of cardiac injury are reviewed, the primary focus of this chapter is to provide clinically useful information for the optimal diagnosis and treatment of these patients.

The number and distribution of cardiac injuries are reflections of the societies in which they occur. With the increasing prevalence of interpersonal violence and the availability of handguns, both the incidence and the lethality of penetrating cardiac injuries have escalated. Additionally, the increased number of endovascular procedures being performed has brought with it a commensurate increase in associated complications. Most of these complications are related to coronary angiography and to coronary stenting, but even noncardiac endovascular procedures may produce injuries to the heart or great vessels within the pericardium. Finally, the rapid growth in the number of motor vehicles has increased both the incidence and severity of blunt thoracic trauma as well. Clearly, skills to diagnose and manage patients with cardiac trauma are essential for providers caring for modern trauma patients.

Penetrating Cardiac Injury

The reported incidence, prevalence, and survival rates following penetrating cardiac injuries vary widely because of differences in study design (autopsy, hospital admission) and location (urban vs. rural, industrialized nation vs. third world country). In a study of 1,198 cases of penetrating cardiac injuries in Durban, South Africa, Campbell and colleagues[1] noted a lethality of 94%, with only a small proportion of patients reaching the hospital alive. Of those who reached the hospital alive, 50% survived. The mechanism of injury was relatively evenly distributed between stab wounds (697) and gunshot wounds (498), and the overwhelming majority of patients with firearm injuries did not reach the hospital alive. Sixty-six patients with stab wounds and four patients with gunshot wounds reached the hospital alive; none of the gunshot-wound patients survived.[1]

A larger study reviewed 20,181 consecutive trauma admissions to a single, urban, Level I trauma center and 6,492 medical examiners' reports from the same city over the same time period.[2] Rhee and colleagues[2] identified 212 penetrating cardiac injuries (1/100,000 person/year) and 1 cardiac injury patient per 210 admissions. The overall survival rate was 19% (9.7% for gunshot wounds and 32% for stab wounds). Most patients (54%) died at the scene. For the 96 patients transported to hospital, there was an overall survival rate of 43% (29% for gunshot wounds and 53% for stab wounds).

Penetrating injuries are most often (80%) confined to one cardiac chamber; injuries to multiple cardiac chambers are associated with mortality rates as high as 97%.[3,4] Most patients with penetrating cardiac trauma sustain their injuries from the front. For this reason, cardiac chambers that are most anterior (i.e., the right ventricle) are injured most frequently, and those that are most posterior (i.e., the left atrium) are injured least often. The right ventricle is injured more frequently than the left ventricle, and left ventricular injuries appear to be more lethal than right ventricular injuries, presumably because of the higher pressures encountered on the left side.[3] The right atrium is injured more frequently than the left. Less frequently injured are the pulmonary artery and the aorta.

Coronary artery injury is infrequently (6%–9%) observed in survivors of penetrating cardiac trauma.[3] This low incidence in survivors may be a reflection of the lethality (90%) of this injury.[5] The left anterior descending artery appears to be the most commonly injured in patients with penetrating cardiac trauma.[1] In addition to injuries to large coronary arteries, direct myocardial injury can occur as a sequela of penetrating injury. Myocardial injury has been detected with electrocardiography in up to 9% of patients with penetrating cardiac trauma.[6]

Missed injuries have significant consequences for all trauma patients, and those with cardiac injury are no exception. In a study by Campbell and colleagues,[1] 20% of patients who died following surgery were found to have a missed injury; in 11% the chamber thought to be injured at surgery was found to be misidentified. Although the vast majority of patients with significant penetrating cardiac injuries will present with cardiac tamponade (80%–90%), a small subset of patients will have delayed tamponade, which can become apparent hours to days after initial presentation.[7]

Injuries to intracardiac structures are less commonly encountered following penetrating cardiac trauma. Intraatrial and intraventricular septal defects are occasionally detected on follow-up echocardiography but are usually small and are well tolerated in the acute setting. The cardiac valves and the conduction system are infrequently injured but represent a potential site for missed injury. Presenti-Ross et al.[8] reported a 4.5% incidence of ventricular septal defects (VSD) following penetrating cardiac injury. Duque et al.[6] reported a 7.9% incidence of VSD and a 7.1% incidence of valvular lesions as well as complete (1.1%) and partial (4.9%) bundle branch block

in a cohort of penetrating cardiac injury survivors evaluated 1 year following injury. Repair of these infrequent sequelae from months to years after cardiac trauma has been reported. A high index of suspicion must be maintained to detect these occult injuries. An echocardiogram should be obtained in patients who have sustained full-thickness penetrating cardiac injury to exclude valvular or septal injury. Electrocardiograms (ECGs) should be obtained to evaluate for conduction abnormalities.

Diagnosis

Patients with penetrating cardiac injuries often present in extremis with a history of chest wall or upper abdominal stab wounds or missile injuries. However, some patients may enjoy a brief period of relative hemodynamic stability and then decompensate en route, on arrival at the emergency department, or shortly thereafter. Intubation and the vasorelaxation associated with anesthetic agents can precipitate hemodynamic collapse. Increases in blood pressure associated with resuscitation can renew intrapericardial bleeding, leading to tamponade and subsequent decompensation. For these reasons, the management of such patients hinges on rapid and accurate diagnosis followed by appropriate therapy.

Aside from a history of penetrating injury to the chest with guns, knives, or other sharp objects, a physical examination is useful. Patients with penetrating injury at or above the costal margin, including the epigastrium, or between the nipples and those with a suspected trajectory of missile through the mediastinum should be assumed to have not only a cardiac injury but also potential injury to aerodigestive structures within the mediastinum as well. Beck's triad, consisting of muffled heart sounds, engorged neck veins, and hypotension, has been the historical hallmark of pericardial tamponade. However, neck vein distension may not be present in profoundly hypovolemic patients. Additionally, the evaluation of neck veins and muffled heart sounds in the busy and noisy emergency department is fraught with difficulty. For this reason, more objective diagnostic testing has proved useful.

Most patients with penetrating cardiac injuries should have a portable chest x-ray if their hemodynamic status permits.[9] Entry and exit wounds should be marked with radiopaque markers; paper clips are useful in this regard. A chest radiograph can demonstrate not only pneumothorax and hemothorax but also an enlarged cardiac silhouette. It should be noted that only small amounts (300 to 400 cc of blood) are required to produce hemodynamically significant tamponade in an otherwise normal pericardium. For this reason, findings of pericardial fluid may not be dramatic on chest x-ray.

The use of emergency ultrasonography—FAST (focused assessment with sonography for trauma)—

performed by acute care physicians has gained popularity in recent years. This modality of ultrasound can be useful in the diagnosis of pericardial tamponade. Handheld echocardiography of the pericardium can be carried out in a matter of seconds, provides useful feedback about the presence or absence of pericardial fluid, and can assess cardiac function and evaluate cardiac filling pressures. Rozycki and colleagues[10] evaluated 261 patients with penetrating chest wounds. They reported 225 (86%) true negatives, 29 (11%) true positives, 7 (2.7%) false positives, and no false negatives. This resulted in a sensitivity of 100% and a specificity of 97%.

We believe that echocardiography is a useful adjunct for the diagnosis of penetrating cardiac injury. Either handheld echocardiography by the acute care surgery team or more formal echocardiography, either transthoracic (TTE) or transesophageal (TEE), performed by specialized providers can result in the rapid diagnosis of pericardial tamponade. High-quality images interpreted by trained personnel allow for the determination of the hemodynamic significance of pericardial fluid collections. Small pericardial fluid collections without hemodynamic significance must be differentiated from clinically significant blood collections. The precise logistics required to obtain echocardiograms on trauma patients will need to be tailored to each institution.

Computed tomography (CT) scanning is useful in the evaluation of penetrating thoracic trauma. Computed tomography scanning can detect not only pericardial blood but also blood that accumulates in the pleural space. This is important as penetrating cardiac wounds combined with defects in the pericardium will often not have significant pericardial fluid collections, the blood having traveled into the pleural space. Unfortunately, hemodynamically unstable patients with penetrating thoracic trauma are not best served by transport to the CT scanner. These patients benefit from the speed and proximity of emergency department echocardiography.

Cardiac Tamponade

Some authors have advocated pericardiocentesis for the diagnosis of blood in the pericardium following a suspected penetrating cardiac injury. At our institution, we have not found this to be a useful modality, and it often confuses the clinical picture. In the somewhat chaotic setting of the emergency department, with a patient who is unstable or receiving cardiopulmonary resuscitation, it is often difficult to blindly enter the pericardium safely. Additionally, the accidental passage of the pericardiocentesis needle into the ventricular cavity can occur in this setting. For these reasons we do not feel that pericardiocentesis is a useful diagnostic tool for penetrating cardiac injury.

Subxiphoid pericardial window has been advocated as a method for evaluating the pericardium. We have found this to be useful, and our preferred venue for this maneuver is in the operating theater where a positive pericardial window can be converted to a full sternotomy for treatment of intrapericardial pathology. The patient must be hemodynamically stable for transport for this approach to work. Additionally, a subxiphoid window is easily performed as an extension of laparotomy in patients who are already being treated for intraabdominal injury.

Thoracoscopy has been utilized for the evaluation of pericardial blood. Morales and colleagues[11] utilized thoracoscopy in 108 hemodynamically stable patients with penetrating injury near the heart but without signs of cardiac injury. Hemopericardium was identified in 33 patients (32%), and the sensitivity, specificity, and accuracy were 100%, 96%, and 97%, respectively. Patients with pericardial blood were converted to thoracotomy or sternotomy for management.[11] When echocardiography is not available or inconclusive, thoracoscopy may be a useful modality to identify patients with pericardial blood.

Open surgical exposure to the pericardium has been advocated as a diagnostic maneuver to evaluate for the presence of pericardial blood. This can be accomplished in the trauma bay via a left anterior lateral thoracotomy. This incision can be performed rapidly with simple instruments, and the pericardium can then be entered with a linear incision along the lateral pericardium, taking care not to injure the phrenic nerve. Some limitations of this incision are apparent in that right-sided cardiac structures are difficult to evaluate and repair. Additionally, the left lung must be retracted to facilitate exposure. Temporary control of bleeding can be obtained, and, if required, the incision can be extended across the sternum and converted into a clamshell-type incision. This approach provides adequate exposure of the entire mediastinum. This rapid and relatively straightforward approach is best suited for patients with severely impaired hemodynamics or those who have arrested.[12]

Sternotomy provides excellent exposure to the heart and great vessels. This exposure requires some form of sternal splitting, ideally with a sternal saw, but this can also be accomplished, albeit more slowly, with a Lebsche knife. Our preference is to transport the patient to the operating theater where personnel and equipment are available to facilitate this approach. Sternotomy for the diagnosis of intrapericardial injury may be considered somewhat aggressive. However, for patients with a high index of suspicion for injury, those with equivocal findings on imaging studies, and those undergoing other procedures in the operating theater, sternotomy allows us to confidently evaluate and treat any intrapericardial pathology. The incision is well tolerated by patients, and we have not experienced deep sternal would infections despite a lack of absolute sterility in some emergent cases.

Venue

Management of cardiac injuries is best performed in the operating room. The reasons for this preference are numerous and include better lighting, access to instruments and sutures specific to cardiac surgery, capability for cardiopulmonary bypass if required, and personnel familiar with cardiac surgery. The principle drawback of this approach is that it requires time to prepare the operating room and to transport patients to the operating room. The delay incurred with this approach will vary from institution to institution, and for this reason each practitioner must develop a strategy that works best in his or her specific work environment. Often the operating room can be made ready for patients with suspected cardiac injuries while they are being evaluated or are still in transit to the hospital.

Exposure

The optimal incision for the management of cardiac injury is one that provides rapid relief of tamponade and access to the injured cardiac structure(s) so that repair can be carried out. As discussed earlier, sternotomy provides optimal exposure to the heart and great vessels as well as to the pulmonary hila. For this reason, sternotomy is our incision of choice for penetrating cardiac injury provided that we are able to transport the patient to the operating room. Left anterolateral thoracotomy is our incision of choice in the emergency department, as it is easy to perform, does not require special equipment, and is rapid.

Once the sternum is divided, the mediastinal fat and thymic tissue are divided and the pericardium is opened. A tense, blue pericardium full of blood can often be difficult to grasp with forceps and must be opened with a knife. Scissors can then be used to extend the pericardial opening down to the diaphragm and up over the aorta. Care must be used so as not to injure the innominate vein as it crosses the midline over the aorta.

Once the pericardium has been opened, clotted blood must be evacuated. Pericardial "stay" sutures can then be placed to facilitate exposure. Although often obvious, the site of injury may in some cases be difficult to recognize immediately. A minority of patients will have temporarily sealed the site of injury caused by hypotension, hypovolemia, or the compressive effects of clot within the pericardium. When the injury is not immediately apparent, the pericardial space must be searched systematically until the injury is located. If injury is not seen on the anterior surface of the right ventricle, right atrium, or great vessels, the left ventricle should be evaluated. This is facilitated by loosening the right-sided pericardial stay sutures, tilting the operating table to the patient's right, and placing one or more warm, wet laparotomy sponges behind the left ventricle. This will serve to expose the left ventricle without undue compressive or rotational force and will preserve hemodynamics. This maneuver will also facilitate exposure to the left atrial appendage.

Most penetrating cardiac injuries can be managed with direct pressure. This can be either digital or with a sponge to compress the site of bleeding. Care must be taken not to further injure the damaged myocardium or to compromise cardiac filling with excessive pressure. By manually controlling bleeding, the anesthesia team is allowed time to "catch up" with the resuscitation, adequate surgical help can be obtained, and equipment can be prepared for definitive repair.

Repair Technique

Once the site of cardiac injury is identified, appropriate suture material should be chosen. Thin cardiac structures such as the atria, the aorta, and the pulmonary artery are best managed with relatively small sutures, such as nonabsorbable 4-0 monofilament with or without pledgets. Thicker structures such as the left ventricle require larger sutures, our preference being pledgeted No. 2 braided, nonabsorbable sutures. Choice of needle is critical as well; for ventricular injury we prefer a large, thin, half-circle needle. Suturing must be precise and not result in additional cardiac injury. The best chance for successful repair is the initial repair, and care should be taken to optimize conditions for the first attempt.

Injuries adjacent to coronary arteries require special care. Attention must be taken so that coronary blood flow is not impaired or occluded by the repair suture. This is facilitated by placing mattress sutures underneath the coronary artery using pledgets on either side. Pledgets can be of either Teflon or pericardium.

Coronary Injuries

Penetrating injuries involving coronary arteries can be managed in a variety of ways. Small coronary arteries and veins that supply small areas of myocardium can be ligated without undue consequence. Larger branch coronary arteries must be either repaired or reconstructed with coronary artery bypass grafting. Bypass grafting using saphenous vein or other suitable conduits such as the internal mammary arteries can be used. Saphenous vein is usually the more appropriate choice in the acute setting, as it can be harvested relatively quickly. Use of the internal mammary artery is theoretically possible for left anterior descending artery injury but requires time to harvest, and the mammary artery may be compromised by the initial chest wall injury. Grafting can be accomplished with the use of either cardiopulmonary bypass or "off pump." Reconstruction of coronary arteries can be technically challenging and is facilitated by the involvement of individuals familiar with the practice of coronary artery bypass grafting.

Destructive Injuries

Finally, large injuries resulting in the destruction of myocardium are difficult to repair. These injuries often follow gunshot wounds to the heart or penetrating injuries with large objects. These injuries cannot be simply repaired by direct suturing but often require patching. This is best accomplished with large pieces of Dacron or cardiovascular felt material, but Goretex and other synthetic materials are equally effective. As with smaller injuries, the best chance for success is on the first attempt at repair. Continued unsuccessful attempts to reconstruct the heart will result in progressive destruction of more tissue and escalating difficulty in eventually accomplishing hemostasis. We have found that direct pressure by one surgeon to control the majority of bleeding while a second surgeon places multiple mattress sutures around the defect is effective. The sutures are then brought up through the patch, and the patch is brought down over the defect and tied in place. This has proved successful for even large destructive injuries with tissue loss, including injuries to both ventricles.

Numerous topical hemostatic agents have been utilized as an adjunct to control bleeding in cardiac injury. Although we have found these agents useful for the control of oozing from injured myocardium, we do not advocate their use for injury to epicardial vessels or for the treatment of full-thickness cardiac injuries. We feel that suture repair provides definitive hemostasis of these injuries and is less vulnerable to failure secondary to progressive coagulation abnormalities, elevations in cardiac chamber pressure, or mechanical dislodgement during the cardiac and respiratory cycle.

Following any kind of pericardial repair, we recommend placement of multiple drains within the pericardium. Additionally, an opportunity should be made to assess for defects in the pericardium resulting in pooled blood in the left or right pleura, as well as the evaluation of associated pulmonary injuries. We routinely open the left and right pleura to look for injury and evacuate any blood that is present. Drains are placed in the pleural spaces as needed. We have rarely thought that placement of postoperative pacing wires is necessary, with the exception being injury to the right coronary artery, where pacing wires would be a reasonable adjunct. The heart should be palpated, and any significant thrill should be evaluated with echocardiography either in the operating room or immediately thereafter.

Follow-Up

In the immediate postoperative period, patients should be managed in a manner akin to all other postoperative trauma patients. Close monitoring of urine output, blood pressure, and other markers of resuscitation is important. A check for additional injuries must be carried out with a secondary survey.

Following myocardial injury, an elevation in troponin will be expected. A small percentage of patients with penetrating cardiac injuries will have a myocardial infarction and an area of ischemia. If evidence of progressive myocardial ischemia or infarction is suspected, electrocardiogram, serum enzymes, and echocardiogram follow up is warranted with appropriate treatment based on these studies. Malignant arrhythmias are uncommon in patients with cardiac injury but should be treated if they compromise cardiac performance. Premature atrial and ventricular beats are common but rarely have clinical implications.

Patients who have sustained penetrating cardiac injuries should have a follow-up echocardiogram. This is because of the small number of septal defects and valvular injuries that are present following penetrating cardiac injury. Many of these injuries are innocuous, but a small percentage will require future attention.

Finally, patients who have had large amounts of blood evacuated from the pericardial space and repair of cardiac injuries will often develop inflammatory pericarditis following surgery. In almost all cases, this can be treated effectively with nonsteroidal antiinflammatory drugs (provided renal function is good). Electrocardiographic changes including diffuse ST-segment elevation often accompany acute pericarditis. These findings can often appear distressingly similar to changes seen with acute myocardial infarction, but their global nature can help differentiate them from ischemic changes.

Factors Affecting Prognosis

Outcomes following penetrating cardiac injury have been extensively studied. Results differ in large part because of variability of the population studied. Studies that have included patients found dead at the scene and those that have included medical examiner cases have in general found higher mortality rates than those reporting on only those patients who arrive at the hospital. Additionally, factors such as prehospital transport times, study environment, and sophistication of both the emergency medical system and the hospital trauma service all affect outcomes.

Despite the above limitations, several general conclusions can be reached. Patients with stab wounds have superior outcomes than those sustaining firearm injuries. This has been found to be true in studies including medical examiner cases and those restricted to only those victims who are transported to the hospital. Rhee and colleagues[2] reported an overall survival rate of 19% (9.7% for gunshot wounds and 32% for stab wounds), and for those patients transported to the hospital, a

TABLE 25.1. Penetrating cardiac trauma: demographics and outcomes.

Study	Study population	Number (overall survival)	Gunshot wound (GSW) No./% (% survival)	Stab wound (S) No./% (% survival)	Hypotension No./% (% survival)	No blood pressure No./% (% survival)	EDT* No./% (% survival)
Rhee et al.,[2] 1998	Population (Level I + medical examiners)	212 (19%) 116 dead at scene	123/58% (12% overall, 29% hospital)	89/42% (33% overall, 53% hospital)	84/88% (36%)	60/50% (18%)	58/60% (31%) S: 36% GSW: 14%
Asensio et al.,[3] 1998	Urban Level I trauma center	105 (33%)	68/65% (16%)	37/35% (65%)	n/a	66/63% (86%)	71/68% (14%)
Mittal et al.,[14] 1999	Urban Level II trauma center	80 (65%)	36/45% (47%)	44/55% (80%)	55/69% (48%)	14/17% (36%)	31/39% (22%) S: 42% GSW: 11%
Campbell et al.,[1] 1998	Urban hospital + medical examiner	1,198 (2.9%) (1,128 dead at scene)	494/44% (0%)	700/56% (53%)	n/a	n/a	n/a
Tyburski et al.,[4] 2000	Urban Level I trauma center	302 (41%)	148/49% (23%)	154/51 % (58%)	n/a	27/9% (19%)	152/50% (13%) S: 59 (20%) GSW: 93 (0%)

*EDT, emergency department thoracotomy.

survival rate of 43% (29% for gunshot wounds and 53% for stab wounds) was noted. The improved survival following stab wounds compared with gunshot wounds has been reported in various geographic settings[1,13] and among diverse patient populations. Additionally, patients with vital signs on arrival and those who are stable enough to be transported to the operating room for surgery fare better.[3,14] These findings are summarized in Table 25.1. Additional factors that have been associated with poor outcomes include multiple cardiac chamber injuries, associated extrathoracic injuries, cardiac tamponade, coronary artery injury, need for aortic cross clamping, left ventricular injury, delay in operative intervention, high injury severity score (ISS) and low Glasgow Coma Score (GCS).[1,3,4,14]

Pearls of Penetrating Thoracic Trauma

1. Echocardiography should be used liberally.
2. The first attempt at repair of a cardiac wound has the best chance of success.
3. A sternotomy in the operating room will provide excellent exposure to all cardiac injuries.
4. Emergency room thoracotomy can be life saving for this patient group, especially patients with stab wounds.

Blunt Cardiac Injury

The precise incidence of blunt cardiac injury is less well characterized than that of penetrating cardiac trauma. Although rare, blunt thoracic trauma resulting in injury to the coronary arteries or heart valves or frank rupture of cardiac chambers is relatively easy to define. Myocardial injury or myocardial contusion is less well defined. Despite multiple attempts, it has been difficult to arrive at a consensus regarding what precisely constitutes "myocardial contusion." This may explain the wide range in incidence of myocardial injury (20% to 75%) reported in the literature.[15,16] Because of the difficulty in defining myocardial contusion, emphasis has shifted from definition of injury to identifying patients who are at risk to develop adverse sequelae of myocardial injury, such as arrythmias and impaired ventricular function. These strategies are addressed later in this chapter.

The American Association for the Surgery of Trauma (AAST) has developed an organ injury scale for cardiac injury. Using the AAST guidelines, echocardiography, and surgical or autopsy findings, Lancey and Monahan[17] reviewed 3,000 consecutive trauma admissions and identified 47 who met these criteria. Motor vehicle crashes were responsible for 85% of the injuries, and of these only 15% were wearing a seatbelt. The average ISS was 27.8, and the overall mortality rate was 31.9%. Factors associated with mortality included elevated organ injury score or ISS, shorter time to diagnosis, cardiac tamponade, cardiac rupture, lack of vital signs on admission, and injury to other major organ systems.[17]

Falls and workplace injuries are also associated with blunt cardiac injury. An autopsy series by Turk and Tsokos[18] included 61 falls, and the authors noted a 54% incidence of cardiac injury. In 16 victims (26%), cardiac injury was thought to be the cause of death, with chamber rupture (ventricular 48%, atrial 57%) the dominant mechanism.[18] Because thoracic trauma is associated with extrathoracic injuries in 70% to 90% of cases, patients must be evaluated in this context.

Less frequently blunt cardiac injuries are incurred during recreational activities. Although most of these low-energy injuries are not life threatening, sudden cardiac death following seemingly innocuous chest wall trauma has been reported and is termed "commotio cordis."[19] First described in 1932, approximately 70 cases have been reported in the literature. The pathophysiology is incompletely understood but appears to be related to the location and timing of the blow in relation to the cardiac cycle. Patients are frequently young, and their chest wall architecture may also contribute to the pathophysiologic response. Regardless of the precise mechanism, outcome is uniformly poor, with only 10% of patients surviving.

Diagnosis

Blunt trauma can cause cardiac injury by direct compressive force, torsional force, or overpressurization of the cardiac chambers. This can result in myocardial contusion and injury to the cardiac chambers, the valves, or, in rare cases, the coronary arteries. The diagnosis and management of these specific injuries are discussed in this section.

General principles of trauma care including the "ABCs" should be followed for patients who have sustained significant blunt force injury to the chest. Chest wall injuries, including flail segments, sternal fractures, and scapular fractures, are associated with severe blunt force trauma to the thorax. Unfortunately, these external stigmata are neither specific nor sensitive markers for particular intrathoracic injuries. Diagnostic tests in the context of clinical judgment are required to precisely diagnose intrathoracic pathology. Injuries that produce damage to the aorta, great vessels, and other noncardiac mediastinal structures often produce significant cardiac injury as well. The corollary is also true: patients with cardiac injury must be thoroughly evaluated for noncardiac thoracic trauma.

Imaging

Routine chest radiographs do not aid in the diagnosis of cardiac contusion. Cardiac enlargement may be present and can represent pericardial blood, may represent mediastinal hematoma, or may be due to magnification of anterior thoracic structures seen with anteroposterior chest x-rays taken at close range. Blood and air in the pleural space or mediastinum are not specific but alert the clinician to the likelihood of injury. Sternal fractures are present in a significant number of patients who have been subjected to blunt thoracic trauma, but the precise significance of this injury in relation to cardiac injury is unclear. In a review of 61 lethal falls, Turk and Tsokos[18] found that sternal fractures were present in 76% of those with cardiac injury and only 18% without cardiac injury. Complex sternal fractures were only seen in those individuals with cardiac injury.[18] Conversely, Rashid et al.[20] reported on a group of 418 patients with blunt chest trauma of whom 29 (7%) had sternal fractures. In this study no association between sternal fractures and the number or severity of other thoracic injuries was found.[20]

A small percentage of patients will have pneumopericardium following blunt thoracic trauma. This can be suspected in patients who have sustained significant blunt thoracic trauma and who have a new murmur detected. Crepitus from subcutaneous air may also be present. Diagnosis is established with either chest radiographs or CT scanning. This entity is usually self-limiting but in rare cases can cause "tension pneumopericardium." The pathophysiology is similar to the compressive syndrome of cardiac tamponade more commonly observed with blood in the pericardium, and treatment is required if compressive symptoms are present.[21] Injury to the aerodigestive tract must be suspected and evaluated in patients with pneumopericardium.

Thoracic CT scanning can detect the sequelae of cardiac injury, such as pericardial fluid, and CT scanning of the chest can be extremely useful in the management of blunt thoracic trauma patients with an enlarged cardiomediastinal silhouette on chest x-ray.[16] Pericardial fluid can be differentiated from periaortic or perispinal hematomas and thus guide further diagnostic and therapeutic interventions. Some authors have reported on the utility of CT scanning for the detection of blunt coronary artery injuries.[22] Additionally, CT scanning with intravenous contrast has been used to identify atrial appendage injury.[16]

Myocardial Contusion

Although difficulties persist in defining exactly what constitutes myocardial contusion, progress has been made in determining which patients are at risk for adverse events following blunt force injury to the chest. Those patients with obvious disruption of cardiac chambers, damage to cardiac valves or coronaries, or those with pericardial blood require urgent attention. The vast majority of patients sustaining blunt thoracic injury will have some degree of myocardial contusion without clear anatomic injury. This can range from elevations of cardiac enzymes with no clinical significance to profound ventricular dysfunction and arrythmias. Several strategies have emerged for identifying those patients in this subgroup who require further monitoring, additional diagnostic tests, and possibly interventions.

Cardiac Enzymes

Although the initial use of serum markers such as CPK-MB to evaluate patients with suspected myocardial contusion was disappointing, more success has been achieved with serum troponin measurements. Several studies have demonstrated that using troponin levels with or without electrocardiograms can safely rule out significant myocardial injury.[23,24] Velmahos and colleagues[24] evaluated 333 patients with significant blunt thoracic trauma using both serum troponin I level and ECG at admission and 8 hours after arrival. Only one patient with an initially normal ECG and normal troponin I level developed abnormalities later. The authors found that combining ECG and troponin I data yielded a sensitivity and negative predictive value of 100%. Unfortunately, the specificity was only 71% and the positive predictive value only 34%. This strategy allowed them to exclude 131 (40%) of their initial 333 patients from further workup of treatment related to their myocardial contusion.

Troponin I levels have been found to correlate with the degree of ventricular impairment following blunt thoracic trauma. In this regard, troponin I may be a biologic marker for estimating the quantity of myocardial damage. Rajan and Zellweger[25] were able to demonstrate a statistically significant association between troponin levels and both ventricular impairment and the occurrence of postinjury arrhythmias. Although different authors have used different threshold levels to define what precisely constitutes an abnormal level in a trauma patient, troponin measurements appear useful to exclude the diagnosis of cardiac contusion and to roughly quantify the degree of injury present.

Blunt Coronary Artery Injury

Coronary artery injury after blunt chest trauma is exceedingly rare. The left anterior descending artery is injured most commonly, the right coronary less frequently, and only two reports of traumatic circumflex artery injury exist.[26] Patients with acute traumatic coronary injury have a high probability to suffer myocardial infarction because chronic collaterals have not developed. Patients with ischemic changes on ECG should have serial troponin levels obtained and be monitored in an appropriate setting with attention to arrhythmia detection and treatment. Echocardiograms to look for wall motion abnormalities should be obtained and cardiac catheterization utilized when indicated. Coronary artery injuries may be either occlusions or dissections, and the majority can be treated percutaneously with stenting. Coronary artery bypass grafting may be required in some cases.

Blunt Valvular Injury

Cardiac valve injury is also uncommon following blunt chest trauma. Injury can be caused by sudden increases in intracardiac chamber pressure and can result in dysfunction in the atrioventricular valves (mitral and tricuspid) because of injury of the chordae, papillary muscles, or leaflets themselves. Dysfunction of the semilunar valves (aortic, pulmonic) occurs when the leaflets themselves are injured or when there is traumatic dissection of the vessel wall leading to loss of leaflet support, lack of proper coaptation, and subsequent regurgitation. The presence of a new murmur following chest trauma should be evaluated by echocardiography, either TTE or TEE. Although valvular injury is often immediately apparent following blunt thoracic trauma, intervals of as long as 12 years have been reported from the time of thoracic injury to the time of diagnosis.[27]

Follow-Up for Blunt Cardiac Injury

Long-term follow up of patients who have sustained myocardial contusion does not appear necessary. Lindstaedt et al.[15] evaluated 118 patients with cardiac contusion, and patients were reevaluated at 3- and 12-month intervals with electrocardiography, bicycle exercise testing, and echocardiography. Seventeen patients had wall motion abnormalities immediately following injury; 10 of the abnormalities were present at 3 months and 4 persisted to 12 months. One patient developed mural thrombus in an akinetic wall segment, but no other new echocardiographic findings were noted. The authors concluded that for asymptomatic patients long-term follow-up evaluation following blunt thoracic trauma is not indicated.[15]

Our current practice is to obtain electrocardiograms and measure troponin I cardiac enzymes for all patients who have sustained significant blunt thoracic injury. Patients with normal baseline and 8-hour electrocardiograms and troponin I levels are thought to need no further treatment. Patients with abnormal enzyme levels, electrocardiograms, arrhythmias, or hypotension undergo echocardiography and monitoring in the intensive care unit.[28] Central venous and pulmonary artery catheters are used as indicated in patients with myocardial injury. Inotropic agents are used judiciously as they have the potential to be proarrhythmic.

Pearls of Blunt Thoracic Trauma

1. Patients with blunt thoracic trauma often have extrathoracic injuries.
2. Patients with normal ECGs and troponin at admission and 8 hours after admission are extremely unlikely to develop late problems.
3. Patients with significant blunt thoracic trauma should have a CT scan of the chest.
4. Emergency room thoracotomy is unlikely to salvage patients without vital signs.

Special Circumstances

Iatrogenic Endovascular Cardiac Injury

Although infrequent, cardiovascular complications of endovascular procedures can be life-threatening.[29,30] Cardiac tamponade has been identified in malpractice suits as the second most common adverse outcome associated with central vascular catheters. In an analysis of 110 lawsuits involving alleged misplacement or mismanagement of central vascular catheters, 16 (20%) were found to be associated with cardiac tamponade and 13 (81%) of the 16 patients died.[31] In addition to central venous catheters, iatrogenic injury and cardiac tamponade secondary to vena cava filter procedures[32] and balloon dilation of the superior vena cava[33] have been reported. The diagnosis of cardiac tamponade was made early in the majority of patients, either clinically or with imaging techniques such as echocardiography or chest radiography. In some cases the diagnosis of cardiac tamponade was delayed for several days. In these cases, patients developed tamponade either from delayed hemorrhage in the pericardial space or from the infusion of fluid into the pericardial space or mediastinum via malpositioned catheters.

Although the likelihood of arterial puncture when attempting central venous catheter puncture can be reduced by using ultrasound imaging guidance, this technique will not impact the rate of cardiac tamponade caused by catheter misplacement in the central circulation. The diagnosis of pericardial tamponade should be entertained for patients with hemodynamic instability following central venous catheter placement. Additionally, follow-up chest radiographs before using central venous lines can also help reduce the problems associated with malpositioned central catheters and should be the standard of care when appropriate. Unfortunately, in the acute care setting with a patient who is already hemodynamically unstable, or in the operating theater, radiographic studies are cumbersome to obtain; therefore clinical judgment or echocardiography must be relied on. Treatment of great vessel or cardiac injury secondary to

central venous catheter placement should be managed like all other cardiac traumas as described elsewhere in this chapter.

Another potential source for iatrogenic cardiac injury is percutaneous cardiovascular procedures with venous access procedures resulting in right atrial, right ventricular, or left atrial injury following transseptal puncture. Percutaneous coronary interventions can result in injury or even rupture of the coronary arteries. These injuries are rare but can result in not only life-threatening interpericardial hemorrhage but also cardiac ischemia in the distribution of the disrupted coronary artery. These injuries can be diagnosed rapidly with the imaging equipment in a cardiac catheterization laboratory; coronary angiography can be used to demonstrate extravasation of dye from the coronary arteries, and echocardiography can demonstrate the presence of fluid within the pericardial space. Cardiac injuries incurred in the cardiac catheterization suite should be managed as all other penetrating cardiac injuries and are discussed elsewhere in this chapter. Coronary injuries often require either coronary artery bypass grafting or, at minimum, coronary vein plasty to reconstruct distal flow. In the case of a life-threatening hemorrhage, coronary ligation can be employed as a last resort.

Transmediastinal Gunshot Wounds

Patients who have sustained transmediastinal gunshot wounds represent a unique diagnostic challenge. Patients who are hemodynamically unstable must undergo emergent operation. In patients who are hemodynamically stable, excluding injury to any of the vulnerable mediastinal structures (aerodigestive, cardiac, vascular, etc.) can prove difficult. Initially these patients were thought to require multiple overlapping modalities to exclude injury to the numerous structures contained within the mediastinum. Bronchoscopy, esophagoscopy, echocardiography, a barium swallow, angiography, and other modalities have all been touted as "required" to exclude injury. More recently, contrast-enhanced CT scanning of the chest has been advanced as a single diagnostic test to exclude injury in stable patients following transmediastinal gunshot wounds.

A study by Stassen and colleagues[34] evaluated 22 patients with transmediastinal gunshot wounds and identified seven patients with injury of whom two eventually required surgical intervention. Of the remaining patients without normal CT scans, none required further interventions, and the authors concluded that CT scanning was able to exclude injury.[34] Other reports have supported this approach with the caveat that patients who develop hemodynamic instability must undergo additional workup (angiography, echocardiography) even if the CT scan is normal.[35]

Cardiopulmonary Bypass

Cardiopulmonary bypass can facilitate repair of cardiac and aortic injury. In addition, cardiopulmonary bypass has been advocated by some to serve as a resuscitative modality for hypotensive critically injured patients. Its use as a rewarming modality has proven effective in the resuscitation of severely hypothermic patients. Extracorporeal membrane oxygenation (ECMO) has been employed to augment gas exchange in trauma patients with severe impairment of pulmonary function, but the utility of this application remains unclear. Although cardiopulmonary bypass has several attractive features, it is not without complications. It requires complex equipment and personnel to operate. Cardiopulmonary bypass requires anticoagulation, and it produces a systemic inflammatory response that may exacerbate the physiologic abnormalities present in severely injured trauma patients. For this reason the potential utility of cardiopulmonary bypass must be carefully evaluated for each patient.

For cardiac trauma patients, cardiopulmonary support can be divided into two general roles: first, as support for patients refractory to conventional resuscitative measures and, second, as a tool for either the acute or delayed reconstruction of cardiac injuries. As an acute resuscitative tool, cardiopulmonary bypass has not emerged as an effective therapy. For patients with unresponsive cardiogenic shock and cardiac injury, Baker and colleagues[13] attempted to salvage four patients with cardiopulmonary bypass and were unable to salvage any. They did have better success using cardiopulmonary bypass to facilitate repair of complex cardiac injuries in patients who were not yet in extremis.

In summary, cardiopulmonary bypass is useful for the repair of complex cardiac injuries to the heart chambers, valves, and coronary arteries but has limited if any value as an adjunct to resuscitation in and of itself, with the exception of patients requiring rewarming from profound hypothermia. Additionally, in the vast majority of patients with intracardiac injury (valvular, septal), the patient can be stabilized and undergo reconstructive cardiac surgery or catheter-based procedures at a more optimal time.[8,27,37]

Pearls of Cardiopulmonary Bypass

1. Facilitates repair of destructive multichamber cardiac injuries.
2. Allows for rewarming of hypothermic patients but does not appear to assist in the salvage of hemodynamically unstable patients.
3. Requires time, specialized equipment and personnel, and anticoagulation to use.

Critique

This is a classic presentation for a postpericardiotomy syndrome (Dressler), which is often a self-limiting pericarditis. There is no indication that this is a pyogenic pericarditis or that it is an associated pericardial effusion. With persistent pain and friction rub, the patient should be given indomethacin, a nonsteroidal antiinflammatory agent.

Answer (A)

References

1. Campbell N, Thomson S, Muckart J, Meumann C, Middelkoop IV, Botha J. Review of 1198 cases of penetrating cardiac trauma. Br J Surg 1998; 85:1737–1740.
2. Rhee P, Foy H, Kaufmann C, et al. Penetrating cardiac injuries: a population-based study. J Trauma 1998; 45(2):366–370.
3. Asensio J, Bern J, Demetriades D, et al. One hundred five penetrating cardiac injuries: a 2-year prospective evaluation. J Trauma 1998; 44(6):1073–1082.
4. Tyburski J, Astra L, Wilson R, Dente C, Steffes C. Factors affecting prognosis with penetrating wounds of the heart. J Trauma 2000; 48(4):587–591.
5. Wall J, Mattox K, Baldwin J. Acute management of complex cardiac injuries. J Trauma 1997; 42:905.
6. Duque H, Florez L, Moreno A, Jurado H, Jaramillo C, Restrepo M. Penetrating cardiac trauma: follow-up study including electrocardiography, echocardiography, and functional test. World J Surg 1999; 23:1254–1257.
7. Enriquez S, Fernadez C, Entem F, Garagarza J, Duran R. Delayed pericardial tamponade after penetrating chest trauma. Eur J Emerg Med 2005; 12(2):86–88.
8. Presenti-Rossi D, Godart F, Dubar A, Rey C. Transcatheter closure of traumatic ventricular septal defect: an alternative to surgery. Chest 2003; 123(6):2144–2145.
9. LeBlang S, Dolich M. Imaging of penetrating thoracic trauma. J Thorac Imaging 2000; 15(2):128–135.
10. Rozycki G, Feliciano D, Ochsner M, et al. The role of ultrasound in patients with possible penetrating cardiac wounds: a prospective multicenter study. J Trauma 1999; 46(4):543–552.
11. Morales C, Salinas C, Henao C, Patino P, Munoz C. Thoracoscopic pericardial window and penetrating cardiac trauma. J Trauma 1997; 42(2):273–275.
12. Gao J, Gao Y, Wei G, et al. Penetrating cardiac wounds: principles for surgical management. World J Surg 2004; 28:1025–1029.
13. Mandal A, Sanusi M. Penetrating chest wounds: 24 years experience. World J Surg 2001; 25(9):1145–1149.
14. Mittal M, McAleese P, Young S, Cohen M. Penetrating cardiac injuries. Am Surgeon 1999; 65:444–448.
15. Lindstaedt M, Germing A, Lawo T, et al. Acute and long-term clinical significance of myocardial contusion following blunt thoracic trauma: results of a prospective study. J Trauma 2001; 52(3):479–485.

16. Wicky S, Wintermark M, Schnyder P, Capasso P, Denys A. Imaging of blunt chest trauma. Eur Radiol 2000; 10:1524–1528.

17. Lancey R, Monahan T. Correlation of clinical characteristics and outcomes with injury scoring in blunt cardiac trauma. J Trauma 2003; 54(3):509–515.

18. Turk E, Tsokos M. Blunt cardiac trauma caused by fatal falls from height: an autopsy-based assessment of the injury pattern. J Trauma 2004; 57(2):301–304.

19. Perron A, Brady W, Erling B. Commotio cordis: an underappreciated cause of sudden cardiac death in young patients: assessment and management in the ED. Am J Emerg Med 2001; 19(5):406–409.

20. Rashid M, Ortenwall P, Wikstrom T. Cardiovascular injuries associated with sternal fractures. Eur J Surg 2001; 167:243–248.

21. Ladurner R, Qvick L, Hohenbleicher F, Hallfeldt K, Mutschler W, Mussack T. Pneumopericardium in blunt chest trauma after high-speed motor vehicle accidents. Am J Emerg Med 2005; 23:83–86.

22. Braatz T, Mirvis S, Killeen K, Lightman N. CT diagnosis of internal mammary artery injury caused by blunt trauma. Clin Radiol 2001; 56:120–123.

23. Salim A, Vemahos G, Jindal A, et al. Clinically significant blunt cardiac trauma: role of serum troponin levels combined with electrocardiographic findings. J Trauma 2001; 50(2):237–243.

24. Velmahos G, Karaiskakis M, Salim A, et al. Normal Electrocardiography and serum troponin I levels preclude the presence of clinically significant blunt cardiac injury. J Trauma 2003; 54(1):45–51.

25. Rajan G, Zellweger R. Cardiac troponin I as a predictor of arrhythmia and ventricular dysfunction in trauma patients with myocardial contusion. J Trauma 2004; 57(4):801–808.

26. Naseer N, Aronow W, McClung J, et al. Circumflex coronary artery occlusion after blunt chest trauma. Heart Dis 2003; 5(3):184–186.

27. Reiss J, Rassouk A, Kiev J, Bansal R, Bailey L. Concomitant traumatic coronary artery and tricuspid valve injury: a heterogeneous presentation. J Trauma 2001; 50(5):942–944.

28. Nagy K, Krosner S, Roberts R, Joseph K, Smith R, Barrett J. Determining which patients require evaluation for blunt cardiac injury following blunt chest trauma. World J Surg 2001; 25:108–111.

29. Forauer A, Dasika N, Gemmete J, Theoharis C. Pericardial tamponade complicating central venous interventions. J Vasc Intervent Radiol 2003; 14(2):255–259.

30. Hohlrieder M, Oberhammer R, Lorenz I, Margreiter J, Kuhbacher G, Keller C. Life-threatening mediastinal hematoma caused by extravascular infusion through a triple-lumen central venous catheter. Anesth Analg 2004; 99:31–35.

31. Domino K, Bowdle T, Posner K, Spitellie P, Lee L, Cheney F. Injuries and liability related to central vascular catheters. Anesthesiology 2004; 100:1411–1418.

32. Hsin S, Luk H, Lin S, Chan H, Tsou M, Lee T. Detection of iatrogenic cardiac tamponade by transesophageal echocardiography during vena cava filter procedure. Can J Anesth 2000; 47(7):638–641.

33. Brown K, Getrajdman G. Balloon dilation of the superior vena cava (SVC) resulting in svc rupture and pericardial tamponade: a case report and brief review. Cardiovasc Intervent Radiol 2005; 28:372–376.

34. Stassen N, Lukan J, Spain D, Miller F, Carrillo E, Richardson J. Reevaluation of diagnostic procedures for transmediastinal gunshot wounds. J Trauma 2002; 53(4):635–638.

35. Nagy K, Roberts R, Smith R, et al. Trans-mediastinal gunshot wounds: are "stable" patients really stable? World J Surg 2002; 26:1247–1250.

36. Baker J, Battistella F, Kraut E, Owings J, Follette D. Use of cardiopulmonary bypass to salvage patients with multiple-chamber heart wounds. Arch Surg 1998; 133(8):855–860.

37. Golbasi Z, Cicek D, Ucar O, et al. Traumatic ventricular septal defect and mitral insufficiency after a Kebab's Shish wound to the chest. Eur J Echocardiogr 2001; 2:203–204.

26
Thoracic Aorta

Peter I. Ellman and Irving L. Kron

Case Scenario

An 18-year-old woman who just recently received her driver's license is involved in a head-on collision. Upon arrival to the trauma bay, she is alert and complaining of chest pain. The patient is hemodynamically stable. Physical examination is unremarkable with the exception of precordial tenderness. Diagnostic workup confirms a traumatic aortic rupture. Which of the following would be the most appropriate management approach?

(A) Thoracotomy
(B) Intraaortic balloon pump
(C) Endovascular stenting
(D) Antihypertensive therapy and monitoring
(E) Observation only

The two major entities that would require the expertise of the acute care surgeon are thoracic aortic injuries and aortic dissections, although the therapeutic armamentarium is expanding to include nonoperative management and less invasive intervention (e.g., endovascular stent placement).

Blunt Aortic Trauma

History and Incidence

Before the advent of the internal combustion engine, blunt aortic injury (BAI) was a rare phenomenon. However, it now is the second most common cause of death in blunt force trauma.[1] Currently, patients involved in car and motorcycle accidents make up a majority of the cases.[2,3] This is not to say that BAI did not exist before the development of motorized transportation. The anatomist Andreas Vesalius was first to report on trau-

matic injury to the aorta, which had manifested as a post-traumatic aortic aneurysm in 1557.[4] However, it would take another 400 years before this problem could be treated. The first reported successful repair was performed by Klassen in 1958, but, interestingly, before that had occurred, it was thought that attempts to repair a traumatically transected aorta may cause more harm than good.[5,6] In the last 20 years a number of advancements have made the repair of BAI not only possible, but something that can be performed with a high degree of success.

Approximately 1% of patients presenting with signs of blunt chest trauma will have an aortic injury.[2,3] Overall, BAI is a relatively uncommon process, occurring about 8,000 times per year in North America.[7] Blunt aortic disruption carries with it high morbidity and mortality rates. Given that an estimated 80% to 85% of these patients will die at the scene, approximately 1,000 people are brought to hospitals alive every year.[2,4] Accidents involving motor vehicles including drivers, passengers and pedestrians, as well as falls from heights greater than 3 meters, make up the majority of cases.[2,4,8] More recently, airbags have been ascribed to injuries occurring in accidents involving cars moving at a slow speed.[9–11]

Etiology and Pathogenesis

Although there are a number of theories as to how blunt force aortic disruption occurs, there is currently no consensus on the pathophysiologic causes. The mechanism of blunt injury to the great vessels is still unclear, and to date it has been difficult to replicate BAI in the laboratory setting. Because injury often occurs at the isthmus, many believe the cause of blunt injury to be rapid deceleration and a shear force caused by the relative mobility of the aorta just adjacent to a fixed point.[12–19] Others postulate that these deceleration forces are not great enough to create an injury. Instead, they believe the injury could be caused by compression of the vessel between bony structures or by severe intraluminal hypertension during the traumatic event.[20–22] In a canine model this "osseous pinch" has been demonstrated to transect the media and intima of the aorta.

A number of different mechanisms of injury have been implicated in BAI. Fabian et al.,[2] in the largest prospectively gathered study on BAI to date, demonstrated that within the group of people who had been in automobile accidents, 62% of BAIs were from head-on collisions and 28% were from other vectors. Another study found that 58% of BAIs were caused by head-on collisions and 42% were from broad side collisions.[23] Falls, crushing injuries, and blasts also are less frequent causes. Clearly, however, it appears that high kinetic energy and rapid deceleration are common to all causes.

Interestingly, when one looks at the anatomic portion of the aorta that is injured, there is a difference in the distribution in autopsy series compared with surgical series. In autopsy series, commonly the aortic isthmus is involved, occurring about 50% of the time.[4,23–25] Approximately 20% involve the ascending aorta, and 20% involve the descending aorta. Conversely, in surgical series the isthmus is involved about 80% of the time, and the ascending aorta is involved much less frequently.[2,26–31] There is some advantage to having the disruption in the region of the isthmus, potentially because of the ability of the periadventitial tissue to prevent free rupture. Typically the aorta is transected transversely, and a complete transaction is more common than a partial transaction.[32,33]

Clinical Presentation and Initial Management

Most patients with BAI will have recently been in a motor vehicle accident or a fall. This patient will usually present with multiple traumatic injuries, and thus one should always have a high index of suspicion in that setting. From 25% to 50% of these patients will have a traumatic injury that will involve the central nervous system.[2,28,33–35] If patients are stable, awake, and conversant, they may describe symptoms such as dyspnea or back pain. However, patients will usually have a number of distracting injuries that make it difficult to understand any physical complaints. From 19% to 58% will have associated lung injuries.[28,33–35] From 35% to 65% will have rib fractures, about 20% will have splenic injuries, and approximately 70% will have some sort of extremity injury. Advanced trauma life support (ATLS) protocol will guide much of the care during the first 24 hours with these patients, and generally neurologic injuries and bleeding (intraabdominal, retroperitoneal, or thoracic) will need to be dealt with expeditiously and will take priority over issues regarding the thoracic aorta. In a way, the problems within the patient will be triaged, and the most deadly problems will be dealt with in the proper prioritized order.

Although it is clearly difficult for the paramedics to know a patient has a great vessel injury, there are a number of prehospital interventions that can be counterproductive to the care of a patient with a thoracic aortic injury. The application of MAST trousers creates the effect of aortic cross clamp and has actually been shown to increase the chance of death.[34,35] Additionally, excessive fluid resuscitation can increase mortality rates as well as other complications.[24]

When the patient reaches the trauma bay, standard ATLS protocol should be followed. The airway should be secured if need be, breathing assessed, and circulation assessed, with the placement of large-bore catheters to allow for resuscitation. The patient should be exposed and log rolled. A good neurologic examination should be done at this time, before any sedation or pain medications are given, and preferably a neurosurgeon should be present to document any disability. During this initial evaluation and stabilization, chest and pelvis x-rays should be obtained. Extremity fractures should be splinted and stabilized if present. Attempts to get a better understanding of the mechanism of injury should be made, as there are a number of particular risk factors that will increase the suspicion of BAI. These involve motor vehicle crash greater than 50 km/hr, no seatbelt, ejection from the vehicle, a broken steering wheel, pedestrian versus motor vehicle, head-on or side-impact car collision, falls from horses, crush injuries, and falls from heights of 30 ft or more. With regard to the physical examination, patients may have shortness of breath, cardiac murmurs, fractured sternum or bruise, hoarseness, back pain, or a difference in the blood pressures of the lower and upper extremities.[21,36–41]

Diagnostic Studies

Early in the resuscitation, a standard anteroposterior chest x-ray should be obtained. This, along with the mechanism of injury, can give a number of clues to increase the suspicion of BAI (Figure 26.1). With regard to the chest x-ray, there are a number of findings that are traditionally associated with blunt aortic disruption (Table 26.1).[42] The most reliable of these signs is a widened mediastinum, which may be present 85% of the time, and loss of the aortic knob.[2,42]

Although these findings can increase the suspicion of a great vessel injury, a chest x-ray does not have the diagnostic sensitivity to rule out aortic injury.[38,42–45] Thus, other radiographic studies will be needed to make a definitive diagnosis of BAI. Aortography, helical computed tomography (CT) scanning, and transesophageal echocardiography (TEE) are all used and are good tests for the evaluation of BAI.

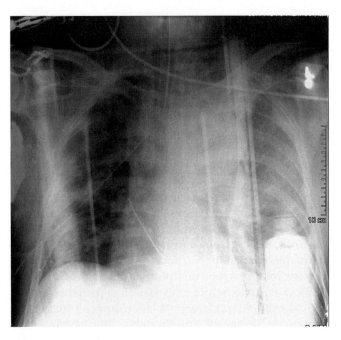

FIGURE 26.1. An x-ray of a patient with blunt aortic injury demonstrating widened mediastinum and loss of the aortopulmonary window.

Aortography has traditionally been considered the gold standard test for the evaluation of aortic injuries, but this is becoming less the case in many centers. It is still, however, the test against which all other tests are compared because its sensitivity and specificity approach 100%.[46] However, it has number of disadvantages, and because of them, most medical centers now use spiral CT as the primary means of ruling out aortic rupture.[44] Per-

TABLE 26.1. Chest x-ray findings associated with blunt aortic disruption.

Fractures
• Sternum
• Scapula
• Multiple left ribs (flail chest)
• Clavicle in multisystem trauma patients

Mediastinal clues
• Obliteration of the aortic knob contour
• Widening of the mediastinum >8 cm
• Depression of the left main stem bronchus
• Loss of paravertebral pleural stripe
• Calcium layering at the aortic knob
• Deviation of nasogastric tube in the esophagus
• Lateral displacement of the trachea

Lateral chest x-ray
• Anterior displacement of the trachea
• Loss of the aortic and pulmonary window
• Other findings
• Apical pleural hematoma
• Massive left hemothorax
• Obvious blunt injury to diaphragm

forming an aortogram takes time and manpower, requires an interventional radiology team, and in some medical centers requires the patient to be brought to the angiography suite—away from the relative safe haven of the operating room or intensive care unit. It is not uncommon for a patient to exsanguinate and die in the angiography suite.[38,47,48] Complications include contrast reactions, renal insufficiency, groin hematomas, and pseudoaneurysms. Given all of these problems, aortography is being used less frequently as a primary means of assessing aortic injury. It clearly has a role for the stable patient who has an equivocal helical CT study. In our institution, we will use aortography for patients who are stable and have equivocal helical CT scans. If the patient is unstable, we plan on using TEE in the operating room as a confirmatory test.

Helical CT scanning is currently the best first test to evaluate for BAI in a stable patient. It offers a number of advantages over aortography without giving up too much in the way of sensitivity or specificity; thus, in most centers helical CT scanning has become as the primary means of ruling out BAI. Some medical centers have now made helical CT the definitive test for BAI without the need for further tests, such as aortography or TEE.[43,49–51] The speed with which the test can be done, its sensitivity and specificity, and the ease of interpretation make spiral CT a superior test to all three in the initial evaluation of a possible traumatic aortic rupture. Many of these patients also will need an abdominal CT scan to evaluate for intraabdominal trauma, thus making spiral CT even more efficacious. The sensitivity and negative predictive value of the test are approximately 100%.[43,45,52,53] The specificity and positive predictive value range between 50% and 89%. Findings that are indicative of traumatic aortic disruption include wall thickening, extravasations of contrast, filling defects, paraaortic hematoma, intimal flaps, mural thrombi, pseudoaneurysm, and psuedocoarctation (Figure 26.2).[44] False-positive results can occur because of a ductus diverticulum, but this will usually be present in the absence of an intimal irregularity or mediastinum hematoma. If the study is equivocal then more studies with a higher specificity will need to be done, such as TEE or aortography.

Transesophageal echocardiography, like other forms of sonography, is operator dependent. There is a variability in the literature with regard to reports of the sensitivity and specificity of TEE, with some reports suggesting 100% accuracy and others suggesting a sensitivity of only 60%.[46,52,54–56] However, in experienced hands it can be a highly accurate way to diagnose BAI, particularly in a patient who is already in the operating room for a lapartotomy. One advantage TEE has over helical CT scanning is that it is portable and can be performed in an unstable patient. Thus, in our center, if a patient with a high index of suspicion for BAI is unstable and requires

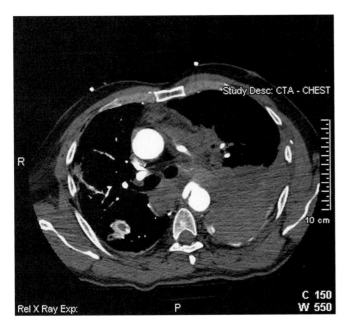

FIGURE 26.2. This CT scan demonstrates the disruption in the descending aorta, as well as periaortic blood and hemothorax.

laparotomy, we will plan on performing TEE in the operating room. Contraindications clearly include patients with oropharyngeal, esophageal, or severe maxillofacial injuries, as well as concomitant cervical spine injuries.

Management

After the initial period of resuscitation some critical decisions will need to be made. The stability of the patient will largely dictate management (Figure 26.3). Because these patients will often have multiple injuries rather than an isolated injury to their aorta, management can often be complicated. Unstable patients will likely have abdominal or pelvic bleeding. Patients requiring laparotomy should be brought to the operating room, and intraoperative TEE can be performed to rule out aortic injury. Patients with pelvic bleeding with the need for angiographic embolization can undergo thoracic aortography in the interventional suite at the time of embolization (see the algorithm in Figure 26.3).

Currently, the standard of care is immediate thoracotomy and aortic repair for stable patients who do not require concomitant laparotomy, craniotomy, or pelvic stabilization. There are a number of comorbid factors that make an open repair a relative contraindication, including pulmonary contusions (thus going on single lung ventilation may not be possible), abdominal bleeding, and nervous system injuries. These patients should be stabilized before attempts are made for open repair. A stable patient with aortic injury should have an expedient preoperative workup that includes a head and abdominal CT. As stated before, relief of space-occupying lesions in the brain and treatment of intraabdominal hemorrhage take precedence over the repair of aortic injuries. The logic behind this is that they are more likely to lead to death than the aortic injury in this situation. After these issues have been dealt with, the patient's stability and overall status should be assessed. If a patient appears to be exsanguinating from the aorta, clearly this should be dealt with immediately. If not, after a laparotomy it is probably best to return the patient to the

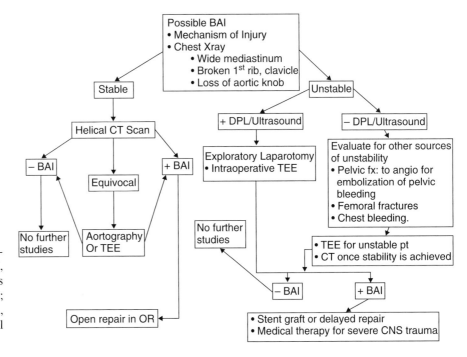

FIGURE 26.3. An algorithm for the management of blunt aortic injury. BAI, blunt aortic injury; CNS, central nervous system; CT, computed tomography; DPL, diagnostic peritoneal lavage; OR, operating room; TEE, transesophageal echocardiography.

intensive care unit where he or she can be stabilized and then brought back within the next 24 to 48 hours for aortic repair.

Patients who are unstable will most likely have multiple traumatic injuries and are unable to withstand the additional stress of an open repair. Traditionally these patients were stabilized in the intensive care unit and open repair is done within the first 48 to 72 hours after the traumatic event. Operative results have been fraught with relatively high rates of paralysis and death in this patient population. In recent years endovascular stent grafting has emerged as a potential option for these patients. It has been highlighted that endovascular stent grafting is safe and effective in the short term and is particularly advantageous for patients who have significant other injuries who would otherwise not be stable enough for an open repair.[57,58] Some medical centers are now using endovascular repair regardless of the severity of other injuries.[59] It should be noted that most reports are anecdotal, with relatively small numbers, but the results are encouraging.[57-59] Given the relative rarity of this phenomenon, a multiinstitutional prospective trial over a number of years would most likely be needed to objectively compare open repair with endovascular stent grafting. In the short term, it appears that the risk of paralysis is also lower with this method. Although the rates of paralysis of open repair are in the range of approximately 10%, there has yet to be a report of paraplegia after the use of endovascular stent grafts in the acute treatment of BAI.[59] Early mortality may also be lower, with rates being between 0% and 16%.[57-60] However, it should be noted that long-term data do not exist. With regard to complications, sometimes it may be necessary to cover the left subclavian artery, which may cause left arm ischemia.[57] In this event, an extraanatomic bypass (such as a carotid–subclavian bypass) can be performed. In summary, stent grafting is currently not the standard of care for all patients, but it clearly has a role for patients who are not stable enough to undergo a thoracotomy. However, it is entirely conceivable that this will surpass open repair as the standard of care for all patients in the future, given all of its advantages.

One issue that should be of concern with this patient population is blood pressure. High blood pressure increases the risk for rupture and should be avoided. Reduction of the change in pressure over the change in time reduces wall stress significantly and has been shown to reduce the in-hospital aortic rupture rates. Pain and blood pressure should be controlled to a target systolic pressure of approximately 110 mm Hg, starting with morphine and an intravenous beta-blocker such as esmolol. If target pressures cannot be achieved with these interventions, sodium nitroprusside should be added. The advantage of using esmolol and sodium nitroprusside is that they have a relatively short half life.

Operative Technique

Before the operation starts, the patient should undergo a complete set of laboratory studies, should be typed and crossed for at least 2 U, and other blood products such as platelets, cryoprecipitate, and fresh-frozen plasma should be readily available. A cell saver should be employed as well. The cardiologists should be alerted, as they will be needed for intraoperative TEE, which should be considered for all patients unless contraindicated. A double-lumen tube or single-lumen tube with left bronchial blocker should be used, as single right lung ventilation allows optimal exposure of the aorta. Throughout the preoperative workup, as well as during the operation, blood pressure control should be paramount, as a hypertensive episode could result in free rupture before the repair begins.

Right femoral and right radial arterial lines should be obtained for monitoring both upper and lower extremity perfusion. The left groin should be prepped and prepared for possible left heart bypass. Large-bore intravenous access and a pulmonary artery catheter should be placed. Temperature, electrocardiogram, and oxygen saturation should all be continuously monitored. A nasogastric tube should be placed and the stomach emptied, followed by the removal of the nasogastric tube so that a TEE probe can be placed. The patient should then be placed in a right lateral decubitus position with the table flexed. A standard fourth interspace posterolateral thoracotomy offers good exposure to the aortic isthmus and proximal descending aorta. Heparinization is relatively contraindicated for intracranial hemorrhage and lung injury.

Some sort of lower extremity perfusion should probably be employed when performing this repair. Historically, patients undergoing this procedure could expect about a 10% chance of permanent lower extremity paralysis after repair of BAI.[2,26,30,31,38,61] For years surgeons have used a "clamp and sew" technique for repair of these injuries, and it is thought that the lack of oxygenated blood to the distal aorta during a clamp and sew repair was one of the factors that led to this rather high level of paralysis. Many surgeons have adopted some sort of lower extremity perfusion method. There is good evidence to suggest this technique, particularly when clamp times are greater than 30 minutes, leads to lower rates of paralysis.[2,62] Moreover, combined short cross-clamp times with lower body perfusion can significantly decrease the incidence of paralysis.[2,61,62] Thus, in most medical centers, the clamp and sew technique has fallen by the wayside in favor of lower extremity bypass. However, it should be noted that some have also had low paraplegia rates using simple cross-clamping techniques,[26,27] and that simple aortic cross-clamping is warranted in a few discrete circumstances. Any patient who is actively bleeding and there is no time to employ lower body perfusion will require simple aortic cross clamping. Additionally, in some circumstances, such as lack of training or hardware to employ lower body perfusion methods, simple aortic cross-clamping may be the only option. Again, if clamp times are kept to less than 30 minutes the risk of paraplegia is relatively low.

Partial left heart bypass shunts blood from the left atrium to the lower body via the distal thoracic aorta or left femoral artery.[64,65] This method has been demonstrated to be very effective, as one review of five published series demonstrated no paraplegia in 58 patients.[66] We prefer to use this technique. It is achieved by placing a 16- to 20-F cannula in the left atrium through the left inferior pulmonary vein to provide inflow into a pump, which in turn pumps to the distal aorta—preferably as proximal as possible or in the femoral artery. The technique serves a number of purposes: it unloads the left heart and allows better control of proximal blood pressure at the time of cross clamping, it maintains lower body perfusion, and it gives the surgeon good control of the intravascular volume. Ventricular arrhythmias are problematic given that the heart still perfuses the upper body and brain.

Right atrial to femoral artery partial bypass is another method that can be employed. This system is done essentially entirely from the groin. A long venous catheter is passed via the left common femoral vein into the right atrium using a guidewire technique. The femoral artery is also cannulated for the perfusion of blood from the pump, which can be used with or without an oxygenator. The distinct advantage to this modality is that it gives the surgeon the opportunity to go on full bypass, which is relevant in the case of arch injury or ventricular arrhythmias. Moreover, if there are issues with the ability of the patient to oxygenate well on the right lung because of injury or intrinsic disease, this is advantageous.

Once the chest is opened, single lung ventilation should be employed. If the patient cannot be adequately ventilated on the right lung alone, then cardiopulmonary bypass should be instituted. The mediastinal pleura should be incised along the anterior surface of the proximal left subclavian artery. The left subclavian should then be encircled with a tape. Dissection should be carried out on the aortic arch, starting lateral to the vagus nerve and carried out proximal to the left common carotid, as this is usually the point needed for proximal aortic control in most cases. Great care should be taken during this dissection to avoid injury or excessive stretching of the phrenic or vagus nerves. The aortic arch between the left common carotid and the left subclavian artery is then encircled with tape. The distal aorta is controlled by dissection of the overlying pleura and encircling it with a tape (Figure 26.4).

If left heart bypass is to be employed, it is done at this point. The left inferior pulmonary vein is dissected ante-

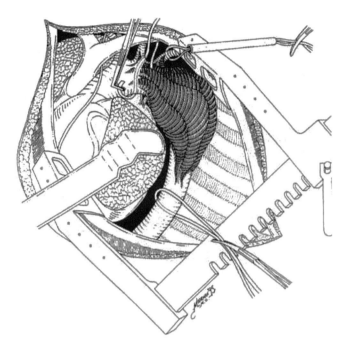

FIGURE 26.4. The surgeon's view (left thoracotomy). After the left lung is deflated and retracted anteriorly, the plane is developed between the left carotid and left subclavian arteries and is encircled with a vessel loop. There is also a vessel loop passed around the distal aorta. A Rommel tourniquet is also placed on the left subclavian artery for control. (Reprinted with permission from Miller OL, Calhoon JH. Acute traumatic aortic transection. In Kaiser LR, Kron IL, Spray TL, eds. Mastery of Cardiothoracic Surgery. Philadelphia: Lippincott-Raven Publishers, 1998.)

riorly, and a purse string suture is placed. Arterial cannulation is performed through the distal aorta (by direct cannulation through a purse string suture) or femoral artery (by Seldinger technique). The inferior pulmonary vein is then cannulated, and bypass is instituted. Once the blood pressure is stable, the left subclavian, proximal, and distal aortas are clamped in respective succession.

At this point the periaortic hematoma is entered, and the extent of the injury is identified (Figure 26.5). Although it is sometimes possible to primarily repair the aorta, it is usually best to debride the torn edges and place a short interposition graft (we prefer to use Dacron).[2,26–28,30,67–70] The graft is sewn using a running 3-0 or 4-0 polypropylene suture with the proximal anastomosis performed first, followed by the distal anastomosis (Figure 26.6). After completion of the anastomosis, the distal clamp should be removed, followed by the proximal aortic and then the left subclavian. The patient should then be weaned off of bypass and heparin reversed. Double lung ventilation should be reinstituted, the chest closed, and the patient taken back to the cardiac intensive care unit.

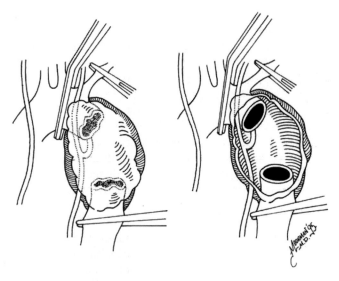

FIGURE 26.5. The hematoma is opened, and the edges of the aorta are debrided. (Reprinted with permission from Miller OL, Calhoon JH. Acute traumatic aortic transection. In Kaiser LR, Kron IL, Spray TL, eds. Mastery of Cardiothoracic Surgery. Philadelphia: Lippincott-Raven Publishers, 1998.)

Complications and Outcomes

For patients who arrive alive at the hospital with traumatic rupture of the aorta, there is still approximately a 30% mortality rate.[2,31] It should be noted, however, that those who are hemodynamically stable and can undergo a planned repair will have about a 14% mortality rate.[2]

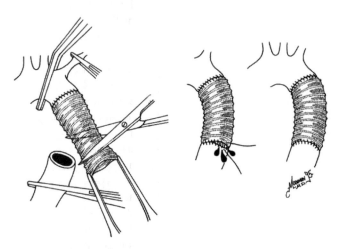

FIGURE 26.6. After completing the proximal anastomosis, the graft is trimmed to an appropriate length, and the distal anastomosis is performed. De-airing and back bleeding through the distal anastomosis should be done after releasing the proximal clamps and before releasing the distal clamp to avoid embolization. (Reprinted with permission from Miller OL, Calhoon JH. Acute traumatic aortic transection. In Kaiser LR, Kron IL, Spray TL, eds. Mastery of Cardiothoracic Surgery. Philadelphia: Lippincott-Raven Publishers, 1998.)

Those patients who are in extremis or who have ruptured aortas will have mortality rates that approach 100%.[2] One third of all patients will die before repair can be performed, and, of the remaining two thirds of patients who die, about one half will die during the repair and one half after the repair. Paralysis in patients who have open repairs occurs approximately 10% of the time.[31] However, the institution of lower extremity perfusion appears to be lowering the rates of paraplegia when cross-clamp times exceed 30 to 35 minutes.[2,31,62,71] There are no reports thus far of any patients who have suffered paralysis after endovascular stent grafting.

Complications that are directly caused by the operation itself in addition to paraplegia include recurrent laryngeal nerve injury and suture line aneurysms; these occur relatively infrequently. Such patients often have multiple injuries, and thus there are a number of complications that may not be directly caused by the aortic repair of itself. Thus the postoperative care of these patients will often be complex, because the trauma of the operation itself will be superimposed on the rest of the injuries the patient has sustained. Pneumonia is the most common complication and occurs at a rate of 20% to 30%.[2,30,33,72,73] This is due in large part to the thoracic injuries often sustained, such as pulmonary contusions, broken ribs, and hemothoraces, as well as prolonged time spent on a ventilator in the intensive care unit. Other complications include renal failure, sepsis, empyema, and abdominal abscess.[2,30,33,73]

To summarize, BAI is a postindustrial age phenomenon. With increases in population and the use of motor vehicles, the incidence will only increase over time. Most people who suffer from BAI will not live to make the trip to the hospital. Those patients who do make it to the hospital, on the other hand, will now have good odds of having their aorta repaired with ever-decreasing chances of suffering any long-term sequelae from the operation. The standard of care in most hospitals today is open repair with some form of lower extremity perfusion, given the increased risk of paralysis with clamp and sew techniques for operations greater than 30 minutes. It is likely that the use of endovascular stent grafts will continue to increase over the next decade, as early results suggest that this is potentially a better alternative to open repair because of the ability to obviate a thoracotomy and decrease the risk of paralysis. Long-term data are necessary to establish whether or not it is indeed better than open repair.

Aortic Dissection

History and Incidence

Sennertus[74] is generally given credit for being the first to describe the dissection process, which he did in the mid-seventeenth century. Approximately 100 years later, Morgani[75] described a number of cases in which blood penetrated the layers of the aortic wall. In 1802, Maunoir[76] provided a more detailed description of the process and is credited with giving the process the name "dissection." The first surgical attempts to intervene in this process were performed by Gurin[77] in 1935, when he performed a fenestration procedure to alleviate ischemia caused by malperfusion. About 20 years later DeBakey[78] was the first to repair a type B aortic dissection, which he repaired by excising the diseased portion of the descending aorta and anastomosing the ends primarily. The first reported repairs of type A dissection were done by Hufnagel and Conrad[79] by means of excising the torn aorta, reuniting the proximal and distal ends, and primarily anastomosing the vessel in an end-to-end fashion.[79] However, this method was replaced by the use of a prosthetic graft, which was introduced by Cooley and DeBakey and is still used today.

Aortic dissection is the most frequently diagnosed lethal condition of the aorta.[80–82] Interestingly, it occurs nearly three times as frequently in the United States as does rupture of an abdominal aortic aneurysm.[83] The incidence is about 5 to 30 cases per 1 million people per year.[84] More than 60% are Stanford type A dissections.[85] Men are more frequently affected, with the ratio ranging from 2:1 to 5:1, depending on the series.[86–88] The incidence, however, is related to the prevalence of risk factors (Table 26.2), with hypertension being the most common factor among patients.[85,89]

TABLE 26.2. Risk factors for thoracic aortic dissection.

Genetic/congenital
• Connective tissue disorders
• Ehlers-Danlos syndrome
• Marfan syndrome
• Turner syndrome
• Anatomic abnormalities
• Bicuspid aortic valve
• Congenital aortic stenosis
• Polycystic kidney disease
• Coarctation of the aorta

Acquired
• Hypertension
• Smoking, dislipidemia, cocaine/crack
• Aortitis
• Cystic medial disease of the aorta
• Iatrogenic
• Atherosclerosis
• Thoracic aortic aneurysm
• Trauma
• Pharmacologic
• Hypervolemia (pregnancy)
• Pheochromocytoma
• Sheehan syndrome
• Cushing syndrome

Etiology and Pathogenesis

Aortic dissection by definition is the development of a false lumen between the layers of the media. Because a number of pathologic processes lead to dissection, it is unlikely that a single disease process explains the phenomenon. It is probably best to think of the etiologies of aortic dissection as those that are genetic connective tissue disorders and those that are acquired.

Marfan syndrome, Ehlers-Danlos syndrome, and familial forms of thoracic aneurysm and dissection are the three major forms of inherited connective tissue disorders known to affect the arterial walls and are associated with aortic dissection. Marfan syndrome is the most prevalent connective tissue disorder, inherited in an autosomal dominant pattern of inheritance with an incidence of approximately 1 in 7,000. The genetic defect results in defective fibrillin in the extracellular matrix, and this can have protean manifestations in multiple organ systems. Over 100 mutations in the fibrillin-1 gene have been identified in people with this disorder, and the penetrance of the disease is variable; there are therefore many different phenotypic variations. However, one thing that is thought to be common among people with aortic wall involvement is the dedifferentiation of vascular smooth muscle cells. This is thought to be caused by enhanced elastolysis of aortic wall components given the defective fibrillin in the extracellular matrix.[90] It is also thought that the enhanced expression of metalloproteinases in vascular smooth muscle cells of patients with Marfan syndrome promotes fragmentation and elastolysis.[91] Like Marfan syndrome, annuloaortic ectasia and familial aortic dissection also have mutations in the fibrillin gene. Bicuspid and unicommisural aortic valves are also risk factors for development of aortic dissection.[92]

Ehlers-Danlos syndrome (EDS), like Marfan syndrome, has a number of genetic abnormalities that are manifest in a number of different phenotypes. The disease is a result of a defect in collagen, like Marfan syndrome, a crucial element in the extracellular matrix, and is manifest by skin extensibility, joint hypermobility, and tissue fragility.[93] It is estimated to occur in approximately 1 in 10,000 births. There are six major types, but aortic involvement is seen primarily in autosomal dominant EDS type IV, also known as "vascular EDS."[93] The disorder is caused by both quantitative and qualitative defects in type III collagen. Interestingly, patients with vascular EDS often have little skin hyperextensibility; however, the skin is thin, translucent, and feels soft. These patients can exhibit poor wound healing and bruisabilty, and patients with vascular EDS are at risk for vascular complications manifest by arterial rupture, tears, or dissection in arteries throughout the body. Arteries in the thorax and abdomen are involved approximately 50% of the time, and extremities are involved 25% of the time.[93–98] Because arteriography can lead to complications in this population, noninvasive means should be used in the diagnosis of dissection.

With regard to acquired conditions, chronic hypertension is the most common condition associated with aortic dissection. Of note, hypertension is found in more than 75% of cases. It is thought that hypertension causes intimal thickening, fibrosis, and fatty acid deposition, and the extracellular matrix undergoes degradation, apoptosis, and elastolysis. Both of these mechanisms can lead to an intimal disruption, usually at the edge of plaques.[99] Moreover, the resultant necrosis of smooth muscle cells and fibrosis of the elastic structures of the vessel wall decrease the compliance of the aortic wall to pulsatile forces, making it more vulnerable for the development of dissection.[100]

Iatrogenic dissection can be caused by a number of procedures involving the aorta, such as any catheterization procedure, aortic root, and/or cannulation for cardiopulmonary bypass, aortic cross clamping, as well as any surgical procedure performed on the aorta.[92,101–103] Thus, surgeons must always have dissection in the backs of their minds when complications of unknown etiology arise after these procedures.

Another theory is that aortic dissections are the result of the creation of an intramural hematoma caused by bleeding from vasa vasorum. This has been put forth because about 20% of patients with acute aortic dissection are found to have an intramural hematoma.[1,104–106] Intramural hematomas rarely regress, and involvement in the ascending aorta is an indication for acute surgery because there is a significant risk of rupture as well as propagation and involvement of the coronary ostia.[104,107]

Clinical Presentation

The diagnosis of acute aortic dissection requires a high level of clinical suspicion. It should be considered in the setting of severe unrelenting chest pain that comes on suddenly. This pain is present in most patients, and this is usually the first time they have experienced such pain. The pain is usually in the midsternum for ascending aortic dissection and in the interscapular region for descending aortic dissection. Classically, the pain is described as "ripping" or "tearing," and it is constant. In the largest prospective study performed to date on patients with aortic dissection, severe chest pain of abrupt onset was the most common complaint, occurring in 73% of patients.[85] Patients may also present with syncope alone, with no other signs of symptoms.[108–112] Patients may also have signs or symptoms related to malperfusion of limbs, brain, or other organs. Abdominal pain and an increase in lactate may indicate involvement of the celiac trunk or the mesenteric artery. Oliguria or anuria may indicate involvement of the renal arteries. Risk factors include

primary hypertension, the presence of aneurysmal disease of the aorta, and, less commonly, a genetic connective tissue disorder.

Patients can present in any number of ways, from stable with a tachycardia to severe hypotension. Pulse deficits can be present in up to 40% of patients and are associated with higher morbidity and mortality rates and poorer outcomes.[113] Abnormal perfusion of the upper extremities can indicate that there is ascending aortic involvement, whereas abnormal perfusion of the lower extremities suggests distal involvement. It is also crucial at the time of presentation to obtain a thorough neurologic examination, as abnormalities are present in up to 35% of acute type A dissections.[113] Hypotension may be due to aortic rupture, acute aortic regurgitation, pericardial tamponade, or myocardial infarction.[85,110,111] On physical examination, a diastolic murmur or muffled heart sound may be heard. With tamponade, jugular venous distension and pulsus paradoxus may be present. Loss of breath sounds, particularly on the left side, can be indicative of left-side hemothorax. Stroke may occur but is infrequent, occurring in less than 5% of patients with acute type A dissection. Loss of perfusion to lumbar or intercostal arteries may result in spinal cord ischemia and paraplegia.

Diagnostic Studies

At the time of presentation, along with the stabilization of the patient, blood tests, electrocardiogram, and chest x-ray should be obtained. Complete blood count, serum electrolytes, myocardial enzymes, blood type and screen, liver function tests, myoglobin, lactic acid, and coagulation studies should be obtained. The electrocardiogram will reveal ischemic changes in approximately 17% of acute type A dissections and in 13% of type B dissections, as well as left ventricular hypertrophy in people with long-standing hypertension.[85] Myocardial infarction is relatively rare, occurring approximately 3% of the time.[85] The chest x-ray will be abnormal in up to 90% of patients with acute dissection, although a normal x-ray cannot rule out dissection. Classic features include a widened mediastinum, rightward tracheal displacement, irregular aortic contour with loss of the aortic knob, an indistinct aortopulmonary window, and a left pleural effusion.

If there is a high clinical suspicion of dissection at this point based on the presentation, the physical examination, and the chest x-ray, care should be expedited to verify that dissection has occurred. The primary modalities used now are CT and echocardiography. These modalities are fast and accurate, which gives them the advantage over magnetic resonance imaging and aortography. It is common to require the use of two imaging modalities to diagnose aortic dissection.[85,114]

Helical CT is now the most frequently utilized first test to diagnose acute aortic dissection, comprising approximately 61% of all first studies.[85,114] It has high sensitivity and specificity for the detection of all types of aortic dissection, approaching an accuracy of 100%.[115,116] When performed as CT angiogram, arch vessel involvement can be identified with a greater than 95% accuracy rate.[115] Diagnosis requires two or more channels separated by an intimal dissection flap. Other findings that can be diagnostic include a hyperattenuating intima, delayed enhancement of a false lumen, and hematomas in the mediastinum, pericardium, or pleura.

Transesophageal echocardiography is the second most frequently used study for diagnosing acute aortic dissection, being used approximately 33% of the time.[85,114] It is the most commonly used secondary study, comprising approximately 56% of secondary studies done. Transesophageal echocardiography may be a more appropriate imaging modality for patients who are unstable and cannot be brought safely to the CT scanner. Patients can be brought to the operating room, sedated, and have TEE. The sensitivity, specificity, and positive and negative predictive values all approach 100% in experienced hands.[117] This study is more operator dependent than CT, although there is a slight risk of causing aortic rupture when doing the study. Making the diagnosis requires visualization of an echogenic surface separating two distinct lumens, repeatedly, in more than one view, and differentiated from normal surrounding cardiac structures. The true lumen is identified by expansion during systole and collapse in diastole. Color Doppler can also aid in distinguishing flow in the false lumen from thrombosis.

Aortography traditionally has been held as the gold standard for the diagnosis of aortic dissection; however, this has been supplanted by CT and echocardiography. The International Registry of Acute Aortic Dissection (IRAD) found that aortography comprised only 4% of the first studies performed, but comprised 17% of the secondary confirmatory studies.[85,114] The need for skilled personnel and the fact that it is an invasive test make it less advantageous than CT or echocardiography. The advantages of aortography include the ability to perform catheter-based interventions in the setting of acute type B dissections with evidence of mesenteric ischemia. However, the use of stent grafts is not yet the standard of care, but they are increasingly being used in this patient population. In our medical center, aortography is used only in the setting of equivocal findings of CT scan or echocardiography.

Magnetic resonance imaging is extremely accurate in the diagnosis of aortic dissection, as the images obtained can yield details of the aorta, pericardium, and surrounding structures. It has not yet become widely available, and in the emergent setting it is not yet a highly used modality.

Classification and Management Decisions

Patients with acute aortic dissection will essentially fall into one of two categories: those who need an urgent operation and those who do not (Figure 26.7). The decision to operate is largely based on the anatomic portion of the aorta that has undergone dissection. These anatomic areas can best be described by either the

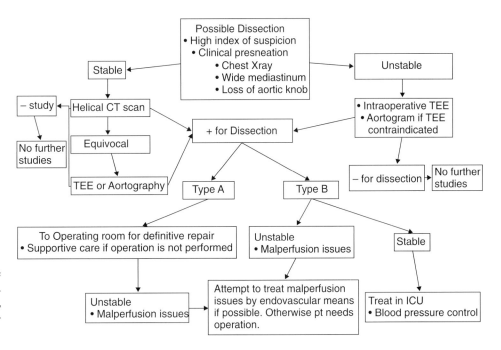

FIGURE 26.7. An algorithm for the management of aortic dissection. CT, computed tomography; ICU, intensive care unit; TEE, transesophageal echocardiography.

DeBakey or the Stanford classification system. The DeBakey system classifies patients into four types. Type I includes dissections that involve the proximal aorta, the aortic arch, and the descending thoracic aorta. Type II involves only the ascending aorta. Type IIIa involves the descending thoracic aorta, and type IIIb involves the descending thoracic as well as the abdominal aorta (Figure 26.8A). The Stanford system only has two classified types of dissection: A and B. Stanford type A involves the ascending aorta, and type B involves only the descending aorta (Figure 26.8B). This classification system is helpful to the surgeon in that type A dissections should receive an operation, whereas type B dissections can usually be medically managed. Because of this practicality, the Stanford classification system is the one most often used by practicing cardiac surgeons when describing aortic dissections.

The natural history of acute type A aortic dissection carries with it high morbidity and mortality rates, as approximately 50% will be dead within 48 hours.[118] Moreover, after the onset of symptoms, there is a 1% to 2% rise in mortality rate per hour.[85] The most common causes of death are aortic rupture, stroke, visceral ischemia, and cardiac tamponade.[110,119] Thus, the primary goal of surgery is to avoid aortic rupture into the pericardium or pleural space. Although the presence of a type A dissection alone is an indication for surgery, there are a number of contraindications to surgery. Age over 80 years is a relative contraindication, as there are few reported survivors in this age group. Neurologic sequelae are a relative contraindication to surgery. Patients who are comatose or obtunded will most likely not improve with surgery. However, stroke and paraplegia are not absolute contraindications. It should be noted that although the dissection may extend into the descending aorta (DeBakey type I), the replacement of the ascending aorta can result in the correction of any malperfusion issues that were caused by dissection. Interestingly less than 10% will have obliteration of the false lumen, although most malperfusion deficits will be corrected after repair. If the repair of the ascending aorta does not result in a correction of malperfusion deficits, other interventions are necessary.

Although type B dissection is less lethal than type A dissection, it can still be associated with a 30-day mortality rate of 10%.[85] Moreover, patients who have evidence of malperfusion manifested by ischemic lower extremities, renal failure, or visceral ischemia may have mortality rates as high as 25% at 30 days. Uncomplicated type B dissection should be treated medically, as approximately 75% of patients with acute type B dissection can be effectively treated in this fashion. More than one half can be managed medically for the rest of their lives.[120] There are, however a number of indications for operat-

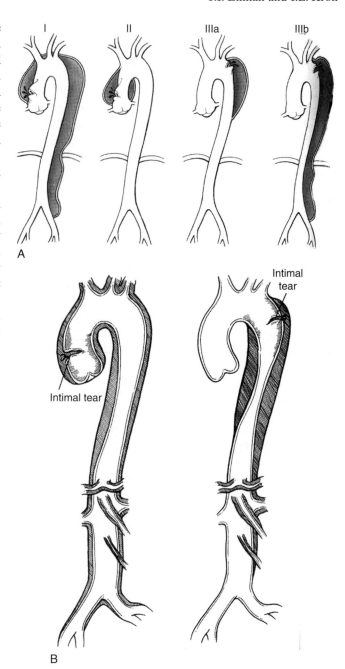

FIGURE 26.8. **(A)** The DeBakey classification system. Type I involves the proximal aorta, arch, and descending aorta. Type II involves the ascending aorta exclusively. Type IIIa involves only the thoracic aorta distal to the left subclavian artery, and type IIIb involves the abdominal aorta as well. (Reprinted with permission of The McGraw Hill Companies from Green R, Kron IL. Aortic dissection. In Cohn LH, Edmunds LH, eds. Cardiac Surgery in the Adult. New York: McGraw-Hill, 2003.). **(B)** The Stanford classification system. (Reprinted with permission from Gardner TJ. Acute aortic dissection. In Kaiser LR, Kron IL, Spray TL, eds. Mastery of Cardiothoracic Surgery. Philadelphia: Lippincott-Raven Publishers, 1998.)

ing on type B dissections, namely, rupture, visceral or limb malperfusion, dissection expansion, and failure of medical management. Factors that may favor early operation include the presence of Marfan syndrome, a large false aneurysm, arch involvement, and presumed medical compliance issues.[121] The acute care and stabilization of these patients should be maximized. Thus, it is extremely important to diagnose the dissection early as well as its type.

Cardiac and vascular surgeons as well as interventional radiologists have developed, and continue to develop, techniques that are useful for patients with descending aortic involvement with both type A and type B dissections. Although type A dissections can only be definitively treated by open cardiac surgery, peripheral vascular malperfusion can occur, and these complications can be dealt with by interventional techniques. Type B malperfusion issues or dissection propagation can be treated definitively by interventional techniques. Slonim et al.[122] have published one of the larger retrospective studies of endovascular techniques at Stanford for patients suffering from ischemic complications with acute aortic dissection. Over a 6-year period, 40 patients (32 male and 8 female) underwent percutaneous treatment for peripheral ischemic complications of 10 type A and 30 type B acute aortic dissections. All type A dissections that were surgically repaired (9/10) were repaired before the interventional procedure was performed. Thirty of these patients had renal, 22 had leg, 18 had mesenteric, and 1 had arm ischemic complications. Fourteen patients were treated with stenting of either the true or the false lumen combined with balloon fenestration of the intimal flap, 24 with stenting alone and 2 with fenestration alone. They were able to successfully revascularize 93% of these patients. There were nine procedure-related complications. Because ischemic complications are associated with a high mortality rate, they had a 30-day mortality rate of approximately 25%. There were 5 late deaths (17%) in the remaining 30 patients. Techniques can range from fenestration of a false lumen to create a communication with the true lumen to the use of covered stents to enter to a false lumen or the use of noncovered stent grafts to enlarge a compressed true lumen. The use of stent grafts as definitive therapy for a type B dissection is growing in acceptance, and early results are encouraging.[123] Flow can be restored in up to 90% of vessels obstructed by aortic dissection.[124–126] Many medical centers are now utilizing these strategies in the setting of both complicated and uncomplicated descending aorta dissection. It is conceivable that over time interventional techniques will replace open techniques for the treatment of type B dissections, as well as malperfusion complications with type A and type B dissections.

The initial medical management will be guided by the stability of the patient. The unstable patient belongs in the operating room. In the operating room stabilization, resuscitation, or acute care surgery can take place with echocardiography occurring concurrently to aid in the diagnosis. Any procedure should preferentially be done on an anesthetized patient, as hypertension due to stress can cause rupture or propagation of the dissection.

If the patient is stable, blood pressure control should be measured in both arms and kept with a systolic pressure between 90 and 110 mm Hg. The avoidance of hypertension is predicated on two issues: first, shear stress on the aorta is decreased by minimizing the rate of rise of aortic pressure to decrease the dissection propagation. Second, aortic wall stress is lowered by decreasing systolic blood pressure. If a patient is in pain, analgesics should be used first. After that, nitroprusside will help to get the pressure down quickly, and the addition of esmolol will decrease pulse pressure.

Operative Technique for Type A Dissection

The only curative therapy that currently exists for type A dissection is open surgery. However, only 72% of patients presenting with type A aortic dissection will undergo surgery.[85] Age (>80 years old is generally considered the relative number, although a fit 80-year-old person could conceivably tolerate the operation), other comorbidities, death, or refusal to undergo surgery are the main reasons why people do not have the operation who have a type A dissection. Approximately 15% of patients will have concomitant coronary artery bypass surgery, 9% will require a total arch replacement, 10% a partial arch replacement and 15% will need valve repair or replacement.[85]

Preparation should include the single endotracheal tube for operations through a median sternotomy and double-lumen tubes if the procedure is to be performed through a left thoracotomy. The patient should have central venous access with a pulmonary artery catheter, as well as radial arterial lines and a femoral arterial line to continually assess peripheral perfusion. Anesthesia cardiology should be employed to help with transeophageal echocardiography. Temperature can be measured through a Foley catheter and a nasopharyngeal probe. The skin should be widely prepped, including the axillary and femoral arteries to allow for all cannulation options. A cell saver should be employed, as blood loss can be substantial in these procedures. The patient should be typed and crossed for at least 2 U of blood, and preparations should be made to have fresh-frozen plasma, platelets, and cryoprecipitate available.

There are a number of options for arterial and venous cannulation for cardiopulmonary bypass. The choice will depend on a number of issues. There is still controversy regarding which femoral artery to cannulate, but we prefer the right because it usually supplies the true lumen. Alternatively, the axillary artery can be used effectively after a graft is anastomosed to it.[127] Venous cannulation is usually through the right atrium using a two-stage venous cannula. A left ventricular vent is necessary in the setting of aortic valve incompetence and should be placed through the right superior pulmonary vein or rarely through the left ventricular apex wall. For type B dissections, partial left heart bypass, as in the case of acute aortic disruption, has replaced the clamp and sew technique.

During the repair of a type A dissection, one must decide on the manner in which the brain will be protected. This can be achieved by deep hypothermia or continued perfusion, be it antegrade or retrograde. If deep hypothermia is to be used, it is thought that up to 14 minutes of circulatory arrest is acceptable at a temperature of 25°C and up to 31 minutes at 15°C.[128] However, for longer periods of time at 15°C, one sees a higher incidence of neurologic sequelae, being as high as 60% at 60 minutes. Thus, for complex repairs that will require longer than 30 minutes, cerebral perfusion should probably be used. Retrograde cerebral perfusion can be done through a bicaval cannula, with reversal of flow occurring through the superior vena cava cannula. It can also be done in a dual-stage manner, with the placement of a retrograde coronary sinus catheter into the superior vena cava through a purse string suture. Selective antegrade perfusion can be accomplished by placing cannulae in the innominate and the left common carotids through the ostia from the inside of the aorta once it is open. The left subclavian should be occluded to avoid back flow, and pressure should be approximately 50 to 70 mm Hg. The cannulae are removed just before completing the anastomosis of the brachiocephalic vessels to the vascular graft, at which time cardiopulmonary bypass may be reinstituted.

After sternotomy, other modifications of the incision can be performed such as a supraclavicular, cervical, or trapdoor incision to gain exposure to the brachiocephalic vessels or the descending thoracic aorta if need be. The dissection should be carried out first on the distal arch, taking care not to injure the left vagus nerve with its recurrent branch and the left phrenic nerve.

An open distal repair is the procedure of choice (Figure 26.9). After placing a clamp on the mid ascending aorta and cardiac arrest is achieved, the aorta proximal to the clamp is opened. At this point, the aortic valve should be evaluated as systemic cooling occurs. The valve usually can be resuspended. If the sinuses are not dilated, then the aorta is transected 5 to 10 mm distal to the sinotubular ridge.

If there is a dissection that involves the root the intima of the coronary, ostia may or may not be involved. If they are not involved, a repair of the sinotubular junction can be performed, reuniting the dissected aortic layers

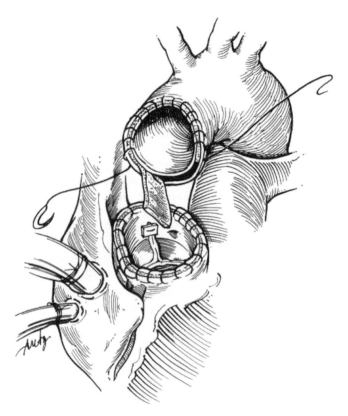

FIGURE 26.9. In most cases an open distal repair is performed. The native aortic valve can usually be repaired and resuspended. The layers of the aorta are repaired with a piece of felt placed in between (both proximally and distally). An interposition graft is then used to complete the repair. (Reprinted with permission from Gardner TJ. Acute aortic dissection. In Kaiser LR, Kron IL, Spray TL, eds. Mastery of Cardiothoracic Surgery. Philadelphia: Lippincott-Raven Publishers, 1988.)

between one or two strips of Teflon felt using 3-0 or 4-0 Prolene suture. A minimal disruption of the coronary ostia can be repaired primarily using a 5-0 or 6-0 suture. If the coronary ostium is circumferentially dissected and aortic root replacement is necessary, an aortic button should be excised and the layers reunited. The coronary button should then be reimplanted into the vascular graft. Aortocoronary bypass should be performed only when the coronary ostium is not reconstructable.

Aortic valve insufficiency is common in these patients, but the valve can be preserved in most patients.[85] The mechanism is usually caused by the loss of commissural support of the valve leaflets. This is repaired first by placing pledgeted 4-0 Prolene sutures to reposition each of the commisures at the sinotubular ridge, followed by a layer of Teflon felt placed circumferentially to reunite the dissected aortic root layers. Some have used Bioglue between the layers of the aorta prior to suture repair of the sinotubular ridge. If the valve cannot be spared, a formal replacement of the valve and the ascending aorta should be performed using a composite valve graft or homograft. The valve is implanted using horizontal mattress 2-0 Tycron sutures. The left coronary button should be implanted into the graft first, and then the right coronary button implanted after the graft is clamped and placed under pressure to allow for the proper anatomic position of the right coronary button.

Once the core temperature reaches approximately 20°C, perfusion is discontinued for a brief period of circulatory arrest. The aortic clamp on the mid ascending aorta is released, and the intima of the aortic arch is inspected and then repaired. If the intima is intact, the distal anastomosis is performed; the graft is then cannulated, de-aired, and clamped for resumption of cardiopulmonary bypass. If the intima is not intact, a hemiarch reconstruction should be performed. The integrity of the brachiocephalic vessel intima and ostia should be inspected from the inside of the aorta. If they are intact, they can be implanted as a Carrel patch into a vascular graft after repair (Figure 26.10). If, however, the dissection involves individual vessels, repair will be needed for the individual vessels, and then they will be implanted into the graft or to short interposition grafts if the dissection extends past the origin of the arteries.

If the ascending aorta cannot be cross clamped because of fear of rupture, the patient is cooled to 20°C and circulatory arrest should be employed. The aorta should be opened, and the distal anastomosis performed. As before, the graft should be cannulated, de-aired, and proximally clamped and cardiopulmonary bypass reinstituted. Because a cross clamp is not applied, the left ventricle must be decompressed once fibrillation starts during systemic cooling to prevent distension and irreversible myocardial injury. During the rewarming period, the proximal ascending aortic repair should be completed.

If the dissection is limited to the ascending aorta or to the proximal arch away from the origin of the brachio-

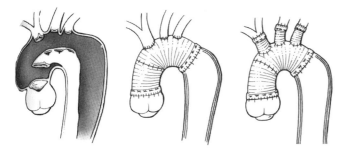

FIGURE 26.10. If the dissection involves the arch vessels, an arch repair is needed. This can be performed by Carrel patch or by anastomosing each vessel to the graft individually. If the dissection involves the origins of the vessels, then short interposition grafts can be utilized in the repair. (Reprinted with permission of The McGraw Hill Companies from Green R, Kron IL. Aortic dissection. In Cohn LH, Edmunds LH, eds. Cardiac Surgery in the Adult. New York: McGraw-Hill, 2003.)

cephalic vessels, an alternative repair can be performed. This entire procedure can be done without requiring deep hypothermia and circulatory arrest. Antegrade perfusion can be performed through the distal arch or the right subclavian artery, or retrograde perfusion through the femoral artery is another alternative. After an aortic cross clamp is applied just proximal to the innominate artery, the ascending aorta is resected to include the inferior aspect of the arch. The layers of the dissected aorta proximal to the clamp are then reunited if necessary. The proximal reconstruction is then performed.

Technique for Type B Dissection

The ideal position for the repair of a type B dissection is right lateral decubitus position. The pelvis should be positioned in such a way that the femoral vessels are accessible. A double-lumen endotracheal tube should be employed. A posterolateral thoracotomy through the fourth intercostal space will allow for good access to the aorta. If, however, there is extension of the dissection into the abdomen with resultant visceral malperfusion, a thoracoabdominal incision should be employed.

Repair of a type B dissection has many similarities to an open repair for BAI. Given the relatively high rates of paralysis reported (about 20%[129]), there are a few strategies that should be employed when performing this operation. The same tenets discussed with regard to lower extremity perfusion in the repair of BAI hold true here as well. Also, given the possibility that disruption of the intercostal arteries can be a contributing factor to paralysis, one should try to replace as little of the descending aorta as possible.

Once the aorta has been exposed, the repair of a descending aortic dissection is similar to that discussed for repair of an aortic disruption. A plane should be developed between the left subclavian and left common carotid arteries and the left subclavian encircled with umbilical tape and Rommell tourniquet. As before, the left vagus and recurrent laryngeal nerves should be identified and preserved during the course of the dissection. The descending aorta should be dissected, and, if left heart bypass is to be employed via the left inferior pulmonary vein, a 4–0 Prolene purse string should be placed posteriorly. After the patient is heparinized a 14-F cannula should be placed into the left inferior pulmonary vein and another cannula placed in the femoral artery. Left heart bypass should then be instituted at flow rates between 1 and 2 L/min. The left subclavian artery is controlled by the Rommell tourniquet, and clamps are placed on the aorta between the left subclavian artery and left common carotid as well as distally. Arterial pressures should be between 100 and 140 mm Hg by right radial artery and greater than 60 mm Hg by the femoral artery. The aorta should then be opened longitudinally, and bleeding from intercostal arteries can be controlled by figure of 8 suture ligation. The aorta should be transected just distal to the origin of the left subclavian artery and the proximal anastomosis of the graft performed using a 3-0 Prolene suture with or without Teflon felt strips. Once the proximal anastomosis is complete the proximal clamp is released and repositioned on the graft. The integrity of the anastomosis should then be inspected. The distal aorta should now be inspected and repaired, with either Teflon felt or glue. The distal anastomosis should then be performed, clamps released, and left heart bypass terminated. We recommend directly repairing anything larger than a 14-F hole left in the femoral artery from cannulation.

Outcomes and Complications

Acute aortic dissection is associated with an in-hospital mortality rate of approximately 27%.[85] However, there are a number of important factors that play into the outcomes of patients who have acute aortic dissection. Patients with type A dissection who do not undergo surgery have the highest mortality rates (58%), followed by type B patients who had surgery (31%), type A patients who had surgery (26%), and type B patients who were treated medically (11%) (Figure 26.11). The higher rate of mortality for patients with type B dissection who undergo surgery versus those with type A is most likely because the patients who undergo surgery for type B dissection often are sicker with malperfusion or rupture.

Age also is a risk factor for both types A and B dissection.[109,111,130] Patients older than 70 years with type A

dissection will have mortality rates of approximately 43% compared with those who are younger than 70 years, who have mortality rates of 28%.[110] Likewise, patients older than 70 years with type B dissection can expect morality rates of approximately 16% vs. 10% for those younger than 70 years.[111]

Other factors that are considered significant risk factors for mortality in patients with type B dissection include the "deadly triad" of hypotension/shock, absence of chest/back pain on presentation, and branch vessel involvement.[109] We have found preoperative shock to be the most important risk factor for repair of type A aortic dissection. Suzuki and colleagues[109] hypothesize that the absence of chest or back pain is probably associated with higher mortality rates because of a delay in diagnosis. This is an important observation because it runs contrary to the classic clinical picture of "tearing" chest or back pain.

End-organ malperfusion is one of the most common complications seen in patients with aortic dissection, and it is associated with a high level of morbidity and mortality. This is caused by compression of the true lumen of the branch vessel by the false lumen. It occurs in 16% to 30% of all cases of type A dissection.[132–136] Repairs of an aortic dissection associated with malperfusion have mortality rates as high as 89%.[137] Organs that are commonly affected include the kidneys and the gut, and there can be involvement of both the upper and lower extremities. The coronary arteries can be involved, and neurologic involvement due to carotid artery involvement can also be seen. Some authors believe that expeditious definitive repair of a type A dissection should supersede any attempts to treat malperfused organs, as the repair of the dissection itself often fixes both the proximal aorta and the vessel that is malperfused.[133–136] Others suggest an alternate strategy whereby endovascular techniques are used to treat the organs or extremities that are malperfused, followed by aortic repair.[137] As the endovascular techniques, as well as treatment pathways to expedite interventional therapy, advance, we may see this method adopted by more surgeons, as it is clear that the systemic inflammatory response that occurs because of ischemia creates a poor setting for major surgery. However, it should also be noted that a person with a type A dissection is at imminent risk for rupture or propagation, and time spent working on malperfusion issues may result in negative outcomes.

Actuarial survival rates for all patients with acute aortic dissection are approximately 55%, 37%, and 24% after 5, 10, and 15 years, respectively, for type A dissections and 48%, 29%, and 11% for type B dissections.[138] Long-term survival rates for all patients who undergo surgery for aortic dissection are approximately 80% at 5 years and 60% at 10 years.[139] These rates are similar for both patients with type A and type B dissections. The inci-

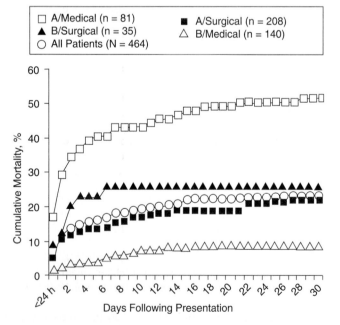

FIGURE 26.11. Thirty-day mortality rates for patients with aortic dissection. (Reprinted with permission from Hagan et al.[85])

dence of late reoperation (dissection related) increases with time, with almost 25% of all patients requiring reoperation by 10 years; again, there was no significant difference among patients with different types or acuity of dissection.[139] Significant independent risk factors for late death included stroke, chronic renal dysfunction, remote myocardial infarction, and operation. Younger age, site of intimal tear (arch tears having higher risk), and cardiac tamponade have a significantly higher likelihood of late reoperation.

To summarize, although mortality rates have improved over the past 40 years, acute dissection of the aorta has a high rate of morbidity and mortality.[140] Because early in the process the development of complications decreases the chances of a positive outcome, a high index of suspicion is needed to diagnose this problem so that proper therapy can be instituted. Helical CT scanning has allowed for improvement in the speed with which dissection can be diagnosed and is now the best first test for this disease. The standard of care for type A dissection is surgical repair. Type B dissections should be treated medically, with surgery or endovascular therapy reserved for complications. Although traditionally type A dissections presenting with malperfusion issues, as well as type B dissections complicated by impending rupture or malperfusion, were indications for emergent surgery, endovascular techniques from fenestration to definitive stent graft repairs are emerging as potential alternatives to open surgical repair.

Critique

With a documented aortic rupture, definitive management would necessitate a thoracotomy to repair the aortic injury. For the patient who has significant comorbidities or associated severe head and pulmonary injuries, intensive care unit monitoring and aggressive antihypertensive therapy would be an appropriate temporizing measure. The role of endovascular stenting is still controversial given that intraluminal stents can (1) migrate, (2) have an associated endoleak, and (3) require lifetime surveillance. Its use should be under strict protocol. There is never a role for observation only. Also, the insertion of an intraaortic balloon pump is contraindicated.

Answer (A)

References

1. Smith RS, Chang FC. Traumatic rupture of the aorta: still a lethal injury. Am J Surg 1986; 152(6):660–663.
2. Fabian TC, Richardson JD, Croce MA, et al. Prospective study of blunt aortic injury: multicenter trial of the American Association for the Surgery of Trauma. J Trauma 1997; 42(3):374–383.
3. Gavant ML, Flick P, Menke P, Gold RE. CT aortography of thoracic aortic rupture. AJR Am J Roentgenol 1996; 166(4):955–961.
4. Parmley LF, Mattingly TW, Manion WC, Jahnke EJ Jr. Nonpenetrating traumatic injury of the aorta. Circulation 1958; 17(6):1086–1101.
5. Steinberg I. Chronic traumatic aneurysm of the thoracic aorta: report of five cases, with a plea for conservative treatment. N Engl J Med 1957; 257(19):913–918.
6. Passaro E Jr, Pace WG. Traumatic rupture of the aorta. Surgery 1959; 46:787–791.
7. Mattox KL. Fact and fiction about management of aortic transection. Ann Thorac Surg 1989; 48(1):1–2.
8. Duhaylongsod FG, Glower DD, Wolfe WG. Acute traumatic aortic aneurysm: the Duke experience from 1970 to 1990. J Vasc Surg 1992; 15(2):331–343.
9. Brown DK, Roe EJ, Henry TE. A fatality associated with the deployment of an automobile airbag. J Trauma 1995; 39(6):1204–1206.
10. Pillgram-Larsen J, Geiran O. [Air bags influence the pattern of injury in severe thoracic trauma.] Tidsskr Nor Laegeforen 1997; 117(17):2437–2439.
11. Dunn JA, Williams MG. Occult ascending aortic rupture in the presence of an air bag. Ann Thorac Surg 1996; 62(2):577–578.
12. Sevitt S. Traumatic ruptures of the aorta: a clinico-pathological study. Injury 1977; 8(3):159–173.
13. Greendyke RM. Traumatic rupture of aorta; special reference to automobile accidents. JAMA 1966; 195(7):527–530.
14. Butcher HR Jr, Jaffe BM. Treatment of aortoiliac arterial occlusive disease by endarterectomy. Ann Surg 1971; 173(6):925–932.
15. Butcher HR Jr. The elastic properties of human aortic intima, media and adventitia: the initial effect of thromboendarterectomy. Ann Surg 1960; 151:480–489.
16. Stapp JP. Human tolerance to deceleration. Am J Surg 1957; 93(4):734–740.
17. Jackson FR, Berkas EM, Roberts VL. Traumatic aortic rupture after blunt trauma. Dis Chest 1968; 53(5):577–583.
18. Sevitt S. The mechanisms of traumatic rupture of the thoracic aorta. Br J Surg 1977; 64(3):166–173.
19. Coermann R, Dotzauer G, Lange W, Voigt GE. The effects of the design of the steering assembly and the instrument panel on injuries (especially aortic rupture) sustained by car drivers in head-on collision. J Trauma 1972; 12(8):715–724.
20. Crass JR, Cohen AM, Motta AO, Tomashefski JF Jr, Wiesen EJ. A proposed new mechanism of traumatic aortic rupture: the osseous pinch. Radiology 1990; 176(3):645–649.
21. Cohen AM, Crass JR, Thomas HA, Fisher RG, Jacobs DG. CT evidence for the "osseous pinch" mechanism of traumatic aortic injury. AJR Am J Roentgenol 1992; 159(2):271–274.
22. Cohen AM, Crass JR. Traumatic aortic injuries: current concepts. Semin Ultrasound CT MR 1993; 14(2):71–84.

23. Feczko JD, Lynch L, Pless JE, Clark MA, McClain J, Hawley DA. An autopsy case review of 142 nonpenetrating (blunt) injuries of the aorta. J Trauma 1992; 33(6): 846–849.

24. Arajarvi E, Santavirta S, Tolonen J. Aortic ruptures in seat belt wearers. J Thorac Cardiovasc Surg 1989; 98(3):355–361.

25. Rabinsky I, Sidhu GS, Wagner RB. Mid-descending aortic traumatic aneurysms. Ann Thorac Surg 1990; 50(1):155–160.

26. Razzouk AJ, Gundry SR, Wang N, del Rio MJ, Varnell D, Bailey LL. Repair of traumatic aortic rupture: a 25-year experience. Arch Surg 2000; 135(8):913–919.

27. Sweeney MS, Young DJ, Frazier OH, Adams PR, Kapusta MO, Macris MP. Traumatic aortic transections: eight-year experience with the "clamp-sew" technique. Ann Thorac Surg 1997; 64(2):384–389.

28. Hilgenberg AD, Logan DL, Akins CW, et al. Blunt injuries of the thoracic aorta. Ann Thorac Surg 1992; 53(2):233–239.

29. Kieny R, Charpentier A. Traumatic lesions of the thoracic aorta. A report of 73 cases. J Cardiovasc Surg (Torino) 1991; 32(5):613–619.

30. Cowley RA, Turney SZ, Hankins JR, Rodriguez A, Attar S, Shankar BS. Rupture of thoracic aorta caused by blunt trauma. A fifteen-year experience. J Thorac Cardiovasc Surg 1990; 100(5):652–661.

31. von Oppell UO, Dunne TT, De Groot MK, Zilla P. Traumatic aortic rupture: twenty-year metaanalysis of mortality and risk of paraplegia. Ann Thorac Surg 1994; 58(2):585–593.

32. McBride LR, Tidik S, Stothert JC, et al. Primary repair of traumatic aortic disruption. Ann Thorac Surg 1987; 43(1):65–67.

33. Schmidt CA, Wood MN, Razzouk AJ, Killeen JD, Gan KA. Primary repair of traumatic aortic rupture: a preferred approach. J Trauma 1992; 32(5):588–592.

34. Kirsh MM, Behrendt DM, Orringer MB, et al. The treatment of acute traumatic rupture of the aorta: a 10-year experience. Ann Surg 1976; 184(3):308–316.

35. Sturm JT, Billiar TR, Dorsey JS, Luxenberg MG, Perry JF Jr. Risk factors for survival following surgical treatment of traumatic aortic rupture. Ann Thorac Surg 1985; 39(5):418–421.

36. Clark DE, Zeiger MA, Wallace KL, Packard AB, Nowicki ER. Blunt aortic trauma: signs of high risk. J Trauma 1990; 30(6):701–705.

37. Gundry SR, Williams S, Burney RE, Cho KJ, Mackenzie JR. Indications for aortography in blunt thoracic trauma: a reassessment. J Trauma 1982; 22(8):664–671.

38. Kram HB, Wohlmuth DA, Appel PL, Shoemaker WC. Clinical and radiographic indications for aortography in blunt chest trauma. J Vasc Surg 1987; 6(2):168–176.

39. Sturm JT, Perry JF Jr, Olson FR, Cicero JJ. Significance of symptoms and signs in patients with traumatic aortic rupture. Ann Emerg Med 1984; 13(10):876–878.

40. Trachiotis GD, Sell JE, Pearson GD, Martin GR, Midgley FM. Traumatic thoracic aortic rupture in the pediatric patient. Ann Thorac Surg 1996; 62(3):724–732.

41. Vlahakes GJ, Warren RL. Traumatic rupture of the aorta. N Engl J Med 1995; 332(6):389–390.

42. Cook AD, Klein JS, Rogers FB, Osler TM, Shackford SR. Chest radiographs of limited utility in the diagnosis of blunt traumatic aortic laceration. J Trauma 2001; 50(5):843–847.

43. Fabian TC, Davis KA, Gavant ML, et al. Prospective study of blunt aortic injury: helical CT is diagnostic and antihypertensive therapy reduces rupture. Ann Surg 1998; 227(5):666–677.

44. Gavant ML. Helical CT grading of traumatic aortic injuries. Impact on clinical guidelines for medical and surgical management. Radiol Clin North Am 1999; 37(3):553–574, vi.

45. Demetriades D, Gomez H, Velmahos GC, et al. Routine helical computed tomographic evaluation of the mediastinum in high-risk blunt trauma patients. Arch Surg 1998; 133(10):1084–1088.

46. Sturm JT, Hankins DG, Young G. Thoracic aortography following blunt chest trauma. Am J Emerg Med 1990; 8(2):92–96.

47. Eddy AC, Nance DR, Goldman MA, et al. Rapid diagnosis of thoracic aortic transection using intravenous digital subtraction angiography. Am J Surg 1990; 159(5):500–503.

48. LaBerge JM, Jeffrey RB. Aortic lacerations: fatal complications of thoracic aortography. Radiology 1987; 165(2):367–369.

49. Wilson D, Voystock JF, Sariego J, Kerstein MD. Role of computed tomography scan in evaluating the widened mediastinum. Am Surg 1994; 60(6):421–423.

50. Mirvis SE, Shanmuganathan K, Buell J, Rodriguez A. Use of spiral computed tomography for the assessment of blunt trauma patients with potential aortic injury. J Trauma 1998; 45(5):922–930.

51. Melton SM, Kerby JD, McGiffin D, et al. The evolution of chest computed tomography for the definitive diagnosis of blunt aortic injury: a single-center experience. J Trauma 2004; 56(2):243–250.

52. Vignon P, Boncoeur MP, Francois B, Rambaud G, Maubon A, Gastinne H. Comparison of multiplane transesophageal echocardiography and contrast-enhanced helical CT in the diagnosis of blunt traumatic cardiovascular injuries. Anesthesiology 2001; 94(4):615–622.

53. Parker MS, Matheson TL, Rao AV, et al. Making the transition: the role of helical CT in the evaluation of potentially acute thoracic aortic injuries. AJR Am J Roentgenol 2001; 176(5):1267–1272.

54. Smith MD, Cassidy JM, Souther S, et al. Transesophageal echocardiography in the diagnosis of traumatic rupture of the aorta. N Engl J Med 1995; 332(6):356–362.

55. Kearney PA, Smith DW, Johnson SB, Barker DE, Smith MD, Sapin PM. Use of transesophageal echocardiography in the evaluation of traumatic aortic injury. J Trauma 1993; 34(5):696–703.

56. Saletta S, Lederman E, Fein S, Singh A, Kuehler DH, Fortune JB. Transesophageal echocardiography for the initial evaluation of the widened mediastinum in trauma patients. J Trauma 1995; 39(1):137–142.

57. Orford VP, Atkinson NR, Thomson K, et al. Blunt traumatic aortic transection: the endovascular experience. Ann Thorac Surg 2003; 75(1):106–112.

58. Ahn SH, Cutry A, Murphy TP, Slaiby JM. Traumatic thoracic aortic rupture: treatment with endovascular graft in the acute setting. J Trauma 2001; 50(5):949–951.

59. Ott MC, Stewart TC, Lawlor DK, Gray DK, Forbes TL. Management of blunt thoracic aortic injuries: endovascular stents versus open repair. J Trauma 2004; 56(3):565–570.

60. Fujikawa T, Yukioka T, Ishimaru S, et al. Endovascular stent grafting for the treatment of blunt thoracic aortic injury. J Trauma 2001; 50(2):223–229.

61. von Oppell UO, Dunne TT, De Groot KM, Zilla P. Spinal cord protection in the absence of collateral circulation: meta-analysis of mortality and paraplegia. J Cardiol Surg 1994; 9(6):685–691.

62. Katz NM, Blackstone EH, Kirklin JW, Karp RB. Incremental risk factors for spinal cord injury following operation for acute traumatic aortic transection. J Thorac Cardiovasc Surg 1981; 81(5):669–674.

63. Pate JW, Gavant ML, Weiman DS, Fabian TC. Traumatic rupture of the aortic isthmus: program of selective management. World J Surg 1999; 23(1):59–63.

64. Szwerc MF, Benckart DH, Lin JC, et al. Recent clinical experience with left heart bypass using a centrifugal pump for repair of traumatic aortic transection. Ann Surg 1999; 230(4):484–492.

65. Fullerton DA. Simplified technique for left heart bypass to repair aortic transection. Ann Thorac Surg 1993; 56(3):579–580.

66. Read RA, Moore EE, Moore FA, Haenel JB. Partial left heart bypass for thoracic aorta repair. Survival without paraplegia. Arch Surg 1993; 128(7):746–752.

67. Plume S, DeWeese JA. Traumatic rupture of the thoracic aorta. Arch Surg 1979; 114(3):240–243.

68. Turney SZ, Attar S, Ayella R, Cowley RA, McLaughlin J. Traumatic rupture of the aorta. A five-year experience. J Thorac Cardiovasc Surg 1976; 72(5):727–734.

69. Zeiger MA, Clark DE, Morton JR. Reappraisal of surgical treatment of traumatic transection of the thoracic aorta. J Cardiovasc Surg (Torino) 1990; 31(5):607–610.

70. Wallenhaupt SL, Hudspeth AS, Mills SA, Tucker WY, Dobbins JE, Cordell AR. Current treatment of traumatic aortic disruptions. Am Surg 1989; 55(5):316–320.

71. Hunt JP, Baker CC, Lentz CW, et al. Thoracic aorta injuries: management and outcome of 144 patients. J Trauma 1996; 40(4):547–556.

72. von Kodolitsch Y, Schwartz AG, Nienaber CA, et al. Clinical prediction of acute aortic dissection. Arch Intern Med 2000 160(19):2977–2982.

73. Kodali S, Jamieson WR, Leia-Stephens M, Miyagishima RT, Janusz MT, Tyers GF. Traumatic rupture of the thoracic aorta. A 20-year review: 1969–1989. Circulation 1991; 84(5 Suppl):III-40–46.

74. Sennertus D. Cap. 42. Op Omn Lib 1650; 5:306.

75. Morgagni G. De dedibus et causis moroborum. Venetiis, 1761.

76. Maunoir J. Memoires Physiologiques et Pratiques sur L'aneurysme et la Ligature des Arteres. Geneva: J.J. Pashoud, 1802.

77. Gurin D. Dissecting aneurysms of the aorta: diagnosis and operative relief of acute arterial obstruction due to this cause. NY State J Med 1935; 35:1200.

78. DeBakey ME, Cooley DA, Creech O, Jr. Surgical considerations of dissecting aneurysm of the aorta. Ann Surg 1955; 142(4):586–612.

79. Hufnagel CA, Conrad PW. Direct repair of dissecting aneurysms of the aorta. Circulation 1962; 25:568–572.

80. Ponraj P, Pepper J. Aortic dissection. Br J Clin Pract 1992; 46(2):127–131.

81. Kouchoukos NT, Dougenis D. Surgery of the thoracic aorta. N Engl J Med 1997; 336(26):1876–1888.

82. Pate JW, Richardson RL, Eastridge CE. Acute aortic dissections. Am Surg 1976; 42(6):395–404.

83. Coady MA, Rizzo JA, Goldstein LJ, Elefteriades JA. Natural history, pathogenesis, and etiology of thoracic aortic aneurysms and dissections. Cardiol Clin 1999; 17(4):615–635, vii.

84. Khan IA, Nair CK. Clinical, diagnostic, and management perspectives of aortic dissection. Chest 2002; 122(1):311–328.

85. Hagan PG, Nienaber CA, Isselbacher EM, et al. The International Registry of Acute Aortic Dissection (IRAD): new insights into an old disease. JAMA 2000; 283(7):897–903.

86. Hirst AE Jr, Johns VJ Jr, Kime SW Jr. Dissecting aneurysm of the aorta: a review of 505 cases. Medicine (Baltimore) 1958; 37(3):217–279.

87. Wilson SK, Hutchins GM. Aortic dissecting aneurysms: causative factors in 204 subjects. Arch Pathol Lab Med 1982; 106(4):175–180.

88. DeBakey ME, McCollum CH, Crawford ES, et al. Dissection and dissecting aneurysms of the aorta: twenty-year follow-up of five hundred twenty-seven patients treated surgically. Surgery 1982; 92(6):1118–1134.

89. Spittell PC, Spittell JA Jr, Joyce JW, et al. Clinical features and differential diagnosis of aortic dissection: experience with 236 cases (1980 through 1990). Mayo Clin Proc 1993; 68(7):642–651.

90. Lesauskaite V, Tanganelli P, Sassi C, et al. Smooth muscle cells of the media in the dilatative pathology of ascending thoracic aorta: morphology, immunoreactivity for osteopontin, matrix metalloproteinases, and their inhibitors. Hum Pathol 2001; 32(9):1003–1011.

91. Segura AM, Luna RE, Horiba K, et al. Immunohistochemistry of matrix metalloproteinases and their inhibitors in thoracic aortic aneurysms and aortic valves of patients with Marfan's syndrome. Circulation 1998; 98(19 Suppl):II-331–338.

92. Larson EW, Edwards WD. Risk factors for aortic dissection: a necropsy study of 161 cases. Am J Cardiol 1984; 53(6):849–855.

93. Germain DP. Clinical and genetic features of vascular Ehlers-Danlos syndrome. Ann Vasc Surg 2002; 16(3):391–397.

94. Mattar SG, Kumar AG, Lumsden AB. Vascular complications in Ehlers-Danlos syndrome. Am Surg 1994; 60(11):827–831.

95. Lauwers G, Nevelsteen A, Daenen G, Lacroix H, Suy R, Frijns JP. Ehlers-Danlos syndrome type IV: a heterogeneous disease. Ann Vasc Surg 1997; 11(2):178–182.

96. Freeman RK, Swegle J, Sise MJ. The surgical complications of Ehlers-Danlos syndrome. Am Surg 1996; 62(10):869–873.

97. Cikrit DF, Miles JH, Silver D. Spontaneous arterial perforation: the Ehlers-Danlos specter. J Vasc Surg 1987; 5(2): 248–255.

98. Beighton P, Horan FT. Surgical aspects of the Ehlers-Danlos syndrome. A survey of 100 cases. Br J Surg 1969; 56(4):255–259.

99. Nienaber CA, Eagle KA. Aortic dissection: new frontiers in diagnosis and management: Part I: from etiology to diagnostic strategies. Circulation 2003; 108(5):628–635.

100. Stefanadis CI, Karayannacos PE, Boudoulas HK, et al. Medial necrosis and acute alterations in aortic distensibility following removal of the vasa vasorum of canine ascending aorta. Cardiovasc Res 1993; 27(6):951–956.

101. Januzzi JL, Sabatine MS, Eagle KA, et al. Iatrogenic aortic dissection. Am J Cardiol 2002; 89(5):623–626.

102. von Kodolitsch Y, Simic O, Schwartz A, et al. Predictors of proximal aortic dissection at the time of aortic valve replacement. Circulation 1999; 100(19 Suppl):II-287–294.

103. Pieters FA, Widdershoven JW, Gerardy AC, Geskes G, Cheriex EC, Wellens HJ. Risk of aortic dissection after aortic valve replacement. Am J Cardiol 1993; 72(14):1043–1047.

104. Nienaber CA, von Kodolitsch Y, Petersen B, et al. Intramural hemorrhage of the thoracic aorta. Diagnostic and therapeutic implications. Circulation 1995; 92(6):1465–1472.

105. O'Gara PT, DeSanctis RW. Acute aortic dissection and its variants. Toward a common diagnostic and therapeutic approach. Circulation 1995; 92(6):1376–1378.

106. von Kodolitsch Y, Csosz SK, Koschyk DH, et al. Intramural hematoma of the aorta: predictors of progression to dissection and rupture. Circulation 2003; 107(8):1158–1163.

107. Ide K, Uchida H, Otsuji H, et al. Acute aortic dissection with intramural hematoma: possibility of transition to classic dissection or aneurysm. J Thorac Imaging 1996; 11(1):46–52.

108. Svensson LG, Hess KR, Coselli JS, Safi HJ, Crawford ES. A prospective study of respiratory failure after high-risk surgery on the thoracoabdominal aorta. J Vasc Surg 1991; 14(3):271–282.

109. Suzuki T, Mehta RH, Ince H, et al. Clinical profiles and outcomes of acute type B aortic dissection in the current era: lessons from the International Registry of Aortic Dissection (IRAD). Circulation 2003; 108(Suppl 1):II-312–317.

110. Mehta RH, O'Gara PT, Bossone E, et al. Acute type A aortic dissection in the elderly: clinical characteristics, management, and outcomes in the current era. J Am Coll Cardiol 2002; 40(4):685–692.

111. Mehta RH, Bossone E, Evangelista A, et al. Acute type B aortic dissection in elderly patients: clinical features, outcomes, and simple risk stratification rule. Ann Thorac Surg 2004; 77(5):1622–1628.

112. Januzzi JL, Isselbacher EM, Fattori R, et al. Characterizing the young patient with aortic dissection: results from the International Registry of Aortic Dissection (IRAD). J Am Coll Cardiol 2004; 43(4):665–669.

113. Bossone E, Rampoldi V, Nienaber CA, et al. Usefulness of pulse deficit to predict in-hospital complications and mortality in patients with acute type A aortic dissection. Am J Cardiol 2002; 89(7):851–855.

114. Eagle KA. Current management in aortic dissection: data from the International Registry for Aortic Dissection (IRAD). Eur Heart J 1999; 20(Suppl):A3827.

115. Yoshida S, Akiba H, Tamakawa M, et al. Thoracic involvement of type A aortic dissection and intramural hematoma: diagnostic accuracy—comparison of emergency helical CT and surgical findings. Radiology 2003; 228(2):430–435.

116. Sebastia C, Pallisa E, Quiroga S, Alvarez-Castells A, Dominguez R, Evangelista A. Aortic dissection: diagnosis and follow-up with helical CT. Radiographics 1999; 19(1):45–60, 149–150.

117. Erbel R, Engberding R, Daniel W, Roelandt J, Visser C, Rennollet H. Echocardiography in diagnosis of aortic dissection. Lancet 1989; 1(8636):457–461.

118. Anagnostopoulos CE PM, Kittle CF. Aortic dissections and dissecting aneurysms. Am J Cardiol 1972; 30: 263.

119. von Kodolitsch Y, Schwartz AG, Nienaber CA. Clinical prediction of acute aortic dissection. Arch Intern Med 2000; 160(19):2977–2982.

120. Elefteriades JA, Lovoulos CJ, Coady MA, Tellides G, Kopf GS, Rizzo JA. Management of descending aortic dissection. Ann Thorac Surg 1999; 67(6):2002–2009.

121. Miller DC. The continuing dilemma concerning medical versus surgical management of patients with acute type B dissections. Semin Thorac Cardiovasc Surg 1993; 5(1):33–46.

122. Slonim SM, Miller DC, Mitchell RS, Semba CP, Razavi MK, Dake MD. Percutaneous balloon fenestration and stenting for life-threatening ischemic complications in patients with acute aortic dissection. J Thorac Cardiovasc Surg 1999; 117(6):1118–1126.

123. Iannelli G, Piscione F, Di Tommaso L, Monaco M, Chiariello M, Spampinato N. Thoracic aortic emergencies: impact of endovascular surgery. Ann Thorac Surg 2004; 77(2):591–596.

124. Ince H, Neinaber, CA. The concept of interventional therapy in acute aortic syndrome. J Card Surg 2002; 17:135–142.

125. Nienaber CA, Fattori R, Lund G, et al. Nonsurgical reconstruction of thoracic aortic dissection by stent-graft placement. N Engl J Med 1999; 340(20):1539–1545.

126. Dake MD, Kato N, Mitchell RS, et al. Endovascular stent-graft placement for the treatment of acute aortic dissection. N Engl J Med 1999; 340(20):1546–1552.

127. Sabik JF, Nemeh H, Lytle BW, et al. Cannulation of the axillary artery with a side graft reduces morbidity. Ann Thorac Surg 2004; 77(4):1315–1320.

128. McCullough JN, Zhang N, Reich DL, et al. Cerebral metabolic suppression during hypothermic circulatory arrest in humans. Ann Thorac Surg 1999; 67(6):1895–1921.

129. Coselli MD JS, LeMaire MD SA, Poli de Figueiredo MD P, Luiz, Kirby MD RP. Paraplegia after thoracoabdominal aortic aneurysm repair: is dissection a risk factor? Ann Thorac Surg 1997; 63(1):28–36.

130. Mehta RH, O'Gara PT, Bossone E, et al. Acute type A aortic dissection in the elderly: clinical characteristics, management, and outcomes in the current era. J Am Coll Cardiol 2002; 40(4):685–692.

131. Long SM, Tribble CG, Raymond DP, et al. Preoperative shock determines outcome for acute type A aortic dissection. Ann Thorac Surg 2003; 75(2):520–524.

132. Borst HG, Laas J, Heinemann M. Type A aortic dissection: diagnosis and management of malperfusion phenomena. Semin Thorac Cardiovasc Surg 1991; 3(3):238–241.

133. Fann JI, Sarris GE, Mitchell RS, et al. Treatment of patients with aortic dissection presenting with peripheral vascular complications. Ann Surg 1990; 212(6):705–713.

134. Lauterbach SR, Cambria RP, Brewster DC, et al. Contemporary management of aortic branch compromise resulting from acute aortic dissection. J Vasc Surg 2001; 33(6):1185–1192.

135. Cambria RP, Brewster DC, Gertler J, et al. Vascular complications associated with spontaneous aortic dissection. J Vasc Surg 1988; 7(2):199–209.

136. Girardi LN, Krieger KH, Lee LY, Mack CA, Tortolani AJ, Isom OW. Management strategies for type A dissection complicated by peripheral vascular malperfusion. Ann Thorac Surg 2004; 77(4):1309–1314.

137. Deeb GM, Williams DM, Bolling SF, et al. Surgical delay for acute type A dissection with malperfusion. Ann Thorac Surg 1997; 64(6):1669–1677.

138. Fann JI, Smith JA, Miller DC, et al. Surgical management of aortic dissection during a 30-year period. Circulation 1995; 92(9):113–121.

139. Haverich A, Miller DC, Scott WC, et al. Acute and chronic aortic dissections—determinants of long-term outcome for operative survivors. Circulation 1985; 72(3 Pt 2):II-22–34.

140. Fann JI, Smith JA, Miller DC, et al. Surgical management of aortic dissection during a 30-year period. Circulation 1995; 92(9 Suppl):II-113–121.

27
Diaphragm

Michel B. Aboutanos, Thérèse M. Duane, Ajai K. Malhotra, and Rao R. Ivatury

Case Scenario

A 29-year-old man presents to the emergency department with a 2-week history of worsening shortness of breath. The patient is alert and hemodynamically stable. Physical examination documents decreased breath sounds at the left base. Chest x-ray demonstrates a dense opacity in the base of the left lung field, along with a large air–fluid level. A computed tomography scan of the chest and abdomen confirms a diaphragmatic hernia. The patient's only other hospitalization was for a left thoracoabdominal stab wound. He recalls having a computed tomography scan done at that time and being discharged the next day. Which of the following would be the most appropriate intervention?

(A) Esophagogastroscopy
(B) Laparoscopy
(C) Celiotomy
(D) Thoracostomy
(E) Expectant management

Diaphragmatic injuries, from blunt as well as penetrating trauma, present numerous challenges in management to the emergency general surgeon. Potential pitfalls in dealing with these management dilemmas can only be minimized by a high index of suspicion. This chapter summarizes the current concepts in this area and briefly addresses other emergencies related to the diaphragm.

Anatomic and Physiologic Considerations

The diaphragm is a dome-shaped, circumferential muscular organ around an aponeurotic sheath called the "central tendon" that separates the abdominal and thoracic cavities. Arching from the first through third lumbar vertebrae posteriorly, the diaphragm attaches to the ribs laterally and to the posterior aspect of the lower sternum. The crura of the diaphragm decussate to form the aortic and esophageal hiatus to transmit the aorta, thoracic duct, the azygos vein, the esophagus, and the vagi. The caval hiatus transmits the inferior vena cava at about the eighth thoracic vertebral level. The undersurface of the diaphragm is closely related to the liver, spleen, stomach, and left kidney. Multiple branches from the aorta, pericardiophrenic arteries, and intercostals supply the diaphragm. The phrenic nerves innervate the diaphragm arising from the third through the fifth cervical roots.

The diaphragm is an important respiratory muscle with a large excursion from the fourth to the eighth intercostal spaces during inspiration and expiration: a fact of vital importance in trauma. This movement of the diaphragm creates a dynamic change in the abdominal cavity and contributes to the "intrathoracic" abdomen (Figure 27.1). Abdominal structures in this area may be injured with wounds of the lower chest situated at or below the nipple line.

Physiologically, the diaphragm, by its motion, creates negative intrathoracic pressure that enhances the tidal volumes generated by the lung. In this function, the diaphragm has more contribution than the rib cage. One study analyzed with magnetic resonance imaging (MRI) the respiratory-related motion of the chest wall and showed linear correlation among instantaneous lung volume, lung cross-sectional area, and motion of the diaphragm and rib. The exception was lower anteroposterior (AP) diameter of the rib cage. The slope(s) of the linear regression line at the anterior diaphragm were significantly smaller than at the middle and posterior parts during maximal deep breathing, but these are approximately five times that of AP motion of the upper rib cage.[1]

The diaphragm also plays a major role in the venous return to the right heart. Inspiration will enhance both

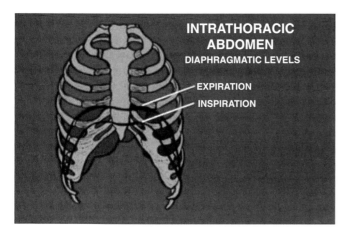

INTRATHORACIC ABDOMEN
DIAPHRAGMATIC LEVELS
— EXPIRATION
— INSPIRATION

FIGURE 27.1. Intrathoracic abdomen created by the wide excursion of diaphragm during inspiration and expiration.

superior (SVC) and inferior (IVC) vena cava blood flows because of the decreased right atrial pressure produced by the fall in intrathoracic pressure. However, inspiration can also increase abdominal pressure caused by the descent of the diaphragm. Robotham and Takata[2] suggested that the abdominal venous compartment can be viewed as either a capacitor (zone III abdomen) or as a collapsible Starling resistor (zone II abdomen). This dual nature of the abdominal venous bed can explain how an inspiratory increase in abdominal pressure can increase IVC flow with hypervolemia but decrease IVC flow with hypovolemia. Increases in abdominal pressures produced by active diaphragmatic descent can increase the total IVC venous return by enhancing the splanchnic IVC flow under relatively hypervolemic conditions but decrease the total IVC venous return by impeding the nonsplanchnic IVC flow under hypovolemic conditions. The authors evaluated changes in total IVC flow as well as regional splanchnic and nonsplanchnic IVC flows by use of ultrasound flow probes placed around the thoracic and subhepatic abdominal IVC during phrenic nerve stimulation (PNS) in anesthetized open-chest dogs.[3] With the abdomen closed (n = 6), PNS under hypervolemic conditions increased the total IVC flow by enhancing the splanchnic IVC flow, with a transient decrease in the nonsplanchnic IVC flow. Under hypovolemic conditions, PNS initially increased the total IVC flow but later decreased the total IVC flow by reducing the nonsplanchnic IVC flow, associated with a venous pressure gradient in the IVC across the diaphragm ($p < 0.05$), consistent with development of a vascular waterfall.

Herniation of abdominal contents into the thoracic cavity after rupture of the diaphragm is related to the tremendous pressure gradient generated by the sudden thrust of kinetic energy on the dome of the diaphragm, leading to rupture and thoracic migration of the abdominal viscera into the thoracic cavity. Of interest is the observation that, in a patient mechanically ventilated with positive pleural pressure, this gradient may not be existent. Intrathoracic migration may not occur, and the diaphragmatic rupture may be missed.

Blunt Diaphragmatic Injuries

History

Traumatic diaphragmatic rupture was first described in the Renaissance by Sennertus in 1541.[4] Blunt rupture of the diaphragm with gastric incarceration was described in 1579 by the French surgeon Ambroise Paré. He performed an autopsy on a stone mason who sustained a severe abdominal trauma 3 days before his demise. Paré found a severely distended stomach present into the thorax. Through a serious of autopsies, Paré described the consequences of diaphragmatic injuries secondary to blunt abdominal trauma.[5,6]

Incidence

Incidences of blunt diaphragmatic injuries have been reported as low as 0.8% and as high as 7%.[7,8] Blunt trauma accounts for 10% to 30% of traumatic diaphragmatic ruptures (TDRs) in North American series from urban trauma centers.[9] In studies from U.S. community hospitals and in Western European series, blunt trauma account for most TDRs.[9,10] Whether because of underdiagnosis, underreporting, true congenital weakening, or effective and protective buffering by the liver, injuries to the right diaphragm are less common than to the left diaphragm, with a reported ratio range of 3–25 to 1.[11–14] In a recent review of 65 patients with traumatic rupture of the diaphragm, Mihos et al.[15] reported left-sided ruptures in 43 patients (66%) that resulted mainly from blunt trauma (86%). Similar results were reported by Shah et al.[5] in a review of 980 patients; left-sided rupture was reported in 68.5% of patients.

Mechanism

Blunt diaphragmatic injuries result from motor vehicle collisions and falls from heights.[16,17] Direct force applied to the abdomen during a motor vehicle collision leads to acute increase in intraabdominal pressure (IAP) and rupture of the diaphragm. The buffer effect of the liver leads to a lower incidence of right versus left diaphragmatic ruptures.[18,19] Overpressure of the abdominal cavity also may explain the 30% to 55% association between pelvic fractures and diaphragmatic rupture. The severe forces required to cause a pelvic fracture are associated with increased IAP and the resultant diaphragmatic weakening and rupture.[20]

Associated injuries

Blunt diaphragm injuries rarely occur alone and are frequently associated with other significant thoracic, abdominal, pelvic, extremity, and central nervous system injuries.[15,16,22] Meyers and McCabe[23] describe a 40% associated incidence of pelvic fractures in patient with blunt diaphragmatic injuries. Other associated thoracoabdominal injuries included hepatic and splenic injuries (25%) and thoracic aortic tears (5%).

In a series of 52 blunt diaphragmatic injuries reviewed by Ilgenfritz and Stewart,[24] blunt thoracic injuries (multiple rib fractures and pneumothoracies) accounted for the highest associated injuries (90%). Long bone fractures and closed head injuries accounted for associated incidences of 75% and 42%, respectively. The associated intraabdominal injuries included splenic injuries (60%), liver injuries (35%), and kidney, pancreas, and small bowel injuries (10% to 12%).

Associated injuries are more common with right diaphragmatic ruptures. Boulanger et al.[25] reported a 100% incidence of intraabdominal injuries associated with ruptures of the right diaphragm compared with a 77% incidence with left diaphragmatic ruptures.

Diagnosis

The diagnosis of blunt diaphragmatic injuries is very difficult even with the highest index of suspicion. Before the current diagnostic modalities were available, most were diagnosed intraoperatively or postmortem. The rate of initially missed diaphragmatic injuries in conservatively managed patients ranges from 12% to 66%.[4,26,27] In the largest reported series (160 patients) of blunt diaphragmatic ruptures from six university medical centers in Canada, the diaphragmatic rupture was diagnosed preoperatively in only 37.1% of patients operated on for reasons other than the diaphragmatic rupture itself.[16] Over 42% of diaphragm injuries are diagnosed during exploratory laparotomy for other injuries.[27] Delayed diagnosis is associated with increased morbidity and mortality.[28–30] A mortality rate as high as 40% can occur when diagnosis is delayed until visceral herniation and strangulation have occurred.[31] Acute symptoms (respiratory compromise, failure to wean from mechanical ventilation) and chronic symptoms (persistent abdominal pain) resulting in significant morbidity have also been described.[10]

The antemortem diagnosis of a traumatic diaphragmatic hernia was established by Bowditch[32] in 1853. Five criteria were established: (1) prominence and immobility of the left thorax, (2) displacement of the cardiac area of dullness to the right, (3) absence of breath sounds over the left thorax, (4) presence of bowel sounds in the left

TABLE 27.1. Clinical manifestation of diaphragmatic injuries.

Symptoms	Physical examination
Thoracic	
Dyspnea/cyanosis	Diminished chest expansion
Orthopnea	Decreased breath sounds
Chest pain	Tympany to percussion
Referred scapular pain	Presence of bowel sounds
	Rib fractures
	Hemopneumothorax
Abdominal	
Localized upper quadrant pain	Localized tenderness
Diffuse abdominal pain	Diffuse tenderness
	Guarding/rebound
	Progressive abdominal distention

thorax, and (5) tympani to percussion in the left chest. Most blunt diaphragmatic injuries, however, do not manifest these criteria.

The clinical manifestation can vary also from absent symptomology upon presentation to severe shock. Beal and McKennan[33] described blunt diaphragmatic injury as a morbid injury. In their series, 54% of the patients presented in severe shock (systolic blood pressure <70 mm Hg) with 81% requiring urgent airway interventions. The symptoms of blunt diaphragmatic injury are listed in Table 27.1.

History and mechanism of injury can be vital for raising the index of suspicion for diaphragmatic injury. Falls from great heights, crush injuries, and lateral impacts in motor vehicle collisions are associated with higher incidences of blunt diaphragmatic injury.[17,34] A recent study found that knowledge of collision kinematics (vehicular intrusion ≥30 cm and delta-V ≥40 kph) combined with identified visceral (splenic) and orthopedic injuries (pelvic fractures) can generate a sensitivity greater than 85% for detecting diaphragmatic injuries.[17]

To date there is no definitive radiologic tool for diagnosis of the occult diaphragmatic insult. The radiologic diagnosis relies on the demonstration of visceral herniation rather than the actual visualization of the diaphragmatic tear. The current modalities used include chest x-rays, thoracoabdominal computed tomography (CT) scanning, sonography, diagnostic peritoneal lavage, upper and lower gastrointestinal contrast studies, liver scintigraphy, contrast or air peritoneography, and MRI.[35–39]

The initial chest x-rays may show visceral herniation, elevation of the diaphragm, loss of the diaphragmatic shadow, irregularity of the apparent contour of the diaphragm, or a pleural effusion.[40] The presence of a nasogastric tube in the left chest cavity is pathognomonic for left diaphragmatic rupture and gastric eventration into the left thorax (Figure 27.2). However, in an estimated 30% to 50% of patients with diaphragmatic

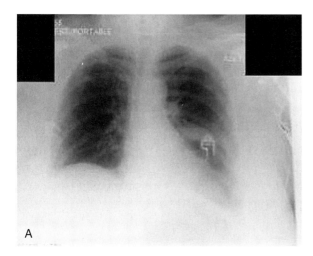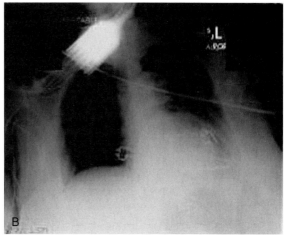

FIGURE 27.2. (A,B) Chest x-ray showing gastric shadow (A) and intragastric Dobhoff tube (B) above the diaphragm in the left chest.

injuries, the initial x-rays are read as normal.[41,42] Demetriades et al.[43] reported a 13% accuracy of chest x-ray. Many other injuries can also mimic diaphragmatic injuries such as pulmonary contusion, hemopneumothorax, or congenital eventration.[44]

For stable patients, contrast studies (upper gastrointestinal series or barium enema) have proved valuable in both acute and chronic situations.[10,21,45] However, such studies are helpful only when visceral herniation through the diaphragmatic injury has occurred.

Computed tomography is currently the diagnostic modality of choice for stable patients with blunt thoracoabdominal injuries. The diagnostic accuracy of CT scans for evaluation of blunt diaphragmatic injuries, however, is variable and often disappointing, especially when typical chest x-ray findings are absent.[46–48] Guth et al.[27] reported a 0% sensitivity for CT scan in detecting right-sided diaphragmatic rupture. It remains to be seen whether the advent of helical (spiral) CT with three-dimensional reconstruction can enhance its diagnostic utility for blunt diaphragmatic injuries.

The use of ultrasound was reported to be helpful mainly for blunt rupture of the right hemidiaphragm. The bare area of the liver may be seen herniating through the discontinuance of the diaphragmatic tear, or the edge of the tear can be identified as a flap between fluid covering both diaphragmatic surfaces.[35,49,50] Its value, however, remains operator dependent. The use of MRI for the diagnosis of blunt diaphragmatic injury has been reported in only a few studies.[39,51] Its usefulness is restricted to stable and chronic patients.

Together with thoracoscopy, laparoscopy has become the diagnostic tool of choice for diaphragmatic injuries compared with other nonoperative modalities.[10,15,49,52–54] The role of laparoscopy has been more defined, however,

for penetrating injuries. Thoracoscopy is mainly helpful in the chronic situation or when abdominal injuries have been ruled out. Tension pneumothorax is the main potential complication of laparoscopy for patients with diaphragmatic injuries.

Treatment

As mentioned above, delayed diagnosis is associated with significant morbidity and mortality, including cardiorespiratory compromise and visceral obstruction and strangulation.[28] All patients with diaphragmatic injury should undergo prompt repair.

Acute blunt diaphragmatic injury is generally repaired using an abdominal approach, with abdominal exploration and repair of any associated visceral injuries (Figure 27.3). Chronic or delayed diagnostic injury is usually repaired via a thoracic approach, where retracted tissues and adhesions are easier to handle. Ultimately, the personal preference of the surgeon should dictate which approach is used.[11] A combined approach may be required in the face of extensive hazardous adhesions and chronic visceral eventration.

There are multiple approaches for the repair of the diaphragm. Primary repair is usually carried out in one or two layers depending on the size and integrity of the tissue, with a nonabsorbable monofilament suture such as 2-0 polypropylene (Figure 27.4). In the face of significant tissue loss, the diaphragm can be reconstructed with a prosthetic nonabsorbable material such as Marlex mesh.[21] Although minimal infectious complications have been reported with this approach, the risk of infection is not negligible especially in the presence of abdominal or thoracic contamination.[21,53] In this scenario, the use of autologous tissue such as a omentum, tensor fascia lata,

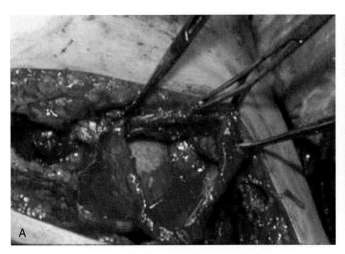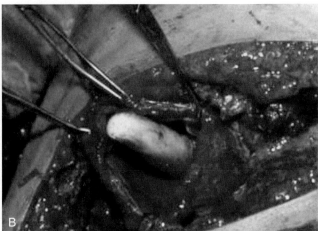

FIGURE 27.3. **(A,B)** Diaphragmatic laceration as seen from the thorax.

or a latissimus dorsi flap may be preferable.[55] The use of biologic tissue grafting material such as AlloDerm (human acellular tissue matrix; Life Cell Corp.) may also be of great benefit.[56]

Transposition of the diaphragm to a higher intercostal space was described by Bender and Lucas[57] for the repair of massive diaphragmatic injuries with chest wall defect. This type of injury is less common in blunt trauma.

With rapid advancement in video technology and technical expertise, there is inevitable progression toward the use of laparoscopy as a therapeutic tool in the selective management of stable patients with abdominal trauma. This is especially true with regard to diaphragmatic repair. The largest initial experience with therapeutic

laparoscopy was reported in 1997 by Zantut et al.,[58] when 26 of 28 patients had successful therapeutic procedures (16 diaphragmatic repair, 6 hepatic repair, 3 gastrostomy repair, and 1 cholecystectomy).

In summary, blunt diaphragmatic ruptures are often missed on initial evaluation. A high index of suspicion is needed. The ruptures are usually associated with other severe injuries. Delayed diagnosis is associated with increased morbidity and mortality. Together with thoracoscopy, laparoscopy has become the diagnostic tool of choice for diaphragmatic injuries. Patients with diaphragmatic injuries should undergo prompt repair. There are multiple approaches for the repair of the diaphragm.

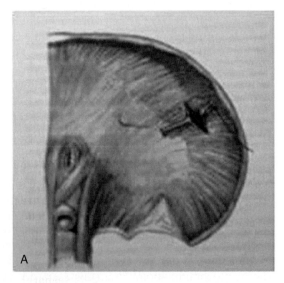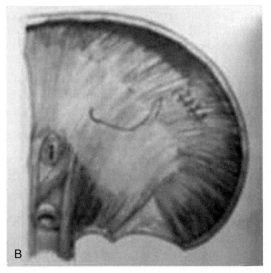

FIGURE 27.4. **(A,B)** Repair of the diaphragm in two layers. (Reprinted from Ivatury RR, Cayten CG, eds. The Textbook of Penetrating Trauma. Baltimore: Williams & Wilkins, 1996.)

Penetrating Injuries to the Diaphragm

Incidence

Diaphragmatic injury can occur after both blunt and penetrating trauma. The rate of injury after a penetrating thoracoabdominal trauma ranges from 0% to 67%.[59,60] The cause of the penetration seems to affect the frequency of the injury, as shown by Murray et al.[61] They looked exclusively at left-sided penetrating thoracoabdominal injuries and found a 42% incidence of diaphragmatic injury with 59% of these from gunshot wounds (GSW) and 32% from stab wounds. Regardless of the cause, the rate of asymptomatic injuries is quite high.

This type of injury was found to be underdiagnosed in a number of series.[60–62] Chen and Wilson[62] evaluated 62 patients with diaphragm injuries of whom 45 had suffered a penetrating trauma. Of these patients, only 17 (27%) had a suspected injury. Stylianos and King[63] did routine celiotomy for 20 patients with anterior stab wounds and found that 10 of them had an isolated diaphragm injury and only 7 had a negative celiotomy. Finally, a group from UCLA found that 26% of their patients had an occult diaphragm injury.[61] Because of the frequency and the insidiousness of its presentation, emphasis must be placed on appropriate and timely diagnosis.

Diagnosis

One must always be concerned about a diaphragm injury when treating a patient with a thoracoabdominal wound. The ability to diagnose such an injury has remained a quandary for trauma surgeons. Options for diagnosis include observation, radiography, operative exploration via either the chest or abdomen, or a minimally invasive approach.

There tends to be little role for simple observation for patients who are at risk for a diaphragm injury after penetrating trauma, given the possible associated injuries to the pleural and peritoneal cavities. Films are frequently needed to evaluate for hemothoraces or pneumothoraces secondary to penetration of the pleural space. Moreover, some sort of evaluation is necessary to rule out intraabdominal trauma. Therefore, studies have focused on the most accurate and efficient methods of evaluating a patient for diaphragm injuries.

In 1984 Miller et al.[42] reviewed their experience with diaphragmatic injuries of which they had 93 penetrating and 9 blunt insults. They found that 40 patients had normal chest x-rays and 20% of patients with a penetrating trauma had a falsely negative diagnostic peritoneal lavage. Because of these findings and the associated injury rate of 87%, they recommended immediate laparotomy for all penetrating trauma to the tho-

racoabdominal region. Other authors[64,65] also suggested that diaphragmatic injury should be suspected in all patients with penetrating as well as blunt injury of the chest and abdomen and particularly of the epigastrium and lower chest. The presence of such an injury should be excluded before the termination of the exploratory procedure. Also, diaphragmatic injury should be suspected in patients with roentgenographic abnormalities of the diaphragm or lower lung field following trauma.

Recently there has been an appreciation for the impact of negative exploration in trauma patients. Ivatury et al.[54] retrospectively reviewed 657 laparotomies for penetrating trauma and found that 78 of these had no injuries. More important, most of the negative laparotomies (44.8%) were from wounds in the lower chest and upper abdomen, with three fourths of these resulting from stab wounds. To avoid these negative explorations other methods of evaluation have been studied.

Radiographs

Plain radiographs have been used over the years to evaluate patients for diaphragmatic injury with varying success. In 1988, Demetriades et al.[43] looked at 163 patients with penetrating trauma to the diaphragm and found the chest x-ray to be diagnostic in only 13% of patients, abnormal but not diagnostic in 76% of patients, and completely normal in 11% of patients. Those patients diagnosed early had a mortality rate of 3.2% versus 30% for those diagnosed late, emphasizing the importance of timely identification of injury. More recently, Shackleton et al.[66] found that in the 25 cases they reviewed of both blunt and penetrating trauma, patients with penetrating injury usually had findings that suggested embarrassment of the diaphragm that would prompt further investigation. Overall it seems that plain radiographs are inadequate to provide conclusive evidence of a diaphragmatic injury after penetrating trauma. The majority of these patients have ambiguous findings,[43,65–67] and others have noted that interventions such as positive pressure ventilation interfere further with the ability to diagnose this problem.[68]

Despite the inaccuracy of chest radiographs, very little has been done to look at other radiographic modalities. Early studies with ultrasound have been disappointing. Udobi et al.[69] prospectively evaluated focused assessment with sonography for trauma (FAST) after penetrating abdominal trauma. Of the 75 stable patients who were included, 13 had false-negative studies. Three of these patients had diaphragm injuries that were not identified by ultrasound. There are two studies from the RA Cowley Shock Trauma Center that lend some credence to using both CT and MRI,[70,71] but their numbers are small and as yet the data can be interpreted as preliminary at best.

Thoracoscopy

Minimally invasive surgery has found a role in this diagnostic dilemma. Thoracoscopy has been studied since the
early 1990s and has consistently been found to be both
accurate and safe.[72–76] In a preliminary study by Ochsner
et al.,[72] 14 patients were evaluated, with 9 patients having
an injury identified. Smith et al.[73] had a slightly larger
series of 24 patients of whom 22 suffered from penetrating trauma, and 5 injuries were identified. Other studies
during this time frame[74] had consistent results, with all of
these citing a low rate of complications involved in this
minimally invasive approach.

   More recently, Freeman et al.[76] published the largest
series to date about the use of video-assisted thoracoscopic surgery (VATS) after penetrating chest trauma.
They reviewed 171 patients who underwent a VATS of
whom 60 patients had a diaphragm injury. Not only were
they able to accurately diagnose these injuries, but they
did so with few complications. Moreover, they identified
five independent risk factors for diaphragm injuries,
including abnormal chest x-ray, right-sided entrance
wound, entrance inferior to the nipple line, velocity,
mechanism of injury, and associated intraabdominal
injuries. Based on this review, they developed an algorithm to incorporate these factors that would decrease
the rate of missed diaphragm injuries with the selective
use of thoracoscopy (Figure 27.3A).

Laparoscopy

Laparoscopy provides another minimally invasive
alternative to thoracoscopy for the evaluation of the
diaphragm. Ivatury and colleagues[77] in the Bronx pioneered the use of laparoscopy and helped to define its
role in the evaluation of diaphragm injuries. Their initial
focus was on its ability to eliminate a number of negative
laparotomies. In 1993 they evaluated 100 hemodynamically stable patients by laparoscopy.[77] A total of 43
patients had no peritoneal penetration, divided between
stabs (22) and GSWs (21). Similar to their previous trial,[54]
75% of these patients studied had thoracoabdominal or
epigastic injuries. More importantly, all 17 patients
with diaphragm lacerations were accurately identified at
the time of laparoscopy just as they had been in the
previous trial (Figure 27.5).[54] The benefits of this less
invasive approach were then confirmed in 1994
when they prospectively evaluated 38 patients using
laparoscopy.[78] In this series, over 60% of the patients had
nonpenetration of the peritoneal cavity. Those patients
who were able to avoid a laparotomy had a significantly
lower hospital stay than those who underwent
exploratory laparotomy for nonpenetrating GSW, and
there were no laparoscopic related complications in this
series.[78]

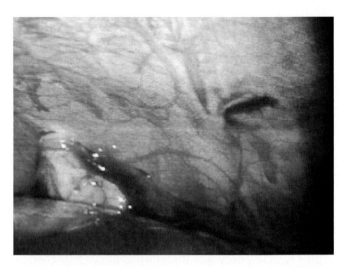

FIGURE 27.5. Laparoscopic view of the diaphragmatic
laceration.

   Since Ivatury and colleagues identified the benefits of
laparoscopy in penetrating trauma to the abdomen,
others have evaluated it more specifically for those
injuries to the thoracoabdominal region. Surgeons at the
University of Southern California had impressive findings when laparoscopy was used for all thoracoabdominal penetrating injuries[79] and just trauma to the left lower
chest.[80] The sensitivity for identifying diaphragm injuries
was 83%,[79] and the incidence of occult injuries was 24%
for left-sided trauma.[80] Ertekin et al.[81] demonstrated a
higher percentage of diaphragm injuries with 100% sensitivity and specificity with its use. McQuay and Britt[82]
had a lower incidence in their series, but almost three
fourths of their patients were spared a formal laparotomy. All groups had minimal complications with this
technique (Table 27.2).

Exploration

Other methods of diagnosis for penetrating trauma
include degrees of exploration. Examples of this are

TABLE 27.2. Outcomes after laparoscopy.

	No. of patients	Percent diaphragm injuries	Percent major complications	Missed diaphragm injuries
Murray et al.[80,88]	110	24	0.5	0
Ivatury et al.[77]	100	30	0	0
Zantut et al.[58]	510	40	0	0
Ertekin et al.[81]	22	81.8	0	0
McQuay and Britt[82]	80	27.5	0.125	0

digital exploration, diagnostic peritoneal lavage (DPL), and open laparotomy. Far less has been written about the former two options than the last. One study looked at the value of digital exploration of left-sided stab wounds to the area of the diaphragm to see if it could reliably identify these injuries.[83] Eighty-two patients who did not have an immediate indication for celiotomy had their wound digitally explored by the attending surgeon. The patient went on to laparotomy if an injury was identified and to thoracoscopy if no lesion was found. This method had a sensitivity of 96%, a specificity of 83.3%, and a positive predictive value of 91% and a negative predictive value of 93.7%. Although these results are promising, they have yet to be replicated.

DeMaria et al.[84] evaluated the role of DPL with penetrating anterior abdominal trauma to see if it could avoid open laparotomy when complemented by laparoscopy. They prospectively compared patients who had no indication for immediate laparotomy and divided them into DPL followed by laparoscopy and possible laparotomy and DPL followed by laparotomy. They found DPL to be reliable, with 11 of 12 patients with positive results requiring surgical repair and 16 of 26 with negative results not requiring intervention. Based on these findings, they recommend DPL as the initial study and only proceed to laparoscopy if this is positive because a number of patients with positive DPLs did not require any type of repair. The caveat to this study was for thoracoabdominal wounds, because the false-negative rate resulted from missed diaphragm injuries. Therefore, although DPL may be valuable for other areas of the abdomen, this study lends credence to the need for laparoscopic evaluation for thoracoabdominal wounds.

Unless other indications are present for exploration, there is very little role for either thoracotomy or laparotomy to look for diaphragm injury. In fact, Simon et al.[85] reviewed their use of laparoscopy over the years and found that its use in penetrating trauma increased from 8.7% to 16% from 1995 to 2000. For stab wounds alone the rate increased to 27%. Simultaneously, their negative laparotomy rate decreased. Once they diagnosed this injury they repaired four patients via the laparoscope. Options for treatment are as wide ranging as those for diagnosis.

Treatment

Observation

Recently an animal model was used to look at the natural history of stab wounds to the diaphragm.[86] Eight pigs had a 1.5- to 2-cm incision made in each diaphragm, one to the muscular portion and one to the tendinous area on the other side. The surgeons reevaluated these wounds at 6 weeks and found that those to the muscular portion of

the diaphragm had all healed spontaneously. Only one defect remained in the tendinous portion of the diaphragm. Based on these findings, they thought it unnecessary to pursue invasive measures to assess the status of the diaphragm.

The previous study is limited to only stab wounds, and it is unlikely that these results could be extrapolated to GSWs as well because those injuries tend to be more disruptive, particularly for higher caliber bullets. The other concern is whether similar results would be found with humans. Observation for these injuries has been inadvertent secondary to missed injuries to the diaphragm. Therefore, we do not know how many patients suffer from these injuries but are never identified. It is only the complications such as incarceration and strangulation through these defects that come to the attention of the practitioner. Because these problems carry high morbidity and mortality rates, it remains prudent to repair diaphragm injuries at the time of diagnosis.

Minimally Invasive Approach

With the increased use of the laparoscope and thoracoscope in the diagnosis of diaphragm injuries, it follows that more attempts will be made to repair these injuries with the less invasive approach when other indications for open exploration are not present. A concern regarding this approach is whether these repairs are as sturdy as those achieved with the standard open repair. Two swine models were studied in an attempt to answer this question. Kozar et al.[87] compared histology and bursting strength measurements of 2-cm lacerations to the diaphragm that were treated with open suture repair, laparoscopic repair by suture, staple, or patch. After 6 weeks of healing all methods had similar histologic healing and burst strength. The patch resulted in less inflammation and greater fibroblastic proliferation.

Murray et al.[88] conducted a similar study with pigs by looking at histologic appearance, macroscopic inspection, and tensile strength. They evaluated 30 lacerations and repaired them by open suturing, laparoscopic suturing, or stapling technique. Again, no differences were found in any of the parameters measured. Both of these groups concluded that open and laparoscopic repair demonstrated similar healing so the approach should be based on surgical skill.

Although there have been case reports since 1994 of penetrating diaphragm injuries being repaired laparoscopically,[89,90] few include only penetrating trauma victims. In the series by Simon et al.,[85] even though they utilized laparoscopy more than in the past for penetrating trauma, they still repaired only four injuries via this technique. Matthews et al.[91] reported on a series of 17 patients, with 8 having penetrating trauma. Only 13 were repaired via the laparoscope, and 4 were converted to open. The 4 patients requiring open technique all suffered from a blunt trauma. The 8 penetrating trauma victims were successfully repaired with the laparoscope, with no documented recurrence at a mean follow-up period of 7.9 months. Zantut et al.,[58] in a multicenter experience, described the role of therapeutic laparoscopy in 1997.

A little more has been published on thoracoscopic repair. In 1993, Smith et al.[73] used this technique successfully in the repair of four out of five diaphragm lacerations, and there were no postoperative complications. In a larger series, Martinez et al.[60] looked at only penetrating trauma patients and identified 35 with diaphragm injuries. Stab wounds caused 80% of these injuries. All of these patients were successfully repaired thoracoscopically without complications.

Another option in the spectrum of repairs is the laparoscopy-assisted repair. This method has been described by Shaw and colleagues.[92] Their series included 25 patients with attempted repair, 24 with a stab wound and 1 with a blunt injury. The procedure was unsuccessful in a stab victim secondary to distension of bowel. The operation uses a 10-mm camera in the supraumbilical region and a 4-cm left subcostal incision for access to the injury. Retraction hooks elevate the upper wound, and the repair is performed using running 1-0 nylon sutures under direct camera visualization. The 24 successful procedures were completed in an average time of 61 minutes, with an average postoperative hospital stay of 2.29 days.

Open Approach

Of all the treatment options, the gold standard still remains an open repair. With the surgeon's increased proficiency with minimally invasive techniques this may change, but for now it remains the safest option. These injuries may be approached via either the thorax or the abdomen. For patients who have an acute injury, the most reasonable option is abdominal exploration to allow for evaluation of the intraabdominal structures.[93] For those patients who have a chronic injury it seems that the technique is based on personal preference. In an extensive review of the literature it seems that the overwhelming preference is a laparotomy.[94]

Acute injuries to the diaphragm may be fixed using interrupted figure-of-eight or horizontal mattress sutures with a 2-0 nonabsorbable material. A two-layer closure is an option for defects longer than 2 cm. The inner layer is an interlocking horizontal mattress suture reinforced by a running 3-0 nonabsorbable suture. For chronic injuries care must be taken to reduce the hernia and perform adhesiolysis. Otherwise the repair is similar. For either situation, larger defects may require a mesh patch to be placed and sutured with 2-0 polypropylene, taking care not to place it in a contaminated field.[93]

Outcomes

Morbidity

Morbidity from diaphragm injuries can be divided into complications of the acute phase or consequences of the chronic phase. During the initial hospitalization it may be from technical problems at the time of repair or from the associated injuries at the time of the trauma. Failure of a repair or a disruption of a suture line is clearly an untoward sequela of the diaphragmatic injury. However, associated injuries may range from a small pneumothorax with little associated morbidity to an organ injury with some morbidity to a major vessel injury with significant morbidity. It is often difficult to attribute perioperative problems directly to the diaphragm itself. In series that evaluated only penetrating trauma, complication rates were as high as 52% and included wound infections, subdiaphragmatic abscess, respiratory insufficiency, hypotension, small bowel obstruction, and bronchopleural fistula.[76,80,82]

Chronic phase morbidity results from unrecognized injury to the diaphragm. This tends to be a greater problem for blunt trauma victims, who have a greater likelihood of being observed than penetrating trauma patients, who usually undergo a more invasive evaluation. Leppaniemi and Haapiainen[59] studied only stab victims and found a 4% rate of missed injuries that resulted in herniation of intraabdominal contents that required repair. Although most studies include both blunt and penetrating trauma, complications from a missed injury are similar. Reber et al.[95] identified 10 missed injuries in both of these populations, with all of them resulting in herniation of intraabdominal contents. These hernias presented 20 days to 28 years after the trauma, with 80% of them located on the left side.

Herniation can result in significant symptoms of pulmonary compromise and intermittent obstruction. The most feared sequela is incarceration with strangulation of the contents. Sullivan[96] looked at 53 such cases and found that 80% presented within 3 years of injury, with the colon being the most common organ involved. Not only morbidity but mortality as well can be significant in these situations.

Mortality

Death can result from the initial trauma or from long-term complications from missed injury. Mortality rates for penetrating trauma range from 0% to 42%. As with morbidity, mortality results primarily from associated injuries. Williams et al.[97] reviewed 731 patients with trauma to the diaphragm. Both blunt and penetrating injuries were included, with shotgun wounds having the highest mortality at 42%. They found that predictors of

FIGURE 27.6. Algorithm for diagnosis of penetrating chest trauma to identify diaphragm injuries. (Reprinted with permission of the Society of Thoracic Surgeons from Freeman et al.[76])

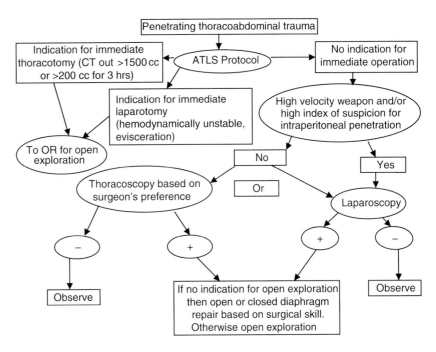

mortality included blood transfusions of greater than 10 U, revised trauma score, and need for thoracotomy. Therefore, they emphasized early identification of associated injuries and control of bleeding to improve survival.

Accurate mortality rates are difficult to assess for chronic disruption of the diaphragm. First, most of the missed injuries are secondary to a blunt cause, and, second, they may not be identified as directly resulting in death. In a small series of 10 patients with both blunt and penetrating trauma with delayed diagnosis of their injury, there was a 10% mortality rate.[95] In a larger series of 50 patients of whom 27 suffered a penetrating trauma, there was a 2% mortality rate.[98] In this study, two patients had a perforated viscus at the time of repair, and one of the deaths was secondary to postoperative perforation. Clearly, it is beneficial to identify these injuries at the time of the trauma to prevent such complications.

Conclusions

Given this review, it seems prudent to consider a diaphragm injury for any patients with penetrating thoracoabdominal wounds because the incidence can be quite high. History and physical examination alone are inadequate to make this diagnosis, and current radiographic techniques are too inaccurate to be relied on safely to exclude this diagnosis. For patients without another indication for exploration, thoracoscopy is a reasonable option when the injury is higher in the chest and from a low-velocity mechanism or when intraabdominal injuries are thought unlikely. Laparoscopy is a better

choice when one has a high index of suspicion for an intraperitoneal injury and can be done safely with the elimination of a large number of laparotomies. These diagnostic and therapeutic considerations were recently summarized.[99]

Treatment is dependent on surgical skill. Closed and open repairs are equivalent in their strengths and outcomes. Therefore, if a patient does not require an open exploration for other reasons, then repair via a scope is a good option. Despite the animal data suggesting that most of these will heal, such has not been shown in humans, and the complications from missed injuries should prompt repair when these injuries are identified.

Morbidity and mortality rates are closely related to the associated injuries. Standard trauma protocols should be followed to care for these victims so that all injuries can be adequately addressed. With aggressive early intervention these patients can expect good outcomes with minimal complications. Figure 27.6 provides an algorithm for the approach to these patients.

Surgical Emergencies Related to Hiatal Hernia

Hiatal hernia is defined as herniation of part or whole of the stomach into the chest through the esophageal hiatus. It is classified into three types depending on the position of the gastroesophageal (GE) junction. The most common (80%) is type I, also called sliding hiatal hernia. In this type, the GE junction rises into the chest to varying heights, dragging the proximal parts of greater and lesser curvatures. The next most common (15%) is

TABLE 27.3. Surgical emergencies associated with hiatal hernias.

Emergencies associated with complications of acid reflux
  Hemorrhage caused by erosive esophagitis and/or ulceration
  Hiatal hernia ulcer perforation
  Esophageal stricture with esophageal dilatation and atony

Emergencies associated with mechanical complication
  Acute gastric volvulus

type II, also called rolling or paraesophageal hiatal hernia. In this type, the position of the GE junction remains intraabdominal, while parts or all of the fundus and body herniate into the chest through the esophageal hiatus to lie adjacent to the distal esophagus. The least common (5%) is the mixed type, or type III, and has elements of both type I (herniation upward of the GE junction with parts of the stomach) and type II (herniation of parts of the fundus and body to lie adjacent to the esophagus within the chest). The fundamental pathophysiology involved in the formation of hiatal hernia is the structural weakness of the phrenoesophageal membrane.

The complications associated with hiatal hernia, which may present as an emergency requiring intervention, can broadly be divided into two categories (Table 27.3). First are complications arising from interference with the lower esophageal sphincteric mechanism allowing reflux of stomach acid into the lower esophagus. These are more common with type I hernias and include esophagitis and ulceration, which can cause upper gastrointestinal hemorrhage, ulcer perforation with resultant mediastinitis with or without peritonitis, and stricture formation with dilatation and atony of the proximal esophagus. Second are complications related to the abnormal mobility of the stomach making it prone to volvulus. These mechanical complications are more often associated with type II hernias.

Upper Gastrointestinal Hemorrhage

The presentation and management of upper gastrointestinal hemorrhage have been dealt with elsewhere in this book. The specific problems associated with bleeding caused by severe reflux esophagitis, or from a peptic ulcer situated within the herniated stomach, are presented here.

Approximately 3% of all upper gastrointestinal hemorrhages are caused by either severe erosive esophagitis or a deeply penetrating esophageal ulcer.[100] Ulcers are most often found in association with Barrett's epithelium and are typically located at the junction of gastric columnar and esophageal squamous epithelium. Hemorrhage due to either of these causes is rarely massive and usually self-limiting. In the rare event that the bleeding fails to stop spontaneously, endoscopic therapy is the initial treatment of choice and has a fairly high success rate.[101]

Following cessation of the hemorrhage, aggressive medical therapy with endoscopic surveillance to ensure healing is recommended. When the cause is an ulcer within the hiatal hernia, efforts to exclude malignancy and appropriate therapy for the Barrett's epithelium should be undertaken after the acute hemorrhage has been controlled.

In the extremely rare situation when the bleeding cannot be controlled by endoscopic means, emergent surgery is indicated. Surgery in such situations is fairly difficult because of the relative inaccessibility of the lesion and the severe inflammation and dense adhesions that maybe present. When planning for the surgery, it is important to consider the site of the ulcer, as an ulcer high up in the chest may prove to be inaccessible through a laparotomy. If it is known that the ulcer is fairly high, consideration should be given to approach the lesion through a left posterolateral thoracotomy. Even when the lesion is accessible from the abdomen, the patient should be draped in a fashion that a thoracotomy can rapidly be performed either separately or by converting the laparotomy incision into a thoracoabdominal incision.

Once the bleeding lesion is located, the actual procedure will depend on the hemodynamic status of the patient, the degree of concern for malignancy, and the presence or absence of Barrett's esophagus. In the ideal situation with a patient relatively stable, patient dissection to release all adhesions and to free the distal esophagus should be performed. Once the esophagus and the herniated stomach are freed, if there is significant concern for malignancy or advanced Barrett's disease, appropriate resection should be performed. If the concern for malignancy is low, and no Barrett's changes are known to be present, oversewing of the bleeding ulcer followed by an appropriate antireflux procedure should be performed. In the latter situation, if dissection is extremely difficult, an acceptable method is to cut around the deeply adherent ulcer and exclude the ulcer by closing the esophagus or stomach as the case maybe and completing the procedure with an appropriate antireflux procedure. The wrap of the antireflux procedure can be utilized to buttress the suture line of the hollow viscus closure.[102] When the patient is hemodynamically unstable, the least surgery to control the bleeding should be performed. This usually consists of opening the organ and oversewing the bleeding lesion. In some cases it maybe necessary to return in 24 to 48 hours and perform a resection or antireflux procedure.

Hiatal Hernia Ulcer Perforation

Peptic ulcers associated with a hiatal hernia may be found within the herniated stomach or at the part of the stomach that traverses the hiatus. The latter ulcer is thought to occur because of ischemia produced at this spot by the displacement of the stomach. Perforation of such ulcers is an exceedingly rare event, with only case reports found in the literature.[103] Such perforations through the wall of the viscus may occur insidiously, with the ulcer first becoming adherent to and then penetrating into adjacent mediastinal organs of the cardiovascular or respiratory systems.[104,105] These may give rise to findings such as spontaneous pneumopericardium.[106] Less often reported are free perforations resulting in mediastinitis and/or peritonitis.[103] For patients with peritonitis, the diagnosis will usually be made at the time of surgery. In the absence of peritonitis, the patients usually present with features of an intrathoracic catastrophe and are often treated for medical conditions.

Whether the diagnosis is made at the time of surgery or preoperatively, the principles of management are similar to those outlined earlier for bleeding ulcer within a hiatal hernia. However, the adhesions in cases of acute or chronic perforation may be even more dense and hence surgery more difficult. Morbidity and mortality rates of such an event are very high because of the diagnostic delay and technical difficulty.

Acute Gastric Volvulus

The normal stomach is held in position by attachments at the cardia and pylorus and peritoneal folds, with the vessels traversing them, over both curvatures. The normal stomach cannot be made to rotate through 180° unless these attachments are either stretched or absent. The most common acquired defect that results in the lengthening of these attachments and hence makes the stomach prone to volvulus is hiatal hernia, especially type II. Most cases of volvulus associated with hiatal hernia are of the organoaxial type where the axis of rotation runs from the cardia to the pylorus, and most cases are anterior. Although most cases of volvulus associated with a hiatal hernia are chronic, acute volvulus can occur, usually after a large meal.

The presentation of an acute volvulus can be fairly dramatic. Borchardt,[107] who first described the condition in 1904, emphasized three principal features: (1) severe pain in the epigastrium associated with distension, (2) vomiting followed by inability to vomit and continued retching, and (3) inability to pass a nasogastric tube. It is thought that the process is initiated by pyloric occlusion resulting in violent vomiting typical of a high occlusion. As the stomach rotates, the cardia too gets occluded, which causes the later retching and inability to vomit and retch. As both ends of the stomach are occluded, the patient develops a closed-loop obstruction, which can cause massive distension and interference with the vascular supply of the organ. Three additional features were later added to this classic description: (1) minimal abdominal signs if most of the stomach is in the thorax,

(2) abdominal and/or chest radiograph showing a gas-filled organ in the lower chest, and (3) obstruction of the stomach on contrast radiography. In a series of 25 patients with acute volvulus, gangrene of the stomach was found in 7 (28%). Gangrene was heralded by bleeding, cardiorespiratory distress, and shock.[108]

Acute volvulus can at times be reduced by simple passage of a nasogastric tube, although in most cases, as noted above, nonpassage of the tube is one of the presenting features. In such situations urgent operation is essential to prevent the disastrous complication of strangulation and gangrene. At the time of surgery, in the absence of strangulation and if the patient is stable, the volvulus should be reduced, and a definitive procedure for the hiatal hernia, usually including an antireflux procedure, should be carried out. If the patient's condition is deemed unstable, the reduced stomach should be held in place by some form of gastropexy, the simplest of these being a gastrostomy. When gastric necrosis has taken place, resection will have to be performed, the extent of which is dictated by the extensiveness of the necrosis.

Because acute gastric surgery for gangrene carries high morbidity and mortality rates, the traditional recommendation has been that elective corrective surgery for type II hernias should be performed to prevent this complication from occurring, even if the hiatal hernia itself is causing minimal or no symptoms. However, this view has recently been challenged. In a study presented to the American Surgical Association, Stylopoulos and associates[109] pointed out that the available surgical literature and the Nationwide Inpatient Sample Database do not support routine elective repair of asymptomatic paraesophageal hernias. Their analysis suggested that prophylactic surgery would be more beneficial than "watchful waiting" for only one of five 65-year-old patients.

In summary, both traumatic and nontraumatic conditions of the diaphragm present challenges to the acute care surgeon. A well-informed surgeon will utilize the various diagnostic and therapeutic options to reduce their associated morbidity and mortality rates.

Critique

With documentation of a diaphragmatic hernia and the fact that it is the delayed (3 years) sequela of a previous injury (left thoracoabdominal penetrating wound), definitive management is now required. This is obviously a missed diaphragmatic injury that should have been found and repaired, and the abdominal cavity should have been thoroughly explored at the time of the original injury. The thoracoabdominal area (from the nipples to the costal margins) has been called the "ultimate blind spot," because no conventional diagnostic study (helical CT scan, ultrasound, MRI, or diagnostic peritoneal lavage) can reliably rule out a diaphragmatic injury. Therefore, celiotomy was the preferred management for these injuries, particularly on the left side. However, Ivatury and others highlighted the advantage of laparoscopy in diagnosing the penetrating diaphragmatic injuries. If a diaphragmatic injury is discovered, then the patient undergoes a celiotomy for a formal abdominal exploration. (It is not recommended that such an exploration be done laparoscopically for fear of missing an intraabdominal injury.) Because it is 3 years after the index injury, a thoracostomy would be the best approach to repair this diaphragmatic hernia because of better exposure and ease of repair compared with a transabdominal approach. In the acute care setting, a transabdominal approach should be the preferred choice because full abdominal exploration would be required. After 3 years, there should be no clinically significant intraabdominal injury.

Answer (D)

References

1. Kondo T, Kobayashi I, Taguchi Y, Ohta Y, Yanagimachi N. A dynamic analysis of chest wall motions with MRI in healthy young subjects. Respirology 2000; 5(1):19–25.
2. Robotham JL, Takata M. Mechanical abdomino/heart/lung interaction. J Sleep Res 1995; 4(S1):50–52.
3. Takata M, Robotham JL. Effects of inspiratory diaphragmatic descent on inferior vena caval venous return. J Appl Physiol 1992; 72(2):597–607.
4. Reber PU, Schmied B, Seiler CA, et al. Missed diaphragm injuries and their long-term sequelae. J trauma 1998; 44(1):183–188.
5. Shah R, Sabanathan S, Mearns AJ, et al. Traumatic rupture of diaphragm. Ann Thorac Surg 1995; 60:1444–1449.
6. Hamby WB. The Case Reports and Autopsy Records of Ambroise Paré. Springfield, IL: Charles C Thomas, 1960; 50–51.
7. Rodriguez-Morales G, Rodriguez A, Shatney CH. Acute rupture of the diaphragm in blunt trauma: analysis of 60 patients. J Trauma 1986; 26:438–444.
8. Rosati C. Acute traumatic injury of the diaphragm. Chest Surg Clin North Am 1998; 8(2):371–379.
9. Johnson CD. Blunt injuries of the diaphragm. Br J Surg 1988; 75:226–230.
10. Patselas T, Gallagher E. The diagnostic dilemma of diaphragm injuries. Am Surg 2002; 68:633–639.
11. Hood RM. Traumatic diaphragmatic hernia. Ann Thorac Surg, 1971; 12:311–324.
12. Bekassy SM, Dave KS, Wooler GH, et al. "Spontaneous" and traumatic rupture of the diaphragm: long-term results. Ann Surg 1973; 177:320–324.
13. Gravier L, Freeark RJ. Traumatic diaphragmatic hernia. Arch Surg 1963; 86:363–373.
14. Andrus CH, Morton JH. Rupture of the diaphragm after blunt trauma. Am J Surg 1970; 119:686–693.
15. Mihos P, Potaris K, Gakidis J, et al. Traumatic rupture of the diaphragm: experience with 65 patients. Injury 2003; 34:169–172.
16. Bergeron E, Clas D, Ratte S, et al. Impact of deferred treatment of blunt diaphragmatic rupture: a 15-year experience in six trauma centers in Quebec. J Trauma 2002; 52(4):633–640.
17. Reiff D, McGwin G, Metzger J, et al. Identifying injuries and motor vehicle collision characteristics that together are suggestive of diaphragmatic rupture. J Trauma 2002; 53(6):1139–1145.
18. Desforges G, Strieder JW, Lynch JP, et al. Traumatic rupture of the diaphragm. J Thorac Surg 1957; 34:779–799.
19. Andrus C, Morton JU. Rupture of the diaphragm after blunt trauma. Am J Surg 1970; 119:686–693.
20. Grage T, Maclean L, Campbell G. Traumatic rupture of the diaphragm. Surgery 1959; 46:669–681.
21. Wilson RF, Walt AJ, eds. Management of Trauma: Pitfalls and Practice, 2nd ed. Baltimore: Williams & Wilkins, 1996.
22. Feliciano DV, Moore EE, Matox KL, eds. Trauma, 3rd ed. Stanford, CT: Appleton-Lange, 1996.
23. Meyers BF, McCabe CJ. Traumatic diaphragmatic hernia. Ann Surg 1993; 218:783–790.
24. Ilgenfritz FM, Stewart DE. Blunt trauma of the diaphragm: a 15 county private hospital experience. Am Surg 1992; 58:334–339.
25. Boulanger BR, Milzman DP, Rosati C, et al. A comparison of right and left blunt traumatic diaphragmatic rupture. J Trauma 1993; 35:255–260.
26. Murray JG, Aioli E, Cruden JF, et al. Acute rupture of the diaphragm due to blunt trauma: diagnostic sensitivity and specificity of CT. AJR Am J Roentgenol 1996; 166(5): 1035–1039.
27. Guth AA, Pachter HL, Kim U. Pitfalls in the diagnosis of blunt diaphragmatic injury. Am J Surg 1995; 170:5–9.
28. Spann JC, Mariachi FE, Wait M. Evaluation of video assisted thoracoscopic surgery in the diagnosis of diaphragmatic injuries. Am J Surg 1995; 170:628–631.
29. Arak T, Solheim K, Pillgram-Larsen J. Diaphragmatic injuries. Injury 1997; 28:113–117.
30. Brasel KJ, Borgstrom DC, Meyer P, et al. Predictors of outcome in blunt diaphragmatic rupture. J Trauma 1996; 4:484–487.
31. Gouin A, Garson AA. Diagnostic problems in traumatic diaphragmatic hernia. J Trauma 1974; 14:20–31.
32. Bow ditch HI. Diaphragmatic hernia. Buffalo Med J 1853; 9(1):65.
33. Beal SL, McKennan M. Blunt diaphragmatic rupture: a morbid injury. Arch Surg 1988; 123:828–832.
34. Kearney PA, Ohana SW, Burney RE. Blunt rupture of the diaphragm: mechanism, diagnosis, and treatment. Ann Emerg Med 1989; 18:1326–1330.
35. Kim HH, Shin YR, Kim KJ, et al. Blunt traumatic rupture of the diaphragm: Sonographic diagnosis. J Ultrasound Med 1997; 16:593–598.

36. Mansouri KA. Trauma to the diaphragm. Chest Surg Clin North Am 1997; 7:373–383.

37. Killeen KL, Mirvis SE, Shanmuganathan K. Helical CT of diaphragmatic rupture caused by blunt trauma. AJR Am J Roentgenol 1999; 173(6):1611–1616.

38. Shapiro MJ, Heifer E, Durham M, et al. The unreliability of CT scans and initial chest radiographs in evaluating blunt trauma-induced diaphragmatic rupture. Clin Radiol 1996; 51:27–30.

39. Shanmuganathan K, Mirvis SE, White CS, et al. MR imaging evaluation of hemidiaphragms in acute blunt trauma: experience with 16 patients. AJR Am J Roentgenol 1996; 67:397–402.

40. Carter BN, Goosefish J. Traumatic diaphragmatic hernia. AJR Am J Roentgenol 1951; 65:56–72.

41. Shapiro MJ, Heifer E, Durham M, et al. The unreliability of CT scans and initial chest radiographs in evaluating blunt trauma induced diaphragmatic rupture. Clin Radiol 1996; 51:27–30.

42. Miller L, Bennett EV, Root HD, et al. Management of penetrating and blunt diaphragmatic injury. J Trauma 1984; 24:403–409.

43. Demetriades D, Kakoyiannis S, Parekh D, et al. Penetrating injuries of the diaphragm. Br J Surg 1988; 75:824–826.

44. Hood RM. Injuries involving the diaphragm. In Hood RM, Boyd AD, Culliford AT, eds. Thoracic Trauma. Philadelphia: WB Saunders, 1989; 267–289.

45. Payne JH, Yellin AE. Traumatic diaphragmatic hernia. Arch Surg 1982; 117:18–24.

46. Worthy SA, Kang EY, Hartman TE, et al. Diaphragmatic rupture: CT findings in 11 patients. Radiology 1995; 194(3):885–888.

47. Jones TK, Walsh JW, Maull KI. Diagnostic imaging in blunt trauma of the abdomen. Surg Gynecol Obstet 1983; 157:389–398.

48. Toombs BD, Sandler CM, Lester RG. Computed tomography of chest trauma. Radiology 1981; 140:733–738.

49. Nau T, Seitz H, Mousavi M, Vecsei V. The diagnostic dilemma of traumatic rupture of the diaphragm. Surg Endosc 2001; 15:992–996.

50. Somers JM, Gleeson FV, Flower CDR. Rupture of the right hemidiaphragm following blunt trauma: the use of ultrasound in diagnosis. Clin Radiol 1990; 42:97–101.

51. Mirvis SE, Keramati B, Buckman R, et al. MR imaging of traumatic diaphragmatic rupture. J Comput Assist Tomogr 1988; 12:147–149.

52. Kurata K, Kubota K, Oosawa H, et al. Thoracoscopic repair of traumatic diaphragmatic rupture. Surg Endosc 1996; 10:850–851.

53. Martin I, O'Rourke N, Gotley D, et al. Laparoscopy in the management of diaphragmatic rupture due to blunt trauma. Aust N Z J Surg 1998; 68:584–586.

54. Ivatury RR, Simon RJ, Weksler B, et al. Laparoscopy in the evaluation of the intrathoracic abdomen after penetrating injury. J Trauma 1992; 33:101–109.

55. Edington HD, Evans S, Sindelar WF. Reconstruction of a functional hemidiaphragm with use of omentum and latissimus dorsi flaps. Surgery 1989; 105:442–445.

56. Hirsch EF. Repair of an abdominal wall defect after a salvage laparotomy for sepsis. J Am Coll Surg 2004; 198(2):324–328.

57. Bender JS, Lucas CE. Management of close-range shotgun injuries to the chest by diaphragmatic transposition: case reports. J Trauma 1990; 30:1581–1584.

58. Zantut L, Ivatury R, Smith S, et al. Diagnostic and therapeutic laparoscopy for penetrating abdominal trauma: a multicenter experience. J Trauma 1997; 42(5):825–831.

59. Leppaniemi A, Haapiainen R. Occult diaphragmatic injuries caused by stab wounds. J Trauma 2003; 55:646–650.

60. Martinez M, Briz JE, Carillo EH. Video thoracoscopy expedites the diagnosis and treatment of penetrating diaphragmatic injuries. Surg Endosc 2001; 15:28–33.

61. Murray JA, Demetriades D, Cornwell EE 3rd, et al. Penetrating left thoracoabdominal trauma: the incidence and clinical presentation of diaphragm injuries. J Trauma 1997; 43:624–626.

62. Chen JC, Wilson SE. Diaphragmatic injuries: recognition and management in sixty-two patients. Am Surg 1991; 57:810–815.

63. Stylianos S, King TC. Occult diaphragm injuries at celiotomy for left chest stab wounds. Am Surg 1992; 58:364–368.

64. Symbas PN, Vlasis SE, Hatcher C Jr. Blunt and penetrating diaphragmatic injuries with or without herniation of organs into the chest. Ann Thorac Surg 1986; 42(2):158.

65. Wiencek RG Jr, Wilson RF, Steiger Z. Acute injuries of the diaphragm. An analysis of 165 cases. J Thorac Cardiovasc Surg 1986; 92(6):989–993.

66. Shackleton KL, Stewart ET, Taylor AJ. Traumatic diaphragmatic injuries: spectrum of radiographic findings. Radiographics 1998; 18:49–59.

67. Adegboye VO, Ladipo JK, Adebo OA, et al. Diaphragmatic injuries. Afr J Med Med Sci 2002; 31:149–153.

68. Karmy-Jones R, Carter Y, Stern E. The impact of positive pressure ventilation on the diagnosis of traumatic diaphragmatic injury. Am Surg 2002; 68:167–172.

69. Udobi KF, Rodriguez A, Chiu WC, Scalea TM. Role of ultrasonography in penetrating abdominal trauma: a prospective clinical study. J Trauma 2001; 50:475–479.

70. Chiu WC, Shanmuganathan K, Mirvis SE, et al. Determining the need for laparotomy in penetrating torso trauma: a prospective study using triple-contrast enhanced abdominopelvic tomography. J Trauma 2001; 51:860–869.

71. Mirvis SE, Shanmuganathan K. MR imaging of thoracic trauma. Magn Reson Imaging Clin North Am 2000; 8:91–104.

72. Ochsner MG, Rozycki GS, Lucente F, et al. Prospective evaluation of thoracoscopy for diagnosing diaphragmatic injury in thoracoabdominal trauma: a preliminary report. J Trauma 1993; 34:704–710.

73. Smith RS, Fry WR, Tsoi EK, et al. Preliminary report on videothoracoscopy in the evaluation and treatment of thoracic injury. Am J Surg 1993; 166:690–695.

74. Uribe RA, Pachon CE, Frame SB, et al. A prospective evaluation of thoracoscopy for the diagnosis of penetrat-

ing thoracoabdominal trauma. J Trauma 1994; 37:650–654.

75. Nel JH, Warren BL. Thoracoscopic evaluation of the diaphragm in patients with knife wounds of the left lower chest. Br J Surg 1994; 81:713–714.

76. Freeman RK, Al-Dossari G, Hutcheson KA, et al. Indications for using video-assisted thoracoscopic surgery to diagnose diaphragmatic injuries after penetrating chest trauma. Ann Thorac Surg 2001; 72:342–347.

77. Ivatury RR, Simon RJ, Stahl WM. A critical evaluation of laparoscopy in penetrating abdominal trauma. J Trauma 1993; 34:822–828.

78. Ivatury RR, Simon RJ, Stahl WM. Selective celiotomy for missile wounds of the abdomen based on laparoscopy. Surg Endosc 1994; 8:366–370.

79. Ortega AE, Tang E, Froes ET, et al. Laparoscopic evaluation of penetrating thoracoabdominal traumatic injuries. Surg Endosc 1996; 10:19–22.

80. Murray JA, Demetriades D, Asensio JA, et al. Occult injuries to the diaphragm: a prospective evaluation of laparoscopy in penetrating injuries to the left lower chest. J Am Coll Surg 1998; 187:626–630.

81. Ertekin C, Onaran Y, Guloglu R, et al. The use of laparoscopy as a primary diagnostic and therapeutic method in penetrating wounds of lower thoracal region. Surg Laparosc Endosc 1998; 8:26–29.

82. McQuay N Jr, Britt LD. Laparoscopy in the evaluation of penetrating thoracoabdominal trauma. Am Surg 2003; 69:788–791.

83. Morales CH, Villegas MI, Angel W, et al. Value of digital exploration for diagnosing injuries to the left side of the diaphragm caused by stab wounds. Arch Surg 2001; 136:1131–1135.

84. DeMaria EJ, Dalton JM, Gore DC, et al. Complementary roles of laparoscopic abdominal exploration and diagnostic peritoneal lavage for evaluating abdominal stab wounds: a prospective study. J Laparoendosc Adv Surg Tech A 2000; 10:131–136.

85. Simon RJ, Rabin J, Kuhls D. Impact of increased use of laparoscopy on negative laparotomy after penetrating trauma. J Trauma 2002; 53:297–302.

86. Shatney CH, Sensaki K, Morgan L. The natural history of stab wounds of the diaphragm: implications for a new management scheme for patients with penetrating thoracoabdominal trauma. Am Surg 2003; 69:508–513.

87. Kozar RA, Kaplan LJ, Cipolla J, et al. Laparoscopic repair of traumatic diaphragmatic injuries. J Surg Res 2001; 15:164–171.

88. Murray JA, Cornwell EE 3rd, Velmahos GC, et al. Healing of traumatic diaphragm injuries: comparison of laparoscopic versus open techniques in an animal model. J Surg Res 2001; 100:189–191.

89. Frantzides CT, Carlson MA. Laparoscopic repair of a penetrating injury to the diaphragm: a case report. J Laparoendosc Surg 1994; 4:153–156.

90. Gonzalez-Rapado L, Collera-Rodriguez SA, Perez-Esteban M, et al. Diaphragmatic hernia caused by penetrating injury: emergency laparoscopic reconstruction. Rev Gastroenterol Mex 1997; 62:281–283.

91. Matthews BD, Bui H, Harold KL, et al. Laparoscopic repair of traumatic diaphragmatic injuries. Surg Endosc 2003; 17:254–258.

92. Shaw JM, Navsaria PH, Nicol AJ. Laparoscopy-assisted repair of diaphragm injuries. World J Surg 2003; 27:671–674.

93. Thal ER, Provost DA. Traumatic rupture of the diaphragm. In Nyhus LM, Baker RJ, Fischer JE, eds. Mastery of Surgery, 3rd ed. Boston: Little, Brown and Company, 1997; 686–693.

94. Asensio JA, Demetriades D, Rodriguez A. Injury to the diaphragm. In Mattox KL, Feliciano DV, Moore EE, eds. Trauma. New York: McGraw-Hill, 2000; 603–632.

95. Reber PU, Schmied B, Seiler CA, et al. Missed diaphragmatic injuries and their long-term sequelae. J Trauma 1998; 44:183–188.

96. Sullivan RE. Strangulation and obstruction in diaphragmatic hernia due to direct trauma. J Thorac Cardiovasc Surg 1966; 52:725–784.

97. Williams M, Carlin AM, Tyburski JG, et al. Predictors of mortality in patients with traumatic diaphragmatic rupture and associated thoracic and/or abdominal injuries. Am Surg 2004; 70:157–163.

98. Mattila S, Jarvinen A, Mattila T, et al. Traumatic diaphragmatic hernia. Report of 50 cases. Acta Chir Scand 1977; 143:313–318.

99. Ivatury RR. Laparoscopy and thoracoscopy in penetrating thoraco-abdominal injuries. Eur Surg 2005; 37(1):19–27.

100. Laine L. Upper gastrointestinal hemorrhage. West J Med 1991; 155:274–279.

101. Rockey DC. Gastrointestinal bleeding. In Feldman M, Friedman LS, Sleisenger MH, eds. Gastrointestinal and Liver Disease, 7th ed. Philadelphia: Saunders, 2002; 211–248.

102. Stabile BE, Stamos MJ. Gastrointestinal bleeding. In Zinner MJ, Schwartz SI, Ellis H, eds. Maingot's Abdominal Operations, 10th ed. Stamford, CT: Appleton & Langer 1997; 289–313.

103. Rakic S, Hissink RJ, Schiff BW. Perforation of gastric ulcer associated with paraesophageal hernia causing diffuse peritonitis. Dig Surg 2000; 17:83–84.

104. Riepe G, Braun S, Swoboda L. Perforation into the heart—a rare complication of stomach ulcer in hiatal hernia. Chirurg 1998; 69:475–476.

105. Trojan I, Imre J, Kulka F. Gastro-pulmonary fistula as an unusual late complication of a hiatal hernia. Thoraxchir Vasik Chir 1971; 19:152–154.

106. Alvarez L, Blondiau JV, Scherpings P, et al. Pneumopericardium: a race against time! Case report and literature review. Rev Med Brux 1996; 17:143–146.

107. Borchardt M. Zur pathologie und therapie des magenvolvulus. Arch FJ Chir 1904; 74:243.

108. Carter R, Brewer LA, Hinshaw DB. Acute gastric volvulus. Am J Surg 1980; 140:99–106.

109. Stylopoulos N, Gazelle GS, Rattner DW. Paraesophageal hernias: operation or observation? Ann Surg 2002; 236:492–500.

28
Abdominal Wall

Jeffrey A. Claridge and Martin A. Croce

Case Scenario

An 82-year-old nursing home patient undergoes emergency intervention for an acute abdomen. Patient stated that the only thing that relieved the pain was flexion of her right thigh. Exploration confirmed strangulate bowel resulting from intestinal herniation. Which abdominal wall/pelvic hernia usually presents as an intestinal obstruction of unknown origin?

(A) Femoral hernia
(B) Lumbar hernia
(C) Umbilical hernia
(D) Spigelian hernia
(E) Obturator hernia

Anatomy

In-depth knowledge of the anatomy and innervation of the abdominal wall is crucial to all facets of abdominal surgery. The emergency surgeon must have a thorough knowledge of abdominal wall anatomy.

The abdomen is the portion of the body bounded above by the diaphragm and continuing into the pelvis below the plane of the pelvic inlet. A trauma surgeon defines the abdominal cavity as beginning below the level of the nipples because a penetrating injury here can violate the diaphragm and injure intraabdominal organs, which can be seen as high as the fifth intercostal space. The abdominal wall is bordered above by the cartilages of the seventh to twelfth ribs and by the xiphoid process of the sternum. Inferiorly, the abdominal wall boundaries are the bones of the pelvis and the inguinal ligament. The prominent iliac crest forms the upper limit of the region of the hip; the curve of the crest ends ventrally in the anterior superior spine of the ileum, which is an important anatomic landmark that can be easily palpated. The

inguinal ligament stretches between the pubic tubercle and the anterior superior iliac. This ligament is the rolled-under inferior margin of the aponeurosis of the external abdominal oblique muscle. In the groin, this is the anatomic separation between the abdominal wall and the lower extremity. Three vertical lines are visible on the anterior abdominal wall and extend from the pubic tubercles to the costal margin. The linea alba is the central line that marks the aponeurotic junction between the two rectus muscles. Two linea semilunares define the lateral margins of the rectus muscles. For simplicity and localization of pain the division of the abdomen into quadrants provides a convenient reference. Such quadrants are defined in relation to the vertical line of the linea alba and to an imaginary transverse plane through the umbilicus.

The abdominal wall is made up of many layers of skin, fat, fascia, and muscle. A scalpel blade or bullet must penetrate multiple layers to enter the innermost layer of the peritoneum. These layers are illustrated in Figure 28.1 and are slightly different depending on the location of the abdomen and relation to the arcuate line (Table 28.1). Being able to identify the layers is crucial to reapproximation of tissue edges and healing of wounds. Furthermore, knowledge of the different layers allows for the creation of complex closures and reconstruction. The understanding of tissue planes and the different physiologic properties of the layers allows for the understanding of many infectious processes. The skin is the outermost layer followed by subcutaneous fat, followed by Scarpa's and then Camper's fascia. These layers may be involved in some types of necrotizing soft tissue infections and allow for rapid spread of organisms. The next layers are muscle and aponeurotic sheaths. The muscles of the abdominal wall comprise two groups, anterolateral and posterior. The posterior muscle is the quadratus lumborum. The anterolateral muscles include two vertical muscles, rectus abdominus and pyramidalis, and three thin muscular layers, which alternate in their fiber

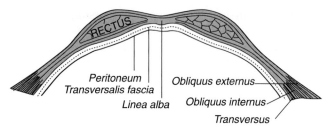

FIGURE 28.1. Layers of the abdominal wall on cross section. (Adapted from Townsend C. Beauchamp RD, Evers BM, Mattox K. Sabiston Textbook of Surgery, 17th ed. Philadelphia: WB Saunders, 2004, with permission from Elsevier.)

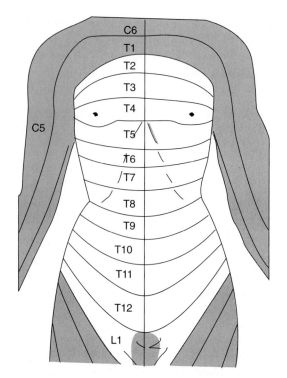

FIGURE 28.2. Segmental innervation of the anterior chest and abdominal wall.

direction. These are the external abdominal oblique, internal abdominal oblique, and transversus abdominus muscles, which have extensive aponeurotic insertions. Their aponeuroses form a sheath for the rectus abdominus and pyramidalis muscles. The alternation in the direction of their muscles and aponeuroses adds strength to the abdominal wall. This also allows for muscle-splitting techniques to be used to enter the abdomen, avoiding transecting muscle and minimizing tissue damage. A muscle-splitting technique versus a muscle-dividing technique has been shown to decrease postoperative pain and increase patient mobility.[1] Knowledge of the muscular anatomy of the abdominal wall and use of muscle-splitting techniques can be useful for emergent surgeries, including appendectomy, open cholecystectomy, and hernia repairs. The innermost layer is the peritoneum, which is separated from the innermost muscle layer of the transversus abdominus. In between these two layers is the preperitoneal space, and it has varying amounts of fat within. Anatomic recognition and knowledge of this

space is crucial to many hernia repairs, which are discussed later in this chapter.

The innervation of the muscles of the abdominal wall is by ventral rami of spinal nerves thoracic seven through lumbar four. This is the same segmental sequence that provides the cutaneous nerves in the region (Figure 28.2). The nerves of the anterior abdominal wall muscles are the intercostal nerves seven through eleven and the subcostal, iliohypogastric, and ilioinguinal nerves. The innermost layer of the abdominal wall, the parietal peritoneum, is richly innervated and very sensitive. Unlike the visceral peritoneum the parietal peritoneal surfaces sharply localize painful stimuli to the site of its origin.

Evaluation of Abdominal Wall

A large number of patients will require evaluation of the abdomen secondary to abdominal pain or traumatic injury. It has been estimated that 5% to 10% of all emergency department visits, or 5 to 10 million patients, with abdominal symptoms present to emergency departments yearly.[2] Another study demonstrated that up to 25% of patients in the emergency room have abdominal pain.[3]

Physical examination of the abdomen always begins with inspection. Specific attention should be paid to scars, hernias, masses, abdominal wall defects, and location of

TABLE 28.1. Layers of the abdominal wall from superficial to deep.

Location in relation to arcuate line	Layers from superficial to deep
Cranial to arcuate line	Skin, Camper's fascia (fatty layer of superficial fascia), Scarpa's fascia (membranous layer of superficial fascia), deep fascia, external abdominal oblique aponeurosis, anterior layer of internal abdominal oblique aponeurosis, rectus abdominus, posterior layer of internal abdominal oblique aponeurosis, transversus abdominus aponeurosis, transversalis fascia, extraperitoneal fat, parietal peritoneum
Caudal to arcuate line	Skin, Camper's fascia (fatty layer of superficial fascia), Scarpa's fascia (membranous layer of superficial fascia), deep fascia, external abdominal oblique aponeurosis, internal abdominal oblique aponeurosis, transversus abdominus aponeurosis, rectus abdominus, transversalis fascia, extraperitoneal fat, parietal peritoneum

injuries. Traditionally, palpation of the abdomen is the next phase of the abdominal examination. Following inspection is auscultation, especially for a patient with acute abdominal pain. The examiner can gently listen to the abdomen without causing any discomfort. This may gain the patient's trust and give him or her more time to relax to allow for further evaluation and palpation. Auscultation of the abdomen gives information about the presence and quality of bowel sounds. A quiet abdomen generally indicates an ileus, whereas hyperactive bowel sounds with high-pitched rushes and tinkles are more characteristic of a mechanical bowel obstruction. One should also listen for the presence of bruits as a marker of vascular disease. Gentle palpation with the stethoscope at the end of the auscultatory phase of the physical examination may elicit information regarding tenderness of the patient's abdominal wall. This portion of the examination is the point at which the examiner can transition into the palpation phase of the abdominal examination.

Palpation should begin with gentle pressure away from the point of abdominal discomfort. The examiner should observe the patient's facial expression for signs of pain or discomfort. The detection of increased muscle tone during palpation is referred to as "guarding," which may be voluntary or involuntary. Involuntary guarding is more concerning for peritonitis. The guarding may also be generalized or it may be localized. The location of pain on the abdominal wall can aid the clinician in making the diagnosis (Figure 28.3). Another sign of peritonitis is rebound tenderness. The last step of the abdominal exam-

ination is percussion. When gentle percussion elicits tenderness, it indicates inflammation and has the same implication as rebound tenderness. Percussion of the abdominal wall may demonstrate tympani as found in bowel obstruction, or it may demonstrate percussive dullness and evidence of fluid in ascites.

Hernias

Simply put, a defect in the normal anatomy of the abdominal wall is the cause of a hernia. The decision to operate emergently or urgently on a patient with a hernia depends on the presentation of the patient. A call to the emergency room or medical intensive care unit to evaluate a patient who is septic and has a large scrotal hernia that worries the nonsurgical colleagues should not immediately prompt operative intervention. The physician should be able to elicit hernias by palpation as well as by asking the patient to perform maneuvers to increase intraabdominal pressure. A valsalva maneuver, or asking the patient to stand if able, is often sufficient.

There are many types of hernias, some of which are discussed later in this chapter, and recognition of which hernias need to be fixed acutely is critical. In general, a hernia that cannot be reduced is termed an "incarcerated hernia" and should be repaired immediately. The concern is that bowel is being strangulated within the incarcerated hernia. Signs that make this more ominous are tenderness during palpation of the hernia, redness around the hernia, fever, tachycardia, and leukocytosis. Furthermore, the signs of a bowel obstruction in the presence of an incarcerated hernia warrant acute surgical intervention. Waiting to operate in this scenario adds morbidity to the procedure. Kulah et al.[4] evaluated 385 consecutive acute care surgeries for incarcerated external hernia. They demonstrated that inguinal and umbilical hernias were most common, at 75% and 13%, respectively. Additionally, they reported that older age, presence of coexisting diseases, and duration of symptoms were associated with negative outcomes.

There are also hernias that are difficult to reduce and may take effort or require sedation to be reduced. If these patients do not have signs of bowel obstruction, fever, elevated white blood count, tachycardia, or evidence of local inflammation, an emergent operation is not generally indicated. However, this is a hernia that is clearly symptomatic and in our opinion should be operated at the next convenient opportunity. The timing of this is usually the next working day during the elective schedule.

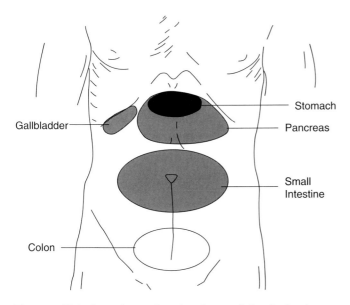

FIGURE 28.3. Location of pain from abdominal viscera. (Adapted from Townsend C. Beauchamp RD, Evers BM, Mattox K. Sabiston Textbook of Surgery, 17th ed. Philadelphia: WB Saunders, 2004, with permission from Elsevier.)

Groin Hernias

Groin hernias are the most common of all abdominal wall hernias. Their exact prevalence is unknown. However, studies have estimated that the lifetime risk of inguinal hernia repairs is 27% for men and 3% for women.[5]

Groin hernias have been classically described and classified on the basis of the clinical presentation of the hernia sac. Thus, they were described as a direct inguinal hernia, an indirect inguinal hernia, both direct and indirect hernia (pantaloon hernia), or femoral hernia. Now that hernias are often repaired from a posterior approach this classification is less relevant, because only the neck of the hernia sac and the parietal defect can be seen. Fruchaud[6] introduced the concept that groin hernias all share the common feature of emerging or beginning in a single weak area he termed the "myopectineal orifice" (MPO). The MPO is a bony muscular framework that is bridged and bisected by the inguinal ligament. The inguinal ligament serves as the dividing line separating inguinal from femoral hernias and defines the medial border of the orifice of the femoral canal. The femoral vessels and the spermatic cord transverse the MPO. The integrity of the MPO depends on the strength of the transverse fascia, which is the innermost muscle layer. Failure of the transverse fascia to retain the peritoneum is the fundamental cause of all hernias of the groin.

Operating in an acute setting on a hernia is generally more difficult and has been shown to have higher complications rates.[5,7] Arenal et al.[8] demonstrated that both increased age and need for acute care surgery were associated with increased mortality. Patients who present with incarcerated groin hernias have been shown in studies[9,10] to be older, have higher American Society of Anesthesiologists scores, and have a high incidence of femoral hernias. Furthermore, inguinal hernia incarceration was shown to be associated with increased morbidity and mortality. If the patient has an incarcerated hernia, the surgeon must evaluate the contents to ensure its viability. Thus, this needs to be kept in mind if the hernia is either intentionally or spontaneously reduced after anesthesia and muscle relaxants. The decision about which type of operation to perform depends on many factors. There are several options for approaching and repairing a groin hernia.

In general, there are two established approaches for repairing a groin hernia. There is an anterior and a posterior approach. There are multiple techniques to each approach. The anterior approach was traditionally used to repair without prosthetic material. The four most popular repairs are the Marcy hernioplasty, the Bassini hernioplasty, the Shouldice hernioplasty, and the Cooper's ligament hernioplasty.

With the Marcy hernioplasty, the deep inguinal ring is tightened and returned to normal size by the placement of one or two permanent monofilament sutures. These sutures are placed medially in the transverse aponeurotic arch and laterally in the iliopubic tract or femoral sheath.

For the Bassini hernioplasty, Bassini divided the floor of the inguinal canal, which is a step that is omitted by some surgeons. This is a three-layer repair that consists of approximating the internal oblique abdominal muscle, the transverse abdominal muscle, and the transverse fascia to the inguinal ligament and iliopubic tract.

With the Shouldice hernioplasty, the floor of the inguinal canal is repaired by imbrication of the innermost fascial layer of the abdominal wall. Suturing begins at the pubic tubercle. The iliopubic tract is fastened to the undersurface of the transverse aponeurotic arch, with a single running suture that is run to the deep internal ring and then run back to approximate the free edge of the transversalis to the shelving edge of the inguinal ligament. The internal oblique abdominal muscle being sutured to the inguinal ligament is described in Shouldice's repair, but is a step that is not uniformly done.

With the Cooper's ligament hernioplasty (McVay-Lotheissen repair), the repair consists of attaching the transverse aponeurotic arch to Cooper's ligament, the medial side of the femoral sheath, and the anterior femoral sheath with interrupted sutures. This repair addresses the three areas that are most vulnerable for herniation in the MPO, the deep inguinal ring, Hesselbach's triangle, and the femoral canal. Therefore, the Cooper's ligament repair is used to manage femoral hernias and large indirect and direct inguinal hernias. The suture affixing the transverse aponeurotic arch to the medial edge of the femoral sheath is called the "transition suture." Relaxing incisions along the rectus sheath are mandatory.

Anterior prosthetic hernioplasty has become increasingly popular. The reason for the increase in popularity is in part because of some of the criticisms of the classic repairs. It is well accepted that considerable experience is required to obtain excellent results using the classic repairs. A classic repair is also thought to be inadequate for recurrent hernias, especially if it was repaired with a classically described technique initially. The largest criticism is that these classic repairs produce tension, and the problems of continued tissue deterioration and strain are not addressed. The most popular version of the anterior prosthetic hernioplasty is the Lichtenstein's tension-free hernioplasty. The repair consists of a polypropylene patch laid over the posterior wall of the inguinal canal. The patch is tailored with a slit or keyhole for the spermatic cord. The prosthesis should extend 1.5 to 2.0cm medial to the pubic tubercle and well lateral to the deep inguinal ring. The patch is sutured securely medially to the pubic tubercle and to the inferior shelving edge of the inguinal ligament inferiorly. It is then sutured superiorly to the underside of the rectus sheath and conjoint tendon. Another type of repair using mesh involves using a mesh plug, which is placed in the hernia defect.

These mesh techniques can also be modified for a posterior preperitoneal approach. This preperitoneal space is a logical site in which to implant a prosthesis. The prosthetic material is held in place by intraabdominal pressure. The preperitoneal space for repair of groin hernia is best approached with an abdominal incision. This allows for excellent exposure without the dissection of the inguinal canal.

Over the past decade there has been an increase in the use of laparoscopic techniques for groin hernia repairs. The two most common techniques for laparoscopic inguinal hernia repair both involve the insertion of mesh into the preperitoneal space. One is referred to as the "transabdominal preperitoneal" approach and the other is referred to as the "totally extraperitoneal" approach.

It is important to understand the different types of hernia repairs; however, for the emergency surgeon, it is more important to identify patients who need emergent operations. Although most hernia repairs are performed electively,[5] there are certainly times when groin hernias need emergent/urgent repair. The indication for emergent/urgent repair of groin hernia is mainly incarceration of the hernia. A nonreducible groin hernia needs to be operated on as soon as possible. The findings at the time of the operation will dictate the type of repair that can and should be performed. Thus, knowledge of various types of procedures is crucial to emergency general surgeons. At this time our opinion is that an incarcerated hernia is a relative contraindication to a laparoscopic approach. Without advanced laparoscopic skills, laparoscopic techniques are contraindicated if the patient exhibits any signs of bowel obstruction or strangulation with an incarcerated hernia. The main rationale for this is as follows. A systematic review (McCormick Cochrane Database) demonstrated that laparoscopic repair techniques have similar recurrence rates in elective cases and may have minimal improvements in return to function and less pain. The Veterans Administration study,[11] however, demonstrated a higher percentage of recurrence and an increase in complications with laparoscopic inguinal hernia repair.

Additionally, laparoscopic surgery requires that all patients get general anesthesia. For patients who are acutely ill, as is often the case in dealing with acute care surgical situations, the option of local or regional anesthetic technique is attractive. Furthermore, if the patient has distended loops of bowel, visualization may be difficult and pneumoperitoneum may be dangerous in an acutely ill patient. Finally, if there is a high suspicion of strangulation and a question of bowel viability, gross contamination with perforation or bowel resection would make the use of prosthetic mesh unwise. One may, however, consider using the laparoscope in the event of the bowel being reduced without it being evaluated

during open repairs. This is only practical if there are no signs of bowel distention.

When the surgical team has deemed that the patient has an incarcerated groin hernia, it should be treated promptly. Kurt et al.[12] demonstrated that although men may have a higher incidence of groin hernia incarceration, women have a higher incidence of bowel compromise requiring resection. Additional risk factors for patients needing bowel resection were patients with femoral hernias and age older than 65 years. Fluid resuscitation should begin immediately if the patient shows signs of dehydration and/or illness from prolonged bowel obstruction. Intravenous access and resuscitation should take no more than a couple of hours. The operating room is also a great place to continue resuscitation. A delay in repairing/correcting the underlying etiology of the illness will likely harm the patient. We favor either a preperitoneal approach using a lower transverse abdominal incision or a classic anterior inguinal incision. When operating, one must make a diligent effort to assess the contents of the hernia sac. The difficulty in this is getting control of the neck of the hernia before reducing it. Evaluation of the contents for necrosis is crucial. If necrosis is discovered or bowel is determined to be not viable, it should be resected. There may already be perforation and local inflammation/infection. In any of these later cases synthetic mesh is not indicated. We would recommend primary repair. If a defect was extremely large and it could not be closed, there are options of using other materials. Vicryl mesh is one option. This will reabsorb and may lead to recurrence, but in the face of infection it is a better option than placing synthetic permanent mesh. Other options are discussed later in this chapter and include biomaterials such as Surgisis (Cook Inc.) and acellular cadaveric dermis (AlloDerm, LifeCell Corporation, Branchburg, NJ).

Other Abdominal Wall Hernias

Ventral Hernias

"Ventral hernias" in this chapter refer to umbilical, periumbilical, parastomal, Spigelian, epigastric, and incisional hernias. The large incisional hernia or planned ventral hernia is discussed later in this chapter.

True umbilical hernias are rare in adults. They are common in infants and usually close without surgical treatment. However, repair is indicated in infants if the hernia is greater than 2 cm in diameter and in all children whose umbilical hernia is still present at 3 to 4 years of age. These seldom need emergent repair and can be dealt with electively. However, adults with periumbilical hernias require repair. Strangulation of the colon, small bowel, and especially omentum is not uncommon. Epigastric hernias occur between the decussating fibers of the linea alba above the umbilicus. Spigelian hernias are relatively rare ventral hernias that occur along the semilunar lines lateral to the rectus abdominal muscle and usually below the umbilicus. Incisional hernias are defects secondary to breakdown along a previous fascial closure. These can be midline or anywhere an abdominal incision can be. A parastomal hernia is a hernia near an ostomy. Regardless of the type of hernia, all but parastomal hernias of the aforementioned hernias can be approached with a similar thought process. Parastomal hernias are discussed separately.

The indication to operate on ventral hernias in a nonelective setting is incarceration. If the patient has a nonreducible mass, he or she should be scheduled for repair. For the same reasons as mentioned earlier, we recommend open repair for symptomatic incarcerated hernias. However, if the patient has no evidence of bowel obstruction or the hernia contents were reduced, laparoscopy is a viable option.

At the time of operation, the contents of the hernia sac need to be evaluated for ischemic changes. Often the omentum is incarcerated, and it can be reduced during the procedure when the sac is opened. If bowel is in the hernia sac, it must be carefully inspected for evidence of ischemia or necrosis. Often it may have some venous congestion and show signs of inflammation. If it is viable it should "pink up" after it is reduced. If it has clear areas of necrosis or perforation, it should be resected. A Richter's hernia is a hernia that may have a partial segment of incarcerated bowel. This may create a small area of necrosis without signs of obstruction. Likewise, ischemic or necrotic omentum needs to be resected. After the contents of the hernia sac are reduced, the hernia sac should be excised and the fascial edges should be identified and dissected free from sac, surrounding connective tissues, or other adhesions. It is important to debride the fascial edges to healthy tissue, because reapproximation of scar will lead to a recurrent hernia. Clearly identifying and visualizing 1 cm of fascia circumferentially around the defect is crucial to properly repairing these hernias. If the hernia is small and not a recurrent hernia, it can be closed with nonabsorbable sutures. Larger hernias are best treated with a prosthetic closure. There are many techniques used to describe the closures of small primary defects (vest over pants imbrication, interrupted simple sutures, multiple figure-of-eight sutures, and continuous suture closures). The key concept is tension-free reapproximation of healthy fascia. Thus, sutures should be placed and tied to reapproximate and not strangulate the tissues.

Arroyo et al.[13] demonstrated that the use of prosthetic closure was superior to primary closure for umbilical defects. They demonstrated a recurrence rate of 11% with suture closure versus a 1% recurrence with mesh ($p =$ 0.0015). A contraindication to the placement of synthetic mesh is exposure of bowel contents. When resection is needed, primary repair can be performed if there is little to no tension. An attractive alternative is the use of biologic mesh material. There are numerous reports in the literature advocating the utility of these products.[14,15] There are multiple methods for securing the mesh, including overlay, underlay, and sandwich-type techniques. If laparoscopy is the method of surgery, the mesh underlay technique is the method to be used for repair.

Parastomal Hernias

A parastomal hernia is a hernia that occurs in proximity to an ostomy. Paracolostomy hernias are more common than paraileostomy stomas. This is likely because of the size of the defect created at the time of the initial surgery. In addition, these hernias are more likely to occur when the stoma emerges through the semilunar lines rather than through the center of the rectus abdominal muscle. Thus, most fascial defects and hernias are lateral to the ostomy. However, they can occur anywhere in relation to the ostomy.

In our experience, parastomal hernias seldom need emergent repair. However, there are several reasons to include them in this text. One, like all hernias, they can cause bowel obstruction secondary to incarceration of bowel. A second reason, and perhaps the more important reason, is that emergent general surgeons and trauma surgeons may see a higher proportion of these hernias. Trauma situations and emergent general situations increase the frequency of ostomies. Additionally, the ostomies are created at the end of a long case and may need to be performed rapidly. Hernias have also been demonstrated to be more common after acute care surgery.[16] Often these patients are critically ill and have prolonged recovery times and likely poor wound healing. Thus, besides taking care to create the ostomy correctly, knowledge of how to address the complications of them is important to emergency general surgeons.

The decision of when to operate on a parastomal hernia depends on the symptoms and the type of patient presenting. If the patient is presenting with symptomatic incarceration and/or complete bowel obstruction, emergent surgical intervention is needed. Parastomal hernias may also cause chronic problems with maintenance of the ostomy. Patients may have a change in bowel habits and have intermittent obstruction requiring dilation and/or frequent irrigation of the ostomy. More commonly, correct seating and fit of the appliance may be difficult. These more chronic problems can be dealt with on an elective basis. The second issue of deciding when to address the parastomal hernia depends on the type of patient. For the patient with a temporary ostomy it seems wise to wait for the resolution of the initial etiology before it is repaired. The patient with a permanent ostomy can be repaired electively.

There are a variety of methods to repair parastomal hernias. The best method is clearly either moving the ostomy to a different site or taking the ostomy down and returning the continuity of the gastrointestinal tract. If the ostomy is temporary, it is likely that the ostomy was present for only a short time and the defect is small. Thus, this can often be repaired with simple sutures and reapproximation of superior fascial edges to inferior fascial edges. If the ostomy is permanent and can be moved to a second site, this is advised. The site should be marked preoperatively with the patient wearing normal clothes. The site should be within the center of the rectus muscle and not in a skin crease. Observe the patients' abdomen when they stand and sit. Also observe where the patients wear their pants, as they may have a preference on the location based on how they wear their clothes.

Again, marking preoperatively is very important. Abdominal exploration via a midline incision before taking the ostomy down is advisable as this will allow for reduction of the hernia and facilitate freeing the ostomy from the abdominal wall. At this time we recommend repairing the defect. If it is small and it can be closed with minimal tension, consider primary repair. Otherwise, mesh may be needed to reinforce the closure. Synthetic material is not recommended if bowel contents were spilled. Biologic material is an attractive alternative to synthetic mesh, especially in the face of contamination. After the hernia defect is closed the new ostomy can be created in the preoperatively marked position. The skin at the previous ostomy site should be left partially open to allow adequate wound care.

When moving the ostomy is not an option, there are techniques for hernia repair. Two techniques are described in the literature. One is described by Leslie[17] in which the incision is made away from the stoma. The skin and subcutaneous tissue are dissected from the abdominal wall and reflected to expose the bowel and fascial defect. The defect is closed with sutures and a piece of mesh is placed anteriorly over the repair with a slit in it to be positioned around the bowel. If a large amount of undermining a dead space occurred during dissection, a closed suction drain is recommended. Sugarbaker[18] described a technique that repairs the hernia from within the abdomen and also uses mesh. The availability of biologic mesh products now allows the surgeon to consider using them in the repair of parastomal hernias. The advantage of biologic meshes is that they are not permanent, minimizing the chances of bowel erosion. Their collagen matrices allow for ingrowth of tissue, and they appear to be relatively resistant to infection.

Abdominal Wall Trauma

Blunt abdominal wall trauma seldom causes injury to the abdominal wall that requires surgical intervention. However, the presence of obvious abdominal wall trauma needs to trigger concern of internal injuries. A well-described injury pattern is that caused by a rapid deacceleration injury while wearing a lapbelt. A red or line abrasion may be seen across the lower abdomen, and the patient may have a lumbar Chance fracture. In this situation the clinician needs to have a high clinical suspicion for intraabdominal injury—especially bowel or mesenteric tears. Wotherspoon et al.[19] demonstrated a higher risk of intestinal injury in patients with an abdominal seatbelt sign. These injuries can also cause a large amount of shearing injury leading to a large soft tissue injury. These injuries can be difficult to manage and may involve multiple trips to the operating room for debridement.

Penetrating abdominal wall trauma is a very common problem faced by the emergency trauma surgeon. As mentioned earlier, the abdominal cavity can begin just below the nipples. Thus patients with lower penetrating chest wounds must have their abdomen evaluated for intraabdominal injury. If the pleura cavity has been violated, the diaphragm must be evaluated. The two main groups of penetrating injuries are stab and gunshot wounds. Patients with gunshot wounds to the abdomen require emergent laparotomy with few exceptions. Their incidence of significant abdominal injury is approximately 80%. On the other hand, patients with stab wounds have a lower abdominal injury rate (about 33%) when a mandatory laparotomy policy is employed. Thus, gunshot and stab wounds necessitate different management schemes. Evaluation of anterior stab wounds is straightforward and illustrated in Figure 28.4. If the anterior fascia is violated, further inspection is needed. The wound should be locally explored, unless intraabdominal injury is obvious. Lidocaine should be injected for local exploration. The entire wound tract must be evaluated. If there is anterior fascia violation or the wound cannot be locally explored fully, the patient needs further intraoperative exploration. Diagnostic peritoneal lavage is not indicated and in this scenario has been shown to be unreliable for penetrating trauma. If there is violation of the fascia but no clear evidence of intraabdominal injury, the surgeon may either observe the patient or perform laparoscopy. If the peritoneum is intact, the laparoscope can be withdrawn and the procedure ended. If there are no other injuries the patient can be safely discharged to home. Our practice is to convert to an open exploration if the laparoscope demonstrates peritoneal violation. If laparoscopy is not available a small midline incision can be made to evaluate for peritoneal violation. The incision can be extended for further exploration if necessary.

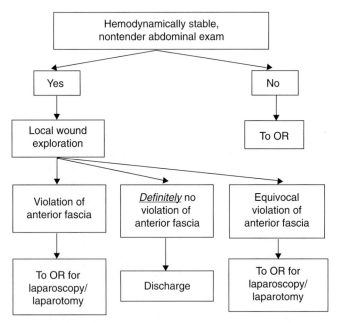

FIGURE 28.4. Algorithm of treatment for penetrating abdominal wound.

Some centers have advocated observation and serial examinations for knife stab wounds. A delay in diagnosis of bowel injuries has been demonstrated to increase morbidity.

Another diagnosis that will confront the emergency surgeon is a rectus sheath hematoma. Patients with rectus sheath hematomas are more commonly women. Patients complain of abdominal pain and may have anemia. Causes include local trauma, straining associated with defecation, coughing, sneezing, and spontaneous. Often patients are receiving anticoagulation therapy. In the literature there are numerous reports of rectus sheath hematoma presenting or masquerading as numerous other conditions, including abruptio placenta,[20] sigmoid diverticulitis,[21] and appendicitis.[22,23]

Ultrasound has been advocated by some as a procedure to assist in the diagnosis of rectus sheath hematoma.[24,25] A method of classification using computed tomography (CT) scan was proposed by Berna et al.[26] and demonstrated three types of hematomas. Type I was a minimal hematoma. Types II and III were moderate and severe hematomas, respectively, and required hospitalization. Anticoagulation is associated with larger hematomas. Patients with larger hematomas likely need transfusion of packed red blood cells and coagulation factors. These patients may present with signs and symptoms similar to patients with an acute abdomen. Both CT scan and ultrasound may be able to assist in the diagnosis. However, it is likely that CT scan is more readily available has fewer user errors. A CT scan may also offer more information about a patient with abdominal pain.

However, the advantage of ultrasound is that it is less costly and is very appropriate, especially for women.

Most rectus sheath hematomas do not require surgery. If there is evidence of ongoing bleeding after correction of a patient's coagulopathy, surgery is indicated. Free fluid in the abdomen is also a sign that the hematoma has ruptured and thus less likely to tamponade. The surgery involves an incision over the hematoma and evacuation of the hematoma. Often the bleeding vessel cannot be identified. We recommend dissecting more inferiorly and ligating the inferior epigastric artery. Although not a common diagnosis, rectus sheath hematomas should be considered in the differential diagnosis for a patient with acute lower abdominal pain. This is especially important if the patient is receiving anticoagulation therapy, as there have been fatalities reported secondary to rectus sheath hematomas.[27] Judicious use of laparotomy is prudent.

Abdominal Compartment Syndrome

Definition

Abdominal compartment syndrome (ACS) is caused by increased intraabdominal pressure that results in pathologic changes. Normal intraabdominal pressure is typically less than 15 mm Hg. The technique to measure intraabdominal pressure with intravesicular pressure monitoring was well described by Kron et al.[28]

The cardiovascular, pulmonary, and renal systems appear to be the most sensitive to the changes in abdominal compartment pressure. The cardiovascular system is affected mainly by reduction in venous return. Thus, decreasing both preload and cardiac output will further exacerbate the shock condition. The pulmonary system is affected secondary to the increase in intraabdominal pressure, causing elevation of the diaphragms. This transmits into higher intrathoracic pressures and subsequent alveolar hypoventilation, leading to subsequent increase in carbon dioxide and acidosis. Hypoxia may also be present, as there is collapse of more alveolar tissue and interparenchymal edema. The renal system is also affected by the increase in intraabdominal pressure. Studies have demonstrated direct effects of increased pressure on the kidney parenchyma and subsequent decrease in glomerular filtration rate.[29] Furthermore, the decrease in cardiac output further leads to a decrease in glomerular filtration rate and low urine output. Patients with closed head injuries also suffer from increased abdominal pressure with increased intracranial pressures. This increase in intracranial pressures is often exacerbated by hypoxia, hypercapnia, decreased venous return, and hypotension.

There is no absolute number at which a patient has ACS; however, an intraabdominal pressure greater than

25 mm Hg measured via bladder pressures is considered elevated. Thus an intraabdominal pressure >25 mm Hg with presence of the above-mentioned pathophysiology defines ACS. Primary ACS has been well recognized by trauma surgeons for many years. Primary ACS is seen often after damage-control operations and occurs in patients with intraabdominal and pelvic pathologies. Secondary ACS is a syndrome now recognized to be caused by conditions outside the abdominal and/or pelvic cavity. Secondary ACS is seen in patients with severe shock needing massive resuscitation.

Etiology

There are many causes of ACS. All patients with ACS are critically ill and carry a significant mortality risk. Abdominal compartment syndrome is most often described in patients with massive abdominal or pelvic hemorrhage. It typically occurs after laparotomy when the fascia is closed and the patient has ongoing blood loss and edema. Other conditions that can lead to ACS are pancreatitis, abdominal burns, and ischemia/reperfusion injury to the bowels. The term "secondary ACS" has been coined to refer to ACS in the absence of abdominal or pelvic pathology and caused by edema and ascites in the presence of shock. This can occur septic shock as patients need large volumes of fluid and develop leaky capillaries that cause massive bowel edema. This can be seen as shock bowel on CT scan (Figure 28.5). Whatever the etiology, the common factor is the abdominal wall and mainly the more restrictive fascia, except in burn where the skin plays a large restrictive role. Like other areas of the body such as extremities, heart within the pericardium, and brain within the cranial vault, the abdomen is enveloped within a closed space. An increase in volume in a closed space leads to an increase in pressure and subsequent pathology.

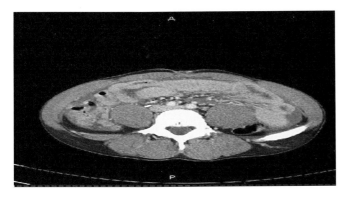

FIGURE 28.5. Computed tomography scan showing evidence of shock bowel.

Treatment

Once the diagnosis is made the decision to intervene should be immediate. Depending on the physical set up of the intensive care unit and operating room the abdomen may be opened at bedside. A midline laparotomy should be performed as soon as possible. The patient's physiologic disarray should begin to correct itself immediately. The most immediate physiologic change that is noticed is a rapid decrease in peak airway pressures. The fascia should be opened from approximately 3 to 4 cm below the xiphoid to a couple of centimeters above the pubic symphysis. If the patient already has a midline incision, simple opening of the incision is usually all that is required. Again, the results of releasing the tension of the abdomen are immediate and often impressive. Fluid and intestines will spring from the wound; thus our bias is to perform this procedure in the operating room. If bleeding or hemorrhage is the etiology, good illumination is paramount. A scrub nurse and access to vascular instruments are also important.

After the abdomen has been opened and hemostasis is ensured, quick exploration for injuries is warranted. The amount of irrigation is one of personal choice. There are multiple methods to "close" the abdomen to prevent evisceration and control fluid loss. These methods are discussed next.

Being able to identify patients at risk for developing ACS would be beneficial, because the mortality of ACS is reported to be between 25% and 75 %.[30] Additionally, an open abdomen is clearly associated with increased morbidity, longer hospital stays, and increased health care costs.

Closure of the Abdominal Wall and/or Skin

In this section we discuss three areas. The first is the decision to close skin. The second is the decision to close fascia and how to manage an open abdomen. The third is the long-term management of the open abdomen and the resultant ventral hernia.

Skin Closure

There are generally three types of closure, which are primary closure, secondary closure, and tertiary closure. Primary or first-intention closure is the most common and can be used for clean wounds. These wounds are immediately closed and usually with the most simple sutures. They can also be closed immediately with skin grafts or flap closures. Secondary closure involves no active intent to seal the wound. These wounds are left open and allowed to heal via contraction and

TABLE 28.2. Surgical wound classification.

Wound class	Definition	Accepted range of infection
I, Clean	Uninfected operative wound in which no inflammation is encountered and the respiratory, alimentary, genital, or urinary tract is not entered. In addition, clean wounds are primarily closed and, if necessary, drained with closed drainage. Operative incisional wounds that follow blunt trauma should be included in this category if they meet criteria	1%–5%
II, Clean contaminated	An operative wound in which the respiratory, alimentary, genital, or urinary tracts are entered under controlled conditions and without unusual contamination. Specifically, operations involving the biliary tract, appendix, vagina, and oropharynx are included in this category, provided no evidence of infection or major break in technique is encountered	3%–11%
III, Contaminated	Open, fresh, accidental wounds. In addition, operations with major breaks in sterile technique or gross spillage from the gastrointestinal tract and incisions in which acute, nonpurulent inflammation is encountered are included in this category	10%–17%
IV, dirty infected	Old traumatic wounds with retained devitalized tissue and those that involve existing clinical infection or perforated viscera. This definition suggests that the organisms causing postoperative infection were present in the operative field before the operation	>27%

reepithelialization. These wounds are seen most commonly when there is a high level of bacterial contamination. Tertiary closure is also commonly referred to as "delayed primary closure." Generally this involves closing an open wound after several days when the tissue bed is clean and the bacterial counts are low. Additionally there is an increase in phagocytes in the wound over the next several days. Thus, it is thought that these wounds can be best closed at around days four to six postoperatively. If this is done, the wound must be watched carefully and should be closed loosely.

The emergent surgeon needs to determine which wounds to close. The risk of closing all wounds is of course infection. An infection of the wound can lead to fascial breakdown and wound dehiscence. Likewise, all wounds should not be left open, as dressing changes lead to discomfort and increased resource utilization. Thus, one needs to have a logical approach to deciding how and when to close the skin. The core issue deals with determining the risk of developing a surgical site infection (SSI).

Classically, four types of wounds have been described.[31] These are clean, clean contaminated, contaminated, and dirty. A description of each and the accepted infection rates are given in Table 28.2. The National Nosocomial Infection Surveillance System (NNIS) has modified this system to include evaluation of the risk factors of long procedure time (>75th percentile), the presence of a contaminated or dirty wound, and an American Society of Anesthesia (ASA) score of 3or higher. The number of risk factors is associated with a percent risk of SSI (Table 28.3).[32] Although these numbers are important for determining overall risk factors for developing SSI, they do not necessary apply to emergent surgery. By definition an emergent surgery increases the ASA score and also an E

is added (for emergency), thus increasing the risk of worse outcomes for such patients. Additionally, patients requiring emergent surgery are more likely to have addition risk factors, including need for blood transfusions and poor glucose control, and are more likely critical care patients. These factors all increase the risk of SSI.

In general, our recommendation is to err on keeping the skin open and reduce the morbidity of a SSI. An SSI in a critically ill patient can be a devastating complication. Open skin wounds usually heal quickly and can be closed by delayed primary closure. All clean and clean contaminated wounds should be able to be closed. The skin wounds that are contaminated or dirty are routinely left open. There are a variety of techniques described to minimize the wound size and hopefully speed the healing process of secondary intention. Sections of the wound can be closed or reapproximated with staples and wicks left in for 2 to 3 days after which they can be removed. If the wound looks clean at that time, some advocate using steristrips to close the small defects, and others let these areas heal by secondary intention. If the wound looks like it is draining or infected, the staples can be removed. Others

TABLE 28.3. National Nosocomial Infection Surveillance System score and risk for surgical site infections (SSIs).

No. of risk factors	Risk of SSIs
0	1.5
1	2.9
2	6.8
3	13.0
Risk factors	Procedure time >75th percentile, contaminated or dirty wound, ASA >3

ASA, American Society of Anesthesia.

advocate leaving the entire wound open and beginning frequent dressing changes the following day. The decision of which technique is best to use is not addressed in the literature and largely depends on personal experience and preference.

The key principles to remember are that the wound that is at higher risk for SSI needs to have the skin left widely open to allow for drainage and that midline abdominal wounds mainly heal from side to side, not vertically. Cosmesis, although important, is not the critical issue for the emergent surgical patient. A wound that has to be reopened or dehisces will also result in worse cosmesis than a wound that heals well with secondary intention. There is minimal to no cosmetic difference in abdominal wounds that are closed with delayed primary closure and primary closure.

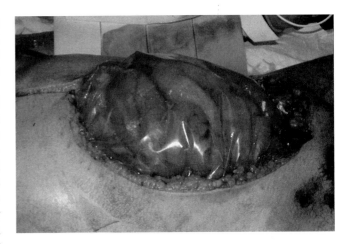

Figure 28.6. Use of radiograph cassette to temporarily cover the abdomen.

The Decision to Close Fascia and Subsequent Management of the Open Abdomen

The decision to close fascia in our opinion is very straightforward. The fascia should be left open in all patients with ACS. Patients who will need reexploration within the next 24 to 48 hours should also have their fascia left open. These patients may be coagulopathic and require packing or have had damage-control surgery and need to have their gastrointestinal continuity returned. The last major reason not to close patients is when there is concern of developing ACS. Numerous studies have been performed to identify patients at risk for developing ACS.[30,33–36] The risk factors that have been identified in trauma patients have been high injury severity scores, increased serum lactate levels, increased base deficits, and blood transfusions.[34] Raeburn et al.[36] demonstrated that increased peak airway pressures were predictive of developing ACS for patients who have had a damage-control operation. If the abdomen is tight it should not be closed, especially in patients who have required a large amount of fluid resuscitation and/or who need ongoing resuscitation. Similar to closing the skin, we recommend erring on the side of keeping the abdomen fascia open. Any fascial closure under tension is a recipe for disaster.

There are a variety of methods used to cover the intestines and manage the open abdominal wound. One technique of closure involves applying numerous towel clips to the skin to reapproximate the skin edges. It is very quick and requires about two towel clips for each 3 cm of incision. There are several situations when doing this may be advantageous. If the patient is extremely ill and needs to be taken off the operating table, quick application of numerous towel clips to the skin is an excellent choice. This may be appropriate for patients who are becoming extremely coagulopathic and cold. If all surgical bleeding

has been addressed, it is crucial to get such patients to the intensive care unit for continued resuscitation with products and warming. This technique allows for easy abdominal packing as well. Towel clipping is also useful for patients with pelvic bleeding or other indications for an arteriogram. The disadvantage of the technique is that abdominal fluid may leak from the abdomen and be challenging for nursing. Another potential disadvantage is that it may not open the abdomen enough to prevent ACS.

Another technique involves suturing a clear drape or covering to the skin. This drape may be a split open 3-L intravenous bag or a sterile cassette cover (for radiographs) (Figure 28.6). We recommend not suturing the material to the fascia to minimize ischemia and injury to the abdominal fascia. This method can be employed when the abdominal fascia needs to remain open and the patient needs a planned return to the operating room in the next 24 to 48 hours. The advantage of this technique is that it allows for inspection of the abdominal contents and it can be done relatively quickly. The disadvantage is that material needs to be sewn to the skin and fluid may leak around it. This leakage is problematic for fluid balance and can increase skin irritation.

Yet another technique involves creating a vacuum covering over the intestines. We simply use a nonadhesive plastic drape (10-10 3M drape) with fenestrations cut in them, two blue towels sandwiched with two large, flat closed-suction drains, and an adhesive bio dressing on top (Figure 28.7). The drains then need to be hooked up to low continuous suction.

Concerns with this technique include the application of suction and the risk of fistula caused by an improperly placed nonadhesive drape. Another disadvantage is that the dressing needs to be changed at least every 3 days in the operating room. The advantages of this technique are

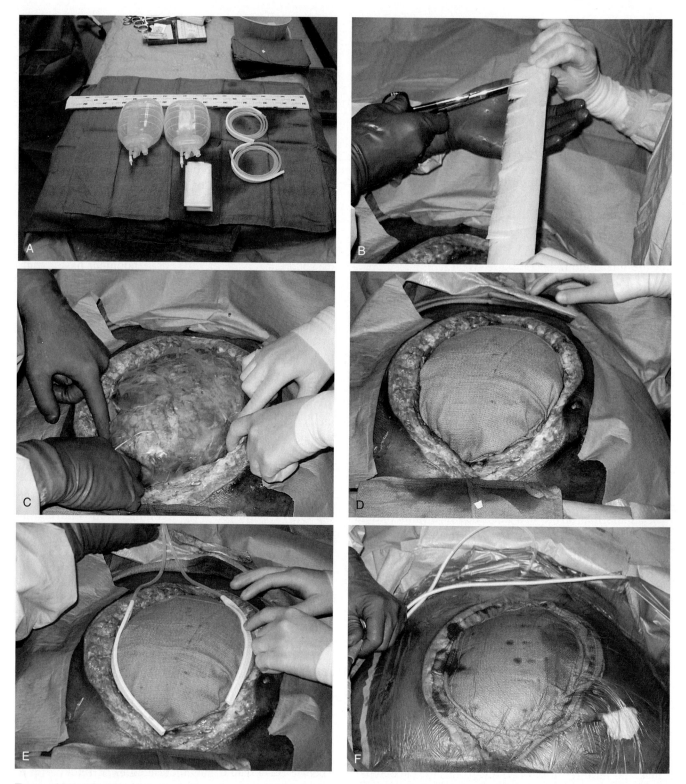

FIGURE 28.7. **(A)** Materials needed to create a vacuum dressing (VAD): two JP drains, a 10-10 drape (sterile nonadhesive plastic drape), two sterile blue towels, and adhesive bio-occlusive drape. **(B)** Fenestrations are cut into the 10-10 drape. **(C)** The fenestrated 10-10 drape is then place over the bowels and tucked under the abdomen. **(D)** This process is then repeated with a blue towel over the 10-10 drape. **(E)** Two large flat JP drains are placed. **(F)** A sterile blue towel is then place over the wound and an adhesive dressing is placed. The JP drains are then hooked to low continuous suction.

that it is quick and inexpensive, especially by avoiding commercially made products. Fluid management is generally good. The active suction and removal of fluid may allow for possible closure of the fascia. We advocate bringing the patient to the operating room every 3 days to change the dressing, wash out the abdomen, and assess for possible closure. If a feeding tube has not already been placed, it can be at any time pending surgeon preference. Care should be taken to place the feeding tube lateral from the midline to facilitate occlusive vacuum dressing (VAD) changes. At the time of the VAD change we opt to place Vicryl mesh to the fascia if the wound can still not be closed with minimal tension.

The last technique involves sewing Vicryl mesh to the fascia. This contains the abdominal organs while relieving the intraabdominal pressure. We recommend using woven Vicryl sewn 360° around the abdominal defect. The sutures should be placed directly to the fascia with healthy bites approximately 1 cm apart. The mesh acts to contain the abdominal contents while holding some of the integrity of the fascia. Over the following days attention should be paid to pulling the fascia back together, which can be done by suturing the center of the mesh together. After the edema has improved, some patients can be brought back to the operating room for formal fascial closure. In the event that the patient needs follow-up surgery or a second look, the mesh can be cut in the midline, especially if primary closure is still not an option at the time of surgery. After a period of time, usually 2 to 3 weeks, the patient can be returned to the operating room. We have previously demonstrated that the fistula rate is higher in patients who are grafted after 3 weeks.[37] At that time the patient should have a healthy bed of granulation under the fascia. The mesh should be removed and the abdomen irrigated gently off and then covered with a split-thickness skin graft. We typically harvest from the anterior thigh and mesh the skin 2:1 or 3:1 for large defects.

Both of the techniques of VAD and utilizing Vicryl mesh have utility and have some success of being able to close the fascia primarily. Unfortunately, a large number of patients will leave with a planned ventral hernia. This can be very large and will likely get larger with time.

The Planned Ventral Hernia

As mentioned, planned ventral hernias can be large and can be associated with a hostile abdomen. Additionally, these patients have recovered from a severe illness. The timing of definitive reconstruction needs to be based on these issues. The patient should have had time for convalescence to allow for an increase in endurance, muscle strength, and nutrition. This process for seriously ill patients often takes several months. Furthermore, time is needed for healing within the abdominal cavity and

for remodeling of scar tissue and adhesions. However, waiting too long is fraught with complications as well. These hernias will enlarge, and often the patient will gain further weight, thus leading to further separation of fascia and loss of abdominal domain. The grafted skin over the abdomen should be soft and separate from the underlying viscera. Our recommendation is to ideally perform the surgery between 6 and 12 months. These defects can be closed with placement of permanent synthetic mesh, placement of a newer biologic mesh, component separation, or a combination of these techniques. Our preference is to do a modified components separation; hernias have been demonstrated to recur in 5% of patients with this technique.[37] The technique is described in Figure 28.8.

In summary, patients with open abdomens have a high incidence of morbidity and mortality. Recognizing ACS and knowledge of the management options for these patients combined with diligent care can clearly save lives and return people to a normal functional status.

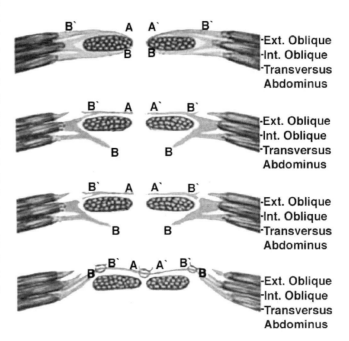

FIGURE 28.8. Modified components separation technique for abdominal wall reconstruction. The top panel shows the normal anatomy above the arcuate line. The posterior rectus sheath is mobilized from the rectus muscle, and the external oblique fascia is divided. The internal oblique component of the anterior rectus sheath is divided down to the arcuate line. The repair is completed by suturing the medial border of the posterior sheath (B) to the lateral border of the anterior sheath, (B′) with approximation of the medial portion of the anterior sheath (A to A′) in the midline. (Reprinted with permission from Jernigan et al.[37] Copyright © Lippincott Williams & Wilkins.)

Critique

The obturator hernia tends to occur in thin, frail elderly women. The preoperative diagnosis is usually an intestinal obstruction of unknown origin. The obturator foramen is the largest foramen in the body. It is formed by the ischial and pubic rami. The foramen is located in the anterolateral pelvic wall. With the exception of a small area, it is closed by the obturator membrane. The obturator canal, a 3-cm tunnel, begins in the pelvis at the defect in the obturator membrane. It passes obliquely downward and ends in the obturator region of the thigh. Usually, preperitoneal connective tissue and fat enters the pelvic orifice of the obturator canal—the prehernia stage. The final stage occurs when there is entrance of an organ, usually the ileum. Pain extending down the inner surface of the thigh to the knee is not uncommon. This pain is often relieved by flexion of the ipsilateral thigh (Howship-Romberg sign). For acute care intervention, a midline vertical abdominal incision is usually the approach made for definitive management.

Answer (E)

References

1. Baguley PE, de Gara CJ, Gagic N. Open cholecystectomy: muscle splitting versus muscle dividing incision: a randomized study. J R Coll Surg Edinb 1995; 40(4):230–232.

2. Graff LGT, Robinson D. Abdominal pain and emergency department evaluation. Emerg Med Clin North Am 2001; 19(1):123–136.

3. Cordell WH, et al. The high prevalence of pain in emergency medical care. Am J Emerg Med 2002; 20(3):16165–9.

4. Kulah B, et al. Emergency hernia repairs in elderly patients. Am J Surg 2001; 182(5):455–459.

5. Primatesta P, Goldacre MJ. Inguinal hernia repair: incidence of elective and emergency surgery, readmission and mortality. Int J Epidemiol 1996; 25(4):835–839.

6. Fruchaud H. Le Traitement Chirurgical des Hernies de L'Aine Chez L'Adulte. 1956.

7. Richards SK, Vipond MN, Earnshaw JJ. Review of the management of recurrent inguinal hernia. Hernia 2004; 8(2):144–148.

8. Arenal JJ, et al. Hernias of the abdominal wall in patients over the age of 70 years. Eur J Surg 2002; 168(8/9):460–463.

9. Alvarez C. Open mesh versus laparoscopic mesh hernia repair. N Engl J Med 2004; 351(14):1463–1465.

10. Alvarez Perez JA, et al. Emergency hernia repairs in elderly patients. Int Surg 2003; 88(4):231–237.

11. Neumayer L, et al. Open mesh versus laparoscopic mesh repair of inguinal hernia. N Engl J Med 2004; 350(18):1819–1827.

12. Kurt N, et al. Risk and outcome of bowel resection in patients with incarcerated groin hernias: retrospective study. World J Surg 2003; 27(6):741–743.

13. Arroyo A, et al. Randomized clinical trial comparing suture and mesh repair of umbilical hernia in adults. Br J Surg 2001; 88(10):1321–1323.

14. Buinewicz B, Rosen B. Acellular cadaveric dermis (Allo-Derm): a new alternative for abdominal hernia repair. Ann Plast Surg 2004; 52(2):188–194.

15. Hirsch EF. Repair of an abdominal wall defect after a salvage laparotomy for sepsis. J Am Coll Surg 2004; 198(2): 324–328.

16. Mingoli A, et al. Incidence of incisional hernia following emergency abdominal surgery. Ital J Gastroenterol Hepatol 1999; 31(6):449–453.

17. Leslie D. The parastomal hernia. Surg Clin North Am 1984; 64(2):407–415.

18. Sugarbaker PH. Prosthetic mesh repair of large hernias at the site of colonic stomas. Surg Gynecol Obstet 1980; 150(4):576–578.

19. Wotherspoon S, Chu K, Brown AF. Abdominal injury and the seat-belt sign. Emerg Med (Fremantle) 2001; 13(1):61–65.

20. Ramirez MM, Burkhead JM 3rd, Turrentine MA. Spontaneous rectus sheath hematoma during pregnancy mimicking abruptio placenta. Am J Perinatol 1997; 14(6):321–323.

21. Klingler PJ, et al. Rectus sheath hematoma clinically masquerading as sigmoid diverticulitis. Am J Gastroenterol 2000; 95(2):555–556.

22. Lohle PN, et al. Nonpalpable rectus sheath hematoma clinically masquerading as appendicitis: US and CT diagnosis. Abdom Imaging 1995; 20(2):152–154.

23. Bober SE, et al. Rectus sheath hematoma simulating appendiceal abscess. J Ultrasound Med 1992; 11(4):179–180.

24. Cervantes J, et al. Ultrasound diagnosis of rectus sheath hematoma. Am Surg 1983; 49(10):542–545.

25. Klingler PJ, et al. The use of ultrasound to differentiate rectus sheath hematoma from other acute abdominal disorders. Surg Endosc 1999; 13(11):1129–1134.

26. Berna JD, et al. Rectus sheath hematoma: diagnostic classification by CT. Abdom Imaging 1996; 21(1):62–64.

27. Ducatman BS, Ludwig J, Hurt RD. Fatal rectus sheath hematoma. JAMA 1983; 249(7):924–925.

28. Kron IL, Harman PK, Nolan SP. The measurement of intra-abdominal pressure as a criterion for abdominal re-exploration. Ann Surg 1984; 199(1):28–30.

29. Doty JM, et al, Effects of increased renal parenchymal pressure on renal function. J Trauma Inj Infect Crit Care 2000; 48(5):874–877.

30. Balogh Z, et al. Both primary and secondary abdominal compartment syndrome can be predicted early and are harbingers of multiple organ failure. J Trauma Inj Infect Crit Care 2003; 54(5):848–861.

31. Mangram AJ, et al. Guideline for prevention of surgical site infection, 1999. Hospital Infection Control Practices Advisory Committee. Infect Control Hosp Epidemiol 1999; 20(4):250–280.

32. Culver DH, et al. Surgical wound infection rates by wound class, operative procedure, and patient risk index. National

Nosocomial Infections Surveillance System. Am J Med 1991; 91(3B):152S–157S.

33. Balogh Z, et al. Supranormal trauma resuscitation causes more cases of abdominal compartment syndrome. Arch Surg 2003; 138(6):637–643.

34. Ivatury RR, et al. Intra-abdominal hypertension after life-threatening penetrating abdominal trauma: prophylaxis, incidence, and clinical relevance to gastric mucosal pH and abdominal compartment syndrome. J Trauma Inj Infect Crit Care 1998; 44(6):1016–1023.

35. McNelis J, Marini CP, Simms HH. Abdominal compartment syndrome: clinical manifestations and predictive factors. Curr Opin Crit Care 2003; 9(2):133–136.

36. Raeburn CD, et al. The abdominal compartment syndrome is a morbid complication of postinjury damage control surgery. Am J Surg 2001; 182(6):542–546.

37. Jernigan TW, et al. Staged management of giant abdominal wall defects: acute and long-term results. Ann Surg 2003; 238(3):349–357.

29
Foregut

Philip E. Donahue

Case Scenario

A 45-year-old international business man is taken emergently to the operating room because of an acute abdomen and demonstration of free air under the diaphragm on chest x-ray. Surgical exploration reveals a perforated proximal body gastric ulcer. This patient has had no history of peptic ulcer disease and has been, essentially, free of health-related problems. Which of the following should be the operative plan of choice?

(A) Truncal vagotomy and pyloroplasty
(B) Truncal vagotomy and antrectomy
(C) Highly selective vagotomy
(D) Omental buttress repair (Graham patch)
(E) Subtotal gastrectomy

Urgent and emergent foregut problems pose unique challenges for patients, physicians, and surgeons in every community on a daily basis. As portrayed on weekly television, the action-hero doctors and nurses become larger than life in their assumed roles, combining accurate diagnosis with an efficient remedy or operation, all packaged into 60 minutes of advertisements and intense activity. Television outcomes, of course, are usually very, very palatable and acceptable to all participants, in contrast to real-life situations where many things are unclear and many outcomes less than perfect. In the real world of surgical practice, everyone's complaints must be evaluated cautiously while initiating stabilization and treatment maneuvers.

The initial responders and emergency facility staff, most of whom are nonsurgeons, must make sophisticated judgments about the type of problem as well as the focus and sequence of investigations; surgeons, by virtue of training and experience, are expected to have an answer to the following questions: Does this problem, with or without a diagnosis, require surgical intervention? Which operation should be performed? What will happen after the operation? Emergency room personnel and surgeons evaluate and treat urgent and emergent conditions; their decisions are made in prospect, with incomplete datasets, attempting to achieve the best possible outcomes with patients presenting in whatever condition exists. This chapter is dedicated to these heroes of the sick and needy.

The physician, the ultimate historian, provides insights that make an individual patient's complaints understandable (whether in prospect or retrospect).[1] This chapter's goal is to assist focused investigation and interventions for diseases affecting the hollow organs just above or beneath the diaphragm, collectively referred to as the "foregut." As there is no consensus about the "best" and most cost-effective approach to testing for many of these conditions, the views expressed are quite subjective, reflecting the view of an experienced surgeon with a lifetime of direct experience with the worst of these conditions. Experience suggests that failure to intervene often leads to death, whereas an urgent intervention can sustain life and function. The surgeon, by virtue of his or her knowledge of the natural history of disease entities, is expected to recommend the most appropriate intervention in an individual circumstance. Furthermore, in dire circumstances, the general surgeon is the only one who can best estimate the overall risks and benefits of aggressive interventions.

If the material in this chapter is helpful to either patients or treating physicians, then a useful purpose will have been served in its preparation. This has been my hope in preparing this chapter.

Foregut Symptoms

The foregut structures have a limited capacity for demonstrating that they are not well and few ways of showing their loss of normal function. Stimuli from an individual visceral structure (e.g., stomach) travel to and are interpreted by the brain, a remote central processing unit (CPU) that interprets stimuli with reference to previous life events as it determines the relevance of the current condition. Because most of us have limited experience with serious emergencies, our CPU often cannot identify the source or magnitude of the problem.

The general symptoms of nausea, vomiting, pain, and discomfort in the abdomen are typical complaints caused by increased pressure within hollow organs; these symptoms are mediated through a combination of afferent vagus nerve pathways that traverse the brain stem nuclei and nerve impulses from the thoracolumbar autonomic nervous system. When bleeding, obstruction, or perforation is present, any observer can recognize the need for immediate attention. Other foregut symptoms are unpredictable and nonspecific, leading experienced examiners to avoid conclusions about the etiology or prognosis of specific events until all possible information is available. The overlapping patterns of signs and symptoms are completely consistent with the innervation of these organs, whose central connections are clustered within a few millimeters of the brain stem.[2,3]

Esophagus, Esophagogastric Junction, Stomach, Duodenum

The swallowing tube is the site of intense activity during a 24-hour cycle of activities, conducting saliva and swallowed materials through its 10-inch length. Although many of the problems that present for evaluation seem to be acute, the retrospective analysis often suggests otherwise because patients do not present themselves (as a rule) for the evaluation of possible problems or vague symptoms and because some symptoms, such as those associated with obstruction, may not become apparent until the process is quite advanced. Urgent signs or symptoms, therefore, often indicate an advanced state in the natural history of the disease process.[4,5] Overt signs and symptoms of esophageal disease may include pain, odynophagia (painful swallowing), dysphagia, and drooling and are readily linked to the swallowing tube. Similarly, prompt regurgitation of swallowed food or liquid has an obvious relation to an abnormality in the swallowing process. In contrast, more subtle symptoms such as solid food intolerance, altered sleeping position, or retrosternal discomfort may occur as a result of many possible disorders, several of which will be investigated before inflammation, ulceration, or obstruction of the esophagus comes to the fore in the differential diagnosis. Often, the physician as well as the patient is so relieved that cardiac disease appears unlikely that the investigation of other possible causes is postponed indefinitely. As

it happens, that may be a big mistake, which is often abundantly clear in retrospect.

Evaluation

The initial evaluation and sequence of testing are determined by the particular complaints and condition of the patient. For example, if dysphagia includes symptoms such as choking and immediate return of swallowed material, an oropharyngeal lesion may be responsible, as opposed to dysphagia with substernal or subxiphoid discomfort, which is more typical of distal esophageal problems such as gastroesophageal reflux.[4] In contrast to obstructive lesions, which often have characteristic features, the source of perforation or bleeding is usually not apparent before the initiation of treatment. When bleeding or perforation is suspected, the acute physiologic response can be dramatic, and supportive measures are initiated before the diagnostic process begins.[6,7]

Proximal esophageal lesions, including cricopharyngeal achalasia and ingested foreign bodies, cause difficulty swallowing immediately, with prompt choking and/or regurgitation. Distal esophageal conditions, including tumors, diverticula, and esophageal achalasia, cause dysphagia within minutes of swallowing, with or without regurgitation. Regurgitation, the aboral transit of swallowed esophageal content, is characterized by bland taste and substantial saliva admixture and occurs at unpredictable intervals after swallowing. If the normal esophagus is acutely occluded, a relatively small volume (50 to 100cc) will cause immediate regurgitation promptly after swallowing; a distended esophagus, in contrast, may contain several hundred cc of semisolid content, without a definite pattern of regurgitation after ingestion of food or liquid. Any patient with dilated esophagus is prone to regurgitate from time to time, because any abrupt change in intrathoracic pressure results in a similar change in intraluminal content.

Weight loss in conjunction with complaints of regurgitation reinforces the serious nature of the complaint, is not an early symptom as a rule, and does not of itself predict whether the underlying cause is malignant or benign. Chest pain, when present, is categorized according to its nature as sharp, dull, heavy, crushing, or burning; because of the possible causes, chest pain demands cautious evaluation. Some descriptions of chest pain are incredibly unique, depending on the individual's command of language and expression. Pains that radiate to the neck, jaw, or left arm may be angina pectoris; those that are aggravated by deep breath may be due to the pleural inflammation associated with pneumonia or to perioperative inflammation in postoperative patients.

Unfortunately for the patient, all of these may be caused by esophageal perforation as well; elimination of the first three possibilities, or wrongful interpretation of the source of pleural effusion, may have fatal consequences if an esophageal perforation is present.[8]

Burning pain with or without accompanying regurgitation is suggestive of gastroesophageal reflux (GER); when this symptom is relieved by antisecretory medications, an inferential diagnosis of GER is suggested. Pain that is sharp, radiating to the back, or with a marked crescendo–decrescendo pattern is not typical of GER, suggesting increased pressure within a hollow viscus. When chest pains or discomfort are caused by GER, the term "atypical" reflux is used to highlight this etiologic mechanism for a problem that is quite severe at times, mimicking acute coronary occlusion. Another variety of pain may be caused by trapped gas and liquid content in an incarcerated segment and is relieved by spontaneous (or induced) vomiting or by gastric intubation; if accompanied by symptoms of GER, the diagnosis of paraesophageal hernia or gastric volvulus is suggested.

Severe and unrelenting pain, especially back pain, is a serious concern that demands investigation. Just as constant headache demands a computed tomography (CT) scan of the head, continuous and severe back pain demands a CT scan to rule out aortic aneurysm, dissection, or perforation. Previous operations such as fundoplication may cause deep subxiphoid pain as well as shoulder pain presumably due to the stout sutures placed in the diaphragm for repair of the hiatus hernia. Although the foregoing statements are true, the observer relies on the combination of prior experience and instinct in evaluating the causality; the choice of observation, invasive testing, or intervention is a matter of judgment, and the consequences of missed perforation can be catastrophic.[9,10]

Because the foregut is composed of hollow organs with an inner mucosa and outer muscular layers, the diseases that occur are limited to a relatively small group of signs and symptoms related to erosion or inflammation of the lining mucosa, increased intraluminal pressure, or obstruction of aborad flow of intestinal contents. Tables 29.1 through 29.4 highlight the classes of disease that affect the foregut organs, arranged according to the presenting symptom. The illustrations of the surgical procedures were chosen to illustrate the breadth of surgical techniques employed to treat these foregut diseases. Although more complete and comprehensive illustrations can be found in specialty textbooks of surgery, there is a new alternative for viewing images of these surgical conditions: web-based search engines such as Google Image and Web-Medicine for immediate access to images for each condition. The world of medical education continues to show dramatic change.

Obstruction

Obstruction of the swallowing tube is a result of inflammatory, neoplastic, degenerative, and acquired conditions (Table 29.1). Whatever the cause, whether a foreign body, inflammatory stricture, mucosal outpouching, or neoplastic growth, the patient requires prompt attention because dehydration, pulmonary aspiration, or other consequences will undoubtedly follow. When a foreign body such as a piece of meat is responsible, the condition is both obvious and identifiable as acutely related to swallowed material; a synonym of this condition ("steakhouse syndrome") is both accurate and descriptive. If the patient is a child, there may be other dramatic overtones related to the terror and uncertainty that accompany difficulty swallowing, with intermittent choking and gasping for breath.

At times, the onset of obstruction creeps to "center stage" inapparently, because symptoms do not occur until 90% of the esophageal lumen is blocked. Whatever the cause, esophageal obstruction from intrinsic or extrinsic disease is a serious problem that requires prompt evaluation and treatment.

The source of the pain is always at the heart of the interaction with the patient, and this is quite true of the patient with an obstruction of the esophagus. At the

TABLE 29.1. Causes of foregut obstruction.

Intrinsic disease, congenital or acquired	Extrinsic disease
Achalasia	Bone diseases
Pylorospasm	Osteophyte
Antral web	Disk space abscess
Annular pancreas	
Benign and malignant tumors	Foreign body
Leiomyoma	Peach pits (esophagus)
Gastrointestinal stromal tumor	Dentures
Duplication cyst	Toys, coins
	Swallowed meat, hair, vegetables
	Bezoar, trichobezoar, phytobezoar
Types II and III hiatus hernia	Pericardial cyst
Gastric volvulus	
Diverticulum	Vascular lesions
Epiphrenic	Dissecting aneurysm
Intraluminal (duodenal)	Aortic aneurysm
	Mesenteric artery syndrome
Carcinoma	Pancreatic disease
Squamous cell (esophagus)	Pseudocyst
Adenocarcinoma (cardia, stomach, duodenum)	Abscess
	Annular pancreas
Peptic ulcer/stricture	
Gastroesophageal junction	
Gastric outlet	
Blunt trauma	
Intramural hematoma of duodenum	

beginning of the interaction, there is no guarantee that the complaint is due to an esophageal source, and the practitioner must always consider the heart and major vessels as possible sources of the problem; for this reason every patient requires a complete physical examination, with special attention to the cardiovascular and pulmonary systems. A rapid pulse, abnormal pulse amplitude in upper extremities, enlarged heart, or other abnormalities should be sought and may have a direct bearing on the final diagnosis. For most adults an electrocardiogram (ECG) and chest x-ray are the first studies performed, and these studies provide extremely useful information for the practitioner. If the ECG does not reveal an acute myocardial problem (ST-T segment changes typical of severe ischemia, acute myocardial infarction, or unusual findings such as peaked T waves, which require immediate attention), the source of the pain can be sought beginning with an oral contrast examination. The findings may include complete obstruction without passage of contrast and prompt regurgitation of swallowed material; this is typical of a high obstruction at the level of the cricopharyngeus muscle. Other findings include restricted passage of contrast with deformity of the esophageal wall or distortion of the normal contour of the esophagus by a mass such as a tumor, enlarged lymph node, or extrinsic mass. The x-ray findings will determine the next step in diagnosis, with specific approaches chosen on an ad hoc basis.[11,12]

Differential Diagnosis

Swallowed objects are the most commonly encountered obstructions, including pieces of meat, toys, dentures, and fruits. The patient complains of dysphagia, drooling, and inability to swallow and usually relates a gradual progression of symptoms. The progression from first symptoms to near-complete obstruction may be relatively short, whereas the natural history of the lesion, which includes the asymptomatic period, is much longer.

The severity of the complaint can be assessed directly by evaluating the response to questions about weight loss, presence and frequency of regurgitation, and other symptoms such as choking, coughing, and episodes of aspiration. The patient with drooling (difficulty tolerating saliva) or who cannot tolerate liquids has a high-grade obstruction and requires urgent evaluation. Although underlying intrinsic diseases such as stricture, carcinoma, anatomic abnormalities (whether congenital or acquired) may ultimately be responsible for the patient's condition, foodstuffs that become impacted in a narrowed swallowing tube are often the cause of an immediate and dramatic increase in the patient's degree of discomfort and distress. Needless to say, investigation of the difficulty must proceed without delay.[6,13–15] The spectrum of possible findings and sometimes bizarre situations that physi-

cians, radiologists, endoscopists, and surgeons encounter is limitless and truly amazing.

Physical Examination

When obstruction is suspected, the clinician will examine the head and neck for obvious abnormalities, especially edema, enlarged lymph nodes, or signs of distended neck veins. The status of the esophageal lumen can be evaluated only indirectly by physical examination (auscultation), and other diagnostic tests such as x-rays and endoscopic examinations are usually required to achieve a diagnosis. Auscultation of a normal swallowing "gurgle" in the subxiphoid location can occasionally avoid a hurried transfer to a diagnostic facility for a patient who claims to be in terrible straits, because a typical sound in the subxiphoid space 12 to 15 seconds after swallowing virtually excludes severe obstruction, favoring hysteria or emotional distress as the explanation for the symptoms. Most patients will require a more sensitive study, such as barium meal or endoscopic examination with biopsy, to reach a diagnosis, and either can be performed with a reasonable expectation of success in diagnosis. The choice of diagnostic procedure is purely a matter of judgment and resource availability.[16]

Endoscopic Examinations

Flexible endoscopic examination allows simultaneous diagnosis and treatment and is an ideal approach for acutely symptomatic patients who have just eaten a meal. Often the limiting factor in performing endoscopy is the ability of the patient to relax and cooperate; for most adults conscious sedation will suffice for the performance of the procedure, whereas for infants a general anesthetic may be necessary.

The endoscopic appearance of foreign bodies is usually readily apparent to a trained endoscopist, and there are several ways of dealing with specific items. A piece of meat or steak impacted at the gastroesophageal junction can be fragmented piecemeal or sometimes pushed into the gastric cavity; dentures, sharp objects, coins, and thermometers are removed with the assistance of overtubes, pouches, or other devices as the situation demands. Sharp objects pose particular problems when they have eroded into contiguous structures, and a sharp piece of metal impinging on a large vascular structure in the thorax can pose serious potential problems. Surgical procedures, however, are employed only for those patients with a specific remediable problem and are not indicated in all cases. That having been said, it is not at all rare for an experienced surgeon to decide that acute care surgical intervention is necessary if specific indicators are present; nonsurgeons sometimes misinterpret the definitive approach of experience and judgment for hyperaggressive treatment, which does not allow time for conservative measures. In this modern world of practice, all possible issues must be addressed, and all possible participants in decisions must be kept informed as to the why and how of decision making. Because serious medical and surgical problems usually have a definite risk of death and disability, none of us takes these matters lightly; however, we are surgeons, and we are the ones who know that even radical procedures can be done with a reasonable expectation of a good outcome.[17] Often, the best outcome is available only to the patient operated before developing complications related to hospital care.

The endoscopist often discovers unusual pathology that has been surprisingly silent before the current disease episode, including far advanced benign or malignant conditions such as advanced adenocarcinoma. A near-complete obstruction, interestingly, does not imply the presence of cancer; for example, if the stomach can be entered with only mild to moderate resistance, achalasia of the esophagus might be present and can be confirmed by postoperative esophageal manometry. If the stomach cannot be entered with the endoscope, the next step will be performance of a contrast study (esophagram) as well as a CT scan; occasionally, a distended stomach that cannot be entered via endoscopic routes must be decompressed by other means.[12]

As shown in Table 29.1, there are several possible findings, ranging from foreign body (dentures, foodstuffs, bezoars) to far-advanced malignancy, whether the lumen being visualized is in the esophagus, stomach, or duodenum. As a rule, a specific therapeutic maneuver is not performed at the initial endoscopic procedure unless there is additional information available to the endoscopist; for example, for a patient with previously diagnosed esophageal cancer, the endoscopist might insert a stent to facilitate swallowing. Alternatively, if the patient has had previous treatment for ulcer disease, and narrowing of the gastric outlet is observed, balloon dilation of the pyloric channel might be performed. Endoscopic techniques are very attractive and have profound utility for specific patients and compare favorably with traditional surgical approaches in some cases.

When endoscopy reveals a tapering stricture without mucosal deformity, inflammation, or obvious tumor, the stomach either can or cannot be intubated and the undersurface of the stricture examined. Is this typical achalasia, pseudoachalasia, stricture, or incarcerated paraesophageal hernia (type I or type II)? The endoscopist will perform biopsies of the mucosa in or near the strictured or narrowed segment. The esophagram may show a "bird's beak" deformity, suggestive of achalasia of the esophagus, whereas the CAT scan will demonstrate enlarged periesophageal lymph nodes if present, with or without massive deformity of the wall of the esophagus or stomach, or a mass lesion involving the retroperitoneal aorta and diaphragm. These typical findings of advanced carcinoma do not change the need for an intervention but must be considered in the construction of a treatment plan; at all times, keep the patient's family informed of the possible outcomes.

Radiographic Studies

Many patients present via the emergency room and often have x-rays performed as part of the initial examination. When an obstruction is present, there are a number of possible findings, depending on the site of the obstruction, including air–fluid levels in the chest, mediastinum, or abdomen, or other abnormalities such as absence of the usual air–fluid level beneath the diaphragm. Other possible x-ray findings are case specific, for example a retroanastomotic (Peterson) hernia causing gaseous distention of the afferent limb following Billroth II gastrectomy, can be evaluated on an ad hoc basis by the surgeon. Similarly, other CT scan findings can trigger additional diagnostic steps on the one hand or obviate further procrastination in others.[18]

Compared with the uncertainties and deliberations of the preoperative period, including the agonizing uncertainties attendant to decisions to proceed with surgery, the conduct of the surgical procedure is relatively uncomplicated. The incision is selected with respect to the target organ and the anticipated operation.

Diverticula

Hypopharyngeal Diverticulum (Zenker's Diverticulum)

The outpouching of mucosa occurs through a potential weak spot in the posterior wall of the hypopharynx as a result of poorly coordinated swallowing between the hypopharynx and the cricopharyngeus muscle. The true incidence of hypopharyngeal diverticula is unknown, but they can become quite large without causing symptoms. The corrective procedure is most often performed via an anterior neck incision parallel to the anterior border of the left sternocleidomastoid muscle; if the diverticulum presents on the right side, a right-sided incision is made along the sternocleidomastoid muscle. The surgical procedure must include myotomy of the cricopharyngeus muscle, because the clinical syndrome is caused by dysfunction (relaxation abnormality) of this muscle; the diverticulum itself is either ignored (when very small, ~1 to 2 cm in greatest dimension), inverted and suspended from the anterior cervical fascia (moderate sized, ~2 to 4 cm), or excised (large, >4 cm in greatest dimension).

Myotomy is performed in a similar fashion as myotomies elsewhere, as described (vide infra) regarding achalasia of the esophagus.

Epiphrenic Diverticulum

Epiphrenic diverticula occasionally present with complete obstruction of the esophagus, and operation is performed in an urgent fashion. More often, the presenting complaints are less dramatic, consisting of dysphagia, weight loss, or regurgitation. For at least 50 years, surgeons have recognized that diverticula can develop as a consequence of motility disorders (viz., achalasia and others) and that the myotomy distal to the neck of the diverticulum is at least as important as treatment of the diverticulum itself.

The approach to the diverticulum is dictated by the experience and judgment of the surgeon; 10 years ago most surgeons utilized a thoracotomy performed via the seventh or eighth left interspace. Presently, the success of transabdominal laparoscopic diverticulectomy and myotomy has become apparent, and this approach will eventually be practiced in most cases. In contrast to the hypopharyngeal diverticula, sac excision is necessary in all cases; surgical staplers are extremely useful in the mediastinum with either a transthoracic or transabdominal approach. Intraoperative endoscopy is occasionally very useful for determining the precise location of the neck of the diverticulum and to verify that sufficient dissection has been performed. The dissection of the diverticulum aims to allow division of the neck of the diverticulum without any narrowing of the esophageal lumen; stapling devices can be applied with a large bougie within the esophagus (50 F–tapered tip) to avoid constriction of the lumen. The same bougie can be used to distend the lumen of the esophagus during myotomy.

Intraluminal Duodenal Diverticulum (Recanalization Failure in the Duodenum)

Intraluminal duodenal diverticula can be observed in infants, children, or adults and occur in the juxtaampullary duodenum. Diagnosis is the major hurdle for this condition, and surgical removal of the diverticulum is the appropriate treatment. Whether an endoscopic, laparoscopic transabdominal approach, or traditional open surgical procedure is chosen, the end result will be satisfactory as long as duodenal narrowing is not created and the biliary and pancreatic ducts traversing ampulla of Vater are not injured. In such cases, a catheter placed into the gallbladder for pre- and postexcision cholangiograms can provide immediate confirmation regarding the presence or absence of unimpeded flow of contrast through the ampulla and into the duodenal lumen.

Achalasia of the Esophagus

The diagnosis of achalasia is usually but not always well established when the patient comes to the attention of the surgeon. Younger patients are sometimes not recognized for years because the esophagram may not be typical of achalasia or because the physician in charge does not think of performing a simple esophageal motility test. Occasionally a motility examination cannot be completed, and the surgeon must operate on the patient without a preoperative motility test; in such cases the typical history, x-ray, or combination of circumstances suffice to justify the performance of an operation. Of course, patient and family (as well as the medical chart) must have been informed and the reasons for performing an operation without a complete workup documented.

Most surgeons utilize the transabdominal approach for myotomy. The abdominal approach allows extension of the myotomy onto the anterior wall of the stomach for 1.5 to 2.0 cm; this approach results in a more effective myotomy, because some of the gastric muscle (gastric sling fibers) are affected similarly as the lower esophageal sphincter muscles in achalasia. In addition, most surgeons perform a limited antireflux operation after a complete esophageal myotomy to mitigate the symptomatic effects of gastroesophageal reflux should it occur postoperatively.[19,20]

The myotomy is performed with a hook cautery device, cold knife, or other means such as bipolar shears or harmonic scalpel. The aim is to divide the various muscle layers that prevent the passing of esophageal contents toward the stomach. After first gaining access to the submucosa, the surgeon patiently dissects the muscles away from the submucosa, attempting to avoid entering the lumen of the esophagus. If mucosal perforation does occur, it is important that it be recognized at the time, because repair can be conveniently performed without side effects; unrecognized perforation, on the other hand, can lead to mediastinitis or peritonitis with its attendant serious risks (Figures 29.1 through 29.3).[21]

Hiatus Hernia

Large hiatus hernias can obstruct the esophagus and/or stomach at times, especially when portions of the stomach have herniated through the esophageal hiatus to reside in the mediastinum. The type II and type III hiatus hernia can be complicated by incarceration and strangulation of the stomach, although the precise incidence of this complication is not known and a subject of debate. Often the initial problem noted is an abnormal air–fluid level on a chest x-ray, a finding that leads quickly to other diagnostic tests or to urgent surgery depending on the condition of the patient. If the patient is asymptomatic, then an endoscopic examination might provide definitive evidence of the presence of the hernia by demonstrating the orifice of the herniated portion of stomach adjacent to the esophagogastric junction. Usually the location of the diaphragm and the diaphragmatic hiatus can be established during endoscopy, and any rugal folds extending

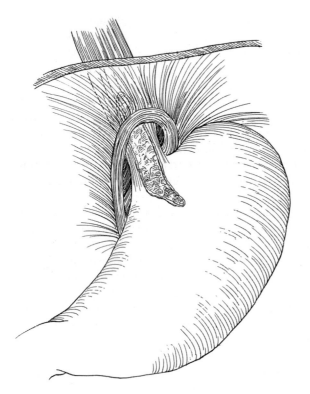

FIGURE 29.1. Modified Heller myotomy. The esophagocardiomyotomy extends for 6cm on the esophagus and 1–2cm on the cardia of the stomach, including the sling fibers of the proximal stomach. The proximal extent of the myotomy is several centimeters above the crural sling of the esophageal hiatus. (Reprinted from Donahue PE, Horgan S, Liu Katherine J-M, Madura JA, Floppy Dor fundoplication after esophagocardiomyotomy for achalasia. Surgery 2002; 132:712–723, with permission from Elsevier.)

above the diaphragm are evidence of a paraesophageal hernia. Although large hernias are very obvious, it is sometimes difficult to identify small hernias endoscopically.

Esophageal motility studies and prolonged esophageal pH monitoring are not routinely necessary because they are unreliable when the stomach is displaced into the thorax. The basic principles of operative technique are hernia sac excision, reduction of the incarcerated organs, and repair of the diaphragmatic defect.[22]

Minimally Invasive Surgery

The initial surgical approach for all hiatus hernias is by minimally invasive means when possible. Surgeons have debated the merits of transthoracic versus transabdominal surgical approaches for years, but most modern surgeons prefer the transabdominal route, which provides better exposure and allows a more precise reduction of the hernia and repair of the esophageal hiatus.

Transdiaphragmatic Approach to the Distal Esophagus

The division of the diaphragm from the hiatus toward the xiphoid process, popularized by Pinotti et al., has simplified the exploration of the lower mediastinum at open surgery. Entry into the mediastinum along the right or left crus is often a gateway to the mediastinal esophagus during reoperative surgery that can help avoid injury to the esophageal wall and allow direct visualization of the esophagus above the points of fixation from previous operations.

Laparoscopic surgeons have demonstrated the feasibility of the transabdominal approach and have reported success in well over 90% of the cases. There is still no consensus about the incidence of "short" esophagus and, by extension, the need for esophageal lengthening procedures. Also, there is debate about the necessity of a routine antireflux operation and the role of prosthetic mesh for reinforcement of the hiatus repair or bridging

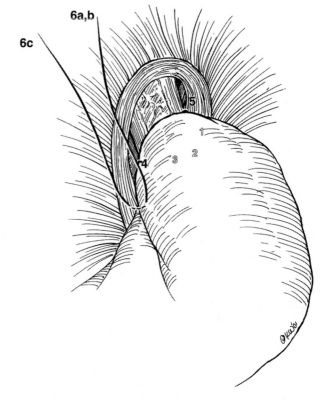

FIGURE 29.2. Fixation of Dor fundopexy. The gastric fundus is folded over the site of the myotomy and anchored to the right and left crus and to the edges of the myotomy at fixation points (numbers 1–6). (Reprinted from Donahue PE, Horgan S, Liu Katherine J-M, Madura JA, Floppy Dor fundoplication after esophagocardiomyotomy for achalasia. Surgery 2002; 132:712–723, with permission from Elsevier.)

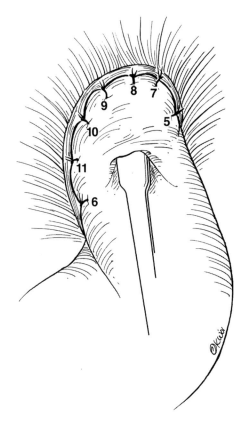

FIGURE 29.3. Completed Dor fundoplication. The fundus is sutured to the arch of the esophageal hiatus to prevent later herniation of the fundus into the thorax. (Reprinted from Donahue PE, Horgan S, Liu Katherine J-M, Madura JA, Floppy Dor fundoplication after esophagocardiomyotomy for achalasia. Surgery 2002; 132:712–723, with permission from Elsevier.)

of diaphragmatic defects. Since most hiatus hernias can be repaired without mesh, and, because there are occasional complications caused by mesh erosion or infection, experienced surgeons utilize mesh selectively.[23,24]

Transthoracic Versus Transabdominal Approach

Surgeons have usually debated the relative merits of transthoracic versus transabdominal surgical approaches from the biased approach of their trade guild, with thoracic surgeons favoring the former and general surgeons reporting success with the latter. Lately, the availability of the laparoscopic tools has made this discussion moot, because almost all surgeons employ the laparoscopic approach.

The transabdominal approach allows more precise reduction of the stomach and more accurate reconstruction of the esophageal hiatus; the transthoracic approach does allow complete esophageal mobilization and removal of the hernia sac but sacrifices the precise reconstruction of the hiatus. Gastroplasty, a technique for allowing fundoplication to reside beneath the diaphragm,

is employed if the esophagus is so short that it still resides intrathoracically despite wide mobilization and can be performed by either approach. There are several technical ways of creating the Collis gastroplasty, including ingenious combinations of stapling devices such as a transgastric end-to-end anastomosis followed by a GIA stapler placed parallel to the lesser curve, intersecting the anastomosis donut hole to create a "neoesophagus." These have been supplanted by the simpler wedge resection of the gastric fundus followed by placation of residual stomach, performed with intraluminal bougie via laparoscopy.[24]

Esophageal shortening is rarely encountered, partially because of the use of more effective antacid medications that avoid or reduce the incidence of transmural inflammation leading to stricture and shortening; in our clinic in Chicago the need for esophageal lengthening is unusual, perhaps because we have learned that the issue of shortening cannot be assessed until mediastinal dissection and sac reduction from mediastinum has been completed.

The Role of Fundoplication

The role of routine fundoplication after reduction of paraesophageal hernia remains controversial. Most patients with paraesophageal hiatal hernias do not have reflux symptoms preoperatively; furthermore, patients repaired with reduction of the hernia, sac excision, and reconstruction of the esophageal hiatus do not have gastroesophageal reflux postoperatively, as a rule. On the other hand, because patients with the esophagus trapped above the diaphragm will have abnormal pH studies, younger surgeons are apt to recommend fundoplication as a routine maneuver; in addition, partial or total fundoplication may reduce the chance of postoperative recurrence of hernia. Whether routine use of mesh reinforcement of the esophageal hiatus repair is indicated remains controversial; with or without reinforcement, some of the repairs will recur, and, depending on the method of categorizing severity or extent of recurrence, the incidence of recurrence may be quite high.

Peptic Stricture of the Esophagus

Esophageal strictures are most often caused by gastroesophageal reflux disease (GERD) and are often symptomatic only in reference to the reflux component. The patient often compensates for the presence of stricture by avoiding those foods that characteristically cause a swallowing problem. The incidence of dense stricture at the gastroesophageal junction has diminished dramatically in the 25 years following the introduction of the first effective histamine receptor antagonists (H$_2$RBs) and proton pump inhibiting agents (PPIs). Because the aggressive effects of acid and pepsin on the gut mucosa have been greatly ameliorated by effective treatments, the complication of stricture is seen only when a patient cannot take medicine for one of several reasons or when the patient has surfaced from an underserved medical area where drugs were unavailable.

Optimal treatment of peptic stenosis is debated by physicians and surgeons. Surgeons know that fundoplication performed before stricture formation has better results and that long-standing inflammation can lead to failure of esophageal propulsion (motor failure) and the need for esophageal resection.

Nissen Fundoplication

The completed wrap must be at least 1.0cm long, and at least two sutures (2–0 silk or nylon) are required. Sutures include the anterior and posterior shoulders of the fundic wrap, resulting in a 360° wrapping of the distal esophagus; an intraluminal bougie (50 to 60F) is placed to prevent a too-tight fundoplication as we described 28 years ago.[25] Fundoplication works to prevent reflux by the mass effect of the plicated fundus, as opposed to active squeezing or augmentation of the lower esophageal sphincter. To achieve a tension-free (floppy) fundoplication in Chicago, furthermore, it is often necessary to divide the short gastric vessels.

Closure of Esophageal Hiatus

Permanent sutures (2–0 silk or nylon) are used for hiatus closure. Figures-of-eight or Teflon-pledgeted sutures are often used, with or without mesh reinforcement according to the surgeon's preference.[23]

Obstructing Mass Lesions: Esophagus, Stomach, and Duodenum

In the presence of Foregut obstruction the timing and specific nature of the intervention are always a matter of judgment which depends upon a host of specific factors. The patient's condition and comorbidities, as well as the availability of specific diagnostic and therapeutic alternatives, are among the important considerations. Most of the benign conditions that afflict patients can be dealt with effectively at the first operation; when a malignant lesion has been identified, the usual goal of complete excision and reconstruction may be modified according to individual circumstances, including the site, size, and extent of the primary lesion. For bulky tumors at the gastroesophageal junction or the body of the stomach, the resection is sometimes postponed until neoadjuvant therapy can be performed, because dramatic changes in the extent of tumor are sometimes observed.[26] At present, the first operation performed might be incisional

biopsy of the mass followed by a feeding jejunostomy, providing an avenue for nutritional support until the most appropriate treatment can be chosen. There is still a role, however, for radical resection of large tumors of the proximal stomach that encroach on the gastroesophageal junction, arising from either the gastric wall or retroperitoneum.

The operation of total gastrectomy is usually performed, with reconstruction by means of a Roux-en-Y jejunal loop, with or without a pouch at the esophagojejunal anastomosis. The use of stapling devices (viz., CEEA stapler, United States Surgical Corporation) has simplified the performance of the esophageal anastomosis, which can be accomplished much more rapidly than the conventional hand-sewn anastomosis.

Obstructing Duodenal Ulcer (Peptic Stricture of Gastric Outlet)

For adult patients, the onset of episodic vomiting, especially after solid food intake, and other signs of gastric outlet obstruction can be insidious. There is a normal tendency to minimize symptoms at times, especially by those adults dealing with other responsibilities who have little time to think about their own situation in an objective fashion. When a person has a history of peptic ulcer disease, the possibility of pyloric channel ulcer or stenosis of a fibrotic pyloric ring must be considered, and appropriate tests to establish the diagnosis are performed. Radiographic studies are often the first test obtained and reveal a large stomach with or without large amounts of residual undigested food; if a CT scan has been obtained, the absence of enlarged lymph nodes suggests but does not guarantee a benign cause of obstruction. Endoscopic biopsy has a 95% sensitivity for discovery of adenocarcinoma and should be performed preoperatively whenever possible.

Gastric Resection Versus Pyloroplasty? Open Surgery Versus Laparoscopic Exploration?

The abdomen is explored by laparoscopic means or via a midline incision and the site of obstruction directly inspected. If the surgeon can identify carcinomatosis or other signs of unresectable cancer, then formal laparotomy can often be avoided in favor of a laparoscopic palliative procedure; when the laparoscopic examination does not reveal the source of obstruction, the next operative maneuver is conversion to laparotomy, because surgeons' hands and fingers can identify induration and inapparent palpable thickening in areas not directly accessible with the laparoscope.

If an obstructing duodenal ulcer is seen, the operation of choice is a matter of preference, with experienced surgeons preferring one of the following approaches:

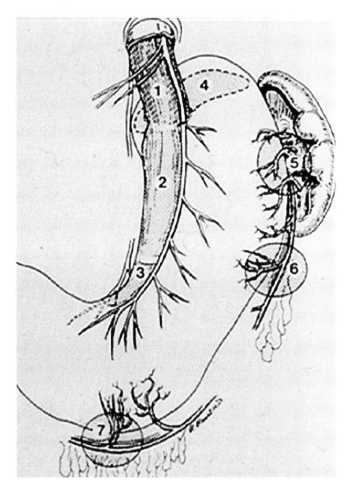

which were substantially changed in the same period, are now rarely necessary as a result of the discovery of effective antisecretory medications. In our own medical center the incidence of advanced ulcer has decreased dramatically, as it has elsewhere; previously, there were 200 to 300 ulcer operations per year, and at present there are less than 25; our fathers in surgery, students of the antrectomy and vagotomy, would be amazed at the current statistics after the introduction of antibiotic treatments for *Helicobacter* species.[29–31]

I believe, and most of my colleagues believe, that a vagotomy of some type still has a role for patients with severe ulcer disease; of course, the unstable patient is another matter. Occasionally, a partial gastrectomy without vagotomy will be performed, depending on the situation; a type IV gastric ulcer, rarely encountered in the modern world of digestive surgery, for example, is an ideal candidate for the Pauchet gastrectomy (Figures 29.5 and 29.6), which incorporates the ulcer in the tongue of

FIGURE 29.4. Areas of vagotomy. These seven sites or "areas" contain preganglionic vagus nerves that innervate the stomach. The original highly selective vagotomy included sites 1–3, whereas the extended highly selective vagotomy also included sites 4, 6, and 7. (Reprinted from Skandalakis LJ, Donahue PE, Skandalakis JE. The vagus nerve and its vagaries. Surg Clin North Am 1993; 73(4):769–784, with permission from Elsevier.)

subtotal gastrectomy, vagotomy (truncal or highly selective) with antrectomy or pyloroplasty (Heineke Mikulicz, Finney, or Jaboulay), or gastroenterostomy. (Highly selective vagotomy with pyloroplasty or gastroenterostomy is a highly effective operation for pyloric stenosis caused by ulcer, with a very low incidence of sequelae such as postvagotomy gastric atony or alkaline gastritis observed with other procedures.) The type of vagotomy is a matter of choice, but my favorite remains the highly selective vagotomy, with or without a drainage procedure depending on the presenting problem; with modern techniques, this procedure (when performed with the assistance of harmonic scalpel dissection) adds 15 minutes to the operation and achieves the goal of permanently reducing acid output (Figure 29.4; see also Figures 29.11 through 29.14).[27,28]

Techniques of gastrectomy have not changed much in the past 50 years. Vagotomy techniques (see Figure 29.4),

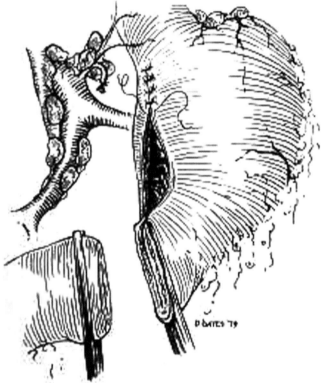

FIGURE 29.5. Rotation gastrectomy, 1. Gastric ulcers near the gastroesophageal junction cannot be included in a conventional gastrectomy but can be included with a free-hand technique that spares uninvolved portions of the stomach (anterior gastric wall in this case). The resulting lesser curve suture line "rotates" posteriorly as the clamps are removed, making the term "rotation gastrectomy" literally correct. (Reprinted with permission from Donahue PE, Nyhus LM. Surgical excision of gastric ulcers near the gastroesophageal junction. Surg Gynecol Obstet 1982; 155:85–88.)

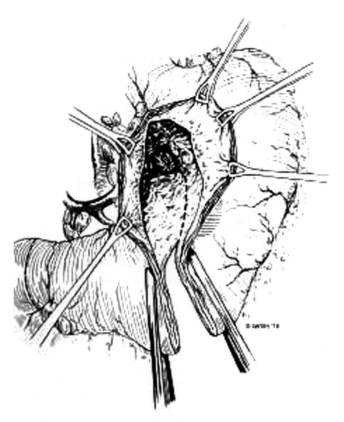

FIGURE 29.6. Rotation gastrectomy, 2. As the dissection proceeds, clamps on the cut edges of the stomach control bleeding, and a stout suture (2–0 Vicryl, general closure needle) allows approximation of tissues, which often have substantial inflammation and edema. (Reprinted with permission from Donahue PE, Nyhus LM. Surgical excision of gastric ulcers near the gastroesophageal junction. Surg Gynecol Obstet 1982; 155:85–88.)

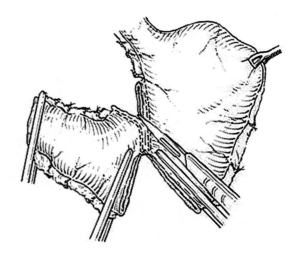

FIGURE 29.7. Schoemaker approach—complete antrectomy. The removal of 25% to 40% of the distal stomach includes a portion of the lesser curvature shown to include gastrin-producing tissue; this maneuver, once thought physiologically important, is really most useful in facilitating tubularization of the gastric remnant. (Reprinted with permission from Wastell C, Corliss D, Nyhus LM. Gastric ulcer. In Wastell C, Donahue PE, Nyhus LM, eds. Surgery of the Esophagus, Stomach, and Small Intestine, 5th ed. Boston: Little Brown & Co., 1995, pp 469–483.)

Pyloric Stenosis (Neonates)

Gastric outlet obstruction in neonates may be a result of pyloric stenosis, a disease of unknown etiology occurring mostly in males less than 6 months of age. The specific physical findings of a palpable lump in the right subcostal

lesser curvature. Although the indications for resections are limited, there are still patients who require traditional and extensive surgical resections. My only concern at present is that there is insufficient time and opportunity to train the next generation of surgeons regarding these matters.

When a possible cancer is present, resection is planned with a goal of a 5 cm margin from the tumor. Whether the reconstruction is performed ad modem Billroth I or Billroth II, antecolic versus retrocolic, isoperistaltic versus retroperistaltic, with inverting or everting suture lines, is of no import in a modern world; all of the techniques work as long as a leak is avoided (Figures 29.7 through 29.10). The "angle of sorrows" suture of the three-cornered junction of the anterior and posterior gastric wall and the duodenum/jejunum is still an important one, because it inverts the tissues prone to ischemic necrosis postoperatively. Although it may not be physiologically necessary to effect complete removal of gastric antral tissue along the lesser curve in this era of modern pharmacotherapy, a tubular gastric remnant is still required for subsequent anastomosis.[31–33]

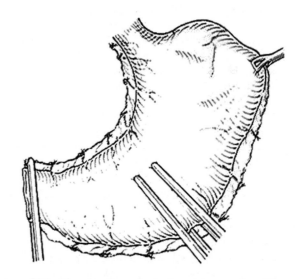

FIGURE 29.8. Planning the extent of gastric resection. The positions of the clamps can be placed according to the surgeon's plan of operation and can be shifted several centimeters in either direction without substantial effects on outcome. (Reprinted with permission from Wastell C, Corliss D, Nyhus LM. Gastric ulcer. In Wastell C, Donahue PE, Nyhus LM, eds. Surgery of the Esophagus, Stomach, and Small Intestine, 5th ed. Boston: Little Brown & Co., 1995, pp 469–483.)

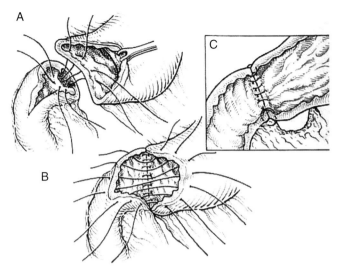

FIGURE 29.9. Penetrating ulcers—Suture technique. Gastroduodenostomy occasionally provides a challenge in the presence of scarified posterior duodenal wall, or disparity in size between the stomach and duodenum. (Reprinted with permission from Wastell C, Corliss D, Nyhus LM. Gastric ulcer. In Wastell C, Donahue PE, Nyhus LM, eds. Surgery of the Esophagus, Stomach, and Small Intestine, 5th ed. Boston: Little Brown & Co., 1995, 469–483.)

margin area may be subtle, but the sonographic demonstration of a typical thickened muscle segment at the distal stomach is sometimes diagnostic.

Surgical treatment of this disorder is aimed at dividing the thickened muscle that surrounds the gastric outlet; medical treatment with per-mouth or intravenous atropine sulfate given before meals is also effective. Pyloromyotomy (Ramstedt procedure) can be performed surgically or via laparoscopic incision and is dramatically effective in relieving the gastric outlet obstruction. Because the underlying mucosa is normal, there is no need to enter the lumen of the gastrointestinal tract when performing pyloromyotomy; inadvertent entry is repaired with suture closure, similar to mucosal perforations performed during esophageal myotomy.

Duodenal Obstruction

Nonpeptic stenosis of the duodenum occurs in adults as a result of neoplasm or other conditions ranging from superior mesenteric artery syndrome to pancreatic pseudocyst. The most common of these is pancreatic cancer, which leads to obstruction of the second or third part of the duodenum, leading to vomiting and inability to eat solid foodstuffs. In contrast, adenocarcinoma of the duodenum is often discovered in the investigation of a patient with anemia or occult gastrointestinal bleeding. In either circumstance, the disease is far advanced when

discovered, and wide resection of the duodenum is the usual remedy.

Intramural hematoma after blunt injury occurs in younger adults and children as a result of blunt injuries to the duodenal wall sustained during trauma, athletic events, or other activities. The disease is a curiosity that is amenable to a relatively minor surgical procedure, incision of the wall of the duodenum (near the ligament of Treitz) and evacuation of the submucosal hematoma.

Superior mesenteric artery syndrome is an acquired condition that occurs after rapid weight loss and is not unusual in patients who are immobilized after trauma or various orthopedic procedures that require long immobilization. Several recent cases reported after laparoscopic gastric bypass illuminate yet another possible cause of this condition.

Internal Hernia

One of the common occurrences after gastric bypass is the internal hernia of a loop of jejunum utilized to drain the gastric segment. The end result is an internal hernia that causes obstruction to flow, and, because it occurs in the morbidly obese, the ordinarily vague signs and symptoms of compromised intestinal viability are magnified. The CT scan provides a means of making the diagnosis but can usually be employed only for those weighing less than 350 pounds.

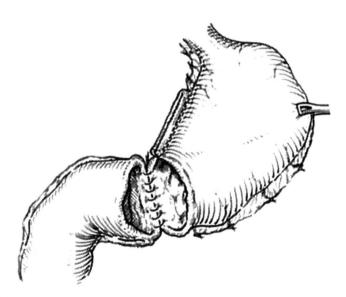

FIGURE 29.10. Gastroduodenostomy. The gastroduodenostomy is performed with two layers, with special attention at the three-corner junction at the lesser curve of the stomach and the duodenum. This "angle of sorrows" is at particular risk for leaks because of its vascularization. (Reprinted with permission from Wastell C, Corliss D, Nyhus LM. Gastric ulcer. In Wastell C, Donahue PE, Nyhus LM, eds. Surgery of the Esophagus, Stomach, and Small Intestine, 5th ed. Boston: Little Brown & Co., 1995, 469–483.)

Perforation

Perforation of the foregut has great potential for serious morbidity (Tables 29.2 and 29.3). Failure to diagnose and treat perforation can lead to death or profound morbidity, and all practitioners will be challenged with this problem during their career. The sequelae of perforation vary according to the site and to the acuity of symptoms that ensue; as in all matters pertaining to the human body, there is great variation among individuals and their reactions to a given stimulus, and no two perforations are alike. Free perforation, contained perforation, forme-fruste perforation, microscopic perforation: all of these terms describe details that affect the severity of the presentation. As surgeons we are called on to have a higher level of excellence than physicians in providing definitive treatment for this condition; as a result, the recommendations we make for care in a given situation must be heavily weighted with the issue of patient safety. Therefore, surgical procedures, often the safest approach, are frequently part of our recommendation. When nonoperative treatment has an approximate 50% chance of success, the chance for successful operative procedure may be substantially diminished by the "watchful waiting." One circumstance in which watchful waiting can be considered is in the individual with pneumoperitoneum or pneumomediastinum following upper gastrointestinal endoscopy, with or without biopsy, who has no evidence of peritoneal irritation, fever, or physical distress. Knowing that gaseous insufflation of air is sometimes followed by a dissection of air into the retroperitoneum, abdomen, or mediastinum without morbid sequelae, the clinician may adopt a waiting attitude for 12 to 24 hours only if a contrast study of esophagus, stomach, and duodenum does not show extravasation of contrast.

TABLE 29.2. Sources of foregut bleeding.

Intrinsic disease	Extrinsic disease
Mucosal inflammation	Portal hypertension
Reflux esophagitis	Splenic vein thrombosis
Gastritis	Cirrhosis of liver
Duodenitis	
Hiatus hernia strangulation	
	Disk space infection
Diverticulum	Dissecting aneurysm
Carcinoma	Aortoenteric fistula
Squamous cell	Graft infection
Adenocarcinoma	Mycotic aneurysm
Intramural tumor	Pancreatic disease
Leiomyoma	Pseudocyst
Gastrointestinal stromal tumor	Abscess/splenic aneurysm
	Splenic vein thrombosis

TABLE 29.3. Causes of perforation: esophagus, stomach, and duodenum.

Intrinsic disease	Extrinsic disease
Esophagitis	Iatrogenic perforation
Gastroesophageal reflux disease	Endoscopy (rigid/flexible)
Peptic ulcer	Dislocated gastrostomy tube
	Stent insertion
Hiatus hernia	Foreign bodies (dentures)
Incarcerated Morgagni hernia	Orthopedic hardware
Gastric volvulus	Missiles/gunshot wounds
Epiphrenic diverticulum	Dissecting aneurysm
Hypopharyngeal diverticulum	Pseudoaneurysm
Boerhaave syndrome	Graft infection
	Mycotic aneurysm

Diagnosis and Management

The diagnosis of perforation is made when a patient has one or more symptoms associated with pain, distress, or altered consciousness and is found to have physical signs or findings consistent with perforation of a hollow viscus. In practical terms, the spectrum of complaints is quite wide, ranging from minimal discomfort in the neck, chest, back, or abdomen to those of excruciating discomfort involving the entire peritoneal cavity.

Physical signs of perforation are nonspecific, consisting of primary or secondary signs of peritonitis or infection if these conditions are present. Primary signs of peritonitis such as involuntary muscle guarding and peritoneal irritation might be diffuse or localized depending on the site of the perforation and whether or not the perforation has been contained or "walled off" by contiguous organs resulting in a "forme-fruste" perforation. When inflammation of the neck or abdominal wall is seen, with or without subcutaneous crepitation caused by air or gases, the condition of advanced sepsis is usually present except if the cause is endoscopic insufflation. The interpretation of abnormal signs and symptoms, as usual, requires sophisticated judgment and interpretation.

Radiographic signs of perforation include the presence of extraluminal air, as seen in the upright chest x-ray or CT scan or extravasation of oral contrast material during a CT scan of the chest or abdomen or during an upper gastrointestinal contrast study. Extraluminal gas or contrast material is never normal, and every instance requires cautious interpretation; however, every instance does not mandate surgical intervention.

Esophagus

Almost every case of esophageal perforation can lead to a fatal outcome if not recognized and treated appropriately. The most common types of perforation are caused by diagnostic or therapeutic maneuvers, and endoscopic procedures account for the majority of these. Stenting of esophageal malignancy, submucosal resection of high-grade dysplasia or early esophageal cancer, and pneumatic dilation of esophageal achalasia are the most common endoscopic procedures, although sclerotherapy of bleeding esophageal varices, snare excision of esophageal tumors, and others have also been reported.

The proximal esophagus is at risk during endotracheal intubation, when the stylus or the endotracheal tube itself can enter the wall of the esophagus. The patient with unrecognized perforation might have swelling or subcutaneous emphysema in the neck (or supraclavicular fossa), fever, pain, or other evidence of cervicofacial inflammation. Once subcutaneous crepitations have been recognized, the onus is on the practitioner to respond in an appropriate way. Perforation in mid or distal esophagus occurs most commonly after dilation of a benign or malignant stricture or after pneumatic dilation (disruption) of the lower esophageal sphincter in achalasia of the esophagus. With the advent of self-expanding stents to maintain the esophageal lumen patency, the incidence of perforation is less than the 5% to 10% incidence reported with rigid stents that required extensive dilation before insertion. Pneumatic dilation in patients with achalasia has a 3% to 5% incidence of perforation, which can convert a simple outpatient procedure into a life-threatening medical and surgical emergency.

Spontaneous perforation of the esophagus, the Boerhaave syndrome, is the prototype of the unrecognized esophageal leak, which was described over 200 years ago. Despite awareness of the syndrome, individuals with "emetogenic vomiting" still pose serious diagnostic challenges for clinicians; up to 50% of patients forget or deny that they vomited, and affected individuals are often in desperate straits, thought to have aspiration pneumonia or cardiac disease because of substantial pleural effusions, obliterated costophrenic angles, and other nonspecific signs of disease. Remember: *No patient is too sick to have an esophagram.* (This single sentence can help every young reader of this chapter to save at least one of his or her patients' lives over the course of a medical career.) Patients with large pleural effusions may have an unrecognized esophageal perforation, and liberal use of oral contrast material can help the clinician to make a diagnosis of an occult esophageal perforation, which cannot be treated successfully without control of the esophageal leak by resection, repair, exclusion, or diversion.[10]

The surgical treatment of perforation depends on the clinical condition of the patient and all pertinent findings related to the illness. When pneumatic dilation of the esophagus is the cause, some physicians recommend conservative treatment; on balance, however, trained surgeons know that a precise Heller myotomy can be done simultaneously with closure of an iatrogenic perforation and will perform it in the acute setting when possible. The use of nonoperative treatment for pneumatic dilator–induced perforation is potentially dangerous, possibly leading to fatal sepsis; if the patient is encouraged to use this "wishful" treatment, then the hour of opportunity for definitive surgery might be lost.

Gastric and Duodenal Perforation

Gastric perforation occurs because of ulceration of the mucosal and muscular lining of the stomach and was frequently caused by peptic ulcer disease before the advent of modern antibiotic treatments versus *Helicobacter* species and proton pump inhibitors. At present, most perforations are related to injudicious ingestion of nonsteroidal antiinflammatory agents as a remedy for arthritis or other rheumatoid conditions. Other causes are foreign bodies, caustic agents, erosion by contiguous organs (such as edge of diaphragm), or ischemic necrosis resulting from incarceration or strangulation of the gastric wall. The forme-fruste perforation is one in which surrounding tissues "wall off" the site of the impending perforation, providing protection from diffuse peritonitis; in contrast, a perforation that liberates acid and pepsin into the peritoneal cavity quickly elicits the typical response of a perforated ulcer: peritonitis, involuntary guarding of the abdominal wall, and prostration.

Treatment of free perforation consists of lavage of the peritoneal cavity, removing all digestive ferments from contact with the abdominal contents. The hole in the stomach must be closed either by direct suture or by omental patch. Alternatively, gastric resection is performed for some large/chronic gastric ulcers, depending on the circumstances at the time of perforation. When cancer of the stomach or duodenum is suspected as a cause of the perforation, a frozen section diagnosis can be very useful in establishing the need for a resection versus simple patch closure of the perforation site.

If the perforation is within 1.0 cm of the pylorus (either proximal or distal), the causal factor(s) may include acid hypersecretion, analgesic-associated injury, or ischemia related to drug ingestion. The specific treatment of such lesions may include closure alone and/or closure with pyloroplasty if pyloric stenosis is present. Vagotomy of truncal or highly selective type is sometimes indicated, depending on the operating surgeon and the specific patient's conditions. My choice is the highly selective vagotomy with pyloric reconstruction (vide supra). Because proton pump inhibitors and antibiotics effective against *Helicobacter pylori* are widely available, the optimistic view of best possible treatment is sometimes stated as "closure of the perforation followed by long-term antibiotic treatment and antisecretory medications." This simplistic view, however, does not address the issues surrounding *Helicobacter* species–negative ulcerations of the stomach and duodenum or provide satisfactory long-term management for those whose ulcers recur during treatment. Because the numbers in both categories are up to 50% of the patients seen, there is a rationale for a "definitive" procedure at the first operation, especially if that operation can be performed with minimal morbidity. Many of the patients we see with acute perforations have had ulcer disease for years and present with a relatively short history of abdominal pain; because the bacterial species associated with gastric perforations are largely not as pathogenic as those associated with colonic perforations, a pyloric reconstruction with highly selective vagotomy can be easily performed with reasonable expectation of quick recovery and minimal morbidity. When patients are moribund or have extensive comorbidities, a simple omental patch is performed, with full realization that sometimes a pyloric stenosis will remain in the postoperative period.

If a foreign body perforation (e.g., chicken bone, sewing needle) is observed, simple closure of the perforation is employed.

Bleeding

Upper gastrointestinal hemorrhage (UGIH) occurs with regularity in all clinical settings; the death rate and the incidence of problems caused by ulcer increase with each decade in the population at large.[34] Endoscopic diagnosis and management (Table 29.4) are the keystone of effective care, because 90% of bleeding sites can be identified and more than 70% managed successfully. Surgery, often considered the intervention of last resort, can be

life saving when other alternatives have been unsuccessful; surgeons must recognize those situations when urgent surgery is necessary. Experienced surgeons are vital participants in the multidisciplinary team of caregivers for patients with gastrointestinal bleeding.

Sentinel Bleeding

When major blood vessels such as the aorta and named major branches erode into the intestine, they do so with a characteristic pattern in which the first bleeding episode is of a limited nature, allowing the medical team to organize its resources before performing corrective surgery. The common sources for sentinel bleeding are aneurysms of the aorta or major visceral structures; pseudoaneurysms related to infection of an aortic graft; or garden-variety mycotic aneurysms of the aorta or its branches. Extraintestinal bleeding sources, including vascular malformations, pseudoaneurysms of the splanchnic circulation including late sequelae of pancreatic necrosis and infections of vascular prostheses, or coagulopathic states are of great interest and are managed individually and are not further mentioned herein. Other lesions that cause massive bleeding infrequently, such as submucosal tumors, are generally not life threatening and are managed according to the same treatment strategy.

Mallory-Weiss Tears

Mallory-Weiss lesions contribute to nearly 10% of all upper gastrointestinal bleeding episodes and are still

TABLE 29.4. Control of Hemorrhage from Esophagus, Stomach, and Duodenum.

Bleeding Site	Endoscopic Rx	Surgical Treatment
Esophageal ulcer GERD	Coagulation, Injection	Fundoplication (reflux prevention) oversewing (rarely necessary)
Tear—Mallory Weiss	Coagulation, Injection	Shunt, TIPS, Liver Transplantation
Esophageal varices	Sclerosis, banding	Resection (best), Oversew (poor risk), Truncal Vagotomy optional
Gastric ulcer, Types I–IV require individual assessment	Coagulation	Oversew ulcer plus Highly Selective Vagotomy (occasional)
	Injection (vessels <1.5 mm diameter)	Resection (subtotal gastrectomy)
	Clip Application	Appropriate operation
Acute Gastric Ulcers	Coagulation Injection	Splenectomy (splenic vein thrombosis) or Shunt (portal hypertension)
Gastric Cancer	Coagulation, Injection	
Gastric Varices	Cyanoacrylate glue injection	
Anastomotic Bleeding	Coagulation Injection	Oversew (rarely necessary)
	Clip Application	
Duodenal Ulcer	Coagulation, Injection (vessels <1.5 mm diameter)	Individualized Treatment: Oversewing only *or* with Vagotomy (Truncal or Highly Selective) Resection (pyloric ring or antrum) Pyloroplasty Antrectomy (occasionally)
Aortoenteric fistula	not effective	Resection of infected graft/aneurysm by vascular graft or bypass, close enteric site without tension (no resection)
Hemosuccus pancreaticus	not effective	Embolization of bleeding vessel Ligation/resection of pancreatic vessels in addition to treatment of the primary pancreatic pathology
Duodenal Diverticula	Coagulation, Injection	Oversew Edge (occasionally necessary)

common causes of massive bleeding. Most will stop bleeding spontaneously. The shearing forces associated with abrupt changes in intragastric pressure cause the mobile portion of the gastric wall to be propelled toward the oropharynx The relatively fixed posterior wall of the cardia and gastroesophageal junction act as a fulcrum for this pressure, so that the gastric wall tears longitudinally. These tears disrupt small arterial branches of the gastric wall, which results in persistent bleeding. Vomiting either does not occur or is underreported in up to 50% of cases. The Mallory lesion is quite amenable to control with either injection or hemoclips applied via the endoscope, and surgical treatment is very unusual (vide infra).

Varices of Esophagus or Stomach

Hemorrhage from varices may be suspected by the past medical history if the patient has known cirrhosis, past history of hepatitis, or other problems. The diagnosis may also be suggested by stigmata of portal hypertension, jaundice, or results of previous endoscopic examinations. When bleeding varices are encountered, prompt endoscopic treatment is indicated; whether sclerosant of endoscopic banding is used is purely a matter of judgment. When varices are discovered incidentally, medical treatments to lower portal pressure is definitely indicated in the postendoscopic period. All patients treated for bleeding varices should be treated with broad-spectrum antibiotics and beta-blocking agents postoperatively; somatostatin is also widely prescribed during the acute variceal bleeding episode because it lowers splanchnic blood flow.

Ulcers of the Stomach and Duodenum

The absence of previous subjective symptoms of ulcer is curious but well established in patients of any age with ulcer for a number of reasons, including visceral insensitivity to early mucosal lesions. Other factors that may be involved in determining whether an ulcer causes symptoms are chronicity, location, and stage of healing. The high-risk ulcer (for ongoing or recurrent bleeding) has a visible vessel or pulsating hemorrhage in the ulcer base; tubular structures protruding above the surface of the ulcer are not vessels, but are casts of platelet debris and are deposited circumferentially around the orifice of a bleeding vessel. Without therapy, persistent bleeding or re-bleeding occurs in more than 50% of patients versus 20% or less if endoscopic treatment is applied.

Bleeding ulcers with a pulsatile bleeding vessel are the greatest risk factor for continued or recurrent bleeding. The success of endoscopic treatment is reflected by the disappearance of major bleeding as an indication for urgent surgery in most medical centers. Low-risk ulcers are those with a clean fibrin base; these lesions do not require hospitalization for successful treatment. Ulcers without a visible vessel or active bleeding site have a low rate of re-bleeding. At present, there is renewed interest in the prognostic value of outpatient (emergency room–based) endoscopy to screen patients with UGIB. Those with clean ulcers have been observed for a short period of time and discharged from the emergency room without substantial morbidity.

Do not forget or omit pulse oximeter application. A pulse oximeter is applied to the fingertip or earlobe of the patient early in the resuscitation effort. If desaturation is noted, administration of oxygen is indicated. Continued desaturation in a patient who is actively bleeding is an indication for endotracheal intubation. The ability to monitor hemoglobin oxygen saturation is a major clinical advance despite the occasional difficulties with false alarms and sensor application.

Regarding *response to intravenous fluid*, if the hypotensive patient has minimal or no elevation in blood pressure in response to the first 1,000 cc, a second liter of Ringer's lactate solution is administered over the next 10 to 15 minutes. If there is still no response in blood pressure, the presence of massive bleeding, cardiogenic shock, and congestive heart failure must be considered. Most patients will demonstrate an increase in blood pressure by the completion of the second liter of intravenous fluid. The endoscopic investigation is deferred until the response to resuscitation is determined.

A small percentage of patients will bleed so massively that transfer to the operating room while continuing the resuscitation is indicated. The typical lesion causing this degree of hemorrhage would be a ≥2 mm arterial vessel or an aortoenteric fistula. The urgency of the situation is reflected by an instability in the vital signs, with marked hypotension and tachycardia after several liters of fluid resuscitation. In this situation, the endoscopic examination is often best deferred until the patient is intubated and partially anesthetized. (This situation is analogous to the patient with penetrating trauma and massive bleeding. The operating room is an ideal [and the only appropriate place] to deal with a patient who is bleeding to death.)

Endoscopic Examination

The endoscope is inserted into the oropharynx while the examiner completes digital exploration of the mouth to ensure that there is no loose tooth or denture that may become dislodged during the procedure. The scope is cautiously advanced toward the upper sphincter, which is located between 15 and 20 cm beyond the incisors. The endoscope is allowed to pass through when the examiner is sure that there is no Zenker's diverticulum. Again, no topical anesthetics are recommended because they compound the risks of aspiration pneumonitis The gag reflex is manually "fatigued" by the sustained pressure of the index finger of the endoscopist on the base of the tongue. After the endoscope has passed the upper esophageal sphincter (cricopharyngeus muscle), the examiner makes the usual cautious inspection of the tube as the endoscope is advanced toward the stomach. Valuable information will be obtained during this examination. Positive findings include lesions within the esophagus that may be identified as sources of bleeding. These include esophageal inflammation, ulcers, tumors, or tears of the gastroesophageal junction that extend into the esophagus. Alternatively, the absence of important potential sources of bleeding may be established.

When the stomach of a bleeding patient is entered, there are two problems: orientation and avoidance of blood clot; if the incisura or gastroesophageal junction can be seen, the endoscope can be advanced toward the gastric outlet. Often the source of bleeding is seen through the pylorus; once the pylorus has been traversed, the bulb and second and third portions of the duodenum can be sequentially distended and examined.

Endoscopic Interpretation

Chronic peptic ulcer of the stomach or duodenum has a mucosal defect, a whitish fibrinous base, or a deformity in the gastric contour. Clot is a constant challenge because active bleeding and clot formation can frustrate any examination, but, if a visible vessel can be identified, an endoscopic modality (injection of dilute epinephrine solution, heater probe, or endoscopic clip) can be used to prevent further bleeding. The bleeding episodes seen in patients with chronic pancreatitis may cause confusion particularly if hemosuccus pancreaticus is the cause of intermittent episodes of hematemesis or hemorrhagic shock. The typical patient has had complicated pancreatitis in the recent past and would be seen to have blood squirting from the ampulla. One group of patients of particular interest are those with a history of vascular or endoscopic prosthesis. Late infection with fistula formation is a known complication after these procedures, and a negative endoscopic examination can be an indication for surgical intervention in some circumstances.

Operative Treatment

Esophagus

If bleeding is from esophageal varices, the modern approach is to control bleeding by pharmacologic and/or endoscopic means. The role for acute care portocaval shunt has disappeared given the widespread availability of transjugular intrahepatic portocaval. If a bleeding esophageal ulcer is found, with or without esophagitis, shunt fundoplication should be performed. with simultaneous intraoperative coagulation of the worst bleeding

points. Esophagotomy or resection is not usually required for control of bleeding unless a particularly difficult Mallory-Weiss tear at the gastroesophageal junction is encountered; endoscopic techniques are usually 80% to 95% effective, and surgery is reserved for patients whose bleeding cannot be controlled nonoperatively.[35-37] Remember to include conventional medical treatments after the endoscopic treatment, or preventable relapse might occur; also, remember that a surgically correctable bleed can never be addressed by hand-wringing and protestations of nonoperability. Variceal bleeding continues to pose challenges that are very complex, and the role of urgent surgical treatment is indeed limited; nonvariceal sources of hemorrhage require individualized management.[38-40]

Gastritis

There is a role for near-total gastrectomy with Roux-en-Y reconstruction for ligation of all blood vessels to the stomach and (apparently) for vagotomy and pyloroplasty, depending on the preference of the surgeon and the condition of the patient. Once 6 to 12 U of blood have been given, an operation can be justified, fully recognizing that mortality risk is high but also recognizing that nonintervention is fatal. Increasingly with older patients, there is no clear indication which approach is best, but for patients with intact brain and loving relatives, there is a role for aggressive surgical intervention; the availability of minimally invasive surgical procedures is definitely an advance in this regard.

Gastric Ulcers

Resection remains the best overall therapy for gastric ulcers. The amount of stomach removed is variable, but vagotomy is not required unless the ulcer is a "secondary" or Dragstedt ulcer. High ulcers present a challenge but can be approached if the principle of Schoemaker and Pauchet is followed, as herein described.

Type I Gastric Ulcer

The most effective treatment for a type I gastric ulcer is a 50% resection performed with or without truncal vagotomy; vagotomy is indicated if there is some evidence of previous duodenal ulcer or typical ulcer deformity of the pylorus. Billroth I gastrectomy has been performed since 1881 and has been a consistent favorite since then. Schoemaker proposed in 1911 that tubularization of the gastric remnant be performed to allow complete excision of the gastric antrum, which sometimes extends cephalad along the lesser curve of the stomach. Billroth II gastrectomy, anastomosis of the gastric remnant to the jejunum, is technically easy in most cases and preferred by many surgeons. The essential part of this procedure is the avoidance of too-long an afferent limb and the avoidance of either acute or chronic afferent loop problems. Kelling and Madlener proposed that gastric ulcers be treated by removal of the distal stomach, leaving an ulcer base in situ in the proximal stomach and thereby avoiding the hazards of performing proximal resections. The options for type IV gastric ulcers include total gastrectomy, wedge excision with vagotomy and drainage, or the Pauchet procedure (the rotation-gastrectomy; see Figures 29.5 and 29.6). Oversewing the bleeder/perforation combined with vagotomy and pyloroplasty is preferable for the patient at high risk of death and complications.

Types II and III Gastric Ulcer

If the patient has a type II ("combined") gastric ulcer or pyloric channel ulcer, a vagotomy and pyloroplasty is indicated because hyperacidity is prominent in these patients. The higher recurrence rate resulting from truncal vagotomy for gastric ulcer and potential for development of gastric atony and increased duodenogastric reflux make the highly selective vagotomy the preferred choice of some surgeons. The standard approach, however, for a chronic gastric ulcer remains gastric resection as presented elsewhere in this text.

Type IV Gastric Ulcer

The high gastric ulcer can be effectively removed by a conservative distal resection, which is somewhat similar to the rotation gastrectomy alluded to previously. When removing a high lesion, it may be necessary to have the tongue of lesser curvature extend into the distal gastroesophageal junction. In such a case, the use of a Roux-en-Y jejunal limb offers a convenient way for both preserving and reconstructing the gastric remnant. In all cases, total gastrectomy is the last choice of operation for a benign disease.

Marginal Ulcers Following Previous Operations

Marginal ulcers following previous operations are caused by incomplete vagotomy or by a combination of alkaline reflux gastritis and gastric inflammation. When bleeding is present, the ulcer must be excised; the choice of reconstruction is individual.

Duodenal and Pyloric Channel Ulcers

Pyloroplasty with vagotomy is the operation of choice. There is still a role for duodenotomy with oversewing of the bleeding followed by highly selective vagotomy (Figures 29.11 through 29.14). Resection is not necessary as a general rule and has neither intrinsic nor essential benefit because the overall morbidity of resection overshadows the benefit of low ulcer recurrence rate. Limit-

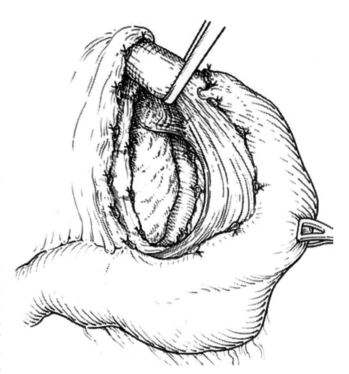

FIGURE 29.11. Gastropancreatic fold. The posterior gastric artery is shown after areas 1–3 have been divided and is easily approached via the lesser curvature. Harmonic scalpel dissection is very useful in this location with either laparoscopic or open surgical techniques. (Reprinted with permission from Donahue PE, Richter HM, Liu K, Anan K, Nyhus LM. Experimental basis and clinical application of extended highly selective vagotomy. Surg Gynecol Obstet 1993; 176:39–49.)

ing the operation to oversewing of the bleeding site followed by aggressive pharmacologic management of the ulcer seems painfully conservative from my perspective, given the ease of performing highly selective vagotomy with modern techniques.

In conclusion, surgical education and practice are at an historic crossroads defined by the intersection of "reasonable" and traditional standards as applied to the breadth and depth of surgical practice. The general surgeons of America are now in an "orphan" category, responsible for most of the acute problems that afflict individuals but not able to control the circumstances of practice in which they find themselves. Foregut emergencies, for example, arise from time to time in all treatment facilities. The general surgeon is expected by virtue of tradition, training, and experience to handle these problems expeditiously according to a reasonable degree of medical and surgical skill. At this time, however, it is not clear that the training programs are producing individuals who are capable of providing this degree of care.

Academic medical centers have a number of engines to which the respective departments are harnessed. Deans, department heads, and many respected educators

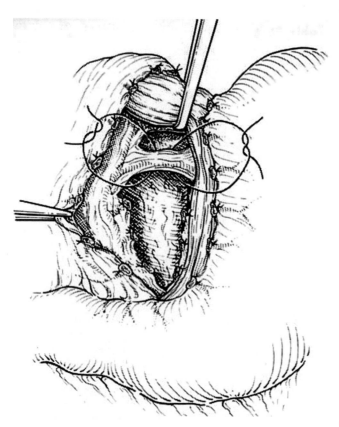

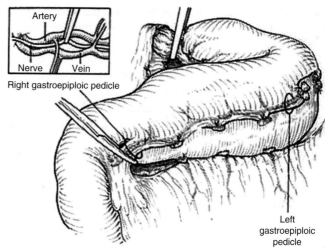

FIGURE 29.13. Gastroepiploic nerves. The right gastroepiploic nerve is by far the most important contributor to acid secretion of the greater curvature nerves. At open surgery, the nerve itself (or its multiple branches) can be separately identified; at laparoscopy, the entire right gastroepiploic pedicle is divided. (Reprinted with permission from Donahue PE, Richter HM, Liu K, Anan K, Nyhus LM. Experimental basis and clinical application of extended highly selective vagotomy. Surg Gynecol Obstet 1993; 176:39–49.)

FIGURE 29.12. Proximal lesser curve dissection. The lesser curve near the gastroesophageal junction is clearly identified with care to avoid perforation of the esophageal or gastric wall. (Reprinted with permission from Donahue PE, Richter HM, Liu K, Anan K, Nyhus LM. Experimental basis and clinical application of extended highly selective vagotomy. Surg Gynecol Obstet 1993; 176:39–49.)

have issues such as maintenance of class size, excellence, and graduate achievement. Surgeons in many if not all medical centers are cash cows, and substantial amounts of their time must be addressed to amassing funds for malpractice policies. What about surgical research? Why are the standards for surgical faculty different from those for medical faculty? The answer: "The matter is unclear at this time." Surgeons have not had ample opportunity to devise practice systems that are reasonable and balanced; however, they want to keep their "lights on" and their office staff employed. Does this imply that patients will be asked to have procedures that are not necessary, not indicated, or unproven?

Graduates of programs are immediately positioned in a queue of maintenance of excellence and certification, which, although unclear and ill-defined, cannot be ignored. In this environment, patients have come to expect perfect outcomes, and plaintiffs' lawyers cruise offshore, awaiting any invitation to look for compensable injury.[41] Life is not as perfect for surgeons as it once was

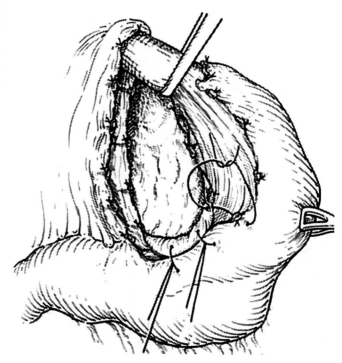

FIGURE 29.14. Serorraphy. Suture approximation of the anterior and posterior gastric wall has a protective effect and prevents the reinnervation effect. In addition, it "looks" right. (Reprinted with permission from Donahue PE, Richter HM, Liu K, Anan K, Nyhus LM. Experimental basis and clinical application of extended highly selective vagotomy. Surg Gynecol Obstet 1993; 176:39–49.)

or as it appears to have been in retrospect. We will continue to practice, however, as long and as "smartly" as we can. The general surgeons of the land will continue to provide the best possible care and must continue to seek better outcomes and more effective treatment strategies.[42,43]

Many of the procedures illustrated and discussed in this chapter are not performed ordinarily by surgeons without special exposure to and experience with advanced surgical techniques; how will surgeons with this type of experience be trained in the future? Are the leaders of American surgery satisfied that they are producing the best types of practitioners for the future? Although the answer is unclear, the problems discussed in this chapter are real and will continue to occur, and I sincerely hope that my words will help some patients and providers to deal with these difficult problems.[44,45]

Critique

A perforated stomach ulcer is a gastric cancer until proven otherwise. However, this patient's ulcer was later determined to be benign. Nevertheless, the operative management in this case should be appropriately aggressive, and the patient needs to undergo a subtotal gastrectomy with the remaining portion being a remnant of the proximal stomach. Irrespective of the *Helicobacter pylori* status, which would likely not be known in this case, such an operative plan would be definitive management for this type of ulcer (benign or malignant). Subsequent tests will determine whether this patient is *H. pylori* positive and requires medical management.

Answer (E)

References

1. Laine L. Evidence-based medicine: clinical judgment is required. Gastroenterology 2003; 124(7):1726.
2. Sugitani A, Donahue PE, Doyle MD, Anan K, Nyhus LM. The ipsilateral organization of the afferent nerves to the stomach. J Surg Res 1993; 54:212–221.
3. Skandalakis LJ, Donahue PE, Skandalakis JE. The vagus nerve and its vagaries. Surg Clin North Am 1993; 73(4):769–784.
4. Donahue PE, Schlesinger PK, Richter HM, Liu KJ-M, Attar B, Madura JA. Surgical physiology of esophagogastric junction—efficacy of selective testing. Hernia 2000; 4:212–218.
5. Portale G, Peters JH, Hsieh CC, et al. Esophageal adenocarcinoma in patients < or =50 years old: delayed diagnosis and advanced disease at presentation. Am Surg 2004; 70(11):954–958.
6. Eroglu A, Kurkcuogu IC, Karaoganogu N, Tekinbas C, Yimaz O, Basog M. Esophageal perforation: the importance of early diagnosis and primary repair. Dis Esophagus 2004; 17(1):91–94.
7. Shimizu Y, Kato M, Yamamoto J, Nakagawa S, Komatsu Y, Tsukagoshi H, Fujita M, Hosokawa M, Asaka M. Endoscopic clip application for closure of esophageal perforations caused by EMR. Gastrointest Endosc 2004; 60(4):636–639.
8. Ghanem N, Altehoefer C, Springer O, Furtwangler A, Kotter E, Schafer O, Langer M. Radiological findings in Boerhaave's syndrome. Emerg Radiol 2003; 10(1):8–13.
9. Ertekin C, Alimoglu O, Akyildiz H, Guloglu R, Taviloglu K. The results of caustic ingestions. Hepatogastroenterology 2004; 51(59):1397–1400.
10. Orlando R, Lirussi F. Bile leakage and resultant bile peritonitis during or after diagnostic laparoscopy: an unpredictable event. Endoscopy 2004; 36(12):1115–1118.
11. Mularski RA, Sippel JM, Osborne ML. Pneumoperitoneum: a review of nonsurgical causes. Crit Care Med 2000; 28(7):2638–2644.
12. Nosher JL, Bodner LJ, Girgis WS, Brolin R, Siegel RL, Gribbin C. Percutaneous gastrostomy for treating dilatation of the bypassed stomach after bariatric surgery for morbid obesity. AJR Am J Roentgenol 2004; 183(5):1431–1435.
13. Lam EC, Brown JA, Whittaker JS. Esophageal foreign body causing direct aortic injury. Can J Gastroenterol 2003; 17(2):115–117.
14. Tomaselli F, Maier A, Sankin O, Pinter H, Smolle J, Smolle-Juttner FM. Ultraflex stent—benefits and risks in ultimate palliation of advanced, malignant stenosis in the esophagus. Hepatogastroenterology 2004; 51(58):1021–1026.
15. Von Rahden BH, Becker I, Stein HJ. Esophageal perforation by portions of a wild boar. Zentralbl Chir 2004; 129(4):314–316.
16. Del Genio A, Rossetti G, Napolitano V, Maffettone V, Renzi A, Brusciano L, Russo G, Del Genio G. Laparoscopic esophagectomy in the palliative treatment of advanced esophageal cancer after radiochemotherapy. Surg Endosc 2004; 18:1789–1794.
17. Williams C, McHenry CR: Unrecognized foreign body ingestion: an unusual cause for abdominal pain in a healthy adult. Am Surg 2004; 70(11):982–984.
18. Abadir JS, Cohen AJ, Wilson SE. Accurate diagnosis of infarction of omentum and appendices epiploicae by computed tomography. Am Surg 2004; 70(10):854–857.
19. Donahue PE, Teresi M, Patel S, Schlesinger PK: Laparoscopic myotomy in achalasia: intraoperative evidence for myotomy of the gastric cardia. Dis Esophagus 1999; 12(1):30–36.
20. Richards WO, Torquati A, Holzman MD, Khaitan L, Byrne D, Lutfi R, Sharp KW. Heller myotomy versus Heller myotomy with Dor fundoplication for achalasia: a prospective randomized double-blind clinical trial. Ann Surg 2004 Sep; 240(3):405–415.
21. Donahue PE, Horgan S, Liu KJ, Madura JA. Floppy Dor fundoplication after esophagocardiomyotomy for achalasia. Surgery 2002 Oct; 132(4):716–723.
22. Lee R, Donahue PE. Paraesophageal hernia. In Cameron JL, ed. Current Surgical Therapy, 6th ed. St. Louis, Mosby Year Book, 2001, pp 41–46.

23. Targarona EM, Bendahan G, Balague C, Garriga J, Trias M. Mesh in the hiatus. A controversial issue. Arch Surg 2004; 139:1286–1296.

24. Terry ML, Vernon A, Hunter JG. Stapled-wedge Collis gastroplasty for the shortened esophagus. Am J Surg 2004; 188(2):195–199.

25. Donahue PE, Bombeck CT, Samelson S, Nyhus LM. The floppy Nissen fundoplication: effective long-term control of pathologic reflux. Arch Surg 1985; 120:663–668.

26. So JB, Yam A, Cheah WK, Kum CK, Goh PM. Risk factors related to operative mortality and morbidity in patients undergoing emergency gastrectomy. Br J Surg 2000; 87(12): 1702–1707.

27. Donahue PE. Parietal cell vagotomy versus vagotomy-antrectomy: ulcer surgery in the modern era. World J Surg 2000; 24(3):264–269.

28. Donahue PE, Yoshida J, Richter HM, Liu K, Bombeck CT, Nyhus LM. Proximal gastric vagotomy with drainage for obstructing duodenal ulcer. Surgery 1988; 104(4):757–764.

29. Kozoll DD, Meyer KA. Effects of treatment on morbidity and mortality in massively bleeding gastroduodenal ulcers. Arch Surg 1964; 89:250–265.

30. Kozoll DD, Meyer K. Effects of surgery on morbidity and mortality in acute gastroduodenal perforations. Am J Surg 1962; 103:577–594.

31. Donahue PE. Massive gastrointestinal bleeding. In Wastell C, Nyhus LM, Donahue PE, eds. Surgery of the Esophagus, Stomach and Small Intestine, 5th ed. Boston: Little Brown and Company, 1995, pp 642–654.

32. Blackshaw GR, Stephens MR, Lewis WG, Paris HJ, Barry JD, Edwards P, Allison MC. Prognostic significance of acute presentation with emergency complications of gastric cancer. Gastric Cancer 2004; 7(2):91–96.

33. Kasakura Y, Ajani JA, Mochizuki F, Morishita Y, Fujii M, Takayama TJ. Outcomes after emergency surgery for gastric perforation or severe bleeding in patients with gastric cancer. Surg Oncol 2002; 80(4):181–185.

34. Everhart JH, ed. Peptic Ulcer Disease. Digestive Diseases in the United States: Epidemiology and Impact. National Digestive Diseases Data Working Group. U.S. Dept. HHS, NIH Publication No. 91–1447, May 1994, pp 357–407.

35. Kubba AK. Endoscopic injection for bleeding peptic ulcer: a comparison of adrenaline alone with adrenaline plus human thrombin. Gastroenterology 1996; 111:623–628.

36. Hsu PI, Lo GH, Lo CC, Lin CK, Chan HH, Wu CJ, Shie CB, Tsai PM, Wu DC, Wang WM, Lai KH. Intravenous pantoprazole versus ranitidine for prevention of rebleeding after endoscopic hemostasis of bleeding peptic ulcers. World J Gastroenterol 2004; 10(24):3666–3669.

37. Gurleyik E. Changing trend in emergency surgery for perforated duodenal ulcer. J Coll Physicians Surg Pak 2003; 13(12):708–710.

38. Barkun A, Fallone CA, Chiba N, Fishman M, Flook N, Martin J, Rostom A, Taylor A. Nonvariceal Upper GI Bleeding Consensus Conference Group. A Canadian clinical practice algorithm for the management of patients with nonvariceal upper gastrointestinal bleeding. Can J Gastroenterol 2004; 18(0):605–609.

39. Carbonell N, Pauwels A, Serfaty L, Fourdan O, Levy VG, Poupon R. Improved survival after variceal bleeding in patients with cirrhosis over the past two decades. Hepatology 2004; 40(3):652.

40. Rubenstein JH, Eisen GM, Inadomi JM. A cost-utility analysis of secondary prophylaxis for variceal hemorrhage. Am J Gastroenterol 2004;99(7): 1274–1288.

41. Vukmir RB. Medical malpractice: managing the risk. Med Law 2004; 23(3):495–513.

42. Bellomo R, Goldsmith D, Uchino S, Buckmaster J, Hart G, Opdam H, Silvester W, Doolan L, Gutteridge G. Prospective controlled trial of effect of medical emergency team on postoperative morbidity and mortality rates. Crit Care Med 2004; 32(4):1071–1072.

43. Calland JF, Adams RB, Benjamin DK Jr, O'Connor MJ, Chandrasekhara V, Guerlain S, Jones RS. Thirty-day postoperative death rate at an academic medical center. Ann Surg 2002; 235(5):690–698.

44. Morris JA Jr, Carrillo Y, Jenkins JM, Smith PW, Bledsoe S, Pichert J, White A. Surgical adverse events, risk management, and malpractice outcome: morbidity and mortality review is not enough. Ann Surg 2003; 237(6):844–852.

45. Dawson EJ, Paterson-Brown S. Emergency general surgery and the implications for specialization. Surgeon 2004; 2(3): 165–170.

30
Small Intestine

Juliet Lee, Todd Ponsky, and Jeffrey L. Ponsky

Case Scenario

A 60-year-old jazz singer, with no history of surgery, is being seen for intestinal obstruction. Computed tomographic scan demonstrates an intussusception of the terminal ileum. In addition to optimal resuscitation, which of the following, at this time, should be the "management?

(A) Expectant management
(B) Hydrostatic reduction by enema
(C) Enteroclysis
(D) Laparoscopy and surgical reduction
(E) Segmental resection

The small bowel is a complex organ involved in the digestion and absorption of nutrients, secretion and immunologic and neuroendocrine functions. The basis of many of its activities is the intestinal epithelium. Crypt cells function in secretion of mucus and neuroendocrine substances and differentiate into primarily absorptive enterocytes. The main secretion by the crypt cells is an isotonic fluid that provides lubrication. The epithelium also provides a barrier against ingested foreign substances, noxious stimuli, and luminal bacteria. Disruption of this barrier by luminal toxins, bacterial or ingested, can lead to bacterial translocation. In addition to the barrier function, plasma cells within the lamina propria of the small bowel secrete immunoglobulin A (IgA). Brush border hydrolases function in the digestion of proteins and carbohydrates into monosaccharides, disaccharides, and amino acids that can be readily used by enterocytes. Pancreatic lipase secreted into the duodenum is responsible for digesting triglycerides. The triglyceride breakdown products are then solubilized by bile and enter micelles for eventual absorption.

Because the small bowel is intricately involved in multiple processes, loss of small bowel can be deleterious to patient survival. Any process that damages or compromises the viability of the epithelium and mucosal barrier may put the patient at risk for significant morbidity or mortality. Ischemia can directly injure this barrier, leading to bacterial translocation. This may result from complete bowel obstruction or vascular occlusion to the small bowel. Perforation can cause spillage of enteric contents and incite the elaboration of multiple inflammatory mediators and cascades. Acute or chronic injury to the epithelium may lead to hemorrhage with subsequent life-threatening hemodynamic instability. This chapter provides an overview of surgical emergencies of the small bowel, including presentation, diagnostic workup, and treatment.

Obstruction

Small bowel obstruction (SBO) continues to be one of the most common, long-term postoperative complications and is most often a result of adhesions. Obstruction may also result from an internal hernia, inguinal hernia, femoral hernia, or ventral hernia. The third most common cause of SBO in adults is tumor. Although primary small bowel tumors are rare causes of bowel obstruction, intraperitoneal metastasis from other organs may lead to an obstruction. Obstruction may also result from acute inflammation from inflammatory bowel disease or from strictures caused by chronic inflammation.

Diagnosis

The presence of SBO is usually suspected by history and physical examination, but abdominal radiographs may help to confirm the diagnosis. Particular attention should be paid to time since the patient last had flatus or a bowel movement, the presence of nausea or vomiting, surgical history, point tenderness on abdominal examination, evidence of peritonitis, and presence of an abdominal wall hernia or mass or a mass on rectal examination. Three plain films, abdominal flat and upright and chest x-ray, should be obtained early. Air–fluid levels on the upright abdominal plain film, dilated loops of small bowel, and absence of colonic air suggest an SBO. Absence of all of these makes the diagnosis of SBO unlikely, and patients with some distal air or the presence of flatus may have a partial SBO. A dilated colon is suggestive of a colonic obstruction, and a barium enema should be ordered. If the plain radiographs are inconclusive, a computed tomography (CT) scan with oral and intravenous contrast should be obtained. Several studies have suggested that routine CT scans of patients with SBO may improve outcomes by predicting early which patients will require surgical intervention. Findings on CT such as a "transition zone" of dilated to decompressed bowel, a closed loop obstruction, or thickened or ischemic-appearing bowel may direct the surgeon toward early operative intervention.

The CT scan may also help demonstrate the etiology of the obstruction such as a hernia, intraabdominal mass, or involvement of the small bowel with intraperitoneal mesh that may be helpful in planning the operation if surgical intervention is deemed necessary. Several studies have also suggested that oral gastrografin may have a therapeutic effect and reduce the number of necessary operations.[1–9]

Treatment

Initial management of an SBO should be directed at early resuscitation. This involves insertion of two large-bore intravenous lines, initiation of isotonic fluid at resuscitative rates, and insertion of a urinary catheter for strict monitoring of urine output and adequacy of resuscitation. Fluid resuscitation should begin with a large fluid bolus if severe dehydration is suspected. Serum electrolytes should be measured and monitored at daily intervals, and abnormalities should be corrected. Patients who have been vomiting often will have a hypokalemic, hypochloremic, metabolic alkalosis. The white blood cell count should be checked. Although a leukocytosis may indicate a compromised loop of bowel, it must be realized that severe dehydration may lead to a falsely elevated white blood cell count, and this should be rechecked after rehydration.

Placement of a nasogastric (NG) tube has been a cornerstone of the management of SBO for decades. Recently, however, the use of an NG tube for these patients has become controversial. Many place NG tubes in all patients with SBOs with the understanding that the tube may help aspirate swallowed air as well as foregut secretions and thereby prevent further perpetuation of bowel dilatation. It has been suggested that limiting further bowel dilatation will allow the inflamed loop of

bowel to heal. In most cases placement of an NG tube provides the only chance of resolving the obstruction nonoperatively.[10–13] Occasionally, patients presenting with a partial SBO, without nausea or vomiting, may resolve without NG tube placement.

Although 80% of SBOs will resolve without operative intervention, the principal issue is deciding when operative intervention is indicated. The classic teaching suggests that complete SBOs should undergo surgical intervention and that partial SBOs can usually be observed, but this differentiation is often inconclusive. The reasoning behind this teaching is that, unlike partial SBOs, complete SBOs resolve only about 20% of the time.

Ultimately, the decision to operate is based on the intention to prevent small bowel ischemia or perforation. This may come about as the intraluminal pressure increases so that capillary blood flow is compromised. Small bowel ischemia may present with exquisite abdominal pain, point abdominal tenderness, peritonitis, a leukocytosis, or evidence of ischemia on radiography. Plain films may show the classic thumbprinting that suggests pneumatosis intestinalis, and CT scans may show thickened loops of small bowel. Other CT findings of ischemia include bowel wall that enhances with intravenous contrast. A metabolic acidosis should also be of concern, especially given that these patients usually have a metabolic alkalosis from vomiting. Diffuse peritonitis on examination or free air on plain films suggests perforation and warrants immediate celiotomy.

Patients who have no evidence of ischemia or perforation may be observed expectantly. Although failure of resolution will require surgical intervention, there is debate regarding the duration of time to wait before intervening. Most surgeons will decide to explore if there has been no clinical improvement after 24–48 hours. Patients who have had no prior surgery are usually obstructed from tumor or hernia, and spontaneous resolution is unlikely. Such patients should be considered for surgery earlier in their course.

Surgical correction of SBO usually involves lysis of adhesions, "unkinking" of the obstructed loop, and a possible resection of compromised bowel. The surgeon should be prudent when entering the peritoneal cavity, as this is a common pitfall of the operation. Loops of small bowel are often adherent to the midline, making this step of the operation particularly risky for causing small bowel enterotomies. To minimize the risk of enterotomy, the incision should be started superior or inferior to the previous scar in order to enter into virgin territory. The entire small bowel should be examined as there may be more than one point of obstruction. Any loop of small bowel that appears compromised should be resected. Assessing for loss of bowel motility, color, mesenteric pulses by palpation or Doppler, or fluorescein staining

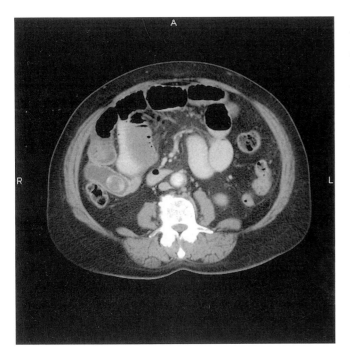

Figure 30.1. Gallstone ileus. Gallstone (lower left) visible as intraluminal foreign body with dilated loops of small bowel.

may help to determine viability. If there is doubt, the abdomen can be closed, and a second-look operation can be performed in 24 hours. A second look with a laparoscope is sometimes feasible. Significant bowel dilatation may make abdominal wall closure difficult. Occasionally an obstructed loop of small bowel may not be easily dissected free and an enteroenterostomy may be necessary to bypass the obstruction. Milking the intraluminal contents either proximally toward the NG tube or distally into the large bowel may facilitate abdominal wall closure. Some surgeons place a sterile, bioresorbable adhesion barrier such as Seprafilm® (Genzyme Biosurgery, Cambridge, MA), which contains sodium hyaluronate and carboxymethylcellulose and has been shown by some studies to reduce the incidence of adhesion formation. There have been several recent reports describing favorable outcomes with laparoscopic lysis of adhesions.[14–20] Although large prospective randomized trials will be needed, preliminary results suggest decreased length of stay, decreased postoperative morbidity, shortened postoperative ileus, and no difference in the intraoperative complication rate.[15]

An NG tube is usually left in place postoperatively and discontinued with return of bowel function. Patients frequently require significant volume resuscitation postoperatively following a major lysis of adhesions. Depending on the extent of bowel dilatation, these patients may have a prolonged ileus.

Most SBOs result from adhesions, hernias, or tumor, but there are other rare causes of obstruction. Intussusception is occasionally seen in adults as a cause of obstruction. Unlike children with intussusception, who can usually be managed nonoperatively, adults with intussusception should undergo surgical exploration as the lead point may be a tumor. Primary small bowel tumors, inflammatory bowel disease, gallstone ileus, and ingested foreign bodies are all rare causes of SBO. Gallstone ileus is a rare cause of SBO in which a fistula between the gallbladder and the duodenum allows for large gallstones to pass into the small bowel and cause obstruction, usually at the ileocecal valve. Evidence of SBO with coexistent pneumobilia on abdominal plain film radiograph is pathognomonic for gallstone ileus, although this can also be seen on CT scan (Figure 30.1). Midgut volvulus may also occur in adults as a result of congenital malrotation or of adhesions and is a surgical emergency because the entire small bowel may become infracted.

Perforation

Small bowel perforation is a surgical emergency. The most common cause is perforation of a duodenal peptic ulcer. Small bowel perforation may also result from an SBO, small bowel ischemia, small bowel neoplasms, ingested foreign body, trauma, or iatrogenic cause.

Diagnosis

Patients who have free perforations of their small bowel will usually develop frank peritonitis. Patients will often complain of generalized abdominal pain that suddenly worsened and note exquisite pain with movement. A detailed history is paramount in helping both to make the diagnosis and to plan the operation. Any history of peptic ulcer disease or gastritis, long-standing aspirin or non-steroidal antiinflammatory (NSAID) use, or postprandial pain suggests a perforated peptic ulcer. Vital signs may show tachycardia and fever. Although blood pressure may be high initially secondary to pain, the onset of a severe systemic inflammatory response may lead to hypotension. Leakage of air or succus into the peritoneal cavity will usually lead to immediate peritonitis, and these patients will have a rigid, tender abdomen with rebound tenderness and pain with movement or percussion. Any of these signs on physical examination should warrant immediate chest x-ray and flat and upright abdominal x-rays to confirm the diagnosis. Free air under the diaphragm on the chest x-ray indicates perforation, and patients should be taken directly to the operating room for celiotomy. These patients should all undergo prompt resuscitation with isotonic fluid, NG tube placement, and intravenous antibiotics.

Treatment

The treatment of a perforated peptic ulcer is most often urgent celiotomy although some have suggested selective nonoperative management. Patients who are hemodynamically stable, without frank peritonitis, and who have evidence of a sealed perforation by an upper gastrointestinal or CT scan may occasionally be managed nonoperatively.[21–23]

The patient's history may help predict which type of incision to make. For patients with a history suggestive of peptic ulcer disease, for example, an upper midline incision may be most appropriate. The bowel should be examined from the cardia of the stomach to the peritoneal reflection of the sigmoid colon. Any perforation of the duodenum should be loosely approximated, and a Graham patch should be performed using any well-vascularized tissue such as omentum. For patients who are hemodynamically stable and are currently being treated medically for ulcer disease, consideration should be made for a definitive acid-reducing operation, such as a vagotomy with antrectomy or highly selective vagotomy. Alternatively, if patients are unstable, vagotomy and pyloroplasty may be performed. The abdomen should be irrigated and a closed suction drain placed in the area of the perforation. These patients should be started on intravenous proton pump inhibitors postoperatively and eventually started on long-term oral therapy. Some surgeons are now advocating laparoscopic surgery for perforated peptic ulcers.[24–30] Since the discovery of *Helicobacter pylori* and its role in the development of peptic ulcer disease, medical therapy directed at destroying this bacteria has significantly evolved. These newer medications have been so successful that surgical therapy for peptic ulcer disease has become much less common.

Other causes of small bowel perforations include mesenteric ischemia, small bowel tumors, and inflammatory bowel disease. These patients will usually require a small bowel resection.

An important cause of small bowel perforation that should be mentioned is an iatrogenic enterotomy or a leaking small bowel anastomosis. This presents a major challenge to diagnosis because most of the findings seen with small bowel perforations are the usual postoperative findings, specifically, abdominal pain, abdominal tenderness, fever, tachycardia, leukocytosis, free peritoneal air, and free peritoneal fluid. An anastomotic leak or enterotomy should be considered for postoperative patients who have an unusually significant amount of postoperative pain, tenderness, fever, tachycardia, or leukocytosis following an abdominal operation.

Gastrointestinal Bleeding

Gastrointestinal bleeding remains a cause of significant morbidity and mortality. In the small bowel, causes of hemorrhage include diverticulosis, angiodysplasia, neoplasm, and ulcer disease. Angiodysplasia and neoplasm are uncommon causes of bleeding from the small bowel. The etiology of ulceration of the small bowel includes ingested medications (NSAIDs), segmental vascular compromise, Crohn's disease, infections such as tuberculosis and syphilis, and rare neoplasms such as gastrinoma. More commonly, ulcerations are noted in the setting of duodenal peptic ulcer disease related to increased acid production in the duodenum and infection with *H. pylori*. Although any diverticulum of the small bowel may cause bleeding, a Meckel's diverticulum is the most common congenital diverticulum of the small bowel. Massive hemorrhage is more common in the pediatric population, but can also occur in adults.

The diagnosis of a small bowel bleed distal to the ligament of Treitz is difficult to diagnose as this region is often out of reach of most endoscopes and is difficult to visualize on angiography. Although duodenal ulcers can usually be visualized by upper endoscopy and a nuclear medicine examination may detect a Meckel's diverticulum, other small bowel lesions may not be visualized until the time of surgery. This may involve palpation of the entire small bowel along with intraoperative endoscopy. The advent of virtual imaging and capsule endoscopy may more readily diagnose lesions in the small bowel.[31,32]

Peptic Ulcer Disease

Peptic ulcer disease occurs frequently and accounts for 50% of the cases of severe upper gastrointestinal bleeding.[33] Fortunately, most cases are self-limited. Prompt resuscitation and early endoscopy are the mainstays of therapy.

Diagnosis

Patients will often present with a history of aspirin or NSAID use, alcohol use, and vague upper abdominal pain or a history of ulcer disease and previous treatment with H_2 blockers or proton pump inhibitors. Patients may also complain of melena or bright red blood per rectum in the case of a brisk upper gastrointestinal bleed; others may present with frank hematemesis or coffee ground emesis. An NG tube should be placed in order to localize bleeding. Clear or nonbloody aspirate does not definitively rule out an upper gastrointestinal bleed. A bile-stained aspirate confirms that there is no source of bleeding up to the second portion of the duodenum. Bloody contents or coffee grounds should be aspirated and lavaged. Ongoing bleeding may be assumed if the aspirate fails to clear with lavage or if there is active bloody drainage.

Endoscopy should be employed early in the course of acute upper gastrointestinal bleeding because of its diagnostic and therapeutic capabilities. Endoscopy may visualize the duodenal ulcer and discern whether there is a high risk of rebleeding. Endoscopic findings include no evidence of active bleeding with a clean ulcer base, active bleeding, adherent clot to the ulcer, or a visible vessel with no associated inflammation or ulcer (Dieulafoy's lesion).[34,35]

Therapy

The immediate care of the patient with acute gastrointestinal bleeding should include assessment of the airway and breathing followed by placement of two large-bore intravenous lines and institution of isotonic volume resuscitation. Patients who are obtunded and unresponsive should have the airway protected with intubation. Supplemental oxygen, whether through nasal cannula, face mask, or mechanical ventilation, will improve oxygen delivery. Laboratory values should be examined, including hemoglobin and hematocrit, coagulation profile, and type and cross for type-specific units of blood.[36]

Endoscopy will usually localize and visualize the duodenal lesion and be potentially therapeutic. In fact, the advances in endoscopy have decreased the necessity of surgical intervention for many cases of duodenal ulcer bleeding. In 1989, a National Institutes of Health consensus study examined the various types of interventions for bleeding. Early surgical involvement was essential in the event that endoscopic measures were not successful. Heater probe and bipolar cautery appeared to be the most effective hemostatic techniques. Other studies have found monopolar coagulation to be more efficacious, especially for high-risk ulcers.[37] Endoscopic features that appear to be predictive of rebleed include a visible vessel, an adherent clot, and arterial spurting or oozing. Approximately 10% to 15% of bleeding duodenal ulcers will rebleed. The decision to treat these patients with repeat endoscopy versus surgery should be made on an individual basis. For patients who are thought to be poor operative risks, attempt at angiographic control with embolization of the bleeding vessel should be considered.[38,39]

Most patients who undergo repeated endoscopic treatment ultimately require surgical intervention. Surgical intervention should be considered strongly for patients who continue to rebleed and who have already received massive transfusions; for upper gastrointestinal bleeds, greater than 6 U of packed red blood cell transfusion is generally considered massive. Endoscopic localization is extremely helpful in planning surgery. At surgery, a lon-gitudinal incision over the pylorus is made with extension onto the duodenum and the antrum of the stomach. The ulcer base and vessel may be oversewn. The gastroduodenal artery is frequently the involved vessel. A three-point stitch should be placed superior, inferior, and medial to the bleeding site. This allows for proximal and distal control of the bleeding vessel, and the medial stitch will occlude the transverse pancreatic branch. Other options include vagotomy and antrectomy or vagotomy and pyloroplasty. The decision to pursue more extensive surgery and resection depends on the patient's hemodynamic stability and history of treatment for ulcer disease.

Meckel's Diverticulum

Meckel's diverticulum is the most common congenital intestinal diverticulum, with a reported incidence of 0.3% to 2.5% in autopsy studies. Although symptomatic Meckel's diverticulum can mimic appendicitis, or result in obstruction, hernia, or intussusception, the most common presentation is massive gastrointestinal hemorrhage. This is caused by heterotopic gastric mucosa, which causes adjacent ileal ulceration and bleeding.

Diagnosis

Symptomatic bleeding from Meckel's diverticulum most often occurs in the pediatric population, but can also present in adults.[40,41] Patients will often have brisk bright red blood per rectum. After a massive upper gastrointestinal bleed and bleeding from a colonic source are ruled out, a bleeding scan may identify the source of bleeding in the small bowel. This study is sensitive, but not specific for Meckel's diverticulum. A better nuclear medicine scan is the Tc-99m pertechnetate Meckel's scan, which localizes to the gastric mucosa of the diverticulum and is reported to be 90% accurate.[42,43] An angiogram may be able to detect a persistent vitellointesinal artery or demonstrate a characteristic blush, early venous return, or arterial abnormality, These studies, however, are often technically difficult and require cannulation of distal ileal arteries.

Treatment

By definition, Meckel's diverticulum identified as a source of bleeding constitutes a symptomatic Meckel's diverticulum and should be treated by surgery. Simple excision may be adequate provided that the lumen is not narrowed. In the setting of gastrointestinal bleeding, a small bowel resection is usually required because of chronic ulceration of the ileal mucosa secondary to heterotopic gastric mucosa and surrounding inflammation.

Mesenteric Ischemia

Mesenteric ischemia is a challenging diagnosis, and a delay in diagnosis often leads to significant morbidity. Time is of the essence in acute mesenteric ischemia, as mortality is related to the extent of small bowel infarction. One must have a high index of suspicion and include this diagnosis in the differential in any patient who presents with an acute abdomen.

Acute mesenteric ischemia may be due to embolic disease, thrombotic occlusion, nonocclusive disease, and mesenteric venous thrombosis. Emboli occur most commonly in the setting of atrial fibrillation with left ventricular clot. Most clots lodge in the jejunal and middle colic branches. A smaller number will lodge at the take-off the superior mesenteric artery.[44] Thrombosis occurs as a result of long-standing atherosclerosis of the mesenteric ostia. Patients may have a chronic history of intestinal angina but may also present acutely with abdominal pain. The presentation may also be subacute and less dramatic than n embolic phenomenon. During times of shock, blood is shunted away from the splanchnic circulation to maintain perfusion to the heart and brain, and there is no vascular obstruction. The first abnormality is that blood is shunted away from the mucosa, leading to loss of epithelial integrity and bacterial translocation. Progressive local vasoconstriction and spasm lead to necrosis. Such patients are often obtunded and are difficult to evaluate.[45] Venous thrombosis may present less dramatically than embolic arterial occlusion. Abdominal pain may be vague and nonspecific. Patients are often found to have a hypercoagulable state. Areas of infarction may be segmental with skip lesions throughout the bowel.[46]

Diagnosis

Mesenteric ischemia presents as a wide spectrum of disease from mucosal injury and bacterial translocation to transmural disease and frank necrosis leading to systemic inflammatory response syndrome and sepsis. Patients present with severe abdominal pain. The classic description of "pain out of proportion to physical examination" should prompt further investigation into ischemia as the etiology of the abdominal pain. The pain is often associated with nausea, vomiting, or diarrhea. Early in the course, the abdomen may appear benign and soft. However, as the ischemia progresses, the bowel may become dilated, leading to abdominal distention, decreased bowel activity, and frank peritonitis as the inflammation irritates the parietal peritoneum.

Laboratory values may help to corroborate the suspicion of ischemia such as leukocytosis, lactic acidosis, and an elevated anion gap. Ultrasound is often only helpful at identifying the main branches of the superior mesenteric artery and vein and portal vein. Distal branches are difficult to visualize. Computed tomography of the abdomen demonstrates signs of ischemia. Free air or free fluid along with thickened loops of small bowel may indicate ischemic bowel that has already progressed to perforation. Other signs of ischemia include hyperemia of the wall characterized by enhancement with intravenous contrast, pneumatosis intestinalis, and inflammatory stranding within the mesentery and around the bowel loops. Intravenous contrast is imperative to demonstrate the branches of the mesenteric vessels. Branches can be traced distally on CT and demonstrate filling defects consistent with embolus or thrombus.[47-50] Angiography remains the gold standard for the diagnosis of mesenteric ischemia where clot and occlusion can be demonstrated. In addition, "pruning" of the vessels is consistent with nonocclusive disease.

Treatment

In the case of nonocclusive mesenteric ischemia, treatment is generally nonoperative and should be directed against the underlying cause such as a low flow state due to cardiogenic or hypovolemic shock. Surgery should be reserved for patients with signs of peritonitis. Because this process is complex and usually occurs in critically ill patients with other organ system failure or dysfunction, the prognosis is grim.

Mesenteric venous occlusion often occurs in the setting of a hypercoagulable state and other conditions such as portal hypertension, cirrhosis, and pancreatitis. Most patients are treated nonoperatively unless there are signs of peritonitis. Patients are treated with aggressive resuscitation, critical care supportive measures, and anticoagulation. Patients who are treated operatively may require second-look laparotomy to assess bowel viability. Fibrinolytic therapy is not usually recommended, and thrombectomy is not successful, in general. Collateral outflow usually develops, and veins recanalize.

Surgery is the best chance for survival for patients with acute ischemia caused by arterial occlusion. If there is frank necrosis and infarction throughout the distribution of the superior mesenteric artery, no surgical therapy should be pursued, as the likelihood of survival is minimal. If there are patchy areas of ischemia, the superior mesenteric artery may be exposed and thromboembolectomy performed. A patch angioplasty may be necessary to repair the artery.[51] If there are segmental areas of intestinal necrosis, they can be resected and primary anastomosis performed.[52] Areas of bowel that are questionable should not be resected, and a second-look operation should be performed at 24 to 48 hours to assess viability. For patients who are poor operative candidates, catheter-directed thrombolysis is a possibility.[53-55] Surgical back-up for these patients is essential for progressive signs of ischemia. It should be noted that once the ischemic bowel has been addressed, patients may continue to have hemodynamic instability. This is caused in part by the reperfusion phenomenon. Free radicals can be perfused back into the mesenteric and systemic circulation once perfusion is restored to the intestine. This process alone can cause multiorgan system failure.

Critique

Intussusception has to be considered in any patient who presents with an intestinal obstruction. With computed tomography confirmation, operative intervention is imperative. Segmental resection of the proximal portion (intussusception) and the adjacent distal bowel (intussuscipiens) is required. Hypertrophied Peyer's patch is the usual lead point—not a malignant neoplasm; however, such determination is usually made postoperatively. In the pediatric population, confirmation of an intussusception would require an attempt at hydrostatic reduction by an enema.

Answer (E)

References

1. Choi HK, Chu KW, Law WL. Therapeutic value of gastrografin in adhesive small bowel obstruction after unsuccessful conservative treatment: a prospective randomized trial. Ann Surg 2002; 236:1–6.
2. Assalia A, Schein M, Kopelman D, Hirshberg A, Hashmonai M. Therapeutic effect of oral gastrografin in adhesive, partial small-bowel obstruction: a prospective randomized trial. Surgery 1994; 115:433–437.
3. Fevang BT, Jensen D, Fevang J, et al. Upper gastrointestinal contrast study in the management of small bowel obstruction—a prospective randomised study. Eur J Surg 2000; 166:39–43.
4. Chen SC, Lin FY, Lee PH, Yu SC, Wang SM, Chang KJ. Water-soluble contrast study predicts the need for early surgery in adhesive small bowel obstruction. Br J Surg 1998; 85:1692–1694.
5. Fevang BT, Jensen D, Svanes K, Viste A. Early operation or conservative management of patients with small bowel obstruction? Eur J Surg 2002; 168:475–481.
6. Chung CC, Meng WC, Yu SC, Leung KL, Lau WY, Li AK. A prospective study on the use of water-soluble contrast follow-through radiology in the management of small bowel obstruction. Aust N Z J Surg 1996; 66:598–601.
7. Blackmon S, Lucius C, Wilson JP, et al. The use of water-soluble contrast in evaluating clinically equivocal small bowel obstruction. Am Surg 2000; 66:238–244.
8. Cox MR, Gunn IF, Eastman MC, Hunt RF, Heinz AW. The safety and duration of non-operative treatment for adhesive small bowel obstruction. Aust N Z J Surg 1993; 63: 367–371.
9. Donckier V, Closset J, Van Gansbeke D, et al. Contribution of computed tomography to decision making in the management of adhesive small bowel obstruction. Br J Surg 1998; 85:1071–1074.
10. Gowen GF. Long tube decompression is successful in 90% of patients with adhesive small bowel obstruction. Am J Surg 2003; 185:512–515.
11. Gowen GF. Decompression is essential in the management of small bowel obstruction. Am J Surg 1997; 173:459–460.
12. Gowen GF, DeLaurentis DA, Stefan MM. Immediate endoscopic placement of long intestinal tube in partial obstruction of the small intestine. Surg Gynecol Obstet 1987; 165:456–458.
13. Gowen GF. Endoscopic decompression in partial small bowel obstruction. Am J Surg 1985; 149:252–257.
14. Franklin ME Jr, Gonzalez JJ Jr, Miter DB, Glass JL, Paulson D. Laparoscopic diagnosis and treatment of intestinal obstruction. Surg Endosc 2004; 18:26–30.
15. Chopra R, McVay C, Phillips E, Khalili TM. Laparoscopic lysis of adhesions. Am Surg 2003; 69:966–968.
16. Kirshtein B, Roy-Shapira A, Lantsberg L, Mandel S, Avinoach E, Mizrahi S. The use of laparoscopy in abdominal emergencies. Surg Endosc 2003; 17:1118–1124.
17. Reissman P, Spira RM. Laparoscopy for adhesions. Semin Laparosc Surg 2003; 10:185–190.
18. Sato Y, Ido K, Kumagai M, et al. Laparoscopic adhesiolysis for recurrent small bowel obstruction: long-term follow-up. Gastrointest Endosc 2001; 54:476–479.
19. Wullstein C, Gross E. Laparoscopic compared with conventional treatment of acute adhesive small bowel obstruction. Br J Surg 2003; 90:1147–1151.
20. Suzuki K, Umehara Y, Kimura T. Elective laparoscopy for small bowel obstruction. Surg Laparosc Endosc Percutan Tech 2003; 13:254–256.
21. Gul YA, Shine MF, Lennon F. Non-operative management of perforated duodenal ulcer. Ir J Med Sci 1999; 168: 254–256.
22. Marshall C, Ramaswamy P, Bergin FG, Rosenberg IL, Leaper DJ. Evaluation of a protocol for the non-operative management of perforated peptic ulcer. Br J Surg 1999; 86:131–134.
23. Jordan PH Jr, Morrow C. Perforated peptic ulcer. Surg Clin North Am 1988; 68:315–329.
24. Seelig MH, Seelig SK, Behr C, Schonleben K. Comparison between open and laparoscopic technique in the management of perforated gastroduodenal ulcers. J Clin Gastroenterol 2003; 37:226–229.
25. Mehendale VG, Shenoy SN, Joshi AM, Chaudhari NC. Laparoscopic versus open surgical closure of perforated duodenal ulcers: a comparative study. Indian J Gastroenterol 2002; 21:222–224.
26. Lau WY. Perforated peptic ulcer: open versus laparoscopic repair. Asian J Surg 2002; 25:267–269.
27. Arnaud JP, Tuech JJ, Bergamaschi R, Pessaux P, Regenet N. Laparoscopic suture closure of perforated duodenal peptic ulcer. Surg Laparosc Endosc Percutan Tech 2002; 12:145–147.

28. Kaiser AM, Katkhouda N. Laparoscopic management of the perforated viscus. Semin Laparosc Surg 2002; 9:46–53.

29. Lagoo SA, Pappas TN. Laparoscopic repair for perforated peptic ulcer. Ann Surg 2002; 235:320–321.

30. Siu WT, Leong HT, Law BK, et al. Laparoscopic repair for perforated peptic ulcer: a randomized controlled trial. Ann Surg 2002; 235:313–319.

31. Lewis B, Goldfarb N. Review article: the advent of capsule endoscopy—a not-so-futuristic approach to obscure gastrointestinal bleeding. Aliment Pharmacol Ther 2003; 17:1085–1096.

32. Pennazio M, Santucci R, Rondonotti E, et al. Outcome of patients with obscure gastrointestinal bleeding after capsule endoscopy: report of 100 consecutive cases. Gastroenterology 2004; 126:643–653.

33. van Leerdam ME, Vreeburg EM, Rauws EA, et al. Acute upper GI bleeding: did anything change? Time trend analysis of incidence and outcome of acute upper GI bleeding between 1993/1994 and 2000. Am J Gastroenterol 2003; 98:1494–1499.

34. Barkun A, Bardou M, Marshall JK. Consensus recommendations for managing patients with nonvariceal upper gastrointestinal bleeding. Ann Intern Med 2003; 139:843–857.

35. Pais SA, Yang R. Diagnostic and therapeutic options in the management of nonvariceal upper gastrointestinal bleeding. Curr Gastroenterol Rep 2003; 5:476–481.

36. Huang CS, Lichtenstein DR. Nonvariceal upper gastrointestinal bleeding. Gastroenterol Clin North Am 2003; 32:1053–1078.

37. Soon MS, Wu SS, Chen YY, Fan CS, Lin OS. Monopolar coagulation versus conventional endoscopic treatment for high-risk peptic ulcer bleeding: a prospective, randomized study. Gastrointest Endosc 2003; 58:323–329.

38. Ljungdahl M, Eriksson LG, Nyman R, Gustavsson S. Arterial embolisation in management of massive bleeding from gastric and duodenal ulcers. Eur J Surg 2002; 168:384–390.

39. Toyoda H, Nakano S, Takeda I, et al. Transcatheter arterial embolization for massive bleeding from duodenal ulcers not controlled by endoscopic hemostasis. Endoscopy 1995; 27:304–307.

40. Happe MR, Woodworth PA. Meckel's diverticulum in an adult gastrointestinal bleed. Am J Surg 2003; 186:132–133.

41. Higaki S, Saito Y, Akazawa A, et al. Bleeding Meckel's diverticulum in an adult. Hepatogastroenterology 2001; 48:1628–1630.

42. Dolezal J, Vizd'a J, Bures J. Detection of acute gastrointestinal bleeding by means of technetium-99m in vivo labelled red blood cells. Nucl Med Rev Cent East Eur 2002; 5:151–154.

43. Lin S, Suhocki PV, Ludwig KA, Shetzline MA. Gastrointestinal bleeding in adult patients with Meckel's diverticulum: the role of technetium 99m pertechnetate scan. South Med J 2002; 95:1338–1341.

44. Cleveland TJ, Nawaz S, Gaines PA. Mesenteric arterial ischaemia: diagnosis and therapeutic options. Vasc Med 2002; 7:311–321.

45. Trompeter M, Brazda T, Remy CT, Vestring T, Reimer P. Non-occlusive mesenteric ischemia: etiology, diagnosis, and interventional therapy. Eur Radiol 2002; 12:1179–1187.

46. Bradbury MS, Kavanagh PV, Bechtold RE, et al. Mesenteric venous thrombosis: diagnosis and noninvasive imaging. Radiographics 2002; 22:527–541.

47. Kirkpatrick ID, Kroeker MA, Greenberg HM. Biphasic CT with mesenteric CT angiography in the evaluation of acute mesenteric ischemia: initial experience. Radiology 2003; 229:91–98.

48. Lee R, Tung HK, Tung PH, Cheung SC, Chan FL. CT in acute mesenteric ischaemia. Clin Radiol 2003; 58:279–287.

49. Wiesner W, Khurana B, Ji H, Ros PR. CT of acute bowel ischemia. Radiology 2003; 226:635–650.

50. Segatto E, Mortele KJ, Ji H, Wiesner W, Ros PR. Acute small bowel ischemia: CT imaging findings. Semin Ultrasound CT MR 2003; 24:364–376.

51. Park WM, Gloviczki P, Cherry KJ Jr, et al. Contemporary management of acute mesenteric ischemia: factors associated with survival. J Vasc Surg 2002; 35:445–452.

52. Char DJ, Cuadra SA, Hines GL, Purtill W. Surgical intervention for acute intestinal ischemia: experience in a community teaching hospital. Vasc Endovasc Surg 2003; 37:245–252.

53. Calin GA, Calin S, Ionescu R, Croitoru M, Diculescu M, Oproiu A. Successful local fibrinolytic treatment and balloon angioplasty in superior mesenteric arterial embolism: a case report and literature review. Hepatogastroenterology 2003; 50:732–734.

54. Savassi-Rocha PR, Veloso LF. Treatment of superior mesenteric artery embolism with a fibrinolytic agent: case report and literature review. Hepatogastroenterology 2002; 49:1307–1310.

55. Sternbergh WC 3rd, Ramee SR, DeVun DA, Money SR. Endovascular treatment of multiple visceral artery paradoxical emboli with mechanical and pharmacological thrombolysis. J Endovasc Ther 2000; 7:155–160.

31
Liver and Biliary Tract

Spiros P. Hiotis and Hersch L. Pachter

Case Scenario

You are asked to see a 32-year-old intensive care unit patient in the medical service who is febrile and lethargic with a history, according to her husband—a self-proclaimed recluse—of shaking chills and who needs evaluation and possible management. With the exception of hospitalization for childbirth (youngest child is 1 year old), the patient has no known medical problems. On physical examination, the patient is jaundice and has right upper quadrant tenderness. There is no rebound tenderness. The patient was recently started on pressors to achieve hemodynamic stability. Pertinent positive laboratory results include an alkaline phosphatase level of 600, a total bilirubin level of 6 (direct –4.5), and a white blood cell count of 15,000. The patient has been receiving full-spectrum antibiotics for 36 hours. Which of the following recommendations should your acute care surgical consultation render?

(A) Change of antimicrobial agents
(B) Emergency cholecystectomy
(C) Computed tomography directed at biliary drainage
(D) Endoscopy
(E) Continuation of current management plan

One of the challenges for the acute care surgeon is the management of hepatic and biliary emergencies. The anatomic complexities of this system, along with the ever-present potential for both bleeding and infectious complications, make staged or definitive treatment a risky undertaking.

Anatomy

The Couinaud description of segmental liver anatomy based on portal venous inflow has led to safer surgical approaches for resection in addition to other procedures. An intimate knowledge of the liver's segmental anatomy is essential to the successful outcome of both elective and acute care surgery of the liver.[1–4]

Portal venous inflow divides the liver into its anatomic right and left lobes. The right lobe is divided into an anterior sector, which is based on the right anterior sectoral branch of the portal vein and consists of segments 5 and 8; and the posterior sector, which is based on the right posterior sectoral branch of the portal vein and consists of segments 6 and 7. In contradiction, the anatomic left lobe of the liver is composed of three different areas based on somewhat less ordered portal venous inflow. Segment 4, sometimes referred to as the "medial segment of the left lobe" by radiologists, is located between the gallbladder bed and the falciform ligament. Portal inflow to segment 4 is largely supplied by two segmental portal venous branches, which usually develop as small branches off the main left portal vein. The left lateral segment is composed of segments 2 and 3, both of which are supplied by highly predictable branches of the main left portal vein. Segment 1 is also referred to as the "caudate lobe" and is a somewhat independent component of the anatomic left lobe. This unusual liver segment straddles the inferior vena cava in a horseshoe-like configuration and is supplied by highly variable portal venous inflow, often based on the main left portal vein but sometimes on the right vein.

As they enter the liver parenchyma, major biliary ducts and hepatic arterial structures follow the direction of portal venous inflow. Thus a thorough knowledge of the patient's portal venous anatomy will also lend familiarity to biliary ductal and hepatic arterial anatomy. These structures are all invested in a fascial sheath, which develops as Glisson's capsule invaginates into the liver parenchyma during embryogenesis. Portal structures are easily distinguished on ultrasonography because of this dense hyperechoic fascial layer that surrounds them. Hepatic venous structures are not surrounded by a similar dense layer of connective tissue and thus can be easily distinguished from portal structures on ultrasonography.

Hepatic venous drainage of the liver is based on three major hepatic veins and is not generally variable between patients. The right hepatic vein has an independent origin off of the inferior vena cava and travels in between segments 7 and 8 in its cephalad location to segment 6 in its caudad location. Contrary to the right hepatic vein, the middle and left hepatic veins share a common origin off the inferior vena cava. The middle hepatic vein travels in diagonal direction through segment 4 and into segments 8 and 5. The left hepatic vein travels from its origin into the left lateral segment. Surgical approaches based on extrahepatic or intrahepatic hepatic venous outflow control require a precise knowledge of hepatic venous anatomy, as inadvertent injuries to these structures can result in exsanguinating hemorrhage or major venous air embolism within a very short period of time.

Physiology

An in-depth analysis of hepatic and biliary physiology is beyond the scope of this chapter. The focus, therefore, relates only to issues pertinent to the surgeon involved in the rapid evaluation of hepatic function in an acute care setting.

The functional capacity of a patient's liver can easily be evaluated with four relatively simple and rapid blood tests: prothrombin time, total bilirubin, albumin, and platelet count. Although many variables can often lead to abnormalities in any of these studies, hepatic synthetic compromise in the otherwise well-nourished patient may become readily apparent by an elevation of the prothrombin time and a decrease in serum albumin. Normal blood clotting, usually measured by the prothrombin time, depends on clotting factors synthesized exclusively by the liver. An unexplained elevation in prothrombin time may be reflective of an underlying diseased liver with impaired synthetic functional capacity.[5] Additionally, when serum albumin, which is also exclusively synthesized by the liver, is noted to be less than 3.0 mg/dL in a well-nourished patient, suspicion should be raised that inherent hepatic synthetic capability of the liver is compromised.[6]

Elevations in a patient's total bilirubin level can occur because of a myriad of physiologic disturbances. Many of these can be hematologic, hepatic, or biliary in origin.

Patients with underlying cirrhosis and compromised liver function will often experience a long-standing elevation in their total bilirubin level as a result of a limited ability to conjugate bilirubin, a process that occurs within hepatocyte cytoplasm. Hyperbilirubinemia secondary to underlying abnormal hepatocyte function manifests itself as a combined elevation of both conjugated and unconjugated (direct and indirect) bilirubin. This abnormality is not usually accompanied by a proportional increase in the serum alkaline phosphatase level. However, elevations in the total bilirubin level resulting from biliary obstruction are predominated by increased levels of the direct bilirubin and are usually accompanied by elevated serum alkaline phosphatase levels.[7]

Decreased platelet counts are often reflective of portal hypertension and may provide some of the earliest clues to the patient with unsuspected cirrhosis. Portal hypertension of any etiologic origin results in increased pressure within the portal, splenic, and superior mesenteric veins. Over time, this pressure increase leads to hypersplenism and subsequent splenic sequestration of platelets. Any patient with suspected underlying liver disease and an unexplained platelet count of less than 100,000 should be considered cirrhotic until proven otherwise. Hepatobiliary surgery for such patients, whether elective or urgent in nature, carries with it a significantly increased risk for perioperative morbidity and mortality.[8–10]

Technology

Few surgical specialties have benefited more from recent technological advances than the field of hepatobiliary surgery. An almost exponential improvement in imaging technology has allowed for an increased accuracy with which liver and biliary anatomy can be evaluated in the preoperative, intraoperative, and nonoperative settings. High-speed spiral computerized tomography (CT) scanners, magnetic resonance imaging (MRI) with emphasis on cholangiopancreatography (MRCP), endoscopic and intraoperative cholangiography (open or laparoscopic), and ultrasonographic technology have revolutionized our ability to precisely image the liver and biliary system, simplifying our understanding of the liver's complex segmental anatomy. Additional semi-invasive imaging modalities such as transhepatic cholangiography have provided a "road map" enabling surgeons to both plan and effectuate a more accurate approach to the liver and biliary tree.[11–18]

Moreover, technological advances have also led to the discovery of sophisticated surgical tools, which have become essential in the modern hepatobiliary operating room. Parenchymal dissection with the ultrasound aspirator (CUSA), tissue link sealing dissector, harmonic scalpel, and Hydro Jet allow for a more precise and safer division of hepatic parenchyma and thereby better visualization of major vascular structures before their division. Other instruments such as the argon beam coagulator facilitate cauterization of a wide field of transected liver substance, greatly enhancing the surgeon's ability to control liver hemorrhage without need for suturing. Finally, new tools for hepatic ablation, such as cryoablation and radiofrequency ablation probes, create opportunities for destruction of specific pathologic areas within the liver without necessitating formal surgical extirpation.[19]

Infections

Hepatic Pyogenic Abscess

Hepatic abscesses result from bacterial infection of the hepatic parenchyma. Because of the firm, solid nature of the liver's substance, bacterial infections of this organ progress to walled-off spherical areas within which liquefied necrotic material is contained. Hepatic abscesses are, therefore, generally composed of fluid-filled central regions that are surrounded by a wall of inflammatory cells, predominantly polymorphonuclear cells (PMNs), and minimal fibrosis.

The etiology of hepatic abscess is related to the route of entry by bacterial organisms. Historically, the most common source of liver abscess occurred secondary to complications of acute appendicitis. In the past, patients with unrecognized or untreated appendicitis frequently developed pyelophlebitis of the portal venous system, with subsequent formation of liver abscess and ensuing sepsis. The widespread use of antibiotics globally has all but eliminated pyelophlebitis as a cause of hepatic abscess. In the new millennium, most hepatic abscesses are related to trauma, cholangitis, intraabdominal infections, and cryptogenic causes.[20] The organisms responsible for pyogenic liver abscess are often those commonly found in the gastrointestinal tract and skin flora. These include the Gram-negative bacilli *Escherichia coli* and *Klebsiella*, anaerobes such *Bacteroides* and *Clostridium* species and Gram-positive cocci such as *Enterococcus*.[21] Culture and Gram stain studies of fluid aspirated or drained directly from a liver abscess are more informative in identifying the offending organism than usual multiple blood cultures taken. Once the organism is identified, appropriate antimicrobial therapy should immediately be directed at the responsible bacteria.[22,23]

Most patients with hepatic abscesses initially present with fever, tachycardia, leukocytosis, and abdominal pain. Although mild symptomatology in the initial period is common, eventual progression to sepsis with hemodynamic compromise can occur in the untreated or inadequately treated patient. As with all abscesses, the mainstay of treatment for hepatic abscesses is drainage. Initial treatment should be attempted through a minimally invasive image-guided percutaneous technique (Figure 31.1). This method has been highly successful when abscesses are unilocular (Table 31.1[24–30]). These techniques require the availability of an experienced interventional radiology team and can be safely performed with local anesthesia with or without intravenous sedation.

Image guidance can usually be accomplished rapidly with transabdominal ultrasonography because of the ease in identifying fluid-filled hypoechoic cavities within the relative hyperechogenicity of normal liver parenchyma. Computed tomography guidance for catheter drainage of liver abscess is seldom necessary but can be used as an alternative to ultrasound guidance. Liver abscesses are easily imaged by both noncontrast and contrast-enhanced CT scans. However, contrast-enhanced CT scans are preferred as they provide clearer images and facilitate identification of major portal and hepatic venous structures, thereby reducing the risk of procedure-related vascular injuries.

The goal of any drainage procedure is twofold: (1) accomplish complete drainage of all abscess fluid and (2) provide sufficient quantities of fluid aspirate for microbiology studies. Some liver abscesses, even when technically accessible by interventional techniques, cannot be completely drained percutaneously because of high viscosity of abscess fluid. Patients for whom percutaneous drainage is not technically possible should be promptly taken to the operating room for surgical drainage. Additionally, open surgical drainage is reserved for those instances when failure of the percutaneous method has occurred or when the abscess is multilocular.[31] Surgical drainage can be achieved equally well via a laparoscopic or open approach. Familiarity with intraoperative ultrasound is essential for proper localization of liver abscesses not readily apparent by inspection or palpation alone. These difficulties become more apparent during a laparoscopic approach and stress the extreme importance of laparoscopic ultrasonography if complete drainage is to be achieved. Simple incision and fenestration of fluid collections within the liver with placement of closed suction drains is adequate. Formal surgical resection of liver containing the abscess is seldom necessary and should strongly be discouraged in the acute setting. Hepatic resection, when necessary, should be reserved for refractory infections and performed by highly experienced hepatobiliary surgeons. Antibiotics in addition to drainage are an important component in the management of these patients. It should be stressed, however, that antibiotics alone are inadequate for definitive treatment of these patients.

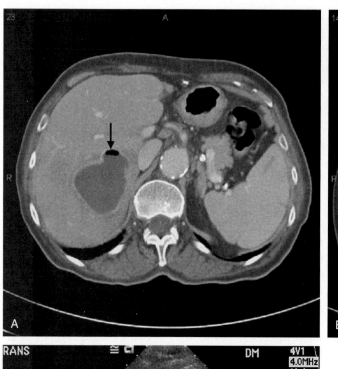

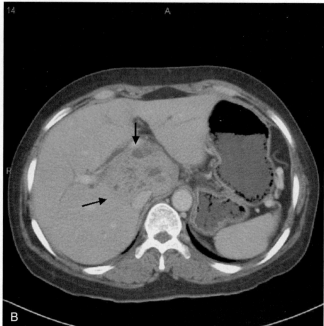

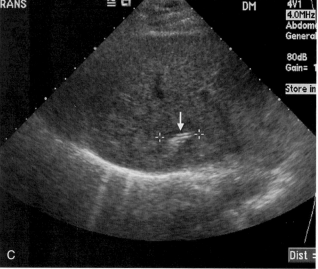

FIGURE 31.1. **(A)** Computed tomography scan with intravenous contrast demonstrating the presence of a uniloculated hepatic pyogenic abscess with gas in segment 6 (arrow). **(B)** A multiloculated abscess (arrows) in the caudate lobe of a different patient. **(C)** Transabdominal ultrasound showing an indwelling catheter in a hepatic abscess (arrow) that was placed percutaneously under ultrasound guidance.

TABLE 31.1. Success rate of percutaneous abscess drainage from selected large published series including at least 100 patients.

Study	Success rate	No. of patients
Goletti et al.[27]	88%	200
Brolin et al.[24]	76%	119
Voros et al.[28]	92%	185
Lang et al.[25]	77%	136
Gerzof et al.[30]	74%	125
Ch et al.[29]	97%	101
van Sonnenberg et al.[26]	90%	101

Cholangitis

Cholangitis is a potentially lethal bacterial infection and is often related to underlying stasis in the biliary ductal system. Patients with cholangitis present with fever, leukocytosis, and right upper quadrant pain.[32–34] Additional symptoms seen in early sepsis include tachycardia and tachypnea. Rapid progression to "suppurative cholangitis" (pus under pressure in the biliary tree) with concomitant septic shock and life-threatening hemodynamic collapse is common in patients with untreated cholangitis, underscoring the importance of prompt diagnosis, resuscitation, and institution of broad-spectrum intravenous antibiotics followed by rapid decompression of the ductal system.[35]

Gram-negative bacilli, particularly, *Escherichia coli*, *Klebsiella*, and the *Proteus* species are most often responsible for biliary infections, necessitating intravenous antibiotics with excellent Gram-negative coverage.[36,37] Antibiotic therapy should be started immediately for any patient with the potential for cholangitis and should not be delayed until positive cultures are obtained or hemodynamic deterioration becomes manifest. The antibiotic of choice should be one that is predominantly excreted in bile, such as ciprofloxacin. Initially, double coverage of Gram-negative organisms seems to provide an excellent early treatment strategy, which can be modified when exact speciation has been ascertained.[38–40]

As with all pyogenic infections, drainage is the mainstay of treatment for patients with cholangitis and underlying biliary obstruction. Depending on the hemodynamic status of the patient, underlying etiology of biliary stasis, and location of biliary obstruction, percutaneous transhepatic cholangiography (PTC) and endoscopic retrograde cholangiopancreatography (ERCP) with sphincterotomy are appropriate methods of drainage (Figure 31.2). Endoscopic retrograde cholangiopancreatography is a less invasive approach than PTC. It is particularly effective for patients with choledocholithiasis or distal common bile duct obstruction caused by periampullary tumors. For these patients, ERCP not only provides diagnostic images but can be therapeutic as well. Placement of distal biliary stents in patients with periampullary malignancies and sphincterotomy with stone retrieval in patients with choledocholithiasis can provide immediate decompression when purulence under pressure exists within the biliary tree.[41]

Percutaneous transhepatic cholangiography is often reserved for patients with high biliary obstruction (above the bifurcation of the common hepatic duct) and for patients for whom ERCP is either not available or not technically feasible. Technical difficulties that commonly preclude ERCP include an inability to cannulate the ampulla of Vater or a complete low common bile duct obstruction that prevents the retrograde introduction of a catheter through the ampulla. Most experienced interventional radiologists are capable of accessing the biliary tree through either the right or the left biliary ductal system when the need arises. Simple aspiration of bile for microbiology studies as well as external catheter placement can be easily and very rapidly performed. If the patient has exhibited any signs of hemodynamic instability at any time, then further manipulation of the obstructing mechanism, at this juncture, should be discouraged. With evidence that hemodynamic stability has returned, and sufficient antibiotic level has been achieved, additional advanced technological maneuvers can then be

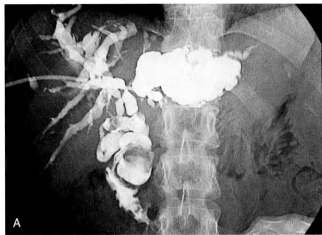

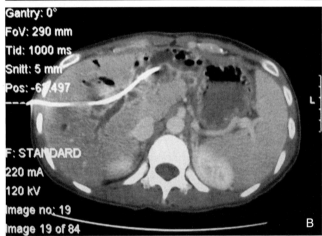

FIGURE 31.2. Percutaneous transhepatic cholangiography (PTC) **(A)** and computed tomography scan **(B)** of a patient with proximal and distal biliary strictures and multiple indwelling biliary stones. This patient presented with massive dilatation of the biliary ductal system, especially involving the left ductal system. A PTC catheter was placed into the left duct via the right duct, facilitating adequate decompression.

employed. These include balloon dilatation of biliary strictures and placement of external biliary stents, which can then be internalized, or self-expanding internal biliary stents.

With the advances in the aforementioned technologies, surgical procedures in the acute setting for management of patients with cholangitis have become increasingly uncommon. However, surgical management is still an important tool for patients for whom less invasive techniques are either not possible or unavailable. Laparoscopic or open surgical procedures provide equivalent results. The method of choice, however, should depend on the individual expertise of the operating surgeon. Patients with biliary sepsis managed surgically in the acute setting should undergo the least complicated and most rapid procedure possible to establish biliary drainage and to obtain bile for culture and Gram stain. At surgery, the initial maneuver is to expose the common bile duct so that instantaneous drainage can be accomplished. No attempt should be made to approach the gallbladder in contemplation of performing a cholecystectomy first and draining the common bile duct secondarily. Drainage is usually accomplished by the placement of a T tube in the common bile duct above the level of obstruction. This maneuver alone is often adequate for definitive surgical management. If at any point during the operation the patient exhibits signs of sepsis or hemodynamic instability, surgery should be immediately terminated after a drain has been placed in the bile duct. The patient should be rapidly closed and brought to a critical care unit for further resuscitation and close monitoring. On the other, if an elevated temperature, leukocytosis, and abnormal liver function tests are the only signs of cholangitis in the absence of "pus" under pressure in the common bile duct in the patient with choledocholithiasis, then cholecystectomy, intraoperative cholangiography (IOC), and common bile duct exploration (CBDE) may be safely undertaken. Internal drainage established by a biliary–enteric anastomosis is strongly discouraged in the acute setting. Patients with cholangitis and infected bile have a compromised ability to tolerate lengthy surgical procedures and carry a significantly increased risk for anastomotic leak and biliary fistula formation.[34,42]

Parasitic

Parasitic diseases of the liver and biliary tract are important worldwide epidemiologic problems. However, these diseases rarely present as acute life-threatening surgical emergencies in Western medical centers. Parasitic hepatobiliary diseases can be subclassified according to the underlying infectious organism.

Amoebiasis is caused by *Entamoeba histolytica*, and hepatic infections manifest themselves as amoebic liver abscess. These organisms reside in the lower gastrointestinal tract and reach the liver parenchyma through the portal venous system. The initial presentation is frequently accompanied by fever, leukocytosis, and abdominal pain. Computed tomography scanning and MRI can provide accurate imaging characteristics of amoebic abscesses, but these tests are sometimes unnecessary as ultrasonography may suffice.[43,44] Transabdominal ultrasound usually reveals a thick-walled hypoechoic fluid collection, which is characteristic for amoebic abscess. Additionally, serum serology studies are invaluable in establishing the correct diagnosis of an amoebic abscess. The treatment of hepatic amoebiasis is nonsurgical, and the overwhelming majority can successfully be managed with an intravenous course of metronidazole.[45–47] Percutaneous aspiration of amoebic abscess should only be performed when (1) the patient is not responding to conventional antibiotic therapy and (2) the diagnosis is uncertain and there is a need to determine whether a pyogenic process is present.

Hydatid disease is caused by the *Echinococcus* species and occurs most commonly in areas with large populations of sheep, which have been identified as the natural animal host. Hydatid cysts of the liver do not usually result in clinical situations requiring emergency care but rather develop over a prolonged period of time. The diagnosis is based on serum serology and imaging studies, which include ultrasonography, CT, and MRI.[48–51]

Liver fluke diseases are caused by *Clonorchis sinensis* or *Fasciola hepatica* organisms. These infections develop after ingestion of contaminated fish or sheep feces, respectively. Clinical manifestations of both diseases include recurrent episodes of cholangitis. Evaluation with serologic or stool studies, liver function tests, and imaging by ultrasound or CT have all been useful in establishing the correct diagnosis. Treatment is primarily medical in nature, and surgical management is required only for patients who develop associated biliary strictures, stones, or malignancy.

Calculus Disease of the Gallbladder and Common Bile Duct

Cholelithiasis, cholecystitis, and choledocholithiasis are responsible for a considerable proportion of surgical emergencies that are dealt with by the general surgeon. Four manifestations of cholelithiasis and choledocholithiasis encompass the spectrum of severe complications that commonly occur as a result of stones in the biliary tree: cholecystitis, biliary obstruction, pancreatitis, and gallstone ileus.

Cholecystitis

Cholecystitis is an inflammatory disease of the gallbladder that develops secondary to obstruction of the cystic duct. This disease is associated with gallstones in 95% of cases and less often can present as "acalculous cholecystitis." Patients at risk for acalculous cholecystitis are diabetics, those who have sustained major abdominal trauma, and patients who have been on nothing-by-mouth status for prolonged periods of time. Biliary stasis in a nonemptying gallbladder leads to an acute inflammatory process that, left untreated, can progress to severe infection, gallbladder wall infarction, and subsequent gangrene.[52] Acute cholecystitis manifests initially as right upper quadrant pain accompanied by fever and leukocytosis. Signs of early sepsis such as tachycardia and tachypnea sometimes accompany the initial presentation.

Physical examination reveals tenderness to palpation in the right upper quadrant that is exacerbated by deep inspiration, referred to as "Murphy's sign." Initial evaluation with complete blood count, serum electrolytes, and liver function tests is appropriate. Initial radiographic evaluation almost always consists of transabdominal ultrasound. Findings of pericholecystic fluid or a thickened gallbladder wall are classically associated with acute cholecystitis.[53] Most experienced ultrasound technicians can often elicit an ultrasound "Murphy's sign" by placing the probe directly over the gallbladder fundus. Most patients who develop acute cholecystitis present with a normal-diameter common bile duct and no common duct stones. It should be noted, however, that ultrasound is notoriously unreliable in detecting stones at the distal one-third of the common bile duct because of a confluence of shadows in the vicinity of the duodenum. Ductal dilatation, on the other hand, is readily apparent on routine ultrasonography.

When the diagnosis is uncertain, additional useful information may be obtained by further studies. For example, patients who present with jaundice and a dilated common bile duct in addition to cholecystitis should undergo a more extensive workup. A variety of diagnostic tools are available, including nuclear medicine hepatobiliary scan, CT with intravenous contrast, MRCP, or ERCP.[54,55]

The traditional approach to management of acute cholecystitis has been to promptly operate on the patient, preferably within 48 hours of the onset of symptoms. Definitive surgical management includes a planned cholecystectomy with intraoperative cholangiography, when feasible, or common bile duct exploration when indicated. For the most part, these procedures can be performed equally well via laparoscopic or open surgical method, depending on the surgeon's level of expertise.[56,57] Prompt cholecystectomy is associated with the most favorable outcome and has gained widespread acceptance over a delayed surgical approach involving treatment with antibiotics followed by interval cholecystectomy 4 to 6 weeks later.[58–61] Several retrospective studies comparing immediate versus delayed cholecystectomy have suggested that the treatment failure and rehospitalization rates for patients managed with delayed cholecystectomy is high. When there has been a delay beyond 48 hours in establishing the diagnosis or for patients with severe comorbidities who are at high risk for immediate surgery, interval cholecystectomy may provide a safer option. The risk for intraoperative complications is increased when cholecystectomy is attempted several days following the onset of symptoms. This increased risk is due to technical difficulties associated with the exacerbation of the inflammatory process and the associated fibrosis in the areas of dissection. Under these circumstances, clear identification of the cystic duct in relation to the common bile duct and

the relationship of medial wall and fundus of the gallbladder to both the common bile duct and the common hepatic duct can be extremely difficult. In this setting, these vital structures become prone to inadvertent injury. These patients are better served by continued antibiotic therapy and interval cholecystectomy at a later date when the acute inflammatory process has subsided. If these high-risk patients do not demonstrate a marked improvement within 48 hours of the initiation of intravenous antibiotics, percutaneous placement of a cholecystostomy tube to decompress the gallbladder may become necessary.[62]

Percutaneous cholecystostomy tube placement should be accomplished under ultrasound or CT guidance, both of which facilitate catheter insertion in a safe and reliable manner. When interventional radiology support is not available, open cholecystostomy tube placement under local anesthesia through a limited open incision is an excellent alternative. The surgeon's success with this approach can be enhanced by ultrasound when performed either at the bedside or in the operating room. Patients with indwelling cholecystostomy tubes who subsequently improve clinically and become candidates for tube removal should first be evaluated with a contrast study through the cholecystostomy tube. The tube should not be removed if (1) the cystic duct is occluded or (2) stones are seen in either the gallbladder or the common bile duct. Under these circumstances, premature tube removal may result in significant recurrent bouts of acute cholecystitis.

Biliary Obstruction

In Western societies calculi in the common bile duct usually originate in the gallbladder. Less common is the formation of common bile duct stones de novo as a result of stasis, foreign body irritation (i.e., secondary to parasites), and stricture. Patients who present with ductal stones, especially those confined to the lower biliary tract, often develop jaundice. These patients can pose diagnostic and therapeutic challenges, and proper management often involves a multidisciplinary approach.

Patients with choledocholithiasis whose initial presentation is accompanied by jaundice frequently are noted to have dilated ducts. Dilated intrahepatic and extrahepatic bile ducts can reliably be detected by transabdominal ultrasonography. The detection of stones within the common bile itself, however, with the exception of a free floating stone in the mid or proximal duct, is marginal at best. Computed tomography scanning and MRCP may play a role in eliminating a distal malignancy as the cause of the extrahepatic obstruction.[63]

Traditionally, patients were managed with cholecystectomy, intraoperative cholangiography, and common bile duct exploration. With the increased success of endoscopic techniques, most medical centers now advocate an approach based on preoperative ERCP, sphincterotomy accompanied by stone extraction, and clearance of the common bile duct.[64–68] Successful preoperative ERCP with clearance of the common bile duct followed by laparoscopic cholecystectomy obviates the need for common bile duct exploration.

Although many surgeons have acquired the laparoscopic skills necessary for common bile duct exploration either transcystically or directly through a choledochotomy, most surgeons lack this expertise. At this juncture, only two options are available to the operating surgeon: (1) conversion to an open surgical approach with traditional CBDE and (2) completion of the laparoscopic cholecystectomy and postoperative ERCP, sphincterotomy, and stone extraction.

Pancreatitis

Gallstone pancreatitis is a common complication of cholelithiasis and, if inappropriately treated, can lead to serious and even lethal complications. The pathophysiology of gallstone pancreatitis involves passage of stones through the ampulla of Vater where they occlude the orifice of the pancreatic duct, most often by edema. Less often a stone becomes impacted at the ampulla of Vater distal to a common channel between the common bile duct and the pancreatic duct. In both instances, pressure within the obstructed pancreatic duct increases, leading to an acute inflammatory response and pancreatitis. Gallstone pancreatitis should be suspected in any patient presenting with acute pancreatitis and gallstones. These patients invariably present with extremely high amylase and lipase levels, which usually plateau over the next 24 to 48 hours.[69,70] Ranson's prognostic criteria are helpful in objectively evaluating the severity of pancreatitis in the initial presentation and 48 hours following admission (Table 31.2). After appropriate fluid resuscitation a CT scan should be performed to assess the degree of pan-

TABLE 31.3. Balthazar computed tomography (CT) grading system for acute pancreatitis.

Grade	CT finding
A	Normal pancreas
B	Pancreatic enlargement
C	Pancreatic and/or peripancreatic fat inflammation
D	Single peripancreatic fluid collection
E	Two or more fluid collections and/or retroperitoneal air

creatitis present (Table 31.3). If the CT scan fails to reveal radiographic evidence of severe pancreatitis (Balthazar grade B or less) laparoscopic cholecystectomy and intraoperative cholangiography can safely be performed at any time.[71–73] On the hand, if severe pancreatitis is noted (Balthazar grade C or higher), surgical intervention should be deferred and a conservative approach with bowel rest and total parenteral nutrition begun.[74,75] For patients with gallstone pancreatitis who present with persistent abdominal pain and abnormal liver function tests, an emergency ERCP, sphincterotomy, and stone extraction should be performed as soon as possible.[66,76,77] What appears less clear is the appropriateness of ERCP for the patient with mild to moderate pancreatitis. Sharma's metaanalysis of randomized controlled trials examining the role ERCP and sphincterotomy in acute biliary pancreatitis revealed that morbidity and mortality were reduced by this approach. Ricci et al.,[78] reflecting the European approach, believe that regardless of the severity of pancreatitis, ERCP and sphincterotomy should initially be performed in all instances and then followed by laparoscopic cholecystectomy. This approach has not uniformly been accepted because of the risk of exacerbating acute pancreatitis by injecting a high-volume bolus of contrast material into the pancreatic duct.

Gallstone Ileus

Gallstone ileus, an uncommon complication of chronic cholecystitis, results in mechanical small bowel obstruction. With multiple bouts of acute and chronic cholecystitis and the ensuing inflammatory process, the gallbladder becomes walled off by the duodenum. As the process repeats itself, fistulization between these two hollow viscous organs occurs, providing a pathway for the migration of gallstones into the intestinal tract. Gallstones are usually trapped in the distal ileum or at the ileocecal valve, resulting in a mechanical small bowel obstruction (rather than the misnomer "ileus"). A plain abdominal x-ray may classically demonstrate dilated small bowel loops with air–fluid levels in addition to pneumobilia, air in the biliary tree (Figure 31.3). Appropriate management dictates prompt surgical intervention to relieve the small bowel obstruction.[79] At laparotomy,

TABLE 31.2. Ranson prognostic criteria for acute pancreatitis.

Parameter	Value
At admission	
Age	>55 years
White blood cell count	>16,000/μL
Serum glucose	>11 mmol/L
Alanine aminotransferase	>350 IU/L
Aspartate aminotransferase	>250 IU/L
During initial 48 hours	
Hematocrit	Decrease of more than 0.10
Blood urea nitrogen	Increase of more than 5 mg/dL
Calcium	<2 mmol/L
PaO_2	<60 mmol/L
Base deficit	>mmol/L
Fluid sequestration	>6 L

FIGURE 31.3. **(A)** Plain abdominal radiographs demonstrating small bowel dilatation, pneumobilia, and a radiopaque stone in the pelvis of a patient with gallstone ileus. **(B)** Computed tomography scans from the same patient clearly demonstrates pneumobilia and localizes the stone in the small bowel lumen.

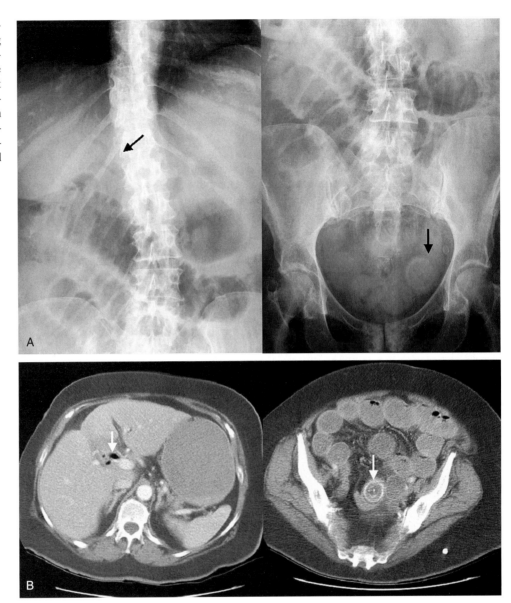

the point of obstruction is readily apparent, but multiple, often nonobstructing stones may have entered the gastrointestinal tract in up to 30% of patients. A complete and thorough evaluation of the entire small bowel becomes mandatory. Calculi found proximal to the area of obstruction should be milked upward into an area of normal bowel and extracted via a small longitudinal enterotomy that can be closed transversely.

Bowel resection is seldom necessary and is reserved only for patients with coexisting ischemia of the small bowel. Cholecystectomy and repair of the cholecystoduodenal fistula should usually be discouraged at the initial operation.[80–82]

Neoplasms

Surgical emergencies related to underlying neoplasms most commonly include tumor rupture with free hemorrhage into the greater peritoneal cavity, central tumor necrosis with abscess formation, and biliary obstruction secondary to invasion or extrinsic compression of major biliary ducts. Tumor rupture can occur in patients with either benign or malignant lesions, but abscesses and biliary obstruction are usually sequelae of malignant tumors. Each of these difficult problems requires multidisciplinary expertise for appropriate management.

Tumor Rupture

Free rupture of hepatic tumors into the peritoneal cavity can result in life-threatening hemorrhage and can pose complex and difficult management issues. Although relatively uncommon, patients with any underlying solid liver mass of significant size (>5cm) are at risk for rupture, hemorrhage, and subsequent shock. Some benign tumors are also associated with an increased risk of rupture, and, along with their counterpart malignant lesions, tumor size is considered to be a significant risk factor. Hepatic adenoma, for example, often develops in women taking oral contraceptive pills and carries a higher risk for rupture than other benign liver lesions; the pathophysiology behind the propensity for hepatic adenomas to rupture is presently unknown (Figure 31.4).[83] Giant hepatic hemangiomas also carry an elevated risk for

tumor rupture. Hemangiomas are classified as giant when their greatest diameter exceeds 5cm. Risk for rupture and other symptoms in patients with these highly vascular tumors is thought to increase proportionally with tumor diameter.[84] Any large malignant lesion can similarly rupture into the peritoneal cavity. Hepatocellular carcinoma is the most common hepatic malignancy associated with hemoperitoneum, but other malignancies, including intrahepatic Cholangiocarcinoma, metastatic adenocarcinoma, and metastatic carcinoid tumor have also been known to rupture into the peritoneal cavity.[85–87]

The clinical presentation in patients with tumor rupture is always intimately associated with abdominal pain, tachycardia, a dropping hemoglobin level, and eventual hypotension. A history of blunt trauma to the abdomen followed by the onset of symptoms is usually noted. Some patients describe very subtle blunt injury

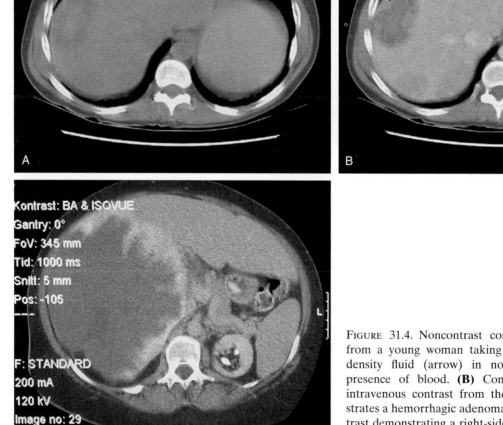

FIGURE 31.4. Noncontrast computed tomography scan (A) from a young woman taking oral contraceptive pills. High-density fluid (arrow) in noncontrast image suggests the presence of blood. (B) Computed tomography scan with intravenous contrast from the same patient clearly demonstrates a hemorrhagic adenoma (arrow). (C) CT scan with contrast demonstrating a right-sided giant hepatic hemangioma in a different patient.

before symptoms; for example, a patient whose automobile hits a bump in the road suddenly develops abdominal pain and comes directly to the emergency room.[83] Evaluation with complete blood count often reveals a severe normocytic anemia. Ultrasonography reveals free peritoneal fluid and usually confirms the presence of a liver mass. Computed tomography scanning with intravenous contrast is the preferred diagnostic modality for assessment of patients with suspected rupture of a hepatic tumor. A CT scan with contrast (1) demonstrates the extent of subcapsular hematoma; (2) allows for the distinction between ascites and free blood in the peritoneal cavity by assessing the Hownsfeld units of the fluid (>25 Hownsfeld units usually indicates the presence of blood); (3) determines the presence or absence of a "contrast blush," the hallmark of active hemorrhage; (4) identifies the exact point of hemorrhage and its relationship to major vascular and biliary structures; and (5) provides the means by which definitive control of the bleeding can be achieved through angioembolization.

The initial management of the patient with a ruptured liver tumor should include resuscitation with intravenous fluids and transfusion of blood products when necessary through large-bore intravenous catheters, followed by prompt transport of the patient (accompanied by a physician) to the angiography suite.[88] Hepatic angiography, in this instance, has a dual purpose: (1) to determine the presence of ongoing hepatic arterial or portal venous bleeding and its precise location and (2) to provide the necessary access by which selective angioembolization can arrest bleeding. Several appropriate materials are available to interrupt arterial inflow, including metallic coils, Avitene, Gelfoam, polyvinyl alcohol (PVA) beads, autologous clot, and Bioglue (Figure 31.5).

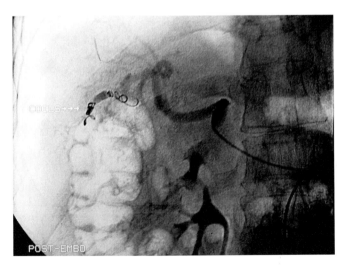

FIGURE 31.5. Postembolization angiogram of a patient with right-sided hepatocellular carcinoma. Metallic coils were used to occlude arterial inflow into this large hypervascular tumor.

Angioembolization is not always effective in controlling hemorrhage, and in such instances operative intervention may be unavoidable.[89] The most common indication for surgical management is hemodynamic instability despite all available nonoperative strategies. To achieve optimal results it would be prudent, when feasible, to have an experienced hepatobiliary surgeon present, as a rapid hepatic resection may become necessary. Emergency resection in the face of ruptured liver tumors is a highly complex and difficult procedure and is often associated with inordinately high morbidity and mortality rates. Operative intervention, if necessary, should not be approached laparoscopically. An open surgical approach is preferred, as it affords maximal exposure of the liver and represents the safest method with which to promptly control the ongoing hemorrhage. Complete resection with negative margins is not necessarily an appropriate goal in an acute care situation. For critically ill patients who are exsanguinating, the immediate objective must always be to promptly gain control of hemorrhage and then rapidly terminate any further surgery. If indicated, temporary packing, rapid towel clip closure, and planned reexploration or transfer to a facility with greater expertise in this area may be life-saving.

Abscess

Hepatic tumors that have grown to a significantly large size can go on to develop central necrosis. This feature is essentially a unique characteristic of malignancies and is almost never observed in benign neoplasms.[90] Even highly vascular malignancies such hepatocellular carcinomas can outgrow their arterial inflow, resulting in areas of necrosis. Tumor necrosis is best delineated by radiographic imaging studies that include intravenous contrast. Both CT and MRI with intravenous contrast can readily demonstrate the presence of necrosis within otherwise viable hepatic neoplasms. On rare occasion, necrotic tumors can become secondarily infected and undergo abscess formation. Once an abscess has formed, therapeutic intervention is always necessary.

Abscesses associated with liver cancers may warrant treatment plans that differ from management of their counterparts not associated with cancer. For patients with otherwise resectable tumors who exhibit mild signs of sepsis, giving intravenous antibiotics to sterilize the bloodstream followed by complete resection seems to be a reasonable approach. For patients with severe infections, not controllable with antibiotics alone, percutaneous drainage of the abscess may become necessary to achieve resolution of the infection before resection. Important considerations in formulating an individualized treatment plan include the risk of seeding the extrahepatic space with tumor cells along the percutaneous drainage route. A second consideration is the juxtaposed risk of proceeding with a formal liver resection for a patient with an unresolved infection.[91–93] This situation can pose difficult management dilemmas, and definitive decisions regarding treatment are often best made after an informed and detailed discussion with the patient.

Biliary Obstruction

Obstruction of biliary outflow secondary to hepatic, biliary, or periampullary malignancies is a commonly seen problem. The etiology of malignant biliary obstruction mimics the incidence of each tumor within a particular geographic region. In the United States and western European countries, adenocarcinoma of the pancreas is the most common cause of malignant biliary obstruction. In East Asian countries with endemic hepatitis B–positive populations, hepatocellular carcinoma is a more likely cause.

Malignant biliary obstructions can be classified according to their anatomic location in either the proximal biliary tree or distal bile duct. Although the clinical presentation may be similar in both instances, definitive treatment varies greatly.

Distal biliary tract obstruction secondary to an underlying malignancy is likely to be caused by one of four common primary periampullary tumors: (1) pancreatic adenocarcinoma, (2) distal bile duct cholangiocarcinoma, (3) periampullary carcinoma, and (4) duodenal adenocarcinoma. Other less likely possibilities include locally advanced gastric and colon cancer and a variety of metastatic carcinomas invading the porta hepatis. Classically the patient presents with painless jaundice, although in reality many patients actually present with upper abdominal or back pain. Patients also frequently describe weight loss, decreased appetite, and fatigue. Jaundiced patients are commonly evaluated initially with basic blood tests, including liver function tests and transabdominal ultrasound. All patients found to have a dilated common bile duct and a suspected periampullary mass on ultrasound must next be evaluated with CT scan with intravenous contrast or MRCP (Figure 31.6). Axial imaging studies are essential in delineating the relationship between the tumor, the common bile duct, and the surrounding blood vessels.[94,95] The proximity to an underlying neoplasm and patency of the portal vein and its branches, superior mesenteric artery, and common hepatic artery are crucial variables in determining potential resectability. Axial imaging studies are also very helpful in determining the presence of distant disease or lymphatic involvement, which usually precludes resection for cure.

Patients who present with malignant distal biliary obstruction and a resectable tumor without metastases should not be immediately referred for endoscopic or percutaneous biliary drainage procedures unless the

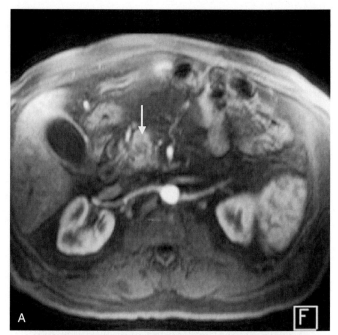

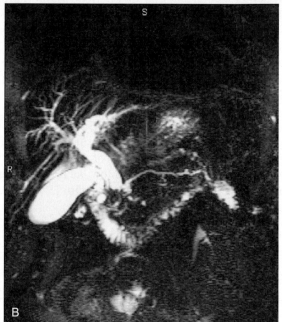

FIGURE 31.6. **(A)** Magnetic resonance image with intravenous contrast demonstrating a mass in the head of the pancreas (arrow) with decreased signal intensity, suggestive of neoplasm. **(B)** Magnetic resonance image with emphasis on cholangiopancreatography demonstrating a double duct sign in a patient with biliary obstruction secondary to a malignant neoplasm in the head of the pancreas.

predominant clinical picture is consistent with cholangitis and ongoing sepsis. When definitive resection can be offered within a reasonable period of time (1 week), there is justification in allowing biliary obstruction to continue until resection and a surgical biliary–enteric reconstruction can be accomplished. This approach is strengthened by the following theoretical advantages: (1) the cost and risks of a potentially unnecessary procedure are avoided; (2) indwelling biliary stents produce peri-ampullary inflammatory changes that may increase the difficulty of resection; and (3) a foreign body in the biliary tree can lead to contamination of a previously sterile compartment.[96]

Patients for whom complete resection cannot be offered within a reasonable period of time should be managed with early ERCP and stent placement or PTC.[97] Operative biliary bypass procedures for patients who are not candidates for complete resection are currently discouraged. Avoidance of surgical biliary bypass procedures has been extensively documented in the literature. Several retrospective studies on this topic have definitively demonstrated that patients with unresectable peri-ampullary malignancies have a median survival time of less than 12 months and thus will subsequently require only a minimal number of stent changes during that period of time. Moreover, only a fraction of patients managed with nonoperative biliary drainage will fail and ultimately require a surgical bypass.[98–100] An exception to this approach is the patient who presents with an unresectable periampullary malignancy along with biliary and gastric outlet obstruction. For such patients prompt operative intervention is justified to reconstruct both gastric and biliary drainage.

Patients with proximal biliary obstruction often pose a more difficult problem than those with distal obstruction. Common etiologies for proximal biliary obstruction include proximal cholangiocarcinoma and hepatocellular carcinoma. Evaluation with liver function tests and ultrasound is appropriate in the initial period. Computed tomography with contrast or MRI is essential in the diagnostic work up of these patients. Most hepatobiliary surgeons would not advocate prompt surgical management without anatomic delineation of the proximal biliary tree and its relationship to the area of obstruction. Although often helpful for diagnostic purposes, ERCP is of limited therapeutic value in cases of high malignant biliary strictures because of the technical difficulty involved in advancing stents across a high stricture via an endoscopic approach. Percutaneous transhepatic cholangiography is more likely to provide both important diagnostic information and a portal for further therapeutic maneuvers. Technical challenges in performing adequate PTC in these patients relate to the involvement of the right, left, or bilateral biliary trees. Protection from cholangitis and sepsis is relatively straightforward by the placement of an external drain above the level of obstruction. In some instances both right and left catheter placement may be necessary to achieve complete decompression for lesions situated at the bifurcation of the main hepatic ducts. After an initial period of decompression with external

drainage, the drainage stent can then be internalized, allowing for free flow of bile into the duodenum. Resectability is ultimately determined by several factors: (1) the absence of extrahepatic disease, (2) the relationship of the tumor to major surrounding vascular structures, (3) the ability to spare an adequate amount of functional hepatic parenchyma, and (4) the technical feasibility of constructing a biliary enteric anastomosis.

Portal Hypertension

Cirrhosis of the liver secondary to any underlying etiology results in increased pressure within the portal venous system. The pathophysiology responsible for portal hypertension is related to increased resistance in small central veins that results from parenchymal fibrosis.[101,102] Similar changes also occur in patients with major hepatic venous outflow obstruction, such as those with Budd-Chiari syndrome. The common sequelae of portal hypertension are numerous and include varices, hypersplenism, and thrombocytopenia. Variceal hemorrhage is the most life-threatening complication in the acute setting, and it can lead to extraordinarily difficult management issues. Although varices can develop in a number of anatomic locations, esophageal and gastric varices are most common.

Esophageal variceal hemorrhage manifests initially as hematemesis, and patients with bleeding esophageal varices can lose massive quantities of blood in a very brief period of time. Prompt diagnosis and treatment are essential. Several diagnostic modalities such as CT and angiography are useful in detecting the presence of esophageal varices in the elective setting.[103] Upper endoscopy, however, remains the most useful diagnostic tool in both the elective and acute setting. Endoscopy with direct visualization of varices is highly accurate and also provides the opportunity for treatment of bleeding varices by banding or direct injection of sclerosing agents.[104,105] Endoscopy in patients with bleeding esophageal varices must be approached with extreme caution as hemorrhage can be exacerbated by the mechanical stress on the wall of the esophagus during the procedure. Although endoscopic therapy is effective in the setting of minimal or no hemorrhage, it is marginally useful as a therapeutic maneuver in the patient with massive hemorrhage.

Treatment of the patient with significant acute variceal hemorrhage must be aggressive and rapidly implemented. Resuscitation with intravenous fluid, transfusion of blood products, and correction of underlying coagulopathy are obvious initial measures. These patients may deteriorate rapidly with the sudden onset of hemodynamic collapse, often with little warning. The unpredictable nature of the patient with active esophageal variceal bleeding would mandate that they be monitored in a critical care unit. In addition to giving a somatostatin analog (octreotide), once the diagnosis of esophageal variceal hemorrhage is definitively established, placement of a Sengstaken-Blakemore (SB) tube can be life saving.[106] Proper placement of an SB tube requires some familiarity with the device.[107] These tubes are modified nasogastric tubes that contain two separate balloons: a long esophageal balloon along its shaft and a spherical gastric balloon at its end. Each of these balloons is insufflated separately, and balloon pressure must be measured carefully during insufflation. The underlying design of the SB tube is based on insufflation of the esophageal balloon to a pressure high enough to occlude variceal blood flow but low enough to avoid pressure necrosis of the esophagus (24 to 45 mm Hg). The gastric balloon is insufflated before the esophageal balloon, and it serves to facilitate gentle traction along the gastric cardia, which is held with a counterweight at the patient's bedside. Extreme care must be taken to avoid inadvertent insufflation of the gastric balloon within the esophagus, as a catastrophic esophageal blowout can result. The tubes are uncomfortable, and adequate sedation of the unobtunded patient is necessary. It has been our practice to intubate all patients requiring the insertion of an SB tube to prevent aspiration.

Sengstaken-Blakemore tube placement in addition to other effective nonoperative measures such as beta blockade and intravenous pitressin serve only as temporizing measures for patients with portal hypertension.[108,109] Definitive long-term treatment requires reduction of portal venous hypertension via a portal-systemic shunt. Two successful approaches may be employed, depending on institutional expertise: (1) surgical portal-caval shunt and (2) interventional transjugular portal-systemic shunt (TIPSS).[110] Despite the controversy regarding which of the two methods is superior overall, both have proven highly effective at controlling hemorrhage in the setting of acute variceal bleeding.

Many surgical variations for portal-caval shunting, including an end-to-side portal-caval shunt, side-to-side portal-caval shunt, or the prosthetic interposition H-graft technique, have been used with success. The latter surgical approach is the only one to have been compared with TIPSS in a randomized prospective study. Rosemurgy and colleagues[111–113] have reported on their extensive experience with both surgical H-graft shunts and TIPSS. In their prospective experience, results with surgical portal-caval shunting were slightly superior than those with TIPSS. The data provided by Rosemurgy notwithstanding, most tertiary care centers perform far more TIPSS procedures than surgically created portal-caval shunts. As expertise, ease, and success by interventional radiologists in TIPSS insertion increase, this approach

would seem to outweigh the marginal benefits and the associated morbidity of an operative portal-caval shunt.[114,115]

Hemobilia

Hemobilia is rare condition that most commonly occurs as a result of either trauma to the liver or iatrogenic injury. Other less likely etiologies include rupture of neoplasm or arterial-venous malformation with hemorrhage into the biliary tree. Endoscopy may play a useful role in establishing the correct diagnosis if blood is seen coming from the ampulla of Vater. In most instances, further diagnosis and management should be made with angiography and angioembolization when feasible. Angiography provides essential diagnostic information by localizing the source of hemorrhage. Following localization, selective hepatic arterial embolization is usually highly effective in controlling hemorrhage.[116,117]

Operative intervention, however, may be necessary for patients with hemodynamic instability secondary to ongoing hemorrhage not controlled by embolization. Surgery is predicated upon suture ligation of bleeding vessels within the hepatic parenchyma or resection of the segment(s) within which hemorrhage has been localized. These procedures are difficult and require an intimate familiarity with complex hepatobiliary surgical techniques.

Critique

The constellation of symptoms and findings is strongly suggestive of a suppurative cholangitis. Further diagnostic screening would probably confirm a dilated and blocked distal common bile duct (choledocholithiasis). The intervention that this critically ill patient should undergo, at this time, is an endoscopic retrograde cholangiography, with removal of a lodged stone in the common bile duct. A cholecystectomy and further evaluation of the biliary radicals can be performed at another time when the patient has recovered from this acute problem.

Answer (D)

References

1. Couinaud C. Liver anatomy: portal (and suprahepatic) or biliary segmentation. Dig Surg 1999; 16:459–467.
2. Botero AC, Strasberg SM. Division of the left hemiliver in man—segments, sectors, or sections. Liver Transplant Surg 1998; 4:226–231.

3. Strasberg SM. Terminology of liver anatomy and liver resections: coming to grips with hepatic Babel. J Am Coll Surg 1997; 184:413–434.

4. Jung G, Krahe T, Krug B, Hahn U, Raab M. Delineation of segmental liver anatomy. Comparison of ultrasonography, spiral CT and MR imaging for preoperative localization of focal liver lesions to specific hepatic segments. Acta Radiol 1996; 37:691–695.

5. Amitrano L, Guardascione MA, Brancaccio V, Balzano A. Coagulation disorders in liver disease. Semin Liver Dis 2002; 22:83–96.

6. Roe PG. Liver function tests in the critically ill patient. Clin Intensive Care 1993; 4:174–182.

7. Moseley RH. Evaluation of abnormal liver function tests. Med Clin North Am 1996; 80:887–906.

8. Lauterburg BH. Assessment of liver function prior to hepatic resection. Swiss Surg 1999; 5:92–96.

9. Shaked A, Nunes FA, Olthoff KM, Lucey MR. Assessment of liver function: pre- and peritransplant evaluation. Clin Chem 1997; 43:1539–1545.

10. Blendis L, Wong F. The hyperdynamic circulation in cirrhosis: an overview. Pharmacol Ther 2001; 89:221–231.

11. Fenchel S, Fleiter TR, Merkle EM. Multislice helical CT of the abdomen. Eur Radiol 2002; 12(Suppl 2):S5–S10.

12. Delgado Millan MA, Deballon PO. Computed tomography, angiography, and endoscopic retrograde cholangiopancreatography in the nonoperative management of hepatic and splenic trauma. World J Surg 2001; 25:1397–1402.

13. Brink JA. Contrast optimization and scan timing for single and multidetector-row computed tomography. J Comput Assist Tomogr 2003; 27(Suppl 1):S3–S8.

14. Mortele KJ, McTavish J, Ros PR. Current techniques of computed tomography. Helical CT, multidetector CT, and 3D reconstruction. Clin Liver Dis 2002; 6:29–52.

15. Nelson RC, Spielmann AL. Liver imaging with multidetector helical computed tomography. J Comput Assist Tomogr 2003; 27(Suppl 1):S9–S16.

16. Reddy SI, Grace ND. Liver imaging. A hepatologist's perspective. Clin Liver Dis 2002; 6:297–310, ix.

17. Ros PR, Mortele KJ. Hepatic imaging. An overview. Clin Liver Dis 2002; 6:1–16.

18. Vauthey JN, Rousseau DL Jr. Liver imaging. A surgeon's perspective. Clin Liver Dis 2002; 6:271–295.

19. Shankar S, van Sonnenberg E, Silverman SG, Tuncali K. Interventional radiology procedures in the liver. Biopsy, drainage, and ablation. Clin Liver Dis 2002; 6:91–118.

20. Huang CJ, Pitt HA, Lipsett PA, et al. Pyogenic hepatic abscess. Changing trends over 42 years. Ann Surg 1996; 223:600–609.

21. Pereira FE, Musso C, Castelo JS. Pathology of pyogenic liver abscess in children. Pediatr Dev Pathol 1999; 2:537–543.

22. Barakate MS, Stephen MS, Waugh RC, et al. Pyogenic liver abscess: a review of 10 years' experience in management. Aust N Z J Surg 1999; 69:205–209.

23. Moore SW, Millar AJ, Cywes S. Conservative initial treatment for liver abscesses in children. Br J Surg 1994; 81: 872–874.

24. Brolin RE, Nosher JL, Leiman S, Lee WS, Greco RS. Percutaneous catheter versus open surgical drainage in the treatment of abdominal abscesses. Am Surg 1984; 50:102–108.

25. Lang EK, Springer RM, Glorioso LW III, et al. Abdominal abscess drainage under radiology guidance: causes of failure. Radiology 1986; 159:329–336.

26. van Sonnenberg E, Wittich GR, Casola G, et al. Percutaneous drainage of infected and noninfected pancreatic pseudocysts: experience in 101 cases. Radiology 1989; 170:757–761.

27. Goletti O, Lippolis PV, Chiarugi M, et al. Percutaneous ultrasound-guided drainage of intra-abdominal abscesses. Br J Surg 1993; 80:336–339.

28. Voros D, Gouliamos A, Kotoulas G, Kouloheri D, Saloum G, Kalovidouris A. Percutaneous drainage of intra-abdominal abscesses using large lumen tubes under computed tomographic control. Eur J Surg 1996; 162:895–898.

29. Ch Yu S, Hg Lo R, Kan PS, Metreweli C. Pyogenic liver abscess: treatment with needle aspiration. Clin Radiol 1997; 52:912–916.

30. Gerzof SG, Johnson WC, Robbins AH, et al. Expanded criteria for percutaneous abscess drainage. Arch Surg 1985; 120:227–232.

31. Sharma MP, Dasarathy S, Sushma S, Verma N. Long term follow-up of amebic liver abscess: clinical and ultrasound patterns of resolution. Trop Gastroenterol 1995; 16:24–28.

32. Carpenter HA. Bacterial and parasitic cholangitis. Mayo Clin Proc 1998; 73:473–478.

33. Sinanan MN. Acute cholangitis. Infect Dis Clin North Am 1992; 6:571–599.

34. Nahrwold DL. Acute cholangitis. Surgery 1992; 112:487–488.

35. Kimmings AN, van Deventer SJ, Rauws EAJ, Huibregtse K, Gouma DJ. Systemic inflammatory response in acute cholangitis and after subsequent treatment. Eur J Surg 2000; 166:700–705.

36. Rerknimitr R, Fogel EL, Kalayci C, Esber E, Lehman GA, Sherman S. Microbiology of bile in patients with cholangitis or cholestasis with and without plastic biliary endoprosthesis. Gastrointest Endosc 2002; 56:885–889.

37. Sheen-Chen S, Chen W, Eng H, et al. Bacteriology and antimicrobial choice in hepatolithiasis. Am J Infect Control 2000; 28:298–301.

38. Karachalios GN, Zografos G, Patrikakos V, Nassopoulou D, Kehagioglou K. Biliary tract infections treated with ciprofloxacin. Infection 1993; 21:262–264.

39. Gumaste VV. Antibiotics and cholangitis. Gastroenterology 1995; 109:323–325.

40. Sung JJ, Lyon DJ, Suen R, et al. Intravenous ciprofloxacin as treatment for patients with acute suppurative cholangitis: a randomized, controlled clinical trial. J Antimicrob Chemother 1995; 35:855–864.

41. Siegel JH, Rodriquez R, Cohen SA, Kasmin FE, Cooperman AM. Endoscopic management of cholangitis: critical review of an alternative technique and report of a large series. Am J Gastroenterol 1994; 89:1142–1146.

42. Lee WJ, Chang KJ, Lee CS, Chen KM. Surgery in cholangitis: bacteriology and choice of antibiotic. Hepatogastroenterology 1992; 39:347–349.

43. Balci NC, Sirvanci M. MR imaging of infective liver lesions. Magn Reson Imaging Clin North Am 2002; 10:121–135, vii.

44. Barreda R, Ros PR. Diagnostic imaging of liver abscess. Crit Rev Diagn Imaging 1992; 33:29–58.

45. Fujihara T, Nagai Y, Kubo T, Seki S, Satake K. Amebic liver abscess. J Gastroenterol 1996; 31:659–663.

46. Hughes MA, Petri WA Jr. Amebic liver abscess. Infect Dis Clin North Am 2000; 14:565–582, viii.

47. Sharma MP, Dasarathy S. Amoebic liver abscess. Trop Gastroenterol 1993; 14:3–9.

48. Pedrosa I, Saiz A, Arrazola J, Ferreiros J, Pedrosa CS. Hydatid disease: radiologic and pathologic features and complications. Radiographics 2000; 20:795–817.

49. Gunay K, Taviloglu K, Berber E, Ertekin C. Traumatic rupture of hydatid cysts: a 12-year experience from an endemic region. J Trauma 1999; 46:164–167.

50. Bartoloni C, Tricerri A, Guidi L, Gambassi G. The efficacy of chemotherapy with mebendazole in human cystic echinococcosis: long-term follow-up of 52 patients. Ann Trop Med Parasitol 1992; 86:249–256.

51. De Rosa F, Teggi A. Treatment of *Echinococcus granulosus* hydatid disease with albendazole. Ann Trop Med Parasitol 1990; 84:467–872.

52. Sakai Y. Images in clinical medicine. Emphysematous cholecystitis. N Engl J Med 2003; 348:2329.

53. Yusoff IF, Barkun JS, Barkun AN. Diagnosis and management of cholecystitis and cholangitis. Gastroenterol Clin North Am 2003; 32:1145–1168.

54. Fayad LM, Holland GA, Bergin D, et al. Functional magnetic resonance cholangiography (fMRC) of the gallbladder and biliary tree with contrast-enhanced magnetic resonance cholangiography. J Magn Reson Imaging 2003; 18:449–460.

55. Gore RM, Yaghmai V, Newmark GM, Berlin JW, Miller FH. Imaging benign and malignant disease of the gallbladder. Radiol Clin North Am 2002; 40:1307–1323, vi.

56. Johansson M, Thune A, Blomqvist A, Nelvin L, Lundell L. Management of acute cholecystitis in the laparoscopic era: results of a prospective, randomized clinical trial. J Gastrointest Surg 2003; 7:642–645.

57. Kitano S, Matsumoto T, Aramaki M, Kawano K. Laparoscopic cholecystectomy for acute cholecystitis. J Hepatobiliary Pancreat Surg 2002; 9:534–537.

58. Bhattacharya D, Senapati PS, Hurle R, Ammori BJ. Urgent versus interval laparoscopic cholecystectomy for acute cholecystitis: a comparative study. J Hepatobiliary Pancreat Surg 2002; 9:538–542.

59. Papi C, Catarci M, D'Ambrosio L, et al. Timing of cholecystectomy for acute calculous cholecystitis: a meta-analysis. Am J Gastroenterol 2004; 99:147–155.

60. Senapati PS, Bhattarcharya D, Harinath G, Ammori BJ. A survey of the timing and approach to the surgical management of cholelithiasis in patients with acute biliary pancreatitis and acute cholecystitis in the UK. Ann R Coll Surg Engl 2003; 85:306–312.

61. Serralta AS, Bueno JL, Planells MR, Rodero DR. Prospective evaluation of emergency versus delayed laparoscopic cholecystectomy for early cholecystitis. Surg Laparosc Endosc Percutan Tech 2003; 13:71–75.

62. Byrne MF, Suhocki P, Mitchell RM, et al. Percutaneous cholecystostomy in patients with acute cholecystitis: experience of 45 patients at a US referral center. J Am Coll Surg 2003; 197:206–211.

63. Haroun A, Hadidi A, Tarawneh E, Shennak M. Magnetic resonance cholangiopancreatography in patients with upper abdominal pain: a prospective study. Hepatogastroenterology 2003; 50:1236–1241.

64. Raraty MG, Finch M, Neoptolemos JP. Acute cholangitis and pancreatitis secondary to common duct stones: management update. World J Surg 1998; 22:1155–1161.

65. Himal HS. Common bile duct stones: the role of preoperative, intraoperative, and postoperative ERCP. Semin Laparosc Surg 2000; 7:237–245.

66. Hammarstrom LE, Andersson R, Stridbeck H, Ihse I. Influence of bile duct stones on patient features and effect of endoscopic sphincterotomy on early outcome of edematous gallstone pancreatitis. World J Surg 1999; 23:12–17.

67. Yao LQ, Zhang YQ, Zhou PH, Gao WD, He GJ, Xu MD. Endoscopic sphincterotomy or papillary balloon dilatation for choledocholithiasis. Hepatobiliary Pancreat Dis Int 2002; 1:101–105.

68. Brooks AD, Mallis MJ, Brennan MF, Conlon KC. The value of laparoscopy in the management of ampullary, duodenal, and distal bile duct tumors. J Gastrointest Surg 2002; 6:139–146.

69. Cohen ME, Slezak L, Wells CK, Andersen DK, Topazian M. Prediction of bile duct stones and complications in gallstone pancreatitis using early laboratory trends. Am J Gastroenterol 2001; 96:3305–3311.

70. Meek K, de Virgilio C, Murrell Z, et al. Correlation between admission laboratory values, early abdominal computed tomography, and severe complications of gallstone pancreatitis. Am J Surg 2000; 180:556–560.

71. Balthazar EJ, Robinson DL, Megibow AJ, Ranson JH. Acute pancreatitis: value of CT in establishing prognosis. Radiology 1990; 174:331–336.

72. Balthazar EJ. Complications of acute pancreatitis: clinical and CT evaluation. Radiol Clin North Am 2002; 40:1211–1227.

73. Balthazar EJ. Acute pancreatitis: assessment of severity with clinical and CT evaluation. Radiology 2002; 223:603–613.

74. Pisters PW, Ranson JH. Nutritional support for acute pancreatitis. Surg Gynecol Obstet 1992; 175:275–284.

75. Ranson JH, Rifkind KM, Roses DF, Fink SD, Eng K, Spencer FC. Prognostic signs and the role of operative management in acute pancreatitis. Surg Gynecol Obstet 1974; 139:69–81.

76. Barkun AN. Early endoscopic management of acute gallstone pancreatitis—an evidence-based review. J Gastrointest Surg 2001; 5:243–250.

77. Kaw M, Al-Antably Y, Kaw P. Management of gallstone pancreatitis: cholecystectomy or ERCP and endoscopic sphincterotomy. Gastrointest Endosc 2002; 56:61–65.

78. Ricci F, Castaldini G, de Manzoni G, et al. Treatment of gallstone pancreatitis: six-year experience in a single center. World J Surg 2002; 26:85–90.

79. Lobo DN, Jobling JC, Balfour TW. Gallstone ileus: diagnostic pitfalls and therapeutic successes. J Clin Gastroenterol 2000; 30:72–76.

80. Doko M, Zovak M, Kopljar M, Glavan E, Ljubicic N, Hochstadter H. Comparison of surgical treatments of gallstone ileus: preliminary report. World J Surg 2003; 27:400–404.

81. Reisner RM, Cohen JR. Gallstone ileus: a review of 1001 reported cases. Am Surg 1994; 60:441–446.

82. Zuegel N, Hehl A, Lindemann F, Witte J. Advantages of one-stage repair in case of gallstone ileus. Hepatogastroenterology 1997; 44:59–62.

83. Suarez-Penaranda JM, de la Calle MC, Rodriguez-Calvo MS, Munoz JI, Concheiro L. Rupture of liver cell adenoma with fatal massive hemoperitoneum resulting from minor road accident. Am J Forensic Med Pathol 2001; 22:275–277.

84. Hotokezaka M, Kojima M, Nakamura K, et al. Traumatic rupture of hepatic hemangioma. J Clin Gastroenterol 1996; 23:69–71.

85. Yoshida H, Onda M, Tajiri T, et al. Treatment of spontaneous ruptured hepatocellular carcinoma. Hepatogastroenterology 1999; 46:2451–2453.

86. Sonoda T, Kanematsu T, Takenaka K, Sugimachi K. Ruptured hepatocellular carcinoma evokes risk of implanted metastases. J Surg Oncol 1989; 41:183–186.

87. Vergara V, Muratore A, Bouzari H, et al. Spontaneous rupture of hepatocellular carcinoma: surgical resection and long-term survival. Eur J Surg Oncol 2000; 26:770–772.

88. Sato Y, Fujiwara K, Furui S, et al. Benefit of transcatheter arterial embolization for ruptured hepatocellular carcinoma complicating liver cirrhosis. Gastroenterology 1985; 89:157–159.

89. Shimada R, Imamura H, Makuuchi M, et al. Staged hepatectomy after emergency transcatheter arterial embolization for ruptured hepatocellular carcinoma. Surgery 1998; 124:526–535.

90. Sarmiento JM, Sarr MG. Necrotic infected liver metastasis from colon cancer. Surgery 2002; 132:110–111.

91. Huang SF, Ko CW, Chang CS, Chen GH. Liver abscess formation after transarterial chemoembolization for malignant hepatic tumor. Hepatogastroenterology 2003; 50:1115–1118.

92. Kim W, Clark TW, Baum RA, Soulen MC. Risk factors for liver abscess formation after hepatic chemoembolization. J Vasc Intervent Radiol 2001; 12:965–968.

93. Song SY, Chung JW, Han JK, et al. Liver abscess after transcatheter oily chemoembolization for hepatic tumors: incidence, predisposing factors, and clinical outcome. J Vasc Intervent Radiol 2001; 12:313–320.

94. Yeh TS, Jan YY, Tseng JH, et al. Malignant perihilar biliary obstruction: magnetic resonance cholangiopancreatographic findings. Am J Gastroenterol 2000; 95:432–440.

95. Georgopoulos SK, Schwartz LH, Jarnagin WR, et al. Comparison of magnetic resonance and endoscopic retrograde cholangiopancreatography in malignant pancreaticobiliary obstruction. Arch Surg 1999; 134:1002–1007.

96. Marcus SG, Dobryansky M, Shamamian P, et al. Endoscopic biliary drainage before pancreaticoduodenectomy for periampullary malignancies. J Clin Gastroenterol 1998; 26:125–129.

97. Lai EC, Lo CM, Liu CL. Endoscopic stenting for malignant biliary obstruction. World J Surg 2001; 25:1289–1295.

98. Espat NJ, Brennan MF, Conlon KC. Patients with laparoscopically staged unresectable pancreatic adenocarcinoma do not require subsequent surgical biliary or gastric bypass. J Am Coll Surg 1999; 188:649–657.

99. Lillemoe KD, Cameron JL, Hardacre JM, et al. Is prophylactic gastrojejunostomy indicated for unresectable periampullary cancer? A prospective randomized trial. Ann Surg 1999; 230:322–330.

100. Sohn TA, Lillemoe KD. Surgical palliation of pancreatic cancer. Adv Surg 2000; 34:249–271.

101. MacMathuna P, Vlavianos P, Westaby D, Williams R. Pathophysiology of portal hypertension. Dig Dis 1992; 10(Suppl 1):3–15.

102. McCormick PA, Jenkins SA, McIntyre N, Burroughs AK. Why portal hypertensive varices bleed and bleed: a hypothesis. Gut 1995; 36:100–103.

103. Hoefs JC, Jonas GM, Sarfeh IJ. Diagnosis and hemodynamic assessment of portal hypertension. Surg Clin North Am 1990; 70:267–289.

104. Celinska-Cedro D, Teisseyre M, Woynarowski M, Socha P, Socha J, Ryzko J. Endoscopic ligation of esophageal varices for prophylaxis of first bleeding in children and adolescents with portal hypertension: preliminary results of a prospective study. J Pediatr Surg 2003; 38:1008–1011.

105. Yoshikawa I, Murata I, Nakano S, Otsuki M. Effects of endoscopic variceal ligation on portal hypertensive gastropathy and gastric mucosal blood flow. Am J Gastroenterol 1998; 93:71–74.

106. Teres J, Cecilia A, Bordas JM, Rimola A, Bru C, Rodes J. Esophageal tamponade for bleeding varices. Controlled trial between the Sengstaken-Blakemore tube and the Linton-Nachlas tube. Gastroenterology 1978; 75:566–569.

107. McCormick PA, Burroughs AK, McIntyre N. How to insert a Sengstaken-Blakemore tube. Br J Hosp Med 1990; 43:274–277.

108. Sokucu S, Suoglu OD, Elkabes B, Saner G. Long-term outcome after sclerotherapy with or without a beta-blocker for variceal bleeding in children. Pediatr Int 2003; 45:388–394.

109. Schiedermaier P, Koch L, Stoffel-Wagner B, Layer G, Sauerbruch T. Effect of propranolol and depot lanreotide SR on postprandial and circadian portal haemodynamics in cirrhosis. Aliment Pharmacol Ther 2003; 18:777–784.

110. Gusberg RJ. Distal splenorenal shunt—premise, perspective, practice. Dig Dis 1992; 10(Suppl 1):84–93.

111. Rosemurgy AS 2nd, Bloomston M, Zervos EE, et al. Transjugular intrahepatic portosystemic shunt versus H-graft portacaval shunt in the management of bleeding varices: a cost-benefit analysis. Surgery 1997; 122:794–800.

112. Serafini FM, Zwiebel B, Black TJ, Carey LC, Rosemurgy AS 2nd. Transjugular intrahepatic portasystemic stent shunt in the treatment of variceal bleeding in hepatocellular cancer. Dig Dis Sci 1997; 42:59–65.

113. Rosemurgy AS, Serafini FM, Zweibel BR, et al. Transjugular intrahepatic portosystemic shunt vs. small-diameter prosthetic H-graft portacaval shunt: extended follow-up of an expanded randomized prospective trial. J Gastrointest Surg 2000; 4:589–97.

114. McCormick PA, Dick R, Chin J, et al. Transjugular intrahepatic portosystemic stent-shunt. Br J Hosp Med 1993; 49:791–797.

115. Boyer TD. Transjugular intrahepatic portosystemic shunt: current status. Gastroenterology 2003; 124:1700–1710.

116. Pachter HL, Hofstetter SR. The current status of non-operative management of adult blunt hepatic injuries. Am J Surg 1995; 169:442–454.

117. Pachter HL. Is a conservative approach justified in penetrating liver injury? HPB Surg 1995; 8:205–208.

32
Pancreas

Juan A. Asensio, Patrizio Petrone, and L.D. Britt

Case Scenario

You are asked to evaluate a patient who was admitted for alcohol-induced pancreatitis. The patient has had a smoldering course despite aggressive resuscitation and is, currently, febrile and toxic while receiving broad-spectrum antimicrobial therapy. Physical examination demonstrates midepigastric tenderness on moderate palpation. Computed tomography scan findings are consistent for necrotizing pancreatitis. The white blood cell count has increased from 12,000 to 16,000 over the past 48 hours. Which of the following is the most prudent management plan at this time?

(A) Continued medical management
(B) Peritoneal lavage
(C) Computed tomography—directed biopsy of the necrotic tissue for confirmation of infectious etiology
(D) Celiotomy
(E) Administration of octreotide

The pancreas is a classic example of an organ poorly designed to withstand the ravages of trauma. Located in the inaccessible and dark reaches of the retroperitoneum, injuries to the pancreas are infrequently suspected and often diagnosed late while more apparent injuries to other organs are addressed. Furthermore, as if to add an insult to injury, pancreatic injuries can be missed, even by experienced trauma surgeons. The soft consistency of this organ and its marginal blood supply, which is shared with the duodenum, are not amenable to sound, leak-proof repairs that heal uneventfully. Pancreatic resections, particularly those involving the head, are extremely difficult procedures, especially when performed under the adverse physiologic conditions of shock or exsanguination.

Because it lies against a most unyielding neighbor, the spinal column, the pancreas is extremely susceptible to crush injury. The pancreas, when injured, can be quite an unforgiving organ. Its myriad of enzymatic byproducts, used for digestion, can also cause injury to the host by digesting suture lines used to repair hollow viscera or vascular structures. Repairing or resecting the pancreas is technically challenging, especially at the time of suturing. Its soft consistency is often not amenable to the placement of sutures. Any less than delicate moves during repair or any undue application of force during its mobilization will be met with tearing or bleeding from the gland that can be quite difficult to control.

Pertinent Anatomy for Trauma Surgeons

The pancreas lies transversally in the retroperitoneum across the upper abdomen. It measures between 15 and 20 cm in length, approximately 3 cm in width, and 1 to 1.5 cm in thickness. Its average weight is approximately 90 g, with a normal weight ranging from 40 to 180 g. It is almost triangular in shape and is related to the omental bursa above, the transverse mesocolon anteriorly, and the greater abdominal cavity below. Its motion is relatively limited; therefore, for all practical purposes, it is considered a fixed organ. The pancreas is anteriorly related to the liver, duodenum, pylorus, stomach, and spleen above; the duodenum, jejunum, transverse colon, and spleen below; and at the same level as the transverse colon, mesocolon, and spleen. Posterior to the pancreas and sharing an anatomically intimate relationship are the aorta, inferior vena cava, both right and left renal veins, and right renal artery. The pancreas is also in close proximity to the hilum of the right kidney. The superior mesenteric artery and vein course posterior to the neck of the pancreas, in their groove, and are closely attached to the uncinate process, with the uncinate wrapping around the posterolateral aspect of the vein. The head of the pancreas lies within the concave sweep of the duodenum, with the body directly crossing the spine and angularly directed superiorly and toward the left shoulder, with the tail in close communication with the hilum of the spleen.

The pancreas is arbitrarily divided into five parts: the head, the uncinate process, the neck, the body, and the tail. Although variations in the shape of the pancreas are known, they are of little surgical importance. The head of the pancreas is defined as the portion lying to the right of the superior mesenteric artery and vein. It is located at the level of the second lumbar vertebra in the midline or slightly to the right of it. The head of the pancreas is located to the left of the spinal column in approximately 5% of individuals.[1] It lies nestled in the C-loop of the duodenum and, in conjunction with it, is suspended from the liver by the hepatoduodenal ligament; thus it is firmly fixed to the medial aspect of the second and third portions of the duodenum. The divisory line between the head and the neck is marked anteriorly by a line originating from the portal vein superiorly to the superior mesenteric vein inferiorly. The head of the pancreas is flattened. Its anterior surface is related to the pylorus and transverse colon.

The anterior pancreaticoduodenal arcade parallels the duodenal curvature but is related to the anterior pancreatic surface rather than to the duodenum. Similarly, the posterior surface of the head of the pancreas is related to the hilum and medial border of the right kidney, the right renovascular pedicle, the inferior vena cava and ostia of the left renal vein as it drains into the inferior vena cava, the right crus of the diaphragm, the posterior pancreaticoduodenal arcade, and the right gonadal vein. The distal portion of the common bile duct is usually totally or partially embedded in the pancreatic substance in 85% or lies in a groove behind the pancreatic head in 15% of the cases. An abnormal hepatic or middle colic artery may lie within or behind the head.[2]

The uncinate process of the pancreas is an extension of the lower left part of the posterior surface of the head, usually passing behind the portal vein and the superior mesenteric vessels just anteriorly to the aorta and inferior vena cava. The presence of the uncinate process is variable. It may be absent, or it may completely encircle the superior mesenteric vessels. Knowledge of its presence should always be taken into consideration when planning distal pancreatectomy.

The neck of the pancreas measures approximately 1.5 to 2 cm in length and lies at the level of the first lumbar vertebra. It is fixed between the celiac trunk superiorly and the superior mesenteric vessels inferiorly. It is defined as that portion that overlies the superior mesenteric vessels. Anteriorly, the neck is partially covered by the pylorus. To the right, the gastroduodenal artery gives off the superior pancreaticoduodenal artery. Posteriorly the union of the superior mesenteric and splenic veins forms the portal vein. In general, there are no anterior tributaries to this vessel. However, one or two small veins may enter directly the portal vein, and four to five may enter the superior mesenteric vein. Making contributions to the portal vein from the right are a few short lateral veins, whereas entering the portal vein from the left are both the left gastric and splenic veins and rarely the inferior mesenteric vein.

The body of the pancreas lies at the level of the first lumbar vertebra and is technically defined as that portion of the pancreas that lies to the left of the superior mesenteric vessels. It is triangularly shaped and is related to the fourth portion to the duodenum and the ligament of Treitz. Both superior mesenteric vessels emerge from under the inferior border of the body and pass over the uncinate process of the head of the pancreas. The crossing over of these vessels divides the third and the fourth portions of the duodenum. The superior border of the body of the pancreas is related to the celiac axis and hepatic artery on the right and to the splenic vessels on the left. The splenic artery and vein course along its superior border. The anterior surface of the body of the pancreas is covered by the posterior wall of the omental bursa that separates the pancreas from the stomach. It is also related to the transverse mesocolon that separates into two layers, one leaf covering its anterior and one leaf covering its inferior surface. The middle colic artery emerges from beneath the inferior border of the pancreas to course through the leaves of the mesocolon. The inferior mesenteric vein is close to the distal portion of the inferior border of the body. The posterior surface is in close proximity to the origin of the superior mesenteric artery, left crus of the diaphragm, the left renovascular pedicle, left kidney, and adrenal gland. The tail of the pancreas rises to the level of the twelfth thoracic vertebra. It is quite mobile. This lends for easy mobilization while its tip is closely related to the hilum of the spleen. Along with the splenic vessels, it is covered by the two layers of the splenorenal ligament. There is no true anatomic landmark dividing the body and the tail, nor is there any anatomically defined dividing line as in the case of the head and neck.

The main pancreatic duct of Wirsung originates at the tail of the pancreas at the level of twelfth thoracic vertebra.[3] Throughout its course in the tail and body, the duct lies midway between the superior and inferior margins and slightly more posterior than anterior. The duct of Wirsung and the accessory duct of Santorini lie anterior to the major pancreatic vessels. In the body and tail, 15 to 20 short tributaries enter the duct at almost right angles.[4,5] The superior and inferior tributaries tend to alternate with one another. In addition, the duct of Wirsung may receive a longer tributary draining the uncinate process. In some patients, the duct of Santorini in the head empties directly into the main duct. Upon reaching the head of the pancreas, the duct of Wirsung may or may not join the duct of Santorini. It turns in a caudal and slightly posterior direction before the entrance at the level of the ampulla of Vater, where the duct turns horizontally to join the caudal surface of the common bile duct to enter the wall of the duodenum, usually at the level of the second lumbar vertebra.[6] The duct of Santorini may drain the anterior superior portion of the head of the pancreas by entering either directly into the duodenum at the minor papilla or into the duct of Wirsung. In 60% of the patients, both ducts open into the duodenum, whereas in 30%, the duct of Wirsung carries the entire secretion of the gland, and the duct of Santorini ends blindly. In 10% the duct of Santorini carries the entire secretion of the gland. In this case the duct of Wirsung is small or totally absent.[7]

The arterial blood supply of the pancreas originates from both the celiac trunk and the superior mesenteric artery. The pancreaticoduodenal arterial arcades are constant. They are formed by a pair of superior and inferior pancreaticoduodenal arteries, each bifurcating into anterior and posterior branches to form these arcades. These arcades lie within the pancreas and also supply the duodenum. The gastroduodenal artery arises as the first major branch from the common hepatic artery approximately 1 cm after the common hepatic artery originates from the celiac trunk.[8] It also gives off the right gastroepiploic and subsequently the superior pancreaticoduodenal artery, which bifurcates into both anterior superior and posterior superior pancreaticoduodenal arteries. The anterior superior pancreaticoduodenal artery lies on the anterior surface of the pancreas and gives off 8 to 10 branches to the anterior surface of the duodenum and numerous branches to the pancreas. On the anterior superior surface, it joins the anterior inferior pancreaticoduodenal artery, a branch from the inferior pancreaticoduodenal artery coming from the superior mesenteric artery to form the anterior arcade. The posterior superior pancreaticoduodenal artery can only be seen when the pancreas is mobilized in a cephalad direction to expose its posterior surface. The posterior superior pancreaticoduodenal artery then joins the posterior inferior pancreaticoduodenal artery to form the posterior arcade.

Another very important blood vessel supplying the pancreas is the dorsal pancreatic artery, known by several names, such as the great superior pancreatic artery of Haller, the superior pancreatic artery of Testut, or the supreme pancreatic artery of Kirk (magna pancreatica). It lies posterior to the neck of the pancreas, and its most common origin is from the proximal splenic artery in 39% of the cases. However, it may arise from the celiac trunk, from the hepatic artery, and least frequently from the superior mesenteric artery. The splenic artery is located on the posterior aspect of the body and tail of the pancreas, and it follows a tortuous course above or below the superior margin of the pancreas, giving off many branches. There are from 2 to 10 branches of the splenic artery that supply the body and tail of the pancreas; many of these branches anastomose with the transverse pancreatic artery.

The venous drainage of the pancreas in general parallels the arteries and lies superficial to them. Venous drainage of the pancreas is to the portal vein, the splenic vein, and the superior and inferior mesenteric veins. The portal vein arises from the confluence of the superior mesenteric and splenic veins behind the neck of the pancreas. The portal vein lies behind the pancreas and in front of the inferior vena cava. It can easily be separated from the posterior surface of the pancreas. As a result, the pancreatic neck can be separated from the portal vein with a small risk of bleeding when transecting the neck of the pancreas either to perform a distal pancreatectomy or to gain exposure to the confluence of the portal and superior mesenteric veins, or to either vessels, in an effort to control massive retropancreatic bleeding.[9,10]

Anatomic Location of Injury

An extensive review of the literature to identify the anatomic location of pancreatic injuries yielded 1,024 injuries (Table 32.1). In this review, the most frequent sites of pancreatic injury included a combination of the head and neck, with 378 injuries (37%), and the body, which sustained 352 (34%). The least frequently injured

TABLE 32.1. Anatomic location of injury.

First author (year)	Head and neck	Body	Tail	Multiple
Baker (1963)[11]	13	27	16	
Culotta (1956)[12]	8	5	8	
Jones (1965)[13]	25	37	13	
Anane-Sefah (1975)[14]	20	9	15	6
Babb (1976)[15]	26	28	30	
Campbell (1980)[16]	13	21		
Nilsson (1986)[17]	6	6	11	
Feliciano (1987)[18]	101	21	7	
Leppaniemi (1988)[19]	17	20	6	
Lewis (1991)[20]	131	50		
Gentilello (1991)[21]	11			2
Madiba (1995)[22]	43	63	38	
Asensio (2004)[23]	82	65	79	
Total	378 (37%)	352 (34%)	294 (29%)	23 (3%)

portion of the pancreas was the tail, accounting for 294 injuries (29%). Multiple sites of injury occurred in 23 patients (3%). An anatomic combination of injuries to the head and neck is the most frequent site for both penetrating and blunt trauma. However, with penetrating trauma, injuries are generally distributed throughout the anatomic course of the pancreas. In blunt trauma most injuries occur at the neck of the gland.

Associated Injuries

The pancreas is rarely injured alone. In fact, multiple associated injuries are the rule rather than the exception. This situation is particularly true for both mechanisms of injuries. Isolated pancreatic injuries are usually seen in the form of blunt pancreatic transections. An extensive review of the literature, including a total of 3,679 patients who sustained 8,480 associated injuries, demonstrates that the liver is the most frequently associated organ injured, with a frequency of 19% of the cases. Other commonly associated injured organs include the stomach (15%), spleen (10.5%), colon (8%), and duodenum (8%). Major abdominal venous injuries, to the inferior vena cava and the portal and superior mesenteric veins, were present in 5.5% of the cases. Arterial injuries, to the aorta and superior mesenteric artery, were present in 4.5% of the patients. Thus vascular injuries represent the third most frequent injury seen in association with pancreatic injuries (Tables 32.2 through 32.4).

TABLE 32.2. Associated injuries ($n = 8,480$).

First author (year)	No. of patients	Associated injuries	First author (year)	No. of patients	Associated injuries
Stone (1962)[24]	62	153	Gorenstein (1987)[46]	21	27
Baker (1963)[11]	82	116	Leppaniemi (1988)[19]	43	89
Jones (1965)[13]	77	204	Pachter (1989)[47]	9	7
Salyer (1967)[25]	1	1	Fabian (1990)[48]	65	85
Werschky (1968)[26]	140	109	Flynn (1990)[49]	11	143
Foley (1969)[27]	3	3	Ivatury (1990)[50]	103	220
Sheldon (1970)[28]	59	98	Lewis (1991)[20]	63	63
Bach (1971)[29]	44	45	Gentilello (1991)[21]	10	48
White (1972)[30]	63	123	Cogbill (1991)[51]	74	175
Salam (1972)[31]	4	2	Voeller (1991)[52]	131	280
Yellin (1972)[32]	60	43	Buck (1992)[53]	17	57
Anderson (1974)[33]	70	16	Rosen (1994)[54]	38	80
Anane-Sefah (1975)[14]	50	366	Delcore (1994)[55]	5	30
Babb (1976)[15]	76	174	Madiba (1995)[22]	152	237
Lowe (1977)[34]	6	25	Craig (1995)[56]	13	27
Jones (1978)[35]	300	608	Degiannis (1995)[57]	57	164
Graham (1979)[36]	448	1,215	Degiannis (1996)[58]	48	161
Majeski (1980)[37]	1	2	Smith (1996)[59]	1	5
Stone (1981)[38]	283	961	Akhrass (1997)[60]	72	230
Berni (1982)[39]	54	89	Farrell (1996)[61]	51	96
Cogbill (1982)[40]	44	116	Patton (1997)[62]	154	46
Fitzgibbons (1982)[41]	56	116	Timberlake (1997)[63]	39	81
Oreskovich (1984)[42]	117	117	Young (1998)[64]	62	196
Sims (1984)[43]	44	43	Asensio (2004)[23]	214	720
Wynn (1985)[44]	40	72			
Nowak (1986)[45]	42	116	Total	3,679	8,480

TABLE 32.3. Associated injuries ($n = 8,480$) per organ.

First author (year)	Major vessel	Liver	SB	Colon	Major veins	Stom	BT	Major arteries	Duod	Sp	GU
Stone (1962)[24]		32	7	8	10	35	3	8	13	18	19
Baker (1963)[11]		24	16	9	8	24		3	12	10	10
Jones (1965)[13]		47		12	41	40		6	16	13	16
Salyer (1967)[25]							1		1		
Werschky (1968)[26]		63	21	24	26	61	7	29	31	29	29
Foley (1969)[27]						2	1		2		
Sheldon (1970)[28]		27	8	7		16		3	8	19	10
Bach (1971)[29]		7	1	2	2	8		4	7	7	4
White (1972)[30]	16	22		11		18			14	18	
Salam (1972)[31]											
Yellin (1972)[32]	25	21	5	6	6	21		2		7	7
Anderson (1974)[33]		5	2		4	5		5	16		6
Anane-Sefah (1975)[14]	87	99	28	28		41	18		38	88	38
Babb (1976)[15]	18	23	20	11		35				22	21
Lowe (1979)[34]		3	1	1	4	4	5		5	1	1
Jones (1978)[35]		149	37	56	43	117	4	65	56	67	53
Graham (1978)[36]	29	184	55	73	98	206	20	65	88	136	122
Majeski (1980)[37]							1		1		
Stone (1981)[38]		150	59	46	56	113	26	35	56	70	68
Berni (1982)[39]		28		3	12	10		2	10	19	5
Cogbill (1982)[40]	11	17	8	13		18	4		17	9	10
Fitzgibbons (1982)[41]	9	23	5	11		23			7	9	15
Oreskovich (1984)[42]		7		4	4	3	1			2	
Sims (1984)[43]		23	9	8					14	10	
Wynn (1985)[44]		14	12		10	12		9		13	8
Nowak (1986)[45]		20	8	17	8	26	3	2	13	12	7
Gorenstein (1987)[46]		3	3		2			1	3	3	3
Leppaniemi (1988)[19]	3	18									
Pachter (1989)[47]		1	1	1		2		1			2
Fabian (1990)[48]		19	6	9		21		11	9	12	
Eastlick (1990)[65]		1	1				1		1		
Flynn (1990)[49]		26	12	22		21	8	26		18	19
Ivatury (1990)[50]		37	4	25	23	42	4	18	5	19	15
Lewis (1991)[20]	10	26				17	3		6	12	4
Gentilello (1991)[21]		6	5	6	2	1	6		13		
Cogbill (1991)[51]		26	7	16	4	22		6	4	39	18
Voeller (1991)[52]	37	68	29	34		58				34	30
Buck (1992)[53]		10	5	6	8	9	5	8			
Rosen (1994)[54]		14	10	5		14			3	14	
Delcore (1994)[55]		2	2	1	3		8	1			
Madiba (1995)[22]		59	14	21		58		11	15	22	7
Craig (1995)[56]		5	2					1		4	
Degiannis (1995)[57]		19	32	12	3	24			7	16	
Degiannis (1996)[58]		21	32	12	13	17		1	21	6	2
Smith (1996)[59]		1			1				1		
Akhrass (1997)[60]	7	39	8	14	2	17		3	15	15	1
Farrell (1996)[61]	22	5	5	14	22	5	5	12		4	
Patton (1997)[62]				24					22		
Timberlake (1997)[63]		9	3	4	1	1		7	4	22	13
Young (1998)[64]	23	33	8	21	9	28	7		22	13	19
Asensio (2004)[23]	82	100	49	74	54	105	18	28	78	53	69
Total	379	1,536	540	671	479	1,300	158	374	653	886	651

BT, biliary tree; Duod, duodenum; GU, genitourinary; SB, small bowel; Sp, spleen; Stom, stomach.

TABLE 32.4. Associated injuries ($n = 8,480$).

Organ	No. of injuries	Percentage (%)
Liver	1,536	18.0
Stomach	1,300	15.0
Major vessels	1,232	14.5
Spleen	886	10.5
Colon	671	8.0
Duodenum	653	8.0
Genitourinary	651	8.0
Small bowel	540	6.0
Major veins	479	5.5
Major arteries	374	4.5
Biliary tree/gallbladder	158	2.0
Total	8,480	100

Surgical Techniques

Intraoperative Evaluation and Exposures

Proven or suspected pancreatic injury, coupled with the classic findings of intraabdominal injury, mandates immediate exploratory laparotomy. Abdominal injuries should be explored through a midline incision extending from xiphoid to pubis, followed by a thorough exploration of the entire abdominal cavity. The pancreas should be thoroughly explored. The head, neck, body, and tail should be visualized directly. Intraoperative findings that alert the trauma surgeon to the presence of a pancreatic injury include central retroperitoneal hematoma, proximity injuries, bile staining noted in the retroperitoneum, and edema surrounding the pancreas and lesser sac.[66,67]

The goal of a thorough exploration of all pancreatic injuries is to include or exclude the presence of a major pancreatic ductal injury. There are three basic maneuvers to achieve this goal. A Kocher maneuver is first performed by sharply incising the lateral peritoneal attachments of the duodenum and sweeping the second and third portions medially, utilizing a meticulous combination of sharp and blunt dissection. In the presence of a large retroperitoneal hematoma we recommend that the nasogastric tube be advanced through the pylorus to serve as a guide and thus avoid iatrogenic lacerations of the duodenal wall during dissection. Duodenal mobilization should be extensive to allow for palpation of the head of the pancreas to the level of the superior mesenteric vessels. This maneuver will allow the surgeon to visualize the anterior and posterior aspects of the second and third portions of the duodenum and will also permit exposure of the head and uncinate process of the pancreas and inferior vena cava. If the pericaval tissues are dissected cephalad, the inferior vena cava can also be exposed at its suprarenal location.

The trauma surgeon must determine if the patient possesses an uncinate process. This is absent in approximately 15% of patients. This becomes an important

consideration if the trauma surgeon entertains performing a distal pancreatectomy to the left of the superior mesenteric vessels, as, normally, a resection to the left of the superior mesenteric vessels extirpates approximately 65% of the gland. Although this is an extensive resection, it is not associated with the development of pancreatic exocrine or endocrine insufficiency. However, if the uncinate process is absent, resection to the left of the superior mesenteric vessels will result in extirpation of 80% of the pancreatic mass. Resections of this magnitude have been associated with the development of pancreatic insufficiency and the need for insulin replacement.

The next maneuver to expose the pancreas consists of transection of the gastrohepatic ligament to gain access to the lesser sac. This facilitates inspection of the superior border of the pancreas, including the head and body, as well as the splenic artery and vein as they course along the superior border of the pancreas. Transection of the gastrocolic ligament permits full inspection of the anterior aspect and inferior borders of the gland inclusive of the head, body, and tail. Complex maneuvers for pancreatic exposure include the Aird maneuver, which exposes the posterior aspect of the tail by mobilizing the splenic flexure of the colon and lienosplenic, splenocolic, and splenorenal ligaments. This mobilizes the spleen from a lateral to medial position. When an injury is detected penetrating the anterior surface of the pancreas, the trauma surgeon must evaluate the integrity of the main pancreatic duct, as this is the "sine qua non" of major pancreatic injury. This requires exposure of the posterior aspect of the body and tail of the pancreas. This complex maneuver may be accomplished by sharply transecting the retroperitoneal attachments of the inferior border of the pancreas while elevating the organ cephalad to allow for inspection of the posterior surface, followed by careful bimanual palpation. This maneuver is technically challenging and should be performed with meticulous precision to prevent iatrogenic injury to the superior mesenteric vessels. All of these maneuvers can provide accurate intraoperative assessment of both glandular and ductal integrity.[66-68]

Intraoperative Adjunct Techniques

The use of clinical intraoperative observations such as direct visualization of ductal violations, complete transection of the pancreas, laceration of more than one half of the diameter of the gland, central perforations, and severe lacerations with or without massive tissue disruption can predict the presence of a major ductal injury with a high degree of accuracy. However, there are circumstances in which assessment of the ductal integrity cannot be made. In these cases, intraoperative pancreatography has been recommended as a technique for visualization of the main pancreatic duct.[69,70]

The technique of intraoperative pancreatography consists of intubating the ampulla of Vater through an open duodenotomy and cannulating the main pancreatic duct. Alternatively, but not recommended, the tail of the pancreas can be amputated and the main duct also cannulated via the amputated tail of the pancreas. The duct is then cannulated with a 5-F pediatric feeding tube followed by gentle instillation of 1 to 5 mL of contrast material to radiographically visualize the pancreatic duct and detect any escape of contrast.[71]

Intubating the ampulla of Vater requires the creation of a duodenotomy, unless there is an associated duodenal injury present. Location of the ampulla of Vater may also be very difficult even with an open duodenum. In extreme and rare cases when pancreatography is imperative, a choledochotomy may be performed with passage of biliary probes or Bakes dilators to identify the ampulla. This also carries the risk of iatrogenic injury to the common bile duct and ampulla, as well as the need for placement of a T tube in a generally small common bile duct that can result in biliary leaks and/or fistulas. Similarly, closure of the duodenotomy may predispose the patient to the development of a duodenal leak and/or fistula. An alternative method to intraoperative pancreatography is a cholangiography using a small butterfly needle. This has a very limited but valuable role and should be reserved to assess ductal integrity when injuries have occurred at the head of the pancreas. This adjunct procedure may yield trauma surgeons vital information to determine whether extensive damage exists to the major duct in the head as a criterion for selection of a complex procedure such as pancreaticoduodenectomy.

Injury Classification

All pancreatic injuries must be classified utilizing the American Association for the Surgery of Trauma—Organ Injury Score (AAST-OIS)[72] (Table 32.5). Simpler surgi-

TABLE 32.5. American Association for the Surgery of Trauma—Organ Injury Score (AAST-OIS) for pancreatic injuries.

Grade	Injury	Description
I	Hematoma	Minor contusion without duct injury
	Laceration	Superficial laceration without duct injury
II	Hematoma	Major contusion without duct injury or tissue loss
	Laceration	Major laceration without duct injury or tissue loss
III	Laceration	Distal transection or parenchymal injury with duct injury
IV	Laceration	Proximal* transection or parenchymal injury involving ampulla
V	Laceration	Massive disruption of pancreatic head

*Proximal pancreas is to the patient's right of the superior mesenteric vein.

Source: Reprinted with permission from Moore et al.[72]

TABLE 32.6. Surgical techniques and procedures for pancreatic and pancreaticoduodenal injuries.

Simple drainage
Simple pancreatorrhaphy
Complex pancreatorrhaphy
Distal pancreatectomy (to the left of the superior mesenteric vessels)
Distal pancreatectomy (to the left of the superior mesenteric vessels) with splenic preservation
Extended distal pancreatectomy (to the right of the superior mesenteric vessels)
Extended distal pancreatectomy (to the right of the superior mesenteric vessels) with distal pancreaticojejunostomy
Duodenal diverticularization (vagotomy and antrectomy, gastrojejunostomy, duodenorraphy, T-tube drainage, and external drainage)
Pyloric exclusion
Pancreatoduodenectomy (Whipple's procedure)

cal techniques should be selected for management of the lesser grade injuries while reserving the most complex techniques for the more challenging and severe injuries.

Principles of Injury Management

A large number of surgical techniques have been described (Table 32.6). Approximately 60% of all pancreatic injuries can be treated by external drainage alone. Approximately 70% can be treated by simple pancreatorrhaphy plus drainage. Basic surgical principles, such as debridement to viable tissue, closure of the transected pancreas with staples and/or nonabsorbable sutures, and ligation of the transected pancreatic duct if identified, are the mainstays of successful management of pancreatic injuries.

We strongly recommend that all pancreatic contusions, as well as any capsular lacerations, be managed by simple external drainage with closed suction systems. The capsule of the pancreas should not be closed by itself, as this has been known to lead to the formation of pancreatic pseudocysts. Any injury that lacerates the pancreatic parenchyma should be gently examined to determine whether there is major versus minor ductal involvement. Having excluded this type of injury, we recommend performing simple pancreatorrhaphy utilizing nonabsorbable sutures in order to approximate the edges of the lacerated parenchyma. Pancreatorrhaphy decreases the incidence of leak from pancreatic exocrine secretions and thus the inflammatory process in surrounding tissues.

At times, it may be quite difficult for the trauma surgeon to determine the involvement of the major ductal system. Performing a pancreatorrhaphy in this scenario will not only miss but also undertreat a major ductal injury, increasing the possibility for development of severe postoperative complications. In this scenario, it is necessary to upgrade the injury in order to select more appropriate treatment, which in this case would be pancreatic resection. This decision is simplified if the injury lies to the left of the superior mesenteric vessels, where distal resection, although technically challenging, does not approach the degree of complexity of a resection to the right of the superior mesenteric vessels. If this injury were to lie to the right of the superior mesenteric vessels, the surgeon must consider either draining extensively and accepting the development of a pancreatic fistula with all of the associated complications or performing an extended resection to the right of the superior mesenteric vessels. The other alternative is performing a segmental pancreatic resection followed by pancreaticojejunostomy, which implies accepting the risk of an anastomotic leak. This procedure is problematic and not recommended.

All pancreatic injuries should be drained. Closed suction systems are employed to establish wide pancreatic drainage. External drainage serves to evacuate pancreatic exocrine secretions and to control a pancreatic fistula, should it develop. The placement of closed suction systems decreases the rate of intraabdominal abscess formation as pancreatic secretions are more reliably collected, and excoriation of the skin is thus avoided. Although there is no uniformity as to the length of time that drains must remain in place, we recommend leaving the drains for 7 to 10 days, as any fistulization process should be evident by that time. Drainage should be maintained while the patient resumes oral intake, as it is well known that pancreatic drainage may decrease after 7 days. However, a significant increase in drainage will often occur subsequently after oral intake has been resumed and should alert the trauma surgeon to the possibility of impending complications.

The trauma surgeon must possess a vast of armamentarium of surgical procedures to manage pancreatic injuries. Grade I and grade II injuries occur with a frequency of 60% and 20%, respectively. Grade III injuries represent 15% of all pancreatic injuries, whereas grade IV injuries are uncommon, occurring with a frequency of 5%. It is for these higher grade injuries that the broader armamentarium of complex surgical techniques should be reserved. The conservative approach with adherence to injury grade and management guidelines will produce better results; this includes selecting the least complex surgical procedure to manage the pancreatic injury, conservative but judicious resection, and debridement and control of pancreatic secretions via external drainage.

Special Situations

Pancreaticoduodenal Injuries

Pancreaticoduodenal injuries are fortunately rare. These injuries are most commonly caused by penetrating injury and are frequently associated with multiple concomitant injuries. Patients with higher pancreatic injury severity and associated duodenal injuries of a significant grade should be considered as candidates for more complex pancreaticoduodenal repairs, such as duodenal diverticulization or pyloric exclusion. Pancreatic injuries of grade II or above in association with duodenal injuries caused by severe blunt trauma or missiles, those involving more than 75% of the duodenal wall, those involving the first and second portions of the duodenum or common bile duct, and those associated with delay in repair of more than 24 hours are also candidates.

Other criteria that may lead the surgeon to strongly consider diverticulization or pyloric exclusion include compromised blood supply to the duodenum and associated injury to the head of the pancreas without disruption of the main pancreatic duct or any pancreatic injury associated with a duodenal injury involving more than 50% of the circumference of the duodenum. The main purpose of this procedure is to exclude the duodenum from the passage of gastric contents, thus allowing for a suitable period of time for the duodenal repair to heal, which can be severely threatened by the presence of pancreatic secretions that promote suture line dehiscence.

Pancreaticoduodenectomy was first reported by Whipple et al.[73] in 1935 as a staged procedure. Modifications were subsequently added to refine the procedure now performed routinely. In 1961, Howell and colleagues[74] first performed pancreaticoduodenectomy for penetrating trauma. In 1964, Thal and Wilson[75] first performed pancreaticoduodenectomy as a treatment for patients sustaining severe blunt trauma to the head of the pancreas. These authors reported three patients who underwent pancreaticoduodenectomy and recommended limiting the use of this procedure for patients incurring massive pancreaticoduodenal injuries involving the head of the pancreas. In 1969, Halgrimson and colleagues[76] reported their experience from Vietnam with two patients, operated on a delayed basis, who survived. Foley and colleagues,[27] also in 1969 and based on three blunt trauma patients, described the following indications for pancreaticoduodenectomy:

- Massive uncontrollable bleeding from the head of the pancreas, adjacent vascular structures, or both
- Massive and unreconstructable ductal injury in the head of the pancreas
- Combined unreconstructable injuries of the following:
  - Duodenum and head of the pancreas
  - Duodenum, head of the pancreas, and common bile duct

Before considering pancreaticoduodenectomy, the trauma surgeon must thoroughly assess the extent of injury; we recommend good exposure of both pancreas and duodenum by an initial extensive Kocher maneuver. This should be extensive enough so that the surgeon can palpate the entire head of the pancreas to the level of the superior mesenteric vessels. This allows the surgeon to visualize both anterior and posterior aspects of the second and third portions of the duodenum and will also permit exposure of the head and uncinate process of the pancreas and inferior vena cava. Intraoperative inspection for ductal violation of the main pancreatic duct, complete transection of the head of the pancreas, pancreatic fluid leak, central perforations, and severe lacerations with or without massive tissue disruption can predict the presence of a major pancreatic ductal injury with a high degree of accuracy.

Similarly, meticulous and gentle exploration of the injured head of the pancreas utilizing the finest of malleable retractors will often expose an injured main pancreatic duct. Assessment of the viability of the duodenum is also quite important. Frequently, injuries in the medial aspect of the first and second portions of the duodenum within the C-loop are deemed unreconstructable upon preliminary inspection. However, with further meticulous dissection, utilizing a Kittner dissector and with the help of fine malleable retractors, some are amenable to primary repair. These maneuvers must be carried out systematically to avoid devascularization of both duodenum and head of the pancreas. If the criteria originally described by Foley and later validated by Asensio are met, the trauma surgeon must proceed to pancreaticoduodenectomy.

Pancreaticoduodenectomy is clearly a formidable procedure in critically ill patients. A review of 64 series reported in the literature from 1964 to 2003 yielded 253 patients who underwent pancreaticoduodenectomy (Table 32.7). Subsequently, 75 of these patients died. The tabulated mortality rate for all series reviewed was 30%, which is not at variance with the range of 30% to 40% reported in the literature. Asensio and colleagues,[111] with the largest series of the literature, reported the use of pancreaticoduodenectomy for severe pancreaticoduodenal injuries. In this series they reported 18 patients with severe and unreconstructable injuries of the head of the pancreas and the first or second portion of the duodenum. In addition, these patients also sustained injuries involving the main pancreatic duct, the intrapancreatic portion of the distal common bile duct, and the ampulla of Vater, with devitalization and destruction of the blood supply. Twelve patients lived, for an overall survival rate of 67%. This compares very favorably with the survival rate reported in the literature, which ranges from 64% to 69%, given the severity of the injuries, large blood losses, and largest number of associated abdominal injuries reported to date. However, much remains to be done to improve the high mortality rates for these rare but highly challenging patients.

TABLE 32.7. Experience with pancreaticoduodenectomy in trauma patients.

First author	Year	No. of patients	No. of deaths
Thal[75]	1964	2	1
Walter[77]	1966	1	0
Thompson[78]	1966	2	1
Salyer[25]	1967	1	0
Sawyers[79]	1967	1	0
Wilson[80]	1967	2	0
Brawley[81]	1968	3	0
Werschky[26]	1968	1	1
Pantazelos[82]	1969	1	1
Halgrimson[76]	1969	3	0
Foley[27]	1969	3	0
Gibbs[83]	1970	1	0
Bach[29]	1971	3	0
Nance[84]	1971	5	2
Jones[85]	1971		
Smith[86]	1971	5	2
Salam[31]	1972	4	1
Anderson[87]	1973	2	1
White[30]	1972	5	0
Owens[88]	1973	3	1
Steele[89]	1973	3	3
Sturm[90]	1973	5	2
Anderson[33]	1974	2	1
Yellin[91]	1975	10	6
Anane-Sefah[14]	1975	6	0
Chamber[92]	1975	1	0
Balasegaram[93]	1976	8	5
Heitsch[94]	1976	2	2
Lowe[34]	1977	6	0
Karl[95]	1977	1	1
Hagan[96]	1978	2	2
Graham[36]	1979	6	3
Stone[97]	1979	3	3
Majeski[37]	1980	1	0
Cogbill[40]	1982	1	0
Levinson[98]	1982	1	1
Berni[39]	1982	8	0
Henarejos[99]	1983	1	0
Oreskovich[42]	1984	10	0
Adkins[100]	1984	5	1
Moore[101]	1984	1	0
Fabian[102]	1984	1	1
Sims[43]	1984	2	0
Donahue[103]	1985	1	1
Jones (1971–1978)[104]	1985	12	7
Ivatury[105]	1985	7	3
Smego[106]	1985	1	0
Wynn[44]	1985	3	2
Nowak[45]	1986	1	1
Walker[107]	1986	1	0
Feliciano[18]	1987	13	6
Melissas[108]	1987	1	0
Leppaniemi[19]	1988	3	1
McKone[109]	1988	5	0
Eastlick[65]	1990	1	0
Gentilello[21]	1991	3	1
Heimansohn[110]	1990	6	0
Ivatury[50]	1990	6	2
Delcore[55]	1994	4	0
Degiannis[58]	1996	3	2
Smith[59]	1996	1	1
Young[64]	1998	2	0
Asensio[111]	2003	18	6
Total		253	75 (30%)

Mortality

Pancreatic injuries, as a whole, carry a significant mortality rate. A review of 44 series in the literature dating from 1956 to 1998 reveals rates of 5% to 54%. A total of 4,134 patients were analyzed of which 790 died for a mean mortality rate of 19%. The lowest rate was reported by Babb and Harmon[15] in 1976. Of their 76 patients, 4 died, yielding a mortality rate of 5%. Fifty-five patients (72%) sustained penetrating abdominal injuries of which 28 were gunshot wounds, 4 were shotgun wounds, and 23 were stab wounds. Remarkably, the head of the pancreas was injured in 26 (34% of the patients). There were 180 associated injuries of which 18 (10%) were to major abdominal blood vessels. Seventy-two of the 76 patients survived, and there were 71 major complications. Although this figure is quite remarkable, it is at variance with most other mortality rates reported in the literature and definitely at variance with the literature.

The highest mortality rate was reported by Gentilello et al.[21] in a series of 13 patients of whom 7 died, for a mortality rate of 54%. This series is unique because it includes only patients who experienced severe combined pancreaticoduodenal injuries. In addition, 9 of the 13 patients sustained additional ampullary or distal common bile duct injuries, as well as a significant number of other associated injuries. Only two (15%) sustained major venous injuries, and no major arterial injuries were reported. All 13 patients underwent pancreaticoduodenectomy, including a formal gastrojejunostomy with common bile duct implantation in the jejunal loop and pancreatic duct ligation with no reconstructive pancreaticojejunostomy. Consequently, this series deals with a very critically injured patient population, and its resultant high mortality rate is also at variance with the literature.

Several authors have reported their overall mortality rates separately from the mortality rates caused exclusively by pancreatic injuries. Associated injuries are responsible for the majority of deaths of patients sustaining pancreatic injuries. Five studies that distinguished mortality from associated injuries versus the pancreatic injury itself revealed that out of 586 patients, 134 died, yielding a mortality rate of 23%. Ninety-nine (74%) died of associated injuries, whereas 35 (26%) succumbed secondary to their pancreatic injury. This yields a ratio of associated injuries to pancreatic mortality of 3.5 to 1. These figures were confirmed in an excellent review of pancreatic injuries by Glancy.[112]

Mortality can be analyzed based on several variables. It can be reviewed on a temporal basis and subdivided into early and late mortality. Most early deaths with pancreatic injuries are caused by exsanguination, usually secondary to major associated vascular injuries. In our own review, associated major vascular injuries were the third most common associated injury and certainly the most lethal. These findings are repeatedly born out in the literature.

Graham et al.[113] reported 73 patients who died out of 448 patients, for a 16% mortality rate. Of the 73 deaths, 47 patients (64%) died during the first 24 hours secondary to hemorrhagic shock, prolonged bleeding, hypothermia, coagulopathy, and the sequelae of massive blood replacement. Similarly, Jones, in his first series,[35] consisting of 300 patients, reported 59 deaths of which 26 (44%) occurred within 24 hours. In Jones's subsequent series,[104] consisting of 500 patients, shock was present in 48% of the patients, and their mortality rate was 40% compared with the 4% mortality rate for normotensive patients. Of the 104 patients who died, 89% had experienced a significant period of shock. Fifty died intraoperatively, secondary to uncontrolled hemorrhage. In the series of Patton et al.,[62] 17 of 134 patients (13%) died from massive hemorrhage.

Mechanism of injury is an important determinant of mortality. In 14 series, the mortality rate secondary to shotgun wounds was 51%, whereas injuries from other types of penetrating and blunt trauma incurred mortality rates ranging from 7% to 23%. Similarly, associated injuries and their numbers are also important determinants of mortality rate. It is well known that patients sustaining penetrating trauma are much more likely to have associated injuries. Howell et al.[74] and Stone et al.[38] correlated the presence or absence of one or more associated injuries in patients sustaining pancreatic injuries caused by either mechanism. They noted a significant difference in 297 of 298 patients (99.7%) with penetrating trauma versus only 62 of 70 patients (88.6%) sustaining blunt trauma. The number of associated injuries clearly affected mortality. Graham et al.,[113] Howell et al.,[74] Balasegaram,[114] and Werschky and Jordan[26] in their series totaling 712 patients, reported the mortality rate for patients with zero to one, two to three, and four or more associated injuries as 2.5%, 13.6% and 29.6%, respectively. According to Asensio,[71] factors known to increase mortality rates include associated duodenal and common bile duct injuries. Proximal pancreatic injuries are also related to increases in mortality.

The type of operative intervention employed to manage these patients can also be correlated with mortality. Glancy[112] reviewed eight studies encompassing 1,407 patients in which mortality was correlated with the type of operative procedure. The overall mortality rate in this group of patients was 16.8%. Patients undergoing total pancreatectomy and pancreatic ductal reanastomosis had consistently higher mortality rates: 100% and 50%, respectively. However, this subset of patients was too small to reach any meaningful conclusions.

In 214 patients, Asensio and colleagues[23] reported a mortality rate of 31%. In this series, 20 patients required emergency department thoracotomy. Patients sustaining penetrating injuries incurred a greater period of intraoperative hypotension than those who sustained blunt injury—124 minutes vs. 16 minutes ($p < 0.005$)—and required a larger number of units of blood transfused—

penetrating 11.3 ± 0.9 units vs. blunt 8.5 ± 1.5 units ($p >$ 0.005). Mortality correlated well with the AAST-OIS for pancreatic injuries: grade I, 4%; grade II, 15%; grade III, 37%; grade IV, 66%; and grade V, 82%.

Morbidity

Pancreatic injuries are associated with very high rates of morbidity. Forty series in the literature encompassing 3,898 patients were selected and reviewed because they clearly outlined morbidity figures. Overall, morbidity rates ranged from 11% to 62%, with an average rate of 36.6%. The lowest morbidity rate was reported by Voeller et al.[52] The highest morbidity rate was reported by Campbell and Kennedy.[16]

Pancreatic morbidity is represented primarily by fistulas. The literature shows no uniformity in the definition of a pancreatic fistula. As a matter of fact, prolonged pancreatic drainage is considered as "a way of life" with these injuries. Another conclusion expressed in the literature is that fistula formation may not be a true complication but simply a result of appropriate therapy. Because fistula formation is usually associated with external drainage and the reason for draining is to avoid collection of pancreatic secretions, the presence of a fistula may signify the prevention of a more serious complication such as a pseudocyst. Therefore, does constitute a fistula? In our opinion, any drainage of more than 50 mL that persists longer than 2 weeks with elevated amylase and lipase levels should be considered a fistula.

In our review of the literature, fistulas were identified with an incidence of 14%; pancreatic abscess was the second most frequent complication (8%), and posttraumatic pancreatitis occurred in 4% of the cases. Pseudocysts were identified in 3% of the patients, whereas late hemorrhage occurred with an incidence of 1%. Lumped into the category of "other complications" is exocrine and endocrine insufficiency (4%). It is hard to determine from the literature the true incidence of this complication.

Cogbill et al.,[51] in a retrospective multiinstitutional 5-year study of 74 patients, reported 10 fistulas, for an incidence of 14% in 71 survivors of the initial operation. This figure falls within the range of 3% to 24% reported in the literature. In this series, the maximum daily fistula output ranged from 70 to 1,000 mL. Spontaneous closure of fistulas occurred in 8 (89%) of 9 survivors in a period of time ranging from 6 to 54 days after discovery. Only one patient required surgical reintervention for completion pancreatectomy of the distal remnant 154 days after the initial operation.

Fistulas result in mortality if associated with pancreatic abscesses. The management of pancreatic fistulas consists of careful monitoring of fluid and electrolyte status concomitant with fluid replacement. Protection of the skin at the fistula site is critical in avoiding significant ulceration of the skin secondary to the corrosive effect of the pancreatic enzymes. We recommend the performance of endoscopic retrograde cholangiopancreatography (ERCP) for confirmation and delineation of the fistulous tract, which is most helpful in establishing the cause of the persistent fistula and in formulating the plan for further therapy.

Aggressive parenteral nutrition with absolute gastrointestinal tract rest is the time-tested method to manage these fistulas, along with maintenance of adequate drainage. This represents the gold standard. One alternative tried was enteral nutrition with an elemental diet provided via distal feeding jejunostomy; however, the authors observed in some cases that the fistula output increased significantly in some patients whereas others tolerated enteral nutrition well and without a concomitant increase in the output. Similarly, the authors noted that a very small group of patients can tolerate a low-fat elemental diet orally without an increase in output; this group remains a very small minority of patients. There are certainly no known explanations as to why this small and selected group of patients does well with this management. This is indicative of our lack of knowledge of the many feedback loops at work between both the proximal and distal small bowel and the pancreas.

The long-acting somatostatin analog octreotide acetate has also been used to inhibit pancreatic exocrine secretion.[115] This was originally reported as a helpful adjunct in the management of complications following elective pancreatic procedures. Good results were noticed, with decreasing times to closure of the postoperative fistula. The use of this synthetic analog has been extrapolated as an adjunct in the management of posttraumatic pancreatic fistulas; however, few data exist in the literature documenting its efficacy. We use it consistently and have noted good results in terms of hastening the closure of fistulas.

Pancreatic abscess as a specific infectious complication of pancreatic injury is difficult to define given the large number of associated injuries in pancreatic trauma. The association with either a colon or a duodenal injury results in a 60% rate of abscess formation versus a much lower rate of 10% to 15% for patients without colonic or duodenal injuries. Similarly, Jones[104] reported that 60% of patients with colon injuries in his series developed intraabdominal abscess, but few were related to the pancreatic injury. Graham et al.[36] reported an 8% incidence of abscess formation in his series generally associated with hepatic and colonic injuries but only a 2% incidence of pancreatic-specific abscesses. Cogbill et al.[51] reported intraabdominal abscess formation in 24 of 71 surviving patients, an incidence of 34%. Left upper quadrant abscesses are much more common after distal pancreatectomy than after distal pancreatectomy with splenic preservation. The mainstay of management consists of percutaneous CT-guided drainage. Cogbill et al.[51] reported a 79% success rate with this approach.

Posttraumatic pancreatitis has been defined by Cogbill et al.[51] as an elevated serum amylase level persisting for more than 3 days. The vast majority of posttraumatic pancreatitis results from blunt abdominal trauma. It is treated with nasogastric decompression, bowel rest, and aggressive nutritional support and usually resolves spontaneously. A highly lethal complication of posttraumatic pancreatitis is its evolution into hemorrhagic pancreatitis. This is usually manifested by bloody pancreatic drainage. It carries an extremely high mortality rate, because there is no effective treatment known. The usual scenario demands the return of the patient to the operating room with the hope of controlling the bleeding by either debridement or pancreatectomy; however, this is usually futile. We have tried interventional angiography with mixed results.

Pancreatic pseudocysts generally result from overlooked blunt pancreatic injuries treated nonoperatively. Kudsk et al.[116] documented 22 pseudocysts in 42 patients with blunt pancreatic injuries managed nonoperatively in seven series reported between 1952 and 1983. Graham et al.[36] reported a 2% incidence of pseudocyst formation after penetrating injury. Cogbill et al.[51] reported a 3% incidence of posttraumatic pseudocyst formation. Pseudocyst formation is usually regarded as failure to establish adequate postoperative drainage to manage pancreatic secretions. The presence of a pseudocyst should be considered if there is prolonged elevation of the serum amylase level postoperatively, and it should be aggressively pursued.

All posttraumatic pseudocysts should be investigated with ERCP, which will delineate the status of the duct. This is important in selecting the method of management. If the ductal system is found to be intact, the pseudocyst can be managed with percutaneous drainage. If the pseudocyst has resulted secondary to a missed ductal injury, percutaneous drainage will not provide definitive therapy, and these patients are best managed by reexploration and pancreatectomy or by internal drainage via a Roux-en-Y jejunal limb. On rare occasions endoscopic transpancreatic stenting of the pancreatic duct has been tried successfully.

Posttraumatic hemorrhage can be quite a lethal complication. Both Jones[35] and Graham et al.[36] describe erosion of vessels surrounding the pancreas. This may occur when there has been an inadequate debridement or external drainage and is totally unpredictable. The management consists of returning the patient to the operating room, but this carries a very high mortality rate. We have tried angiographic embolization as a temporizing means before returning the patient to the operating room, as well as for definitive control, with mixed results.

Either exocrine or endocrine insufficiency is unusual after pancreatic injuries. Distal pancreatectomy to the left of the superior mesenteric vessels should leave adequate functioning pancreatic tissue. Jones,[104] in a series of 500

patients, reported 11 patients who had 11.5 to 14 cm of the pancreas resected, or 80% or more of the pancreas, as measured by pathologic examination. Three of these patients subsequently developed pancreatic insufficiency requiring hormonal replacement for life. Balasegaram[93] reported no pancreatic insufficiency after resections of up to 90% of the pancreas. No case of pancreatic insufficiency was reported by Graham et al.,[36] whereas Cogbill et al.[40] reported only one patient who required insulin following an 80% resection.

Pancreatic Emergencies (Nontrauma)*

Complications of acute pancreatitis are the most common problems that an acute care surgeon will encounter. Such complications include biliary pancreatitis, infected or hemorrhagic pseudocyst, necrotizing pancreatitis, and pancreatic abscess. The definitions of term describing pancreatitis are highlighted in Table 32.8.

TABLE 32.8. Definitions of terminology in pancreatitis.

Acute interstitial pancreatitis: A mild, self-limited form of pancreatitis characterized by interstitial edema and an acute inflammatory response without necrosis, local complications, or systemic manifestations such as organ failure

Necrotizing pancreatitis: A severe form of acute pancreatitis characterized by locoregional tissue necrosis and systemic manifestations such as pulmonary, renal, or cardiac failure

Sterile necrosis: Acute pancreatitis leading to tissue necrosis without supervening infection

Infected necrosis: Acute pancreatitis with locoregional tissue necrosis complicated by bacterial or fungal infection

Acute fluid collections: A fluid collection occurring early in the course of acute pancreatitis, located in or near the pancreas, and lacking an epithelial lining or a defined wall of granulation or fibrous tissue

Pancreatic pseudocyst: A pancreatic or peripancreatic fluid collection with a well-defined wall of granulation tissue and fibrosis, absence of an epithelial lining. Pancreatic pseudocysts can arise in the setting of chronic pancreatitis, without the sequela of an episode of necrotizing pancreatitis. One of the common complications of pseudocyst is the development of infection

Pancreatic cysts: A fluid-filled pancreatic mass with an epithelial lining. These may be neoplastic lesions, such as serous cystadenomas or mucinous cystic tumors, or congenital cysts

Pancreatic abscess: A circumscribed intraabdominal collection of pus, usually in proximity to the pancreas, containing little or no pancreatic necrosis, arising as a consequence of necrotizing pancreatitis or pancreatic trauma

Suppurative cholangitis: Bacterial infection within the biliary tree, associated with ductal obstruction, usually from a stone or stricture

Source: Adapted with permission from Bradley E and members of the Atlanta International Symposium. A clinically based classification system for acute pancreatitis. Arch Surg 1993; 128(5):586–590.

---

*This section is reprinted with the kind permission of Springer Science and Business Media from Mulvihill SJ. Pancreas. In Norton JA, Barie PS, Bollinger RR, Chang AE, Lowry SF, Mulvihill SJ, Pass HI, Thompson RW, eds. Surgery: Basic Science and Clinical Evidence. New York: Springer, 2001: 523–526.

Table 32.9. Ranson criteria for assessing severity of acute pancreatitis.

At admission	Within the first 48 hr
Age >55 years	Drop in hematocrit >10%
White blood cell count >16,000/μL	Fluid deficit >4,000 mL
Serum glucose >200 mg/dL (11 mmol/L)	Serum calcium <8.0 mg/dl (<1.9 mmol/L)
Serum lactate dehydrogenase >400 IU/L	Hypoxemia (PO$_2$ <60 mm Hg)
Serum aspartate aminotransferase >250 IU/L	Rise in blood urea nitrogen >5 mg/dL (>1.8 mmol/L)
	Drop in albumin <3.2 g/dL

Source: Reproduced with permission from Ranson JH, Rifkind KM, Turner JW. Prognostic signs and the role of operative management in acute pancreatitis. Surg Gynecol Obstet 1976; 143:209–219.

Clinical and radiographic criteria are used to estimate the severity of pancreatitis. However, Ranson's classification is still the most commonly used criteria (Table 32.9). The mortality rate increases for a patient as more criteria are documented.

With hypovolemia being the most common systemic complication of acute pancreatitis, aggressive resuscitation is an essential component of the management. In the management of acute necrotizing pancreatitis, the indications for surgical management are infected pancreatic necrosis and sterile pancreatic necrosis in which there is persistent necrotizing pancreatitis or fulminant acute pancreatitis.[117]

The surgical intervention required is a necrosectomy or debridement. A component of the treatment armamentarium for acute management of a pancreatic pseudocyst (infected or rapidly expanding) is external drainage. Fortunately, with early intervention and aggressive resuscitation, operative intervention with acute pancreatitis is not common.

Critique

This scenario is, perhaps, the most frequent indication for surgical intervention for a fulminant pancreatitis. With increasing toxicity, even in the absence of documented infection, this patient needs to undergo a celiotomy and surgical debridement of necrotic tissue, along with wide drainage of the pancreatic bed. In a case without the worsening toxicity, CT-directed biopsy to confirm an infectious etiology would be recommended. If there is documentation of air in the retroperitoneum, operative intervention would also be indicated.

Answer (D)

References

1. Kreel L, Sandin B. Changes in pancreatic morphology associated with aging. Gut 1973; 14:962.
2. Baldwin WM. The pancreatic ducts in man, together with a study of the microscopical structure of the minor duodenal papilla. Anat Rec 1911; 5:197.
3. Anacker H. Radiological anatomy of the pancreas. In Anacker H, ed. Efficiency and Limits of Radiologic examination of the Pancreas. Acton, MA: Publishing Sciences Group, 1975.
4. Classen M, Koch H, Ruskin H, et al. Pancreatitis after endoscopic retrograde pancreatography (ERCP). Gut 1973; 14:431.
5. Sivak MV, Sullivan BH. Endoscopic retrograde pancreatography: analysis of the normal pancreatogram. Am J Dig Dis 1976; 51:263.
6. Gross RE. Surgery of Infancy and Childhood. Philadelphia: WB Saunders, 1972.
7. Silen W. Surgical anatomy of the pancreas. Surg Clin North Am 1964; 44:1253.
8. Michels NA. Blood supply of the pancreas and duodenum. In Blood Supply Anatomy of the Upper Abdominal Organs with a Descriptive Atlas. Philadelphia: JB Lippincott, 1995: 236–247.
9. Child CG. The Hepatic Circulation and Portal Hypertension. Philadelphia: WB Saunders, 1954.
10. Gray SW, Skandalakis JE. Embryology for Surgeons. Philadelphia, 1972.
11. Baker RJ, Dippel WF, Freeark RJ, et al. The surgical significance of the trauma to the pancreas. Arch Surg 1963; 86:1038–1044.
12. Culotta RJ, Howard JM, Jordan GL. Traumatic injuries of the pancreas. Surgery 1956; 40:320–327.
13. Jones RC, Shires GT. The management of pancreatic injuries. Arch Surg 1965; 90:502–508.
14. Anane-Sefah J, Norton LW, Eiseman B. Operative choice and technique following pancreatic injury. Arch Surg 1975; 110:161–166.
15. Babb J, Harmon H. Diagnosis and management of pancreatic trauma. Am Surg 1976; 6:390–394.
16. Campbell RC, Kennedy T. The management of pancreatic and pancreaticoduodenal injuries. Br J Surg 1980; 67:845–850.
17. Nilson E, Norby S, Skulman S, et al. Pancreatic trauma in a defined population. Acta Chir Scand 1986; 152:647–651.
18. Feliciano DV, Martin TD, Cruse PA, et al. Management of combined pancreaticoduodenal injuries. Ann Surg 1987; 205:673–680.
19. Leppaniemi A, Haapiainen R, Kiviluoto T, et al. Pancreatic trauma: acute and late manifestations. Br J Surg 1988; 75:165–167.
20. Lewis G, Knottenbelt JD, Jriege JE. Conservative surgery for trauma to the pancreatic head: is it safe? Injury 1991; 3722:372–374.
21. Gentilello LM, Cortez V, Buechter K, et al. Whipple procedure for trauma: is duct ligation a safe alternative to pancreaticojejunostomy? J Trauma 1991; 31:661–668.

22. Madiba TE, Mokoena TR. Favorable prognosis after surgical drainage of gunshot, stab or blunt trauma of the pancreas. Br J Surg 1995; 82:1236–1239.

23. Asensio JA, Petrone P, Roldan G, et al. Operative management and outcome in 214 pancreatic injuries. Trauma surgical procedure and AAST-OIS predict morbidity and mortality. In press.

24. Stone HH, Stowers KB, Shippey SH. Injuries to the pancreas. Arch Surg 1962; 85:187–192.

25. Salyer K, McClelland R. Pancreaticoduodenectomy for trauma. Arch Surg 1967; 95:636–639.

26. Werschky LR, Jordan GL. Surgical management of traumatic injuries of the pancreas. Am J Surg 1968; 116:768–772.

27. Foley WJ, Gaines RD, Fry WJ. Pancreatoduodenectomy for severe trauma to the head of the pancreas and the associated structures: report of three cases. Ann Surg 1969; 170:759–765.

28. Sheldon GF, Cohn LH, Blaisdell FW. Surgical treatment of pancreatic trauma. J Trauma 1970; 10:795–800.

29. Bach RD, Frey CF. Diagnosis and treatment of pancreatic trauma. Am J Surg 1971; 121:20–29.

30. White PH, Benfield JR. Amylase in the management of pancreatic trauma. Arch Surg 1972; 105:158–162.

31. Salam A, Warren WD, Kalser M, et al. Pancreatoduodenectomy for trauma: clinical and metabolic studies. Ann Surg 1972; 175:663–669.

32. Yellin AE, Vecchione TR, Donovan AJ. Distal pancreatectomy for pancreatic trauma. Am J Surg 1972; 124:135:42.

33. Anderson CB, Connors JP, Mejia DC, et al. Drainage methods in the treatment of pancreatic injuries. Surg Gynecol Obstet 1974; 138:587–590.

34. Lowe RJ, Saletta JD, Moss GS. Pancreatoduodenectomy for penetrating trauma. J Trauma 1977; 17:732–741.

35. Jones RC. Management of pancreatic trauma. Ann Surg 1978; 187:555–564.

36. Graham JM, Mattox KL, Vaughan GD III, et al. Combined pancreatoduodenal injuries. J Trauma 1979; 19:340–346.

37. Majesky JA, Tyler G. Pancreatic trauma. Am Surg 1980; 10:593–596.

38. Stone HH, Fabian TC, Satiani B, et al. Experiences in the management of pancreatic trauma. J Trauma 1981; 21:257–262.

39. Berni GA, Bandyk DF, Oreskovich MR, et al. Role of intraoperative pancreatography in patients with injury to the pancreas. Am J Surg 1982; 143:602–605.

40. Cogbill TH, Moore EE, Kashuk JL. Changing trends in the management of pancreatic trauma. Arch Surg 1982; 117:722–758.

41. Fitzgibbons TK, Yellin AE, Maruyama MM, Donovan AJ. Management of the transected pancreas following distal pancreatectomy. Sur Gynecol Obstet 1982; 154:225–231.

42. Oreskovich MR, Carrico CJ. Pancreaticoduodenectomy for trauma: a viable option? Am J Surg 1984; 147:618–623.

43. Sims EH, Mandal AU, Schlater T, et al. Factors affecting outcomes in pancreatic trauma. J Trauma 1984; 24:125–128.

44. Wynn M, Hill DH, Miller DR, et al. Management of pancreatic and duodenal trauma. Am J Surg 1985; 150:327–332.

45. Nowak MM, Baringer DC, Ponsky JL. Pancreatic injuries: effectiveness of debridement and drainage for nontransecting injuries. Am Surg 1986; 52:599–602.

46. Gorenstein A, O'Halpin D, Wesson DE, et al. Blunt injury to the pancreas in children: selective management based on ultrasound. J Pediatr Surg 1987; 22:1110–1116.

47. Pachter HL, Hofstetter SR, Liang HG, et al. Traumatic injuries to the pancreas: the role of distal pancreatectomy with splenic preservation. J Trauma 1989; 29:1352–1355.

48. Fabian TC, Kudsk KA, Croce MA, et al. Superiority of closed suction drainage for pancreatic trauma: a randomized prospective study. Ann Surg 1990; 211:724–730.

49. Flynn WJ, Cryer HG, Richardson JD. Reappraisal of pancreatic and duodenal injury management based on injury severity. Arch Surg 1990; 125:1539–1541.

50. Ivatury RR, Nallathambi M, Rao P, et al. Penetrating pancreatic injuries: analysis of 103 consecutive cases. Am Surg 1990; 56:90–95.

51. Cogbill TH, Moore EE, Morris JA, et al. Distal pancreatectomy for trauma: a multicenter experience. J Trauma 1991; 31:1600–1606.

52. Voeller GR, Mangiante EC, Fabian TC. The effect of a trauma system on the outcome of patients with pancreatic trauma. Arch Surg 1991; 126:578–580.

53. Buck JR, Sorensen VJ, Fath JJ, et al. Severe pancreaticoduodenal injuries: the effectiveness of pyloric exclusion with vagotomy. Am Surg 1992; 58:557–561.

54. Rosen MA, McAninch JW. Management of combined renal and pancreatic trauma. J Urol 1994; 152:22–25.

55. Delcore R, Satuffer JS, Thomas JH, et al. The role of pancreatogastrostomy following pancreatoduodenectomy for trauma. J Trauma 1994; 37:395–400.

56. Craig MH, Talton DS, Hauser CJ, et al. Pancreatic injuries from blunt trauma. Am Surg 1995; 61:125–128.

57. Degiannis E, Levy RD, Potokar LT, et al. Distal pancreatectomy for gunshot injuries of the distal pancreas. Br J Surg 1995; 82:1240–1242.

58. Degiannis E, Levy RD, Velamhos G, et al. Gunshot injuries of the head of the pancreas: conservative approach. World J Surg 1996; 20:68–72.

59. Smith DR, Stanley RJ, Rue LW III. Delayed diagnosis of pancreatic transaction after blunt abdominal trauma. J Trauma 1996; 40:1009–1013.

60. Akhrass R, Yaffe MB, Brandt CP, et al. Pancreatic trauma: a ten-year multi-institutional experience. Am Surg 1997; 63:598–604.

61. Farrell RJ, Krige EJ, Bornman PC, et al. Operative strategies in pancreatic trauma. Br J Surg 1996; 83:934–937.

62. Patton J Jr, Lyden SP, Croce MA, et al. Pancreatic trauma: a simplified management guideline. J Trauma 1997; 43:234–241.

63. Timbelake GA. Blunt pancreatic trauma: experience at a rural referral center. Am Surg 1997; 63:282–286.

64. Young P Jr, Meredith JW, Baker CC, et al. Pancreatic injuries resulting from penetrating trauma: a multi-institutional review. Am Surg 1998; 64:838–844.

65. Eastlick L, Fogler R, Shaftan GW. Pancreaticoduodenectomy for trauma: delayed reconstruction: a case report. J Trauma 1990; 30:503–505.

66. Asensio J, Demetriades D, Berne J, et al. A unified approach to the surgical exposure of pancreatic and duodenal injuries. Am J Surg 1997; 174:54–60.

67. Asensio JA, Demetriades D, Hanpeter DE, et al. Management of pancreatic injuries. Curr Probl Surg 1999; 36(5):325–420.

68. Asensio JA, Petrone P, Roldan G, et al. Pancreatic and duodenal injuries: complex and lethal. Scand J Surg 2002; 91(1):81–86.

69. Kasugai T, Kuno N, Kobayashi S, et al. Endoscopic pancreatocholangiography, I: the normal endoscopic pancreatocholangiogram. Gastroenterology 1972; 63:217.

70. Classen M, Koch H, Ruskin H, et al. Pancreatitis after endoscopic retrograde pancreatography (ERCP). Gut 1973; 14:431.

71. Asensio JA. Operative pancreatograms at 2 AM? In Critical Decision Points in Trauma Care. Proceedings of postgraduate course. Am Coll Surg 1992; 5:55–57.

72. Moore EE, Cogbill TH, Malangoni MA, et al. Organ injury scaling, II: pancreas, duodenum, small bowel, colon and rectum. J Trauma 1990; 30:1427.

73. Whipple AO, Parson WB, Mullins CR. Treatment of carcinoma of the ampulla of Vater. Ann Surg 1935; 102:763–779.

74. Howell JF, Burrus GR, Jordan GL. Surgical management of pancreatic injuries. J Trauma 1961; 1:32–40.

75. Thal AP, Wilson RF. A pattern of severe blunt trauma to the region of the pancreas. Surg Gynecol Obstet 1964; 119:773–778.

76. Halgrimson CG, Trimble C, Gale S, et al. Pancreaticoduodenectomy for traumatic lesions. Am J Surg 1969; 118:877–882.

77. Walter RL, Gaspard DJ, German TD. Traumatic pancreatitis. Am J Surg 1966; 111:364–368.

78. Thompson RJ, Hindshaw DB. Pancreatic trauma. Ann Surg 1966; 163:153–160.

79. Sawyers JL, Carlisle BB, Sawyers JE. Management of pancreatic injuries. South Med J 1967; 60:382–386.

80. Wilson RF, Tagett JP, Pucelik JP, et al. Pancreatic trauma. J Trauma 1967; 7:643–651.

81. Brawley RK, Cameron JL, Zuidema G. Severe upper abdominal injuries treated by pancreaticoduodenectomy. Surg Gynecol Obstet 1968; 126:516–522.

82. Pantazelos HH, Kerhulas AA, Byrne JJ. Total pancreaticoduodenectomy for trauma. Ann Surg 1969; 170:1016–1020.

83. Gibbs BF, Crow JL, Rupnik EJ. Pancreatoduodenectomy for blunt pancreatoduodenal injury. J Trauma 1970; 10:702–705.

84. Nance FC, De Loach DH. Pancreaticoduodenectomy following abdominal trauma. J Trauma 1971; 11:577.

85. Jones RC, Shires T. Pancreatic trauma. Arch Surg 1971: 102:424–430.

86. Smith A, Wolverton W, Wiechert R III, et al. Operative management of pancreatic and duodenal injuries. J Trauma 1971; 11:570–576.

87. Anderson CB, Weisz D, Rodger MR, et al. Combined pancreaticoduodenal trauma. Am J Surg 1973; 125:530–534.

88. Owens M, Wolfman E Jr. Pancreatic trauma: management and presentation of a new technique. Surgery 1973; 73:881–886.

89. Steele M, Sheldon GF, Blaisdell FW. Pancreatic injuries. Arch Surg 1973; 106:544–549.

90. Sturm JT, Quattlebaum FW, Mowlem A, et al. Patterns of injury requiring pancreatoduodenectomy. Surg Gynecol Obstet 1973; 137:629–632.

91. Yellin AE, Rossof L. Pancreatoduodenectomy for combined pancreatoduodenal injuries. Arch Surg 1975; 110:1117–1183.

92. Chamber RT, Norton L, Hinchey EJ. Massive right upper quadrant intra-abdominal injury requiring pancreaticoduodenectomy and partial hepatectomy. J Trauma 1975; 15:714–719.

93. Balasegaram M. Surgical management of pancreatic trauma. Am J Surg 1976; 131:536–540.

94. Heitsch RC, Knutson CO, Fulton RL, et al. Delineation of critical factors in the treatment of pancreatic trauma. Surgery 1976; 80:523–529.

95. Karl HW, Chandler JG. Mortality and morbidity of pancreatic injury. Am J Surg 1977; 134:549–554.

96. Hagan WV, Urdaneta LF, Stephenson SE. Pancreatic injury. South Med J 1978; 171:892–894.

97. Stone HH, Fabian TC. Management of duodenal wounds. J Trauma 1979; 19:334–339.

98. Levinson MA, Peterson SR, Sheldon GF, et al. Duodenal trauma: experience of a trauma center. J Trauma 1982; 24:475–480.

99. Henarejos A, Cohen DM, Moosa AR. Management of pancreatic trauma. Ann R Coll Surg Engl 1983; 65:297–300.

100. Adkins RB Jr, Keyser JE III. Recent experience with duodenal trauma. Am Surg 1984; 5:121–231.

101. Moore JB, Moore EE. Changing trends in the management of combined pancreatoduodenal injuries. World J Surg 1984; 8:791–797.

102. Fabian TC, Mangiante EC, Millis M. Duodenal rupture due to blunt trauma: a problem in diagnosis. South Med J 1984; 77:1078–1082.

103. Donahue JH, Crass RA, Trunkey DD. The management of duodenal and other small intestinal trauma. World J Surg 1985; 9:904–913.

104. Jones RC. Management of pancreatic trauma. Am J Surg 1985; 150:698–704.

105. Ivatury RR, Nallathambi M, Gaudino J, et al. Penetrating duodenal injuries: analysis of 100 consecutive cases. Am J Surg 1985; 2:153–158.

106. Smego DR, Richardson JD, Flint LM. Determinants of outcome in pancreatic trauma. J Trauma 1985; 25:771–776.

107. Walker ML. Management of pancreatic trauma: concepts and controversy. J Natl Med Assoc 1986; 78:1177–1183.

108. Melissas J, Baart GD, Mannel A. Pancreaticoduodenectomy for pancreatic trauma. S Afr Med J 1987; 71:32–34.

109. McKone TK, Bursch LR, Scholten DJ. Pancreaticoduodenectomy for trauma: a life-saving procedure. Am Surg 1988; 54:361–364.

110. Heimansohn DA, Canal DF, McCarthy MC, et al. The role of pancreaticoduodenectomy in the management of traumatic injuries to the pancreas and duodenum. Am Surg 1990; 56:511–514.

111. Asensio JA, Petrone P, Roldan G, et al. Role of the pancreaticoduodenectomy: a rare procedure for the management of complex pancreaticoduodenal injuries. J Am Coll Surg 2003; 197:937–942.

112. Glancy KE. Review of pancreatic trauma. West J Med 1989; 151:45–51.

113. Graham JM, Mattox KL, Vaughan GD III, et al. Traumatic injuries of the pancreas. Am J Surg 1978; 136:744–748.

114. Balasegaram M. Surgical management of pancreatic trauma. Curr Probl Surg 1979; 16:1–59.

115. Buchler M, Friess H, Klempa I, et al. Role of the octreotide in the prevention of postoperative complications following pancreatic resections. Am J Surg 1992; 163: 126–131.

116. Kudsk KA, Temizer D, Ellison EC, et al. Post-traumatic pancreatic sequestration: recognition and treatment. J Trauma 1986; 26:320–324.

117. Werner J, Uhl W, Buchles M, eds. Cameron's Current Surgical Therapy, 8th ed. Philadelphia: Elsevier/Mosby, 2005: 456–469.

33
Spleen

L. D. Britt

Case Scenario

A U.S. exchange student, who recently returned after spending 3 weeks backpacking in some of the remote areas of sub-Saharan Africa, presents to the emergency department complaining of a throbbing headache, fever, and left shoulder pain. The patient denies any recent trauma. She is diaphoretic and hemodynamically labile (blood pressure, 80 mm Hg; pulse, 130) and has a distended abdomen, which is diffusely tender to palpation.

Acute care ultrasonography demonstrates a substantial amount of free fluid in the abdominal cavity. In addition to appropriate resuscitative efforts, which of the following should be the specific management approach at this time?

(A) Computed tomography scan of the abdomen
(B) Arteriography and possible embolization
(C) Admission to the intensive care unit and administration of broad-spectrum antibiotics
(D) Diagnostic peritoneal lavage
(E) Celiotomy

Our knowledge of the spleen has expanded since Aristotle's pronouncement that the spleen possessed mystical properties and that it siphoned off "humors" from the stomach.[1] Galen referred to the spleen as "organum mysterum" (organ of mystery). Mamonides, in the twelfth century, believed that the spleen was an essential organ for life and had a vital physiologic function—the purification of blood. He introduced the concept of blood cleansing by the spleen.[2]

There were some scholars who thought that the spleen was not essential and could be removed with impunity.[3] William Mayo believed that there were no adverse sequelae for a patient as a result of having his or her spleen removed.[4]

In fact, the full spectrum of physiologic functions of the spleen (from removing particulate matter and destroying red blood cells to enhancing the immune process) were not known until recently. The spleen is the primary site of opsonin production and lymphocytic response to antigenic stimulation. Animal experiments performed by Morris and Bullock[5] demonstrated the spleen's pivotal role in preventing infections in rats.

A clinically significant immunodeficiency with increased susceptibility to infections can occur after removal of the spleen.[6,7] Although there were concerns about postsplenectomy infection as was highlighted by Morris and Bullock in their 1919 paper, the landmark article by King and Schumacher[8] confirmed this finding in humans by demonstrating an increased infection rate in infants following splenectomy. This study had a small sample with two of the five patients who underwent splenectomy for congenital hemolytic anemia dying from overwhelming infections. Several other authors have subsequently noted this increased rate of overwhelming sepsis in adults. [9-14]

Postsplenectomy, overwhelming sepsis occurs in up to 0.5% of patients who have undergone splenectomies as a result of trauma and in up to 20% in patients with hematologic disorders that necessitate a splenectomy. The group with the greatest risk for this highly lethal infection is asplenic patients less than 2 years old; mortality rate can be as high as 80% in this cohort. However, the death rate, in general, is extremely low. Singer[15] noted that of the 2,795 patients he reviewed, the death rate for adults was 0.01% and higher for children at 0.58%. Because of a permanent increase in the susceptibility to infections, there was still an appropriate emphasis over the past two decades on splenic conservation, which included nonoperative management of splenic injuries in hemodynamically stable patients and splenic salvage, if possible, when operative intervention is required. Unknowingly, nonoperative management was practiced before the advent of abdominal computed tomography

(CT) scanning for unsuspected splenic injuries that did not result in hemodynamic deterioration. With respect to the role of nonoperative management, controversies still exist, including the following: (1) nonoperative management in the elderly patients, (2) nonoperative management in the neurologically impaired, (3) the need for repeated imaging, and (4) activity after discharge. An injured spleen secondary to blunt trauma in the hemodynamically labile patient is the most frequent reason for emergency operative management of the spleen in the acute setting. However, there are other indications, albeit uncommon, for acute surgical intervention, including spontaneous rupture of the spleen from various infectious etiologies, including mononucleosis, mumps, malaria, and AIDS.[16] Irrespective of the specific etiology (splenic disorder or trauma), acute care surgical intervention will likely be required in the setting of hemodynamic instability secondary to active splenic bleeding.

Clinical Anatomy

Knowledge of the anatomy of the spleen and its anatomic relationships is essential for successful management of splenic injuries or disorders that prompt surgical intervention in the acute care setting and avoidance of iatrogenic complications while operating in the abdominal cavity. The spleen is the single largest mass of lymphoid tissue in the body. However, splenic size can vary during life depending on the amount of contained blood. The embryonic development of the spleen, which begins in the fifth gestational week, is clinically important, for its development from a small cluster of mesenchymal cells is sometimes incomplete, resulting in isolated mesenchymal variants. These isolated remnants develop into accessory spleens. The incidence of accessory spleens is 15% to 20%. With the embryologic origin of the spleen being the dorsal mesogastrium, the location of an accessory spleen is quite variable, and its blood supply ranges from branches of the splenic vessels to independent tributaries from other vascular organs in the abdomen, including the gastroepiploic vessels. There is no documentation that this additional splenic volume can maintain normal splenic function after a splenectomy is performed.

The spleen, with its notched anterior border, lies in the left hypochondrium. With its longitudinal axis bordered by the tenth and eleventh ribs, the normal spleen usually cannot be palpated. The peritoneum envelops the spleen and continues with peritoneal folds to connect the left kidney and stomach by what is known as the "lienorenal" (or "splenorenal") and the gastrosplenic ligaments, respectively. The lienorenal ligament contains the splenic vessels and the tail of the pancreas, which can be in close proximity to the splenic hilum. The gastrosplenic ligament passes from the hilum of the spleen to the greater

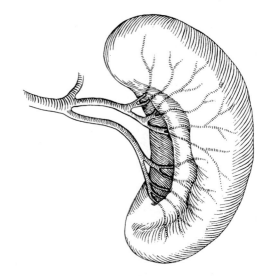

FIGURE 33.1. The splenic artery, the largest branch of the celiac trunk, runs horizontally behind the stomach and along the posterior and superior borders of the pancreas. After crossing anterior to the upper pole of the kidney, the splenic artery divides into segmental (terminal) branches just before entering the hilum. With most splenic lacerations occurring in the transverse plane, this greatly facilitates splenic salvage by allowing the surgeon to perform a more anatomic partial resection. (Reprinted with permission from Britt et al.[38])

curvature of the stomach. This ligament contains the short gastric veins and arteries, along with the left gastroepiploic vessels. Other suspensory ligamentous attachments include the splenophrenic and splenocolic ligaments, which are normally avascular. However, certain disease states, such as myeloproliferative disorders and portal hypertension, can result in vascular development in suspensory ligaments.

The spleen derives its blood supply from the splenic artery and the short gastric vessels (vasa brevia). The splenic artery, a major branch of the celiac axis, also supplies the stomach, greater omentum, and distal pancreas. With the division of the splenic artery into several segmental arteries in the splenic hilum, the resulting segments of the spleen are separated by relatively avascular planes (Figure 33.1). This anatomic configuration allows for partial resection of the spleen.[17,18] The splenic vein is formed by venous tributaries that emerge at the hilum of the spleen. Before joining the superior mesenteric vein to form the portal vein, the splenic vein runs with artery along the dorsal surface of the pancreas in the splenorenal ligament. Up to 40% of the portal blood flow comes from the splenic vein. In addition, there is venous drainage of the spleen through the short gastric veins, which subsequently drain into the left gastroepiploic. The lymphatic vessels drain the capsule and trabeculae and then pass through the pancreaticosplenic lymph nodes and drain into the celiac nodes. The nerves are derived from the celiac plexus and accompany the splenic artery. The spleen acts as a reservoir for blood that can be returned to the circulation. However, there is no active contraction because of the absence of smooth muscle in the splenic capsule. The spleen is relatively large in children because of its pivotal reticuloendothelial function and its role in the production of erythrocytes. Such major functions of the spleen are not required in adulthood. As a result, there is a commensurate decrease in the size, with the normal adult spleen weighing approximately 150 to 170 g. However, certain disease entities (e.g., malaria and infection mononucleosis) can substantially alter with the size and the consistency of the spleen. In addition to the child's spleen being larger, the splenic capsule is thicker and the parenchyma more firm in children.

Function

The normal spleen has both hematologic and immunologic functions. With respect to the former, the human spleen extracts aged and abnormal red blood cells from circulation. Morphologically deformed cells are unable to traverse the splenic circulation before becoming trapped. The spleen also participates in the maturation process of red blood cells by removing nuclear fragments, denatured hemoglobin, iron granules, and surface spurs and pits. In addition, the spleen is an important storage site for platelets and iron.[19] Although the hematologic function is maintained throughout life, the adult spleen has essentially no role in hematopoiesis, unless there is underlying myeloproliferative disorder.

The immunologic responses of the spleen are specific and nonspecific, having both humoral and cell-mediated immune responses. Specifically, the spleen is involved in the immune response to polysaccharide capsules of *Pneumococcus, Haemophilus*, and *Meningococcus* organisms. The differentiation between the red and white pulp is of functional importance. The anatomic design of the red pulp allows for the filtering of old and poorly functioning erythrocytes. The major phagocytic activity of the spleen is attributed to the fixed macrophages within the red pulp, which originates from circulating monocytes. This phagocytic activity is facilitated by the splenic production of opsonins and tuftsin. The juxtapositioned white pulp of the spleen contributes to the immune process by the filtering of antigens by the dendrite cells, with subsequent presentation to the immunocompetent cells. The bacteria are captured in a way to allow exposure of their antigens to the lymphocytes that are located in the white pulp. A quarter of the body's phagocytic activity occurs in the spleen.[20] As discussed earlier, removal of the spleen can result in one of the most potentially fatal complications—overwhelming sepsis postsplenectomy. Fortunately, the true incidence of this potentially lethal complication is

extremely low, especially for adults. It has been estimated that up to 50% of splenic tissue must be preserved in order to have normal splenic function.[21] There has been no documentation that any amount of accessory splenic tissue can prevent or attenuate postsplenectomy overwhelming sepsis.

Indication for Operative Intervention

The indications for surgery of the spleen are included under five categories: trauma, hypersplenism, malignancy, occult or infection related, and incidental to other surgery. In the acute setting, trauma, including iatrogenic injuries, is the major reason for splenic surgery, which often necessitates a splenectomy. Coon[22] highlighted that at least 20% of all splenectomies are actually performed for trauma. However, this percentage increases substantially if iatrogenic injuries are included.

Coon stated that several operations were often associated with iatrogenic injuries, including left nephrectomy (47%); hiatal hernioplasty; left or total colectomy (2%); gastric procedures (2%); and aortic aneurysmectomy (1%). The severity of associated injuries usually determines the mortality rate. An occult or spontaneous splenic rupture can also warrant acute care intervention. Table 33.1 lists some of the likely etiologies. The full spectrum of infections can lead to spontaneous splenic rupture. Infections with bacteria, fungi, viruses, protozoa, spirochetes, and rickeisiae have resulted in occult splenic rupture necessitating operative management. Zingman and Viner[23] reported a high mortality rate from spontaneous splenic rupture.

Although the authors noted some utility with abdominal ultrasonography, the diagnosis of a splenic rupture in this setting is, invariably, made at the time of the acute care laparotomy. Ultrasonography can expeditiously determine that there is an intraabdominal source of bleeding in such a setting. However, using this diagnostic modality to determine a specific solid organ injury is not recommended in the acute care setting.

Since the documentation of a fulminant septic course in a person rendered asplenic initially described by King and Schumacher,[8] the emphasis on the role of nonoperative management of splenic injuries has broadened. In the trauma setting, a nonoperative approach to splenic injuries has become the management of choice for the

TABLE 33.1. Some of the likely etiologies of splenic rupture.

Infection (malaria, mumps, mononucleosis)
Intrasplenic injury
Vascular abnormalities
Infiltrative splenic conditions (amyloidosis)
Primary and metastatic neoplasms

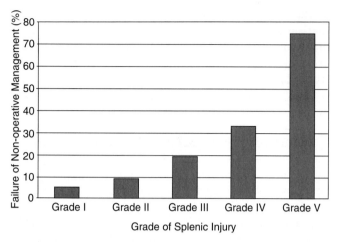

FIGURE 33.2. Multiinternational study: failure rates by grade of injury. (Reprinted with permission from Peitzman et al.[32])

hemodynamically stable patient. [24–27] Such expectant management of splenic injuries is now highly successful in both the pediatric and adult population with a greater than 90% and 80% success rate, respectively. [28–31] A multiinstitutional study was conducted by the Eastern Association of the Surgery for Trauma (EAST).[32] Twenty-seven trauma centers participated, and there were approximately 1,500 adults (>15 years of age) included in this analysis. Thirty-eight percent of the patients went directly to the operating room, with the remaining patients (62%) admitted for nonoperative management. In this cohort of patients, the failure rate of nonoperative management was 10.8%, with an associated mortality rate of 12.6%. Most of the failures of nonoperative management occurred in the first 96 hours (60.9%). Older patients (>55years of age) had a higher rate of failure than those patients <55 years of age. The study also demonstrated a linear relationship between the failure rate and the grade of injury (Figure 33.2). The particular age range in which nonoperative management is not as successful is still debated.[33,34] The liberal use of CT in the diagnostic workup of the blunt trauma patient has greatly facilitated this nonoperative approach for both splenic injuries.[35] Also, the advent of the helical CT scan further improved detection and characterization of splenic pathology.[36]

Even when operative intervention is required, some form of splenic salvage should be considered if the risk/benefit ratio is favorable. Such an effort to preserve the spleen is not a new concept.

On the contrary, splenic repairs, including partial splenectomy and direct suture repair, were reported over a century ago. Today, the concept of splenic salvage has been re-embraced.[37–43] However, each case should be individualized. Preservation is achieved by nonoperative management, splenorrhaphy, or partial splenectomy. For example, a trauma patient who is hemodynamically labile

and undergoing operative intervention should probably not have any attempts to salvage the spleen, particularly if there are other associated injuries. On the other hand, an attempt to achieve splenic preservation is very appropriate if a patient remains hemodynamically stable and if there are no other associated major injuries. Some authors advocate selective arteriography and embolization in an attempt to avoid operative intervention for the patient who has ongoing splenic bleeding.[44–46] Even with successful splenic embolization, the question still remains if splenic immunologic function is fully maintained. Also, this intervention has a failure rate of 13.5% and is associated with several complications, including hemorrhage, infection, and missed injuries.

Operative Management

General

The spleen is one of the most frequently injured solid organs in abdominal and thoracoabdominal blunt trauma. Although most patients can be managed nonoperatively, having an armamentarium of operative options is imperative. With there being more innovative ways of preserving the spleen, what was initially thought to be irreversible injuries of the spleen (e.g., hilar injuries) are now being managed without whole-organ removal. The caveat, which should always be considered when deciding whether to perform a splenectomy or splenorrhaphy, is the ever present patient risk/benefit ratio. For example, for the patient who is hemodynamically labile or has associated intraabdominal injuries, splenectomy will likely be the preferred operative management strategy.

Refractory shock always dictates operative intervention. The particular grade of injury (Table 33.2) does not always correspond with level of intervention. Although arteriography/embolization has a role in the management of splenic emergencies, this approach should not be considered for any patient in refractory shock.

Certain symptoms and physical findings are suggestive of splenic injuries, such as left upper abdominal pain and tenderness or left upper quadrant or lower chest wall abrasions. Also, left lower rib cage tenderness suggests an associated fracture and possible splenic injury.[47] Symptomatology might include left shoulder pain (Kehr's sign), which can occur as a result of irritators (blood or expanding subdiaphragmatic hematoma) of the left hemidiaphragm consistent with an injury or a pathologic process with subdiaphragmatic (e.g., splenic) trauma.

The initial management of any splenic problem necessitating acute surgical intervention includes absolute prioritization, with airway, breathing, and circulation assessments always being the top priorities along with appropriate fluid resuscitation. When possible, obtaining an adequate history from the patient or family members

TABLE 33.2. Organ injury scale: spleen.

Grade*		Injury description
I.	Hematoma	Subcapsular, nonexpanding, <10% surface area
	Laceration	Capsular tear, nonbleeding, <1 cm parenchymal depth
II.	Hematoma	Subcapsular, nonexpanding, 10%–50% surface area; intraparenchymal, nonexpanding. <2 cm in diameter
	Laceration	Capsular tear, active bleeding, 1–3 cm parenchymal depth that does not involve a trabecular vessel
III.	Hematoma	Subcapsular, >50% surface area or expanding; ruptured subcapsular hematoma with active bleeding; intraparenchymal hematoma, <2 cm or expanding
	Laceration	>3 cm parenchymal depth or involving trabecular vessels
IV.	Hematoma	Ruptured intraparenchymal hematoma with active bleeding
	Laceration	Laceration involving segmental or hilar vessel producing major devascularization (>25% of spleen)
V.	Laceration	Completely shattered spleen
	Vascular	Hilar vascular injury that devascularizes spleen

* Advance one grade for multiple injuries to the same organ. Based on most accurate assessment at autopsy, laparotomy, or radiologic study.
Source: Reprinted with the permission of the Organ Injury Scaling Committee of the American Association for the Surgery of Trauma.

and friends is important. Initial laboratory tests should be done, including hemoglobin, hematocrit, arterial blood gases, and unit type and cross-matching for possible use of blood. In general, laboratory tests have limited value in the acute care setting. However, the role of diagnostic imaging cannot be overemphasized. For the hemodynamically labile patient, diagnostic peritoneal lavage (DPL) still has a role, although the focused abdominal sonographic test (FAST) has almost supplanted DPL because of its sensitivity in determining intraperitoneal fluid accumulation in the hemodynamically labile patient.[48]

Abdominal sonography can quickly determine if there is a large amount of fluid in the peritoneal cavity. Such determination of substantial free fluid in the abdominal cavity in a patient who is hemodynamically unstable is hemoperitoneum until proven otherwise and should prompt operative intervention. Abdominal ultrasonography is still operator dependent, and subtle intraabdominal injuries can be missed by all but the most experienced.

As highlighted earlier, CT scanning of the abdomen is the diagnostic modality most often used in the evaluation of the spleen, unless the patient is hemodynamically unstable. The CT scan can help delineate parenchymal disruption of spleen, subscapular hemostasis, splenic abrasions, and splenic artery aneurysms. Also, the demonstration of a hyperdense area (consistent with contrast material) is the so-called blush seeps in the disrupted

parenchyma of the spleen.[49] Such a finding suggests the need for urgent intervention by either an acute care celiotomy or arteriography/embolization.

Because vaccination prophylaxis to meningococcal and streptococcal infection is likely more effective when administered while the spleen is still in the patient, these vaccines should be given before operative intervention, if possible. In addition to optimal resuscitative efforts, the patient undergoing operative management should have preoperative antibiotics. Whether or not antibiotics should be continued postoperatively depends on the operative findings. However, unless there is associated abscess or gross contamination such as feculent spillage, antibiotics should be discontinued after surgery. Also, in preparation for splenic surgery, the stomach should be decompressed with a nasogastric or orogastric tube to facilitate mobilization of the spleen.

Operative Approach

Optimal exposure is always essential to any operative intervention. The incision of choice should be a midline vertical approach with the option of extending the incision cephalad (to the left of the xiphoid). Such an incision allows the surgeon rapid access to other areas of the abdominal cavity to rule out associated injuries. For more elective surgery, the preferred incision may vary; however, the midline vertical approach provides excellent exposure even in the elective, nontraumatic cases requiring access to the spleen. Both the subcostal and transverse incision, as used in more elective cases, can be extended to provide better exposure (Figure 33.3). For example, the Kehr incision has a vertical extension to the xiphoid, which can provide better access for mobilization of large spleens. Nevertheless, in the acute care setting, the midline vertical incision remains the mainstay approach.

After making the appropriate incision and obtaining adequate access into the abdominal cavity, general exploration of the abdominal cavity should be done. This entails the evisceration of bowel in order to pack the four quadrants of the abdomen if a substantial amount of gross blood is encountered in entering the abdomen. Thorough exploration of the abdomen is always prudent after operative stabilization of any massive bleeding. When indicated, control of gross contamination is next after establishing hemodynamic stability. If there is an isolated splenic problem necessitating total or partial splenectomy, then the spleen needs to be mobilized and delivered to the central area of the abdominal cavity and, if possible, onto the abdominal wall for better inspection. Also, this maneuver would facilitate more accurate control of the segmental vasculature at the hilum. Such control is essential when splenorrhaphy or partial splenectomy is being considered. During the

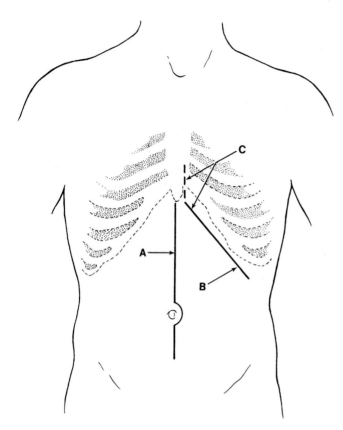

clamps and tied, being careful not to injure the greater curvature of the stomach. In order to bring the spleen onto the abdominal wall, dissection must include mobilization of the tail and part of the body of the pancreas. After adequate mobilization of the spleen, all options are open to the surgeon with respect to splenic preservation (partial splenectomy and splenorrhaphy).

Isolation and control of the main splenic artery is often recommended before mobilization in nontrauma cases in which the spleen is remarkably enlarged. In the trauma setting, compression of the hilar vessels can provide excellent temporary vascular control necessary for optimal management of splenic injuries.

Management Options of Specific Injuries

Unless there is hemodynamic lability, major associated injuries, or a pulverized splenic injury, splenic preservation should be attempted. There is a growing armamentarium of surgical options/adjuncts in an effort to salvage the spleen. The specific approach should be based on the extent of injury. Matching a specific surgical approach to

FIGURE 33.3. The midline vertical incision (A) is the incision of choice for most trauma cases. Such an operative approach provides excellent exposure not only of the spleen but also of the other organs that might require concomitant surgical repair. However, other incisions have been advocated for more elective operations, including the left subcostal (B) with an option for a xiphoid extension (C). The operation should utilize table movement (right-side down/moderate reverse Trendelenburg) when appropriate to enhance the exposure of the spleen. (Reprinted with permission from Britt et al.[38])

mobilization, care should be taken to avoid capsular avulsion. Such mobilization is initiated with the division of anterior and posterolateral peritoneal attachments. It should be noted again that, in most cases, the splenogastric ligament is the only peritoneal attachment that encompasses significant vasculature (i.e., vasa brevia). Unless there is active brisk hemorrhage or the vascular anatomy is obscured by perisplenic hematoma, division of the superior vasa brevia should be performed before medial mobilization of the spleen to prevent an inadvertent capsular avulsion at the superior splenic pole site, which is a common intraoperative complication.

The spleen should always be gently grasped and retracted medially with the surgeon's nondominant hand, as this allows expeditious mobilization and minimizes additional injury to the spleen (Figure 33.4). Division of the splenogastric ligament and all the vasa brevia vessels need to be divided for optimal exposure of the splenic artery. All short gastric vessels should be divided with

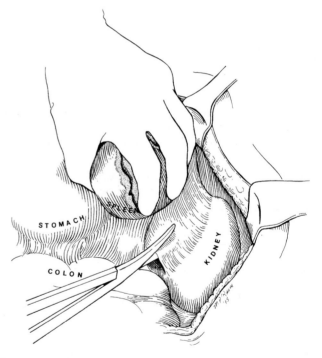

FIGURE 33.4. Mobilization of the spleen should ultimately allow the surgeon to deliver the spleen into the central position of the abdominal cavity. Anterior and posterolateral peritoneal attachments need to be divided to initiate mobilization. Division of the splenogastric ligament and all the vasa brevia vessels will need to be directed for optimal exposure of the splenic artery. Care should be taken not to avulse the splenic capsule. To bring the spleen onto the abdominal wall for optimal evaluation and management, the tail and part of the body of the pancreas need to be mobilized. (Reprinted with permission from Britt et al.[38])

a given injury always depends on the surgeon's technical skills and experience. For grade I and most grade II injuries, a hemostatic agent applied topically along with direct pressure should provide optimal management. In addition, the Argon Beam Coagulator (Bard Electro Medical Systems) is a very useful modality for grade I and some grade II injuries. It is particularly useful for raw surface areas as a result of surgical dissection or subcapsular hematoma decompression. An omental, Teflon, or collagen buttress can also be used with these injuries (Table 33.3). Splenic lacerations can be sutured directly. However, the splenic capsule does not hold sutures well. Pledget materials would be applicable, if this option is chosen.

For grade III and IV injuries, optimal mobilization of the spleen is imperative. Active bleeding can be temporarily controlled by digital compression of the hilar vessels. Once this is accomplished and the full extent of the splenic injury can be assessed, care should be taken to expose the splenic hilar vasculature, particularly when a partial anatomic resection of the spleen is being considered. It should be noted that, because of the spleen's horizontal blood supply and the fact that lacerations usually occur in the transverse plane, an anatomic resection can often be performed if there is segmental damage of the spleen. Ligation of a segment artery that supplies the deeply lacerated region of the spleen will produce the demarcation zone, thus providing an excellent guide for the anatomic resection. The actual dissection of this spleen involves incising the splenic capsule followed by either blunt or sharp dissection into the parenchyma. The finger fracture technique between the index finger and thumb or blunt dissection with the handle of the scalpel (or suction catheter tip) will allow expeditious dissection through the parenchyma (Figure 33.5). The intrasplenic vessels encountered should be selectively ligated with either hemoclips or direct suture ligature.

Severely lacerated spleens involving segmental and/or hilar vessels and extensively denuded splenic capsule can sometimes be successfully managed with mesh wraps.[50,51]

TABLE 33.3. Surgical adjuncts for splenic salvage.

Topical agents
 Fibrin Glue (cryoprecipitate, bovine topical thrombin, and calcium
  chloride)
 Microfibrillar collagen (Avitene)
 Thrombin-soaked gel foam

Wraps and buttresses
 Omentum
 Teflon pledget
 Vicryl mesh

Cautery and dissectors
 Electrocautery
 CUSA ultrasonic cavitator
 Argon Beam Coagulator

Source: Reprinted with permission from Britt et al.[38]

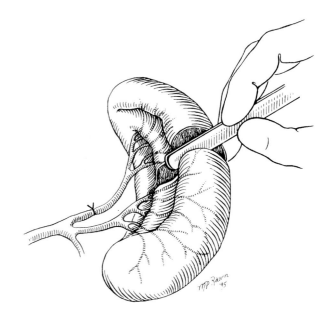

FIGURE 33.5. After the incision of the splenic capsule, division of the splenic parenchyma can be achieved by blunt dissection with the handle of the scalpel (or suction catheter tip). Intrasplenic vessels should be selectively ligated with either hemoclips or direct suture ligature. Appropriate extrasplenic vasculature needs to be ligated if a partial splenectomy is being attempted. (Reprinted with permission from Britt et al.[38])

A woven polyglycolic acid mesh can be fashioned as a "wrap," or jacket, for the injured spleen, with the artery and vein being allowed to exit through a slit in the mesh (Figure 33.6). The wrap is then snugly sutured to encase the spleen and provide the necessary tamponade effect.

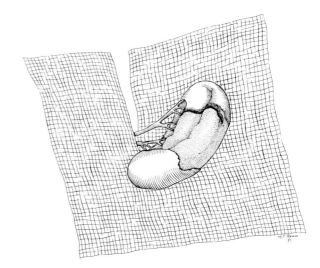

FIGURE 33.6. A woven polyglycolic acid mesh can be fashioned to provide a tamponade wrap for a severely lacerated spleen or a denuded splenic capsule. This is accomplished by snugly fitting the mesh around the spleen and suturing it in place. A slit is made in the mesh wrap to allow the entry and exit of the splenic artery and vein, respectively. (Reprinted with permission from Britt et al.[38])

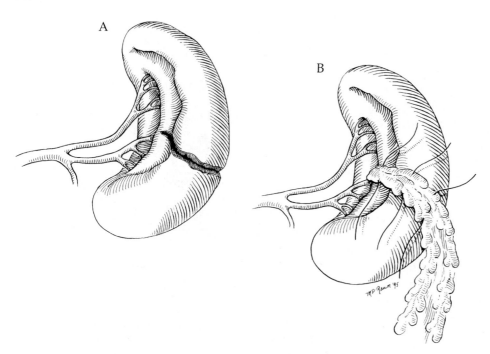

Often, hilar and/or intrasplenic vessels will still require selective ligation before the mesh wrap is applied. The authors have found the omentum to be useful in the preservation of the spleen as a buttress to both deep lacerations (Figure 33.7) and the raw surface area of a splenic remnant status after partial resection (Figure 33.8). With such an assortment of surgical options, splenic salvage should always be the rule and not the exception.

Although the literature is replete with respect to successful laparoscopic splenectomies (complete and partial), there are few indications, if any, for laparoscopic intervention in the emergency setting with acute splenic problems. If splenectomy is performed, the splenic bed or fossa should be initially packed and then carefully examined for residual bleeding; this includes inspecting the short gastric vascular remnants on the greater curvature. The role of autotransplantation of splenic tissue is dubious, at best. The fact that fatal postsplenectomy infections have been reported after splenic autotransplantation should remove all controversy surrounding this issue.[52]

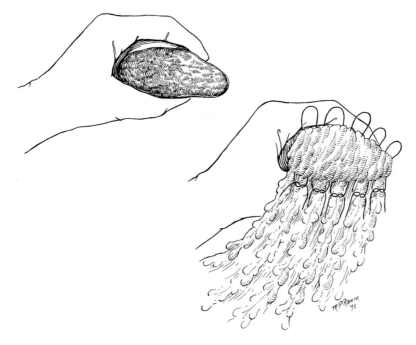

FIGURE 33.8. In addition to the hemostatic advantage, the omentum has phagocytic properties that make it a superb endogenous buttress. (Reprinted with permission from Britt et al.[38])

Drainage

Normally, there is no indication for drainage after the splenic repair or partial splenectomy. Insistence on using postoperative drains after a splenectomy could increase the complication rate, especially for intraabdominal abscess formation. However, closed suction drainage should be used if there is a suspicion of a pancreatic tail injury. Such a drain can usually be removed within 36 to 48 hours if there is no significant output.

Postsplenectomy Complications

In addition to the postoperative complications that can occur after any transabdominal operation (e.g., pulmonary problems), there are some specific complications such as bleeding following a splenorrhaphy or splenectomy that might necessitate reoperation. Such bleeding can occur from the raw surface area after splenorrhaphy or a partial resection, or it could come from the short gastric vessels or the splenic bed. Because of the close proximity of the tail of the pancreas to the splenic hilum, an iatrogenic pancreatic injury can occur with a resulting fistula. Necrosis of the greater curvature of the stomach is a result of clamping a portion of the gastric wall when attempting to clamp the various short gastric vessels. There could be a subsequent leak with fistulization and/or abscess formation. In the asplenic patient, there is a defective immune response to intravascular antigen. However, the immune response is unaltered if the antigens are presented via other routes (e.g., intradermal). With the exception of ongoing hemorrhage in the acute care setting, overwhelming postsplenectomy sepsis (OPSI) is one of the most dreaded complications after a splenectomy. The organisms that have been associated with this fulminant septic process are encapsulated bacteria, including *Streptococcus pneumoniae*, *Hemophilus influenzae* type B, and *Neisseria meningitidis* along with group A *Streptococcus*.[53] The lifetime risk is reported to be 0.026 and 0.052 for adults and children, respectively.[54]

However, the mortality of OPSI is significant and has been reported to be as high as 50%. This specific sepsis complication can progress very rapidly and is refractory to aggressive medical management. Splenic preservation and postsplenectomy prophylaxis vaccines are the best measures to prevent this complication. However, even with this possible lethal complication, there should be no attempts at splenic preservation if the risks to the patient outweigh the benefit of splenic salvage. Although the risk of OPSI is negligible, the asplenic patient is more prone to other infections. Green et al.[55] reported on late septic complications in adults following removal of the spleen.

To summarize, the rationale for splenic preservation and the evolving options of nonoperative management of acute splenic problems are well documented. However, in the acute setting in which a patient is hemodynamically unstable because of splenic injury or spontaneous rupture, the definitive management of choice is operative intervention. Quickly assessing the risk/benefit ratio is imperative before any attempt at splenic preservation.

Critique

Although uncommon, spontaneous rupture of the spleen is known to occur with a malarial infection. It is likely that this student had the required pretravel vaccinations and chemoprophylaxis. Unfortunately, such medical intervention does not confer 100% protection. With this student backpacking in an area endemic for malaria, spontaneous rupture of an enlarged spleen should be considered in the differential. However, a specific diagnosis is not needed given this presentation, because a patient who is diaphoretic and hemodynamically labile with a distended and diffusely tender abdomen presents a surgical emergency. In addition, the free fluid (hemoperitoneum) demonstrated during acute care ultrasonography—focused assessment sonography in trauma (FAST)—confirms the need for surgical intervention. Hemodynamic stability is essential for successful nonoperative management of splenic rupture. This is clearly not the case in this scenario. An acute care celiotomy was performed. There was 2 L of free blood originating from a ruptured, enlarged spleen. Although there are proponents for splenic preservation (even in the setting of malarial splenomegaly and spontaneous rupture), expeditiously performing a splenectomy would be the most prudent option.

Answer (E)

References

1. Aristotle. Parts of Animals, Book III. (Peck AL, trans.) Cambridge, MA: Harvard University Press, 1955.
2. Rosner F. The spleen in the Talmud and other early Jewish writings. Bull Hist Med 1972; 46(1):82–85.
3. Morgenstern L. A history of splenectomy. In Hiatt JR, Phillips EH, Morgenstern L, eds. Surgical Diseases of the Spleen. New York: Springer, 1999: 3.
4. Mayo WJ. Principles underlying surgery of the spleen, with a report on ten splenectomies. JAMA 1910; 54:14.
5. Morris DH, Bullock FD. The importance of the spleen in resistance to infection. Ann Surg 1919; 70:513.
6. Eichner ER. Splenic function: normal, too much and too little. Am J Med 1979; 66(2):311–320.
7. Downey EC, Shackford SR, Fridlund PH, Ninnemann JL. Long-term depressed immune functions in patients splenectomized for trauma. J Trauma 1987; 27(6):661–663.

8. King H, Schumacher HB Jr. Splenic studies. I. Susceptibility to infection after splenectomy performed in infancy. Ann Surg 1952; 136(2):239–242.

9. Lynch AM, Kapila R. Overwhelming postsplenectomy infection. Infect Dis Clin North Am 1996; 10(4):693–707.

10. Sekikawa T, Shatney CH. Septic sequelae after splenectomy for trauma in adults. Am J Surg 1983; 145(5):667–673.

11. Gopal V, Bisno AL. Fulminant pneumococcal infections in "normal" asplenic hosts. Arch Intern Med 1977; 137(11): 1526–1530.

12. Diamond LK. Splenectomy in childhood and the hazard of overwhelming infection. Pediatrics 1969; 43(43):886–889.

13. Holdsworth RJ, Irving AD, Cuschieri A. Postsplenectomy sepsis and its mortality rate: actual versus perceived risks. Br J Surg 1991; 78(9):1031–1038.

14. Robinette CD, Fraumeni JF Jr. Splenectomy and subsequent mortality in veterans of the 1939–45 war. Lancet 1977; 2(8029):127–129.

15. Singer DB: Post-splenectomy sepsis Perspect Pediatr Pathol 1973; 1:285–311.

16. Massad M, Murr M, Razzouk B, Nassourah Z, Sankari M, Najjar F. Spontaneous splenic rupture in an adult with mumps: a case report. Surgery 1988; 103(3):381–382.

17. Dixon JA, Miller F, McCloskey D, Siddoway J. Anatomy and techniques in segmental splenectomy. Surg Gynecol Obstet 1980; 150(4):516–520.

18. Barnhart MI, Lusher JM. Structural physiology of the human spleen. Am J Pediatr Hematol Oncol 1979; 1(4): 311–330.

19. Aster RH. Pooling of platelets in the spleen: role in the pathogenesis of "hypersplenic" thrombocytopenia. J Clin Invest 1966; 45(5):645–657.

20. Stielm ER, Wokim M. The spleen in infection and immunity. In Hiatt JR, Phillips EH, Morgenstern L, eds. Surgical Disease of the Spleen. New York: Springer, 1997: 53.

21. Van Wyck DB, Witte MH, Witte CL, Thies AC Jr. Critical splenic mass for survival from experimental pneumococcemia. J Surg Res 1980; 28(1):14–17.

22. Coon WW. Surgical aspects of splenic disease and lymphoma. Curr Probl Surg 1998; 35(7):543–646.

23. Zingman BS, Viner BL. Splenic complications in malaria: case report and review. Clin Infect Dis 1993; 16(2):223–232.

24. Lally KP, Rosario V, Mahour GH, Woolley MM. Evolution in the management of splenic injury in children. Surg Gynecol Obstet 1990; 170(3):245–248.

25. Malangoni M, Levine AW, Droege EA, Aprahamian C, Condon RE. Management of injury to the spleen in adults. Results of early operation and observation. Ann Surg 1984; 200(6):702–705.

26. Wisner DH, Blaisdell FW. When to save the ruptured spleen. Surgery 1992; 111(2):121–122.

27. Uranus S, Pfeifer J. Nonoperative treatment of blunt splenic injury. World J Surg 2001; 25(11):1405–1407.

28. Nix JA, Costanza M, Daley BJ, Powell MA, Enderson BL. Outcome of the current management of splenic injuries. J Trauma 2001; 50(5):835–842.

29. Haller JA Jr, Papa P, Drugas G, Colombani P. Nonoperative management of solid organ injuries in children. Is it safe? Ann Surg 1994; 219(6):625–628.

30. Schwartz MZ, Kangah R. Splenic injury in children after blunt trauma: blood transfusion requirements and length of hospitalization for laparotomy versus observation. J Pediatr Surg 1994; 29(5):596–598.

31. Cocanour CS, Moore FA, Ware DN, Marvin RG, Duke JH. Age should not be a consideration for nonoperative management of blunt splenic injury. J Trauma 2000; 48(4):606–610.

32. Peitzman AB, Heil B, Rivera L, et al. Blunt splenic injury in adults: multiinstitutional study of the Eastern Association for the Surgery of Trauma. J Trauma 2000; 49(2):177–187.

33. Barone JE, Burns G, Svehlak SA, et al. Management of blunt splenic trauma in patients older than 55 years. Southern Connecticut Regional Trauma Quality Assurance Committee. J Trauma 1999; 46(1):87–90.

34. Harbrecht BG, Peitzman AB, Rivera L, et al. Contribution of age and gender to outcome of blunt splenic injury in adults: multicenter center study of the Eastern Association for the Surgery of Trauma. J Trauma 2001; 51(5):881–895.

35. Williams RA, Black JJ, Sinow RM, Wilson SE. Computed tomography–assisted management of splenic trauma. Am J Surg 1997; 174(3):276–279.

36. Urban BA, Fishman EK. Helical CT of the spleen. Am J Roentgenol 1998; 170(4):997–1003.

37. Pachter HL, Hofstetter SR, Spencer FC. Evolving conception splenic surgery: splenorrhaphy versus splenectomy and postsplenectomy drainage: experience in 105 patients. Ann Surg 1981; 194(3):262–269.

38. Britt LD, Berger J. Splenic repair and partial splenectomy. In Nyhus LM, Baker RJ, Fischer JE, eds. Mastery of Surgery, vol 2, 3rd ed. Boston: Little, Brown & Company, 1997: 1276–1281.

39. Schweizer W, Bohlen L, Dennison A, Blumgart LH. Prospective study in adults of splenic preservation after traumatic rupture. Br J Surg 1992; 79(12):1330–1333.

40. Cogbill TH, Moore EE, Jurkovich GJ, et al. Nonoperative management of blunt splenic trauma: a multicenter experience. J Trauma 1989; 29(10):1312–1317.

41. Feliciano DV, Spjut-Patrinely V, Burch JM, et al. Splenorrhaphy. The alternative. Ann Surg 1990; 211(5):569–580.

42. Morgenstern L, Shapiro SJ. Techniques of splenic conservation. Ann Surg 1979; 114(4):449–454.

43. Dunham CM, Cornwell EE 3rd, Militello P. The role of Argon Beam Coagulation in splenic salvage. Surg Gynecol Obstet 1991; 173(3):179–182.

44. Sclafani SJ, Shaftan GW, Scalea TM, et al. Nonoperative salvage of computed tomography-diagnosed splenic injuries: utilization of angiography for triage and embolization for hemostasis. J Trauma 1995; 39(5):818–825.

45. Moz MF, Spigos DG, Pollak R, et al. Partial splenic embolization, an alternative to splenectomy. Results of a prospective, randomized study. Surgery 1984; 96:694–702.

46. Haan JM, Biffl W, Knudson MM, et al: Improved success in nonoperative management of blunt splenic injuries: embolization of splenic artery pseudoaneurysms. J Trauma 1998; 44:1008–1015.

47. Shweiki E, Klena J, Wood GC, Indeck M. Assessing the true risk of abdominal solid organ injury in hospitalized rib fracture patients. J Trauma 2001; 50(4):684–688.

48. Rozycki GS, Ochsner MG, Jaffin JH, Champion HR. Prospective evaluation of surgeons' use of ultrasound in the evaluation of trauma patients. J Trauma 1993; 34(4):516–526.

49. Omert LA, Salyer D, Dunham CM, Porter J, Silva A, Protetch J. Implications of the "contrast blush" finding on computed tomographic scan of the spleen in trauma. J Trauma 2001; 51(2):272–277.

50. Lange DA, Zaret P, Merlotti GJ, Roin AP, Sheaff C, Barrett JA. The use of adsorbable mesh in splenic trauma. J Trauma 1998; 28(3):269–275.

51. Rogers FB, Baumgartner NE, Robin AP, Barrett JA. Absorbable mesh splenorrhaphy for severe splenic injuries: functional studies in an animal model and an additional patient series. J Trauma 1991; 31(2):200–204.

52. Moore GE, Stevens RE, Moore EE, Aragon GE. Failure of splenic implants to protect against fatal postsplenectomy infection. Am J Surg 1983; 146(3):413–414.

53. Miller JR, Sirenek KR. Overwhelming postsplenectomy infection. J Surg Infect 1997; 3:1, 4–5.

54. Luna GK, Dellinger EP. Nonoperative observation therapy for splenic injuries: a safe therapeutic option? Am J Surg 1987; 153(5):462–468.

55. Green JB, Shackford SR, Sise MJ, Fridlund P. Late septic complications in adults following splenectomy for trauma: a prospective analysis in 144 patients. J Trauma 1986; 26(11):999–1004.

34
Intraabdominal Vasculature

George H. Meier III and Hosam F. El Sayed

Case Scenario

While undergoing an emergency exploratory laparotomy for management of a perforated sigmoid colon and perforated diverticulum, a 62-year-old patient was discovered to have a 5-cm splenic artery aneurysm. The patient's comorbidities include diabetes mellitus, chronic obstructive pulmonary disease, and coronary artery disease angioplasty and stent placement x3 performed 10 months ago. Which of the following is the most prudent management approach for the splenic artery aneurysm?

(A) Construction of a bypass graft
(B) Resection of the aneurysm and splenectomy at the time of the operation
(C) Postoperative placement of an endovascular stent
(D) Aneurysmectomy only
(E) Expectant management

Vascular emergencies occur for only one of two reasons: vessel occlusion or bleeding. Although both have unique features, the ultimate challenge for the vascular specialist is to either restore flow or limit it. This obvious dichotomy influences the approach to the patient as well as the approach to the vessel involved. Anatomy of the vessels is common to both endovascular and open procedures, with access considerations similar independent of the disease process encountered. Despite this, endoluminal approaches rely on continuity of vascular anatomy to the site of intervention, whereas surgical approaches more directly externally access only the vessels involved. The result of this difference is the need for anatomic consideration in planning the procedure, in some cases altering the balance between open and endovascular approaches. If bleeding is the issue, then an endovascular

approach may allow remote access and proximal control when a direct approach for surgery may be dangerous. Similarly, if multiple diseased vessels limit endovascular access, then an open approach, with or without endovascular adjuncts, may be better suited to the patient's needs. These issues will continue to influence individualized management of specific clinical scenarios for vascular emergencies.

Arterial or venous occlusion can occur under several broad categories. The underlying pathophysiology is the critical component, necessitating procedural tasks specific for the pathology responsible. Thrombus can form in situ, or it can lodge remote from the site of its formation. These differences are inherent in the pathology responsible. Treatment will be directed at the source of the thrombus when possible but may require remote treatment as well. For this reason, constant review of the differential diagnosis is needed as new clinical findings are encountered to provide complete, definitive treatment for the patient's occlusion.

With bleeding, the focus of care is on stopping the hemorrhage and repairing the anatomic issue responsible for the bleeding. This may result in an extensive reconstruction, or it may be as simple as repair of a needle puncture. In conjunction with the control of bleeding is the management of any underlying coagulopathy that may have caused or resulted from the hemorrhagic event. Thus, the management of bleeding emergencies also requires an overall perspective, with frequent modifications as clinical data evolve during the patient's care. In bleeding emergencies, endovascular access is rarely a problem because the flow of blood is by definition unrestricted. In many cases, endovascular control and treatment may be advantageous, particularly for complex patients with multiple issues to manage or for anatomically inaccessible locations.

Although arteries and veins have unique physiologies that may mandate altered approaches to treatment, the fundamental objectives remain the same. Venous occlusions are, in general, better tolerated than those in the arterial system because the flow of oxygenated blood is rarely compromised. Nonetheless, venous occlusions can result in altered end-organ physiology because of increased capillary oncotic pressure and stagnant capillary flow. Venous bleeding presents the same challenges as arterial, but the treatment of venous bleeding is often complicated by the issues of coagulopathy and the difficulty of localizing high-volume, low-pressure flow. Fortunately, tamponade of venous bleeding can be an effective clinical strategy, minimizing the need to directly attack venous injury resulting in hematoma.

Acute Mesenteric Ischemia

Anatomy and Pathophysiology

The flow of blood to the intestine and liver is a common source of acute care intervention in many clinical scenarios.[1] Despite the general need for maintained perfusion to the viscera, tolerance to ischemia is variable depending on the specific arteries involved. For instance, liver blood flow is the sum of the portal vein and the proper hepatic artery blood flows. Because both are normally present, the liver can survive a compromise in one source of blood flow. Hepatic artery blood flow is similar to renal blood flow: low-resistance, continuous flow at a constant demand.[2] Superior mesenteric blood flow, on the other hand, is intermittent with increases noted after meals or associated with disease in the other arterial distributions. If the mesenteric blood flow demonstrates a low-resistance pattern, then some physiologic cause must be present. Hepatic artery blood flow is continuous and low resistance unless anatomic disease causes a high-resistance pattern.

Arterial anatomy of the intestines and liver consists of three main arteries: the celiac axis, which gives rise to the common hepatic, splenic, and left gastric arteries; the superior mesenteric artery; and the inferior mesenteric artery. In general, acute ischemia can occur with an occlusion to any of these vessels, but, realistically, only involvement of the superior mesenteric artery will present as acute intestinal ischemia. If acute thrombosis occurs in the setting of chronic disease, the superior mesenteric artery will be involved but generally in association with disease of the other two vessels as well. If an acute embolus to the intestine presents with an acute abdominal emergency, then it will usually be to the superior mesenteric artery. All other arteries in the visceral circulations are much more tolerant of acute occlusion than is the superior mesenteric artery.

Practically speaking, there are two disease processes that lead to acute mesenteric ischemia, with a third arterial diagnosis that is defined by excluding the other two

diagnoses.[3–10] The two main diagnoses are acute mesenteric thrombosis and acute mesenteric embolus. If the mesenteric arteries are not occluded, but simply spastic, then nonocclusive mesenteric ischemia (NOMI), the third diagnosis, may be present. This diagnosis was more common in the past[11,12] and associated with digoxin (a known mesenteric artery vasoconstrictor) therapy. Nonetheless, NOMI can occur in any setting in which overall cardiac compromise leads to low-flow ischemia in the intestinal bed. In this situation, therapy is directed at the underlying cardiac issues once occlusive ischemia is ruled out by arteriography.

Acute mesenteric embolus results in acute ischemia of sudden onset, often associated with an acute urge to defecate.[13,14] These patients can usually give you the time to the minute when this event occurred because of the sudden onset of the symptoms. Most of the time the classic "pain out of proportion to the clinical examination" is the presenting clinical scenario, commonly associated with an underlying cardiac arrhythmia.[6,15] The duration of symptoms is usually short because of the severity of the pain. Most patients will present to the emergency room within 2 hours of the initial event.[16] Anatomically, the superior mesenteric is most commonly involved, with the embolus usually lodging beyond its the origin at the level of the first few major branches. This will usually result in sparing of the proximal jejunum at laparotomy, further reinforcing the diagnosis of embolus. Additionally, multiple clinical and angiographic criteria suggest the diagnosis of an embolic event as outlined in Table 34.1.

As discussed earlier, emboli to other visceral vessels may cause symptoms but are generally better tolerated, with symptoms that may be so vague as to be clinically inconsequential. Segmental infarctions can occur in any organ and have been described in the liver, spleen, colon, and other viscera.[17,18] These emboli are not generally life threatening and may be misdiagnosed in the short term. An underlying cardiac abnormality may be the only clue to the diagnosis, and the liberal use of echocardiography should be encouraged in this setting.

Acute mesenteric arterial thrombosis can also lead to life-threatening intestinal complications, but in this case the history provides many clues.[19–25] Usually, a preexistent unexpected weight loss, postprandial abdominal pain, or "food fear" can be elicited on questioning and should be sought in this patient group. Typically, associated cardiac

TABLE 34.1. Factors suggesting embolus as a diagnosis.

No prior symptoms
Meniscus at the proximal end of the clot
Cardiac rhythm other than normal sinus
No other peripheral vascular disease
History of embolus

TABLE 34.2. Factors suggesting thrombosis as a diagnosis.

History of postprandial abdominal pain
Tapered occlusion at the proximal end of the clot
No history of cardiac arrhythmia
History of vascular disease in other beds
Significant smoking history

or other peripheral vascular disease is present to provide evidence of systemic vascular disease. The onset of ischemia may be more gradual in these patients, but the severity of the pain is just the same. Anatomically, the loss of the final artery supplying the intestine leads to symptoms, and the associated vascular disease makes treatment by any modality more complicated. Although endovascular treatment may be more attractive for this high risk group, the extent of the disease process may preclude it. Diagnostic criteria suggesting thrombosis are outlined in Table 34.2.

The diagnosis of acute mesenteric arterial occlusion requires two elements: a high clinical index of suspicion and an arteriogram. If the diagnosis of mesenteric ischemia is entertained seriously, then arteriography is the diagnostic test of choice.[1,25-30] Other modalities such as magnetic resonance angiography (MRA) or duplex ultrasound may suggest the diagnosis, but the gold standard is early arteriography. In acute ischemia, time is of the essence, and therefore clinical suspicion with early arteriography provides the highest likelihood of a good outcome for patients with acute mesenteric ischemia.

Surgical Management

Once the diagnosis of acute mesenteric ischemia is made, the treatment of the patient requires two independent components: management of the vascular disease and management of the end-organ damage. The authors defer discussion of the management of end-organ damage to associated chapters in this text. The management of the vascular component is the focus of this chapter.

The management of the underlying vascular component is predicated on the diagnosis responsible for the ischemia. Embolic occlusion requires removal of the offending embolus to restore blood flow to the viscera. Acute mesenteric thrombosis requires bypass of the involved segment to restore blood flow. Usually both are approached through a midline laparotomy with a direct approach to the visceral vessels. The presence and severity of intestinal gangrene is not to be assessed until revascularization is complete, because improvement in the bowel can be seen for some time after revascularization.[29,30] Nonetheless, the observations about the pattern of ischemic changes in the bowel can be helpful in defining the diagnosis and treatment needed.

If the diagnosis of acute arterial embolus is obvious clinically, then treatment should be aggressively directed at clearing the embolus and restoring flow.[32] Usually a transverse arteriotomy is sufficient with passage of a Fogarty embolectomy catheter to remove any remote thrombus. Multiple branches may be involved, and arteriography with selective wire-directed embolectomy may be needed. At the conclusion, the artery is usually relatively disease free, and in-flow should be brisk. Angiography should be a routine adjunct to prevent retained thrombus and document the successful treatment of the ischemia.[30]

With acute mesenteric thrombosis, treatment is more complicated, but the end-organ tolerance for ischemia is also greater, secondary to conditioning and collaterals from the chronic underlying ischemia. Nonetheless, a major reconstructive procedure is often required because of the diffuse nature of the atherosclerotic process and the multiple vessels involved. Bypass is the mainstay for acute ischemia due to thrombosis, with the aim being revascularization of at least two vessels. Other modalities such as endarterectomy or reimplantation can be used in selective cases, but for most cases bypass is preferred.[33-35]

The origin of the bypass for acute mesenteric ischemia has been the subject of numerous studies, but currently the preferred in-flow is the supraceliac aorta.[36-39] This segment of the aorta is often spared severe disease and avoids angulation problems associated with retrograde bypass from the iliac artery or the infrarenal aorta. The use of this segment also allows easy use of bifurcated grafts, either vein or prosthetic, to bypass both the celiac and the superior mesenteric circulation. This approach also usually allows the surgeon to avoid cross-clamping the aorta, yielding less morbidity from ischemic compromise to the lower half of the body and associated cardiac issues from the high afterload produced by thoracic aortic cross-clamping. If the infrarenal aorta or iliac artery is used for bypass, care must be taken to avoid kinking of the bypass when the intestines are replaced in the abdominal cavity at closure. This technical issue can be quite problematic and requires attention to detail to avoid graft compromise.

The conduit used for mesenteric bypass varies according to the clinical scenario. Generally, prosthetic material is to be avoided during acute episodes secondary to the risk of contamination associated with bowel resection and restoration of intestinal continuity. Bifurcated vein bypasses, using the saphenous vein in most cases, is the preferred technique in potentially contaminated fields and is the likely conduit used in the acute setting. In many cases a naturally bifurcated vein for bypass can be harvested from the saphenofemoral junction, using the anterior saphenous branch for celiac reconstruction and the main saphenous for the superior mesenteric artery. Obviously, the use of this bifurcation requires that the valves be rendered incompetent and that the vein be used in a nonreversed fashion. If this natural bifurcation is inadequate, two segments of saphenous vein can be used to perform the bypasses. If bowel ischemia is not advanced, and the risk of contamination is low, then it may be appropriate to use prosthetic material. From the supraceliac aorta, a small-diameter aortic bifurcated graft is typically employed to provide limbs for bypass to both the celiac axis and the superior mesenteric artery.

Intraoperatively, several adjuncts may be beneficial to the management of the patient with acute arterial mesenteric ischemia. Initially, both intraoperative and postoperative vasoconstriction can be a significant clinical issue that may limit reperfusion. Experimental studies endorse the routine use of perioperative glucagon to address these concerns.[12,40–44]

Glucagon, a trophic hormone of pancreatic origin, has three actions beneficial to the patient with acute intestinal ischemia. First, glucagon-generated smooth muscle relaxation occurs not only in the arterial wall but also in the bowel muscularis. The ileus thus generated puts the bowel at rest and decreases the overall metabolic and oxygen demands by the intestine, rendering the bowel more tolerant of intestinal ischemia. Second, glucagon is a significant mesenteric vasodilator, preventing reflex vasospasm after reperfusion and minimizing some components of reperfusion injury in the intestine. Finally, glucagon is an independent cardiac inotrope, unrelated to catecholamine levels. As a result, in these patients who are often critically ill, cardiac output can be bolstered by the use of glucagon infusion in this setting. It is our practice to routinely use glucagon in all cases of acute mesenteric ischemia of arterial origin.

Both intra- and postoperatively, pulmonary compromise can be a major issue, requiring high levels of pressure support or positive end-expiratory pressure to maintain oxygenation. These issues arise from unknown factors, probably related to complement activation and fluid sequestration in the lungs. These factors often persist after successful mesenteric reperfusion, resulting in acute respiratory distress syndrome and prolonged ventilatory requirements for these already compromised patients. Similarly, myocardial depression results from the same factors, and cardiac support with inotropes is often the norm. These patients often require prolonged intensive care unit support for their survival,[45] and the breadth of complications associated with these challenging patients is beyond the scope of this discussion.

After revascularization, the natural history of the reconstruction is usually dependent on the underlying cause of the ischemia. If the disease is an isolated embolus and the patient is otherwise healthy aside from the cardiac arrhythmias, then the long-term outcome may be good with systemic anticoagulation. On the other hand, emboli arising from a ventricular aneurysm or valvular heart disease may cause prohibitive mortality because of the underlying disease. Thus, generalized conclusions relative to the prognosis of embolic events is difficult, and the prognosis depends on associated factors related to the cause. For patients with acute arterial thrombosis, the diffuse nature of the vascular process means that disease in associated vascular beds is usually present and the resultant prognosis often poor.

Endovascular Management

Percutaneous management of acute mesenteric ischemia is just beginning to be recognized as a viable alternative to surgical treatment. In this approach, the endovascular tools are not only diagnostic but also therapeutic. The use of angiographic endovascular techniques for the diagnosis of mesenteric ischemia is widely accepted; however, the skills and equipment necessary for therapeutic intervention are just beginning to be available.

Embolic disease presents several unique challenges to endovascular management. First, the clot origin is remote from the treatment site. Therefore, the clot is often mature thrombus with significant contraction and fibrosis, making the clot resistant to thrombolysis and fragmentation. Second, the clot may still be present at the site of origin, increasing the risk of further embolization, especially with the use of systemic doses of thrombolytic agents. Finally, fragmentation of the embolus may have already occurred with the initial event, resulting in the need to treat multiple beds as part of the endovascular procedure. The diagnosis of embolus is suggested by several clinical and angiographic criteria as outlined in Table 34.1.

Perhaps the most critical component relative to treatment of an embolus is the consistency of the clot. Once the diagnosis of an embolus is reached, management requires removal of the embolic obstruction. Several techniques have been suggested either as stand-alone therapy or in combination with thrombolysis (Table 34.3). Although each technique has advantages and disadvantages, the decision of which to use is often determined by the technology available at the time of the procedure and by the participating physician's expertise with the modalities available.

The use of thrombolysis relies on expertise and experience. The diagnosis of mesenteric ischemia is an acute

TABLE 34.3. Endovascular options for percutaneous thrombus treatment.

Suction thrombectomy
Amplatz catheter
Possis AngioJet mechanical thrombectomy catheter
Oasis devices
Laser clot ablation
Bacchus Trellis device

diagnosis with the need to revascularize quickly. For this reason, infusion thrombolysis is seldom indicated. Nonetheless, thrombolysis is often used as an adjunct to mechanical clot removal and anticoagulation.[46–50] The agent of choice today is tissue plasminogen activator (tPA) with doses determined by the clinical scenario. Our current practice limits the use of tPA to about 4 mg during the procedure as an adjunct to endovascular techniques. This dose is contrasted by the recommended systemic dose for acute myocardial infarction of 50 mg over 90 minutes. Obviously the risk of systemic complications is drastically reduced by the directed use of lower doses associated with endovascular treatment.

Our current endovascular tool of choice for embolic treatment is the AngioJet® device from Possis Medical.[47] This device was developed for coronary use, but further redesign has allowed its use in peripheral arteries and veins. The device fragments the clot by alternating high-pressure infusion with rapid suction, removing many fragments of even chronic emboli. Despite the success of this technique, chronic clot is often difficult to fragment to a small enough size to allow easy removal. Combination with thrombolysis allows clot dissolution to augment the mechanical fragmentation, with improvement in thrombolysis as the surface area of the clot increases. In this fashion, most clots can be cleared in a few minutes, making this a valuable technique in high-risk operative settings.

In acute mesenteric thrombosis, the endovascular issues are much different. In thrombosis, the disease often begins at the arterial orifice, sometimes making cannulation of the vessel nearly impossible. Even if cannulation is possible, the obstructive process may preclude luminal treatment, requiring a subintimal approach to revascularization. Finally, the angulation of the visceral arteries may make it challenging to work from any given approach without loss of access. Therefore, the interventionalist must be ready to use both femoral and brachial access to complete the endovascular procedure.

With these caveats, treatment itself has a relatively simple goal: traversing the diseased segment from a normal proximal lumen into a normal distal lumen.[51–57] Once traversal is achieved, the treatment will usually require stent placement due to the chronic disease present. If traversal cannot be achieved, then endovascular treatment is not possible and conventional open surgery should be utilized without delay.

In this regard, a few comments about the use of endovascular therapy are in order. Remember that the ischemic interval is limited before irreversible changes develop, requiring that any endovascular approach be relatively expeditious. If the risk of surgical therapy is high enough, then the endovascular approach may be the only clinical option. Nonetheless, most patients are somewhere in between, making the decisions about when to abort the endovascular approach critical to a successful outcome. Awareness on the part of the interventionalist is critical to this process. If progress is not being made in an endovascular approach, then a surgical alternative should be chosen. In many centers, the use of mobile C-arm technology may allow diagnostic endovascular, therapeutic endovascular, and open surgical treatment to be performed in a single clinical venue, the operating room. In this setting, all modalities can be provided without delays associated with patient transport or preparation time. The decisions as to venue will be different at each institution as the procedures evolve.

Even with successful endovascular intervention, the question remains as to how to monitor end-organ damage. Although conventional open treatment requires laparotomy, successful endovascular treatment can be performed without laparotomy. Therefore, laparotomy may be required independent of endovascular revascularization to assess intestinal viability and the possibility of hemorrhagic conversion of bowel infarctions. Whether in the future laparoscopy can replace laparotomy for the initial assessment or for the second look remains to be determined.[58,59] Some method of visualization of the intestine after endovascular revascularization is essential.

Ischemia Associated with Aortic Dissection

Aortic dissection is a life-threatening entity in its own right, but the complications of the acute dissection are often remote from the origin of the dissection. Although acute hemodynamic issues can lead to direct repair of the origin itself to avoid aortic rupture, cardiac tamponade, or acute cardiac decompensation, delayed intervention may also be required for visceral or lower extremity compromise secondary to the dissection. Type A dissection, originating in the ascending aorta, is an accepted indication for direct aortic repair due to the high incidence of cardiac compromise associated with this diagnosis. Visceral, renal, or lower extremity compromise may occur when these vessels are split in their perfusion between the true arterial lumen and the new false dissection channel. Even with repair of the entry point, this false channel can have multiple reentry points that maintain false lumen flow (Figure 34.1). If the flow is sufficiently compromised, visceral ischemia can develop.

Type B dissection, with a point of entry near the origin of the left subclavian artery in the descending aorta, is more problematic. The mortality rate associated with direct aortic repair in type B dissection is high, and only a minority of patients will develop complications requiring treatment.[60–62] Therefore, the conventional wisdom is surgical treatment of type B dissection only when visceral compromise develops or other local features such as expansion or rupture require it.[63] These patients are primarily treated with aggressive antihypertensive therapy,

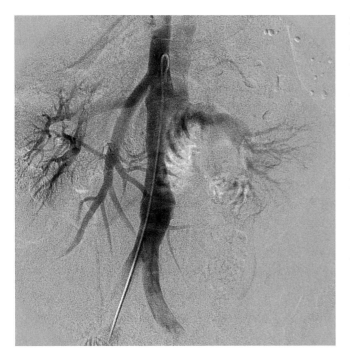

Figure 34.1. Aortic dissection showing multiple reentry points.

and only if end-organ complications develop is surgery performed.

The main concern for these patients is development of visceral, renal, or lower extremity malperfusion. The false lumen commonly encroaches on the true lumen, with variable perfusion to the aortic branches depending on the dissection path. Each dissection is unique, with variable perfusion patterns and perfusion to these branches arising from the true lumen, the false lumen, or both. The challenge in this setting is to maintain organ perfusion without making the situation worse. If the right kidney is perfused from the true lumen and the left is perfused from the false, restoring flow down the true lumen by surgical reconstruction or endograft may render the left kidney ischemic. On the other hand, ischemia to the right kidney may be best treated by directing flow down the true lumen. To effectively treat these patients, an overall map of branch vessel blood flow needs to be created so that vascular compromise can be addressed. Which lumen should be approached in a given situation is dictated by such a flow map.

An alternative to redirecting blood flow as above is the concept of equalizing blood flow and perfusion pressure in the true and false lumens. Although this gives up any option of sealing the true lumen back to the underlying media, it does allow flow from both channels to be legitimized, perfusing organs from both lumens. Because flow can then be maintained from both sides, the channels can then heal independently and visceral compromise is minimized. The most common approach used for this is aortic

fenestration, in which a window is created between the true lumen and the false lumen, usually in the visceral bearing segment, to allow the flow of blood to pass freely between the true and false lumens in this segment.[62–70] In some approaches direct fenestration includes the branches, avoiding persistent hypoperfusion by sealing the flap surgically at the orifice of each ostium. Again, the surgical technique must be individualized to the patient, and fenestrations can be performed at any level from the thoracic aorta to the femoral artery depending on the presentation.

Endovascular options for treatment of complications after aortic dissection are attractive because of the high morbidity rate associated with open surgical fenestration.[69,71–73] Percutaneous fenestration has been performed with a number of techniques.[74] In the most common of these, the septum is traversed with a guidewire so that separate access is obtained to both the true and false lumens, usually from a femoral approach.[75,76] Starting with a small balloon and working toward a large 20- to 30-mm size, the path into the opposite lumen is opened to allow equalization of blood flow. The balloon creates a split that will stabilize with time, and true and false lumen pressures are immediately equalized.[77]

A second technique of endovascular fenestration that is gaining popularity is similar in its access.[78] Once access is gained into both lumens, a small-diameter catheter or guide is passed over both wires together. At the point where the septum is traversed, a scissoring action occurs as the sheath is advanced, using the two wires as the blades of the scissors. The septum can therefore be opened to any degree necessary, although use of this technique near visceral origins holds theoretic danger if the branch origin itself is traversed. This technique can be used in both the thoracic and abdominal aorta as needed.

The direct endovascular approach to the aortic type B dissection is only now beginning to be fully explored as new thoracic stent grafts become available that were specifically designed for this purpose.[79,80] In many patients the pattern of true lumen and false lumen flow is established within minutes of the onset of the dissection, and stent graft coverage of the aortic tear may compromise flow unless adjuvant branch vessel stenting is provided. The ultimate use of aortic stent grafts in acute type B dissection remains under investigation for the foreseeable future.[81]

The final endovascular approach to branch vessel compromise is much more direct. In this technique the object is to stent the vessel compromised into whichever lumen provides blood flow.[61,82] In most cases this is the true lumen, which is being collapsed by the false lumen encroaching on the vessel orifice. There are many technical pitfalls to this approach. In many cases the neo-orifice into the true lumen is often several millimeters away from the former vessel orifice. In these cases the stent has to be placed well into the aortic lumen, sometimes interfering with future endovascular interventions. Nonetheless, success in this technique has been reported, and in high-risk patients this technique may be beneficial.

In conclusion, treatment of type B dissection, in particular, lends itself well to endovascular options. Despite this promise of success in these challenging patients, at the current time all patients undergoing dissection should have their care individualized to their unique anatomy, including a carefully derived flow map to guide any necessary revascularization. The standard of care for type A dissection remains open surgery; the standard for type B dissection remains conservative with intervention reserved for vascular compromise. If peripheral vascular compromise occurs in either type, the compromised flow can be managed with either endovascular or open surgical techniques.

Acute Renal Ischemia

Although the tolerance of the mesenteric circulation of arterial ischemia is intermediate, the tolerance of the renal circulation to arterial ischemia approaches that of the brain in the severity and rapidity of reversible injury. The kidney is one of the few organs in the body that requires a continuous supply of oxygenated blood to avoid ischemic injury. Although the kidney can tolerate some degree of gradual onset chronic ischemia, the lack of collateral connections between the branches of the renal artery makes it intolerant of acute compromise in its blood supply. Generally, the kidney can tolerate about 30 minutes of warm ischemia before irreversible injury begins.[83–85] By 90 minutes of warm ischemia, irreversible damage is complete unless some collateral flow is present. Even shorter periods of ischemia may cause significant renal dysfunction.

As a result of these physiologic limits, the management options in acute renal ischemia are limited. First, the diagnosis of acute renal ischemia in a timely fashion is a challenge, because, by the time a patient arrives in the emergency room with flank pain from renal infarction, the damage is likely irreversible. A high degree of suspicion when the risk of acute ischemia is high is the most important factor. If a patient has been in a sudden deceleration event, such as a fall or motor vehicle accident, then computed tomography (CT) scanning may demonstrate evidence of renal ischemia. If the lesion is isolated without associated injuries, treatment may be possible. In most cases, however, associated injuries preclude either timely treatment or anticoagulation, resulting in nephrectomy in many cases.

Although success with surgical revascularization of renal artery occlusion can be achieved,[86,87] it is rare that revascularization can be performed before irreversible injury to the kidney occurs. In general, embolic occlusions

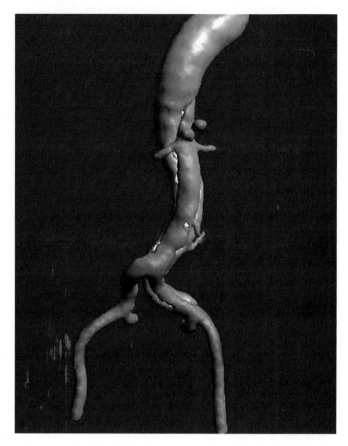

FIGURE 34.2. Three-dimensional computed tomography reconstruction showing the spiral nature of the dissected lumen.

are sudden and the primary therapy should be anticoagulation. With thrombotic occlusions, retrieval of renal function is possible even in a delayed fashion secondary to collateral preservation of renal parenchymal function.[88] The method of surgical revascularization will be determined by local expertise and experience. Direct approaches are preferred by many, whereas extra-anatomic approaches are used by others. The specific revascularization technique is less important than patient selection for revascularization.

The endovascular management of renal artery occlusion is limited by the duration of warm ischemia leading to diagnosis and intervention. If the duration of ischemia exceeds 90 minutes, endovascular options are generally viewed as futile, if not dangerous.[89] Despite this concern, endovascular approaches are often the quickest method of confirming the diagnosis and providing therapeutic management (Figure 34.2) if it will be possible, given the time constraints.

Acute Aortic Occlusion

Although chronic aortic occlusion can develop insidiously without major clinical sequelae, acute aortic occlusion caused by embolus or thrombosis is a true emergency. The development of occlusion must be sudden and uncompensated to develop symptoms, and generally patients can describe the exact moment of onset of symptoms. In any presentation, the risk of significant morbidity and mortality remains secondary to metabolic derangements.[90,91] The aggressive treatment of the underlying disorder is the only possible solution to symptoms.

Typically, the patient with acute aortic occlusion presents to the emergency room with paralysis of the lower extremities and severe pain. Often the patient is mottled from the waist distally with cool pale lower extremities. The patient with acute aortic occlusion appears severely ill at presentation, with the only question being the diagnosis.

The presentation of aortic saddle embolus can be severe and acute or, less commonly, more gradual in onset. Often the presence of a cardiac rhythm other than normal sinus is helpful in suggesting the diagnosis of embolic aortic occlusion. Most patients will deny any history of preexistent symptoms, although there may be a history of previous cardiac issues or arrhythmias.

The therapy is acute intervention by either surgery or endovascular techniques. Typically, surgical intervention is performed by a bilateral femoral approach, using Fogarty embolectomy catheters to simultaneously remove thrombus from the aorta and both iliac systems. Systemic heparin should be given early, as soon as the diagnosis is reached. Distal thrombectomy is necessary because clot propagation is the rule. Thrombolytic infusion may be beneficial in an attempt to improve clearance of distal thrombus but in higher doses may expose the patient to the risk of further embolization from the embolic source as the clot of origin lyses further.

Open aortic surgery is rarely necessary for aortic embolus, but, if the diagnosis is uncertain, aortic reconstruction may be performed. Rarely, direct embolectomy from an aortic approach is needed if the femoral approach fails. As an alternative in this setting, endovascular treatment with kissing stents may fixate any mobile component of the embolus with the stents providing a flow channel to the iliac system. Thrombectomy may then be completed from the femoral approach as outlined above.

If endovascular treatment is undertaken, usually bilateral femoral access is needed for thrombolysis and suction thrombectomy (Figure 34.3). This is often done best in the operating room, as the backup is operative embolectomy. After unilateral access for diagnosis is performed, bilateral retrograde femoral access is obtained for percutaneous thrombectomy and possible thrombolytic infusion. Typically, acute thrombus removal improves the patient clinically, but thrombolysis is often needed secondary to the chronic character of embolic clot. The exact duration of thrombolysis is determined by the clinical situation, but close monitoring is essential (Figure 34.4).

Aortic thrombosis presents in much the same way, with paralysis or paresthesias common. In this presentation, the history of preexistent claudication is important in providing insight into this diagnosis. Many patients with thrombosis will have evidence of atherosclerotic vascular disease in other distributions. Coronary artery disease is common as well, as is a history of tobacco use. These elements emphasize the multisystem nature of management in these complicated patients.

Operative treatment is generally by direct aortic surgery once the diagnosis is reached. Again, early heparin administration is essential to prevent clot propagation. Although a bilateral femoral approach is often the initial step, direct aortic replacement is appropriate operatively once the diagnosis is confirmed. Typically aortobifemoral reconstruction is the norm. In high-risk settings, axillobifemoral reconstruction may be warranted. As with aortic embolus, distal thrombectomy should be performed to remove clot that may have propagated to the femoral systems.

Endovascular treatment of acute aortic thrombosis is possible, again by bilateral femoral approach. As with aortic embolus, treatment is best undertaken in the operating room, thus avoiding delays in revascularization in the event that operative treatment is necessary. Typically, a bilateral femoral approach is undertaken with retrograde access either percutaneously or by open access. Access up both iliac systems to the aorta is achieved, and directed thrombectomy is performed. Adjuvant thrombolysis or percutaneous thrombectomy may be used as well. Once a channel is established, then balloon angioplasty and stenting as appropriate is used to reopen the occluded aorta. Generally an open approach is beneficial because removal of iliac thrombus is safer using an open approach. The clot burden seen in aortic thrombosis is often substantial, making the open approach preferred, even for endovascular treatment.

Other Acute Arterial Occlusions

Any acute arterial occlusion by either embolus or thrombosis of preexistent disease can produce an emergency, and the most common emergencies have been described earlier. In general, the tolerance of the end organ to ischemia, coupled with the vascular bed's ability to form collaterals, defines the tolerance of the tissues involved to ischemia. If the end organ is tolerant, or the vascular bed has alternative supplies of blood flow, then acute care intervention can be averted. The specific clinical situation will define the nature of the intervention and outcome, and every clinical presentation should be evaluated individually for the possibility of arterial ischemia.

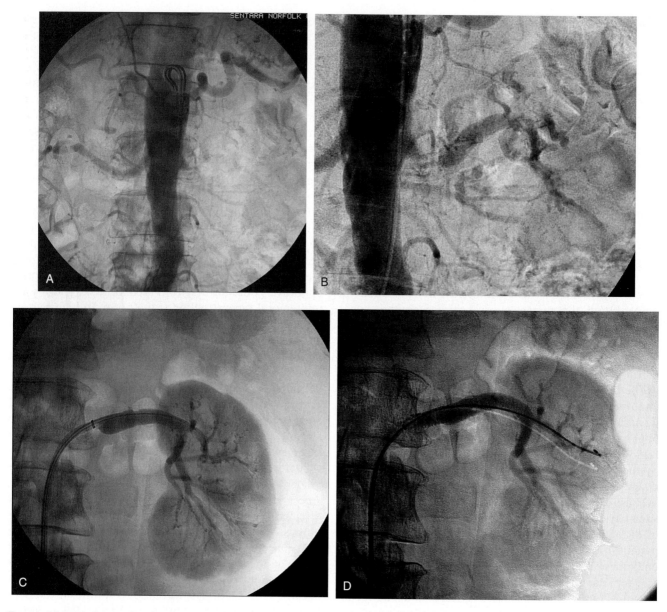

FIGURE 34.3. Endovascular treatment of acute renal artery occlusion. **(A)** Left renal artery filling is absent. **(B)** After AngioJet thrombectomy and tissue plasminogen activator, the distal renal artery is now visible. **(C)** Another view of the distal renal artery. **(D)** Final result after placement of left renal stent.

Acute Venous Occlusions

Although arterial occlusions are consistent emergencies in the acute setting, the clinical presentation of acute venous thrombosis is rarely emergent. Nonetheless, subacute venous thrombosis often presents as an acute clinical event, resulting in acute care treatment despite the delayed onset or diagnosis. The issue is the clinical consequences of the venous thrombosis. When the

patient perceives the clinical situation as acute, he or she seeks attention for that problem. The origins, however, may have occurred over days or even weeks, with the clinical scenario the real emergency. Thus venous events can generate acute care diagnosis and treatment.

In any venous thrombosis, the issue of hypercoagulability becomes a clinical issue. Most patients do not spontaneously form a venous clot without an inciting event such as surgery or trauma. Therefore, any venous throm-

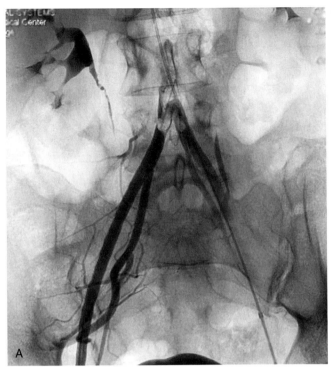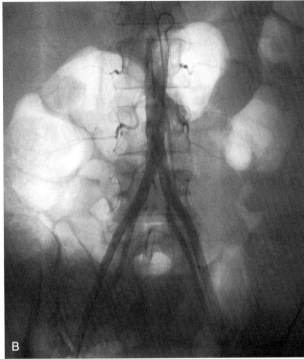

FIGURE 34.4. Endovascular treatment of acute aortic embolus. **(A)** Aortic saddle embolus in 48-year-old female with atrial arrhythmia. **(B)** End result of 12-hour infusion of tissue plasminogen activator.

bosis without an obvious antecedent cause should be suspicious for a hypercoagulable state. Although discussion of this problem is impossible in this limited space, recognizing the associated risk of hypercoagulability is important to the managing physician in any venous thrombotic event, particularly involving the visceral veins.

Acute Mesenteric Venous Thrombosis Including Portal Vein Thrombosis

Acute presentation of mesenteric venous thrombosis for acute care intervention is rare, but the diagnosis of this entity is becoming increasingly common as the use of abdominal CT scans with intravenous contrast increases. In most cases, the diagnosis is happened upon by chance, with the patient presenting with ill-defined gastrointestinal symptoms and the CT scan revealing mesenteric or portal venous thrombosis. In the nonacute setting, anticoagulation with or without thrombolysis is the standard, with surgery reserved for bowel complications.

Spontaneous mesenteric or portal venous thrombosis is rare in the absence of hypercoagulable syndromes, and the remainder usually associated with trauma or infection.[92] In adults the most common causes are cirrhosis or neoplasm, neither an acute event. Management of thrombosis in these venous distributions is expectant, with anticoagulation the standard. Any acute care intervention is

for end-organ complications and is discussed elsewhere. There is no accepted role for open mesenteric venous thrombectomy except in unusual circumstances.

Acute Renal Vein Thrombosis

Even more uncommon than mesenteric venous thrombosis is the diagnosis of acute renal vein thrombosis. Although more common in infancy associated with dehydration and prolonged hypotension,[93] renal vein thrombosis in adults is often associated with various hypercoagulable syndromes. Only with bilateral renal vein thrombosis is an acute event likely, because renal function will otherwise be normal with a single functioning kidney. Nonetheless, the diagnosis of flank pain with or without hematuria, associated with imaging studies demonstrating renal vein thrombosis, raises the possibility of an acute event.

Surgical management of the acutely thrombosed renal vein is mentioned only to condemn its application. Unless by clinical circumstances the diagnosis is made intraoperatively, operative thrombectomy is ill advised because of comorbid conditions that may have contributed to the thrombotic event. Additionally, the duration of renal ischemia from venous congestion is usually ill defined, resulting in uncertain benefit to intervention. Therefore, the risk/benefit ratio is against operative intervention in most situations of renal vein thrombosis.

On the other hand, endovascular intervention carries a much lower morbidity than open surgery in this setting. For this reason, percutaneous venous thrombectomy, with or without thrombolysis, may provide an easy pathway to relief of the venous congestion seen in acute venous thrombosis and is worthwhile to consider for this patient group. The mainstay of therapy remains anticoagulation, and, in the absence of anticoagulation, any venous thrombectomy, percutaneous or open, is likely to fail.

Rarely, acute inferior vena cava thrombosis can mimic the diagnosis of acute renal vein thrombosis. The issues for caval thrombosis are the same, with the additional proviso that edema of the lower extremities will be almost universal in the acute setting. The presence of flank pain associated with significant lower extremity edema of acute onset suggests the diagnosis of renal vein compromise by inferior vena cava obstruction and thrombosis. In this setting the treatment must be directed at both components, and the benefits of thrombolysis are increased secondary to the chronic lower extremity consequences for these patients.

Acute Complications of Aneurysmal Disease

Symptomatic Abdominal Aortic Aneurysm Including Rupture

Rupture is regarded as the most dreaded complication of abdominal aortic aneurysm (AAA) and one of the most fatal acute care surgical conditions of the abdomen. This entity claims at least 15,000 lives annually in the United States.[94] The aim of elective repair of AAA is to avoid this clinical presentation, because the mortality of elective repair averages 6% compared with 48% or more for ruptured aortic aneurysms. The number of ruptured AAA is on the rise because of the increased prevalence of AAA as well as the aging population of the United States.[95] The primary reason for this continued problem is the fact that most patients with a ruptured AAA do not know that they have an aneurysm until the day of rupture. Ruptured AAA is the fifteenth leading cause of death in U.S. males.[96] Sixty percent of patients will die en route to the hospital or before reaching the operating room, resulting in an overall mortality rate approaching 90%.[97]

Etiology and Risk Factors of Aneurysm Rupture

Multiple risk factors are associated with an increased risk of AAA rupture. The most important is the maximum aneurysm sac diameter. Multiple studies have shown that increased aneurysm size is associated with increased risk of rupture. Aneurysms 4.0 to 5.4 cm in diameter have a yearly risk of rupture of 0.5% to 1.0 %. Aneurysms of 6 to 7 cm have a 6.6% risk of rupture yearly, and aneurysms larger than 7 cm have a 19% risk of rupture.[98–100]

Other factors have been implicated in increasing the risk of AAA rupture. Hypertension and chronic obstructive pulmonary disease (COPD) have been found in several studies to be independent risk factors for rupture.[101,102] The explanation for a causative role of hypertension is straightforward based on Laplace's law. The association of COPD with rupture is less straightforward but may relate to a systemic imbalance in proteinase activity affecting both pulmonary and aortic connective tissues.[103] Smoking has also been shown in different studies to be a risk factor for rupture, raising the risk almost fivefold over that for nonsmokers.[104,105] Although in these studies the effects of smoking cannot be separated from the effects of COPD, the significant increased risk of rupture cannot be ignored when counseling patients for smoking cessation. Female gender has been suggested as an independent risk factor for AAA rupture. Women are generally more prone to rupture than men with the same aneurysm diameter.[106,107] This difference might be related to the smaller size of the abdominal aorta in women than in men, but this theory has not been proven.

Other factors related to the AAA itself may also be considered as risk factors for rupture. For example, eccentric saccular aneurysms may represent greater rupture risk than more diffuse cylindrical aneurysms. One analysis based on computer modeling found that wall stress is substantially increased by asymmetric bulge in AAA.[108] The effect of the thrombus in the aneurysm sac is debatable. Some studies suggest that thrombus in the lumen of AAA reduces the tension on the aneurysm wall and hence reduces risk of rupture, but other studies refute this.[109,110] The rate of expansion of the AAA as an independent risk factor for rupture is hard to define. The rate of enlargement of AAA is usually 0.2 to 0.4 mm per year.[111] Some studies have reported that the expansion rate was greater in ruptured than in intact AAA, but the ruptured group had larger AAA diameters, which confounds the conclusions.[112] Other studies found that the absolute AAA diameter rather than the rate of expansion predicted rupture.[113]

Clinical Presentation and Diagnosis

The classic clinical picture of AAA rupture is the triad of acute abdominal pain, hemodynamic instability, and a pulsating abdominal mass. This picture is not always the case, and a high index of suspicion has to be exercised to detect those cases. Actually, only 50% of cases have this classic presentation.[114] Consequently, the diagnosis can be challenging because up to 80% of patients will not have a history of known AAA. Other clinical problems can be with the differential diagnosis, including perforated viscus, enteric ischemia, strangulated hernia, ruptured visceral artery aneurysm, acute aortic dissection, acute cholecystitis, acute pancreatitis, ruptured hepatobiliary tumors, aortic occlusion, and myocardial infarction. Misdiagnosis appeared uncommon and actually occurs in around 10% of cases. Fortunately, virtually all patients who underwent operations for suspected ruptured AAA had other disease entities that benefited from acute intervention.[115]

Nearly all patients will have acute, sudden-onset, unremitting abdominal pain radiating to the back. The pain is usually associated of lightheadedness or collapse because of sudden hypovolemia. If the rupture is in the retroperitoneum against the ureter, pain may be referred to the ipsilateral testicle or groin. Rarely, the aneurysm may rupture into the duodenum, the colon, or the inferior vena cava. The patient will then present with massive gastrointestinal bleeding or high-output congestive heart failure. A pulsatile abdominal mass is usually present if the systolic blood pressure is above 90 mm Hg.

Patients who present with the classic picture who are hemodynamically unstable need no further diagnostic evaluation, and their only chance of survival is expedited operative intervention to stop the bleeding. The diagnostic dilemma is a patient who presents with acute abdominal and back pain with no hemodynamic instability and has a pulsating abdominal mass or a history of AAA disease. These patients may have a symptomatic AAA with no rupture, a contained AAA rupture, or no AAA at all. In this clinical situation, a high-quality CT of the abdomen and pelvis with intravenous contrast is ideal. Computed tomography scanning can diagnose ruptured AAA with an accuracy above 90% (Figure 34.5).[116]

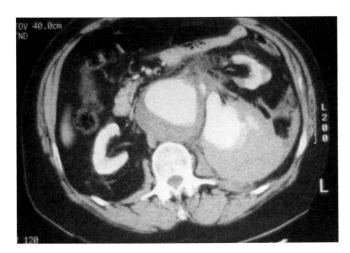

FIGURE 34.5. Computed tomography scan demonstrating ruptured aortic aneurysm with acute false aneurysm laterally.

For these patients CT scan is helpful not only in diagnosing rupture but also in deciding the type and timing of repair of the aneurysm, as is discussed later. Computed tomography is the standard for sizing AAA in preparation for endografts should that modality be deemed suitable for a particular patient. Also, CT may provide other useful information, including the presence of left-sided inferior vena cava, inflammatory aneurysms, associated thoracic aneurysm, or other pathology. All of these may have implications in the management of the aneurysm.

Duplex ultrasound is another modality that is available in many emergency departments and is sometimes used to diagnose AAA rupture. Its main use is the rapid determination of the presence of an AAA, but it cannot reliably distinguish between a ruptured versus a non-ruptured AAA. It is important to stress the fact that ultrasound or CT imaging of hemodynamically unstable patients cannot be justified, even if such imaging studies are readily available in the emergency room. Such patients belong in the operating room.

Management

All patients with ruptured AAA will require operative intervention the aim of which is to stop the bleeding. The management of ruptured AAA includes three phases: preoperative preparation, the operation, and postoperative management.

The Preoperative Phase

The preoperative phase includes two important aspects. The first is determining when to operate; the second is preparing the operating room.

The first issue is when to operate. For patients who are hemodynamically unstable, the operation must be emergently performed after minimal preoperative resuscitation. However, for hemodynamically stable patients the decision on the timing of repair depends on the CT scan findings. For patients with symptoms and contained retroperitoneal rupture detected on CT scan, the treatment is still an acute care procedure, as these patients can rapidly deteriorate and become hemodynamically unstable with much higher mortality and morbidity rates than hemodynamically stable patients. For patients with no CT findings suggestive of rupture, repair of these symptomatic aneurysms can be postponed for up to 24 hours. During this time, the patient's condition is optimized by thorough preoperative preparation, including treatment of comorbid conditions such as diabetes mellitus and cardiac, renal, and pulmonary disease. Precipitous operation for nonruptured but symptomatic AAAs results in an operative mortality rate five times greater than that of the elective procedure.[117]

The second part of the preoperative phase is the preparation for surgery. The duration and thoroughness of this phase depends on the clinical presentation of the patient and the patient's stability. For the unstable patient, the best treatment is to take him or her to the operating room as soon as possible. Large intravenous lines including central lines must be started on the way to the operating room. Arterial lines and central venous catheters are also needed; however, they should not delay the process of taking the patient to the operating room and actually can be inserted during the surgery. Resuscitation should be started with crystalloid lactated Ringer's solution, and typing and cross for blood products must be sent immediately. Many recommend against aggressive preoperative resuscitation with restoration of normal blood pressure, as this can provoke extension of retroperitoneal bleeding and death.[118,119] Most authors recommend keeping the blood pressure in the 50 to 70 mm Hg range, which is enough to support the patient until the surgery yet low enough to avoid excessive ongoing bleeding. Blood product transfusion is withheld until cross-clamping of the aorta has been performed in the operating room.[120] Blood products must be available for use in the operating room, and these should include at least 6 U of packed red blood cells, understanding that more may be needed. Fresh-frozen plasma and platelets should also be available. A general guideline is to transfuse 2 to 4 U of fresh-frozen plasma and 6 packs of platelets for every 8 U of packed red blood cells required.

For the hemodynamically stable patient with CT evidence of contained rupture, the same rules apply. However, in this setting there is more time to place the lines and resuscitate the patient before taking the patient to the operating room for definitive treatment. For the stable patient with no CT evidence of rupture, the operation is not considered as emergent as for the patients in the other categories. Studies show that taking time to optimize both the medical condition of the patient and the operating room staff and resources and then performing the surgery on an urgent basis within the next 24 hours has a much better outcome than performing the surgery on an acute care basis.[121,122]

The Operation

Classically the treatment of ruptured or symptomatic AAA is by open surgery. Now, endovascular techniques are becoming another option of repair for selected patients. In the operating room, the patient must be kept warm and blood products must be available before the incision is made. The patient should be prepped and draped from the suprasternal notch down to the knees. This should be done before induction of general anesthesia, because severe hypotension is anticipated with induction of anesthesia, and the team must be ready to make the skin incision as soon as general anesthesia is induced. A Foley urinary catheter and a nasogastric tube should be standard. The nasogastric tube also helps in identification of the esophagus should supraceliac clamping be needed during the procedure. Some surgeons advocate the placement of an intraaortic balloon through the left brachial artery into the proximal abdominal aorta and inflating it with induction to reduce the risk of hypotension.[118,123]

The usual approach adopted by most surgeons is a long midline incision from the xiphoid to the symphysis pubis entering the peritoneal cavity as quickly as possible. The prime aim of the surgery is to stop the bleeding from the aortic rupture. This can be accomplished by either aortic clamping or the use of intraaortic balloon tamponade. The usual way is to perform supraceliac aortic clamping before approaching the aneurysm. The lesser omentum is opened using cautery; the supraceliac aorta is identified at the level of the diaphragm to the right of the esophagus. Blunt dissection is performed in that area on both sides of the aorta followed by the placement of a long aortic clamp to clamp the aorta side to side. This markedly reduces the bleeding from the ruptured aneurysm, allowing a direct approach to the aneurysm, opening it longitudinally in the infrarenal segment of the aorta and identifying the neck from within the aneurysm.

Distal control of the iliac arteries is usually performed using balloon tamponade, which is much safer than dissecting in that area around both iliac arteries to place external clamps when there is a large hematoma increasing the risk of iatrogenic injury to the ureters or the iliac veins. Back bleeding from the lumbar arteries and the inferior mesenteric artery is controlled by suturing. At this moment, if the neck of the aneurysm below the renal arteries can be dissected free, an infrarenal clamp is placed on the aorta above the aneurysm, and then the supraceliac clamp can be removed. This markedly reduces the visceral ischemia time and reduces the risk of renal failure associated with a prolonged supraceliac clamp time.

When the infrarenal neck cannot be adequately dissected, the proximal anastomosis is performed quickly between the graft and the neck of the aneurysm using a continuous 3–0 Prolene suture. The graft used is usually a Dacron tube graft in 90% of the cases where the distal anastomosis can be performed to the distal aorta above the bifurcation. In cases where associated iliac artery aneurysms are present, a bifurcated graft is used with the distal anastomosis performed to the common iliac or femoral arteries. At this stage, a clamp is applied to the proximal graft, and the aortic clamp is removed. The anesthesiologist must be warned before removal of the aortic clamp, and the clamp should be slowly released after the patient is fully resuscitated with crystalloids and blood products to avoid sudden hypotension that can occur with the sudden release of the proximal clamp. The distal anastomosis is then performed in the same way, and revascularization of both lower extremities is done.

Another but more cumbersome method of bleeding control is balloon tamponade through the aneurysm using a Foley catheter. This method is less effective than the clamping of the aorta, and usually the restoration of blood pressure will dislodge the balloon distally into the wound with loss of control. The method can, however, be used temporarily in cases of free intraperitoneal rupture until proximal aortic control with the clamp is achieved. Heparin is not usually used in these cases as the patients are liable to coagulopathies associated with shock, hypothermia, and massive blood loss and replacement.

Some surgeons advocate the use of a retroperitoneal approach for treatment of AAA rupture.[124] This is achieved through a left retroperitoneal approach, which allows excellent exposure of the proximal abdominal aorta for proximal aortic control. The technique is especially beneficial for patients who have had previous abdominal surgery and intraperitoneal adhesions that will make expeditious exposure of the supraceliac aorta for clamping quite difficult. The technique, however, should be used only by surgeons who have adequate experience with the technique in elective AAA repair before trying to use it in acute care cases.

The use of endovascular stent grafts for the treatment of ruptured AAA is a new trend, and its success has been reported in the literature.[125,126] The technique is attractive because it is minimally invasive with much less hemodynamic and physiologic burden on patients who are already maximally stressed by their illness. The pitfall of the technique is that many of the ruptured aneurysms are anatomically unsuitable for stent graft placement.[127] The technique starts with placement of a guidewire through the left brachial artery into the abdominal aorta in the operating room. A balloon is then inflated in the proximal aorta to stop the bleeding. An aortogram is then obtained to evaluate the anatomy of the aneurysm. If the anatomy is unsuitable for endovascular repair, then open surgery is performed in the usual way.

Postoperative Management

Iatrogenic injury during surgery occurs in about 10% of cases to such structures as the left renal vein, renal artery, iliac veins, vena cava, superior mesenteric vein and artery, inferior mesenteric vein, spleen, and duodenum. Unfortunately these iatrogenic injuries are almost universally fatal because of increased bleeding, prolonged surgery, and direct adverse effects of the injury.[128]

As stated earlier, the overall mortality rate for patients with ruptured AAA is 90%, with most occurring before the operating room. Compared with a mortality rate of around 5% for patients undergoing elective open AAA repair, the mortality rate for patients undergoing acute care aortic repair for AAA rupture is about 50% and around 20% for acute care aortic repair for symptomatic but unruptured AAA. Patients who survive their operation and the perioperative period have an excellent long-term survival rate, similar to that for elective aortic repair.

Major postoperative complications after ruptured AAA repair are common and occur in 50% to 70% of patients. Prolonged respiratory failure requiring mechanical ventilation is the most common, occurring in about 50% of patients who survived their procedure. Many of the complications are caused by the prolonged hypotension, prolonged supraceliac cross-clamping, or a combination of both. Most of these complications have a high mortality rate if they occur. The most common of these complications are renal failure (29%), myocardial infarction (24%), sepsis (24%), and ischemic colitis (10%).[129,130]

Aortoenteric Fistula

The occurrence of a major gastrointestinal bleed after previous aortic grafting is an indication for further imaging to rule out the presence of an aortic enteric fistula. The danger of the undiagnosed aortoenteric fistula is the risk of exsanguinating hemorrhage. Although many patients may have a "herald bleed" before developing a severe hemorrhage, this is not the rule, and any hemorrhage in this setting may prove fatal.[131–133]

Physical findings related to an aortoenteric fistula may be minimal. In general, the presence of heme-positive stool is obvious, with maroon stool or frank blood the common presentation. The bleeding may be subtle in its initial onset, but in most cases by the time of clinical presentation the bleeding will be obvious.

Diagnostic imaging is critical to the diagnosis of aortoenteric fistula. Currently, CT scan with intravenous contrast is the standard for initial evaluation.[134–140] Findings of intravenous contrast in the bowel lumen, an anastomotic false aneurysm, or air around the aortic graft can be evidence of aortoenteric fistula and suggest the need for acute intervention. In some cases arteriography is needed, with the presence of a "nipple" near the bowel indicating a source of the bleeding. With aortoenteric fistula, the treatment is operative, with a limited role for endovascular adjuncts. The treatment is conventional, with aortic closure or reconstruction depending on the clinical situation. Both in situ and extraanatomic reconstructions have been advocated,[141–147] and the choice depends on the clinical scenario encountered.

Ruptured Visceral or Renal Artery Aneurysm

Although visceral artery aneurysms are not uncommon, ruptured visceral and renal artery aneurysms account for a minority of abdominal vascular emergencies.[148,149] Any artery can present with aneurysmal changes, but the hepatic, splenic, and renal arteries seem to be involved more commonly. In many cases the aneurysm is diagnosed as a byproduct of a CT scan done for other intra-abdominal pathology. If the aneurysm is ruptured, then symptoms are common and the aneurysm will usually require emergent treatment. Typically, rupture of visceral and renal artery aneurysms is more common during pregnancy.[150–164]

Treatment of ruptured visceral or renal arteries is by open ligation of the aneurysm once the diagnosis is made. Although reconstruction is possible in many cases, it is generally unnecessary and prolongs the procedure for an otherwise unstable patient. Therefore, the simplest treatment possible is usually the best.

Because revascularization is usually not needed, endovascular approaches have gained favor in recent years.[165–174] Generally, embolization of the aneurysm, or more recently covered stents, has been used to stop the hemorrhage and allow the patient to stabilize. Obviously an endovascular approach is much easier on the patient's recovery, but the object should be on aggressive control of bleeding rather than risking the possibility of incomplete control. The preferred techniques should therefore be institution specific, depending on the expertise available at the treating institution.

Abdominal and Pelvic Vascular Trauma

Trauma is the leading cause of death in Americans aged 44 years and younger. Blunt and penetrating abdominal vascular injuries account for some of the highest mortality rates in trauma patients. Like trauma to any other body region, abdominal and pelvic vascular injuries can result from either blunt or penetrating trauma. A trend toward increasing incidence of penetrating abdominal injuries has been seen in the recent years secondary to increasing civilian violence[175] Most abdominal vascular injuries are caused by penetrating trauma, with fewer resulting from blunt trauma. Abdominal vascular injuries, whether blunt or penetrating, usually occur in severely injured patients with multiple other abdominal and non-abdominal injuries and carry high morbidity and mortality rates.[176] Among patients undergoing laparotomy for blunt trauma, stab wounds, or gunshot wound, 3%, 10%, and 25% respectively have associated abdominal vascular injuries.[177]

As for all penetrating injuries, the degree of tissue destruction depends on the speed, trajectory, and size of the wounding object. The effect of penetrating trauma is generally one of bleeding or the development of traumatic arteriovenous fistula. If an abdominal vessel is injured, bleeding either occurs freely into the peritoneal cavity or is partially or completely contained in the retroperitoneum, allowing a tamponading effect to slow down the bleeding. Any vessel of the abdomen or pelvis can be affected by penetrating injuries. Arteriovenous fistulas may occur with penetrating injuries as well. Fistulas between the hepatic artery and portal vein, mesenteric arteriovenous fistulas, and fistulas between the aorta and vena cava have been reported.[178,179]

Blunt abdominal vascular traumas are much less common than penetrating injuries. They usually develop secondary to motor vehicle crashes or in rural areas.[180] The mechanism of injury includes compression and deceleration injuries. When enough energy is absorbed, avulsion of small vessels and bleeding can occur, usually from ruptured mesenteric branches. Another effect of blunt trauma is stretching the vessel because of deceleration injury that leads to intimal tears, with resultant intimal flaps and vessel thrombosis and occlusion. Sudden deceleration with the continued forward motion of the internal organs is thought to be the mechanism for thoracic aortic injury and proximal occlusion of the renal arteries.[181,182]

Additionally, long bone injury or pelvic fractures can result in bony fragments impinging arteries and veins, leading to internal bleeding from vascular injury. In many cases, these bony injuries once stabilized lead to cessation of internal bleeding and hemodynamic stability. Nonetheless, in some cases, open repair of arterial or venous lacerations is necessary after long bone trauma if the injury is severe enough.

Lately, there has been an increased incidence of iatrogenic abdominal and pelvic vascular injuries that corresponds to the increased used of minimally invasive techniques in various fields of medicine, especially in vascular surgery.[183] These injuries usually result during the use of endovascular techniques especially for therapeutic indications.[184,184] They can also result during spinal surgery,[186,187] laparoscopic abdominal surgery,[188] and sometimes even open abdominal procedures, especially pelvic gynecologic procedures.[189]

Diagnosis and Evaluation

The management of abdominal vascular injuries initially follows the same outline as for the primary and secondary surveys, resuscitation and diagnostic studies that are standards for management of any trauma patient. Frequently, patients with abdominal vascular injuries will present with hemodynamic instability, and a high index of suspicion must be exercised in managing these patients to avoid unnecessary delay in their management. Although the classic signs and symptoms of vascular injury may be present, indirect evidence of injury is more important than direct vascular examination of the abdominal and pelvic vessels because of inaccessibility.

Physical findings of significance include any penetrating injury from the nipple line to the symphysis pubis, a rapidly expanding abdomen, an audible bruit, or asymmetric lower extremity pulses. Importantly, normal vascular examination findings do not exclude the possibility of major abdominal or pelvic vascular injury. The most important point in the preoperative management is aggressive resuscitation with warm crystalloids and blood products to maintain adequate tissue perfusion. Patients should have two wide-bore peripheral lines in the upper extremities with type and cross matching samples sent while the lines are being inserted. All patients should have a nasogastric tube, a Foley urinary catheter, and aggressive hemodynamic monitoring. Patients who are hemodynamically unstable, whether from blunt or penetrating trauma, belong in the operating room, and no time should be wasted in protracted examination and diagnostic studies. For patients who are hemodynamically stable, there is more time for detailed diagnostic studies that will aid in further management.

Patients with penetrating abdominal injuries will still need to go the operating room; however, if they are hemodynamically stable, an abdominal CT scan with contrast is a reasonable diagnostic modality. It is particularly important to assess kidney perfusion and possible renal pedicle injury, which is a very valuable information should a perinephric hematoma be discovered intraoperatively. The exploration of such a hematoma carries a high risk of nephrectomy, so it would be most beneficial to know if exploration of that hematoma is really needed. Also, for a gunshot injury with no exit wound, a flat abdominal x-ray is helpful to locate the missile and determine the possibility of missile embolism in cases of venous injuries.

Blunt traumas of abdominal and pelvic vasculature are more difficult to diagnose in the hemodynamically stable patient. A high index of suspicion is important to detect these injuries. Any patient with abdominal pain, tenderness, abdominal wall hematoma, or seatbelt marks should undergo a CT scan of the abdomen and pelvis with contrast. This is particularly important when renal artery injuries are suspected. The findings include unequal enhancement of both kidneys; loss of enhancement of one kidney suggests the presence of renal artery occlusion with a very high degree of accuracy.[190] Patients with unequal femoral pulses are suspected of having aortoiliac injury. If any of these findings are present on physical or CT examination, arteriography is the next study to be performed. Arteriography in these patients can diagnose significant arterial injuries and can also be therapeutic by implementing endovascular techniques in the possible treatment of those injuries.

Management

The aims of the management of abdominal vascular injuries are first to stop the bleeding and second to restore blood flow to underperfused structures. Any

patient who is hemodynamically unstable with suspicion of an abdominal source must be taken immediately to the operating room for formal abdominal exploration to achieve the above-mentioned goals. Patients who sustained penetrating abdominal traumas still need to go to the operating room for open exploration for diagnosis and management of associated injuries as stated above. Blunt abdominal vascular trauma, depending on the presentation, extent, and pathology of the injury, can be treated in selected patients with endovascular techniques with or without open repair of associated injuries.[191–193] An evolving endovascular role in the treatment of penetrating abdominal vascular trauma as an adjunct to open surgery is also beginning to be reported in the literature.[194]

Operative Management

The first step in the operating room is preparation and draping of the patient. This must include a wide area from the chin to the feet. The reason for the wide field is the possibility that access to the chest, the femoral vessels, and the saphenous veins will needed for grafting. The patient must be prepped and draped before induction of anesthesia so that the team is ready to go quickly into the abdomen in anticipation of possible hypotension with induction.[195] Blood products should be available in the operating room, and O-negative blood must be available if cross-matched blood is not yet available. An autotransfusion device should also be available. Hypothermia is to be avoided by raising the room temperature and using warm intravenous and irrigation fluids and warm blood products. Warming blankets and warm anesthesia circuits are also of help. Antibiotic prophylaxis should be given at this time if not already given in the emergency room.

The abdomen should be entered quickly through a long midline incision from the xiphoid to the symphysis pubis. The primary aim of the procedure is to stop ongoing bleeding, stop any contamination from bowel injury, and repair the injuries. The conventional teaching was to do all of these steps in the same operative procedure; however, the new concept of damage-control surgery has been increasingly used for selected patients.[196,197] This is particularly important for patients with extensive injuries who are exsanguinating, hemodynamically unstable, or, especially , have associated gastrointestinal injuries. In this technique, the aim of the first surgery is to stop the bleeding and contamination, pack the abdomen, and expedite closure. The patient is then returned to the intensive care unit for resuscitation and correction of his or her coagulopathy, hypothermia, and acidosis, and re-exploration is then planned to deal with the specific injuries.

For the hemodynamically unstable patient with free intraperitoneal bleeding or a large expanding, pulsating retroperitoneal hematoma, expedited proximal aortic control is the first step. This can usually be obtained through clamping the supraceliac aorta through the lesser omentum.[198] When there is a large hematoma at the level of the diaphragm, supradiaphragmatic control of the descending thoracic aorta through an added thoracotomy can be helpful.[199]

Endovascular Management

The use of endovascular techniques in the management of vascular trauma in general and particularly in abdominal and pelvic vascular injuries is an evolving field with multiple reports in the literature addressing its utilities and limitations.[191,193,200–203] These techniques are needed because of the inherent limitations of the conventional open surgical techniques for the management of vascular injuries. These limitations include inaccessibility of the vascular lesion, anatomic distortion that results in venous hypertension with excessive bleeding, and the inherent problems with operating in a traumatized and often contaminated field. Furthermore, the presence of multiple trauma or severe medical comorbidities can increase the incidence of surgical complications and mortality.[204]

Endovascular techniques in the management of abdominal and pelvic vascular injuries offer many potential advantages. Angiography can diagnose intimal flap dissections and traumatic arteriovenous fistulas and accurately evaluate the vascular injuries related to gunshot wounds in which more extensive tissue damage is present than anticipated. Embolization techniques for hemostasis have been well studied and are the standard for the management of bleeding from pelvic fractures.[205] Stent grafts can also be used to definitively treat traumatic lesions of the vessels in different vascular beds. Also, endovascular techniques can be used as an adjunct to open surgical management of traumatic vascular injuries by allowing proximal intraluminal vascular control with decreased blood loss and dissection of injured vessels.[206] The concept of using a remote insertion site for the placement of stent grafts away from an operative field contaminated by associated bowel injury is also appealing.[193,207]

Specific Vascular Injuries and Their Management

Abdominal Aortic Injuries

Injuries to the abdominal aorta are usually caused by penetrating trauma, and they carry a high mortality rate because of exsanguination.[208] Occasionally the aortic injury is the result of blunt abdominal trauma with deceleration, such as with seatbelts or falls.[209] The result of the blunt injury can be either rupture or intimal tears with resultant aortic occlusion.

Abdominal aortic injuries are classified into suprarenal or infrarenal injuries. Proximal control of the aorta is the first step in dealing with these injuries. This can be done as previously stated by supraceliac clamping and supradiaphragmatic clamping if needed. Proximal aortic control using an endovascular aortic balloon placed through the brachial or femoral artery may be used in an attempt to prevent the severe hypotensive response to induction of general anesthesia in the setting of hypovolemia that can occur in such patients.[210]

Exposure of the suprarenal aorta is done through medial visceral rotation of the left colon, spleen, stomach, and pancreas. Exposure of the infrarenal aorta is done through incising the posterior peritoneum to the left of the mesentery lateral to the duodenum, taking care not to injure the duodenum, the left renal vein, or the inferior mesenteric artery, which may be difficult to identify in the face of the large hematoma at this area. It is important to move the proximal aortic clamp to the lowest possible level above the injury to avoid the possible renal injury and accentuation of coagulopathy caused by prolonged visceral ischemia from a supraceliac clamp.

The aortic injury is then identified, and adequate debridement is performed to healthy vessel wall. If the defect in the vessel wall is small, it can be repaired primarily; however, a large defect that affects only part of the circumference should be repaired by patch angioplasty using autogenous great saphenous vein or prosthetic material. Although the use of prosthetic material for repair of traumatic vascular injuries has been associated with a low infection rate,[211] it should be used with caution in a contaminated field, and autogenous grafts are preferred whenever possible.[212] If the defect affects the entire circumference of the aorta, repair is done by using an interposition prosthetic graft. Sometimes in the presence of severe contamination, closure of the proximal and distal aortic stumps with the use of an extraanatomic bypass is another reasonable alternative.[213]

Traumatic aortic injuries have been repaired in selected patients recently, with encouraging success rates, using endovascular techniques and stent grafts. They can be used for bleeding aortic injuries, traumatic aortocaval arteriovenous fistulas, and aortic occlusions secondary to intimal tears and dissections.[194,214] They can also be used in conjunction with open surgery to repair the arteries using peripheral unaffected sites away from contaminated fields, thereby avoiding placement of synthetic grafts in these situations.[192,207]

Iliac Vessel Injuries

Injuries of the iliac vessels from both penetrating and blunt injuries, especially those associated with bony pelvis fractures, are usually associated with other visceral injuries, including the urinary tract and the colon.[215]

Another cause is the iatrogenic injury during the performance of endovascular therapeutic procedures with rupture of the iliac arteries during balloon angioplasty and stent placement.[216] The presentation of the injury can be either excessive bleeding or occlusion of the affected iliac vessels. Treatment of these injuries is usually complex and challenging because of the difficult surgical exposure and the associated visceral injuries involved.

During surgery the same operative standards of proximal and distal control are used. Exposure of the iliac arteries is performed through the mobilization of the cecum and distal small bowel on the right and the sigmoid colon on the left. Exposure of the iliac veins can sometimes be challenging and may require division of the right common iliac artery to expose the proximal left common iliac vein and the iliac vein confluence at the inferior vena cava to repair injuries at these sites.[217]

Simple injuries of the iliac vessels can be repaired primarily by lateral arteriorrhaphy or venorrhaphy if they are not accompanied by narrowing of the affected vessels. For more extensive injuries, resection of the affected segment with primary anastomosis is possible if the lost segment is less than 2 cm after mobilization of the ends of the divided iliac arteries. The internal iliac artery can be an excellent graft for short-segment reconstruction. For more extensive injuries requiring long-segment reconstruction, prosthetic grafts are a reasonable alternative, with reports of very low infection rates even in contaminated fields.[215] In cases of severe contamination, both arterial ends are oversewn and the suture lines bolstered within the retroperitoneum with omentum or psoas muscle to prevent disruption of vascular suture lines.[218] In these cases, early revascularization should be attempted by performing extraanatomic bypass if the patient is stable enough to undergo the procedure in the same setting.[215]

Endovascular techniques have been used to treat iliac injuries. These are especially important for the hemodynamically unstable patient with pelvic fracture caused by uncontrolled retroperitoneal bleeding after attempts at stabilizing the pelvis fail to correct the problem. In these cases, arteriography and selective internal iliac branch embolization can be used to rapidly and effectively slow down the bleeding and restore hemodynamic stability because open surgery has very high morbidity and mortality rates.[219] Endovascular use of covered stents is also very effective in the treatment of iatrogenic injuries of the iliac arteries during the performance of therapeutic endovascular procedures.[220]

Inferior Vena Cava Injuries

The inferior vena cava injuries are classified into injuries of the infrarenal, suprarenal, infrahepatic, or retrohepatic portions. Infrarenal injuries occur in one half of the cases.[221,222] Exposure of this segment of the vena cava is performed through mobilizing the right colon and duodenum through an extended Kocher maneuver. Control of the bleeding is achieved by sponge stick or digital compression both above and below the injury or through the use of a side-biting clamp in lateral injuries. Simple injuries can usually be repaired by primary repair. Through-and-through injuries are repaired by extending the anterior injury and repairing the posterior injury from within followed by repair of the anterior one. For extensive infrarenal inferior vena cava injury, the treatment is with either prosthetic grafts or ligation. In cases of severe contamination, ligation is appropriate and is well tolerated by most patients. Lower extremity swelling is inevitable after ligation but can be improved markedly by leg elevation and elastic compression stockings.

Suprarenal and retrohepatic inferior vena cava injuries carry a high mortality rate because of extensive blood loss, difficulty of control and repair, and associated injuries of the renal and hepatic veins. Injuries of these segments mandate repair as ligation is not well tolerated because of severe impairment of the cardiac preload and renal venous hypertension with potential renal failure. The most difficult step in the procedure is obtaining adequate proximal and distal control of the inferior vena cava without severe impairment of the venous return. Clamping of the inferior vena cava above and below the lesion, clamping of the portal vein at the porta hepatis (Pringle maneuver), and clamping of the supraceliac aorta will effectively ensure a dry field for adequate repair. A variety of atriocaval shunts and venovenous bypasses have been used to avoid impairment of the cardiac preload. Although all such techniques have their respective risks, each has allowed occasional successful repair of the injuries.[223] Because of the high mortality rate of retrohepatic inferior vena cava injuries, several studies suggested leaving small retrohepatic hematomas undisturbed in stable patients.[224]

Renovascular Injuries

Renal vascular injuries can result in hemorrhage or occlusion of the renal arteries. Hemorrhage usually results from penetrating injuries, but occlusion is usually caused by blunt abdominal trauma, particularly deceleration injuries where the vessels develop intimal tears, dissections, and subsequent occlusions.[181,182] It is important to diagnose renovascular injuries, as the kidney function becomes severely impaired after 6 hours of warm partial ischemia and after 3 hours of warm total ischemia.[225] The decision to repair or ligate the affected vessel depends on the type of injury, the overall condition of the patient, the associated injuries, the condition of the ipsilateral and contralateral kidney, and the duration of renal ischemia.[226] In most cases of blunt renal artery trauma, repair is not appropriate because of multisystem trauma or delay in diagnosis.

Simple renal artery injuries can be repaired by artery debridement and end-to-end anastomosis. For more extensive injuries, an interposition saphenous vein graft is required. Sometimes, proximal anastomosis of the graft to the aorta is needed. For stable patients, the splenic artery can be used to replace the left renal artery and the hepatic artery can be used to replace the right renal artery. Endovascular techniques have been used successfully to treat renal artery occlusions and dissections.[227,228]

Mesenteric Vascular Injuries

Injuries to the celiac artery can usually be ligated because of excellent collateral flow. On the other hand, injuries to the superior mesenteric artery should always be repaired. Proximal superior mesenteric artery injuries with concomitant duodenal or pancreatic injury are repaired by ligation of the proximal arterial stump and creation of an aorta to superior mesenteric artery bypass. The inferior mesenteric artery can usually be safely ligated except in the rare atherosclerotic patient with large collateral vessels that need to be reimplanted into the aorta. Proximal superior mesenteric vein injuries should be repaired to avoid venous engorgement of the small bowel and possible venous gangrene; however, distal venous injuries can usually be managed by ligation. A second-look laparotomy is generally performed after repair or ligation of mesenteric arterial or venous injuries, as discussed earlier in this chapter.

Portal Region Injuries

Injuries of the portal vein and the hepatic arteries at the porta hepatic are rare and, when present, are often lethal because of the excessive bleeding and the associated severe injuries. Attempts to repair portal vein injuries can be made by ligation. Portal vein ligation carries a mortality rate of almost 90% and repair 42%.[229] Hepatic artery ligation and repair are associated with mortality rates of 58% and 86%, respectively. The cause of mortality is significant blood loss in both injuries. For this reason, whenever possible, portal vein and hepatic artery repair are recommended if no excessive blood loss is associated with the repair. When there is excessive blood loss, early ligation of the injury is advised. In cases of portal vein ligation, excessive fluid requirements postoperatively are anticipated because of sequestration by the congested bowel.

Critique

The mortality rate associated with splenic artery rupture is significant. However, the rupture rate is relatively low, particularly for asymptomatic patients. Considering this patient's numerous comorbidities and the setting of emergency colon surgery, there is no indication for surgical intervention at this time. Even if the patient develops symptomatology, a nonoperative approach, if possible, would be the prudent option.

Answer (E)

References

1. Boley SJ, et al. An aggressive roentgenologic and surgical approach to acute mesenteric ischemia. Surg Annu 1973; 5:355–378.
2. Ginsberg M, Grayson J. Contributions to liver blood flow of the portal vein and hepatic artery. J Physiol 1952; 118(2):16P.
3. Andersson R, et al. Acute intestinal ischemia. A 14-year retrospective investigation. Acta Chir Scand 1984; 150(3): 217–221.
4. Bergan JJ. Recognition and treatment of intestinal ischemia. Surg Clin North Am 1967; 47(1):109–126.
5. Burns BJ, Brandt LJ. Intestinal ischemia. Gastroenterol Clin North Am 2003; 32(4):1127–1143.
6. Hertzer NR, Beven EG, Humphries AW. Acute intestinal ischemia. Am Surg 1978; 44(11):744–749.
7. Jamieson WG. Acute intestinal ischemia. Can J Surg 1988; 31(3):157–158.
8. Marston A, et al. Intestinal ischemia. Arch Surg 1976; 111(2):107–112.
9. Perdue GD Jr, Smith RB 3rd. Intestinal ischemia due to mesenteric arterial disease. Am Surg 1970; 36(3):152–156.
10. Acosta S, Nilsson TK, Bjorck M. D-dimer testing in patients with suspected acute thromboembolic occlusion of the superior mesenteric artery. Br J Surg 2004; 91(8): 991–994.
11. Weil J, Sen Gupta R, Herfarth H. Nonocclusive mesenteric ischemia induced by digitalis. Int J Colorectal Dis 2004; 19(3):277–280.
12. Levinsky RA, et al. Digoxin induced intestinal vasoconstriction. The effects of proximal arterial stenosis and glucagon administration. Circulation 1975; 52(1):130–136.
13. Mimori K, et al. A new approach for acute embolus occlusion of the superior mesenteric artery. Surg Today 1996; 26(11):949–951.
14. Pasupathy S, Sebastian MG, Chia KH. Acute embolic occlusion of the superior mesenteric artery: a case report and discussion of management. Ann Acad Med Singapore 2003; 32(6):840–842.
15. Freund U, Romanoff H, Floman Y. Mortality rate following lower limb arterial embolectomy: causative factors. Surgery 1975; 77(2):201–207.

16. Inderbitzi R, et al. Acute mesenteric ischaemia. Eur J Surg 1992; 158(2):123–126.

17. Carnevale NJ, Delany HM, Cholesterol embolization to the cecum with bowel infarction. Arch Surg 1973; 106(1):94–96.

18. Rosenman LD, Gropper AN. Small intestine stenosis caused by infarction: an unusual sequel of mesenteric artery embolism. Ann Surg 1955; 141(2):254–262.

19. Ridley N, Green SE. Mesenteric arterial thrombosis diagnosed on CT. AJR Am J Roentgenol 2001; 176(2): 549.

20. Shen VS, Pollak EW. Mesenteric arterial thrombosis. A late complication following aortic repair. J Kans Med Soc 1981; 82(5):213–215.

21. Holt PM, Hollanders D. Massive arterial thrombosis and oral contraception. Br Med J 1980; 280(6206):19–20.

22. Rous RC. Mesenteric thrombosis. J S Afr Vet Assoc 1975; 46(1):79–80.

23. Rob C. Stenosis and thrombosis of the celiac and mesenteric arteries. Am J Surg 1967; 114(3):363–367.

24. Sharma BD, Singh RP. Thrombosis of mesenteric artery. (Case report). Indian Pract 1966; 19(4):317–318.

25. Knepper PA, et al. Primary mesenteric thrombosis treated with resection and anticoagulants. Am J Surg 1950; 80(7):937–940.

26. Carrasco D, et al. The value of emergency angiography in the diagnosis and prognosis of acute mesenteric arterial insufficiency. Am J Gastroenterol 1978; 69(3 Pt 1):295–301.

27. Aakhus T. The value of angiography in superior mesenteric artery embolism. Br J Radiol 1966; 39(468):928–932.

28. Boley SJ. Early diagnosis of acute mesenteric ischemia. Hosp Pract (Off Ed) 1981; 16(8):63–71.

29. Boley SJ, et al. Initial results from an aggressive roentgenological and surgical approach to acute mesenteric ischemia. Surgery 1977; 82(6):848–855.

30. Clark RA, Gallant TE. Acute mesenteric ischemia: angiographic spectrum. AJR Am J Roentgenol 1984; 142(3): 555–562.

31. Kaleya RN, Sammartano RJ, Boley SJ. Aggressive approach to acute mesenteric ischemia. Surg Clin North Am 1992; 72(1):157–182.

32. Klempnauer J, et al. Long-term results after surgery for acute mesenteric ischemia. Surgery 1997; 121(3):239–243.

33. Sakaguchi S, et al. Revascularization to prevent postoperative bowel infarction after surgery for acute superior mesenteric artery thromboembolism. Surg Today 2002; 32(3):243–248.

34. Tracy GD. Implant surgery for arterial injury and disease. Med J Aust 1969; 2(2):106–109.

35. Hardy JD. Surgery of the aorta and its branches. Part IV: Occlusive disease of the celiac, superior mesenteric, inferior mesenteric, renal, iliac, femoral, and more distal arteries. Am Pract Dig Treat 1960; 11:317–340.

36. Cho JS, et al. Long-term outcome after mesenteric artery reconstruction: a 37-year experience. J Vasc Surg 2002; 35(3):453–460.

37. Johnston KW, et al. Mesenteric arterial bypass grafts: early and late results and suggested surgical approach for chronic and acute mesenteric ischemia. Surgery 1995; 118(1):1–7.

38. Testart J, et al. Is emergency aorto-superior mesenteric artery by-pass worthwhile? Int Angiol 1992; 11(3):181–185.

39. Hermreck AS, et al. Role of supraceliac aortic bypass in visceral artery reconstruction. Am J Surg 1991; 162(6):611–614.

40. Herrmann-Rinke C, et al. Studies on the viability of the isolated vascularly perfused rat colon. Digestion 1996; 57(5):349–355.

41. Gangadharan SP, Wagner RJ, Cronenwett JL. Effect of intravenous glucagon on intestinal viability after segmental mesenteric ischemia. J Vasc Surg 1995; 21(6):900–908.

42. Schneider JR, et al. Glucagon effect on postischemic recovery of intestinal energy metabolism. J Surg Res 1994; 56(2):123–129.

43. Sardella GL, Bech FR, Cronenwett JL. Hemodynamic effects of glucagon after acute mesenteric ischemia in rats. J Surg Res 1990; 49(4):354–360.

44. Oshima A, et al. Does glucagon improve the viability of ischemic intestine? J Surg Res 1990; 49(6):524–533.

45. Mulherin JL Jr, et al. Management of early postoperative complications of arterial repairs. Arch Surg 1977; 112(11):1371–1374.

46. Tsuda M, et al. Acute superior mesenteric artery embolism: rapid reperfusion with hydrodynamic thrombectomy and pharmacological thrombolysis. J Endovasc Ther 2003; 10(5):1015–1018.

47. Sternbergh WC 3rd, et al. Endovascular treatment of multiple visceral artery paradoxical emboli with mechanical and pharmacological thrombolysis. J Endovasc Ther 2000; 7(2):155–160.

48. Hirota S, et al. Simultaneous thrombolysis of superior mesenteric artery and bilateral renal artery thromboembolisms with three transfemoral catheters. Cardiovasc Intervent Radiol 1997; 20(5):397–400.

49. Badiola CM, Scoppetta DJ. Rapid revascularization of an embolic superior mesenteric artery occlusion using pulse-spray pharmacomechanical thrombolysis with urokinase. AJR Am J Roentgenol 1997; 169(1):55–57.

50. Kwauk ST, et al. Intra-arterial fibrinolytic treatment for mesenteric arterial embolus: a case report. Can J Surg 1996; 39(2):163–166.

51. Wakabayashi H, et al. Emergent treatment of acute embolic superior mesenteric ischemia with combination of thrombolysis and angioplasty: report of two cases. Cardiovasc Intervent Radiol 2004; 27(4):389–393.

52. Bertran X, et al. Occlusion of the superior mesenteric artery in a patient with polycythemia vera: resolution with percutaneous transluminal angioplasty. Ann Hematol 1996; 72(2):89–91.

53. Allen RC, et al. Mesenteric angioplasty in the treatment of chronic intestinal ischemia. J Vasc Surg 1996; 24(3): 415–423.

54. Tytle TL, Prati RC Jr. Percutaneous recanalization in chronic occlusion of the superior mesenteric artery. J Vasc Interv Radiol 1995; 6(1):133–136.

55. Salam TA, Lumsden AB, Martin LG. Local infusion of fibrinolytic agents for acute renal artery thromboembolism: report of ten cases. Ann Vasc Surg 1993; 7(1):21–26.

56. Warnock NG, et al. Treatment of intestinal angina by percutaneous transluminal angioplasty of a superior mesenteric artery occlusion. Clin Radiol 1992; 45(1):18–19.

57. MacFarlane SD, Beebe HG. Progress in chronic mesenteric arterial ischemia. J Cardiovasc Surg (Torino) 1989; 30(2):178–184.

58. Spittler C, et al. Second-look laparoscopy for visceral ischemia facilitated by preinstalled ports. Am Surg 1997; 63(8):732–734.

59. Bickel A, et al. A technique for second-look laparoscopy in the obese patient. J Laparoendosc Surg 1996; 6(2):113–115.

60. Girardi LN, et al. Management strategies for type A dissection complicated by peripheral vascular malperfusion. Ann Thorac Surg 2004; 77(4):1309–1314.

61. Vedantham S, et al. Percutaneous management of ischemic complications in patients with type-B aortic dissection. J Vasc Interv Radiol 2003; 14(2 Pt 1):181–194.

62. Laas J, et al. Management of thoracoabdominal malperfusion in aortic dissection. Circulation 1991; 84(5 Suppl): III20–III24.

63. Oderich GS, Panneton JM. Acute aortic dissection with side branch vessel occlusion: open surgical options. Semin Vasc Surg 2002; 15(2):89–96.

64. Benson WR, Hamilton JE, Claugus CE. Dissection of aorta: report of a case treated by fenestration procedure. Ann Surg 1957; 146(1):111–116.

65. Elefteriades JA, et al. Management of descending aortic dissection. Ann Thorac Surg 1999; 67(6):2002–2019.

66. Elefteriades JA, et al. Fenestration revisited. A safe and effective procedure for descending aortic dissection. Arch Surg 1990; 125(6):786–790.

67. Fann JI, et al. Treatment of patients with aortic dissection presenting with peripheral vascular complications. Ann Surg 1990; 212(6):705–713.

68. Harms J, et al. The abdominal aortic fenestration procedure in acute thoraco-abdominal aortic dissection with aortic branch artery ischemia. J Cardiovasc Surg (Torino) 1998; 39(3):273–280.

69. Lauterbach SR, et al. Contemporary management of aortic branch compromise resulting from acute aortic dissection. J Vasc Surg 2001; 33(6):1185–1192.

70. Okita Y, et al. Surgical strategies in managing organ malperfusion as a complication of aortic dissection. Eur J Cardiothorac Surg 1995; 9(5):242–247.

71. Beregi JP, et al. Endovascular treatment of acute complications associated with aortic dissection: midterm results from a multicenter study. J Endovasc Ther 2003; 10(3):486–493.

72. Fann JI, Miller DC. Endovascular treatment of descending thoracic aortic aneurysms and dissections. Surg Clin North Am 1999; 79(3):551–574.

73. Greenberg R, et al. Aortic dissections: new perspectives and treatment paradigms. Eur J Vasc Endovasc Surg 2003; 26(6):579–586.

74. Clair DG. Aortic dissection with branch vessel occlusion: percutaneous treatment with fenestration and stenting. Semin Vasc Surg 2002; 15(2):116–121.

75. Chavan A, et al. Intravascular ultrasound-guided percutaneous fenestration of the intimal flap in the dissected aorta. Circulation 1997; 96(7):2124–2127.

76. Williams DM, et al. The dissected aorta: percutaneous treatment of ischemic complications—principles and results. J Vasc Interv Radiol 1997; 8(4):605–625.

77. Slonim SM, et al. Percutaneous balloon fenestration and stenting for life-threatening ischemic complications in patients with acute aortic dissection. J Thorac Cardiovasc Surg 1999; 117(6):1118–1126.

78. Beregi JP, et al. Endovascular treatment for dissection of the descending aorta. Lancet 2000; 356(9228):482–483.

79. Duebener LF, et al. Emergency endovascular stent-grafting for life-threatening acute type B aortic dissections. Ann Thorac Surg 2004; 78(4):1261–1267.

80. Lepore V, et al. Endograft therapy for diseases of the descending thoracic aorta: results in 43 high-risk patients. J Endovasc Ther 2002; 9(6):829–837.

81. Rodriguez JA, Olsen DM, Diethrich EB. Thoracic aortic dissections: unpredictable lesions that may be treated using endovascular techniques. J Card Surg 2003; 18(4):334–350.

82. Walker PJ, et al. The use of endovascular techniques for the treatment of complications of aortic dissection. J Vasc Surg 1993; 18(6):1042–1051.

83. Toosy N, et al. Ischaemic preconditioning protects the rat kidney from reperfusion injury. BJU Int 1999; 84(4):489–494.

84. Florack G, et al. Definition of normothermic ischemia limits for kidney and pancreas grafts. J Surg Res 1986; 40(6):550–563.

85. Hoffmann RM, et al. Renal ischemic tolerance. Arch Surg 1974; 109(4):550–551.

86. Cohen DL, et al. Dramatic recovery of renal function after 6 months of dialysis dependence following surgical correction of total renal artery occlusion in a solitary functioning kidney. Am J Kidney Dis 2001; 37(1):E7.

87. de la Rocha AG, Zorn M, Downs AR. Acute renal failure as a consequence of sudden renal artery occlusion. Can J Surg, 1981; 24(3):218–222.

88. Ouriel K, et al. Acute renal artery occlusion: when is revascularization justified? J Vasc Surg 1987; 5(2):348–355.

89. Blum U, et al. Effect of local low-dose thrombolysis on clinical outcome in acute embolic renal artery occlusion. Radiology 1993; 189(2):549–554.

90. Surowiec SM, et al. Acute occlusion of the abdominal aorta. Am J Surg 1998; 176(2):193–197.

91. Busuttil RW, et al. Aortic saddle embolus. A twenty-year experience. Ann Surg 1983; 197(6):698–706.

92. Janssen HL, et al. Extrahepatic portal vein thrombosis: aetiology and determinants of survival. Gut 2001; 49(5):720–724.

93. Verhaeghe R, Vermylen J, Verstraete M. Thrombosis in particular organ veins. Herz 1989; 14(5):298–307.

94. Ernst CB. Abdominal aortic aneurysm. N Engl J Med 1993; 328(16):1167–1172.

95. Graves EJ. Detailed diagnosis and procedures, National hospital discharge survey, 1988. Vital Health Stat 1991; 107:1–239.

96. Desai MM, Zhang P, Hennessy CH. Surveillance for morbidity and mortality among older adults—United States,

1995–1996. MMWR CDC Surveill Summ 1999; 48(8): 7–25.

97. Johansen K, et al. Ruptured abdominal aortic aneurysm: the Harborview experience. J Vasc Surg 1991; 13(2):240–247.

98. Darling RC, et al. Autopsy study of unoperated abdominal aortic aneurysms. The case for early resection. Circulation 1977; 56(3 Suppl):II161–II164.

99. Szilagyi DE, Elliott JP, Smith RF. Clinical fate of the patient with asymptomatic abdominal aortic aneurysm and unfit for surgical treatment. Arch Surg 1972; 104(4):600–606.

100. Mortality results for randomised controlled trial of early elective surgery or ultrasonographic surveillance for small abdominal aortic aneurysms. The UK Small Aneurysm Trial Participants. Lancet 1998; 352(9141):1649–1655.

101. Cronenwett JL, et al. Actuarial analysis of variables associated with rupture of small abdominal aortic aneurysms. Surgery 1985; 98(3):472–483.

102. Foster JH, et al. Comparative study of elective resection and expectant treatment of abdominal aortic aneurysm. Surg Gynecol Obstet 1969; 129(1):1–9.

103. JL, C, Factors increasing rupture risk of small aortic aneurysms. In FJ V, ed. Current Critical Problems in Vascular Surgery, vol 3. St Louis: Quality Medical Publishing, 1991: 234.

104. Sterpetti AV, et al. Factors influencing the rupture of abdominal aortic aneurysms. Surg Gynecol Obstet 1991; 173(3):175–178.

105. Strachan DP. Predictors of death from aortic aneurysm among middle-aged men. The Whitehall study. Br J Surg 1991; 78:401.

106. Brown LC, Powell JT. Risk factors for aneurysm rupture in patients kept under ultrasound surveillance. UK Small Aneurysm Trial Participants. Ann Surg 1999; 230(3):289–297.

107. Brown PM, Zelt DT, Sobolev B. The risk of rupture in untreated aneurysms: the impact of size, gender, and expansion rate. J Vasc Surg 2003; 37(2):280–284.

108. Vorp DA, Raghavan ML, Webster MW. Mechanical wall stress in abdominal aortic aneurysm: influence of diameter and asymmetry. J Vasc Surg 1998; 27(4):632–639.

109. Kushihashi T, et al. [CT of abdominal aortic aneurysms—aneurysmal size and thickness of intra-aneurysmal thrombus as risk factors of rupture.] Nippon Igaku Hoshasen Gakkai Zasshi 1991; 51(3):219–227.

110. Mower WR, Quinones WJ, Gambhir SS. Effect of intraluminal thrombus on abdominal aortic aneurysm wall stress. J Vasc Surg 1997; 26(4):602–608.

111. Lederle FA, et al. Rupture rate of large abdominal aortic aneurysms in patients refusing or unfit for elective repair. JAMA 2002; 287(22):2968–2972.

112. Limet R, Sakalihassan N, Albert A. Determination of the expansion rate and incidence of rupture of abdominal aortic aneurysms. J Vasc Surg 1991; 14(4):540–548.

113. Nevitt MP, Ballard DJ, Hallett JW Jr. Prognosis of abdominal aortic aneurysms. A population-based study. N Engl J Med 1989; 321(15):1009–1014.

114. Wakefield TW, et al. Abdominal aortic aneurysm rupture: statistical analysis of factors affecting outcome of surgical treatment. Surgery 1982; 91(5):586–596.

115. Valentine RJ, Barth MJ, Myers SI, et al. Nonvascular emergencies presenting as ruptured abdominal aortic aneurysms. Surgery 1993; 11:799–803.

116. Weinbaum FI, et al. The accuracy of computed tomography in the diagnosis of retroperitoneal blood in the presence of abdominal aortic aneurysm. J Vasc Surg, 1987; 6(1):11–16.

117. Sullivan CA, Rohrer MJ, Cutler BS. Clinical management of the symptomatic but unruptured abdominal aortic aneurysm. J Vasc Surg 1990; 11(6):799–803.

118. Veith FJ, et al. Endovascular grafts and other catheter-directed techniques in the management of ruptured abdominal aortic aneurysms. Semin Vasc Surg 2003; 16(4):326–331.

119. Ohki T, Veith FJ, Endovascular grafts and other image-guided catheter-based adjuncts to improve the treatment of ruptured aortoiliac aneurysms. Ann Surg 2000; 232(4):466–479.

120. Crawford ES. Ruptured abdominal aortic aneurysm. J Vasc Surg 1991; 13(2):348–350.

121. D'Angelo F, et al. Changing trends in the outcome of urgent aneurysms surgery. A retrospective study on 170 patients treated in the years 1966–1990. J Cardiovasc Surg (Torino) 1993; 34(3):237–239.

122. Shifrin EG, et al. Urgent abdominal aortic aneurysm repair in patients over the age 80. J Cardiovasc Surg (Torino) 1987; 28(2):167–170.

123. Veith FJ, Gargiulo NJ 3rd, Ohki T. Endovascular treatment of ruptured infrarenal aortic and iliac aneurysms. Acta Chir Belg 2003; 103(6):555–562.

124. Chang BB, et al. Can the retroperitoneal approach be used for ruptured abdominal aortic aneurysms? J Vasc Surg 1990; 11(2):326–330.

125. Scharrer-Pamler R, et al. Endovascular stent-graft repair of ruptured aortic aneurysms. J Endovasc Ther 2003; 10(3):447–452.

126. Veith FJ, et al. Treatment of ruptured abdominal aneurysms with stent grafts: a new gold standard? Semin Vasc Surg 2003; 16(2):171–175.

127. Rose DF, et al. Anatomical suitability of ruptured abdominal aortic aneurysms for endovascular repair. J Endovasc Ther 2003; 10(3):453–457.

128. Donaldson MC, Rosenberg JM, Bucknam CA. Factors affecting survival after ruptured abdominal aortic aneurysm. J Vasc Surg 1985; 2(4):564–570.

129. Alric P, et al. Ruptured aneurysm of the infrarenal abdominal aorta: impact of age and postoperative complications on mortality. Ann Vasc Surg 2003; 17(3):277–283.

130. Hatswell EM. Abdominal aortic aneurysm surgery, part I: an overview and discussion of immediate perioperative complications. Heart Lung 1994; 23(3):228–241.

131. Antinori CH, et al. The many faces of aortoenteric fistulas. Am Surg 1996; 62(5):344–349.

132. Dachs RJ, Berman J. Aortoenteric fistula. Am Fam Physician 1992; 45(6):2610–2616.

133. Robbins JA, Ashmore JD. Aortoenteric fistula: diagnosis and management. Dis Colon Rectum 1984; 27(3):196–198.

134. Perks FJ, Gillespie I, Patel D. Multidetector computed tomography imaging of aortoenteric fistula. J Comput Assist Tomogr 2004; 28(3):343–347.

135. Puvaneswary M, Cuganesan R. Detection of aortoenteric fistula with helical CT. Australas Radiol 2003; 47(1):67–69.

136. Roos JE, Willmann JK, Hilfiker PR. Secondary aortoenteric fistula: active bleeding detected with multidetector-row CT. Eur Radiol 2002; 12(3 Suppl):S196–S200.

137. Busuttil SJ, Goldstone J. Diagnosis and management of aortoenteric fistulas. Semin Vasc Surg 2001; 14(4):302–311.

138. Higgins RS, et al. Computed tomographic scan confirmation of paraprosthetic enteric fistula. Am J Surg 1991; 162(1):36–38.

139. Low RN, et al. Aortoenteric fistula and perigraft infection: evaluation with CT. Radiology 1990; 175(1):157–162.

140. Raptopoulos V, Cummings T, Smith EH, Computed tomography of life-threatening complications of abdominal aortic aneurysm. The disrupted aortic wall. Invest Radiol 1987; 22(5):372–376.

141. Saers SJ, Scheltinga MR. Primary aortoenteric fistula. Br J Surg 2005; 92(2):143–152.

142. Cendan JC, Thomas JBT, Seeger JM. Twenty-one cases of aortoenteric fistula: lessons for the general surgeon. Am Surg 2004; 70(7):583–587.

143. Embil JM, Koulack J, Greenberg H. Aortoenteric fistula. Am J Surg 2001; 182(1):75–76.

144. Kuestner LM, et al. Secondary aortoenteric fistula: contemporary outcome with use of extraanatomic bypass and infected graft excision. J Vasc Surg 1995; 21(2):184–196.

145. Rakatansky H. Aortoenteric fistula. N Engl J Med 1993; 329(8):578–579.

146. O'Mara CS, Williams GM, Ernst CB. Secondary aortoenteric fistula. A 20 year experience. Am J Surg 1981; 142(2):203–209.

147. Humphries AW, et al. Complications of abdominal aortic surgery. I. Aortoenteric fistula. Arch Surg 1963; 86:43–50.

148. Chiesa R, et al. Visceral artery aneurysms. Ann Vasc Surg, 2005.

149. Smith JA, Macleish DG, Collier NA. Aneurysms of the visceral arteries. Aust N Z J Surg 1989; 59(4):329–334.

150. Ufberg JW, McNeil B, Swisher L. Ruptured renal artery aneurysm: an uncommon cause of acute abdominal pain. J Emerg Med 2003; 25(1):35–38.

151. Popham P, Buettner A. Arterial aneurysms of the lienorenal axis during pregnancy. Int J Obstet Anesth 2003; 12(2):117–119.

152. Hunsaker DM, Turner S, Hunsaker JC 3rd. Sudden and unexpected death resulting from splenic artery aneurysm rupture: two case reports of pregnancy-related fatal rupture of splenic artery aneurysm. Am J Forensic Med Pathol 2002; 23(4):338–341.

153. Mattar SG, Lumsden AB. The management of splenic artery aneurysms: experience with 23 cases. Am J Surg 1995; 169(6):580–584.

154. Holdsworth RJ, Gunn A. Ruptured splenic artery aneurysm in pregnancy. A review. Br J Obstet Gynaecol 1992; 99(7):595–597.

155. Hidai H, et al. Rupture of renal artery aneurysm. Eur Urol 1985; 11(4):249–253.

156. Garcia CA, Dulcey S, Dulcey J. Ruptured aneurysm of the spinal artery of Adamkiewicz during pregnancy. Neurology 1979; 29(3):394–398.

157. Nathanson SD, Levitt CH, Bremner CG. Ruptured splenic artery aneurysm. S Afr Med J 1974; 48(21):917–918.

158. Thirugnanam A, Sauter KE, Costello AC. Ruptured splenic artery aneurysms: review of literature and presentation of two cases. Vasc Surg 1973; 7(5):269–275.

159. Macfarlane JR, Thorbjarnarson B. Rupture of splenic artery aneurysm during pregnancy. Am J Obstet Gynecol. 1966; 95(7):1025–1037.

160. Burt RL, et al. Ruptured renal artery aneurysm in pregnancy; report of a case with survival. Obstet Gynecol 1956; 7(3):229–233.

161. Tanner FN, Miller HB. Rupture of splenic artery aneurysm during pregnancy; a case report. Nebr State Med J 1955; 40(1):9–11.

162. Poidevin LO. Rupture of splenic artery aneurysm in pregnancy. Med J Aust 1955; 42, 1(25):922–923.

163. Hack RW. Rupture of an aneurysm of the left renal artery during pregnancy. Am J Obstet Gynecol 1953; 65(5):1142–1145.

164. Tennent RA, Starritt A. A case of rupture of aneurysm of the splenic artery during pregnancy. Glasgow Med J 1950; 31(12):465–466.

165. Lookstein RA, Guller J. Embolization of complex vascular lesions. Mt Sinai J Med 2004; 71(1):17–28.

166. Flye MW, et al. Retrograde visceral vessel revascularization followed by endovascular aneurysm exclusion as an alternative to open surgical repair of thoracoabdominal aortic aneurysm. J Vasc Surg 2004; 39(2):454–458.

167. Deshmukh H, et al. Transcatheter embolization as primary treatment for visceral pseudoaneurysms in pancreatitis: clinical outcome and imaging follow up. Indian J Gastroenterol 2004; 23(2):56–58.

168. Parildar M, Oran I, Memis A. Embolization of visceral pseudoaneurysms with platinum coils and N-butyl cyanoacrylate. Abdom Imaging 2003; 28(1):36–40.

169. Atkins BZ, Ryan JM, Gray JL. Treatment of a celiac artery aneurysm with endovascular stent grafting—a case report. Vasc Endovasc Surg 2003; 37(5):367–373.

170. Larson RA, Solomon J, Carpenter JP. Stent graft repair of visceral artery aneurysms. J Vasc Surg 2002; 36(6):1260–1263.

171. Gabelmann A, Gorich J, Merkle EM. Endovascular treatment of visceral artery aneurysms. J Endovasc Ther 2002; 9(1):38–47.

172. Bruce M, Kuan YM. Endoluminal stent-graft repair of a renal artery aneurysm. J Endovasc Ther 2002; 9(3):359–362.

173. Kasirajan K, et al. Endovascular management of visceral artery aneurysm. J Endovasc Ther 2001; 8(2):150–155.

174. Panayiotopoulos YP, Assadourian R, Taylor PR. Aneurysms of the visceral and renal arteries. Ann R Coll Surg Engl 1996; 78(5):412–419.

175. Mattox KL, et al. Five thousand seven hundred sixty cardiovascular injuries in 4459 patients. Epidemiologic evolution 1958 to 1987. Ann Surg 1989; 209(6):698–707.

176. Lim RC Jr, Trunkey DD, Blaisdell FW. Acute abdominal aortic injury: an analysis of operative and postoperative management. Arch Surg 1974; 109(5):706–711.

177. Carrillo EH, et al. Abdominal vascular injuries. J Trauma 1997; 43(1):164–171.

178. Saunders MS, Riberi A, Massullo EA. Delayed traumatic superior mesenteric arteriovenous fistula after a stab wound: case report. J Trauma 1992; 32(1):101–106.

179. Risaliti A, et al. [Arterio-portal fistula. Report of a case and review of the literature.] Minerva Chir 1995; 50(4):399–403.

180. Oller DW, Tutledge R, Clancy T, et al. Vascular injuries in a rural state: a review of 978 patients from a state trauma registry. J Trauma 1992; 32(6):740–745.

181. Randhawa MP Jr, Menzoian JO. Seat belt aorta. Ann Vasc Surg 1990; 4(4):370–377.

182. Haas CA, Spirnak JP. Traumatic renal artery occlusion: a review of the literature. Tech Urol 1998; 4(1):1–11.

183. Nehler MR, Taylor LM Jr, Porter JM. Iatrogenic vascular trauma. Semin Vasc Surg 1998; 11(4):283–293.

184. Modine T, et al. Iatrogenic iliac artery rupture and type a dissection after endovascular repair of type B aortic dissection. Ann Thorac Surg 2004; 77(1):317–319.

185. Laureys M, et al. Percutaneous treatment of iatrogenic iliocaval fistula related to endograft placement for abdominal aortic aneurysm. J Vasc Interv Radiol 2002; 13(2 Pt 1):211–213.

186. Smythe WR, Carpenter JP. Upper abdominal aortic injury during spinal surgery. J Vasc Surg 1997; 25(4):774–777.

187. Lim KE, et al. Iatrogenic upper abdominal aortic injury with pseudoaneurysm during spinal surgery. J Trauma 1999; 46(4):729–731.

188. Fruhwirth J, et al. Vascular complications in minimally invasive surgery. Surg Laparosc Endosc 1997; 7(3):251–254.

189. Bergqvist D, Bergqvist A. Vascular injuries during gynecologic surgery. Acta Obstet Gynecol Scand 1987; 66(1):19–23.

190. Steinberg DL, Jeffrrey RB, Federele MP, et al. The computerized tomography appearance of renal pedicle injury. J Urol 1984; 132:1163.

191. Sternbergh WC 3rd, et al. Acute bilateral iliac artery occlusion secondary to blunt trauma: successful endovascular treatment. J Vasc Surg 2003; 38(3):589–592.

192. Stahlfeld KR, Mitchell J, Sherman H. Endovascular repair of blunt abdominal aortic injury: case report. J Trauma 2004; 57(3):638–641.

193. McArthur CS, Marin ML. Endovascular therapy for the treatment of arterial trauma. Mt Sinai J Med 2004; 71(1):4–11.

194. Ohki T, et al. Endovascular approaches for traumatic arterial lesions. Semin Vasc Surg 1997; 10(4):272–285.

195. Mattox KL, et al. Management of penetrating injuries of the suprarenal aorta. J Trauma 1975; 15(9):808–815.

196. Nicholas JM, et al. Changing patterns in the management of penetrating abdominal trauma: the more things change, the more they stay the same. J Trauma 2003; 55(6):1095–1010.

197. Rotondo MF, et al. "Damage control": an approach for improved survival in exsanguinating penetrating abdominal injury. J Trauma 1993; 35(3):375–383.

198. Sensenig DM. Rapid control in ruptured abdominal aneurysms. Arch Surg 1981; 116(8):1034–1036.

199. Wieneck RG, Wilson RF. Injuries to the abdominal vascular system: how much does aggressive resuscitation and prelaparotomy thoracotomy really help? Surgery 1987; 102:731–736.

200. Taylor PR, Bell RE, Reidy JF. Aortic transection due to blunt trauma: evolving management using endovascular techniques. Int J Clin Pract 2003; 57(8):652.

201. Lyden SP, et al. Common iliac artery dissection after blunt trauma: case report of endovascular repair and literature review. J Trauma 2001; 50(2):339–342.

202. Marin ML, Veith FJ. Clinical application of endovascular grafts in aortoiliac occlusive disease and vascular trauma. Cardiovasc Surg 1995; 3(2):115–120.

203. Sobeh MS, et al. Balloon angioplasty catheters for endovascular tamponade after vascular trauma. Injury 1993; 24(5):355–356.

204. Messina LM, Brothers TE, Wakefield TW, et al. Clinical characteristics and surgical management of vascular complications in patients undergoing cardiac catheterization: interventional versus diagnostic procedures. J Vasc Surg 1991; 13:593–600.

205. Scalea TM, Sclafani S. Interventional techniques in vascular trauma. Surg Clin North Am 2001; 81:1–12.

206. Martin ML, Veith FJ. Transluminally placed endovascular stented graft repair for arterial trauma. J Vasc Surg 1994; 20:299–302.

207. Kramer S, Palmer R, Seifarth H, et al. Endovascular grafting of traumatic aortic aneurysms in contaminated fields. J Vasc Surg 2002; 8:262–267.

208. Accola KD, et al. Management of injuries to the suprarenal aorta. Am J Surg 1987; 154(6):613–618.

209. Lassonde J, Laurendeau F. Blunt injury of the abdominal aorta. Ann Surg 1981; 194(6):745–748.

210. Long JA, et al. [Endovascular aortic balloon catheter occlusion for severe renal trauma.] Prog Urol 2004; 14(3):394–397.

211. Feliciano DV. Abdominal vascular injuries. Surg Clin North Am 1988; 68(4):741–755.

212. Landreneau RJ, Lewis DM, Snyder WH. Complex iliac arterial trauma: autologous or prosthetic vascular repair? Surgery 1993; 114:9–12.

213. Naude GP, et al. Blunt disruption of the abdominal aorta: report of a case and review of the literature. J Vasc Surg 1997; 25(5):931–935.

214. Picard E, et al. Endovascular management of traumatic infrarenal abdominal aortic dissection. Ann Vasc Surg 1998; 12(6):515–521.

215. Carrillo EH, Spain DA, Wilson MA, et al. Alternatives in the management of penetrating injuries to the iliac vessels. J Trauma 1998; 44:1024–1030.

216. Weibull H, Bergqvist D, Jonsson K, et al. Complications after percutaneous transluminal angioplasty in the iliac, femoral and popliteal arteries. J Vasc Surg 1987; 5:681–686.

217. Salam AA, Stewart MT. New approach to wounds of the aortic bifurcation and inferior vena cava. Surgery, 1985; 98(1):105–108.

218. Coselli JS, Crawford ES, Williams TW, et al. Treatment of postoperative infection of ascending aorta and transverse aortic arch, including use of viable omentum and muscle flaps. Ann Thorac Surg 1990; 50:868.

219. Pieri S, Agresti P, Morucci M, De' Medici L, Galluzzo M, Oransky M. Percutaneous management of hemorrhages in pelvic fractures. Radiol Med (Torino) 2004;107(3):241–251.

220. Formichi M, Raybaud G, Benichou H, et al. Rupture of the external iliac artery during balloon angioplasty: endovascular treatment using a covered stent. J Endovasc Surg 1998; 5:37–41.

221. Buckman RF, et al. Injuries of the inferior vena cava. Surg Clin North Am 2001; 81(6):1431–1447.

222. Degiannis E, et al. Penetrating injuries of the abdominal inferior vena cava. Ann R Coll Surg Engl 1996; 78(6):485–489.

223. Roger FB, Reese J, Shackford SR, et al. The use of venovenous bypass and total vascular isolation of the liver in the surgical management of juxtahepatic venous injuries in blunt hepatic trauma. J Trauma 1997; 43:530–533.

224. Posner MC, Moore EE, Greenholz SL, et al. Natural history of untreated inferior vena cava injury and assessment of venous access. J Trauma 1986; 26:698.

225. Lohse JR, Shore RM, Belzer FO. Acute renal artery occlusion: the role of collateral circulation. Arch Surg 1982; 117:801–804.

226. Shackford SR, Sise MJ. Renal and mesenteric vascular trauma. In Bongard F, Wilson SE, Perry MO, eds. Vascular Injuries in Surgical Practice. Norwalk, CT: Appleton & Lange, Norwalk. 1991: 173.

227. Dobrilovic N, Bennett S, Smith C, Edwards J, Luchette FA. Traumatic renal artery dissection identified with dynamic helical computed tomography. J Vasc Surg 2001; 34(3):562–564.

228. Lee JT, White RA. Endovascular management of blunt traumatic renal artery dissection. J Endovasc Ther 2002; 9(3):354–358.

229. Jurkovich GJ, Hoyt DB, Moore FA, et al. Portal triad injuries. J Trauma 1995; 39:426–434.

35
Colon and Rectum

Herand Abcarian

Case Scenario

A 54-year-old patient, while being managed for noso-comial pneumonia, develops an antibiotic-induced colitis (pseudomembranous colitis). Although Flagyl was given orally, the patient becomes febrile and toxic. He is admitted to the intensive care unit and broad-spectrum antibiotics are initiated. Radiographic find-ings are consistent with a toxic megacolon. The patient continues to deteriorate. Which of the following is the most appropriate treatment option?

(A) Limitation of antifungal therapy
(B) Decompressive colonoscopy
(C) Segmented resection
(D) Abdominal colectomy
(A) Administration of a prokinetic agent

Anorectal Disease and Trauma

Abscess

By far the most common anorectal disease requiring acute care surgery is anorectal abscess. Anorectal ab-scesses originate from a cryptoglandular source in the overwhelming majority of cases. Crohn's disease and trauma either external (penetrating injuries) or internal (from ingested sharp objects such as toothpicks or chicken or fish bones) rounds out the causes of anorectal abscess. Depending on the anatomic location of abscess, distal or proximal to the anorectal ring, the presenting symptoms are quite different.

"Lower abscesses," that is, those located distal to the anorectal ring (perianal, ischiorectal, intrasphincteric), are associated with more intense local symptoms, such as pain, swelling, cellulitis, and tenderness, and much less systemic symptoms of fever, chills, and malaise. There-fore, these abscesses are easier to diagnosis and more amenable to emergency incision and drainage in the office or emergency departments. On the other hand, "high abscesses," that is, those located proximal to the anorectal ring (high intramuscular, supralevator), often present with minimal local symptoms, such as vague pelvic or rectal pressure, and more systemic symptoms and may easily be diagnosed as fever of unknown origin and treated with ineffective nonsurgical measures if a careful rectal examination is omitted at the time of first presentation. A high index of suspicion, careful digital rectal examination, and, if needed, often examination under anesthesia are essential for proper and timely sur-gical management of high anorectal abscesses.[1]

The principal treatment of all anorectal abscesses is early, adequate, and dependent drainage. Small super-ficial perianal abscesses can be drained under local anes-thesia using a cruciate incision or unroofed to prevent premature closure of the wound. The drainage incision should be placed as close to the anal canal as possible to shorten the subsequent fistula tract if one develops. Larger abscesses are best drained in the operating room under regional or general anesthesia. Packing the abscess inflicts unnecessary pain on the patients on insertion and withdrawal of the pack. If the abscess is large, multiple radial incisions rather than a long circumanal one should be made, and Penrose drains can be looped and sutured around the skin bridges to maintain postoperative drainage as long as needed.

The natural history of anorectal abscess treated with drainage ranges from complete healing to healing and recurrence to nonhealing with persistent drainage both of which indicates presence of a fistula. Therefore, in selected cases when a fistula is easily identified and there is minimal overlying sphincter muscle, surgeons may elect to perform a primary fistulotomy to complete the treat-ment, minimize morbidity, and shorten the patients' sick days.[2,3] On the other hand, primary fistulotomy in inex-perienced hands carries the risk of unintended extensive sphincterotomy and postoperative fecal incontinence. Therefore, if the surgeon identifies the fistula track but is unsure of its complexity, it is best to insert a thick braided suture or silastic (vessel loop) Seton in the fistulous tract and delay the definitive treatment of the fistula for a later time or refer the patient to a more experienced specialist.[4]

"High" anorectal abscesses must always be drained in the operating room under appropriate anesthesia to allow for careful examination of the abscess cavity in relation to the anal sphincter complex. The abscess may be drained intrarectally or through the ischiorectal fossa but never in both directions simultaneously, because it will invariably result in an iatrogenic extrasphincteric fistula, which is extremely difficult or impossible to cure.[5]

Fournier's gangrene is a very morbid and potentially lethal synergistic infection of the perineal, perianal, scrotal, and vulvar soft tissues that can originate from urologic, gynecologic, or most frequently anorectal sources. The treatment must include immediate resuscitation of the patient, administration of broad-spectrum intravenous antibiotics, and extensive surgical debridement as soon as possible. Any delay in surgery will result in massive invasion of the infection to surrounding tissue, extending into the anterior abdominal wall, gluteal muscles, upper thighs, and external genitalia. Debridement must aggressively remove all necrotic or suspiciously compromised tissues down to bleeding healthy margins. Vulvar, scrotal, and penile skin must be excised if involved, but orchiectomy is almost never necessary. Anal sphincters, although rarely necrotic, should be debrided as needed without concern for subsequent fecal incontinence (Figure 35.1).

The most important surgical principle after the original extensive debridement is a second-look operation in 24 to 48 hours to debride any additional necrotic tissue developed since the first procedure. If the patient remains febrile, a return to the operating room every 48 hours is mandatory to completely debride all compromised tissue and to irrigate the tissues with a jet irrigation system. If urinary tract involvement is documented by retrograde urethrocystography, a suprapubic cystostomy is essential. If the sphincter mechanism is extensively debrided, an open or laparoscopic diverting colostomy will be needed to prevent continued postoperative fecal wound contamination.

A critically important treatment plan for these very sick patients is early institution of total parenteral nutrition and control of the blood sugar level, because up to 50% of these patients are diabetic. The patient should be managed in the intensive care unit until no further trips to the operating room are necessary, and then twice daily whirlpool treatments will be very helpful in their wound care. The role of hyperbaric oxygen in the treatment of Fournier's gangrene remains controversial, but it most

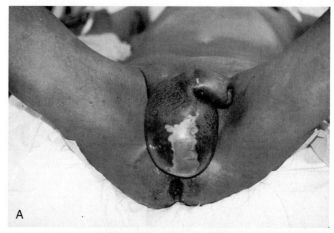

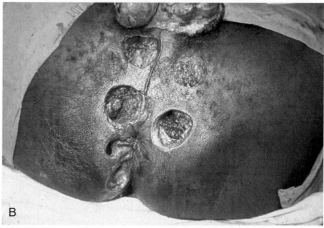

FIGURE 35.1. **(A)** Fournier's gangrene involving bilateral ischiorectal fossa and scrotum. **(B)** Same patient after third surgical intervention. Note scrotal debridement and multiple ischiorectal fossa counterincisions.

certainly should not replace or supercede adequate surgical debridement.[6,7]

Hemorrhoids

Acute care surgery for hemorrhoids is performed for the following conditions.

Thrombosed external hemorrhoids usually occur suddenly and often with no prior history of straining with constipation, diarrhea, or heavy lifting. The painful swelling increases in size for a day or two and can be differentiated from an abscess because of its sharp distant borders, absence of adjacent cellulitis, and close proximity to the anal canal. The swelling and pain will decrease after 96 hours with dissolution of the thrombosis, and the patient may not need any surgical treatment thereafter. When the patient has acute swelling, the best treatment is immediate excision of the thrombosed hemorrhoid under local anesthesia. This is preferable to incision and enucleation of the clot, because the latter procedure leaves the offending hemorrhoidal tissue behind and predisposes to recurrent thrombosis. The incision should not involve the anoderm because it may lead to a subsequent iatrogenic anal fissure.

Bleeding internal hemorrhoid is rarely life threatening and does not require acute care treatment, except in cases of coagulopathy whether caused by disease (liver failure) or medications (anticoagulant therapy). In these instances, immediate injection sclerotherapy is preferable to either hemorrhoidectomy or rubber band ligation. Bleeding hemorrhoids can be injected with 5% phenol in vegetable oil or one of the agents commonly used for injection of esophageal varices, for example, sodium morrhuate or sulfate tetradecyl solution.

Bleeding after hemorrhoidectomy may occur whether an open (Milligram Morgan), closed (Ferguson), or stapled technique is utilized. Early bleeding (within hours of surgery) is rare and is related to technical error and must be treated by returning the patient to the operating room. Delayed bleeding (i.e., after 3 to 7 days) usually results from the suture or staple line separation or from necrosis caused by ischemia. If bleeding is significant with the patient needing to be resuscitated, it is best to reexamine the patient under anesthesia. Most often no active bleeding will be found in the operating room after irrigation and evaluation of the clots. However, it is important to reinforce the apex of the hemorrhoidectomy incision or the staple line anyway to prevent recurrent bleeding.

Bleeding after rubber band ligation is reported to occur in 1 in 200 cases. Bleeding is arterial and will often continue without intervention. The most expeditious way to control this type of bleeding is anoscopic examination, removal of clots, and application of a cotton applicator impregnated with 1/1,000 solution of epinephrine. This causes intense vasoconstriction and stops the bleeding. The open vessel can then be cauterized with silver nitrate or Monsell's solution or even suture ligated if necessary.

Acute hemorrhoidal crisis is a term used to describe incarcerated prolapsed internal hemorrhoids with corresponding doughnut-shaped swelling and even thrombosis of the external hemorrhoids. In early cases, the edema can be reduced by injection of Lidocaine with 1/2,000,000 epinephrine mixed with 150 IU of hyaluronidase, directly into the external hemorrhoids. The dispersion of hyaluronidase immediately reduces the swelling, and the anesthetized external sphincter relaxes, allowing for the reduction of prolapsed internal hemorrhoids. External thrombotic hemorrhoids can then be excised and internal hemorrhoids treated with rubber band ligation. This urgent but conservative care is preferable to acute care hemorrhoidectomy, which under these conditions often leads to excessive excision of anoderm and postoperative anal stenosis.[8] However, if the patient seeks medical attention after tissues necrosis has occurred, an emergent hemorrhoidectomy is needed and care must be taken to leave as much normal anoderm as possible between suture lines to prevent subsequent anal stricture.

Pelvic cellulitis following rubber band ligation of hemorrhoids is a rare but potentially lethal complication of this common office procedure. Typically, patients complain of increasing pain and dysuria on the second or third day after the procedure. These symptoms warrant an acute care examination under anesthesia. Any delay in diagnosis and treatment results in septic shock and death in most cases. In the operating room the grayish necrotic area surrounding the ligated hemorrhoid must be debrided to bleeding, healthy tissue. Broad-spectrum antibiotics and other supportive measures should be instituted as needed.[9,10]

Anal Fissure

Anal fissure rarely requires an acute care operation unless there is an associated low intersphincteric abscess-fistula, which should be treated with unroofing and primary fistulotomy. The procedure of choice for fissures is lateral internal sphincterotomy, and this can always be done on an elective basis. When patients suffer from severe pain, topical application of 0.2% nitroglycerine ointment or 2% Diltiazem® gel may be used to temporize the symptoms until elective surgery can be scheduled.[11]

Pilonidal Cyst-Abscess

Pilonidal cyst-abscess should be drained under local anesthesia as soon as diagnosis is made to prevent unnecessary spread of the infection. The patient can then be taken to the operating room electively for excision of the cyst to prevent recurrent abscess. Acute care primary excision of large pilonidal cyst-abscesses results in very large wounds and prolonged healing time.

Rectal Procedentia (Rectal Prolapse)

Acute care surgery for rectal procedentia is rarely needed. If the patient presents with incarceration, the sphincter mechanism should be infiltrated with dilute lidocaine (0.5%) and epinephrine solution (1/200,000) circumferentially. This causes the external sphincter to relax and allows the prolapse to be reduced with gentle compression. If tissue edema rather than sphincter contraction is the primary reason for incarceration, covering the prolapse with gauze moistened with witch hazel granulated sugar is effective in reducing the swelling. When a neglected procedentia results in strangulation and tissue necrosis, reduction of the tissue, much like strangulated inguinal hernias, is contraindicated. The patient should be

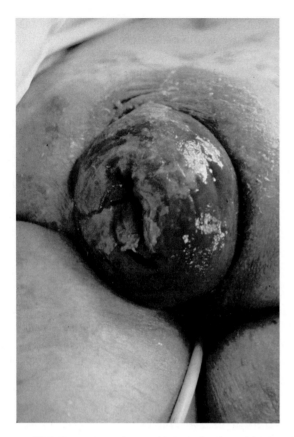

FIGURE 35.2. Incarcerated rectal procedentia with mucosal ischemia and ulceration.

taken to the operating room and undergo an acute care perineal proctectomy and posterior levatorplasty (Prasad modification of the Altemeier procedure) (Figure 35.2).[12] It is very rare that a patient should require abdominoperineal resection of the rectum because the anal sphincter mechanism resists ischemia much more so than the prolapsed rectal wall.

Colorectal Disease and Trauma

Neoplastic Disease

Acute care surgery in colorectal cancer is usually necessary in cases of bleeding, perforation, or obstruction.

Bleeding from colorectal cancer is rarely massive or life threatening and thus necessitating acute care surgery. When the diagnosis of cancer is already established, acute care resection is indicated. Nonoperative measures, including angiographic embolization, should be reserved only for debilitated patients who are considered very poor anesthetic risk. Following acute care resection of the colon for massive bleeding, primary anastomosis is usually feasible due to the cathartic nature of intraluminal bleed. However, if an anastomosis is considered risky (e.g., for a hypotensive patient with unstable vital signs),

an end loop colostomy or end stoma and Hartmann closure of the distal segment may be performed.

Colonic perforation from cancer signifies an advanced stage of the disease and is associated with a poor prognosis. Perforation may occur at the site of the cancer due to deep penetration (T_3–T_4 lesions) or proximal to an obstructing cancer. In either situation, primary resection of the malignant tumor is the procedure of choice, and this may have to be extended to include the proximal perforation (e.g., right hemicolectomy in addition to transverse colon resection for obstructing transverse colon cancer with cecal perforation). Depending on the general condition of the patient, a stoma might be deemed safer than primary anastomosis. In such cases an end loop stoma placing the distal (disfunctioned) limb at the same location as the matured proximal end should be considered. An end loop stoma is preferable to placing the proximal stoma and mucous fistula in separate sites or quadrants, because its closure does not mandate a subsequent laparotomy.[13]

Colonic obstruction is the most often encountered complication of cancer requiring acute care intervention. If the obstruction is incomplete, a slow gradual preparation with cathartics administered orally or via the nasogastric tube may effectively decompress and cleanse the colon in preparation for surgery. For "low" obstructing cancers involving the rectum or rectosigmoid or lower sigmoid colon, a gastrogaffin enema is useful to locate the tumor and soften impacted stool. Afterwards, multiple small-volume enemas can be utilized for retrograde colonic evacuation. Occasionally it is possible to pass a small-caliber Salem nasogastric tube through the obstructing lesion to allow for decompression of air and gentle bowel preparation. This is an old-fashioned alternative to the currently used wall stents that can be deployed in the operating room, gastrointestinal laboratory, or interventional radiologic suite with the aid of fluoroscopy.[14] A wall stent may be used as a temporizing tool to allow the lumen to remain patent in the short term (i.e., preoperative bowel decompression) or for preparation for surgery or long term use (e.g., during preoperative neoadjuvant therapy aimed at downstaging the disease). Alternatively, for individuals with widespread metastases and a very limited life expectancy, wall stents may be deployed as a palliative measure to avoid a colostomy in near dying patients.[15]

Other surgical alternatives might be applicable for patients with obstructed distal cancer and extensive proximal colonic distention. The first is extended colectomy, which often signifies resection of the entire distended colon and ileorectosigmoid anastomosis. This procedure is unsuitable for true obstructing rectal cancers because of the need to anastomose the terminal ileum to the mid or distal rectum. In such cases, despite all efforts in preserving the water-absorbing terminal ileum, the patient may not have the necessary rectal compliance to handle liquid stools and might well end up with fecal incontinence.[16,17] Another alternative is intraoperative colonic lavage followed by primary anastomosis. In this technique the Foley catheter is inserted into the cecum through the appendiceal stump or, in patients with previous appendectomy, via a purse string in the terminal ileum. It is necessary to mobilize both colonic flexures to allow for free flow of the irrigating fluid. The obstructing tumor is resected, and the mobilized end of the proximal colon is moved outside the abdomen and sutured to a drainage tube. After irrigation with 4 to 5 L of saline or lactated Ringer's solution, as the colonic effluent clears, the irrigation is discontinued, the irrigating tube is removed, and a stapled or hand-sewn colocolonic or colorectal anastomosis is performed in the usual fashion. This procedure takes an extra 45 to 60 minutes and is suitable only for good-risk patients. There is an increased incidence of cardiopulmonary complications as well as a high risk of wound infections and intraabdominal abscess.[18,19]

In both surgical alternatives it is mandatory to mobilize both flexures. Mobilization of the splenic flexure in a grossly distended colon increases the risk of splenic injury. Also manipulation of a massively distended cecum with tineal diastases predisposes to intraoperative perforation and fecal contamination. Therefore, it is imperative to decompress the colon with a large-bore needle, trocar, or suction catheter (e.g., Salem nasogastric tube) inserted in the colon through a small colotomy or through the resected appendiceal stump to allow for safe mobilization of the chronically distended colon. Despite these minor difficulties and inherent increase in risk of postoperative infection, extended colectomy or intraoperative colonic lavage are suitable alternatives to a diverting colostomy in many good-risk patients with grossly dilated colons secondary to distal obstruction.

Diverticular Disease

Bleeding secondary to diverticulosis may be massive and life threatening. However, in most cases the bleeding stops spontaneously, only to recur later. The incidence of rebleeding after the first episode is as high as 30% and rises to 50% after a second bleed and up to 80% afterwards. The key to successful management of bleeding diverticulosis is accurate diagnosis, which can be difficult at times. Blind total abdominal colectomy with ileostomy and Hartmann closure of the rectum or ileorectostomy, popular in some institutions in the early 1960s, has been replaced by a standard therapeutic algorithm utilizing endoscopy, bleeding scan, angiography, and surgery (Figure 35.3). In short, after esophagogastroduodenostomy, anoscopy, and rigid or flexible sigmoidoscopy have excluded upper gastrointestinal and anorectal sources of

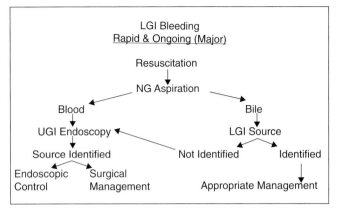
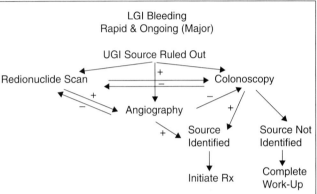
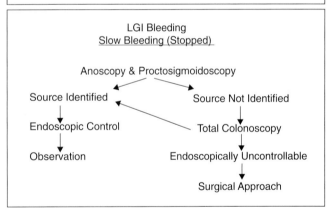

FIGURE 35.3. Lower gastrointestinal (LGI) bleeding: treatment algorithm based on activity and severity of bleeding. NG, nasogastric; Rx, treatment; UGI, upper gastrointestinal.

massive bleeding, the patient should undergo a tagged red blood cell scan, which generally is more sensitive then angiography in localization of bleeding (0.5 mL/min vs. 1 mL/min bleeding).[20] If a radionuclide scan is negative, proceeding with angiography is usually fruitless. However, if the scan is positive, angiography might localize the bleeding point, allowing embolization therapy with coils or Gefoam®. At angiography all three visceral vessels must be studied. Because of the anatomic overlap of hepatic flexure and the duodenum in the nuclear medicine scan, a negative small mesenteric artery injection may miss bleeding from duodenal feeding vessels. If the bleeding site is localized and controlled with embolization, the catheter can be removed or left in place for 24 hours. Angiography can be repeated if the bleeding recurs, and conversely the catheter can be removed if no extravasation is seen by the radiologist and no further clinical bleeding occurs. Immediate colonoscopy during active bleeding has been advocated by Forde but is not popular because of the lack of the required expertise and demand in many institutions. However, if the bleeding stops, the patient can be prepared with polyethylene glycol solution and undergo colonoscopy within a few hours.[21]

If the site of bleeding is localized but the bleeding is not controllable with angiography, then a resection of the appropriate colonic segment is indicated. In such cases, the catheter should be left in and injected with methylene blue during laparotomy to facilitate accurate localization of the bleeding site.[22] Recurrent bleeding during the same hospitalization stay or soon after discharge is managed in a similar fashion. Bleeding occurring weeks or months after cessation of the original bleeding must be reworked up utilizing the same algorithm. If the bleeding stops at the completion of the workup, acute care surgery in not required; however, the patient should be prepared and undergo elective surgery if bleeding has recurred two or three times previously.

Complications of diverticulitis (i.e., obstruction, perforation, and fistulas) need to be addressed surgically. Diverticular obstruction should be treated with bowel rest and intravenous antibiotics. If the obstruction responds to medical management as documented by physical examination, water-soluble enema, or computed tomography (CT) scan, the patient may be prepared and operated electively. If the obstruction does not respond to medical management and the patient requires acute care surgery, the same alternatives discussed for colorectal cancer must be considered, including resection, proximal colostomy and Hartmann closure of rectum, intraoperative lavage and primary anastomosis, or extended colectomy. Madden[23] in the 1960s advocated primary anastomosis with no bowel preparation with excellent results, and reports from the Lahey Clinic comparing three- and two-stage procedures concluded that the hospital stay was shorter and total sick days fewer if primary anastomosis is done in unprepared colon and is protected with proximal diversion.[24] Recent experience with primary closure of colonic injuries has led to reevaluation of mandatory colostomy when the surgeon is facing an obstructed colon filled with stool.

Perforation of the colon secondary to diverticulitis may be classified into (1) perforation with local abscess or (2) perforation with purulent peritonitis or rectal peritonitis. The Hinchey classification adds very little knowledge to the pathophysiology of the complications.

Perforation with local abscess is best treated with CT-guided drainage, intravenous antibiotics, and bowel rest. This modality reduces the incidence of sepsis, avoids the necessity of acute care surgery and colostomy. On the other hand, if the abscess cannot be adequately drained or persists despite drainage or the patient continues to have fever, elevated white blood cell count, persistent abdominal pain, and tenderness beyond 5 to 7 days, urgent surgery should be scheduled without further delay. A sigmoid colectomy and Hartmann procedure with end colostomy is the preferred procedure especially for poor-risk patients.[25] On the other hand, good-risk patients may undergo resection and primary anastomosis with proximal colostomy or intraoperative colonic lavage and primary anastomosis without diversion.

Perforation with purulent or fecal peritonitis should be treated with aggressive resuscitation, intravenous broad-spectrum antibiotics, and acute care surgery. The surgeon is usually faced with massive contamination of the peritoneal cavity in a patient often in poor general condition. In the past, closure of the perforation, drainage of the abscess, and a proximal colostomy, as advocated by Colcock and Stahmann,[26] was the procedure of choice. Continued sepsis was always blamed on poor diversion, and an end colostomy was advocated to accomplish total diversion. However, it is now well understood that continued or recurrent sepsis is caused by continuous leakage of stool left between the colostomy and the colonic perforation site. For this reason, primary resection of the perforated segment and proximal end colostomy and closure of the rectum is preferable in such cases.

The most important technical point to observe during acute care surgery for diverticulitis is avoidance of extensive pelvic dissection below the sacral promontory and division of the rectum at the mid-rectal level. This causes distal retraction of the rectum below the prostate or cervix and makes restoration of colorectal continuity at a later date extremely difficult.

Malignant diverticulitis is a term coined by Morgenstern et al.[27] to describe the invasive spread of infection to adjacent pelvic organs and side walls. This invasion makes identification of surgical planes difficult and contributes to bladder and ureteral injuries. When such cases are suspected by the appearance of diffuse pelvic inflammatory change on preoperative CT scan, perioperative insertion of ureteral catheters is extremely helpful. Even though urerteral catheters do not prevent ureteral injury, they facilitate the intraoperative detection of urethral injury leading to immediate repair. Furthermore, it is recommended that in order to protect the left ureter the standard lateral to medial mobilization of colon (incising the line of Toldt) be abandoned in favor of proximal to distal dissection. In this technique the sigmoid descending junction, often the soft pliable proximal colon, is divided, and the surgeon lifts the colon and begins dissection, well proximal to the phlegmon, separating the colon from the Gerota's fasia and retroperitoneal strictures. Downward continuation of this dissection allows the surgeon to mobilize the colon while leaving the left ureter and the gonadal vessels posteriorly (Figure 35.4). The peritoneal reflexion of Toldt is then opened laterally and the mesocolic vessels ligated and divided medially,

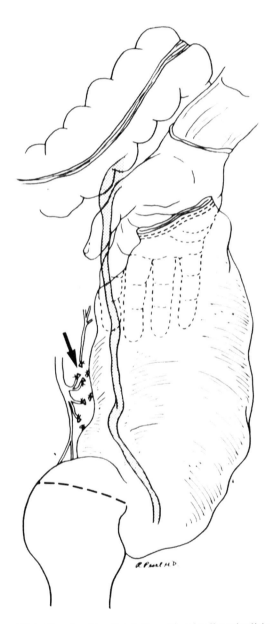

FIGURE 35.4. Proximal to distal dissection in diverticulitis. Note that the colon is stapled and divided proximal to the phlegmon. The surgeon's hand behind the colon and anterior to Gerota's fascia aids in safe dissection of the phlegmon from the retroperitoneum. The left ureter remains posteriorly with the kidney. (Reprinted from Abcarian H. The difficult resection in diverticulitis. Semin Colon Rectal Surg 1990; 1:97–98, with permission from Elsevier.)

resulting in safe mobilization of the colon. The anterior attachment of the sigmoid to bladder dome or the uterus is then "pinched off," allowing access to the normal rectum below. The rectum is stapled off at the level of the sacral promontory and the specimen is removed, avoiding further mobilization or shortening of the rectal stump.[28]

Sigmoid fistulas in diverticulitis are not a cause for acute care surgery. Sigmidovaginal fistulas always occur in women with prior hysterectomy and present with passage of gas or stool per vagina after a bout of diverticulitis. Sigmoidovesical fistulas present with pneumaturia and fecaluria and may result in symptomatic urinary tract infection and sepsis. Under these circumstances the patient should be operated urgently as soon as systemic sepsis is controlled. Surgical intervention includes resection of the involved colonic segment and colorectal anastomosis. The opening in the bladder or vagina is often very small and need not be closed separately. Interposition of omentum between the anastomosis and the vagina or bladder is quite adequate in achieving permanent closure. The bladder should be drained for 7 to 10 days via a Foley catheter, and a cystogram may be done before the Foley catheter is removed, although in most cases this is not necessary.

Finally, it must be pointed out that colocolostomy in diverticular disease results in a much higher recurrence rate than coloproctostomy. Although the presence of diverticula proximal to the anastomosis is of no clinical significance, leaving diverticula in a high-pressure zone distal to the anastomosis leads to a much higher recurrence rate (14% vs. <2%).[29]

Cecal diverticulitis clinically mimics appendicitis and on CT scan may be indistinguishable from perforated cecal cancer. Acute care surgery for right lower quadrant peritonitis caused by perforated cecal diverticulitis almost always necessitates right hemicolectomy and ileotransverse colostomy because of intraoperative confusion of this entity with perforated cecal cancer.

Inflammatory Bowel Disease

Acute care surgery for ulcerative colitis is indicated for massive bleeding or toxic megacolon. Patients with severe colitis unresponsive to medical management often undergo surgery on urgent rather than an acute care basis. Bleeding, although the most common symptom of ulcerative colitis, is rarely massive. Instead, the patient with severe colitis may lose sufficient blood during multiple daily bowel movements to require transfusion every 2 or 3 days. If this pattern continues, the patient should be operated on urgently as an intractable case.

Massive bleeding requiring multiple consecutive transfusions occurs in 3% of patients with ulcerative colitis and warrants acute care surgery. It is important to exclude the rectum as the source of massive bleeding endoscopically either preoperatively or during laparotomy. With the patient in the dorsal lithotomy position, the rectosigmoid junction can be occluded and the rectum examined with a rigid or flexible sigmoidoscope. Exclusion of the rectum as the source of massive bleeding will allow the surgeon to limit the operation to abdominal colectomy, ileostomy, and closure of the rectum rather than the more complicated and morbid acute care total proctocolectomy (Figure 35.5). The latter procedure must be avoided if at all possible to allow for subsequent restorative proctectomy and ileal-pouch anal anastomosis.

Toxic megacolon, a complication of ulcerative colitis, pseudomembranous colitis, and disease of the colon, results from loss of normal colonic motility caused by severe inflammation. This is aggravated by the use of contrast enemas, endoscopic air insufflation, and prescription of narcotics or anticholinergics for abdominal pain. The colon is not massively distended as in Ogilvie's syndrome or volvulus. Rather, there is a segmental dilatation of the colon, usually the transverse colon. The patient may be toxic but the inflammatory response masked or blocked by the use of large doses of intravenous steroids. Progression of colonic dilatation in subsequent plain films of the abdomen, appearance of "thumb printing" signifying deepening ulcerations, and most importantly presence of air in the bowel wall or gas in the portal systems are all ominous signs of impending perforation (Figure 35.6).

Because perforation of the colon increases the morbidity and mortality of the toxic megacolon at least 10-fold, acute care surgery is mandatory if the disease appears to be progressing despite maximal medical therapy. In the absence of objective improvement, surgery should be not be delayed beyond 24 to 48 hours because the patient may not be able to mount sufficient

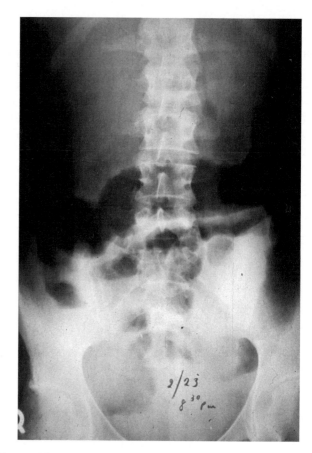

FIGURE 35.6. Plain abdominal radiograph showing toxic megacolon. Note the moderate distention of the transverse colon. "Thumb printing" denotes deep ulceration and impending perforation.

inflammatory response to raise suspicion of impending or existing perforation.

The current acceptable operation for toxic megacolon is total abdominal colectomy, ileostomy, and closure of the rectum (or distal sigmoid mucous fistula). Turnbull et al.[30] advocated ileostomy and multiple blow hole colostomies to avoid manipulation of an extremely dilated and thin-walled colon. This procedure is not performed any longer because patients undergo surgery much earlier than before mostly because of the ileal J pouch anal anastomosis designed by Utsunomiya et al.[31]

Two technical points are notable regarding the abdominal colectomy and ileostomy for massive bleeding or toxic megacolon. First, the ileocolic vessels must be preserved by ligating the feeding vessels of the cecum distal to the main ileocolic artery. This will offer the surgeon the alternative of dividing the superior mesenteric artery distal to the jejunal branches if this vessel is too short to allow pouch anal anastomosis. Second, the rectum should not be mobilized in order to facilitate subsequent dissection during restorative proctectomy, especially in male patients, for whom repeated pelvic dissections increase the likelihood of postoperative sexual dysfunction.

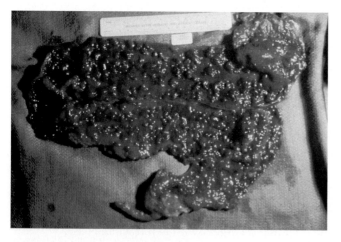

FIGURE 35.5. Proctocolectomy specimen revealing changes typical of ulcerative colitis with foreshortening of the colon and extensive pseudopolyp formation.

Acute care surgery for Crohn's disease is often indicated for perforation or obstruction and rarely for fistulization or bleeding. Perforation may be spontaneous or iatrogenic. The transmural nature of Crohn's disease leads to deep ulcers and fissures, and, unless the bowel is in close contact with the abdominal wall or another intraabdominal organ, spontaneous perforation may occur. However, in most cases perforation is seen immediately or soon after a colonoscopy performed for diagnostic or surveillance purposes and especially when multiple biopsy specimens have been taken.

Diagnosis of Crohn's perforation is easily made on plain abdominal films or by CT scanning. Although at times minute perforations during colonoscopy can be treated nonoperatively, it is unlikely that perforation in a diseased bowel will close spontaneously, and acute care surgery is indicated. At laparotomy, the diseased segment including the perforation must be resected. If the entire colon is diseased, near-total colectomy with ileostomy and sigmoid mucous fistula is preferable. Proctocolectomy must be avoided if at all possible. Depending on the severity of disease within the rectum, subsequent proctectomy for severe disease (including fistulas) or ileorectal anastomosis for mild to moderate proctitis may be recommended, avoiding a permanent ileostomy.

Retroperitoneal perforation of the descending colon may cause an abscess overlying the psoas muscle.[32] This may result in a confusing clinical picture of fever, positive psoas sign, and no significant worsening of gastrointestinal symptoms. Computed tomography–guided drainage of the abscess must be followed by elective colonic resection. Similarly, retroperitoneal perforation or phlegmon on the right side may cause urinary symptoms secondary to inflammatory encroachment, narrowing, or occlusion of the right ureter. Stenting the right ureter to preserve kidney function may then be followed by intense medical treatment or right hemicolectomy to remove the phlegmon. Obstruction secondary to Crohn's disease is caused by progressive impingement and narrowing of the bowel lumen by the transmural inflammation and wall thickening. Symptoms are often insidious and progressive until critical obstruction necessitates acute care treatment. Patients may be treated with nasogastric suction and intravenous fluids, and diagnosis can be made by CT scan or contrast studies. One problem might be diagnosing the acute (inflammatory) from chronic (scarring) stricture. In such cases, an indium- or technetium-labeled white blood cell scan is very helpful for differentiation. An acute inflammatory process is seen as a "hot" spots on the scan, whereas chronic strictures do not "light up."[33]

Acute inflammatory stricture unresponsive to intravenous corticosteroids and antibiotics warrants resection. The resection is limited to the diseased segment in the small bowel to preserve length, but it may encompass a large segment of the colon. Recurrence and leak rates are identical whether the margins of resection are clear or contain microscopic evidence of Crohn's disease. Chronic colonic strictures may be resected; however, small bowel strictures are best treated with a Heinke-Mikulicz–type (for short lesions) or a Finney-type (for long lesions) strictureplasty to preserve small bowel length.[34]

If during surgery internal fistulas are encountered, the diseased bowel is resected, and the opening in the adjacent hollow viscera is debrided and closed primarily. External fistulas such as colocutaneous, rectovaginal, or rectourethral and anorectal fistulas are rarely in need of acute care surgery as are most internal fistulas such as ileoileal, ileocolic, colovesical, colovaginal, and gastrocolic.

Bleeding as an indication for acute care surgery for Crohn's disease is exceedingly rare but may be seen in cases of indeterminate colitis when the anatomic and pathologic findings of ulcerative colitis and Crohn's disease coexist. Treatment for massive bleeding from Crohn's disease is analogous to that for ulcerative colitis.

Colonic Volvulus

Volvulus of the colon is a true surgical emergency that, if untreated, can result in ischemia and necrosis. Sigmoid volvulus accounts for over 80% of colonic volvulus and is commonly seen in elderly or institutionalized patients. Abdominal distension and presence of a "bent inner tube" or "coffee bean sign" on plain films of the abdomen is diagnostic (Figure 35.7). The patient should undergo acute care endoscopy and detortion of the volvulus. If detortion is successful, a chest tube should be placed in the lumen as a splint to prevent recurrence while the patient is being prepared for surgery. On the other hand, if detortion is unsuccessful or there is an endoscopic sign of mucosal ischemia, acute care surgery should be recommended. At surgery the elongated sigmoid colon is resected, and, because of the debilitated condition of most patients, a colostomy is often the safest operation. The two ends of the colon should be brought out through the same abdominal wall opening as the "end-loop stoma" advocated by Prasad and colleagues. The advantage of this type of stoma is that the patient will not have to undergo a second laparotomy for colostomy closure.[35] Cecal volvulus accounts for 15% of all volvuli and may occur as an axial torsion along the ileocolic vessel, which is rarely reduced spontaneously. However, a cecal bascule, folding over the ascending colon, may spontaneously reduce and manifest as intermittent small bowel obstruction. Cecal volvulus can be diagnosed by plane abdominal films showing a gas-filled cecum in the mid abdomen pointing toward the left upper quadrant. Also, the point of twist may be seen as a "bird's beak" during a water-soluble contrast enema study (Figure 35.8).

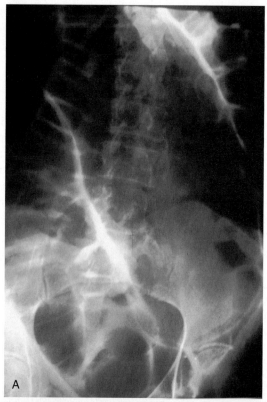

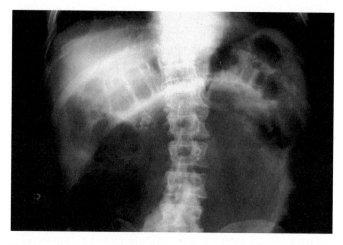

FIGURE 35.8. Plain abdominal radiograph of cecal volvulus demonstrating a large air-filled structure in the mid abdomen extending to the left upper quadrant.

If at laparotomy the cecum is viable and there is no perforation, cecopexy is associated with less complications than right hemicolectomy. Although sutured cecopexy and appendicostomy have been described, it is best to create a peritoneal flap, place it over the cecum, and suture it to the tinea, which technically returns the cecum to its retroperitoneal position.

Volvulus of the transverse colon or flexures is rare (less than 5%) and occurs mostly after the colon has previously mobilized. Diagnosis is missed because of a low index of suspicion. Volvulus of the transverse colon or flexures has a high incidence of recurrence and therefore is often treated with resection rather than fixation.[36]

Ogilvie's Syndrome

Massive colonic distention either spontaneously or associated with other medical conditions may require surgical intervention if it cannot be treated medically. Intravenous neostygmine is usually effective in contracting the colon. Epidural anesthesia has also been used successfully. If medical measures fail, colonoscopic decompression with or without placement of a splinting tube may be curative.[37] However, if decompression fails or distention recurs and the cecal diameter exceeds 10 cm, surgical intervention may be needed. Cecostomy, cecopexy, right transverse colostomy, and right hemicolectomy (when cecal integrity is in question) have all been utilized.

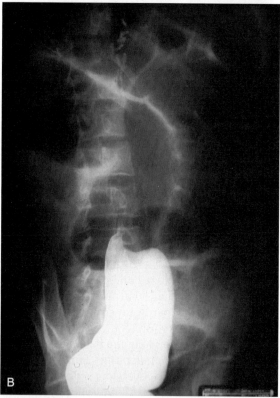

FIGURE 35.7. Plain abdominal radiographs demonstrating **(A)** the "bent inner tube" or "coffee bean" sign typical of sigmoid volvulus and **(B)** a "bird's beak" sign as revealed by contrast enema. Contrast fails to flow cephalad, and there is massive proximal colonic distention.

Ischemic Colitis

Ischemic colitis is an entity totally separate from small bowel ischemia, which is caused by occlusion of superior mesenteric artery by embolus or thrombosis. In ischemic colitis, there is usually a gradual decrease in perfusion of the colon in water shed areas until the ischemia becomes critical, leading to mucosal ulceration, paradoxical bleeding associated with diarrhea, abdominal pain, and tenderness.[38] The exception to this is ischemia caused by aortoiliac bypass, which manifests acutely within a few hours after surgery.[39] Diagnosis is often made with plain abdominal films showing "thumb printing" in the left colon just distal to the splenic flexure. A careful flexible endoscopy study with low air insufflation may demonstrate the demarcation point, and biopsy material may reveal the characteristic hemosiderin-laden macrophages.

It is rare that ischemic colitis requires acute care surgery because of excessive bleeding or perforation unless caused by careless endoscopy. In such cases, resection and proximal colostomy and Hartmann closure of the rectum is advisable because of the uncertainty as to the viability of the resection line. If a severe case of ischemic colitis responds to medical management, the sloughed cast of colonic mucosa may be replaced by fibrosis and result in colonic stricture, which may need subsequent resection for obstructive symptoms.

Colorectal Trauma

Colorectal trauma is one of the most common reasons for acute care colonic surgery in the inner city hospital. Gunshot wounds of the abdomen account for penetrating colon and rectal injuries in 25% to 30% of cases, and stab wounds are associated with a 5% injury rate. In hospitals where penetrating injuries predominate, guns shot wounds account for 70% of colonic perforations and stab wounds for 20%.[40]

Closure of colonic wounds during World War I was associated with a mortality rate of 50%, whereas routine colostomy during World War II reduced the mortality rate to 30%.[41] During the Korean and Vietnam conflicts, mortality rates dropped to 12% to 15%. Civilian penetrating injuries were treated with obligatory colostomy when there was hypotension, over 1 L hemoperitoneum, fecal contamination, major colonic injury, or abdominal wall tissue loss.[42] However, in recent years primary closure of colonic injuries was linked to the Flint colon injury score[43] and later to a penetrating abdominal trauma index (PATI) of less than 25. Using the latter criterion, 50% to 65% of colonic wounds are eligible for primary closure.[44]

A recent survey of trauma surgeons in the United States shows that there is a further trend toward primary closure of penetrating colonic injuries in civilians.[45] A systematic review of primary repairs of penetrating colonic injuries included a metaanalysis of 467 patients randomized in five trials. The PATI scores were similar for primary repair and diversion groups. The hospital stay was shorter for the primary repair group. Also, total complications, infectious complications, abdominal infections with and without dehiscence, and wound complications with and without dehiscence all favored primary repair over fecal diversion.[46]

Finally, acute care surgery may be needed for obstruction caused by impacted colorectal foreign bodies used for autoeroticism or to treat colonic perforation caused by foreign bodies used for criminal sexual assault. Obstruction of the rectum causes negative pressure, preventing easy extraction. In such cases, regional anesthesia is used to relax pelvic floor and sphincter muscles. Three or four well-lubricated Foley catheters are passed transanally above the obstructing foreign body, and air is insufflated through the catheters to break the negative pressure (suction effect). The Foley balloons are then inflated, and, using the catheters as handles, the object is extracted carefully to prevent breakage. A postextraction rigid or flexible sigmoidoscopy is essential to evaluate the extent of colonic mucosal injury and to exclude the presence of perforation. If the object cannot be extracted or if free air is seen in the abdominal films, acute care laparotomy is needed to extract the foreign body through a colotomy and/or repair the colonic perforation.[47]

Critique

With documented toxic megacolon that is refractory to medical management, the only option at this point is an abdominal colectomy with establishment of an end ileostomy and Hartmann procedure. Decompressive colonoscopy is contraindicated, and segmented resection is inadequate treatment of this potentially fatal problem.

Answer (D)

References

1. Abcarian H. Acute suppuration of anorectum. Surg Ann 1975; 8:305–333.
2. McElwain JW, MacLean MD, Alexander RM, et al. Experience with primary fistulotomy for anorectal abscess. A report of 1000 cases. Dis Colon Rectum 1975; 18:646–649.
3. Ramanujam PS, Prasad ML, Abcarian H, et al. Perianal abscesses and fistulas. A study of 1023 patients. Dis Colon Rectum 1984; 7:593–597.
4. Ramanujam PS, Prasad ML, Abcarian H. Role of setons in fistulotomy of the anus. Surg Gynecol Obstet 1983, 157:419–423.
5. Prasad ML, Abcarian H, Read DR. Supralevator abscess: diagnosis and treatment. Dis Colon Rectum 1981; 24:456–462.
6. Abcarian H, Eftaiha M. Floating free-standing anus. A complication of massive anorectal infections. Dis Colon Rectum 1983; 21:287–291.

7. Riseman JA, Zamboni WA, Curtis A, et al. Hyperbaric oxygen therapy for necrotizing fasciitis reduces mortality and the need for debridements. Surgery 1990; 108:847–850.

8. Eisenstat T, Salvati EP, Rubin RJ. The operative management of acute hemorrhoidal disease. Dis Colon Rectum 1979; 22:315–319.

9. Russell TR, Donohue JH: Hemorrhoidal banding. A warning. Dis Colon Rectum 1985; 28:291–296.

10. Quevedo-Bonilla G, Farkas AM, Abcarian H, et al. Septic complications of hemorrhoidal banding. Arch Surg 1988; 123:650–651.

11. Gorfine SR. Treatment of benign anal disease with topical nitroglycerine. Dis Colon Rectum 1995; 38:453–456.

12. Prasad ML, Pearl RK, Nelson RL, et al. Perineal proctectomy, posterior rectopexy and postanal levator repair for rectal prolapse. Dis Colon Rectum 1988; 29:547–552.

13. Prasad ML, Pearl RK, Abcarian H. End-loop colostomy. Surg Gynecol Obstet 1984; 158:1984–1986.

14. Tejero E, Fernandez-Lobato R, Mainar A, et al. Initial results of a new procedure for treatment of malignant obstruction of the left colon. Dis Colon Rectum 1997; 40:432–436.

15. Rey JF, Romanczy KT, Greff M. Metal stents for palliation of rectal carcinoma. A preliminary report on 12 patients. Endoscopy 1995; 27:501–504.

16. Brief DK, Brener BJ, Glenkranz Rl. An argument for increased use of subtotal colectomy in the management of carcinoma of the colon. Ann Surg 1983; 49:66–69.

17. Halevy A, Levi J, Orda R. Emergency subtotal colectomy. A new trend for treatment of obstructing carcinoma of the left colon. Ann Surg 1989; 210:220–224.

18. Foster ME, Johnson CD, Billings PT, et al. Intraoperative antegrade lavage and anastomotic healing in acute colonic obstruction. Dis Colon Rectum 1986; 29:255–259.

19. Thomson WHF, Carter SEC. On table lavage to achieve safe restorative rectal and emergency colonic resection without covering colostomy. 1986; 73:61–64.

20. Winzelberg GG, McKusick KA, Waltman AC, et al. Radionuclide localization of lower gastrointestinal hemorrhage. Radiology 1981; 139:465–469.

21. Forde KA. Colonoscopy in acute rectal bleeding. Gastrointest Endosc 1981; 27:219–222.

22. McDonald ML, Farnell MB, Stanson AW, et al. Preoperative highly selective catheter localization of occult small intestinal hemorrhage with methylene blue dye. Arch Surg 1995; 130:106–110.

23. Madden JL. Treatment of perforated lesions of the colon by primary resection and anastomosis. Dis Colon Rectum 1966; 9:413–416.

24. Hackford AW, Schoetz, Coller JA, et al. Surgical management of complicated diverticulitis. Dis Colon Rectum 1985; 28:317–321.

25. Eisenstat TE, Rubin RJ, Salvati EP. Surgical management of diverticulitis. The role of the Hartmann procedure. Dis Colon Rectum 1983; 26:429–432.

26. Colcock BP, Stahmann FD. Fistulas complicating diverticular disease of the sigmoid colon. Ann Surg 1972; 175:838–846.

27. Morgenstern L, Weiner R, Michael SL. "Malignant" diverticulitis: a clinical entity. Arch Surg 1979; 114:1112–1116.

28. Abcarian H, Pearl RK. A safe technique for resection of perforated sigmoid diverticulitis. Dis Colon Rectum 1990; 33:905–906.

29. Wolff BG, Ready RL, McCarty RL, et al. Effect of sigmoidal resection in progression of diverticulosis. Dis Colon Rectum 1984; 27:645–649.

30. Turnbull RB Jr, Hank WA, Weakly FL. Surgical treatment of toxic megacolon. Ileostomy and colostomy to prepare patients for colectomy. Am J Surg 1971; 122:325–331.

31. Utsunomiya J, Iwana T, Imajo M, et al. Total colectomy, mucosal proctectomy, and ileoanal anastomosis. Dis Colon Rectum 1980; 23:459–465.

32. Lee S-Y, Leonard MB, Beart RW Jr, et al. Psoas abscess: changing patterns of diagnosis and etiology. Dis Colon Rectum 1986; 26:694–698.

33. Nelson RL, Subramanian K, Gasparaitis A, et al. Indium-111 labeled granulocyte scan in the diagnosis and management of acute inflammatory bowel disease. Dis Colon Rectum 1990; 33:451–457.

34. Taschieri AM, Cristaldi M, Elli M, et al. Description of new bowel-sparing technique for long strictures of Crohn's disease. Am J Surg 1997; 173:509–512.

35. Rogers RL, Harford FJ. Mobile cecum syndrome. Dis. Colon Rectum 1984; 69:399–402.

36. Anderson JR, Lee D, Taylor TV, et al. Volvulus of transverse colon. Br J Surg 1986; 68.179–181.

37. Morrisey KP, Cahan AC. Colonoscopic decompression for nonobstructed colonic dilatation. Curr Concepts Gastroenterol 1989; 13:7–10.

38. Longo WE, Ballantyne GH, Gusberg RJ. Ischemic colitis: patterns and prognosis. Dis Colon Rectum 1992; 35:726–730.

39. Brewster DC, Franklin DP, Cambria RP, et al. Intestinal ischemia complicating abdominal aortic surgery. Surgery 1991; 109:447–454.

40. Abcarian H. Trauma to the colon and rectum In Mazier WP, Levien DH, Luchtefeld MA, Senagore AJ, eds. Surgery of the Colon, Rectum and Anus. Philadelphia: WB Saunders Company, 1995:774–777.

41. Ogilvie WH. Abdominal wounds in the western desert. Surg Gynecol Obstet 1944; 78:225–228.

42. Stone HH, Fabian TC. Management of perforating colon trauma. Randomization between primary closure and exteriorization. Ann Surg 1979; 190:430–434.

43. Flint LM, Vitale GC, Richardson JD. The injured colon: relationships of management to complications. Ann Surg 1981; 193:619–623.

44. Moore EE, Dunn EL, Moore JB, et al. Penetrating abdominal trauma index. J Trauma 1981; 21:439–445.

45. Eshraghi N, Mullins RJ, Mayberry CM, et al. Surveyed opinion of American trauma surgeons in management of colon Injuries. J Trauma 1998; 44:93–97.

46. Singer MA, Nelson RL. Primary repair of penetrating colon injuries. A systematic review. Dis Colon Rectum 2002; 45:1579–1587.

47. Abcarian H. Colorectal foreign bodies In Mazier WP, Levien DH, Luchtefeld MA, Senagore AJ, eds. Surgery of the Colon, Rectum and Anus. Philadelphia: WB Saunders Company, 1995:538–540.

36
Urogenital Tract

Nejd F. Alsikafi, Sean P. Elliott, Maurice M. Garcia, and Jack W. McAninch

Case Scenario

A 19-year-old patient is undergoing emergency exploration for a transabdominal gunshot wound. Multiple small bowel enterotomies are found along with a large zone II (perinephric) retroperitoneal hematoma. The hematoma is nonpulsatile and not expanding. The patient is hemodynamically stable. In addition to repair of the intestinal enterotomies, which of the following would be the most appropriate and immediate management step at this time?

(A) Exploration of the zone II retroperitoneal hematoma
(B) Nephrectomy without exploration of hematoma
(C) Stent placement
(D) Establishment of nephrostomy
(E) Expectant management

Infection

Emphysematous Pyelonephritis

Definition

Emphysematous pyelonephritis (EP) refers to a necrotizing parenchymal and perirenal condition that often affects diabetics and other immunocompromised patients. It is associated with poorly functioning kidneys and kidneys which are obstructed. Although the pathophysiology of EP is poorly understood, it is suspected to be caused by organisms that ferment glucose to carbon dioxide. The infection is often life threatening, with mortality rates reported near 40%,[1] and is most commonly associated with *Escherichia coli*, *Klebsiella pneumoniae*, and *Enterobacter cloacae*.

Clinical Presentation

The clinical presentation of EP is not distinct from that of other upper urinary tract infections. Fever, flank pain, and pyuria are common, though, because EP can illicit an intense inflammatory response, an elevated white count, tachycardia, low systolic blood pressures, and other hemodynamic parameters consistent with sepsis.

Diagnosis

The diagnosis is often made radiographically. The single best radiographic test is the abdominal computed tomography (CT) scan, but, although less reliably, plain abdominal radiographs or ultrasonography can also make the diagnosis.[2] Regardless of imaging modality, the characteristic signs of EP are the presence of gas in the renal and perinephric tissues with tissue destruction (Figure 36.1). At times the gas may extend into the renal pelvis and ureter (Figure 36.2).

A radiographic classification has been made regarding the CT appearance of air in patients with EP. Type I EP is characterized by parenchymal destruction with either absence of fluid collection or presence of streaky or mottled gas, whereas type II EP is characterized as either renal or perirenal fluid collections with bubbly or loculated gas or gas in the collecting system.

Management

Once it is clear clinically that the patient has an infection from a urinary tract source, appropriate broad-spectrum antibiotics should be started, urinary tract obstruction should be assessed and relieved, and prompt control of blood glucose should begin. If EP is diagnosed and fails to respond promptly to nonsurgical management, the appropriate treatment is most commonly surgical removal (radical nephrectomy), although for select cases the less aggressive approach of percuteneous nephrostomy tube placement and antibiotics has been successful.[3]

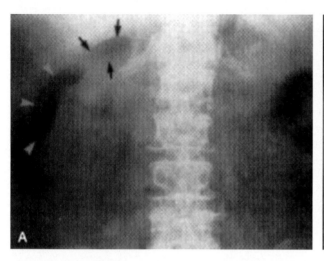 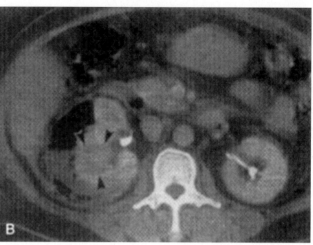

FIGURE 36.1. Emphysematous pyelonephritis. **(A)** Radiograph shows crescent-shaped (arrowheads) and loculated (arrows) gas in the right renal area. **(B)** Computed tomography image obtained after administration of contrast material shows a low-attenuation area (arrowheads) in the right kidney caused by acute pyelonephritis as well as a subcapsular abscess with fluid and bubbly and loculated gas. The patient survived after percutaneous drainage was performed. (A and B reprinted with permission from Wan et al.[5])

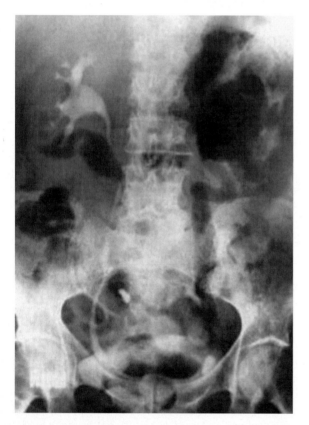

FIGURE 36.2. Emphysematous pyelonephritis. Gas in the left renal and perirenal tissues. The renal pelvis and ureter are also distended with gas. (Reprinted with permission of Elsevier from Grainger & Allison's Diagnostic Radiology: A Textbook of Medical Imaging, 4th ed. New York: Churchill Livingstone, 2001.)

Prognosis

In a recent study by Wan et al., predictors of survival in their cohort of patients with EP included platelet count, serum creatinine level, and the radiologic type of EP. Patients with a platelet count of less than 60,000, a serum creatinine level above 1.4, and radiologic type I EP were significantly more likely to die.[4,5]

Renal and Perirenal Abscess

Definition

Renal abscesses are divided into two types. One type is the renal cortical abscess, which is believed to originate from hematogenous spread of bacteria, most commonly *Staphlococcus aureus* and usually from infected skin, bone, or an endovascular prosthesis.[6] Predisposing factors for cortical abscesses are intravenous drug use and diabetes.

The second type of renal abscess is the corticomedullary abscess, which is believed to be caused by an ascending infection from the bladder. The organisms that cause these abscesses are the typical bacteria that cause lower urinary tract infections, such as *E. coli*, *K. pneumonia*, and *Proteus*. In either case, the renal abscess from the offending organism causes pyelonephritis. If the local immune response cannot adequately control the bacteria, parenchymal destruction and liquification result, leading to microabscess formation, which can coalesce to form either solitary or multiple larger renal abscesses. These abscesses can break through the capsule of the

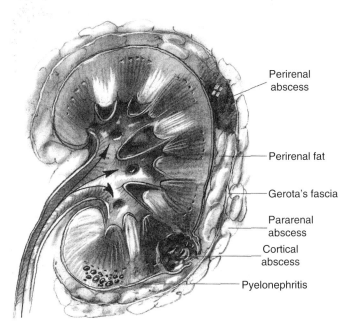

FIGURE 36.3. Anatomic renal infections. (Reprinted from McAninch JW. Genitourinary disorders. In Davis JH. Sheldon GF, eds. Surgery: A Problem Solving Approach, 2nd ed. St. Louis: Mosby, 1995, with permission from Elsevier.)

kidney and extend into perirenal tissues, forming a perirenal abscess (Figure 36.3). Although this may occur, it does so only rarely (in about 10% of renal abscesses); it is more commonly associated with underlying urinary tract abnormalities, such as calculi or obstruction, and with corticomedullary abscesses.[7]

In addition to ascending infections of the urinary tract, perirenal abscesses may be caused by dissemination of infection from other sites, including the liver, gallbladder, pancreas, pleura, prostate, and the female reproductive tract.[8] In some series perirenal abscesses are associated with a 50% mortality rate, but this is primarily because of delayed diagnosis. In a more recent series in which CT scans were used more liberally, the mortality rate from all perinephric abscesses was much less (12%) because of earlier diagnosis and treatment.[9]

Clinical Presentation

Unlike other forms of upper urinary tract infection, patients present with fever, flank pain, and leukocytosis. In small abscesses, localized physical findings are minimal, but in larger abscesses a palpable mass may be detected. Systemic symptoms include lethargy, loss of appetite, and chills associated with fever spikes.

Diagnosis

Urinalysis demonstrates white blood cells 75% of the time, whereas urine cultures identify the causative organism in only a third of cases.[10] Blood cultures, which have

been shown to have a higher correlation with the offending organism, should also be drawn.[11]

The most effective diagnostic study is the renal CT, which shows the most anatomic detail of the kidney and its surrounding organs and can detect abscesses less than 2 cm in size.[12] Classically the abscess appears as a circumscribed region of low attenuation soft tissue surrounded by an inflammatory wall, which appears as a contrast-enhancing rim ("ring sign"). The CT scan also may demonstrate thickening of Gerota's fascia, stranding of perinephric fat, or obliteration of the surrounding soft tissue planes (Figure 36.4).[13]

Ultrasound may also be used, and as it is useful in differentiating an intrarenal lesion as cystic, suppurative, or solid, and it can provide information about renal morphology. Additionally ultrasonography can provide information about the presence of an obstructive uropathy, retroperitoneal or intraabdominal processes, and suppurative renal complications.[14] However, for perirenal abscesses, in one study ultrasound was falsely negative in 36% of cases compared with CT.[15]

Management

Once the diagnosis is established, prompt appropriate intravenous antibiotics should be initiated tailored to blood and urine culture results. For cortical renal abscesses, antistaphylococcal intravenous antibiotics

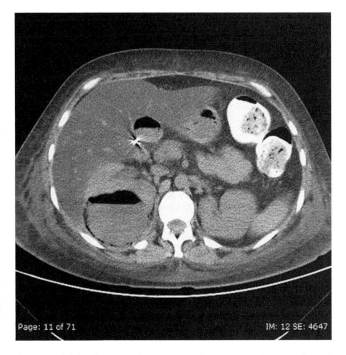

FIGURE 36.4. Computed tomography scan of a perirenal abscess. Notice the air and fluid collection around the right kidney. (Reprinted with permission from Rauschkolb EN, Sandler CM, Patel S, et al. Computed tomography of renal inflammatory disease. J Comput Assist Tomogr 1982; 6:502.)

should be started. Typically the clinical course for these abscesses is that flank pain resolves shortly after the antibiotics are started with a gradual and progressive decrease in fever spikes over the next 5 to 7 days. By 1 week, the fevers should abate. Appropriate oral antibiotics may be started once fevers no longer exist and should be continued for a total of 3 to 4 weeks.

For corticomedullary abscesses, because isolation of the offending organism early in the clinical course may be difficult, broad-spectrum antibiotics are recommended initially (e.g., ampicillin and gentamicin), and more selective intravenous antibiotics should commence once more specific identification is made. For abscesses smaller than 5 cm, percutaneous drainage of the abscess is recommended if the patient shows no improvement after 48 hours of antibiotics. For abscesses larger than 5 cm, percutaneous drainage or open surgical drainage is recommended, as antibiotics alone are often ineffective with abscesses this large. Open surgical drainage is often reserved for patients who have failed percutaneous drainage and antibiotics and for patients with multifocal abscesses, obstructive uropathy, advanced age, or immunocompromised state.[16]

For perirenal abscesses, drainage of the infection is the mainstay of treatment. In addition to antibiotics, percutaneous drainage or open surgical drainage is necessary as antibiotics alone are insufficient.

Pyonephrosis

Definition

Pyonephrosis refers to a condition in which complete or partial upper urinary tract obstruction leads to hydronephrosis that becomes infected. This infected hydronephrosis can result in systemic sepsis and lead to the destruction of renal parenchyma. Timely diagnosis and treatment of pyonephrosis is necessary to avoid irreversible renal damage and clinical deterioration.

The urinary obstruction can be caused by various etiologies, including an obstructing kidney or ureteral stone, a complete or partial ureteropelvic junction obstruction, a ureteral stricture, or other causes.

Clinical Presentation

Patients with pyonephrosis are often persistently febrile, complain of flank pain with or without nausea and vomiting, and appear ill. They often have a markedly elevated white blood cell count and can present in various physiologic stages of sepsis.

Diagnosis

The diagnosis of pyonephrosis is often made by the clinical presentation coupled with a urinalysis strongly posi-

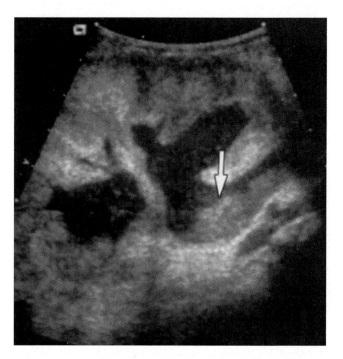

FIGURE 36.5. Sonogram of pyonephrosis. The collecting system is dilated. The calyces are clubbed, and there are numerous echoes in the dependent portion of the pelvis. In view of the clinical findings, this is consistent with pyonephrosis. Kidney; Liver. (Reprinted from Brenner BM. Brenner & Rector's The Kidney, 6th ed. Philadelphia: WB Saunders, 2000, with permission from Elsevier.)

tive for pyuria and bacteriuria. However, if upper urinary tract obstruction is complete, the urinalysis maybe negative for signs of infection or inflammation.

Radiographically, CT and ultrasonography are perhaps the most commonly used modalities because of their high sensitivity to detect hydronephrosis. A CT scan typically shows hydronephrosis with or without dilation of the ureter, depending on the source of obstruction, and signs of inflammation or infection of the renal parenchyma and perirenal tissues. On ultrasound, several patterns are consistent with pyonephrosis: (1) persistent echoes from the inferior portion of the collecting system, (2) a fluid-debris level with dependent echoes that shift when the patient changes position, (3) strong echoes with acoustic shadowing from air in the collecting system, or (4) weak echoes throughout a dilated collecting system (Figure 36.5).[17]

Management

The mainstay of treatment of pyonephrosis is relief of the obstruction, which can often be done adequately by placement of a ureteral stent concomitantly with a urethral catheter, and the administration of appropriate broad-spectrum antibiotics. If the clinical status of the patient does not adequately improve, a percutaneous nephrostomy tube should be considered.

Prostatic Abscess

Definition

Most cases of prostate abscess occur as sequelae to previously inadequately treated acute bacterial prostatitis. Often, such patients report prior treatment for acute bacterial prostatitis, with recurrence of symptoms during or soon after treatment despite initial response to antibiotics. The pattern suggests development of an abscess, as the infection becomes effectively impervious to circulating antibiotics and provides a persistent source of infection and discomfort. Prostate abscesses are often seen in patients with chronic indwelling catheters and in immunocompromised patients: diabetics and patients on hemodialysis. The incidence of opportunistic infections in the prostate gland is well reported among patients who are human immunodeficiency virus 1 (HIV-1) seropositive.[18]

Clinical Presentation

Patients present similar to those with acute bacterial prostatitis, with constitutional symptoms (fever, chills, malaise, arthralgia, and perineal, suprapubic, lower-back, and/or rectal pain) and urinary symptoms (frequency, urgency, and/or dysuria and sometimes with urinary retention caused by swelling of the prostate).[19] Patients may also complain of associated discomfort to the external genitalia. Urinalysis is often notable for presence of white blood cells and occasionally hematuria. Serum leukocytosis can also be present. Digital rectal examination often reveals a tender, swollen gland, but fluctuance is seen in only 16% of patients with prostate abscess.[20]

Diagnosis

Imaging with CT scan or transrectal ultrasound is essential for both diagnosis and treatment.

Management

Prostatic abscesses require drainage in conjunction with antibiotic therapy. Computed tomography imaging or transrectal ultrasound can be used to direct transrectal or transurethral endoscopic drainage.[21] Although transurethral incision and drainage of the abscess is optimal when adequate radiographic guidance is available, transperineal drainage must be considered when the abscess has extended beyond the prostatic capsule or through the levator ani muscle.[22,23] Bacterial prostatitis requires an extended course (minimum 6 weeks) of antibiotic therapy. The antibiotic chosen must have a high degree of prostatic tissue penetrance. Fungal prostatitis

is often treated with a two-agent regimen (amphotericin and flucytosine), with long-term oral fluconazole therapy for persistent or recurrent infections.[16,24] With proper diagnosis and treatment, most cases resolve without significant sequelae.[18]

Acute Prostatitis

Definition

Bacterial infection of the prostate gland can be divided into two categories: acute bacterial prostatitis and chronic bacterial prostatitis. Prostatitis is the most common urologic diagnosis in men younger than 50 years and the third most common urologic diagnosis in men older than age 50 years.

Acute bacterial prostatitis is inflammation of the prostate gland in association with urinary tract infection and, occasionally, generalized sepsis. It is believed that acute bacterial prostatitis is the result of either infected urine refluxing from the bladder into the prostatic ducts or from ascending urethral infection.[25] Edema and hyperemia of the prostate subsequently develop. Chronic prostatitis is rarely associated with fever and is more commonly seen with recurrent urinary tract infections.

The most common cause of bacterial prostatitis is the Enterobacteriaceae family of Gram-negative bacteria, which originate in gastrointestinal flora. *Escherichia coli* is identified in 65% to 80% of infections, and *Serratia, Pseudomonas, Klebsiella,* and *Enterobacter* species account for 10% to 15% of cases.[26] Gram-positive *Enterococcus* species account for 5% to 10% of cases.

Clinical Presentation

Patients usually present with abrupt onset of constitutional symptoms (fever, chills, malaise, perineal/lowerback/rectal pain, arthralgias) and urinary symptoms (frequency, dysuria, urgency, and occasionally urinary retention).[27] Digital rectal examination reveals a tender, swollen gland that is often warm and irregular in shape.

Diagnosis

Serum leukocytosis, pyuria, and hematuria are found in patients with acute prostatitis. Although some advocate microscopic analysis and culture of expressed prostatic secretion (EPS) and a urine sample taken both before and after prostatic massage for a definitive diagnosis, we advocate not performing prostatic massage or urethral catheterization in early-stage acute prostatitis, as there is a risk of seeding bacteria with massage, and the gland can be extremely tender early in the course of infection.

Radiologic imaging is rarely indicated for acute bacterial prostatitis. Select uses include bladder ultrasonography to evaluate for urinary retention and transrectal ultrasound for evaluation of patients who do not respond to conventional therapy.

Treatment

Upon diagnosis, empiric antimicrobial therapy directed at Gram-negative bacteria and enterococci should be initiated immediately and continued until culture results are available. The goal of treatment is thorough and complete eradication of infection within the prostatic tissue so as to prevent progression to chronic prostatitis or prostatic abscess.[28,29] The treatment duration is generally 4 to 6 weeks, utilizing antibiotics with high absorption and penetration into prostate tissue, such as trimethoprim and fluoroquinolones.[30] Patients who show signs of sepsis, have significant comorbidities, are immunocompromised, or are in acute urinary retention are likely best managed with hospitalization and parenteral antibiotics. Acute urinary retention should be managed with suprapubic catheterization, as transurethral catheterization is contraindicated.

Infected Urinary and Genital Prosthetics

Definition

Infection associated with penile prostheses and artificial urinary sphincters is fortunately rare. For both, in reoperative situations and with complex implant situations, the infection rate is slightly higher. Risk of infection can be divided into two categories: perioperative risk, generally manifested as early infection; and postoperative risk, which presents as late infection. In a recently published series, most infections, 56%, occurred within 7 months of implantation, 36% between 7 and 12 months, and only 2.5% after 5 years.[31]

Early infection is more common, and most infections are caused by bacterial seeding at the time of surgery. Diabetes increases the risk of infection by two to three times[32,33] and is well known for increasing the risk of infection by two separate mechanisms: inhibiting the body's natural immune response by inhibiting white blood cell function and damaging small blood vessels, which hampers local wound healing. Additionally, patients with spinal cord injury and chronic steroid use have high rates of infection, ranging from 9% to 30% and 50%, respectively.[34,35] The presence of a foreign body alone causes the amount of bacteria necessary to produce a wound infection to decrease 100-fold.[36]

Clinical Presentation

Infections of penile prostheses and artificial urinary sphincters present with one of two categories of symptoms: subclinical or clinical. The more common of the two types, subclinical infection tend to present only with chronic prosthesis-associated pain and without symptoms of frank infection. These indolent infections account for 80% of prosthesis-associated infections and are more commonly associated with Gram-positive bacteria (S. aureus or S. epidermidis) and usually present on average at 5.75 months after implantation. Staphylococcus epidermidis is the single most common organism found in infected prosthetics and is found in 80% of all reported cases.[23]

Clinical infection, by contrast, manifests with more classic symptoms: fever, erythema, induration overlying the prosthesis, penile pain, and, often, extrusion of the device. These infections account for 20% of infections, usually manifest within 1 month of implantation, and tend to be caused by Gram-negative bacteria, such as Proteus mirabilis, Pseudomonas aeruginosa, E. coli, and Serratia marcescens.[37]

Pain caused by infection of an implanted artificial urinary sphincter is usually localized to the region of the scrotal pump. Infection can also cause the cuff to erode into adjacent tissues, including the urethra. Presenting symptoms include pain and swelling localized to the perineum and scrotum, pain referred to the tip of the penis, recurrent incontinence, and even bloody discharge. Erosion can be confirmed with cystoscopy. When very early, however, erosion of the cuff can also be caused by unrecognized iatrogenic urethral injury or unrecognized anterior urethral thinning at the time of operation. Cuff erosion not associated with infection can occur at any time, but it is most commonly seen at 3 to 4 months after implantation and necessitates removal of the cuff.

Diagnosis

The diagnosis of infection is mainly based on clinical suspicion, as no single radiologic modality has proved reliable in determining most prosthetic infections. For patients without a clear medical history, perineal, scrotal, or inguinal scars or a palpable device within the scrotum can suggest the presence of a prosthesis.

Treatment

In all cases, suspected infection or malfunction of a penile prosthesis or artificial urinary sphincter should prompt urologic consultation. When infection is suspected, broad-spectrum antibiotics should be instituted immediately, and manipulation of prosthetic hardware should be avoided. When the presence of an artificial urinary sphincter is confirmed or suspected, urethral catheterization should never be attempted unless the mechanism has been examined and one is sure that the cuff is deflated. If possible, all catheterization should be deferred to a consulting urologist, who may elect to first evaluate the urethra endoscopically.

When infection of a penile prosthesis is confirmed, surgeons may remove the prosthesis immediately with plans for possible reinsertion 2 to 6 months later or may perform a "salvage procedure" wherein all prosthetic materials are removed, the wound is systematically cleansed with a series of different antiseptic solutions, and a new prosthesis is placed in the surgical site within the same surgical procedure.

Necrotizing Gangrene of the Genitalia and Perineum

Background

Necrotizing soft tissue infections of the genitalia and perineum constitute a urologic emergency, are potentially life threatening, can progress rapidly, and can cause significant morbidity and mortality. Such infections present diagnostic and therapeutic challenges that are best served with an aggressive multidisciplinary teamwork, implementing the expertise of the urologist, reconstructive surgeon, and either general or colon/rectal surgeon as an operative team.

The most frequent sources of necrotizing genital gangrene fall into three categories: anorectal infections, genitourinary infections, and cutaneous injuries (Table 36.1).[38] Among gastrointestinal causes (30% to 50%), perianal, intrasphincteric, and ischiorectal abscesses account for approximately 70%.[32] Necrotizing gangrene has also been associated with minor anorectal procedures such as anal dilation and rectal mucosal biopsy.[39,40] Genitourinary foci of infection account for the second major source of infection (20% to 40%). Underlying urethral

TABLE 36.1. Fournier's gangrene: associated etiologic factors.

Gastrointestinal (50%–70%)
  Anorectal (perianal, intrasphincteric, ischiorectal) abscesses
  Appendicitis
  Carcinoma: sigmoid and rectum
  Herniorraphy
  Hemorroidectomy/rectal mucosal biopsy
  Diverticulitis

Genitourinary (20%–40%)
  Urethral stricture
  Urethral trauma/instrumentation
  Urinary extravasation
  Prostate biopsy/massage
  Indwelling urethral catheter

Cutaneous (20%)
  Skin lesion, bite
  Injection
  Circumcision
  Balanoposthitis
  Penile prosthesis
  Vasectomy

stricture and periurethral infection are the most common causes. Other associated urologic conditions include trauma to the urethra (instrumentation, urethral calculi, indwelling urethral catheters), prostate biopsy/massage, and epididymitis. Cutaneous injuries and infection account for 20% of cases.[32] The dermal source is often minor, such as from insect or human bites. Trauma to superficial soft tissues is another important etiology.

Necrotizing gangrene is more common in men (ratio 10:1). A common etiology in women is abscess of the vulva or Bartholin's gland, which initiates gangrene of the perineum.

Increased prevalence of comorbidities such as diabetes (30% to 60%) and alcoholism (40% to 50%) have been reported.[41,42] It is possible that decreased defense systems and susceptibility to infection from an impaired active immune system contribute to the increased incidence. However, outcomes have not correlated with the presence or absence of the comorbid states.[35,36]

Fulminant infection of the genital and perineal soft tissues spreads along initially subcutaneous, then fascial, planes in a pattern explained by the fascial anatomy of the perineum. Thrombosis of subcutaneous vessels and necrosis of superficial fascia are appreciable histologically.[43] Except in clostridial infections, myonecrosis is rarely encountered.[44] After 4 to 5 days, gangrene is evident as tissue necrosis spreads, normal flora invades the perifascial plane, bacterial overgrowth and synergy ensues, oxygen tension decreases, and at 8 to 10 days necrotic tissue separates by suppuration from underlying ischemic but viable tissue.

Bacteriologic studies reveal that the infections are polymicrobial, with a mean of two to four organisms isolated per patient.[36,45] The organisms most commonly isolated include *Bacteroides*, coliforms, *Streptococcus*, *Staphylococcus*, and *Peptostreptococcus*. Anaerobes, although less frequently isolated, are invariably present.[36,46] Bacterial metabolism may also produce insoluble gases, resulting in subcutaneous emphysema. Bacterial synergy in conjunction with host factors appears to account for the degree of pathogenicity of such low to moderate organisms.[47]

Clinical Presentation

Most cases begin insidiously, with scrotal discomfort and malaise, with the progressive development of fever, chills, and scrotal skin changes (swelling, erythema). However, because the skin can appear relatively normal during the first days, presentation is often delayed (an average 5 days).[48] Pressure necrosis of cutaneous nerves may also cause decreased pain. Signs and symptoms at presentation include pain (100%), swelling (60% to 80%), fever (70%), and crepitus (60% to 70%). Possible systemic manifestations such as toxic shock and altered mental status must be recognized early. A careful history can often elucidate the etiology.

Because of its nonspecific symptoms, indolent course, and often unremarkable cutaneous appearance, necrotizing gangrene of the perineum can often be mistaken for scrotal cellulitis and balanoposthitis.[49] Other conditions that mimic Fournier's gangrene include scrotal abscess and incarcerated hernia.[50] In the later, fulminant phases of the clinical course, the infection may advance rapidly along fascial planes (up to 1 inch/hr), with woody induration of affected tissues, crepitus, and purulent discharge.[51]

Diagnosis

Although necrotizing gangrene of the genitalia and perineum remains a clinical diagnosis, various imaging modalities including plain film radiography, ultrasonography, CT, and magnetic resonance imaging (MRI) are useful in confirming the diagnosis, evaluating the extent of disease, and determining the etiology.[52] Plain films can demonstrate subcutaneous air before crepitus is palpable and, according to one retrospective review, are more sensitive in detection than physical examination.[53] Ultrasound is also quite useful in detecting the presence of subcutaneous gas when not clinically evident. The ultrasonographic appearance is striking: air appears as discrete bright hyperechoic areas with posterior acoustic shadowing. A CT can suggest the extent of the gangrene by delineating thickened soft tissues with surrounding fat stranding and gas dissecting along fascial planes. In addition, the excellent anatomic detail afforded is helpful to diagnose the initial source of infection. Magnetic resonance imaging affords similar advantages, with improved soft tissue resolution.

Laboratory findings are often nonspecific and include leukocytosis (>15,000/μL in 80% of patients), anemia, hypocalcemia (caused by chelation of calcium by bacterial lipases), coagulopathy, hyperglycemia, and hyponatremia.[54]

Treatment

After diagnosis, initial management is aimed at preparation for surgery. Medical therapy has only a limited role. Urologic and/or general surgical consultation is mandatory and should precede any laboratory or imaging results. As sepsis may be present, hemodynamic stabilization and the need for transfusion, invasive monitoring, and ventilatory support should be addressed. Empiric, broad-spectrum antibiotic therapy should be instituted immediately. Typical regimens include ampicillin for streptococci, clostridia, and certain anaerobes; gentamicin for Gram-negative rods; and clindamycin for *Bacteroides* and other anaerobes. Semisynthetic penicillins and third-generation cephalosporins are newer alternatives to aminoglycosides.

Uncertainty in diagnosis should not delay surgical debridement. Examination under anesthesia is easily performed. Operative management consists of complete debridement of all areas with overt necrosis. Incision and drainage of necrotic areas are wholly insufficient, and outcomes are correlated with extent of initial debridement.[55] As skin changes can lead to underestimation of the degree of underlying tissue damage, extensive unroofing of involved areas is necessary. Subsequent procedures are likely to be necessary, and reports have documented a mean of two to four procedures per patient.[56,57]

Other important issues include evaluation of caloric balance and optimal nutritional support. Routine wound care with either saline of Dakin's soaked dressings is important after debridement. Given the common presence of anaerobes in necrotizing infections, hyperbaric oxygen has been used as an adjunctive therapy.[58,59] Clinical evidence supporting its utility is inconclusive.[60]

Prognosis

Reported mortality rates range from 0% to 80%.[31,34] One review of 449 cases yielded an overall mortality rate of 22%.[36] Average hospitalization was 40 days. Early diagnosis, complete debridement of all necrotic tissue, and a surgical multidisciplinary approach are essential for improved outcomes.

Hemorrhage

In urology, there are few conditions that can result in acute life-threatening hemorrhage. These include acute and heavy bleeding from a renal angiomyolipoma and arteriovenous malformation of the kidney.

Angiomyolipoma of the Kidney

Definition

Angiomyolipoma (AML) is a benign mass of the kidney, often associated with tuberous sclerosis syndrome, a neurofibromatosis condition diagnosed with the classic clinical triad of mental retardation, adenoma sebacium, and epilepsy. Although penetrance of these conditions is variable in people with tuberous sclerosis syndrome (TSS), approximately 50% of all people with TSS have AML. Pathologically, as its name implies, AMLs are composed of varying amounts of mature blood vessels, smooth muscle, and fat.

Angiomyolipomas are universally benign masses of the kidney except in rare circumstances, when they can be associated with renal cell carcinoma. In most patients, AMLs are asymptomatic and are stable in size; however, in approximately 10% of patients AMLs can become pro-

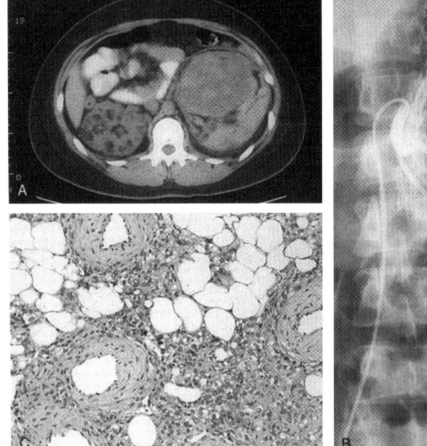

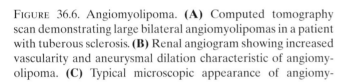

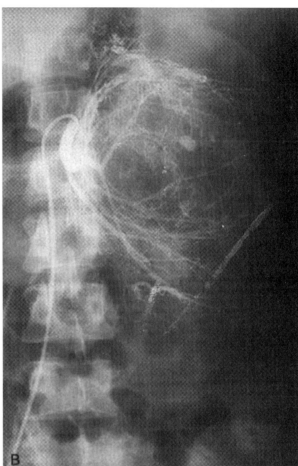

FIGURE 36.6. Angiomyolipoma. **(A)** Computed tomography scan demonstrating large bilateral angiomyolipomas in a patient with tuberous sclerosis. **(B)** Renal angiogram showing increased vascularity and aneurysmal dilation characteristic of angiomyolipoma. **(C)** Typical microscopic appearance of angiomyolipoma with admixture of mature adipose tissue, smooth muscle, and thick-walled blood vessels. (Reprinted from Novick AC, Campbell SC, Renal Tumors. In Walsh PC, Retik AB, Vaughan ED, Wein AJ, eds. Campbell's Urology, 8th ed. Philadelphia: WB Saunders, 2002: 2682, with permission from Elsevier.)

gressively larger and rupture, leading in spontaneous retroperitoneal hemorrhage.[61] Pregnancy appears to increase the risk of hemorrhage from AML.

Clinical Presentation

Typically AMLs are asymptomatic, but they can lead to spontaneous hemorrhage with the common signs or symptoms of flank pain, hematuria, palpable mass, and hypovolemic shock, which can be fatal if not identified and promptly treated.[62,63] Other more subtle presentations of AML include anemia and hypertension.

Diagnosis

Abdominal CT scan has been the most reliable diagnostic imaging modality for AML.[64] The hallmark sign for AML on CT is the presence of fat (confirmed by Hounsfield units ≤10), regardless of amount. The presence of any fat virtually excludes the diagnosis of other renal masses, including renal cell carcinoma, and is considered 100% diagnostic of AML (Figure 36.6).[65] Ultrasonography may also be used, but less reliably. The typical appearance is a well-circumscribed, highly echogenic lesion, often associated with shadowing (renal cell carcinoma rarely shadows).[66] Finally, fat-suppressed images on MRI may be helpful in difficult cases or when CT is contraindicated for other reasons.

Management

In the nonacute setting, management of AML is based on the size of the lesion and on the concomitant risk of hemorrhage. For lesions <4 cm, annual imaging studies (CT or ultrasound) of the lesion is recommended to assess for interval growth. For asymptomatic patients with lesions >4 cm, semiannual imaging versus prophylactic angioablation is recommended (taking into consideration patient age, comorbidities, and other related factors), while for symptomatic patients (bleeding or pain) renal angiography with angioembolization of the AML is the preferred modality. Open nephron-sparing surgery can also be performed for patients who do not respond to angioembolization.

In the acute setting, most patients with acute or potentially life-threatening hemorrhage will require total nephrectomy if explored. If a patient has tuberous sclerosis, bilateral disease, preexisting renal insufficiency, or other medical or urologic disease that could affect future renal function, selective embolization should be considered.[67] In such circumstances, selective embolization can temporize and, in many cases, prove definitive.

Arteriovenous Malformation of Kidney

Definition

An arteriovenous malformation (AVM) of the kidney is a fistula between the arterial and venous systems of the kidney. They are associated with previous injury to the kidney and can be seen in patients with previous renal trauma, percutaneous needle renal biopsies, nephrostomy tube placements, or, rarely, cases of renal cell carcinoma. They have also been recognized in patients with a prior nephrectomy where the renal pedicle in its entirety has been ligated together. In 25% of patients, the AVMs are congenital.

Clinical Presentation

Patients with small renal AVMs are asymptomatic. As the AVMs increase in size, the likelihood for rupture and clinical symptoms increases. Renal AVMs may be the source of microscopic or gross hematuria. Arteriovenous malformations with wide communication may be hemodynamically significant, resulting in a palpable abdominal thrill and murmur, a wide pulse pressures, and an elevated systolic blood pressure. In rare circumstances, AVMs may spontaneously rupture, resulting in a retroperitoneal bleed, with classic signs and symptoms of acute hemorrhage.

Diagnosis

Renal angiography is the single best diagnostic modality for significant AVMs. Computed tomography, ultrasonography, and recently duplex ultrasound with color flow have been helpful in making the diagnosis. If hematuria is a significant sign, cystoscopy is essential in excluding concomitant sources of hematuria from the lower urinary tract.

Management

Small asymptomatic AVMs rarely need treatment as they heal spontaneously. More significant AVMs, which can be visualized angiographically, are reliably treated with renal angioembolization. Those communicating from the main renal artery and vein must be repaired operatively.

Acute Urinary Tract Obstruction

As in the biliary system or the gastrointestinal tract, urinary obstruction results in colicky pain, nausea, and vomiting. These symptoms should prompt one to consider imaging and drainage.

Upper Tract Obstruction

Definition

The most common cause of upper urinary tract obstruction is renal or ureteral urinary lithiasis. Other causes include intraluminal tumor, stricture, extrinsic compression, urothelial polyp, blood clot, and fungal ball. This discussion focuses on renal and ureteral stones; however, many of the principles discussed also apply to other causes of upper urinary tract obstruction.

Clinical Presentation

Essential elements of the history specific to a patient with flank pain include fever, character of pain, nausea, vomiting, chills, and history of kidney stones, urologic surgery, pyelonephritis, diabetes, or other immunodeficiency and medications. The abdomen should be assessed for costovertebral angle tenderness; if present, pyelonephritis should be considered. Without flank tenderness, urinary tract obstruction is more likely the cause of flank pain. The kidneys should be palpated for the presence of a mass. Other abdominal pathology should be ruled out.

Diagnosis

A urinalysis will show microscopic or gross hematuria in >90% of cases of urinary lithiasis. The presence or absence of hematuria does not correlate with the degree of hydronephrosis or with stone size.[68] In the case of pyelonephritis the urinalysis may show bacteria, pyuria, or hematuria; however, exceptions include complete ureteral obstruction or hematogenous rather than urinary source of infection, in which cases lower tract urinalysis will not correlate with upper tract pathology. A urine culture is important in tailoring antibiotic therapy in the case of urinary obstruction; however, one should not wait for urinary culture results to confirm infection before proceeding with drainage of pyonephrosis (obstructed pyelonephritis with purulent upper tract urine). Pyonephrosis requires urgent drainage, as it can lead to severe urosepsis. Broad-spectrum antibiotics should be given before instrumentation.

The serum creatinine level should be measured. In the case of unilateral urinary tract obstruction and a normal contralateral kidney, the serum creatinine level should be unchanged from baseline. A rise in renin secretion from the obstructed kidney will lead to an increased glomerular filtration rate in the unobstructed kidney. Total urine output as well as excretion of metabolic byproducts such as creatinine will be maintained. However, if the baseline renal function is compromised, or in the case of bilateral obstruction or obstruction of a solitary kidney, urinary output will drop and serum creatinine level will rise.[69]

The preferred radiologic method for evaluation of flank pain is a three-phase CT scan—noncontrast, contrast, and delayed images. Noncontrast images allow identification of urinary tract stones. Degree of hydronephrosis can also be assessed on noncontrast images, but this is easier with contrast and delayed images. Contrast images will demonstrate pyelonephritis, renal abscess, and renal mass. Delayed images allow one to follow the course of the ureter down to the bladder: this is rather difficult distally without contrast in the ureter. On contrast and delayed images, one can also estimate the relative function of the kidneys. Reduced enhancement of the renal parenchyma and delayed contrast excretion are consistent with reduced renal function. This can be chronic or acute and can be secondary to obstruction.

Ultrasound and plain film radiography (kidney, ureter, bladder [KUB] x-ray) have limited efficacy in the evaluation of upper urinary tract obstruction or flank pain in the modern CT era.[70] Ultrasound can identify renal masses and abscesses, but it has a high false-negative rate in the diagnosis of acute upper tract obstruction.[71] Furthermore, ultrasound may not visualize the ureter well, and, therefore, although it may show hydronephrosis, it may not show the cause. Likewise, although KUB is a reasonable study for the evaluation of urinary tract stones, it cannot demonstrate hydronephrosis or identify noncalcareous sources of urinary obstruction. Furthermore, it can be difficult to differentiate between urinary stones, fecoliths, and phleboliths on KUB. Computed tomography is the ideal examination for assessment of flank pain. Intravenous plain-film pyelography (IVP) is a reasonable alternative if CT is not available, but it is less sensitive than CT.[72] The combination of ultrasound and KUB is an alternative for the patient with reduced renal function; however, even in this case a noncontrast CT scan would provide more information.

Management

Management should be tailored to the degree of obstruction and the acuity of the situation. In the case of obstruction from a ureteral calculus, the size and location of the stone will also affect management.

TABLE 36.2. Rates of spontaneous stone passage.

Stone location	Stone size (mm)			
	<3	3–4	4–6	>6
Lower ureter	90.8%	53.4%	25.3%	1.7%
Mid ureter	44.4%	26.1%	11.7%	0.8%
Upper ureter	24.3%	14.3%	6.7%	0.4%

Rates of stone passage after 6 weeks are listed and grouped by stone size and location in the ureter at the time of diagnosis.
Source: Reprinted with permission from Hubner et al.[73]

The degree of obstruction can be ascertained from the severity of hydronephrosis and any delay of contrast excretion. An assessment of the clinical acuity includes the presence of fever or sepsis, refractory pain, nausea, or vomiting. Urinary infection behind an obstruction is a urologic emergency. Antibiotics should be administered immediately, and drainage should be accomplished promptly. Pain, nausea, or vomiting that persists after medical therapy should prompt admission for intravenous analgesia, antiemetics, and hydration. If symptoms do not improve shortly, then one should proceed with drainage. In the case of a ureteral calculus, the size of the stone is indirectly proportional to its likelihood of passing. Additionally, the more distal the stone, the more likely it is to pass[73,74] (Table 36.2). It is reasonable to try a course of expectant management for the small distal ureteral stone when pain is well managed and nausea does not preclude adequate oral hydration. Any compromise of renal function from complete unilateral ureteral obstruction will be completely reversible if relieved within 2 weeks. Partial recovery can be expected if obstruction is relieved in 2 to 6 weeks. After 6 weeks, studies suggest renal damage is permanent.[69]

Ideally, obstructing ureteral stones are removed with ureteroscopic lithotripsy at the time of diagnosis. However, when the stone is too large or too proximal or the patient is ill, it is wise to proceed with drainage and forego stone removal until a later date. The drainage procedure of choice should be cystoscopy with placement of an internalized double J ureteral stent. This procedure is done under general anesthesia and has the advantage of being a completely internal drainage system. In contrast, a percutaneous nephrostomy tube can be placed under local anesthesia; however, the patient must learn to care for the external catheter, which can be uncomfortable. There is great debate about which method is safer for the unstable patient with an infected stone and hydronephrosis, as both multiple renal punctures and retrograde injection of contrast can precipitate sepsis.[75–76] On balance, an internal stent should remain the procedure of choice unless the stone appears to be too impacted to permit easy passage of a guidewire. In such cases, the degree of hydronephrosis is often significant, making percutaneous nephrostomy easier.

Prognosis

The prognosis for upper urinary tract obstruction depends on the etiology. In cases of advanced malignancy there may be little chance of reversing the obstruction, only relieving the symptoms of obstruction by drainage with a stent or a nephrostomy tube. In the case of both renal and ureteral stones, there is an excellent chance of removing the cause of obstruction. Utilizing advances in technology such as extracorporeal shock wave lithotripsy and endoscopic therapies, urinary stones can be removed with more than 90% success; however, recurrent stone formation is common.[77–78] The 5-year recurrence rate for all patients with stones is approximately 60% if no medical therapy is given. Diagnostic metabolic evaluation followed by medical and/or dietary intervention can decrease the 5-year recurrence rate to 30%.[79]

Lower Tract Obstruction

Definition

Lower tract obstruction is the blockage of urine anywhere in the outflow tract—from the bladder neck to the urethral meatus. Lower urinary tract obstruction in men is most commonly from benign prostatic hyperplasia (BPH). Other common etiologies include hematuria with clot retention, acute prostatitis (see earlier section), and urethral stricture. Boys, especially newborns, with lower urinary tract obstruction should be evaluated for posterior urethral valves (see later section). Urethral obstruction is rare in women, as the short urethra allows easier passage of obstructing clots and urethral stricture is rare.

Presentation

Although BPH is a chronic disease that leads to progressive obstruction of urinary flow, in its early stages bladder hypertrophy may maintain urinary flow. In some cases the patient may not present to a physician until the bladder decompensates and urinary flow becomes more difficult or stops. The patient will describe a weak urinary stream followed by an inability to void. In some cases there may be overflow incontinence, or the patient may have small frequent voids that do not sufficiently empty the bladder. The patient may complain of suprapubic pain. In the case of hematuria with urine and clot retention, the urine will progress from clear to pink, then red, and finally thick red with clots. The patient may give no history to suggest BPH. Instead, outflow obstruction will occur acutely as clots accumulate in the bladder. In the man complaining of acute onset of dysuria and obstructive symptoms in the absence of significant hematuria, acute prostatitis is a possible etiology. Fever may or may not be present. If the patient describes a history of ure-

thral instrumentation or perineal trauma, the physician must suspect a urethral stricture.

Evaluation

The patient should be questioned as to the acuity of the urinary problems, the degree of hematuria, any history of urinary tract trauma, and the presence or absence of fever. A thorough history of voiding symptoms should include an assessment of the degree of frequency, urgency, hesitancy, nocturia, dysuria, and intermittency of the urinary stream over both the previous 24 hours and the previous year. The bladder may be palpable as high as the umbilicus and is typically tender. Visual inspection of the patient's voided urine for the degree of gross hematuria if present should be followed by laboratory urinalysis and culture. An examination of the genitalia should be done to rule out meatal stenosis or any evidence of prior trauma. A rectal examination should be performed with attention to the size, consistency, and tenderness of the prostate. The normal prostate should be 15 to 20 cc in size and have a firm, uniform consistency. A "rock-hard" prostate suggests advanced prostate cancer, whereas a soft prostate is consistent with acute prostatitis. In the case of hematuria, a cystoscopy and three-phase CT scan will be needed in order to diagnose the cause of the bleeding; however, these tests can be done on an outpatient basis.[80] The etiology of hematuria is beyond the scope of this discussion but can commonly include BPH, urinary stones, and bladder and renal cancer.

Management

Regardless of the etiology of urinary retention, a catheter must be placed to relieve the obstruction. In most cases the catheter can be placed per urethra; exceptions include acute prostatitis and a dense/narrow urethral stricture. In the case of acute prostatitis, the passage of a urethral catheter may lead to bacteremia; therefore, a percutaneously placed suprapubic catheter is preferable. In the case of a complicated urethral stricture that will not accept a catheter, flexible cystoscopy can be performed with passage of a guidewire through the stricture, and then a catheter can be fed over the wire. If this is unsuccessful, then a suprapubic tube should be placed.

If one has difficulty passing a catheter and BPH is suspected based on rectal examination, then one should next try placing an 18-F Coude urethral catheter. The larger diameter of the catheter will help it push its way through the lumen of the prostate. The curved tip will help it negotiate the natural curve of the membranous urethra. The curve at the tip is often in the same direction as the luer lock for the balloon port. As such, when passing a Coude catheter one should keep the balloon port oriented to keep the catheter tip up. The patient should be started on an alpha-blocker to alleviate obstruction from BPH.[81]

The medication takes effect within a few days at which point a voiding trial is done.

Hematuria in and of itself is not an emergency. The degree of blood loss is generally small, and most bleeding will stop spontaneously. The patient should increase oral fluid intake to keep the blood dilute and avoid the formation of blood clots in the bladder. If hematuria is significant enough that the patient is passing clots, the physician should be concerned about more significant blood loss and the possibility of urinary clot retention. A large-bore three-way hematuria urethral catheter should be placed. Aggressive irrigation should be done by hand with a syringe. Once all clots are removed, the urine should be clear. Continuous bladder irrigation should be immediately started to keep the urine clear. If bleeding confined to the bladder cannot be stopped with these conservative measures, other options include endoscopic surgical intervention, chemical fulguration with intravesical instillation of alum, or formalin.[82]

Penile Emergencies

Priapism

Background

Priapism is an uncommon condition of prolonged, usually painful, penile erection, persisting beyond sexual excitement. It is generally classified as primary/idiopathic or secondary. Although the idiopathic type is often initially associated with prolonged sexual excitement, cases of priapism due to the secondary causes are generally unrelated to sexual excitement. Priapism can also be separated hemodynamically into two distinct groups: low-flow, ischemic (veno-occlusive) and high-flow, nonischemic (arterial).

Priapism can occur in all age groups, including the newborn, but its peak incidence is from ages 5 to 10 and from 20 to 50 years. Although the slight majority of presenting cases overall are idiopathic, in the younger aged group priapism is most often associated with sickle cell anemia (42% adults and 62% children with sickle cell disorder eventually develop it) or neoplasm, and in the older age group it is most often associated with pharmacologic agents (Table 36.3).[83,84] Incidence is clearly affected by demography.

Other etiologies of secondary priapism include thromboembolic, neurogenic, neoplastic, infectious, and iatrogenic. The category of iatrogenic etiologies of priapism is extensive and includes a host of medications, and perhaps the most likely cause of priapism to confront physicians currently and in the future is overdosage of intracavernous injection of vasoactive substances for diagnosis or treatment of erectile dysfunction.[85] Ischemic priapism has also been associated with administration of the 20%

TABLE 36.3. Reported priapism-inducing medications.

Antidepressants
  Trazodone
  Fluoxetine
  Sertraline and lithium
  Bupropion

Recreational drugs
  Alcohol
  Cocaine

Antipsychotics
  Clozapine

Psychotropics
  Chlorpromazine

Antianxiety agents
  Hydroxyzine

Tranquilizers
  Mesoridazine
  Perphenazine

Anticoagulants
  Heparin
  Warfarin (Coumadin)

Alpha-adrenergic blocker
  Prazosin

Hormone
  Gonadotropin-releasing hormone (in hypogonadal men)

intravenous fat emulsion (Intralipid) component of total parenteral nutrition. Patients have described recurrent episodes several hours after administration. Proposed mechanisms include direct increase in blood coagulability and fat emboli. Recommendations to avoid such effects include slow-rate administration of 10% fat emulsion, diluted with normal saline.[80,82]

Clinical Presentation

Upon presentation, priapism must be considered a urologic emergency, as it most commonly is associated with ischemia, which, if persisting beyond 4 hours, is a compartment syndrome requiring emergent intervention.

Every case of priapism begins with a physiologic erection, wherein the corpora cavernosa are filled with well-oxygenated blood. In the patient with low-flow (veno-occlusive, ischemic) priapism, there is a failure of the detumescence mechanism from any number of causes: blockage of draining venules, paralysis of the intrinsic detumescence neurologic mechanism at the neurologic or smooth muscle level, excessive neurotransmitters, or prolonged relaxation of intracavernous smooth muscles. Blood gasses begin to show signs of ischemia and acidosis after 4 hours.[80] Pain typically ensues after 4 to 6 hours. These patients usually presents with several hours of painful erection. Typically, only the corpora cavernosa are involved and are tense with congested blood, and associated pain and tenderness result from the direct effects of tissue ischemia and acidosis. The degree of ischemia is a function of the duration of venous occlusion.[80]

The less common high-flow (nonischemic) priapism is usually painless, and the erection is not always fully rigid. High-flow priapism usually occurs secondary to laceration to cavernous artery branches within the corpora cavernosa, from blunt trauma, or from intracavernous injection. When from blunt trauma, onset is typically delayed, as it is often not until vasodilation from nocturnal erections occurs that the damaged arterial branch ruptures, thus resulting in unregulated high penile blood-flow into the cavernosa.[86] In both types, the corpus spongiosum remains soft, and only in rare cases (tricorporal priapism) is it involved.[87]

Priapism can also present as acute, intermittent (recurrent/stuttering) erection.[88] Onset is frequently during nocturnal penile tumescence. Stuttering priapism is characterized by acute, self-limiting transitory veno-occlusive episodes, generally lasting less than 3 hours and occurring most commonly during sleep. This syndrome, although incompletely understood, may develop secondary to an initial ischemic episode, resulting in a functional alteration of the adrenergic and/or endothelial-mediated mechanisms that control penile tumescence and maintain penile flaccidity.[89]

Diagnosis

The diagnosis of priapism is usually based on history and physical examination. Acute low-flow (veno-occlusive) priapism, when lasting several hours, is usually painful because of associated tissue ischemia. In contrast, high-flow (arterial) priapism is usually painless.

Diagnosis is sometimes self-evident when priapism presents in the context of one of the more common associated causes: after perineal trauma (high-flow), sickle cell anemia (low-flow, recurrent), and, perhaps the currently most common cause encountered, intracavernous injection therapy for impotence.

On physical examination, the corpora cavernosa are fully rigid in low-flow priapism and fully to partially rigid in high-flow priapism. Although the cavernosal tissue is tender, the glans and corpus spongiosum are rarely involved.[90]

Our recommended diagnostic approach is illustrated in Figure 36.7. In addition to a thorough history and physical examination, blood and urine samples should be obtained to evaluate for hemoglobin S, leukemia, and urinary tract infection.

Intracavernosal blood gas measurement is highly useful to determine the type of priapism: blood gas values similar to those from venous blood suggest low-flow priapism, and values similar to those of arterial blood

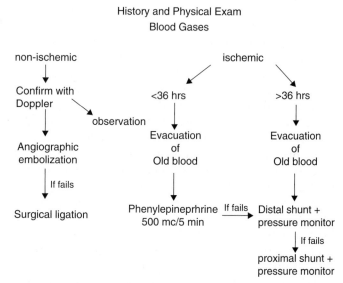

FIGURE 36.7. A practical algorithm for the treatment of priapism. (Reprinted from Walsh PC, Retik AB, Vaughan ED, Wein AJ, eds. Campbell's Urology, 8th ed. Philadelphia: WB. Saunders, 2002, with permission from Elsevier.)

suggest high-flow priapism.[91] Because, by definition, all episodes of priapism begin as high-flow states (physiologic erection), an important caveat to consider is that if cavernosal blood gas measurement (in true low-flow priapism) is done too early, results can be misleading. If any doubt exists during diagnosis, a color-coded duplex ultrasound scan of the cavernous arteries and the corpora cavernosa is often definitive: distended corpora cavernosa with minimal arterial flow is seen with low-flow priapism, whereas a ruptured artery with unregulated blood pooling at the site of injury is often seen in trauma-induced high-flow priapism.[92]

Management

The goal of primary management is to abort the erection so as to relieve pain and to prevent the permanent fibrotic damage to the corpora cavernosa that eventually leads to impotence. Medical management should always be tried before resorting to surgery.

The first line of treatment involves aspiration of the corpora and intracavernosal injection with an alpha-adrenergic agonist. Specifically, the corpus cavernosum on one side of the penile base is aspirated via a 21-gauge butterfly needle on a 60-cc syringe. Following initial aspiration of blood (typically dark, sludge-like blood in low-flow priapism), 250 to 500 µg of phenylephrine (0.5 cc of a diluted solution of 10 mg/ml phenylephrine mixed with 19 cc normal saline) is slowly injected over 5 minutes, and this is repeated until detumescence occurs. Some have described irrigating with a diluted alpha-adrenergic solution.[93] Orally administered terbutaline has been reported to bring detumescence in cases of priapism related to use of intracavernosal injection, although others have found no benefit of terbutaline over placebo.[94,95] Nevertheless, intracavernosal injection with an alpha-adrenergic agonist remains the most effective treatment for low-flow priapism, and it is almost 100% effective if within 12 hours of onset.[80] After 36 hours, however, no patients have been reported to respond to injection with alpha-adrenergics, and all result with some degree of intracavernous fibrosis.[96]

For patients with sickle cell disease, treatment is directed at reducing further sickling: aggressive hydration, oxygenation, and metabolic alkalinization. Aspiration and irrigation of the corpora cavernosa, as described, should be performed as soon as possible.

Recurrent or stuttering priapism is a common problem for patients with sickle cell trait or disease and for nonsickle cell patients with prior episodes of priapism. For patients who wish to remain sexually active, self-injection of an alpha-adrenergic agent such as phenylephrine, as described, can be used.[97] If sexual function is not a concern, nocturnal erections (and the associated recurrence of priapism) can be suppressed with the aid of a gonadotropin-releasing hormone agonist and/or an antiandrogen.[82]

High-flow priapism is best managed by arteriography and embolization of the affected artery; erectile function is usually preserved. Spontaneous resolution of high-flow priapism, with the aid of local ice-packing (causing vasospasm and spontaneous thrombosis of the ruptured artery), has been reported.[93] However, most cases with delayed arterial rupture do not subside spontaneously and ultimately require arteriography and embolization.[83,89] Follow-up imaging with color Doppler is also useful. High-flow priapism itself does not cause impotence, but injury to erectile tissue and associated nerves may result from either the primary injury or the treatment.

Prognosis

Untreated low-flow (ischemic) priapism leads to corporal fibrosis and impotence. Tissue ischemia begins after about 4 hours. Although the overall impotence rate for such patients is reported to be about 50%, almost all regain their previous potency if the erection is aborted within 12 hours of onset.

Early complications of treatment include cellulitic infection and urethral injury from needle puncture, bleeding and hematoma of the penile shaft after aspiration, and side effects from alpha-adrenergic agents (acute hypertension, headache, palpitation, and cardiac arrhyth-

mia). To avoid such potential complications, strict asepsis during corporal aspiration, in addition to administered antibiotics, are recommended. Holding firm pressure at the site of needle aspiration after the needle has been withdrawn will minimize hematoma formation. Blood pressure monitoring during administration of alpha-adrenergic agents is also useful.

Penile Fracture

Diagnosis

Penile fracture refers to a disruption of the tunica albuginea lining the corpora cavernosa (Figure 36.8). As a rule it occurs in the erect penis. During erection the tunica albuginea thins out as it is stretched, making it susceptible to injury. The most common etiology is intercourse, although self-inflicted injuries do occur.[98,99]

Presentation and Evaluation

Patients report hearing a "snap" or "crack" and feeling pain during thrusting. This is followed by rapid detumescence, ecchymosis, and sometimes impressive swelling resulting in an "eggplant deformity" (Figure 36.9). Penile fracture should be differentiated from rupture of the veins and arteries superficial to the tunica albuginea—this leads to ecchymosis and variable amounts of swelling but without a "snapping" sensation or loss of erection. Concomitant injury to the corpus spongiosum occurs in approximately 20% and urethral injury in 3% to 20%.[100,101] Urethrography should be performed if there is blood at the meatus, any degree of hematuria, or obstructive urinary symptoms.

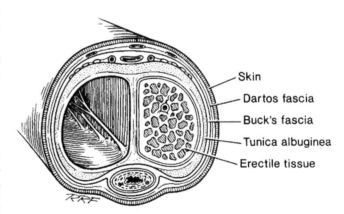

FIGURE 36.8. Anatomy of the fascial layers of the penis. Penile fracture causes disruption of the tunica albuginea with extravasation of blood into the space contained by Buck's fascia. (Reprinted from Lewis RW, Jordan GH. Surgery for erectile dysfunction. In Walsh PC, Retik AB, Vaughan ED, Wein AJ, eds. Campbell's Urology, 8th ed. Philadelphia: WB Saunders, 2002, with permission from Elsevier.)

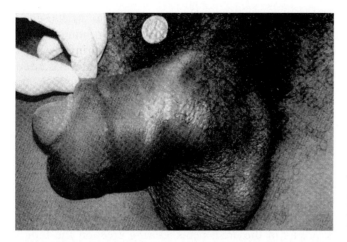

FIGURE 36.9. "Eggplant deformity" characteristic of penile fracture. (Reprinted with permission of Elsevier from Miller KS, McAninch JW. Penile fracture and soft tissue injury. In McAninch JW, ed. Traumatic and Reconstructive Urology. Philadelphia: WB Saunders, 1996.)

Management

Some relief of symptoms is obtained with an ice pack; however, surgical repair should be done as early as possible. It is believed, although not proven, that early evacuation of hematoma and primary closure of the tunical defect minimizes inflammation, fibrosis, and consequent penile curvature. The repair can be accomplished through either a longitudinal incision over the injury or a circumferential subcoronal incision followed by degloving of the penis. The corpus spongiosum and contralateral corpus cavernosum should be inspected to rule out injury. Most urethral tears are minor and can be managed with primary closure over a catheter, urethral catheter drainage alone, or suprapubic cystostomy.[102] Complete transection of the urethra should be debrided, mobilized, and repaired primarily as described elsewhere.[100]

Prognosis

Complications of penile fracture are limited to minimal/moderate penile curvature in 7%. In one series with good follow-up of 170 patients who were repaired surgically, there were no cases of de novo erectile dysfunction.[101]

Acute Scrotum

Torsion

Definition

The acute scrotum can be caused by epididymo-orchitis or torsion of the testes or one of its appendages. Differ-

entiating the two is crucial, as testicular loss because of a missed diagnosis of torsion is one of the more litigious cases in urologic practice.

Presentation

Of all children with acute scrotal pain, 11% to 14% will have epididymitis, 12% to 20% will have testicular torsion, and 54% to 70% will have torsion of one of the appendages. Specifically, the 12- to 18-year-old age group with acute scrotal pain is at most risk, with a 50% to 60% chance of testicular torsion. Older age groups will more likely have epididymo-orchitis as the cause of acute scrotal pain.[101,102] Patients with torsion will report acute onset of intense testicular pain, referred to the abdomen, with nausea and sometimes emesis.

Evaluation

The testicle may be high riding and exquisitely tender. There may be loss of the cremasteric reflex; although a normal cremasteric reflex does not rule out torsion, its absence does make torsion highly likely.[103]

Management and Prognosis

In the cooperative or mildly sedated patient, one may be able to manually detorse the testicle. As the direction of torsion is often medial, the testicle should be detorsed as if opening a book while standing at the patient's feet, that is, the patient's left testicle is rotated clockwise and the right is rotated counterclockwise.[104] As some degree of torsion may persist and retorsion is likely, orchidopexy should still be done on an urgent basis. If signs, symptoms, and age suggest testicular torsion and manual detorsion is unsuccessful, then the scrotum should be immediately explored surgically. Once torsed, testis loss occurs within 6 hours; therefore, ultrasound should be reserved for the patient for whom one has low suspicion of torsion.[104] In the operating room, if the testis is blue or black and color does not return after detorsion, then orchiectomy should be performed. If color returns, the testis should be pexed to the scrotal wall to prevent retorsion. It is common practice to pex the contralateral side at the same time.

Torsion of one of the testicular appendages is not a surgical emergency like testicular torsion, nor does it require antibiotic therapy like epididymitis. In fact, if properly diagnosed, it can be managed with analgesics. However, unless the scrotum is explored or an ultrasound is performed, it can be difficult to differentiate the three entities. In fact, even an ultrasound frequently results in misdiagnosis of testicular appendage torsion as epididymitis. A low threshold for testicular exploration should be maintained.

Epididymitis

Presentation

Epididymitis can occur in the young or old. Infection travels from the urinary tract; left untreated, the infection will progress from epididymitis to epididymo-orchitis.[105] In the young patient it must be differentiated from torsion. In the older patient, subacute scrotal pain is most likely epididymo-orchitis. As in torsion, the testicle and/or epididymis is painful and tender; however, in this case, scrotal pain is more gradual in onset, there is no nausea or vomiting, the testicle is not high riding, and there is associated erythema and edema.

Evaluation

Culturing the epididymal fluid for infection is not practical; however, examination of a urethral swab or midstream urine will generally reveal the offending agent. In sexually active men younger than 35 years of age, the most common etiology is sexually transmitted urethritis. In 10% to 50% of these men a urethral swab will demonstrate Gram-negative intracellular diplococci consistent with gonococcal urethritis; nongonococcal urethritis is caused by *Chlamydia trachomatis* (24% to 85% of all urethritis) or less commonly *Ureaplasma urealyticum* or *Mycoplasma hominis*.[106] Upon investigation, children and older adults will usually be found to have concomitant urinary tract infection with coliform bacteria.

Management

Antibiotic therapy should be based on urinary Gram stain and culture results; however, in general, agents active against coliform bacteria will be appropriate for children and older adults, whereas men younger than 35 years old should be treated for both gonococcal and nongonococcal urethritis. This may include a single dose of ceftriaxone followed by at least 7 days of doxycycline or erythromycin. Alternatively, a fluoroquinolone can be used as a single agent against both types of organisms; however, its activity against nongonoccocal urethritis is not as high as doxycycline or erythromycin.[107] Pain should be managed with narcotics or a nonsteroidal analgesic as appropriate. Bed rest and scrotal elevation is helpful.

Prognosis

Although the infection may be cleared in as few as 7 to 10 days, testicular edema, erythema, and pain will often persist for 2 to 3 weeks. For this reason, many physicians prefer to continue antibiotics for 3 weeks. Epididymitis leads to epididymal scarring, in some cases resulting in tubular obstruction. It is an etiologic factor in spermatocoeles and infertility caused by obstructive azoospermia.[108,109]

Iatrogenic Complications

Operative iatrogenic injuries to the genitourinary system are best categorized as injuries to the ureter, bladder, male urethra, and external genitalia. Renal or renal vascular surgical injuries are rare.

The ureters and urinary bladder are well-protected from injury because of their location in the extraperitoneal cavity. Most intraabdominal surgeries can be performed without encountering these structures. However, pelvic surgery, retroperitoneal surgery, and laparoscopy put the ureters and bladder at risk of injury.

Ureteral Injury

Definition and Background

Because of its size, shape, and location, the ureter is easily mistaken for a blood vessel. A thorough knowledge of the anatomic course of the ureter and the common landmarks for identification and a careful visual inspection of the ureter help avoid injury.

The ureter is approximately 25 to 30 cm in the adult. It arises from the renal pelvis, posterior to the renal vasculature (Figure 36.10). It courses inferiorly in a position posterior and lateral to the gonadal vein, with which it is easily confused. It crosses posterior to the gonadal vein at the level of the iliac vessels. The ureter then crosses anterior to the iliac vessels and courses along the pelvic sidewall. The superior vesicular pedicle crosses anterior to the ureter. The ureter then passes under the vas deferens and into the bladder trigone in the male. In the female, the ureter runs posterior to the uterine vessels in the base of the broad ligament. It then passes only 1 to 2 cm lateral to the upper cervix before inserting into the muscular posterior bladder wall. The proximity of the ureter to the colon, colonic mesentery, rectosigmoid colon, and cervix put it at risk of injury during surgery in these areas, especially when the normal anatomy is altered by the diseased organ. The ureter derives its blood supply from the renal artery and aorta proximally and from branches of the internal iliac artery distally. In general, the blood supply is medial in its cephalad course and lateral caudally. Arterioles then course in the ureteral adventitial sheath (Figure 36.11).

Presentation

The ureter can be injured by resection, laceration, ligation, contusion, electrocautery, Devascularization, and encasement in surrounding fibrosis. Ureteral injury occurs in 1% to 2% (Wolfe) of ureteroscopic procedures; however, with rapid advances in technology and ever smaller ureteroscopes, injuries can be expected to be rare in the modern era. The most common cause on

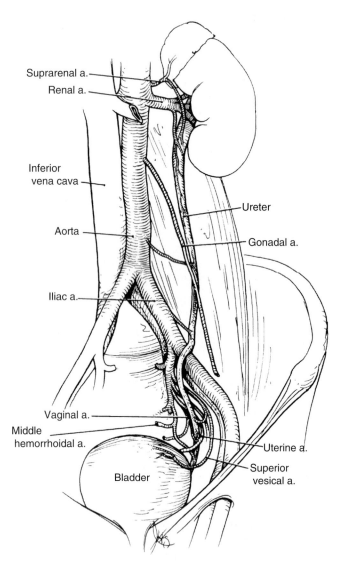

FIGURE 36.10. Anatomy of the retroperitoneum illustrating the course of the ureter. (Reprinted with permission of Elsevier from Coburn M. Ureteral injuries from surgical trauma. In McAninch JW, ed. Traumatic and Reconstructive Urology. Philadelphia: WB Saunders, 1996.)

nonurologic, iatrogenic ureteral injury is gynecologic surgery, accounting for approximately 60% of injuries.[110] Because of the proximity of the female reproductive organs to the ureter, the ureter may be injured at the pelvic brim or as it crosses under the broad ligament close to the cervix. Hysterectomy and cesarean section are associated with a 1% risk of ureteral injury.[111] Ureteral injury may also occur in other pelvic or retroperitoneal surgeries such as abdominoperineal resection (incidence of 0.3% to 5.7%), colectomy, or vascular procedures such as abdominal aortic aneurysm repair and aortofemoral bypass graft.[112] Pelvic or retroperitoneal inflammation and bulky tumors increase the risk of injury.

Evaluation

Injury commonly occurs in areas with altered anatomy or at the limits of exposure; therefore gaining additional exposure and identifying the ureter in an anatomically normal area should be the first steps when encountering a suspected ureteral injury. A vessel loop can then be placed around the ureter and its course followed toward the area in question. The adventitia should be preserved at all times. Gentle compression leads to peristalsis and can aid in identification of the ureter. Additional maneuvers to aid in identifying a ureteral injury include administration of methylene blue (either intravenous or directly into the urinary system), cystotomy, passage of a guidewire and ureteral catheter up the ureter, and, finally, pyelography. Intravenous pyelography is an insensitive indicator of ureteral injury, but retrograde pyelography and computerized tomography are more accurate.[113]

Occasionally, a ureteral injury is not recognized at the time of operation. In these cases the patient may present either acutely with abdominal pain and urosepsis or in a delayed fashion with hydronephrosis. Imaging should be followed by immediate repair or percutaneous nephrostomy and delayed repair, depending on the clinical situation.

Management

Ureteroureterostomy Most ureteral injuries are minor and require either no intervention or simple placement of a ureteral stent for 3 to 6 weeks. Lacerations and

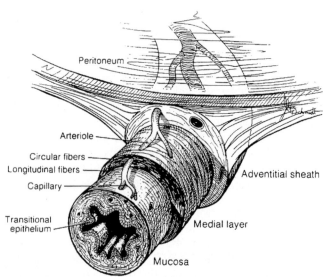

FIGURE 36.11. Layers of the ureteral wall, showing blood supply coursing in the adventitial sheath. (Reprinted with permission of Elsevier from Coburn M. Ureteral injuries from surgical trauma. In McAninch JW, ed. Traumatic and Reconstructive Urology. Philadelphia: WB Saunders, 1996.)

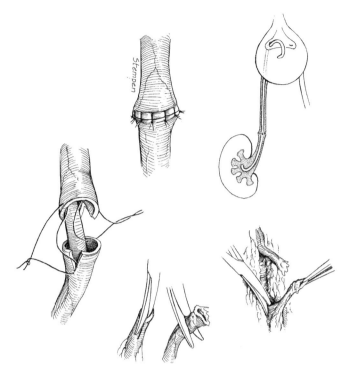

FIGURE 36.12. Technique of ureteroureterostomy. Illustrates principles of mobilization, debridement, spatulation, and anastomosis using fine absorbable suture over an internalized stent. (Reprinted with permission of Elsevier from Presti JC, Carroll PR. Ureteral and renal pelvic trauma: diagnosis and management. In McAninch JW, ed. Traumatic and Reconstructive Urology. Philadelphia: WB Saunders, 1996.)

ligatures result in short injuries. The involved segment should be debrided and the ureter reanastomosed in a tension-free, spatulated fashion over a stent. Conditions in which one would not attempt a primary repair include pelvic ureteral injuries or longer ureteral injuries in which a tension-free anastomosis cannot be achieved (Figure 36.12).

Ureteroneocystostomy Pelvic ureteral injuries are anatomically difficult to repair with a ureteroureterostomy; a ureteroneocystostomy is preferred. Briefly, the proximal free edge of ureter is debrided and spatulated. It is then reimplanted into the dome of the bladder in a tunneled fashion over a stent. If the defect is more cephalad, additional length can be gained by performing a bladder psoas hitch. The contralateral bladder pedicles are divided, and the ipsilateral bladder is pexed to the psoas fascia. The ureter is the reimplanted as described (Figures 36.13 and 36.14).

Transureteroureterostomy Transureteroureterostomy is an option in a mid to distal ureter when there is pelvic pathology that precludes ureteroneocystostomy and ureteroureterostomy. Examples could include gross fecal

soiling in the pelvis or severe scarring that limits the mobility of the bladder. Care should be taken to pass the ureter above the inferior mesenteric artery to avoid kinking. The anastamosis is done in a side-to-side fashion over a stent.

Autotransplant, Boari Flap, and Ileal Ureter Long ureteral defects extending to the proximal ureter will require a complicated repair such as an extended bladder tube flap (Boari flap), ileal ureter, or autotransplant. Consideration should be given to diverting the urine with a nephrostomy and approaching such a long repair at a later time, after a thorough discussion of options with the patient.

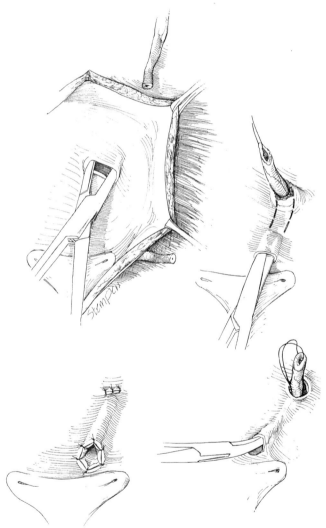

FIGURE 36.13. Technique of ureteroneocystostomy. Illustrates principles of tunneling and interrupted anastomosis using fine absorbable suture. An internalized stent should be placed. (Reprinted with permission of Elsevier from Presti JC, Carroll PR. Ureteral and renal pelvic trauma: diagnosis and management. In McAninch JW, ed. Traumatic and Reconstructive Urology. Philadelphia: WB Saunders, 1996.)

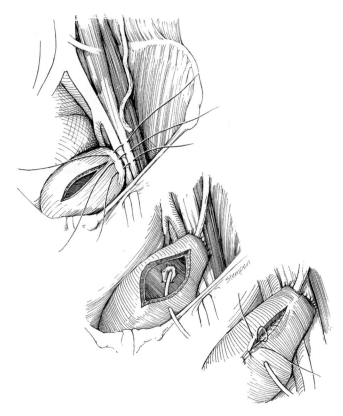

FIGURE 36.14. Technique of psoas hitch ureteroneocystostomy. Care should be taken to identify and avoid the genitofemoral nerve when pexing the bladder to the psoas fascia. (Reprinted with permission of Elsevier from Presti JC, Carroll PR. Ureteral and renal pelvic trauma: diagnosis and management. In McAninch JW, ed. Traumatic and Reconstructive Urology. Philadelphia: WB Saunders, 1996.)

All ureteral repairs should be performed over a double J ureteral stent. Stents range in size from 4.8 to 8 F and from 18 to 30cm. Typically, a 6-F, 24- to 28-cm stent is appropriate, depending on the patient's height. A KUB should be performed after the procedure to confirm stent position. The stent should be removed and a retrograde pyelogram or intravenous pyelogram done 6 weeks later.

Bladder Injury

Definition

As in ureteral injury, the bladder is well protected from injury during intraabdominal surgery; however, during laparoscopy, diagnostic peritoneal lavage, and pelvic surgery the bladder is at risk. Minor bladder injuries are likely underreported as they are often missed. In one review, the mean size of lacerations presenting for repair was 2.5cm (n = 65; range 0.5 to 10). The location of injury was anterior in 40%, posterior in 33%, and dome in 27%.[114]

Presentation

Iatrogenic bladder injury accounts for 14% to 49% of all bladder injuries; external violent trauma accounts for most.[115,116] There is a minority of nontraumatic, noniatrogenic bladder ruptures that occur spontaneously in the intoxicated patient or the augmented bladder.

In one series, iatrogenic bladder injury occurred during gynecologic procedures in 52% to 62%, urologic in 12% to 39%, and general surgery procedures in the remaining 9% to 26%.[117,119] The bladder is at risk during any percutaneous abdominal puncture, during either initial access for laparoscopy or diagnostic peritoneal lavage. When appropriate precaution is used by placing a urinary catheter before beginning the procedure, bladder injury is rare during trocar insertion. Bladder injury represents only 3% of all nonfatal visceral injuries during laparoscopic trocar placement.[117] Bladder injury can also occur during dissection in the pelvis and is most common during hysterectomy, although still occurring in less than 1% of procedures.[118] The bladder is most at risk during dissection off the anterior wall of the uterus and upper vagina.

Evaluation

Bladder injuries are characterized as intraperitoneal and extraperitoneal. Most iatrogenic intraoperative injuries are intraperitoneal. Bladder injury is invariably associated with gross hematuria, and the awake patient may complain of abdominal pain.[119] If the abdomen is not open, then diagnosis should be established by a contrast cystogram. After a scout film, cystograffin is infused through a bladder catheter, and flat and oblique views are taken with the bladder full and then again after emptying. An extraperitoneal rupture is characterized by extravasation of contrast into a confined space, whereas the spread of contrast into the peritoneum gives a more diffuse picture of contrast leakage (Figures 36.15 and 36.16).

Management and Prognosis

Most extraperitoneal bladder injuries can be managed with an indwelling urinary catheter for 2 weeks. Exceptions to this rule include lacerations that involve the bladder neck and lacerations that include the uterus or vagina. All intraperitoneal and complicated extraperitoneal bladder injuries should be repaired via laparotomy and three-layered closure of the bladder with absorbable sutures. Laparoscopic repair is an option as long as a thorough assessment for associated injuries is still possible.[120] As intraoperative bladder injury often occurs during difficult procedures, the ureters should be considered at risk as well and should be evaluated as described in the previous section.

Male Urethral Injuries

Most nontraumatic male urethral injuries are minor. The most common is traumatic urinary catheter placement. If an unsuccessful catheter placement has resulted in blood at the meatus, then a urethral injury should be suspected. At this point one can still proceed with catheter placement, although with caution. An additional attempt or two can be made using a curved tip or Coude catheter with the curve directed superiorly. If this is unsuccessful, then cystoscopy should be considered. Most urethral injuries from catheter placement are limited to the mucosa and will heal over a catheter left in place for 1 week. No further imaging is indicated unless the patient complains of difficulty urinating after catheter removal.

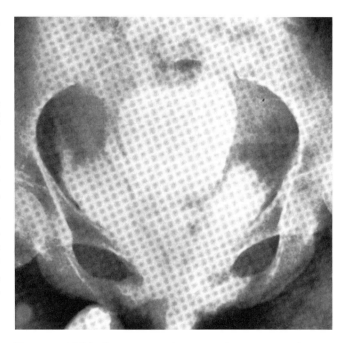

FIGURE 36.16. Cystogram demonstrating extraperitoneal bladder rupture. (Reprinted from Cass AS. Diagnostic studies in bladder rupture: indications and techniques. Urol Clin North Am 1989; 16(2):271, with permission from Elsevier.)

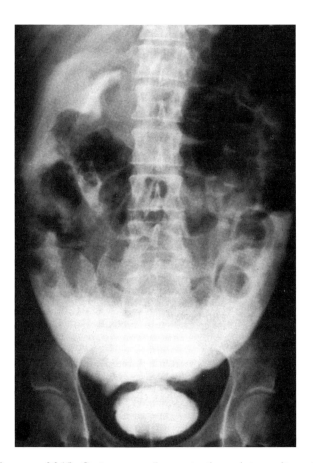

FIGURE 36.15. Cystogram demonstrating intraperitoneal bladder rupture. (Reprinted from Cass AS. Diagnostic studies in bladder rupture: indications and techniques. Urol Clin North Am 1989; 16(2):271, with permission from Elsevier.)

Pediatric Emergencies

Most pediatric urology conditions are nonemergent, although several conditions require appropriate initial management for optimal outcome. Of these conditions, the situations discussed will include circumcision complications, ambiguous genetalia, and posterior urethral valves.

Circumcision Complications

Circumcision is the most commonly performed procedure in the United States and is primarily done for cultural and religious reasons. Although evidence exists that circumcised boys have a decreased incidence of urinary tract infections and penile cancer, in most cases circumcision exposes the young boy to iatrogenic complications leading to penile disfigurement without medical benefit. Circumcision, however, is indicated for patients with infections, phimosis, or paraphimosis and is contraindicated for patients with hypospadias, micropenis, epispadias, and the buried penis.

Minor complications of circumcision include bleeding, wound infection, penile adhesions, removal of too much or too little skin, and injury to the glans, urethra, or penile shaft.[121] Of these complications, the ones that require urgent attention include postoperative bleeding, excision of too much skin, and inadvertent amputation of the glans.

Bleeding postoperatively is usually from a frenular vessel or rarely a large artery or vein in the penile shaft. These bleeds can typically be managed by manual compression or, for more brisk bleeding, silver nitrate sticks, suture ligation, or electric cautery are usually successful.

Excision of excess skin is most commonly a complication in patients who have a buried penis (Figure 36.17). "Buried penis" refers to a penile shaft that is buried below the surface of the prepubic skin because of insufficient attachment of the penile skin to the underlying dartos and Buck's fascia, which allows the penile skin at the base of the phallus to migrate distally toward the glans penis and beyond. Boys with this anatomic variant of penile skin attachment are more prone to complications from circumcision because of the physician's attempt to unconceal the penis by resecting too much "foreskin" that is actually penile shaft skin folded anteriorly. The result is a penis deficient of a large area of penile shaft skin. The best management in these cases is application of antibiotic ointment and adherent gauze the bare penile shaft. Typically reepithelialization occurs and bridges the defect. Skin grafting is rarely necessary.

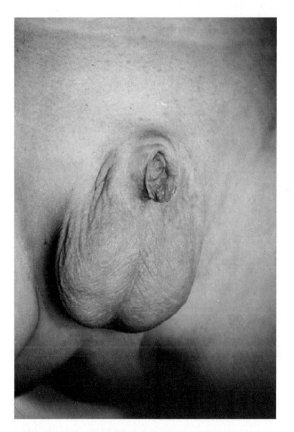

FIGURE 36.17. An illustration of a buried penis. The penis is hidden by the overlying scrotal and pubic tissue. (Reprinted from Williams CP, Richardson BG, Bukowski TP. Importance of identifying the inconspicuous penis: prevention of circumcision complications. Urology 2000; 56(1):140–142, with permission from Elsevier.)

The most feared complication is inadvertent amputation of the glans, which is more apt to occur with use of various circumcision clamps. The most appropriate management is preserving the excised tissue and reimplanting it onto the penile glans with fine suture.[122] Microscopic reattachment is usually beneficial.

Ambiguous Genitalia

Definition

"Ambiguous genitalia" (AG) refers to a constellation of conditions in which the phenotypic sex of the newborn child is not obvious. Ambiguous genetalia can be categorized into four distinct groups: female pseudohermaphrodism, which accounts for 70% of all cases of AG; male pseudohermaphrodism; true hermaphrodism; and mixed gonadal dysgenesis. The reason why AG is an emergency situation is twofold; it is imperative for the new parents emotionally and psychologically to know the sex of their new baby, and congenital adrenal hyperplasia (CAH), the most common form of female pseudohermaphrodism, can be rapidly fatal if not diagnosed in a timely matter.

Congenital adrenal hyperplasia is responsible for approximately 70% of all cases of AG and accounts for greater than 95% of all female pseudohermaphrodism. Deficiencies in 21α-hydroxylase accounts for 90% of all CAH and can result in salt wasting and eventual cardiovascular collapse. The pathophysiology of 21α-hydroxylase deficiency can be best explained by referring to the steroid hormone biosynthetic pathway illustrated in Figure 36.18. The absence of 21α-hydroxylase makes it impossible for the synthesis of mineralocorticoids (aldosterone) and glucocorticoids (cortisol) and shunts the steroid synthetic pathway toward the formation of weak androgens, which result in the virilization of female external genitalia (Figure 36.19). Congenital adrenal hyperplasia caused by 21α-hydroxylase deficiency can also occur in male newborns, although the diagnosis is clinically less obvious because the weak androgens have no effect on the appearance of male external genitalia.

Clinical Presentation

Ambiguous genitalia presents at birth when the genitalia cannot clearly be classified as truly male or female. In patients with the classic form of 21α-hydroxylase deficiency, impaired cortisol and aldosterone production leads to electrolyte and fluid losses, hyponatremia, hyperkalemia, acidosis, dehydration, increased plasma renin, and eventual hemodynamic collapse.

Diagnosis

A practical scheme can be used to evaluate for AG based on the physical examination and the karyotype of the

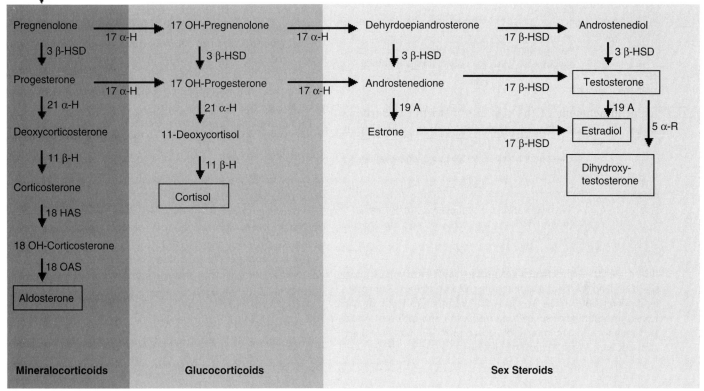

Cholesterol

StAr (20,22 Desmolase)

Pregnenolone	17α-H →	17 OH-Pregnenolone	17α-H →	Dehyrdoepiandrosterone	17β-HSD →	Androstenediol
3β-HSD		3β-HSD		3β-HSD		3β-HSD
Progesterone	17α-H →	17 OH-Progesterone	17α-H →	Androstenedione	17β-HSD →	Testosterone
21α-H		21α-H		19 A		19 A 5α-R
Deoxycorticosterone		11-Deoxycortisol		Estrone	17β-HSD →	Estradiol
11β-H		11β-H				Dihydroxy-testosterone
Corticosterone		Cortisol				
18 HAS						
18 OH-Corticosterone						
18 OAS						
Aldosterone						

Mineralocorticoids   **Glucocorticoids**   **Sex Steroids**

FIGURE 36.18. Pathway of steroid hormone biosynthesis. (Reprinted with permission of The McGraw Hill Companies from Baskin LS. Abnormalities of sexual determination and differentiation. In Tanagho EA, McAninch JW, eds. Smith's General Urology, 16th ed. New York: McGraw Hill, 2004.)

child (Figure 36.20). The diagnosis of 21α-hydroxylase deficiency is made by elevated levels of 17-hydroxyprogesterrerone present in both the urine and blood.

Management

The management of 21α-hydroxylase deficiency is initially the replacement of intravascular volume with normal saline with aggressive monitoring of electrolytes. After the patient is hemodynamically stable, glucocorticoid, mineralocorticoid, and salt replacement is instituted with routine measurements of serum electrolytes, plasma renin levels, and adrenocorticotropic hormone to monitor adequacy of treatment. Discussion of the management of other causes of AG is beyond the scope of this book.

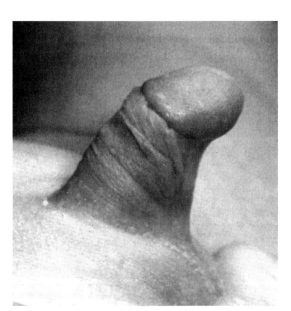

FIGURE 36.19. A female patient with severe masculinization from congenital adrenal hyperplasia. (Reprinted with permission of The McGraw Hill Companies from Baskin LS. Abnormalities of sexual determination and differentiation. In Tanagho EA, McAninch JW, eds. Smith's General Urology, 16th ed. New York: McGraw Hill, 2004.)

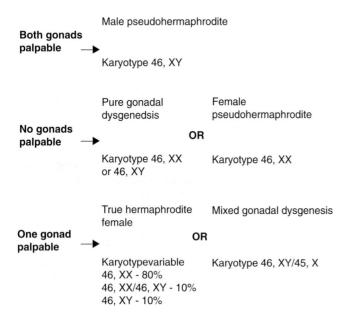

FIGURE 36.20. A practical algorithm for initial workup of intersex based on physical examination and karyotype. (Reprinted with permission of The McGraw Hill Companies from Baskin LS. Abnormalities of sexual determination and differentiation. In Tanagho EA, McAninch JW, eds. Smith's General Urology, 16th ed. New York: McGraw Hill, 2004.)

Posterior Urethral Valves

Definition

Posterior urethral valves are the most common source of urethral obstruction in male newborns and are caused by embryologic remnant membranes that are persistent in the distal prostatic urethra. The membranes behave as one-way valves to obstruct the urinary outlet in varying degrees and can lead to a large, thick-walled bladder with variable degrees of hydronephrosis.

Clinical Presentation

The clinical presentation depends on the degree of obstruction caused by the urethral valves. When the valves cause complete or near-complete obstruction, the newborns are often born with pulmonary hypoplasia because of oligohydramnios in utero, have a distended abdomen, and are anuric or oliguric. A palpable midline mass is typical of a distended bladder. In patients with moderate obstruction, a poor, intermittent, dribbling urinary stream is common. Often failure to thrive is the only significant symptom.

Diagnosis

The diagnosis of posterior urethral valves is most reliably made by renal and bladder ultrasound combined with a voiding cystourethrogram (VCUG). Classic findings on the ultrasound include a large, thick-walled bladder and varying degrees of hydroureteronephrosis. On VCUG, a scalloped, heavily trabeculated bladder with varying degrees of reflux is seen. Additionally a hypoplastic prostate with a large prostatic urethra are common. The valves can occasionally be seen (Figure 36.21).

Management

The acute management of a newborn with posterior urethral valves is prompt urethral catheterization with a 5-F feeding tube. Although the valves can adequately obstruct urine, they are rarely obstructive to the introduction of a catheter. Serum electrolytes and creatinine levels are measured, intravenous fluids are started, and intravenous antibiotics are initiated.

If the serum creatinine level normalizes and the patient is stable, definitive endoscopic fulguration of the valves is recommended. In cases of a high nadir creatinine level, reflux, and less stable clinical status, debate among

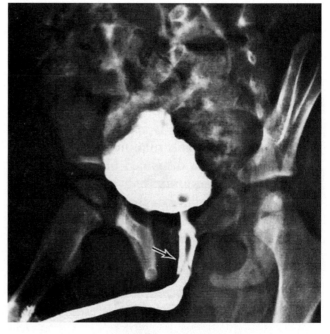

FIGURE 36.21. A patient with posterior urethral valves.

leading authorities continues regarding the optimal management strategy. These strategies include endoscopic fulguration, vesicostomy, and bilateral ureterostomy. In these cases consultation with an experienced pediatric urologist should be obtained.

Critique

All retroperitoneal hematomas (zone I [central], zone II [perinephric], and zone III [pelvic]) resulting from penetrating trauma should be explored. Preexploration vascular control is strongly recommended, if possible. For nonexpanding and nonpulsatile hematomas secondary to blunt trauma, only zone I (central) mandates exploration.

Answer (A)

References

1. Freiha FS, Messing EM, Gross DM. Emphysematous pyelonephritis. Urology 1979; 18:9–12.
2. Michaeli J, Mogle P, Perlberg S, Heiman S, Caine M. Emphysematous pyelonephritis. J Urol 1984; 131:203–208.
3. Chen MT, Huang CN, Chou YH, Huang CH, Chiang CP, Liu GC. Percutaneous drainage in the treatment of emphysematous pyelonephritis: 10-year experience. J Urol 1997; 157(5):1569–1573.
4. Wan YL, Lo SK, Bullard MJ, Chang PL, Lee TY. Predictors of outcome in emphysematous pyelonephritis. J Urol 1998; 159(2):369–373.
5. Wan YL, Lee TY, Bullard MJ, Tsai CC. Acute gas-producing bacterial renal infection: correlation between imaging findings and clinical outcome. Radiology 1996; 198:433.
6. Dembry LM, Andriole VT. Renal and perirenal abscesses. Infect Dis Clin North Am 1997; 11(3):663–680.
7. Yen DH, Hu SC, Tsai J, Kao WF, Chern CH, Wang LM, et al. Renal abscess: early diagnosis and treatment. Am J Emerg Med 1999; 17(2):192–197.
8. Saiki J, Vaziri ND, Barton C. Perinephric and intranephric abscesses: a review of the literature. West J Med 1982; 136:95.
9. Meng MV, Maria LA, McAninch JW. Current treatment and outcomes of perinephric abscesses. J Urol 2002; 168:1227–1240.
10. Edelstein H, McCabe RE. Perinephric abscess: modern diagnosis and treatment in 47 cases. Medicine 1988; 67:118.
11. Anderson KA, McAninch JW. Renal abscesses: classification and review of 40 cases. Urology 1980; 16(4):333–338.
12. Merenich WM, Popky GI. Radiology of renal infection. Med Clin North Am 1991; 75:425.
13. Dalla Palma L, Pozzi-Mucelli F, Ene V. Medical treatment of renal and perirenal abscesses: CT evaluation. Clin Radiol 1999; 54:792.
14. June CH, Browning MD, Smith LP, et al. Ultrasonography and computed tomography in severe urinary tract infections. Arch Intern Med 1985; 145(5):841–845.
15. Edelstein H, McCabe RE. Perinephric abscess: modern diagnosis and treatment in 47 cases. Medicine 1988; 67:118.
16. Siegel JF, Smith A, Moldwin R. Minimally invasive treatment of renal abscess. J Urol 1996; 155(1):52–55.
17. Coleman BG, Arger PH, Mulhern CB Jr, et al. Pyonephrosis: Sonography in the diagnosis and management. AJR Am J Roentgenol 1981; 137:939.
18. Kaplan MS, Wechsler M, Berson MC, et al. Urologic manifestations of AIDS. Urology 1987; 30:441–443.
19. Nguyen HT. Bacterial infections of the urinary tract. In Tanagho EA, McAninch JW, eds. Smith's General Urology. New York: McGraw Hill Co. Inc, 2004: 2218–2220.
20. Weinberger M, et al. Prostatic abscess in the antibiotic era. Rev Infect Dis 1988; 10:239.
21. Barozzi L, et al. Prostatic abscess: diagnosis and treatment. AJR 1998; 170:753.
22. Pai MG, Bhat HS. Prostatic abscess. J Urol 1972; 108: 599–600.
23. Graanados EA, Riley G, Salvador J, et al. Prostatic abscess: diagnosis and treatment. J Urol 1992; 148:80–82.
24. Nickel JC. Evolving management strategies. Urol Clin North Am 1999; 26:743–751.
25. Nickel JC. Prostatitis and related conditions. In Walsh PC, Retik AB, Vaughan ED, Wein AJ, eds. Campbell's Urology, 8th ed. Philadelphia: WB Saunders, 2002: 603–630.
26. Weidner W, Scheifer HG, Brahles E. Refractory chronic bacterial prostatitis: a re-evaluation of ciprofloxacin treatment after a median follow-up of 30 months. J Urol 1991; 146:350–352.
27. Nguyen HT. Bacterial infections of the urinary tract. In Tanagho EA, McAninch JW, eds. Smith's General Urology. New York: McGraw Hill Co. Inc, 2004: 2218.
28. Nickel JC: Antibiotics for bacterial prostatitis. J Urol 2000; 163:1407.
29. Childs S. Current diagnosis and treatment of urinary tract infections. Urology 1992; 40:295.
30. McNaughton-Collins M, Fowler FJ, Elliot DB, et al. Diagnosing and treating chronic prostatitis: do urologists use the four-glass test? Urology 2000; 55:403–407.
31. Lewis RW. Long term results of penile prosthetic implantations. Urol Clin North Am 1995; 22:847–863.
32. Wilson SK, et al. Quantifying risks of penile prosthesis infection with glycosylated hemoglobin. J Urol 1998; 159:1537–1540.
33. Fallon B, Ghanem H. Infected penile prosthesis: incidence and outcomes. Int J Impot Res 1989; 1:175.
34. Wilson SK, Delk JR. Inflatable penile implant infection: predisposing factors and treatment suggestions. J Urol 1995; 153:659–661.
35. Gross AJ, et al. Penile prosthesis in paraplegic men. Br J Urol 1996; 78:262–264.
36. Elek SD, Connin PE. The virulence of Staphylococcus pyogenes for man: the study of the problems of wound infection. Br J Exp Pathol 1957; 38:573–586.
37. Carson CC. Management of prosthesis infections in urologic surgery. Urol Clin North Am 1999; 26:829–839.

38. Lauks SS. Fournier's gangrene. Surg Clin North Am 1994; 74:1339.
39. Cunningham B, Nitavongs S, Shons A. Fournier's syndrome following anorectal examination and mucosal biopsy. Dis Colon Rectum 1979; 22:51.
40. Paty R, Smith AD. Gangrene and Fournier's gangrene. Urol Clin North Am 1992; 19:149.
41. Baskin LS, Carroll PR, Cattolica EV, et al. Necrotising soft tissue infections of the perineum and genitalia. Br J Urol 1990; 65:524.
42. Clayton MD, Fowler JE, Sharifi R, et al. Causes, presentation, and survival of fifty-seven patients with necrotizing fasciitis of the male genitalia. Surg Gynecol Obstet 1990; 170:49.
43. Rea WJ, Wyrick WJ. Necrotizing fasciitis. Ann Surg 1970; 172:957.
44. Weiss G. Pathogenicity of *Bacteroides melaninogenicus* and its importance in surgical infections. Surgery 1943; 13:683.
45. Carroll PR, Cattolica EV, Turzan CW, et al. Necrotizing soft-tissue infections of the perineum and genitalia: etiology and early reconstruction. West J Med 1986; 144:174.
46. Spirnak JP, Resnick MI, Hampel N. Fournier's gangrene: a report of 20 patients. J Urol 1984; 131:289.
47. Finegold SM. Pathogenic anaerobes. Arch Intern Med 1982; 142:1988.
48. Meng MV, McAninch JW. Necrotizing gangrene of the genitalia and perineum. Infect Urol 1999; Sept/Oct:132.
49. Miller JD. The importance of early diagnosis and surgical treatment of necrotizing fasciitis. Surg Gynecol Obstet 1983; 157:197.
50. Cohen MS. Fournier's gangrene. Am Urol Assoc Update Ser. 1986; 5:6.
51. Church JM, Yagahan RJ, Al-Jaberi TM, et al. Fournier's gangrene: changing face of the disease. Dis Colon Rectum 2000; 43:1300–1308.
52. Rajan DK, Scharer KA. Radiology of Fournier's gangrene. AJR Am J Roentgenol 1998; 170:163.
53. Fisher JR, Conway MJ, Takeshita RT, et al. Necrotizing fasciitis: importance of roentgenographic studies for soft-tissue gas. JAMA 1979; 241:803.
54. Ahrenholz D. Necrotizing soft-tissue infections. Surg Clin North Am 1988; 68:199.
55. Kaiser RE, Cerra FB. Progressive necrotizing surgical infections—a unified approach. J Trauma 1981; 21:349.
56. Laor E, Palmer LS, Tolia BM, et al. Outcome prediction in patients with Fournier's gangrene. J Urol 1995; 154:89.
57. Wolach MD, MacDermott JP, Stone AR, et al. Treatment and complications of Fournier's gangrene. Br J Urol 1989; 64:310.
58. Pizzorno R, Bonini F, Donelli A, et al. Hyperbaric oxygen therapy in the treatment of Fournier's disease in 11 male patients. J Urol 1997; 158:837.
59. Riseman JA, Zamboni WA, Ross DO. Hyperbaric oxygen therapy reduced mortality and the need for debridement. Surgery 1990; 108:847.
60. Capelli-Schellpfeffer M, Gerber GS. The use of hyperbaric oxygen in urology. J Urol 1999; 162:647–654.

61. Eble JN. Angiomyolipoma of kidney. Semin Diagn Pathol 1998; 15:21–40.
62. Oesterling JE, Fishman EK, Goldman SM, Marshall FF. The management of renal angiomyolipoma. J Urol 1986; 135:1121–1124.
63. Steiner MS, Goldman SM, Fishman EK, Marshall FF. The natural history of renal angiomyolipoma. J Urol 1993; 150:1782–1786.
64. Lemaitre L, Claudon M, Dubrulle F, Mazeman E. Imaging of angiomyolipoma. Semin Ultrasound CT MR 1997; 18:100–114.
65. Bosniak MA, Megibow AJ, Hulnick DH, et al. CT diagnosis of renal angiomyolipoma: the importance of detecting small amounts of fat. AJR Am J Roentgenol 1998; 151:497–501.
66. Siegel CL, Middleton WD, Teefey SA, McClennan BL. Angiomyolipoma and renal cell carcinoma: US differentiation. Radiology 1996; 198:789–793.
67. Novick AC, Campbell SC. Renal Tumors. In Walsh PC, Retik AB, Vaughan ED, Wein AJ, eds. Campbell's Urology, 8th ed. Philadelphia: WB Saunders, 2002: 2682.
68. Li J, Kennedy D, Levine M, Kumar A, Mullen J. Absent hematuria and expensive computerized tomography: case characteristics of emergency urolithiasis. J Urol 2001; 165(3):782–784.
69. Gulmi FA, Felsen D, Vaughan ED. Pathophysiology of urinary tract obstruction. In Walsh PC, Retik AB, Vaughan ED, Wein AJ, eds. Campbell's Urology, 8th ed. Philadelphia: WB Saunders, 2002: 411–462.
70. Kobayashi T, Nishizawa K, Watanabe J, Ogura K. Clinical characteristics of ureteral calculi detected by nonenhanced computerized tomography after unclear results of plain radiography and ultrasonography. J Urol 2003; 170(3):799–802.
71. Hamm M, Wawroschek F, Weckermann D, Knopfle E, Hackel T, Hauser H, Krawczak G, Harzmann R. Ultrasound versus intravenous urography in the initial evaluation of patients with suspected obstructing urinary calculi. Scand J Urol Nephrol Suppl 1991; 137:45–47.
72. Catalano O, Nunziata A, Altei F, Siani A. Suspected ureteral colic: primary helical CT versus selective helical CT after unenhanced radiography and sonography. AJR Am J Roentgenol 2002; 178(2):379–387.
73. Hubner WA, Irby P, Stoller ML. Natural history and current concepts for the treatment of small ureteral calculi. Eur Urol 1993; 24(2):172–176.
74. Coll DM, Varanelli MJ, Smith RC. Relationship of spontaneous passage of ureteral calculi to stone size and location as revealed by unenhanced helical CT. AJR Am J Roentgenol 2002; 178(1):101–103.
75. Watson RA, Esposito M, Richter F, Irwin RJ Jr, Lang EK. Percutaneous nephrostomy as adjunct management in advanced upper urinary tract infection. Urology 1999; 54(2):234–239.
76. St Lezin M, Hofmann R, Stoller ML. Pyonephrosis: diagnosis and treatment. Br J Urol 1992; 70(4):360–363.
77. Chow GK, Patterson DE, Blute ML, Segura JW. Ureteroscopy: effect of technology and technique on clinical practice. J Urol 2003; 170(1):99–102.

78. Sozen S, Kupeli B, Tunc L, Senocak C, Alkibay T, Karaoglan U, Bozkirli I. Management of ureteral stones with pneumatic lithotripsy: report of 500 patients. J Endourol 2003; 17(9):721–724.

79. Mardis HK, Parks JH, Muller G, Ganzel K, Coe FL. Outcome of metabolic evaluation and medical treatment for calcium nephrolithiasis in a private urological practice. J Urol 2004; 171:85–88.

80. Grossfeld GD, Litwin MS, Wolf JS Jr, Hricak H, Shuler CL, Agerter DC, Carroll PR. Evaluation of asymptomatic microscopic hematuria in adults: the American Urological Association best practice policy—part II: patient evaluation, cytology, voided markers, imaging, cystoscopy, nephrology evaluation, and follow-up. Urology 2001; 57(4):604–610.

81. AUA Practice Guidelines Committee. AUA guideline on management of benign prostatic hyperplasia (2003). Chapter 1: Diagnosis and treatment recommendations. J Urol 2003; 170(2 Pt 1):530–547.

82. Choong SKS, Walkden M, Kirby R. The management of intractable hematuria. BJU Int 2000; 86:951–959.

83. Lue T. Physiology of penile erection and pathophysiology of erectile dysfunction and priapism. In Walsh PC, Retik AB, Vaughan ED, Wein AJ, eds. Campbell's Urology, 8th ed. Philadelphia: WB Saunders, 2002: 1612.

84. Hashmat AI, Rehman J. Priapism. In Hashmat AI, Das S, eds. The Penis. Philadelphia: Lea & Febiger, 1993; 219–243.

85. Elkstrom B, Ollson AM. Priapism in patients treated with total parenteral nutrition. Br J Urol 1987; 59:170.

86. Ricciardi R Jr, Bhatt GM, Cynamon J, et al. Delayed high-flow priapism: pathophysiology and management: J Urol 1993; 149:119–121.

87. Sharpsteen JR, Powars D, Johnson C, et al. Multisystem damage associated with tricorporal priapism in sickle cell disease. Am J Med 1993; 94:289–295.

88. Emond AM, Holman R, Hayes RJ, et al. Priapism and impotence in homozygous sickle cell disease. Arch Intern Med 1980; 140:1434.

89. Levine JF, Saenz de Tejada I, Payton TR, Goldstein I. Recurrent prolonged erections and priapism as a sequela of priapism: pathophysiology and management. J Urol 1991; 145:764–767.

90. Broderick GA, Harkaway R. Pharmacologic erection: time-dependent changes in the corporal environment. Int J Impot Res 1994; 6:9–16.

91. Lue T, Hellstrom WJ, McAninch JW, Tanagho EA. Priapism: a refined approach to diagnosis and treatment. J Urol 1986; 136:104–108.

92. Brock G, Bezra J, Lue T, Tanagho EA. High flow priapism. A spectrum of disease. J Urol 1993; 150:968–971.

93. Sidi AA. Vasoactive intracavernous pharmacotherapy. Urol Clin North Am 1988; 15:95–101.

94. Lowe FC, Jarrow JP. Placebo-controlled study of oral terbutaline and pseudoephedrine in management of prostaglandin E1-induced prolonged erections. Urology 1993; 42:51–54.

95. Govier FE, Jonsson E, Kramer-Levin D. Oral terbutaline for the treatment of priapism. J Urol 1994; 151:878–879.

96. Ilkay AK, Levine, LA. Conservative management of high-flow priapism. Urology 1995; 46:419–424.

97. Steinberg J, Eyre RC. Management of recurrent priapism with epinephrine self-injection and gonadotropin-releasing analogue. J Urol 1995; 153:152–153.

98. Beysel M, Tekin A, Gűrdal M, Yűcebas E, Sengor F. Evaluation and treatment of penile fractures: accuracy of clinical diagnosis and the value of cavernosography. Urology 2002; 60:492–496.

99. Zargooshi J. Penile fracture in Kermanshah, Iran: the long-term results of surgical treatment. BJU Int 2002; 89:890–894.

100. Jordan GH, Schlossberg SM. Surgery of the penis and urethra. In Walsh PC, Retik AB, Vaughan ED, Wein AJ, eds. Campbell's Urology, 8th ed. Philadelphia: WB Saunders, 2002; 3886–3954.

101. McAndrew HF, Pemberton R, Kikiros CS, Gollow I. The incidence and investigation of acute scrotal problems in children. Pediatr Surg Int 2002; 18(5–6):435–437.

102. Mushtaq I, Fung M, Glasson MJ. Retrospective review of paediatric patients with acute scrotum. Anz J Surg 2003; 73:55–58.

103. Nelson CP, Williams JF, Bloom DA. The cremasteric reflex: a useful but imperfect sign in testicular torsion. J Pediatr Surg 2003; 38(8):1248–1249.

104. Sessions AE, Rabinowitz R, Hulbert WC, Goldstein MM, Mevorach RA. Testicular torsion: direction, degree, duration and disinformation. J Urol 2003; 169(2):663–665.

105. Hagley M. Epididymo-orchitis and epididymitis: a review of causes and management of unusual forms. Int J STD AIDS 2003; 14(6):372–377.

106. Berger RE, Lee JC. Sexually transmitted diseases: the classic diseases. In Walsh PC, Retik AB, Vaughan ED, Wein AJ, eds. Campbell's Urology, 8th ed. Philadelphia: WB Saunders, 2002: 671–691.

107. Workowski KA, Levine WC. Sexually transmitted diseases treatment guidelines 2002. Centers for Disease Control and Prevention. MMWR Recomm Rep 2002; 51(RR-6):1–78.

108. Patel PJ, Pareek SS. Scrotal ultrasound in male infertility. Eur Urol 1989; 16(6):423–425.

109. Merino G, Murrieta S, Rodriguez L, Sandoval C, Moran C, Bailon R. Sexually transmitted diseases and related genital pathologies in oligozoospermia. Arch Androl 1993; 31(2):87–94.

110. Payne CK, Raz S. Ureterovaginal and related fistulas. In McAninch JW, ed. Traumatic and Reconstructive Urology. Philadelphia: WB Saunders, 1996; 213–247.

111. Mäkinen J, Johansson J, Tomás C, Tomás E, Heinonen PK, Laatikainen T. Morbidity of 10,100 hysterectomies by type of approach. Hum Reprod 2001; 17:1473–1478.

112. St Lezin M, Stoller ML. Surgical ureteral injuries. Urology 1991; 38(6):497–506.

113. Elliott SP, McAninch JW. Ureteral injuries from external violence: the 25-year experience at San Francisco General Hospital. J Urol 2003; 170:1213–1216.

114. Armenakas NA, Pareek G, Fracchia JA. Iatrogenic bladder perforations: long-term follow-up of 65 patients. JACS 2004; 198(1):78–82.

115. Husmann DA. Diagnostic techniques in suspected bladder injury. In McAninch JW, ed. Traumatic and Reconstructive Urology. Philadelphia: WB Saunders, 1996; 261–268.

116. Dobrowolski ZF, Lipczynski W, Drewniak T, Jakubik P, Kusionowicz J. External and iatrogenic trauma of the urinary bladder: a survey in Poland. BJU Int 2002; 89:755–756.

117. Bhoyrul S, Vierra MA, Nezhat CR, Krummel TM, Way LW. Trocar injuries in laparoscopic surgery. JACS 2001; 192: 677–683.

118. Cosson M, Lambaudie E, Boukerrou M, Querleu D, Crépin G. Vaginal, laparoscopic, or abdominal hysterectomies for benign disorders: immediate and early postoperative complications. Eur J Obstet Gynecol Reprod Biol 2001; 98(2):231–236.

119. Carroll PR, McAninch JW. Major bladder trauma: mechanisms of injury and a unified method of diagnosis and repair. J Urol 1984; 132(2):254–257.

120. Cottam D, Gorecki PJ, Curvelo M, Shaftan GW. Laparoscopic repair of traumatic perforation of the urinary bladder. Surg Endosc 2001; 15(12):1488–1489.

121. Baskin LS, Canning DA, Snyder HM, Duckett JW. Treating complications of circumcision. Pediatr Emerg Care 1996; 12:62.

122. Gluckman G, Stoller M, Jacobs M, Kogan B. Newborn penile glans amputation during circumcision and successful reattachment. J Urol 1995; 153:778.

37
Pelvis

Craig M. Rodner and Bruce D. Browner

Case Scenario

A jockey sustains lower torsopelvic trauma after his horse falls on him while attempting to jump over a hurdle. The patient presents with an obvious crushed pelvis. The patient is hemodynamically stable. A retrograde urethrogram was performed (no urethral injury) followed by cystography that demonstrated an extraperitoneal bladder injury. Further diagnostic evaluation (computed tomography scan) demonstrated no abdominal pathology. The unstable pelvis fracture will require the application of an external fixator. Which of the following is an essential component of this specific management plan?

(A) Diagnostic peritoneal lavage
(B) Laparoscopy
(C) Diverting colostomy
(D) Pelvic angiography
(E) Proctoscopy

Injuries to the bony pelvis can be caused by low- or high-energy trauma. Low-energy injuries usually result in fractures of individual pelvic bones that will not compromise the integrity of the pelvic ring. In contrast, high-energy injuries can disrupt the pelvic ring, potentially shearing posterior veins as well as increasing the potential space in the pelvis for subsequent hemorrhage. In the hemodynamically labile trauma patient, unstable pelvic fractures are of acute concern as bleeding may continue undeterred without a prompt diagnosis and emergent pelvic stabilization. This chapter discusses the breadth of skeletal pelvic trauma with a focus on the evaluation and emergency treatment of pelvic ring injuries.

Anatomy of the Pelvic Ring

To evaluate and treat the fractured pelvis, it is first necessary to understand the osseous and ligamentous anatomy of this complex structure. Stated simply, the pelvic ring is composed of three large bones, the sacrum and two innominate bones, which articulate with the sacrum posteriorly at the sacroiliac joints and with each other anteriorly at the pubic symphysis. The innominate bones themselves are the composite of three bones, the ileum, ischium, and pubis, which fuse during skeletal maturation at the triradiate cartilage.

The skeletal framework of the pelvis alone offers little inherent stability, depending instead on a robust ligamentous architecture to resist deforming forces. The stabilizing structures of the pelvis can be thought of in three anatomic locations: (1) anteriorly, (2) posteriorly, and (3) on the pelvic floor.

Anteriorly, the pubic rami articulate at the hyaline cartilage–covered symphysis pubis. Thick fibrocartilage runs between the rami and is reinforced by the arcuate ligament or inferior pubic ligament. These anterior stabilizing structures contribute some stability to the pelvis, but less than that provided by the posterior ligaments.

Posteriorly, the sacroiliac (SI) ligaments are indeed the strongest and most important contributor to pelvic stability.[1] The SI ligaments act as a posterior tension band to the pelvis, and, if sectioned, the innominate bone can be displaced anteriorly from the sacrum. The SI ligaments are composed of both short and long ligaments. As illustrated in Figure 37.1A, the short ligaments run obliquely from the posterior ridge of the sacrum to the posterior superior and inferior iliac spines, while the long ligaments are oriented longitudinally, coursing from the lateral aspect of the sacrum to the posterior superior iliac spine (PSIS). At the PSIS, the long posterior SI ligaments join the sacrotuberous ligaments from the pelvic floor. The iliolumbar ligaments, as their name suggests, run between the posterior iliac crest and the transverse processes of

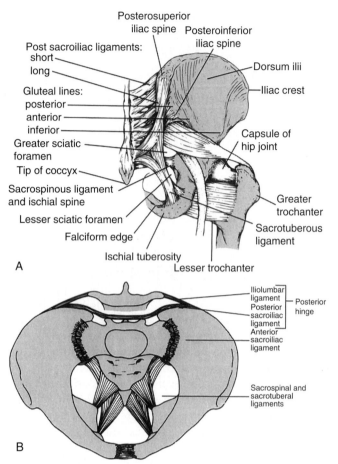

Figure 37.1. **(A)** A posterior-to-anterior view of the pelvis, illustrating the bony attachments of the posterior sacroiliac ligaments (both short and long) and the ligaments of the pelvic floor (sacrotuberous and sacrospinal). **(B)** An axial inlet view of the pelvis, depicting the ligamentous architecture of the pelvic ring. (Reprinted from Browner B, Jupiter J, Levine A, Trafton P, eds. Skeletal Trauma, 3rd ed. Philadelphia: WB Saunders, 2003: 1053, 1057, with permission from Elsevier)

the fourth and fifth lumbar vertebrae. Lumbosacral ligaments course from the transverse process of L5 to the sacral ala.

The ligaments of the pelvic floor, which include the sacrotuberous and sacrospinous ligaments, also contribute to the stability of the bony pelvis. The sacrotuberous ligament is the longer of the two and runs between the posterior aspect of the SI ligaments and the ischial tuberosity, resisting rotational vertical-shearing forces. The sacrospinous ligament is shorter, arising from the lateral edge of the sacrum and coursing more transversely to the ischial spine. This ligament resists external rotation forces applied to the hemipelvis. Figure 37.1B depicts an axial (inlet) view of the pelvis, demonstrating the location of the sacrotuberous and sacrospinal ligaments on the pelvic floor.

As long as the ligamentous architecture of the pelvic ring is intact, particularly posteriorly, the pelvis remains stable. Under normal physiologic conditions, Tile and Hearn[2] demonstrated that, with sitting or standing, the pubic symphysis is under tension and the posterior ligaments are compressed. In contrast, during single stance phase, the symphysis becomes compressed and the posterior ligaments are under tension. With sequential sectioning of these ligaments, Tile and Hearn[2] demonstrated the relative value of each. When just the symphysis was sectioned, mechanical loading of the pelvis showed an anterior diastasis of no more than 2.5 cm, as further spreading was prohibited by the sacrospinous and anterior SI ligaments. When these ligaments were sectioned as well, more than 2.5 cm of diastasis in external rotation was observed; this is an example of a rotationally unstable pelvis. Vertical stability remained, as well as resistance to posterior displacement, in this scenario because of the competence of the posterior SI ligaments and sacrotuberous ligaments. When these ligaments are sectioned, the pelvis not only is rotationally unstable, but it becomes vertically and posteriorly unstable as well.

Pelvic Stability and Mechanism of Injury

"Stable" or "unstable" are terms often employed in describing various pelvic ring injuries. A stable pelvis, stated simply, is one that can withstand normal physiologic forces without undergoing any deformation. In contrast, an unstable pelvis does deform to physiologic forces and can do so rotationally and/or vertically. It is important to note that stability in pelvic trauma is more of a continuum than a black-or-white category. Tile[2–6] has developed a helpful classification system that categorizes pelvic fractures based on the relative stability of the pelvic ring, from those fractures that have a completely intact ring (Tile A) to those with complete rotational and vertical instability (Tile C). Those fractures that partially disrupt pelvic ring stability, but still have some resistance to complete vertical displacement of the hemipelvis, are classified in between the two extremes (Tile B).

The direction and magnitude of the applied force to the pelvis at the moment of injury plays the key role in determining its stability. In general, there are four types of deforming forces: (1) lateral compression, (2) external rotation, (3) anterior posterior, and (4) shearing.

Lateral-Compression Force

Lateral-compressive forces to the hemipelvis cause internal-rotation deformities. This mechanism is the most common etiology of pelvic fractures. During this pattern of injury, the force often impacts on the outer table of the iliac wing in a parallel fashion to the trabeculae of the sacrum. The pubic ramus on the side of the impact may be pushed across the midline, as the hemipelvis "closes in" on its other half. Effectively, this can produce a lateral compression injury on the side of impact and an external rotation injury on the contralateral side, with disruption of the anterior SI ligaments. If the posterior ligaments remain intact, sacral impaction will occur on the side of impact. If, instead, the bone of the sacrum proves to be more resilient than the posterior SI ligaments, these ligaments will tear first. However, overall pelvic ring stability still remains because the sacrotuberous and sacrospinous ligaments of the pelvic floor are not compromised with a lateral-compression force. Although dramatic internal-rotation deformities may occur, even violent forces applied in this manner usually will not produce significant posterior or vertical translation of the hemipelvis.

External-Rotation Force

External-rotation forces applied through the intact femur can potentially tear the hemipelvis away from the sacrum if enough force is present. This injury first causes a disruption of the anterior pelvic ring, by either a lesion at the pubic symphysis or, more rarely, a fracture through the pubic rami. As the external-rotation deforming force continues, the hemipelvis begins to hinge on its robust posterior ligamentous structures. The ligaments of the pelvic floor are compromised and, with more force, the anterior SI ligaments are torn and the hemipelvis springs open like an "open book." The posterior SI ligaments usually remain intact, imparting the pelvic ring with some element of partial stability.

Anterior-Posterior Force

External rotation of the hemipelvis can also be caused by an anterior-posterior force to the pelvic ring. With such an insult, the pelvis can spring open, hinging on its intact posterior ligamentous structures. Although this force may compromise the ligaments of the pelvic floor and even the anterior SI ligaments, the posterior SI ligaments remain intact and thus the ring is vertically stable.

Shearing Force

Shearing forces are usually secondary to high-energy trauma and are applied longitudinally with respect to the axis of the pelvis. They are often the result of falls onto an extended lower extremity, impacts from above, or motor vehicle accidents with force applied through an extended lower extremity against the firewall or floor. Such injuries have the potential to tear the ligamentous restraints of the pelvic floor and the SI complex and, as such, can produce completely unstable pelvic rings. Indeed, unlike the lateral-compression and external-rotation patterns of injury, vertical shearing mechanisms often render the pelvis not only rotationally but also vertically and translationally unstable.

Classification

With the concept of pelvic stability, both partial and absolute, as well as the mechanisms of injury in mind, the classification schemes of pelvic ring fractures become much easier to digest.

Young and Burgess Classification

The Young-Burgess system was developed in 1987 and is based on the mechanism of pelvic ring injury.[7] This classification system is helpful to the treating traumatologist because it alerts him or her to certain pelvic fractures that may carry with them greater morbidity. Young and Burgess divided pelvic fractures into three main categories: (1) lateral-compression injuries, (2) anterior-posterior compression injuries, and (3) vertical shearing injuries.

Lateral Compression

Lateral-compression (LC) forces, as described earlier, produce implosion-type injuries of the hemipelvis. These injuries, which usually result from motor vehicle accidents, were categorized into three subtypes by Young and Burgess (Figure 37.2A). Lateral-compression type I injuries involve a transverse fracture of the pubic ramus, with sacral impaction on the side of the impact. Lateral-compression type II injuries describe those with a posterior iliac wing fracture on the side of the impact with variable amounts of disruption of the posterior ligaments, producing variable degrees of mobility of the anterior hemipelvis to internal-rotation stresses. This injury pattern may be associated with an anterior sacral fracture. Lateral-compression type III injuries describe an LC-I or LC-II injury on the side of impact but a propagation of force to the contralateral hemipelvis that acts as an external-rotation force to that side. This produces the classic "windswept" appearance to the pelvis (internal-rotation deformity on the side of impact, external-rotation deformity on the contralateral side). Pelvic ring disruptions caused by an LC mechanism have a relatively high incidence of associated visceral and traumatic brain injuries compared with others, but a relatively low incidence of pelvic bleeding. Death from an LC pelvic injury would most likely be caused by an associated brain and/or intraabdominal injury.

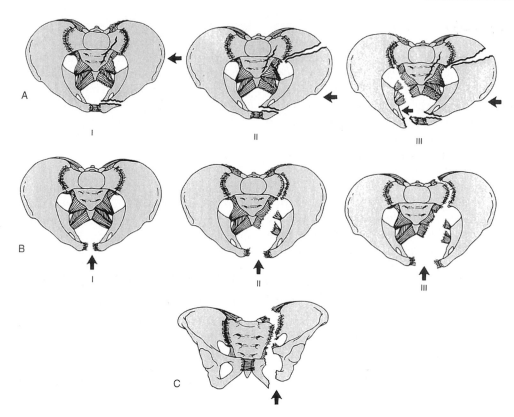

FIGURE 37.2. The Young-Burgess classification7 is based on the mechanism of pelvic ring injury. **(A)** They describe three types of lateral-compression (LC) injuries: LC-I, LC-II, and LC-III. **(B)** Three types of anterior-posterior (AP) compression injuries: AP-I, AP-II, and AP-III. **(C) A** vertical shearing mechanism. (Reprinted from Browner B, Jupiter J, Levine A, Trafton P, eds. Skeletal Trauma, 3rd ed. Philadelphia: WB Saunders, 2003: 1061, with permission from Elsevier.)

Anterior Posterior

Anterior-posterior (AP) forces are produced by direct impact to the hemipelvis, as would be the case in a pedestrian hit by an automobile, or indirectly from a force applied to the lower extremity, resulting in external-rotation injuries, symphyseal diastases, or longitudinal pubic rami fractures. Again, Young and Burgess divided AP injuries into three main categories (Figure 37.2B). Anterior-posterior type I injuries describe those with less than 2.5 cm of symphyseal diastasis in which the posterior ligaments are pristine. Anterior-posterior type II injuries are those with greater than 2.5 cm of symphyseal diastasis with injury to the ligaments of the pubic symphysis, pelvic floor, and the anterior SI ligaments. The SI joint is widened, producing the characteristic open-book hemipelvis with rotational instability (to both internal and external rotation stresses). However, it is important to note that vertical translational stability is maintained because of the integrity of the posterior SI ligaments. Anterior-posterior type III injuries describe those with complete disruption of the pubic symphysis anteriorly, the sacrotuberous and sacrospinous ligaments of the pelvic floor, and SI ligaments posteriorly. Rendering the hemipelvis completely unstable, AP-III pelvic ring disruptions are associated with the highest rate of associated neurovascular injuries and blood loss. Because AP injuries are most closely associated with hemorrhage, they put the patient at markedly higher risk for hypovolemia and shock than do, for example, LC injuries.[7]

Vertical Shear

Vertical forces applied to the pelvis, from falls most commonly, are applied longitudinally to the axis of the hemipelvis. As such, they typically produce a complete shearing of the symphyseal ligaments, pelvic floor ligaments, and the SI complex (Figure 37.2C). Such vertically oriented shearing forces result in complete pelvic ring instability, both rotationally and translationally (cephaloposterior). Like AP-III injuries, vertical shear injuries have a high incidence of hemorrhage and concomitant neurovascular insult. Both completely unstable patterns of pelvic ring disruption, they are distinguished from one other by the direction of causative force.

Combined Mechanical

Young and Burgess proposed a fourth type of pelvic ring injury, which they described as those cause by a combination of forces. The most common type, they submit, is vertical shear and lateral compression.

Tile Classification

Whereas Young and Burgess classified pelvic fractures on the basis of their mechanism of injury, Dr. Tile's system is based solely on the stability of the pelvic ring. He started with three main categories of injury, those that were stable (Tile A), those that were partially stable (Tile B), and those that were completely unstable (Tile C). Completely unstable pelvic ring disruptions are relatively uncommon, even at major trauma centers. Indeed, the literature would suggest that Tile A and B fractures constitute 70% to 80% of the total number of pelvic injuries.[8]

From his basic "A B C" framework of pelvic stability, Tile divided each category into subtypes based on the specific injury pattern. His classification is described below.

Tile A

Tile A fractures do not compromise the stability of the pelvic ring at all. A-1 injuries describe avulsion fractures of the pelvis, and A-2 injuries describe nondisplaced fractures of the pelvic ring, such as those sustained by a direct blow to the innominate bones. A-3 injuries involve transverse sacral or coccygeal fractures.

Tile B

Tile B injuries are rotationally unstable but vertically and translationally stable because of an incomplete disruption of the posterior SI complex. B-1 injuries are of the unilateral external-rotation (open-book) variety, whereas B-2 injuries describe a unilateral internal-rotation deformity (caused, as we have discussed, by a lateral compression force). B-3 injuries describe involvement of both sides of the pelvis, whether it be a bilateral open-book pelvis caused by external-rotation deformities to each hemipelvis, a "windswept" pelvis deformity caused by a lateral-compression force on one side and an external-rotation force on the other, or a bilateral closed-book pelvis caused by lateral-compression forces. They key thing to remember about all of these injury patterns is that, even in the bilateral open-book deformity, there is still only an incomplete disruption of the posterior ligaments. As a result, translational stability of the pelvis is maintained, thus defining the above as Tile B, and not C, injuries.

Tile C

Tile C injuries are both rotationally and translationally unstable because of a complete disruption of posterior pelvic stability. This may be caused by a complete fracture of the iliac wing or the sacrum or by complete tearing of the anterior and posterior SI ligaments. Tile divided his type C injuries into three categories. C-1 injuries are unilateral, with subdivisions delineated for how the posterior instability is achieved: through the iliac wing (C-1.1), the SI joint (C-1.2), or the sacrum (C-1.3). C-2 injuries describe bilateral involvement, with one hemipelvis only rotationally unstable (Tile B type) and the contralateral side completely unstable (Tile C). Finally, C-3 injuries are truly "the worst of the worst," with both sides of the pelvis being rotationally and vertically unstable.

Although memorizing the specific subtypes of each fracture pattern is probably unnecessary for the average traumatologist, it *is* very helpful to keep in mind Tile's general framework when approaching a patient with a pelvic fracture. Trauma surgeons should realize that Tile A fractures are stable and rarely associated with hemodynamic instability and that Tile C fractures are unstable and often associated with hemodynamic instability. Finally, traumatologists should understand that Tile B fractures include both external rotation and internal rotation injuries and that the implications for pelvic volume are quite different in each case: increased in the former (B-1), but decreased in the latter (B-2). These take-home points are delineated in Figure 37.3.

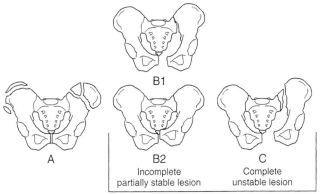

FIGURE 37.3. Tile's classification2–6 is based on the stability of the pelvic ring, dividing pelvic fractures into three main categories: those that are completely stable (Tile A), those that are rotationally unstable but vertically stable (Tile B), and those that are completely unstable (Tile C). Tile B injuries can be of the external rotation (B1) or internal rotation (B2) variety. (Reprinted from Browner B, Jupiter J, Levine A, Trafton P, eds. Skeletal Trauma, 3rd edition. Philadelphia: WB Saunders, 2003: 1062, with permission from Elsevier.)

Evaluation

With an understanding of the anatomy of the pelvic ring and the classification systems used for pelvic ring trauma, we are now ready to discuss evaluation of the trauma room patient with a pelvic fracture. Of course, evaluation involves both a comprehensive history (when possible) and a physical examination, as well as a thorough radiographic evaluation. We discuss each of these elements in turn.

Clinical Evaluation

It is important to note that the evaluation and initial care of the patient with a pelvic ring injury begins before his or her arrival in the trauma room. Indeed, at the scene of the motor vehicle accident or fall, emergency medical personnel who are trained to look for lower extremity deformity, pelvic crepitus or motion, and/or ecchymoses should apply a temporizing splint to individuals with suspected pelvic ring disruption. Several types of splints have been described, from pneumatic military antishock trousers (MAST) to pelvic stabilizing belts. In the event of a true open-book–type pelvic injury, such measures to reduce intrapelvic volume en route to the hospital can be life saving.

Once the patient arrives in the trauma room, stable pelvic fracture or not, he or she should first be assessed according to standard trauma protocol. That is to say, the A B Cs (airway, breathing, and circulation) must always be attended to before focusing on the obvious musculoskeletal deformity there may or may not be. Resuscitative measures should be instituted, usually involving the insertion of two large-bore intravenous lines and the restoration of volume in the unstable patient. If the patient is alert and communicative, obtaining an accurate history of the injury can be invaluable. Low-energy pelvic injuries are produced from falls from a low height (less than 1 meter), as is the case with an elderly person tripping on a throw rug. In contrast, high-energy injuries are usually caused by falls from heights (more than 1 meter), motor vehicle or motorcycle accidents, or crushing injuries.[8] Whereas low-energy pelvic fractures are often isolated, high-energy injuries are frequently associated with other problems, and clinical suspicion must be high to rule out concomitant injuries.

From an orthopedic perspective, a complete head-to-toe evaluation should be performed with a careful assessment of distal neurovascular status and the presence of any subtle open wounds. Palpation of the pelvic brim may reveal crepitus or abnormal motion of the hemipelvis. Compression of the iliac crest may produce abnormal rotation. Vertical traction to an uninjured lower limb can reveal translational instability. Given the high energy

required to produce pelvic ring injuries, it is important to recognize that ipsilateral lower extremity fractures are common. All long bone fractures should be identified and stabilized with splinting or skeletal traction. In the absence of a concomitant lower extremity fracture or dislocation, a salient sign of pelvic ring injury may be a leg-length discrepancy with shortening or rotational deformity of the involved side. Flank or buttock ecchymoses and swelling may be signs of significant pelvic hemorrhage. Palpating the posterior aspect of the pelvis may reveal a defect representing fracture or SI widening. The posterior SI and perineal area must be examined carefully, as a subtle wound on the buttock or in the rectum or vagina may indicate the presence of an open fracture.

Associated Injuries

Injuries to the pelvic ring usually do not happen in isolation and are often part of a constellation of injuries. From 60% to 80% of patients with a high-energy pelvic fracture have additional musculoskeletal injuries.[9] In addition to long bone fractures, injury to the lumbosacral plexus is a common concomitant orthopedic injury, occurring in about 10% of patients. Translationally unstable, Tile C injuries can have a nearly 50% incidence of such accompanying injuries.[10] For any patient with a fractured pelvis, it is also important to be vigilant for signs of genitourinary or, less frequently, bowel injury, as they can also occur concomitantly with high-energy pelvic fractures. Both bladder and urethral injuries have a high incidence rate (>10%) with pelvic trauma.[11] Any blood at the urethral meatus or expression of blood with Foley catheterization is a warning sign of a concomitant genitourinary injury. A rectal examination may reveal a high-riding or "floating" prostate. Concomitant head and intraabdominal injuries are not uncommon with high-energy pelvic trauma and are frequently the cause of death in such patients. Dalal et al.[12] reviewed 343 multi-trauma patients with pelvic ring disruptions and found a significant difference between the causes of death in people with pelvic injuries caused by lateral-compression forces (brain injury) and those caused by anterior-posterior compression forces (visceral organ injury).

Radiographic Evaluation

Before instituting measures to reduce pelvic volume (at least the more invasive ones), it is helpful to know whether the pelvic fracture sustained by the patient has resulted in an increase in pelvic potential space. For example, placing a pelvic C-clamp on the hemodynamically unstable trauma patient with a Tile A or Tile B lateral-compression type injury, in which the pelvis is already imploded onto itself, not only will be ineffective but also may delay the diagnosis of the true source of bleeding. Thus, understanding plain radiographs of the pelvis and their implication for potential pelvic volume and stability is critical.

The standard trauma radiographs include an anterior-posterior chest, a cervical spine film (with an adequate lateral image often viewed as the most important), and an anterior-posterior view of the pelvis. The anterior-posterior pelvis radiograph provides the clinician with an overall sense of the "personality" of the injury: whether it is low or high energy, whether the hemipelvis is internally rotated or externally rotated, and whether there are any stigmata of translational vertical instability. Although anterior lesions, such as a pubic rami fracture or symphyseal displacement, are often obvious, posterior lesions, such as subtle SI joint widening, sacral fractures, iliac fractures, or L5 transverse process fractures, can be more subtle. An avulsion fracture of the transverse process of L5 is especially worrisome as it may indicate an antecedent vertical shearing mechanism producing posterior instability. Avulsion fractures of the sacrum or ischial spine may indicate disruption of the sacrospinous ligament.

To better characterize the nature of the injury, so-called inlet and outlet views should be obtained in every case of pelvic ring trauma. An inlet view is taken with the patient in a supine position and the beam tilted 60° caudally (Figure 37.4A). This view gives a true axial view of

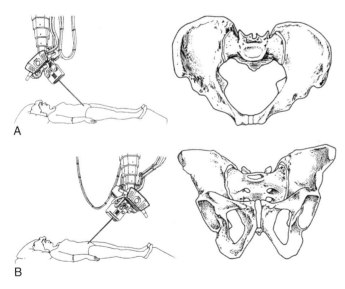

FIGURE 37.4. **(A)** An inlet view of the pelvic ring taken with the patient in a supine position and the beam tilted 60° caudally, giving a true axial view of the sacrum. **(B)** An outlet view is also obtained with the patient supine but with the beam directed 45° cephalad, giving a true anterior-posterior view of the sacrum. (Reprinted with permission from Rockwood CA Jr, Green DP, Bucholz RW, Heckman JD, eds. Rockwood and Green's Fractures in Adults, 4th ed, vol 2. Philadelphia: Lippincott-Raven, 1996: 1599.)

the sacrum and is ideal for looking at anterior to posterior displacement of the hemipelvis through the SI joint, the sacrum, or the iliac wing. An outlet view is also taken with the patient supine but with the beam directed 45° cephalad (Figure 37.4B). This gives a true anterior-posterior view of the sacrum and is therefore well suited to detect vertical displacement or rotatatory abnormalities of the hemipelvis. Dynamic stress push–pull films can also be helpful in evaluating patients with pelvic ring fractures. The most accurate results of such films require general anesthesia and can be useful in determining whether there is truly a component of translational instability in a pelvic ring injury that may appear like a Tile B on nonstress images. Tile[5] defined vertical instability as hemipelvis displacement greater than or equal to 1 cm.

Although acetabular fractures should really be thought of as separate entities from pelvic ring disruptions, these two injuries may be confused by trauma personnel. It is important for trauma teams to recognize that isolated acetabular fractures, while technically pelvic fractures, do not have the same potential for pelvic bleeding that pelvic ring disruptions do. Unless they are associated with an open-book pelvic ring injury, acetabular fractures do not benefit from external stabilization. Nonetheless, it is prudent to discuss the radiographic evaluation of acetabular fractures in this context such that their differences from pelvic ring disruptions can be delineated.

Understanding fracture lines in and around the acetabulum requires not only an anterior-posterior view of the pelvis but also oblique images. These images, often referred to as "Judet views," are composed of two 45° oblique views of the hemipelvis: one with the obturator foramen en face (the so-called obturator oblique view) and one with the iliac wing en face (the iliac oblique). Note that an obturator oblique image of one hemipelvis reveals the iliac oblique of the contralateral side. In evaluating the anterior-posterior pelvis film for an acetabular fracture, one should look at any discontinuities in the iliopectineal line (the inferior three fourths of which marks the anterior column) and the ilioischial line (posterior column). The obturator oblique view brings the anterior column into profile, and the posterior wall of the acetabulum is seen en face. In contrast, the iliac oblique shows the posterior column en face and the anterior wall in profile. Note that in most isolated acetabular fractures, the ligaments of the pubic symphysis, pelvic floor, and SI complex are completely uninvolved, and the pelvic ring remains stable.

Computed tomography (CT) has revolutionized imaging of pelvic ring injuries and offers outstanding visualization of SI widening and subtle fractures of the sacrum. Figure 37.5 illustrates the added fracture detail an axial CT scan image provides compared with plain film. Although performing CT scanning of pelvic ring disruptions has become commonplace and is currently the

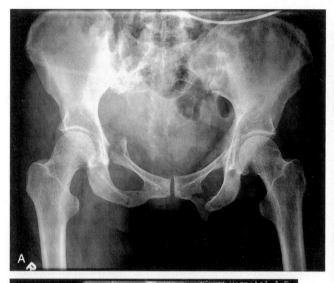

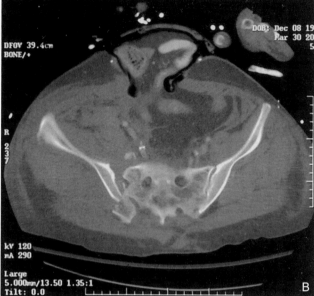

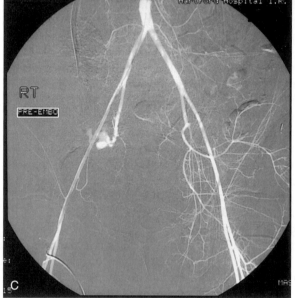

FIGURE 37.5. Ms. C.B. is a pedestrian struck by a motor vehicle. **(A)** Anterior-posterior plain film demonstrates bilateral rami fractures and a right-sided posterior fracture in the sacroiliac (SI) region. **(B)** Axial computed tomography scan more clearly delineates the posterior fracture fragments and degree of SI displacement. **(C)** Angiography demonstrated a right-sided internal iliac artery hemorrhage.

standard of care, obtaining three-dimensional reconstruction images has become possible at many medical centers and provides extraordinary visualization of the pelvis in space (Figure 37.6).

Hemodynamic Status and Emergent Stabilization

It cannot be emphasized enough that as the physical examination is occurring the patient's hemodynamic status must continuously be carefully monitored. Establishing two 14- to 16-gauge intravenous lines in the upper extremity is a good idea to allow for appropriate fluid resuscitation. Avoiding lower extremity access sites is probably wise in the setting of a pelvic ring fracture because of the possibility of damaged venous circulation in that region. If the patient remains hemodynamically unstable, and in the absence of obvious external hemorrhage, internal bleeding must of course be suspected. From a general surgical perspective, the presence of intraabdominal bleeding can be ruled out with either a deep peritoneal lavage (DPL) or, less invasively, an abdominal ultrasound examination at the bedside or a CT scan. In the presence of a disrupted pelvic ring, particularly in those force patterns that produce an external rotation open-book deformity of one or both sides of the pelvis, retroperitoneal hemorrhage must be suspected as well.

Retroperitoneal hemorrhage can be associated with massive loss of a patient's intravascular volume, as the retroperitoneal space can hold up to 4 L of blood volume.

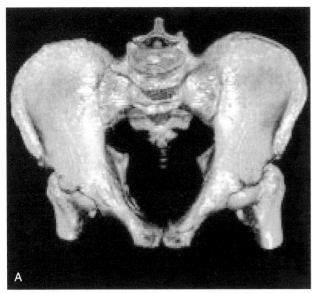

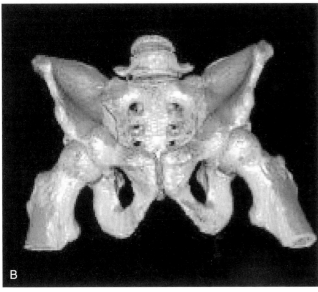

FIGURE 37.6. Three-dimensional reconstruction images of a normal pelvis, with (**A**) inlet and (**B**) outlet projections.

The most common cause of such hemorrhage in the setting of pelvic trauma is a disruption of the venous plexus in the posterior pelvis. Less commonly, but possible, is injury to larger vessels, such as the external or internal iliac. Arterial injury is much less common, and only a small percentage of patients with pelvic fractures require embolization. In a 5-year review of 800 patients admitted to a Level I trauma center with pelvic fractures, Agolini et al.[13] found that only 1.9% required embolization. Unless the potential space is decreased with external stabilization, venous bleeding in the presence of an open-book type of pelvis injury may continue undeterred until the patient is in shock. Thus, the chief determination that the trauma surgeon, in conjunction with the orthopedist,

must make in this context is whether stabilizing the pelvis is appropriate. There are several different options for decreasing retroperitoneal volume emergently, thus helping to tamponade venous bleeding. As mentioned previously, one well-described way to do this is before the patient even arrives in the hospital with the application of MAST. Such pneumatic trousers work by increasing peripheral vascular resistance as well as by physically splinting previously moving fracture fragments. After they are applied en route, MAST should not be removed until intravenous access is established and the patient is in a controlled environment, such as an operating room. Military antishock trousers are not intended for indefinite use, as skin problems and compartment syndromes have been well described with prolonged use.

Often, of course, patients with pelvic ring injuries are not diagnosed in the field, and they arrive in the trauma room without MAST applied. In a hemodynamically unstable patient with an open-book pelvic ring injury, emergent pelvic stabilization can be a matter of life or death. It is important to reiterate that not all pelvic ring fractures will benefit from pelvic stabilization. It makes sense that only lesions that increase the potential space in the pelvis for hemorrhage, such as partially stable open-book fractures (i.e., a Tile B-1 injury) and all completely unstable (Tile C) injuries, would benefit from interventions aimed at reducing pelvic volume. There are several reasonable means to achieve this end, such as wrapping a sheet or placing a compressive strap circumferentially around the pelvis or applying a pelvic clamp or a more traditional anterior external fixator.

Noninvasive pelvic stabilization with a circumferential compression strap has been shown in a biomechanical cadaveric study to be an effective means to achieve reduction of external-rotation type pelvic fractures.[14] Wrapping a sheet around the pelvis can also be effective in closing down anterior symphyseal diastasis. A "bean bag" positioning device can be applied to the flanks of the patient to help reduce pelvic volume as well.[15]

Using skeletal traction through the injured femoral supracondylar region is helpful as an adjunctive measure by pulling the displaced hemipelvis into a more reduced position, helping to tamponade venous bleeding. Tile recommends using 30 pounds of traction through skeletal pins in the distal femur to help maintain pelvic ring disruptions in the reduced position. By hanging weight off the injured extremity, the hemipelvis is given an internal rotation force, thereby closing down anterior diastasis. This is of course most effective in achieving stability if there is integrity to the posterior ligaments. The added benefit of skeletal traction is that it prevents shortening of the hemipelvis in the indefinite period of time between injury and definitive operative stabilization.

Another way to emergently stabilize the pelvis is by applying a pelvic clamp in the emergency room to the

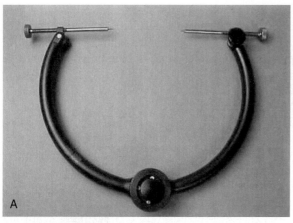
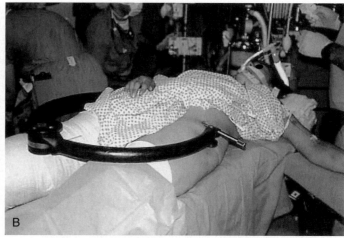

FIGURE 37.7. **(A)** An example of a particular pelvic C-clamp model developed by Dr. Bruce Browner. **(B)** It is easy to access the abdomen or the perineum, depending on which way the clamp is swung.

posterior aspect of the pelvis.[16,17] Application of a pelvic C-clamp is appealing because it can be applied relatively quickly in the emergency room while allowing the trauma surgeon adequate access to the abdomen (Figure 37.7). Pohlemann et al.[18] have described a safe anatomic landmark for pin placement as the region on the lateral aspect of the iliac wing where a palpable "groove" is formed by angulations of the lateral cortex. In general, pin insertion should be in the cancellous bone superior to the acetabulum in the posterior aspect of the pelvis.

Although pelvic C-clamps are in use at many medical centers, the more standard method for controlling unstable pelvic ring injuries remains the application of an anterior external fixator with two or three pins placed in the anterior iliac crest and joined by an anterior frame.[19,20] Although they can conceivably be applied in the emergency room like pelvic C-clamps, anterior fixators are more commonly placed in the operating room. When laparotomies are necessary, the application of these fixators may unfortunately be further delayed.

During the evaluation and resuscitation of the pelvic-fractured patient, the timing of placement of the pelvic stabilization device is sometimes debated. At our trauma center, it is thought that a pelvic C-clamp should be applied initially in all hemodynamically unstable patients with unstable pelvic fractures. Delaying pelvic stabilization to the operating room may allow retroperitoneal hemorrhaging to continue in the interim and puts the patient at unnecessary risk as the trauma room's "golden hour" of resuscitative opportunity elapses. If the patient becomes stable with this simple orthopedic intervention, the need for a laparotomy may be precluded. Trauma surgeons in Europe, who take care of both orthopedic and intraabdominal injuries, also proceed in this fashion, with the application of a pelvic stabilizer being seen as a top priority in the emergency room.[21,22]

Whether the pelvis is stabilized with a C-clamp or an anterior frame, external fixators exert their effectiveness not only by reducing pelvic volume but also by preventing disruption of blood clots. However, such fixators alone do not provide sufficient posterior stabilization if the posterior pelvic ligaments are disrupted. Both pelvic clamps, as well as more traditional external frames, have been shown to restore adequate stability to Tile B, but not Tile C, fractures.[17,23] Using pelvic external fixation in conjunction with skeletal traction through the involved leg may help control vertical instability more effectively, although not completely.

Only if the patient remains hemodynamically unstable despite adequately stabilizing the pelvis and findings on DPL (or abdominal ultrasound or CT scan) are negative should arterial bleeding be assumed and angiography performed. This is a critical point for the trauma team to understand. Because the vast majority of pelvic bleeding originates from venous sources,[24] patients with open-book pelvic ring injuries should be sent to the angiography suite only after the application of a pelvic stabilization device has *failed* to provide hemodynamic stability. In contrast, patients who are hemodynamically unstable with closed-book pelves could be considered for earlier angiography (albeit still after intraabdominal sources of hemorrhage are ruled out). In order to clearly delineate this point, consider the following contrasting cases of Ms. C.B. and Mr. J.W.

Ms. C.B. is a 54-year-old female pedestrian struck by a motor vehicle. She came to the trauma room hemodynamically unstable, despite plain films that showed a relatively closed-book pelvic ring injury (see Figure 37.5A). Not surprisingly, given the nature of her pelvic fractures, Ms. C.B. remained hemodynamically unstable despite emergent application of a compressive pelvic sheet in the trauma room. After abdominal ultrasound was performed and showed no intraabdominal bleeding, the

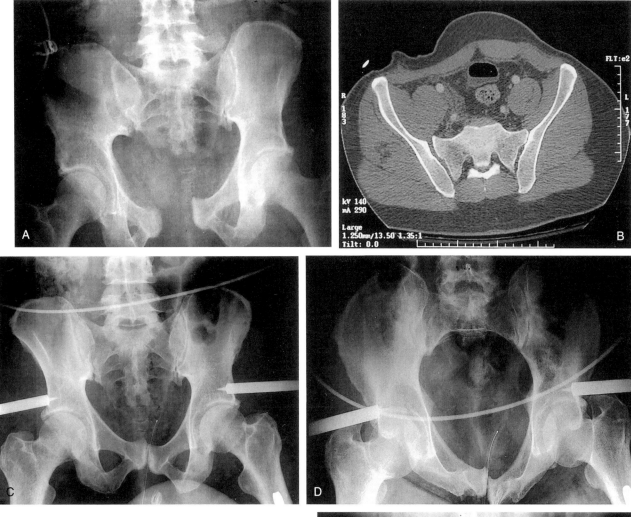

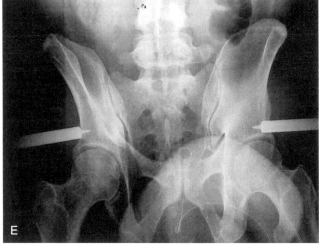

FIGURE 37.8. Mr. J.W. was involved in a head-on motor vehicle accident. **(A)** Anterior-posterior plain film demonstrates approximately 4 cm of symphyseal diastasis, suggesting injury to the ligaments of the pubic symphysis and pelvic floor. The right sacroiliac (SI) joint is widened, implicating injury to the anterior SI ligaments on this side. This characteristic open-book hemipelvis is consistent with a Young-Burgess AP-II or Tile B1 pelvic ring disruption. **(B)** Axial computed tomography scan lends support to this being a Tile B (and not a Tile C) injury, because, although there is right-sided *anterior* SI widening, the *posterior* SI joint spaces are symmetric. Therefore, although the pelvic ring is rotationally unstable, its intact posterior SI ligaments confer to it vertical and translational stability. **(C–E).** Emergent application of a pelvic C-clamp effectively "closed" the pelvic ring, as demonstrated by anterior-posterior (C), inlet (D), and outlet (E) images.

patient was taken urgently to angiography where a right-sided internal iliac artery hemorrhage was identified and successfully embolized (see Figure 37.5C).

Mr. J.W. is a 52-year-old male driver of an automobile involved in a high-speed head-on collision. He too came to the trauma room hemodynamically unstable, but (unlike Ms. C.B.) with radiographic findings of an open-book pelvic ring injury (Figure 37.8A). Rather than rush this patient off to the angiography suite or to the operating room, the traumatologist reviewed his plain films and astutely identified an unstable pelvic ring injury consistent with an AP-type mechanism producing an external-rotation deformity of the hemipelvis. As a result, the orthopedic surgeon was consulted, and a C-clamp was applied to Mr. J.W.'s pelvis within 30 minutes of his arrival to the trauma room. Moments after application of the C-clamp, presumably because of the dramatic reduction of his pelvic volume (Figure 37.8C–E) and subsequent tamponade of venous hemorrhage, J.W.'s heart rate and blood pressure normalized. It is critically important to recognize the folly in taking a patient such as Mr. J.W. to angiography before applying simple pelvic stabilization measures in the trauma room.

Once a patient becomes hemodynamically stable, an additional treatment question must be asked: Does the pelvic ring need to be fixed? To answer this question, the orthopedic surgeon should be consulted—if he or she is not already involved in the case. Through orthopedic consultation, the need for further imaging studies or surgery can be determined. The orthopedist may choose to fix certain fractures in the first day or two, whereas in other instances waiting a couple of weeks may be deemed preferable. Although discussing techniques for definitive fixation of the pelvis is beyond the scope of this chapter, it is important to realize that the orthopedic surgeon has two goals when dealing with unstable pelvic ring injuries. The first goal, to reduce pelvic volume when appropriate, is immediate and can be a matter of life or death. The second goal is to restore the integrity of the pelvic ring and to give the patient the best chance to avoid long-term dysfunction from his or her injury. This involves preventing malunion and nonunion and restoring leg lengths as best as possible. The timing of surgery is dictated by the patient's stability and the condition of the surrounding soft tissues. The specific surgical approach used depends on both the integrity of the skin and the specific fracture pattern needing to be fixed. It is important that traumatologists and orthopedists communicate with each other so that the placement of suprapubic tubes or colostomy pouches, if possible, are not in line with the preferred orthopedic incision.

No discussion of pelvic fractures is complete without mentioning the complications that can result from both the injury itself and the operative treatment. Nerve injury can of course result from either the initial injury or the surgical manipulation. The overall prevalence of nerve injury in patients with pelvic fractures is approximately 10% to 15%.[25] Deep venous thromboses are common after pelvic trauma, in the range of 35% to 50%, and antithrombotic prophylaxis is warranted.[26,27] The incidence of symptomatic pulmonary embolism (PE) is in the range of 2% to 10% and that of fatal PE lower, from 0.5% to 2%. Infection is of course a serious complication, and great care should be taken to avoid operating through damaged skin and subcutaneous tissues. Even in

the best of circumstances, severe pelvic ring disruptions have a profound effect on future quality of life. Although appropriate emergent care may be life saving, lingering pain from more severe fractures is unfortunately quite common.[28]

In summary, unlike most other orthopedic injuries, high-energy trauma to the pelvic ring has the potential to be life threatening. Although it is obvious that the orthopedic surgeon should be well versed in the diagnosis and management of pelvic ring injuries, it is important to recognize the key role that all caregivers have in successfully managing these fractures. All trauma personnel, from the on-the-scene paramedic, to the emergency room physician, to the trauma team leader, must have a high clinical suspicion for these injuries in patients who have been involved in high-energy falls or motor vehicle accidents. Recognizing patients at risk for unstable pelvic fractures, vigilantly monitoring their response to resuscitation, and applying acute pelvic stabilization when it is both appropriate clinically (i.e., in the setting of hemodynamic instability) and radiographically (i.e., in open-book type ring disruptions) can indeed be the difference between life and death.

Critique

Hemorrhage is the leading cause of death directly related to pelvic fractures. Sepsis is the second leading cause of death directly related to a pelvic fracture. Proctoscopy is an essential component in the evaluation of this patient to rule out an associated rectal injury. On occasion, a rectal injury is obvious when digital rectal examination determines that there is a spicule or an edge of fragmented bone penetrating the rectum. If there is evidence of an associated rectal injury, the patient should undergo a colostomy to divert the fecal stream.

Answer (E)

References

1. Vrahas M, Hearn TC, Diangelo D, Kellam J, Tile M. Ligamentous contributors to pelvis stability. Orthopedics 1995; 18:271–274.
2. Tile M, Hearn T. Biomechanics. In Tile M, ed. Fractures of the Pelvis and Acetabulum, 2nd ed. Baltimore: Williams & Wilkins, 1995; 22–36.
3. Tile M. Pelvic ring fractures: should they be fixed? J Bone Joint Surg Br 1988; 70:1–12.
4. Tile M. Classification. In Tile M, ed. Fractures of the Pelvis and Acetabulum, 2nd ed. Baltimore: Williams & Wilkins, 1995; 66–101.
5. Tile M. Acute pelvic fractures I: causation and classification. J Am Acad Orthop Surg 1996; 4:143–151.
6. Tile M. Acute pelvic fractures II: principles of management. J Am Acad Orthop Surg 1996; 4:152–161.

7. Young JW, Burgess AR, Brumback RJ, et al. Pelvic fractures: value of plain radiography in early assessment and management. Radiology 1986; 160:445–451.

8. Gansslen A, Pohlemann T, Paul CH, et al. Epidemiology of pelvic ring injuries. Injury 1996; 27(Suppl 1):S-A13–20.

9. McMurtry RY, Walton D, Dickinson D, et al. Pelvic disruption in the polytraumatized patient. A management protocol. Clin Orthop 1980; 151:22–30.

10. Slatis P, Huittinen VM. Double vertical fractures of the pelvis: a report on 163 patients. Acta Chir Scand 1972; 138:799–807.

11. Colapinto V. Trauma to the pelvis: urethral injury. Clin Orthop 1980; 151:46–55.

12. Dalal S, Burgess AR, Siegel J, et al. Pelvic fracture in multiple trauma: classification by mechanism is key to pattern of organ injury, resuscitative requirements, and outcome. J Trauma 1989; 29:1000–1002.

13. Agolini SF, Shah K, Jaffe J, et al. Arterial embolization is a rapid and effective technique for controlling pelvic fracture hemorrhage. J Trauma 1997; 43:395–399.

14. Bottlang M, Simpson T, Sigg J, et al. Noninvasive reduction of open-book pelvic fractures by circumferential compression. J Orthop Trauma 2002; 16:367–373.

15. Falcone RE, Thomas BW. "Bean bag" pelvic stabilization. Ann Emerg Med 1996; 28:458.

16. Buckle R, Browner BD, Morandi M. A new external fixation device for emergent reduction and stabilization of displaced pelvic fractures associated with massive hemorrhage. J Orthop Trauma 1993; 7:177–178.

17. Ganz R, Krushell RJ, Jakob RP, et al. The antishock pelvic clamp. Clin Orthop 1991; 267:71–78.

18. Pohlemann T, Braune C, Gansslen A, et al. The pelvic emergency clamps: anatomic landmarks for a safe primary application. J Orthop Trauma 2004; 18:102–105.

19. Kellam JF. The role of external fixation in pelvic disruptions. Clin Orthop 1989; 241:66–82.

20. Riemer BL, Butterfield SL, Diamond DL, et al. Acute mortality associated with injuries to the pelvic ring: the role of early patient mobilization and external fixation. J Trauma 1993; 35:671–677.

21. Nerlich M, Maghsudi M. Algorithms for early management of pelvic fractures. Injury 1996; 27(Suppl 1):S-A29–37.

22. Pohlemann T, Bosch U, Gansslen A, et al. The Hannover experience in management of pelvic fractures. Clin Orthop 1994; 305:69–80.

23. Witschger P, Heini P, Ganz R. Pelvic clamps for controlling shock in posterior pelvic ring injuries: application, biomechanical aspects and initial clinical results. Orthopade 1992; 21:393–399.

24. Mucha P Jr, Welch TJ. Hemorrhage in pelvic fractures. Surg Clin North Am 1988; 68:757–773.

25. Weis EB. Subtle neurological injuries in pelvic fractures. J Trauma 1984; 24:983–985.

26. Geertz WH, Code KI, Jay RM, et al. A prospective study of venous thromboembolism after major trauma. N Engl J Med 1994; 331:1601–1606.

27. Buerger PM, Peoples JB, Lemmon GW, et al. Risk of pulmonary emboli in patients with pelvic fractures. Am Surg 1993; 59:505–508.

28. Draijer F, Egbers HJ, Havemann D. Quality of life after pelvic ring injuries: follow-up results of a prospective study. Arch Orthop Trauma Surg 1997; 116:22–26.

38
Lower Extremities

Tina A. Maxian and Michael J. Bosse

Case Scenario

A 28-year-old motorcyclist, who lost control of his bike, is brought to the trauma bay by the emergency medical technicians for evaluation and definitive management of multiple injuries. The patient has been hemodynamically stable throughout his transport and upon arrival. He is alert, oriented, and complaining only of left lower extremity pain. Advanced Trauma Life Support protocol was initiated. In addition to scattered torso abrasions and superficial lacerations of bilateral lower extremities, the patient was found to have an unstable left knee. The involved extremity has no palpable dorsalis pedis and posterior tibial pulses. Plain radiography of the neck and chest demonstrated no obvious injuries. Focused abdominal sonography revealed no fluid accumulation. After life-threatening injuries were ruled out, the knee dislocation was reduced with no return of pulses. What is the most appropriate management plan at this time?

(A) Operative exploration
(B) Expectant (observation) management
(C) Traction application and admission
(D) Arthroscopy
(E) Arteriography

Surgery may be deemed urgent in order to save an extremity or to save the patient's life. Although this chapter deals with treatment of a variety of lower extremity conditions, in all cases, the overall condition of the patient must be kept in mind. In some clinical scenarios, a compromised limb that may be salvageable when occurring in isolation may need to be amputated from a patient in extremis in order to save the patient's life. Always, preservation of the patient's life supercedes preservation of the limb. Additionally, should a patient become unsta-

ble, the surgeon must be prepared to abandon complex procedures and resort to simpler ones, coming back later for staged procedures once the patient is more stable.

Foremost, the surgeon must have a plan before embarking on an emergent procedure, and the goals of that plan should be kept in mind in the operating room. Patients who require emergent surgery may be extremely ill and may not tolerate prolonged procedures. The temptation to do "just a little more" should be resisted, as a short procedure can insidiously, and unintentionally, become a long one if the surgeon is distracted from the goals, resulting in additional and unnecessary physiologic stress on an already sick patient.

Infections

Necrotizing Soft Tissue Infections

The challenge with necrotizing soft tissue infections is in making the diagnosis. For the septic patient with an obviously infected and necrotic limb, the diagnosis is straightforward. The difficulty is identifying the patient with a necrotizing soft tissue infection before it progresses to overwhelming sepsis.[1-4]

Necrotizing soft tissue infections destroy fat, fascia, and even muscle.[2,4,5] They can occur at any age and tend to occur in those who are immunocompromised through advanced or extremely young age, diabetes, or chronic renal failure or in the extremities with local compromise because of peripheral vascular disease or lymphadema.[6,7] Patients may or may not have previous trauma. If present, often the trauma is trivial.

Patients may have cellulitis with pain out of proportion to the apparent involvement. They may or may not have systemic signs or symptoms.[1] Crepitus on examination or subcutaneous air on plain radiographs is virtually pathognomonic.[4] As the infection progresses, the skin involvement changes from a cellulitic appearance to a more necrotic one, with bullae and violaceous skin color changes.[2]

The most common cause of single microbe infection is group A *Streptococcus*; however, necrotizing soft tissue infections may be polymicrobial or may be caused by a myriad of Gram-positive and Gram-negative organisms acting alone.[1–3] Initial treatment is broad-spectrum antibiotics, resuscitation, and support for those patients who are systemically ill and surgical debridement.

Once in the operating room, all signs of infection in the skin, soft tissues, and muscles should be debrided. If the entire extremity is compromised, then a guillotine amputation should be performed at the level that will provide clean margins. The wounds should not be closed. Serial debridements at 24 to 48 hours are required until viable margins are obtained. With massive debridements, early plastic surgery consultation may be advisable in order to obtain appropriate soft tissue coverage. Hyperbaric oxygen therapy has been reported to improve outcome in some small patient series[2,3,8]; however, there are no randomized trials that clearly demonstrate any improved efficacy with its use in necrotizing soft tissue infections. Vacuum-assisted dressings have been of some use in the management of soft tissue infections in limited clinical studies.[9]

Septic Joints

Typically, a septic joint has a painful range of motion, with overlying warmth and erythema. The patient may or may not have systemic symptoms of fever and malaise and an elevated peripheral white blood cell count.[10] Usually, the C-reactive protein and erythrocyte sedimentation rates are elevated.[10–12] The diagnosis of septic arthritis, however, is made through aspiration of the joint fluid, which is then sent for Gram stain, cell count, differential, and crystal analysis (to rule out crystalline arthropathy).[10]

An emergent washout of the joint is usually performed when organisms are seen on the Gram stain, for white cell counts >50,000, and for neutrophil counts >90% of the joint fluid total white blood cell count.[10] Joint irrigation and debridement should be performed emergently to minimize articular cartilage destruction. In children, growth disturbances,[13] such as premature physeal closure or, conversely, complete physeal separations,[14] may result if the joint is not washed out expeditiously. The washout may be arthroscopic or open; there are no clinical data supporting the superior efficacy (or lack thereof) of arthroscopic washout over open arthrotomy.

For infected total joint replacements, the urgency is usually not as great as when a native joint is at risk unless the patient is septic. Infections that occur within the first 2 weeks of joint replacement may be treated with an irrigation and debridement with polyethylene liner exchange, so the surgeon proceeding with such a washout should be sure that the correct components are available.[15,16]

For infections occurring after the first 2 weeks, eradication of the infection is better accomplished with a two-stage procedure consisting of removal of the components and placement of an antibiotic spacer, followed by later reimplantation of new components once the infection has been cleared.[15,16] If the entire prosthesis must be removed, any surgeon entertaining removal of an infected total joint should have all the necessary removal equipment available and should be able to construct an antibiotic spacer with the appropriate levels of antibiotics.[17]

For patients who are truly septic and in extremis due to an infected total knee or infected antibiotic spacer, serious consideration should be given to emergent guillotine above the knee amputation.[18,19] An emergent hip disarticulation or resection arthroplasty would be the equivalent procedure at the hip, but this has been infrequently reported.[20]

The Nontraumatic Ischemic Extremity

The patient with acute limb ischemia will present with some or all of the classic "P's" for ischemia: pain, pulselessness, pallor, poikilothermia, paralysis, and paresthesias. Because this patient group tends to have a history of peripheral vascular disease,[21] handheld Doppler devices should be used to evaluate for pulses when none are palpable.

Preoperatively, one needs to consider the cause and duration of the ischemia, as both play roles in determining the type of surgery required. Embolic events tend to have sudden onset of symptoms, occur in patients with a recent cardiac event (myocardial infarction, new-onset arrhythmia), and may have a minimal history of claudication. Thrombotic events tend to have a vague onset in patients with a history of claudication. The Society for Vascular Surgery–International Society for Cardiovascular Surgery (SVS-ISCVS) has classified acute limb ischemia to facilitate communication and aid with clinical decision making (Table 38.1) for both nontraumatic and traumatic ischemia.[22]

Surgical decision making for this patient population must also take into account the patients' frequent significant comorbidities, especially diabetes mellitus and cardiac and pulmonary conditions.[23,24] If no allergies or other contraindications are present, all patients should be given aspirin and started on a heparin protocol.[21] Basic laboratory tests to evaluate renal function and to determine if acidosis or hyperkalemia are present should be performed.[21] An electrocardiogram to evaluate for arrythmias or myocardial infarction should be obtained, as most embolic phenomena tend to be cardiac in origin.[21,25] The patient should be hydrated.[26] For those facing surgery and with a significant cardiac history, a

TABLE 38.1. SVS-ISCVS clinical categories of acute limb ischemia.

Category	Description	Capillary return	Muscle weakness	Sensory loss	Doppler signals Arterial	Venous
I. Viable	Not immediately threatened	Intact	None	None	Audible, pulsatile flow	Audible
II. Threatened	Reversible if relieved quickly	Slow			No pulsatile flow, inaudible	Audible
a. Marginally	Salvageable if promptly treated		None	Minimal (toes or none)		
b. Immediately	Salvageable with immediate revascularization		Mild, moderate	More than toes, associated with rest pain		
III. Irreversible	Amputation required	Absent (marbling)	Profound (rigor)	Profound (anesthetic)	Inaudible	Inaudible

Source: Adapted from Rutherford RB, Baker D, Ernst C, et al. Recommended standards for reports dealing with lower extremity ischemia: revised version. J Vasc Surg 1997; 26:517–538, with permission from Elsevier.

Swan-Ganz catheter may be necessary for fluid management.[21,26] The level of demarcation on the lower extremity, as well as any neurologic deficits, may give an indication as to the level of obstruction.

For patients with Level I or IIa ischemia with less severe symptoms of a more chronic duration,[24] an attempt at endovascular revascularization may be a reasonable choice. For those with Level III symptoms, prompt amputation may be life saving, with any attempt at revascularization placing the patient at risk from reperfusion injury with renal dysfunction, pulmonary insufficiency, and/or cardiovascular collapse.[27]

For an amputation, the level at which to perform the amputation and whether or not to close the wound become the primary concerns. For an extremely sick patient or when the margins of necrosis are unclear, a guillotine amputation may be best done emergently, with a plan to perform a second look and revision with closure at a later time. If, however, clean, viable flaps are available and the patient is stable, the surgeon may proceed with immediate closure.

For those with Level II ischemia caused by an embolism or thrombus in situ, an open catheter thromboembolectomy is warranted.[21] The femoral artery is exposed and a thromboembolectomy performed taking care not to injure or dissect the vessel. In some cases, exposure below the knee may be performed to gain access to a vessel. After removing the embolus or thrombus, angiography is used to verify patency of the vascular system. If an occlusion persists, a bypass, or even amputation, may be required.[23,28] Distal fasciotomies should be performed for all Level IIb revascularizations.[21]

Compartment Syndrome

A compartment syndrome occurs in an osseofascial compartment when either the volume of the compartment is decreased (as with occlusive dressings or a cast) or the contents of the compartment increase (e.g., postperfusion swelling, hemorrhage). In either scenario, the intracompartmental pressure increases and, if not relieved, eventually exceeds the capillary perfusion pressure, causing ischemia.[29]

A compartment syndrome can occur with crush injuries, burns, and fractures or after revascularization with reperfusion. Compartment syndromes may also occur with open fractures,[30] because, although traumatic wounds may cause tears in the fascia, these tears by no means ensure decompression of the compartments. Compartment syndromes do not have to have a traumatic etiology. Certain drugs (statins) or nutritional supplements (creatine) have also been associated with compartment syndromes.[31] Clotting abnormalities (anticoagulants, hemophilia) may cause excessive bleeding after seemingly innocuous trauma and result in a compartment syndrome.[32,33]

The classic signs and symptoms of a compartment syndrome include pain out of proportion to the injury and uncontrollable pain in a patient who previously was relatively comfortable.[34] Pain may also occur with passive range of motion of the ankle and toes. Compartments are tense on examination. Paresthesias and pulselessness usually occur late and are of no use in early diagnosis.[34,35] In an unconscious patient or a patient with a spinal cord injury, the patient may not be able to communicate or to sense that he or she is in pain. Pain may also be absent in patients with spinal or epidural anesthesia.[36–39] These confounding factors have led to the use of compartment pressure measurements to assist with the diagnosis.

Compartment syndrome is generally taken to exist when compartment pressures are within 30 mm Hg of the diastolic pressure.[34,35] A compartment syndrome may exist with lower pressures in a hypotensive patient,[34] as the hypotension contributes to ischemia. Undoubtedly, patients may have compartment pressures within 30 mm Hg of the diastolic pressure who do not have clinically

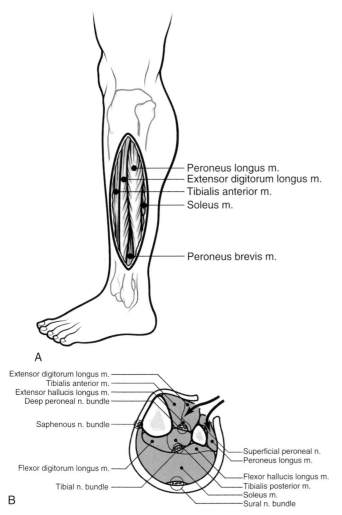

FIGURE 38.1. Lateral fasciotomy incision of the leg. **(A)** Incision after compartment release. **(B)** Path of the surgical release in the transverse plane.

apparent compartment syndromes.[40] The diagnosis needs to be bolstered by clinical examination.

Once the diagnosis of a compartment syndrome is made, the patient should be taken emergently for fasciotomies. The fasciotomies should release the skin and fascia over the muscle. For a two-incision approach in the leg, the lateral incision does not need to be taken proximal to the fibular head or distal to the lateral malleolus: this is a tendonous region, and, consequently, there is no muscle tissue to be decompressed here (Figure 38.1A). Conversely, the fasciotomy incisions should not be minimal dermatomies with subcutaneous release of the fascia. The skin itself may act as a constrictive barrier if not released adequately.[41]

For a two-incision technique in the leg,[42] the lateral incision is centered over the approximate fascial plane between the anterior and lateral compartments, although this may be difficult to identify in obese patients or in a markedly swollen limb. Once the skin is incised, the fascia over the anterior and lateral compartments is released,

taking care to protect the superficial peroneal nerve in the lateral compartment (Figure 38.1B). The medial incision is made posteromedially (Figure 38.2A), taking care to identify and protect the saphenous vein if encountered. The superficial posterior compartment fascia is released; then the muscles are pealed off the posterior aspect of the tibia until the deep posterior compartment is encountered and its fascia released (Figure 38.2B).

To release the compartments of the thigh,[43] a lateral incision is made. The tensor fascia lata is incised (Figure 38.3A). Next, the intermuscular septum between the lateral and posterior compartments is identified and released in order to decompress the posterior compartment (Figure 38.3B). At this point, the medial compartment is reassessed. If it is still tense on clinical examination, or if repeated pressure measurements still indicate elevated pressures, then a separate medial incision is made to release the medial compartment.

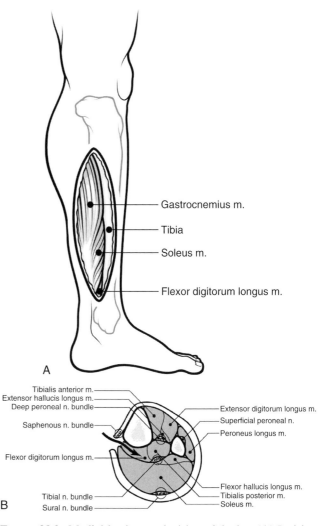

FIGURE 38.2. Medial fasciotomy incision of the leg. **(A)** Incision after compartment release. **(B)** Path of the surgical release in the transverse plane.

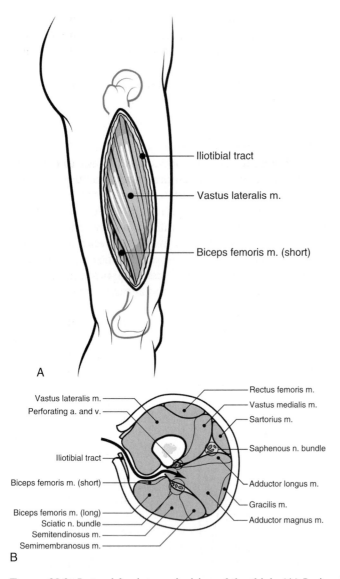

A

B

FIGURE 38.3. Lateral fasciotomy incision of the thigh. **(A)** Incision after compartment release. **(B)** Path of the surgical release in the transverse plane.

Gluteal compartment syndrome, although rare, does occur and is released through an incision similar to a posterior approach to the hip.[36,44] The fascia of the gluteus maximus, gluteus medias, and tensor fascia lata must be released while protecting the neurovascular structures.

Like compartment syndromes of the leg or thigh, those of the foot are characterized by pain, swelling, and elevated intracompartmental pressures,[29,45,46] Generally, to adequately release the interossei and adductor compartments, dorsal incisions are made medial to the second metatarsal and lateral to the fourth metatarsal.[29] Care must be taken to make these incisions in the appropriate locations to avoid necrosis of the skin bridge that can occur if the incisions are made too close together. The medial, superficial, calcaneal, and lateral compartments are decompressed through a medial incision over the

medial side of the calcaneus.[29] Opinions differ, however, on the need to decompress foot compartment syndromes, as the residual deformity associated with the fasciotomies may exceed that of the intrinsic foot contractures.

In all cases, obviously necrotic muscle should be debrided. If the muscle in all compartments is dead, then an amputation to a viable level should be performed. There are extremely limited data demonstrating the efficacy of hyperbaric oxygen therapy in the treatment of compartment syndromes.[47] Vacuum-assisted dressings to fasciotomies have been shown to decrease serum myoglobin levels in a rabbit model of compartment syndrome,[48] but no similar clinical studies with humans have been published to date.

Trauma

Irreducible Dislocations

Irreducible dislocations of the lower extremity are those in which a closed manipulation does not result in joint reduction. The reduction may be blocked by interposed soft tissues or incarcerated fracture fragments. The surgical goals are to remove the blocks to reduction, by open means when necessary, to repair any vascular problems that remain after reduction, and to provide fixation when necessary to keep the joint reduced.

Hip

Irreducible dislocations of the hip can be caused by acetabular fracture dislocations with the head "button holed" through the capsule, large incarcerated fragments contained in the joint (Figure 38.4), or acetabular

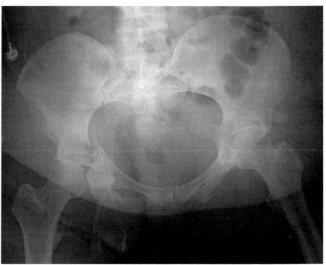

FIGURE 38.4. A radiograph of a hip fracture dislocation with an incarcerated fragment. The fragment is blocking concentric reduction of the right hip.

fracture dislocations accompanied by femoral head fracture. Overall, outcomes for patients with irreducible hip dislocations tend to be poor.[49] Additionally, outcomes related to the hip are worse with longer times to reduction.[50,51]

A surgeon faced with an irreducible dislocation of the hip should be comfortable with complex acetabular surgery before proceeding; otherwise, the patient should be transferred to a surgeon who regularly deals with such surgery. However, if faced with a progressive neurologic deficit or vascular injury, or should a neurovascular deficit occur after a successful, closed reduction, the patient needs emergent open reduction or transfer to a facility with staff capable of performing one.[52–54]

Knee

The irreducible dislocation of the knee is characterized by a skin pucker, representing the medial femoral condyle "button holed" through the capsule.[55–57] Patients with this injury need emergent reduction to avoid skin necrosis, which can cause disastrous long-term results.[57] Open reduction is required if the knee cannot be reduced with closed manipulation under general anesthesia. If a vascular injury is also present, the patient requires emergent repair, as with any vascular injury. For knee dislocations with a normal vascular examination before and after reduction, arteriography does not need to be performed, and the patient may be monitored with serial examinations for the first 48 hours.[58,59] Emergent ligamentous repair is not recommended,[60–62] and the patient may need to be placed in knee-spanning external fixation if the knee is unstable after reduction or if large areas of soft tissue compromise are present that require management and would be inappropriate for treatment in a splint or knee immobilizer.

Ankle and Foot

Irreducible ankle and foot dislocations are most commonly seen in ankle fracture dislocations or in subtalar dislocations. Such injuries require open reductions emergently to reduce tenting on soft tissue or if a vascular injury is present that does not improve with closed manipulation.

Irreducible subtalar dislocations tend to occur with higher energy mechanisms. In one series,[63] one third of subtalar dislocations required open reductions. The key to an open reduction is to identify the direction of the dislocation in order to decide on the surgical approach that will gain access to the structures most likely responsible for blocking the reduction. Soft tissue entrapment blocks reduction in 50% of irreducible reductions. For lateral dislocations, the posterior tibialis, flexor hallucis, or flexor digitalis longus tendons tend to be the blocking

structures.[63] For medial dislocations, the blocking structures tend again to be the tibialis posterior and the flexor digitalis longus or the talar head button holed through the capsules.[63] Bony blocks or capsular incarcerations may also occur in either dislocation direction.

Femoral Neck Fractures in the Young

"Young" is generally defined as less than 50 years of age, although for certain individuals the age to consider urgent reduction of a femoral neck fracture may be extended to 65 years or older. Femoral neck fractures in young patients usually result from high-energy trauma. Fractures resulting from a fall or from minimal trauma (other than displaced stress fractures) occur because the bone is compromised by some metabolic process (e.g., osteoporosis or chronic renal disease). In these cases, fixation may be inadequate, or the patient's condition may be such that definitive treatment is hemiarthroplasty.

The femoral head receives its blood supply through retinacular vessels within the capsule, the metaphyseal bone, and the artery of the ligamentum teres, with the most important contribution coming from the superior retinacular and lateral epiphyseal vessels.[64] In a femoral neck fracture, especially a displaced one, the superior reticular vessels may be disrupted, leaving only the inferior ones. Should these vessels be disrupted as well, the head becomes entirely dependent on the artery of the ligamentum teres, which generally provides only a small contribution in the adult. Accurate, prompt fracture reduction is thought to "unkink" these vessels if they are not torn.

When the femoral neck fracture in a young patient results from high-energy trauma, any life-threatening or limb-threatening injuries should be addressed first. The femoral neck fracture should then be treated, if possible, without compromising the patient's resuscitation, as soon as possible[65] in order to reduce the incidence of avascular necrosis of the head and fracture nonunion.

An attempt at closed reduction may be performed first on a fracture table. Any reduction maneuvers should be gentle so as not to traumatize further the already tenuous blood supply to the femoral head.[66–68] External rotation may tear any remaining inferior retinacular vessels.[64] Gentle traction is applied to the leg. The hip is internally rotated and then abducted.[69,70] The reduction is assessed in two views using fluoroscopy.

If the reduction is anatomic, the surgeon may proceed with fixation, preferably with three, percutaneously placed, cannulated screws. All starting portals should be above the level of the lesser trochanter[71] to avoid stress risers that can lead to iatrogenic subtrochanteric fractures. The screw threads should not cross the fracture site to allow for compression.[70] The screws should be tightened simultaneously to avoid a malreduction. Because posterior comminution tends to be present in most displaced fractures,[72] tightening screws that are more posteriorly located first will cause the fracture to fall into retroversion. For basicervical femoral neck fractures that would require starting portals very close to the lesser trochanter and also cause a relatively large lever arm on the smaller screws, a compression hip screw with a derotation screw should be used for fixation.[73]

Controversy exists as to whether capsulotomy should be performed. Two very small clinical studies showed that if the hip capsule was intact, then intracapsular pressures were elevated.[74,75] In another small study involving human patients,[76] blood flow was shown to be decreased in the femoral head with an intact capsule and elevated capsular pressures. When capsulotomy was performed, the capsular pressure decreased.[76] However, there are no clinical studies that demonstrate that capsulotomy has any effect on patient outcome.

If the reduction is not anatomic after an attempt at closed reduction, then preparation for an open reduction should be made rather than remanipulating the hip and traumatizing its vasculature further.[69] If the surgeon is comfortable with an anterior approach on the fracture table, the patient can be prepped out with attention made to prepping the leg out more anteriorly than is usual when using a fracture table. Otherwise, the patient should be transferred to a radiolucent table.

The anterolateral approach to the hip is used to perform an open reduction.[65,69] The capsulotomy is performed anteriorly and in line with the femoral neck to minimize dissection. The reduction is made and fixation obtained with cannulated screws in the same manner as with closed reduction.

If a femoral shaft fracture complicates the femoral neck fracture, several fixation options have been described: cannulated screws and a retrograde nail, screws with plating, a reconstruction nail, or cannulated screws with an antegrade nail. The reconstruction nail has proved to have the most complications of the device combinations.[77] In general, the femoral neck fracture should take precedence and be fixed first should the patient decompensate and the surgery need to be stopped.[78] The femur fracture can then be treated in traction or with an external fixation until the patient's condition allows definitive fixation.

Vascular Injury

The most important goals in vascular injury management are gaining control of bleeding and maintaining limb viability.[79] When external hemorrhage is present, control of bleeding is initially attempted with direct pressure and packing. In some cases, direct pressure may have to be maintained until operative exposure and control is obtained. Tourniquet use is discouraged, as it causes additionally ischemia and tissue compromise in an already compromised extremity. In a worst case scenario, for an extremely sick patient whose mangled, ischemic limb is only one of multiple traumatic injuries, proceeding with an amputation may be in the best interest of the patient, even though vascular reconstruction may be possible, as a manner of controlling bleeding and avoiding a revascularization insult to the patient. When amputation of a mangled extremity is the obvious surgical option, application of a tourniquet above the injury level can be employed to limit blood loss as the patient is evaluated and prepared for the operating room.

The diagnosis of vascular injury must also be made correctly. Fractures and dislocations should be reduced and splinted and the vascular examination repeated. If the "hard signs" of vascular injury remain, then the patient requires operative treatment[80]: pulselessness, pallor, paresthesia, pain, paralysis, poikilothermia; obvious active arterial hemorrhage; a rapidly expanding, large, or pulsatile hematoma; a palpable thrill or audible bruit; or absent pulses and distal ischemia.

In contrast, the "soft signs" of vascular injury can be managed expectantly,[80,81] which include history of active bleeding at the injury scene; a penetrating wound or blunt trauma in close proximity to a major artery; a small, nonpulsatile hematoma; unexplained neurologic deficit in an extremity; or unexplained shock.

Arteriography should also be used when the patient's injuries are such that it is difficult to discern if the ischemia or lack of motion is caused by a soft tissue, vascular, or nerve injury, especially with fractures, dislocations, or shotgun injuries.[80,82,83] Gunshot wound proximity is not a sensitive indicator of vascular injury in a patient with a normal examination.[84] For older patients with chronic vascular insufficiency and trauma, angiography may need to be used more liberally to rule out vascular injury because of the confusing picture of symptoms.[85]

Compartment syndromes can also cause abnormalities on angiograms.[86] Consequently, when a compartment syndrome is present, fasciotomies should be performed before any vascular exploration is performed and the vascular status reassessed after the fasciotomies are completed. The fasciotomies also decompress the collaterals and venous system, which permits some flow to occur while the repair is being carried out.[83]

Some injuries may be treated within the angiography suite, and, as interventional radiographic techniques improve, the list of treatable conditions continues to expand. Currently, low-flow arteriovenous fistulas, false aneurysms, or branches of larger arteries or vessels in anatomic regions that are difficult to reach surgically can be embolized with coils or balloons.[80] If radiographically diagnosed uncontrollable bleeding is amenable to surgical repair, a balloon may be placed in the angiography suite to control bleeding, with subsequent repair in the operating room.[80] At all times, the team treating a trauma patient in the angiography suite must remain cognizant that the patient is a trauma patient: the patient must be kept warm, procedures must be expedited, and the patient must be closely monitored for declines in hemodynamic or respiratory status.

The Doppler index is of assistance in determining if a vascular injury is present. The distal systolic blood pressure of the injured extremity is divided by the systolic blood pressure in an uninjured extremity. A value less than 0.9 is a significant predictor of an arterial injury[80,82]; however, such measurements may be difficult to make in a multitrauma patient who may not have an uninjured upper extremity or whose fractures or splints in the involved lower extremity may make pressure measurements difficult if not impossible.[87] Duplex ultrasound may also be used to assess the vessels, although this technique requires specialized equipment and personnel that may not be available at all times. When available, imaging of the vessels with this modality in patients with soft signs should be considered.

Systemic or local heparin may be helpful for combined or crush injuries or when a long delay is possible between injury and revascularization.[88] If systemic heparinization is contraindicated because of other injuries, intermittent intraarterial irrigation may be used during revascularization.[88]

Evidence clearly shows that muscle necrosis is present after even as short a time as 3 hours of ischemia.[27] After 6 hours of total ischemia, muscle necrosis is nearly complete.[27] The degree of ischemia that occurs in an injured extremity is not necessarily total, however, and depends on the level of injury, the presence of functioning collaterals, and the degree and duration of shock in which the patient has been.[89] Reperfusion of a cadaveric extremity, however, may very well kill a patient, especially if an entire extremity is reperfused.[27]

Temporary intraluminal shunting should be used when faced with an ischemic limb that requires fracture fixation, extensive soft tissue debridement, or treatment of a life-threatening emergency that will cause delay until the definitive revascularization surgery can be performed.[80,82,90] The priority should be to restore blood flow within 3 to 6 hours; however, such shunts have successfully been left in place up to 52 hours without systemic anticoagulation in damage-control situations.[91]

Once in the operating room, the entire lower extremity to be revascularized should be prepped, as well as the contralateral lower extremity or upper extremity, if grafting is anticipated or a possibility. If extraanatomic grafting is a possibility, the patient should be prepped to the axillae. Any foreign bodies, especially penetrating ones, should not be removed until proximal vascular control has been obtained.[82] The repairs vary as necessary, with extraanatomic grafts usually reserved for repairs in beds with significant mounts of soft tissue injury or infection.[80]

Autogenous grafts are preferred[80,86]; however, synthetic grafts may be used in sites above the knee when no autogenous grafts are available or a large-sized discrepancy may result with an autogenous graft.[80] Synthetic grafts may also be used for an unstable patient who requires a rapid repair to avoid graft harvest.[80,92] In this scenario, however, consideration should be given to temporary shunting followed by definitive repair once the patient is stable. All repairs should be without tension and covered with adequate soft tissue in order to prevent dessication followed by rupture of the graft. Several small studies have documented that vascular repair followed by fracture fixation can be performed in this order with no subsequent disruption or compromise of the vascular repair.[92–94]

Obviously necrotic muscle should be debrided; however, it is important to note that perfused, dead muscle will readily bleed if partially debrided and may lead to significant blood loss, especially if the patient is anticoagulated or coagulopathic. Muscle viability is determined most reliably by contractility, which is tested by lightly touching the muscle with the electrocautery or by briskly striking the muscle. Of note, muscle necrosis of all four compartments of the lower leg should prompt the surgeon to proceed with an amputation.

Once repairs are complete, postrepair arteriography or duplex examination is performed in the operating room, if the patient can tolerate the additional contrast load. In this manner, thrombi or stenosed repairs may be identified and corrected before leaving the operating room.

The remaining subsections cover aspects of revascularization unique to each anatomic region of the lower extremity.

Femoral Artery Injuries

For femoral injuries, the incision is made over the femoral triangle.[80] If proximal access is needed to control bleeding, a second incision may be made in the superior to the inguinal ligament in order to gain proximal control via the external iliac artery.[88] A Fogarty catheter is used to remove clot or thrombus in the vessel before repair, and, ideally, retrograde bleeding is present.[88]

If a graft interposition is required for repair, autologous saphenous vein is harvested. However, in this anatomic region, synthetic grafts may be used. For grossly contaminated wounds or wounds with extensive soft tissue injuries, an extraanatomic repair can be performed, through the posterior soft tissue planes.[88] Intravascular shunts may also be used as a temporizing measure in this anatomic region.[88,92] In a damage-control scenario, with an exsanguinating, dying patient, the femoral artery may be ligated with the knowledge that such a maneuver results in a 50% amputation rate.[88] The proximal profunda femoris may also be ligated if faced with exsanguination.[80]

Intimal flaps, focal narrowing, small, false aneurysm, and arteriovenous fistulas may all be observed and repaired electively if signs of ischemia occur or worsen.[88] Vein repair should also be performed, if possible, as such repairs have been shown to improve the patency of arterial repairs. Also, a more normal distal vascular bed resistance is maintained, and a reduced incidence of chronic venous insufficiency and associated postphlebitic syndrome occurs.[88,95]

Popliteal Artery

Of the arterial injuries to the leg, those to the popliteal artery are the most limb threatening because of the limited collaterals to the foot and leg.[85,86] The popliteal artery divides into the anterior tibial artery and the tibioperoneal trunk, which exists for several millimeters before dividing into the peroneal and posterior tibial arteries. The vein travels close to the artery in this region, which explains the frequency of simultaneous injury to both. The popliteal vein should be repaired at the same sitting as the artery, if possible, to reduce outflow obstruction and to improve limb salvage.[83] Shunts may be difficult to use distal to the knee because of the decreasing size of the vessels.[83]

The patient is placed supine on the operating room table with the hip flexed and abducted. A medial approach is used to the vessels,[83,96] although a posterior approach may be used when a penetrating wound occurs directly posterior.[85] The artery should be debrided to healthy tissue, with an end-to-end repair the most desired result.[85] If more than 2 cm is debrided, then a graft is required. The geniculates should not be divided to mobilize the vessels.[85] Prosthetic grafts should be avoided in this anatomic region, if possible.[86] If an extraanatomic bypass is required, it should be placed out through lateral tissues.[80] If a repair is performed after knee dislocation, the knee may be stabilized with knee-spanning external fixation.

Infrapopliteal Arteries

Three main arteries supply the leg and foot: the anterior and posterior tibial arteries and the peroneal artery. These vessels have a good collateral supply, so, if one vessel is injured, no repair needs to be performed. Should an injured vessel actively continue to bleed, either ligation or embolization may be performed.[80,83] If, however, two of the vessels are injured or the tibioperoneal trunk is injured, then a vascular repair should be performed. Venous injuries in this anatomic region are rarely repaired.[80,83]

A longitudinal incision is used to gain access to the vessel of interest and a Fogarty catheter used to remove any thrombus.[83] These vessels can rarely be repaired primarily and generally require an autogenous saphenous vein graft because of their small size.[83] Shunts are also difficult to use in this region because of the small size of the vessels.[83]

Open Fractures and Open Joints

The classic teaching is that open fractures need to be debrided within 6 to 8 hours as this is thought to be the time it takes for bacteria to multiply to the critical infecting innoculum of 10^5 organisms.[97] The early work determining this was done before antibiotics were used regularly. With the use of antibiotics, the window for washout may be expanded, although there are no randomized, clinical trials proving any of these practices.[98–101]

The key is to diagnose an open fracture correctly and to start the appropriate antibiotics. Our protocol is to use a broad-spectrum cephalosporin to provide antibiotic coverage for Gustilo type I through type IIIB open fractures, with the addition of an aminoglycoside reserved for type IIIC open fractures. For wounds contaminated with soil, fresh water, or "farm wounds," penicillin coverage is added. Wounds are washed out using 1 L of normal saline in the emergency room, a sterile dressing is applied, and the fracture is splinted. This dressing is not removed again until the patient is in the operating room for definitive washout, as such repeat looks increase the infection rate.[102] With the advent of digital photography, consideration should be given to obtaining quick digital photos of wounds in the emergency room to show to team members who arrive later, rather than disturbing the dressings.

The current literature supports washout of an open fracture as soon as is possible, given operating room availability and the patient's condition.[98] For a multiple trauma patient, this may mean going to the intensive care unit for several hours for warming and resuscitation before proceeding to the operating room. One retrospective review of multiple types of open fractures at multiple sites showed no increase in infection or nonunion rates with times up to 13 hours to definitive irrigation and debridement.[99] Data from the Lower Extremity Assessment Project (LEAP) corroborated this result, with the patient's time from injury to admission at the trauma center being the only factor predictive of infection.[100] Another study retrospectively examined low-energy type I open fractures in over 91 patients who received intravenous antibiotics, but only one patient had a formal washout within 12 hours. Some patients received no formal irrigation and debridement, yet no infections were observed in the study.[103]

Once in the operating room, the open fracture must be explored. Dead or heavily damaged skin, especially the traumatic wound edges, should be excised. Nonviable muscle should be excised. The fracture itself should be stabilized with appropriate fixation. If the wound can be closed, there is no hard evidence indicating that it should not be.[101] Currently, a randomized study is underway to determine if closable wounds associated with tibia fractures may be closed primarily versus brought back to the operating room for a repeat washout with secondary closure. Of course, if any tissue, especially muscle, is of questionable viability at the time of the original surgery, or if the wound is extremely contaminated, the patient should be brought back to the operating room in 24 to 48 hours for a second-look procedure.[101] At present, there exist only small clinical studies that suggest vacuum-assisted dressings may be of benefit with traumatic wounds.[104]

The Mangled Extremity

In the emergency room, grossly contaminated wounds should be washed out, wounds packed with sterile dressings, and the extremity splinted. As long as bleeding in the extremity is controlled in this manner, the patient may remain in the splint while being resuscitated in the intensive care unit or while undergoing other life-saving procedures. Temporary intravascular shunts may be placed and left in while the patient undergoes resuscitation or other procedures.[91] For the patient in extremis, a guillotine amputation with control of bleeding may be the best course of action, especially for an ischemic mangled extremity. For the "less ill" patient, vascular repair (if necessary), irrigation and debridement, and skeletal stabilization should be the course of action. The vascular repair should take precedence over skeletal stabilization as discussed in the section on vascular injuries.[92-94]

External fixation is typically the form of stabilization used initially in the management of mangled extremities. External fixators can be rapidly applied and then converted to other forms of fixation once the degree of soft tissue injury becomes fully known. Fixators may be placed in the operating room or the intensive care unit. For fixator placement in the intensive care unit, spot radiographs may be used to determine the approximate levels for pin placement with skin stab incisions made accordingly. This can be especially useful for fixation of the femur where the thigh musculature obscures bony landmarks.

Ideally, the external fixation pins should go through regions where open reduction is not planned later to avoid potential contamination of the tissues and interference with flap placement. Fixators on the femur may be anterior or lateral. Unfortunately, anterior pins violate the quadriceps mechanism but are often the easiest to place, especially in the intensive care unit. Ideally, spanning fixators should have pins into segmental fracture fragments, as the segments will sag otherwise and the entire construct will shorten. One rapid form of spanning fixator that can be applied to the leg uses tibial and calcaneal traction pins that are then connected with a unilateral frame. In extremely ill patients, traction pins alone may be placed. For entire leg involvement, a calcaneal traction pin may be used to provide traction to the lower extremity. Vacuum-assisted dressings may be useful in the management of the soft tissue injuries encountered in mangled extremities[104]; however, there are currently few published data from randomized clinical trials to show improvement in patient outcome with these dressings.[104,105]

The multicenter LEAP study comparing the results of amputation with limb salvage for mangled extremities showed that patient outcome was no different whether limb salvage or amputation was performed.[106] However, the outcomes for patients with early amputations was better than for those whose amputations were performed later.[107] The LEAP study did show, however, that none of the current mangled extremity scoring systems was clinically useful in determining whether a limb should be amputated.[108]

Critique

With there being no immediate life-threatening injuries, the management priority for this patient, at this time, is addressing the obvious acute arterial insufficiency of the involved extremity. This patient should undergo acute care exploration of the popliteal artery, with repair of bypass being the likely surgical option. With there not being multiple levels of injury, arteriography is not *essential* for this particular patient, and such an intervention would delay definitive management and possibly result in irreparable damage. This patient has a popliteal artery injury and needs operative intervention by both vascular and orthopedic surgeons.

Answer (A)

References

1. Wong C-H, Chang H-C, Pasupathy S, Khin L-W, Tan J-L, Low C-O. Necrotizing fasciitis: clinical presentation, microbiology, and determinants of mortality. J Bone Joint Surg Am 2003; 85A:1454–1460.
2. Mills WJ, Swiontkowski MF. Fatal group A streptococcal infection with toxic shock syndrome: complicating minor orthopaedic trauma. J Orthop Trauma 1996; 10:149–155.
3. Takahira N, Shindo M, Tanaka K, Soma K, Ohwada T, Moritoshi I. Treatment outcomes of nonclostridial gas gangrene at a Level I trauma center. J Orthop Trauma 2002; 16:12–17.

4. Elliott DC, Kufera JA, Myers R. Necrotizing soft tissue infections: risk factors for mortality and strategies for management. Ann Surg 1996; 224:672–683.

5. Bisno AL, Stevens DL. Streptococcal infections of skin and soft tissues. N Engl J Med 1996; 334:240–245.

6. Cunningham JD, Silver L, Rudikoff D. Necrotizing fasciitis: a plea for early diagnosis and treatment. Mt Sinai J Med 2001; 68:253–261.

7. Dahl PR, Perniciaro C, Holmkvist K, O'Connor MI, Gibson LE. Fulminant group A streptococcal necrotizing fasciitis: clinical and pathologic findings in 7 patients. J Am Acad Dermatol 2002; 47:489–492.

8. Rocca AF, Moran EA, Lippert FG. Hyperbaric oxygen therapy in the treatment of soft tissue necrosis resulting from a stingray puncture. Foot Ankle Int 2001; 22:318–323.

9. Trent JT, Kirsner RS. Necrotizing fasciitis. Wounds 2002; 14:284–292.

10. Shirtliff ME, Mader JT. Acute septic arthritis. Clin Microbiol Rev 2002; 15:527–544.

11. Jung ST, Rowe SM, Moon ES, Song EK, Yoon TR, Seo HY. Significance of laboratory and radiologic findings for differentiating between septic arthritis and transient synovitis of the hip. J Pediatr Orthop 2003; 23:368–372.

12. Levine MJ, McGuire KJ, McGowan KL, Flynn JM. Assessment of the test characteristics of C-reactive protein for septic arthritis in children. J Pediatr Orthop 2003; 23:373–377.

13. Choi IH, Pizzutillo PD, Bowen JR, Dragann R, Malhis T. Sequelae and reconstruction after septic arthritis of the hip in infants. J Bone Joint Surg Am 1990; 72A:1150–1165.

14. Aroojis A, Johari AN. Epiphyseal separations after neonatal osteomyelitis and septic arthritis. J Pediatr Orthop 2000; 20:544–549.

15. Salvati EA, Gonzalez Della Valle A, Masri BA, Duncan CP. The infected total hip arthroplasty. Instr Course Lect 2003; 52:223–245.

16. Hanssen AD, Spangehl MJ. Treatment of the infected hip replacement. Clin Orthop 2004; 420:63–71.

17. Joseph TN, Chen AL, DiCesare PE. Use of antibiotic-impregnated cement in total joint arthroplasty. J Am Acad Orthop Surg 2003; 11:38–47.

18. Roth A, Fuhrmann R, Lange M, Mollenhauer J, Straube E, Venbrocks R. Overwhelming septic infection with a multi-resistant Staphylococcus aureus (MRSA) after total knee replacement. Arch Orthop Trauma Surg 2003; 123:429–432.

19. Sierra RJ, Trousdale RT, Pagnano MW. Above-the-knee amputation after a total knee replacement. J Bone Joint Surg Am 2003; 85A:1000–1004.

20. Fenelon GCC, von Foerster G, Engelbrecht E. Disarticulation of the hip as a result of failed arthroplasty. J Bone Joint Surg Am 1980; 62B:441–446.

21. Henke PK. Approach to the patient with acute limb ischemia: diagnosis and therapeutic modalities. Cardiol Clin 2002; 20:513–520.

22. Rutherford RB, Baker D, Ernst C, et al. Recommended standards for reports dealing with lower extremity ischemia: revised version. J Vasc Surg 1997; 26:517–538.

23. Nypaver TJ, Whyte BR, Endean ED, Schwarcz TH, Hyde GL. Nontraumatic lower-extremity acute arterial ischemia. Am J Surg 1998; 176:147–152.

24. Eliason JL, Wainess RM, Proctor MC, et al. A national and single institutional experience in the contemporary treatment of acute lower extremity ischemia. Ann Surg 2003; 238:382–390.

25. Kumar SR, Rowe VL, Petrone P, Kuncir EJ, Asensio JA. The vasculopathic patient: uncommon surgical emergencies. Emerg Med Clin North Am 2003; 21:803–815.

26. Tawes RL, Harris EJ, Brown WH, et al. Arterial thromboembolism: a 20-year perspective. Arch Surg 1985; 120:595–599.

27. Blaisdell FW. The pathophysiology of skeletal muscle ischemia and the reperfusion syndrome: a review. Cardiovasc Surg 2002; 10(6):620–630.

28. Feliciano DV. Heroic procedures in vascular injury management: the role of extra-anatomic bypass. Surg Clin North Am 2002; 82:115–124.

29. Fulkerson E, Razi A, Tejwani N. Review: acute compartment syndrome of the foot. Foot Ankle Int 2003; 24:180–187.

30. Blick SS, Brumback RJ, Poka A, Burgess AR, Ebraheim NA. Compartment syndrome in open tibial fractures. J Bone Joint Surg Am 1986; 68A:1348–1353.

31. Sandhu R, Como JJ, Scalea TS. Renal failure and exercise-induced rhabdomyolysis in patients taking performance-enhancing compounds. J Trauma 2002; 53:761–764.

32. Nixon RG, Brindley GW. Hemophilia presenting as compartment syndrome in the arm following venipuncture. Clin Orthop 1989; 244:176–181.

33. Hope MJ, McQueen MM. Acute compartment syndrome in the absence of fracture. J Orthop Trauma 2004; 18:220–224.

34. Whitesides TE, Heckman MM. Acute compartment syndrome: update on diagnosis and treatment. J Am Acad Orthop Surg 1996; 4:209–218.

35. Elliott KGB, Johnstone AJ. Diagnosing acute compartment syndrome. J Bone Joint Surg Am 2003; 85B:625–632.

36. Pacheco RJ, Oxborrow NJ, Weeber AC, Allerton K. Gluteal compartment syndrome after total knee arthroplasty with epidural postoperative analgesia. J Bone Joint Surg Am 2001; 83B:739–740.

37. Price C, Ribeiro J, Kinnebrew T. Compartment syndromes associated with postoperative epidural analgesia. J Bone Joint Surg Am 1996; 78A:597–599.

38. Strecker WB, Wood MB, Bieber EJ. Compartment syndrome masked by epidural anesthesia for postoperative pain. J Bone Joint Surg Am 1986; 68A:1447–1448.

39. Morrow BC, Mawhinney IN, Elliott JRM. Tibial compartment syndrome complicating closed femoral nailing: diagnosis delayed by an epidural analgesic technique-case report. J Trauma 1994; 37:867–868.

40. Janzing HMJ, Broos PLO. Routine monitoring of compartment pressure in patients with tibial fractures: beware of overtreatment. Injury 2001; 32:415–421.

41. Gaspard DJ, Kohl RD. Compartment syndromes in which the skin is the limiting boundary. Clin Orthop 1975; 113:65–68.

42. Mubarak SJ, Owen CA. Double-incision fasciotomy of the leg for decompression in compartment syndromes. J Bone Joint Surg Am 1977;59A:184–187.

43. Tarlow SD, Achterman CA, Hayhurst J, Ovadia DN. Acute compartment syndrome of the thigh complicating fracture of the femur. A report of three cases. J Bone Joint Surg Am 1986 ;68A:1439–1443.

44. Bleicher RJ, Sherman HF, Latenser BA. Bilateral gluteal compartment syndrome. J Trauma 1997; 42:118–122.

45. Perry MD, Manoli A. Foot compartment syndrome. Orthop Clin North Am 2001; 32:103–111.

46. Fakhouri AJ, Manoli A. Acute foot compartment syndromes. J Orthop Trauma 1992; 6:223–228.

47. Bouachour G, Cronier P, Gouello JP, Toulemonde JL, Talha A, Alquier P. Hyperbaric oxygen therapy in the management of crush injuries: a randomized double-blind placebo controlled clinical trial. J Trauma 1996; 41:333–339.

48. Morykwas MJ, Howell H, Bleyer AJ, Molnar JA, Argenta LC. The effect of externally applied subatmospheric pressure on serum myoglobin levels after a prolonged crush/ischemia injury. J Trauma 2002; 53:537–540.

49. McKee MD, Garay ME, Schemitsch EH, Kreder HJ, Stephen DJG. Irreducible fracture-dislocation of the hip: a severe injury with a poor prognosis. J Orthop Trauma 1998; 12:223–229.

50. Yang R-S, Tsuang Y-H, Hang Y-S, Liu T-K. Traumatic dislocation of the hip. Clin Orthop 1991; 265:218–227.

51. Jacob JR, Rao JP, Ciccarelli C. Traumatic dislocation and fracture dislocation of the hip. Clin Orthop 1987; 214:249–263.

52. Jaskulka RA, Fischer G, Fenzl G. Dislocation and fracture-dislocation of the hip. J Bone Joint Surg Am 1991; 73B:465–469.

53. Alonso JE, Volgas DA, Giordono V, Stannard J. A review of the treatment of hip dislocations associated with acetabular fractures. Clin Orthop 2000; 377:32–43.

54. Nerubay J. Traumatic anterior dislocation of hip joint with vascular damage. Clin Orthop 1976; 116:129–132.

55. Siegmeth A, Menth-Chiari W, Amsuess H. A rare case of irreducible knee dislocation in a seventy-three-year-old male. J Orthop Trauma 2000; 14:70–72.

56. Wand JS. A physical sign denoting irreducibility of a dislocated knee. J Bone Joint Surg Am 1989; 71B:862.

57. Hill JA, Rana NA. Complications of posterolateral dislocation of the knee: case report and literature review. Clin Orthop 1981; 154:212–215.

58. Stannard JP, Sheils TM, Lopez-Ben RR, McGwin G, Robison JT, Volgas DA. Vascular injuries in knee dislocations: the role of physical examination in determining the need for arteriography. J Bone Joint Surg Am 2004; 86A:910–915.

59. Kleinberg EO, Crites BM, Flinn WR, Archibald JD, Moorman CT. The role of arteriography in assessing popliteal artery injury in knee dislocations. J Trauma 2004; 56:786–790.

60. Wascher DC. High-velocity knee dislocation with vascular injury. Clin Sports Med 2000; 19:457–477.

61. Scheid DK. Treatment of the multiple ligament injured knee and knee dislocations: a trauma perspective. Instr Course Lect 2003; 52:409–411.

62. Harner CD, Waltrip RL, Bennett CH, Francis KA, Irrang JJ. Surgical management of knee dislocations. J Bone Joint Surg Am 2004; 86A:262–273.

63. Bibbo C, Anderson RB, Davis WH. Injury characteristics and the clinical outcome of subtalar dislocations: a clinical and radiographic analysis of 25 cases. Foot Ankle Int 2003; 24:158–163.

64. Plancher KD, Donshik JD. Femoral neck and ipsilateral neck and shaft fractures in the young adult. Orthop Clin North Am 1997; 28:447–459.

65. Swiontkowski MF, Winquist RA, Hansen ST. Fractures of the femoral neck in patients between the ages of twelve and forty-nine years. J Bone Joint Surg Am 1984; 66A:837–846.

66. Keller CS, Laros GS. Indications for open reduction of femoral neck fractures. Clin Orthop 1980; 152:131–137.

67. Calandruccio RA, Anderson WE. Post-fracture avascular necrosis of the femoral head: correlation of experimental and clinical studies. Clin Orthop 1980; 152:49–84.

68. Frangakis EK. Intracapsular fractures of the neck of the femur. J Bone Joint Surg Am 1966; 48B:17–30.

69. Bosch U, Schreiber T, Krettek C. Reduction and fixation of displaced intracapsular fractures of the proximal femur. Clin Orthop 2002; 388:59–71.

70. Bray TJ. Femoral neck fracture fixation. Clin Orthop 1997; 339:20–31.

71. Asnis SE, Wanek-Sgaglione L. Intracapsular fractures of the femoral neck. J Bone Joint Surg Am 1994; 76A:1793–1803.

72. Scheck M. The significance of posterior comminution in femoral neck fractures. Clin Orthop 1980; 152:138–142.

73. Browner B, Trafton P, Green N, Swiontkowski M, Jupiter J, Levine A. Skeletal Trauma: Basic Science, Management, and Reconstruction, 3rd ed. Philadelphia: Saunders, 2003.

74. Crawfurd EJP, Emery RJH, Hansell DM, Phelan M, Andrews BG. Capsular distension and intracapsular pressure in subcapital fractures of the femur. J Bone Joint Surg Am 1988; 70B:195–198.

75. Stromqvist B, Nilsson L, Egund N, Thorngren K-G, Wingstraad H. Intracapsular pressures in undisplaced fractures of the neck. J Bone Joint Surg Am 1988; 70B:192–194.

76. Harper WM, Barnes MR, Gregg PJ. Femoral head blood flow in femoral neck fractures. J Bone Joint Surg Am 1991; 73B:73–75.

77. Watson JT, Moed BR. Ipsilateral femoral neck and shaft fractures. Clin Orthop 2002; 399:78–86.

78. Swiontkowski MF, Hansen ST, Kellam JF. Ipsilateral fractures of the femoral neck and shaft. J Bone Joint Surg Am 1984; 66A:260–268.

79. Aucar JA, Hirshberg A. Damage control for vascular injuries. Surg Clin North Am 1997; 77:853–862.

80. Weaver FA, Papanicolaou G, Yellin AE. Difficult peripheral vascular injuries. Surg Clin North Am 1996; 76:843–859.

81. Frykberg ER, Dennis JW, Bishop K, Laneve L, Alexander RH. The reliability of physical examination in the evaluation of penetrating extremity trauma for vascular injury: results at one year. J Trauma 1991; 31:502–511.

82. Bandyk DF. Vascular injury associated with extremity trauma. Clin Orthop 1995; 318:117–124.

83. Keeley SB, Snyder WH, Weigelt JA. Arterial injuries below the knee: fifty-one patients with 82 injuries. J Trauma 1983; 23:285–292.

84. Francis H, Thal ER, Weigelt JA, Redman HC. Vascular proximity: is it a valid indication for arteriography in asymptomatic patients? J Trauma 1991; 31:512–514.

85. Frykberg ER. Popliteal vascular injuries. Surg Clin North Am 2002; 82:67–89.

86. Feliciano DV, Herskowitz K, O'Gorman RB, et al. Management of vascular injuries in the lower extremities. J Trauma 1988; 28:319–328.

87. Johansen K, Lynch K, Paun M, Copass M. Non-invasive vascular test reliably exclude occult arterial trauma in injured extremities. J Trauma 1991; 31:515–522.

88. Carrillo EH, Spain DA, Miller FB, Richardson JD. Femoral vessel injuries. Surg Clin North Am 2002; 82:49–65.

89. Reber PU, Patel AG, Sapio NLD, Ris H-B, Beck M, Kniemeyer HW. Selective use of temporary intravascular shunts in coincident vascular and orthopedic upper and lower limb trauma. J Trauma 1999; 47:72–76.

90. Wolf YG, Rivkind A. Vascular trauma in high-velocity gunshot wounds and shrapnel-blast injuries in Israel. Surg Clin North Am 2002; 82:237–244.

91. Granchi T, Schmittling Z, Vasquez J, Schreiber M, Wall M. Prolonged use of intraluminal arterial shunts without systemic anticoagulation. Am J Surg 2000; 180:493–497.

92. Starr AJ, Hunt JL, Reinert CM. Treatment of femur fracture with associated vascular injury. J Trauma 1996; 40:17–21.

93. Drost TF, Rosemurgy AS, Proctor D, Kearney RE. Outcome of treatment of combined orthopedic and arterial trauma to the lower extremity. J Trauma 1989; 29:1331–1334.

94. McHenry TP, Holcomb JB, Lindsey RW. Fractures with major vascular injuries from gunshot wounds: implications of surgical sequence. J Trauma 2002; 53:717–721.

95. Ashworth EM, Dalsing M, Glover JL, Reilly MK. Lower extremity vascular trauma: a comprehensive, aggressive approach. J Trauma 1988; 28:329–336.

96. Muscat JO, Rogers W, Cruz AB, Schenck RC. Arterial injuries in orthopaedics: the posteromedial approach for vascular control about the knee. J Orthop Trauma 1996; 10:476–480.

97. Elek SD. Experimental staphylococcal infections in the skin of man. Ann NY Acad Sci 1957; 65:85–90.

98. Khatod M, Botte MJ, Hoyt DB, Meyer RS, Smith JM, Akeson WH. Outcomes in open tibia fractures: relationship between delay in treatment and infection. J Trauma 2003; 55:949–954.

99. Harley BJ, Beaupre LA, Jones CA, Dulai SK, Weber DW. The effect of time to definitive treatment on the rate of nonunion and infection in open fractures. J Orthop Trauma 2002; 16:484–490.

100. Pollak AN, Castillo RC, Jones AL, Bosse MJ, MacKenzie EJ, Group LS. Time to definitive treatment significantly influences incidence of infection after open high-energy lower-extremity trauma. In Orthopaedic Trauma Association 19th Annual Meeting, Salt Lake City, UT, 2003: 98–100.

101. Weitz-Marshall AD, Bosse MJ. Timing of closure of open fractures. J Am Acad Orthop Surg 2002; 10:379–384.

102. Olson SA, Schemitsch EH. Open fractures of the tibial shaft: an update. Instr Course Lect 2003; 52:623–631.

103. Yang EC, Eisler J. Treatment of isolated type I open fractures: is emergent operative debridement necessary? Clin Orthop 2003; 410:289–294.

104. Webb LX. New techniques in wound management: vacuum-assisted wound closure. J Am Acad Orthop Surg 2002; 10:303–311.

105. Hercovici D, Sanders RW, Scaduto JM, Infante A, Dipasquale T. Vacuum-assisted wound closure (VAC therapy) for the management of patients with high-energy soft tissue injuries. J Orthop Trauma 2003; 17:683–687.

106. Bosse MJ, MacKenzie EJ, Kellam JF, et al. An analysis of outcomes of reconstruction or amputation of leg-threatening injuries. N Engl J Med 2002; 347:1924–1931.

107. Smith DG, Castillo RC, MacKenzie EJ, Bosse MJ, Group LS. Functional outcome of patients who have late amputation after trauma is significantly worse than for those who have early amputation. In Orthopaedic Trauma Association 19th Annual Meeting, Salt Lake City, UT, 2003: 101–102.

108. Bosse MJ, MacKenzie EJ, Kellam JF, et al. A prospective evaluation of the clinical utility of the lower-extremity injury-severity scores. J Bone Joint Surg Am 2001; 83A: 3–14.

39
Hand and Upper Extremities

David T. Netscher and Idris Gharbaoui

Case Scenario

A motorcyclist is brought to the trauma bay after crashing into a parked pick-up truck. He is alert, oriented, and hemodynamically stable. The patient has no intrathoracic or abdominal injuries. He does have extensive abrasions and bruises of his upper extremities, although radiologic evaluation demonstrates no skeletal fractures or dislocation. However, over of the course of 3 hours, the patient complains of increasing numbness and paresthesia of the left forearm. On physical examination, the involved extremity is swollen and very tense, with tenderness over the forearm musculature and paresthesia confirmed over the distribution of the median and ulnar nerves. The patient has a very strongly palpable radial pulse. Which of the following should be the management at this time?

(A) Application of a sequential compression garment
(B) Elevation of the involved extremity and artenography
(C) Three-compartment fasciotomy
(D) Venous Doppler studies
(E) Repeated extremity x-rays

Principles

Treatment Planning

Acute care surgery to the upper extremity may be secondary to trauma or may be from nontraumatic causes such as infections, compartment syndrome, and vascular emergencies. Treatment must be directed at the specific structures damaged—skeletal, tendon, nerve, vessels, and integument.[1] Goals of management in acute care situations are to obtain a healed wound, to preserve motion, and to retain distal sensation. Stable skeletal architecture is essential for effective motion and function of the extremity, and this is established in the primary phase of care. It also results in reestablishing skeletal length, straightening deformities, and correcting compression or kinking of nerves and vessels. Arteries should also be repaired in the acute phase of treatment to maintain distal tissue viability. Similarly, extrinsic compression on arteries must be released emergently such as in compartment pressure problems. In clean-cut type injuries, tendons should be repaired primarily. In situations where there is a chance that tendon adhesions may form, such as with associated fractures, it is often better nonetheless to repair the tendons with preservation of their length and if necessary to perform tenolysis later. However, in open, contaminated, and severe crushing injuries, it is prudent to delay repair of both tendon and nerve injuries.

In sharp, clean-cut wounds primary nerve repair lessens the possibility of nerve end retraction and therefore the need for later nerve graft. Primary repair of nerves should not be performed in situations in which contusion-causing forces have been directed to the nerve (gunshot wounds, power saw injuries, blunt crushing), since the extent of the proximal axonal injury may not be immediately evident. Nerve repair before this is apparent may result in abnormal nerve ends being reattached, negating the chance for return of function.

In severe soft tissue injuries, wound closure may not be immediately possible. However, initial open treatment is directed at preventing infection and protecting critical deep structures by proper dressing and wound management. Adequate debridement is essential, but thereafter appropriate soft tissue coverage must be achieved as soon as possible. The sooner the soft tissue coverage can be achieved, the less likely there will be secondary deformity due to fibrosis and joint contractures. The more rapidly one can start hand therapy, the better the chances of maximizing return of function. The treatment regimen consists of debridement, rigid skeletal fixation, and early soft tissue resurfacing followed by protected range of

615

motion exercises as soon as possible. Early soft tissue reconstruction results in improved function, decreased morbidity, and shortened hospital stay.

Appropriate treatment of acute care situations involving the upper extremity requires knowledge of local and regional anesthesia, use of a tourniquet to provide a bloodless field, correct placement of incisions to minimize later scar contractures, appropriate use of dressings and splints to reduce edema and maintain functional position, and above all a clear knowledge of the unique anatomy of the hand and upper extremity that will not only aide in accurate clinical diagnosis but also enable surgery to be performed safely.

Anesthesia

The choice of general, regional (such as intravenous Bier block or brachial plexus block that includes either supraclavicular or axillary block) or local anesthesia is gov-

erned by the extent and length of the operation.[2,3] An upper arm tourniquet can be used on the unanesthetized extremity with only local anesthetic field infiltration or wrist or digital block for as long as 30 minutes in the relaxed cooperative patient provided the arm is well exsanguinated. After this time tourniquet pain will not permit more extensive local anesthetic procedures. The need to operate in other areas, such as for the harvesting of bone, nerve, tendon, or skin graft, and more extensive surgical procedures will require general anesthesia.

Digital blocks and median, ulnar, and radial wrist nerve blocks are very useful especially for more limited emergency room procedures (Figure 39.1). Digital nerve blocks as a rule should not include epinephrine, which could lead to vasospasm, ischemia, and necrosis, although recent evidence implies the safety of distal blocks using an epinephrine solution. The maximum safe dose of lidocaine is 4 mg/kg.

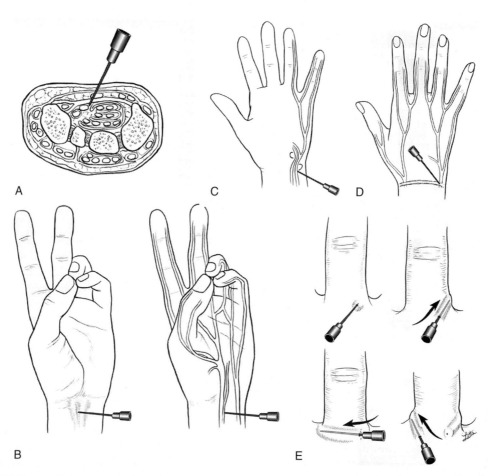

FIGURE 39.1. Median anesthetic block is done by locating the interspace between the palmaris longus and flexor carpi radialis tendons in the distal forearm just proximal to the carpal tunnel. (A) Ulnar nerve block is performed by inserting the injecting needle just proximal to the pisiform and passing deep to the flexor carpi ulnaris tendon. (B–D) A wheal of local anesthetic raised across the dorsum of the wrist will anesthetize the branches of the superficial radial nerve and also the dorsal cutaneous branch of the ulnar nerve. (E) A method of injecting to achieve a digital nerve block.

Tourniquet Application

Clear visualization of all structures in the operative field depends on tourniquet use.[1] Penrose drains, rolled rubber glove fingers, or commercially available tourniquets can be used on digits. Great care is taken in using any constrictive device on digits as narrow bands can cause direct injury to underlying nerves and digital vessels. With use of upper arm tourniquets, the skin beneath the cuff should be protected by several wraps of cast padding. During skin preparation this area must be kept dry in order to prevent blistering of the skin by an inflated cuff over moist padding. The cuff selected should be as wide as the diameter of the arm. Standard pressures used are 250 to 280 mm Hg in adults and 150 to 200 mm Hg in children. As a rule, the cuff should be deflated every 2 hours for 15 to 20 minutes to revascularize distal tissue and to relieve pressure on the nerves locally before reinflating the cuff for more extensive procedures. Exsanguination is performed by wrapping the extremity with a Martin's bandage in all cases except those involving infection or tumors. In these cases, there is a possibility of embolization by mechanical pressure, and so exsanguination should be avoided. Merely elevating the extremity for a few minutes before tourniquet inflation suffices.

Incisions

Incisions should be of the Bruner zigzag or midaxial type or combinations of these in order to avoid motion-restricting scars (Figure 39.2).[1] Any scar dorsal or palmar to the flexion axis of a joint or crossing its axis at 90° can cause contracture across that joint. The juncture of a skin graft and healthy skin is also a potential scar line, and so

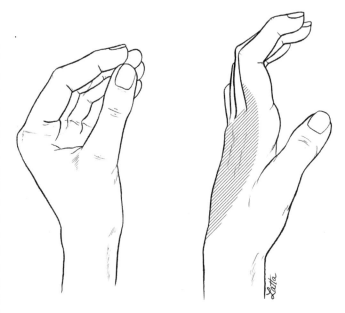

FIGURE 39.3. Edema and swelling tend to accumulate dorsally (cross-hatching), drawing the fingers into extension at the metacarpophalangeal joints.

the design for a margin of the graft should also be planned on the same lines as the incision so as to prevent contractures, even if on occasion this requires removal of small areas of healthy skin. Palmar incisions follow the pattern of the skin creases. Dorsal incisions of the fingers and wrists and also incisions on the forearm may follow longitudinal straight lines.

Dressings and Splints

The purposes of dressings are to protect wounds, absorb drainage, and help splint repaired structures.[4] The first layer should be nonadherent and may contain an antibiotic. The next layer should be soft and bulky and is usually followed by a firmer external wrap. Conforming compression is useful, but constriction is harmful.

Splints should be made to protect only the part necessary and should not prevent motion in the remainder of the extremity. Frequently patients will keep the injured, operated, or infected hand in a flexed wrist position, and this automatically causes the metacarpophalangeal joints to extend, thereby placing the collateral ligaments in their shortest length. Edema fluid is deposited dorsally, and the resulting tightness causes stiff joints (Figure 39.3); thus, a splint that keeps the hand in the "protected" position should extend the wrist 40° to 50°, maintain the metacarpophalangeal joints at 70° of flexion, and maintain the interphalangeal joints in a neutral position (Figure 39.4). Postoperative hand elevation is essential to reduce edema.

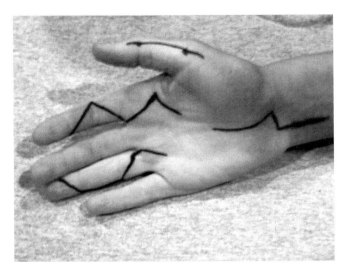

FIGURE 39.2. Placement of incisions for palmar exposure of structures (longitudinal midaxial digital incisions must not be placed volar to joint flexion creases).

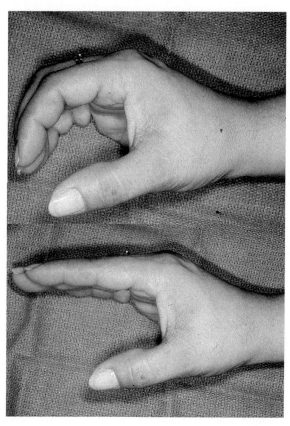

FIGURE 39.4. The "safe" position or "protected" position of the hand (below) differs from the "resting" position of the hand (above). The former is the preferred manner of splinting the injured hand, as it preserves the maximum length of collateral ligaments and minimizes the risk of developing postoperative extension contractures at the metacarpophalangeal joints and flexion contractures at the interphalangeal joints.

Examination and Diagnosis

Observation

Inspection of the resting posture of the hand provides valuable information. A severed flexor tendon is readily diagnosed by the fact that the affected finger does not assume its normal resting position in line with the natural flexion cascade of the adjacent digits (Figure 39.5).[5,6] Extensor tendon injuries might be indicated by a droop at the affected joint. On the other hand, a clawed posture of the little and ring fingers is characteristic of an ulnar nerve injury. Absence of sweating at the fingertips may also imply a nerve injury in that particular distribution. Swelling and erythema may be indicative of a hand infection, and a purulent flexor tenosynovitis will always result in a flexed position of the finger. Rotational and angular deformities of the digits will occur when there are underlying fractures (Figure 39.6).

Neurovascular Examination

An Allen test confirms the patency of the ulnar and radial arteries. Moving two-point discrimination is the most sensitive method of testing for sensory loss and is easily done by using a bent paperclip (Figure 39.7).[5,6] The ends of the paperclip are set 5 to 8mm apart for fingertip pulp testing. Points are aligned along the axis of the finger and moved transversely across the axis. If the test is not reproducible, because the patient is uncooperative, suspicion of nerve injury is simply confirmed by the tactile adherence test in which a plastic pin is passed back and forth gently across the pulp on either side of each finger. Adhesion, caused by sweat, is shown by slight but definite movement of the finger being examined (an anesthetic finger pulp will not sweat).

A knowledge of surface anatomy of nerves helps in the evaluation of a specific lacerating injury (Figure 39.8).[7] The ulnar attachment of the flexor retinaculum is to the pisiform and hook of hamate, and radial attachment is to the scaphoid and ridge of trapezium. The median nerve passes through the carpal tunnel between these landmarks. It provides sensation to the thumb, index finger, middle finger, and radial half of the ring finger. The palmar cutaneous branch of the median nerve arises from its radial aspect 5 to 6cm proximal to the wrist and provides sensation to the palmar triangle. The ulnar nerve is on the radial side of the pisiform and passes to the ulnar side of the hook of the hamate in its passage through Guyon's canal. It provides sensation to the little finger and ulnar half of the ring finger, while the dorsal branch of the ulnar nerve (arising proximal to the wrist and curving dorsally around the head of the ulna) supplies the same digits on their dorsal aspect. The superficial radial sensory nerve emerges from under the brachioradialis in the distal forearm and divides into two or three branches

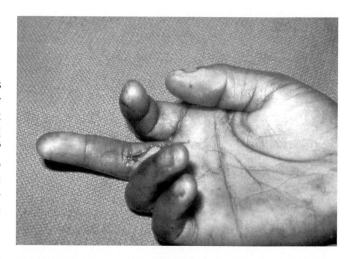

FIGURE 39.5. Flexor tendon injury to the middle finger is readily diagnosed by the resting posture of that digit, which does not assume the natural resting flexion "cascade" of the adjacent fingers.

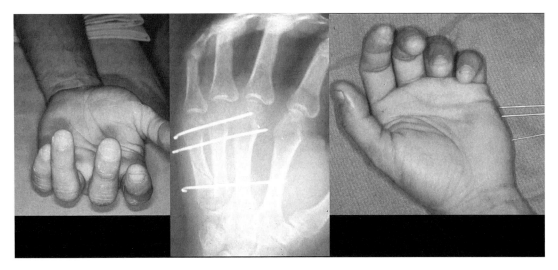

FIGURE 39.6. **(Left to right)** Rotational deformity is seen with the fingers flexed. This is secondary to a spiral fracture of the middle finger metacarpal. Closed reduction of the fracture and percutaneous pinning show restoration to normality of the previous deformity.

proximal to the radial styloid, which proceed in a subcutaneous course across the "anatomic snuffbox" to innervate the skin of the dorsum of the first web space. The number of fingers served by each nerve may vary. As an absolute rule, however, the palmar surfaces of the index and little fingers are always served by the median and ulnar nerves, respectively (Figure 39.9).

With regard to the motor supply of the nerves,[7] the ulnar nerve serves the hypothenar muscles, interossei, ulnar two lumbricals, adductor pollicis, and deep head of the flexor pollicis brevis. The median nerve serves abductor pollicis brevis, opponens pollicis, radial two lumbricals, and superficial head of the flexor pollicis brevis. In summary, the median nerve supplies all of the extrinsic digit flexors and wrist flexors (except the flexor digitorum profundus to the ring and little fingers and the flexor carpi ulnaris, which are supplied by the ulnar nerve) and all the thumb intrinsic muscles (except the adductor pollicis, supplied by the ulnar nerve). The ulnar nerve innervates all the interossei, all the lumbricals (except the radial two, supplied by the median nerve), and the adductor of the thumb. The radial nerve supplies all of the wrist, finger, and thumb long extensors. There are two muscle tests that may provide one with an absolute diagnosis of median and ulnar nerve injury. The motor function of the abductor pollicis brevis tests the median nerve. With the hand flat and facing palm up, the patient is asked to touch with the thumb the examiner's fingers held directly over the thenar eminence (Figure 39.10A). The flexor digiti minimi muscle function tests the motor supply of the ulnar nerve: In the same hand position, the patient is asked to raise the little finger vertically, flexing the metacarpophalangeal joint to a 90° angle with the interphalangeal joints straight (Figure 39.10B).

Musculoskeletal Examination

Tendons are individually tested for integrity.[7] Flexion at the distal joints of the thumb and fingers (Figure 39.11A,B) respectively confirms integrity of the flexor pollicis longus and flexor digitorum profundus. Testing of flexor digitorum superficialis tendons is more complex (Figure 39.11C). It is not possible to flex the ulnar three distal interphalangeal (DIP) joints independently of one another because of the common origin of the profundus tendons; therefore, two of the three are fixed in extension by the examiner, and the patient is asked to bend the third. This movement will be produced by the flexor digitorum superficialis and occurs at the proximal interphalangeal (PIP) joint. In one third of normal patients, the superficialis cannot produce little finger flexion. In half of these, there is a common origin with the ring finger, and

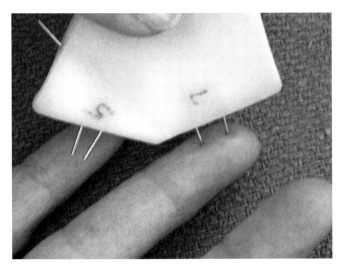

FIGURE 39.7. Testing of two-point sensory discrimination. (This test can also be simply done by bending up the ends of a paperclip.)

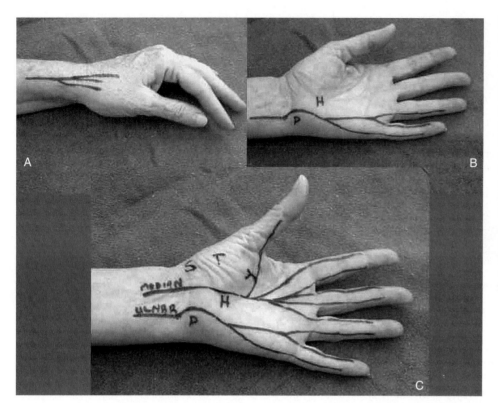

FIGURE 39.8. **(A)** Surface landmarks of the superficial radial nerve as it crosses the "anatomic snuffbox." **(B)** The ulnar nerve passes through Guyon's canal between the pisiform (P) and hook of hamate (H) bone landmarks. **(C)**The transverse carpal ligament forms the roof of a carpal tunnel and spans between the scaphoid (S) and trapezium (T) on the radial side and between the pisiform (P) and hook of hamate (H) on the ulnar side. The median nerve travels through the carpal canal before dividing into the digital branches and the recurrent motor branch to the thenar muscles.

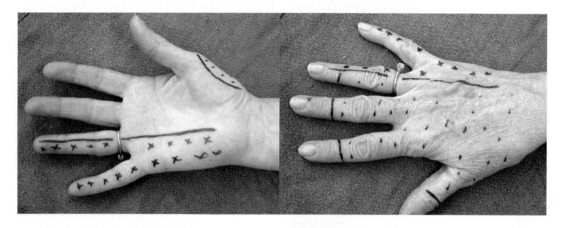

FIGURE 39.9. Sensory distribution of the ulnar nerve (×), radial nerve (–), and median nerve (•) to the hand.

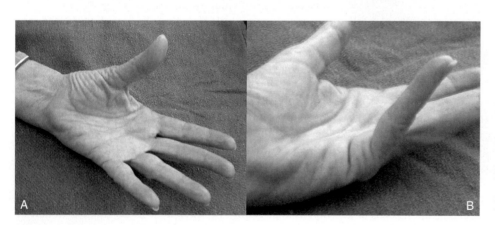

FIGURE 39.10. **(A)** Palmar abduction of the thumb tests the median muscle innervation. **(B)** Flexion of the little finger at the metacarpophalangeal joint is performed by innervation of the hypothenar muscles (flexor digiti minimi) by the ulnar nerve.

FIGURE 39.11. **(A)** Flexor pollicis longus is tested by thumb intraphalangeal joint flexion. **(B)** Flexor digitorum profundus flexes the distal intraphalangeal joint while the rest of the finger is stabilized and prevented from flexing. **(C)** Testing of the flexor digitorum superficialis to the middle finger is done by holding the other three fingers out in extension and the middle finger flexes at the proximal interphalangeal joint. **(D)** Long extensors of the fingers are tested by placing the hand flat on an examining surface and then elevating the specific finger from that surface.

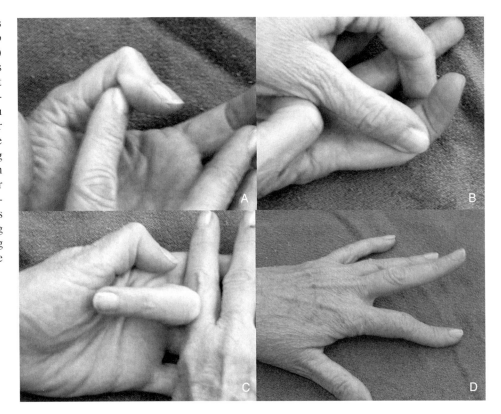

so flexion will occur if the ring finger is permitted to flex simultaneously. More infrequently, there is no profundus tendon to the little finger, and the superficialis inserts into both the middle and distal phalanges.

The long and short extensors and long abductor of the thumb can be tested by asking the patient to extend the thumb against gentle resistance while the tendons are individually palpated. The long extensors of the fingers are tested by asking the patient to extend against gentle resistance applied to the dorsum of each proximal phalanx (Figure 39.11D).

Special Investigations

Radiographs are obtained in almost every case.[8] These will help in diagnosis and evaluation of fractures and also in investigation of foreign bodies (Figure 39.12). Multiple

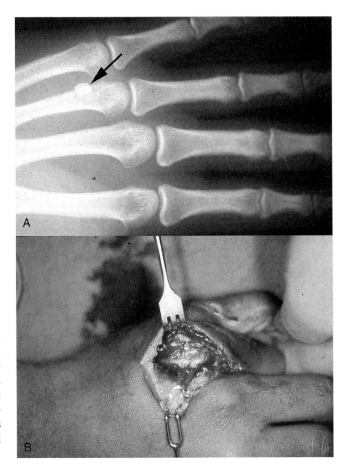

FIGURE 39.12. This patient had a seemingly innocuous dorsal hand laceration and refused to offer any potentially incriminating history about the mechanism of injury. **(A)** A radiograph showed a radiodense foreign object directly overlying the metacarpophalangeal joint (arrow). **(B)** Upon surgical exploration of that joint, an assailant's broken off tooth (arrow) was found imbedded in the articular cartilage of the distal metacarpal.

radiographic views of the affected part are frequently required to define the pathology. Glass is frequently visualized on plain radiographs and if not seen but suspected, is clearly visualized by computed tomography (CT) or magnetic resonance imaging (MRI).[9,10] If plastic is painted, it may be seen on routine radiographs; otherwise, it is only poorly visualized on CT scan but clearly seen with MRI. Wood foreign bodies are detected by CT or MRI but not by routine radiography.[9,10.]

Various stress radiographic views and cineradiography are useful for demonstrating dynamic wrist instability patterns (particularly scapholunate separation).[8] Arthrography detects ligamentous tears by extravasation of contrast material between the radiocarpal, distal radioulnar, and midcarpal joints. Magnetic resonance imaging may detect triangular fibrocartilage tears. Radionuclide bone scanning may be helpful, and focal uptake may be seen in phase III in osteomyelitis, but for the hand false-positive scans are seen because of close proximity of soft tissue infections to the bones. "Occult" wrist fractures may be localized by increased radionuclide uptake, but a false-positive test may occur with ligamentous injuries.[8] Computed tomography may be the best modality for diagnosing suspected carpal fractures that are not seen on routine radiographs.

Wrist arthroscopy is a recently introduced diagnostic and therapeutic modality for a number of wrist problems, particularly for disorders of the triangular fibrocartilage. Minimally invasive surgery with arthroscopic guidance has added a new dimension to the treatment of acute wrist disorders, including scaphoid and distal radius intraarticular fractures.

Patients with ischemic problems usually require noninvasive vascular studies. Doppler pressure measurements help to localize the site of the lesion. Angiography should be done in the presence of a vasodilator (such as Priscoline or nitroglycerin) or axillary block in order to differentiate apparent vessel occlusion from vasospasm. Subtraction radiographs with magnification help to improve the detail and definition of the vascular study (particularly in the distal forearm and hands).[6,8]

Fingertip and Nailbed Injuries

All patients presenting with nailbed injuries must have radiograms.[11] An underlying distal phalangeal fracture must have appropriate protective splinting, reduction to improve alignment if necessary, and occasional internal fixation if the fracture is unstable. Internal fixation is most frequently provided by simply placing a longitudinal 0.028-inch Kirschner wire. Appropriate antibiotics are administered, as technically the fractures are open.

The least severe injury of the dorsum of the fingertip is a nailbed hematoma. If seen early, the hematoma can be decompressed by perforating the nail plate after administration of a digital local anesthetic block.[11] Most fingertip and nailbed injuries can be managed with digital block anesthesia and placement of a Penrose drain at the base of the finger as a tourniquet. If the nail plate is split, the nail should be gently removed to examine the underlying nailbed. Suture repair of the nailbed is done by using loupe magnification and a 6-0 catgut suture. Stellate nailbed injuries must be meticulously repaired after appropriate wound irrigation and cleansing. Once the nailbed has been repaired, it is best to place the thoroughly cleaned nail back into the nail fold where it both serves as a rigid splint for an underlying distal phalangeal fracture and prevents adhesions from forming between the adjacent surfaces of the nail fold, which might lead to an unsightly "split" nail deformity. If a piece of nailbed is missing, the undersurface of the avulsed nail plate should be examined. The missing piece may still be adherent to the nail, and it can be gently removed and replaced as a nailbed graft. If the missing piece of nailbed cannot be retrieved, the defect may be treated by obtaining a split nailbed graft from an adjacent nail or from a toenail bed. More severe dorsal fingertip injuries can be resurfaced by using a reverse cross-finger subcutaneous flap as described by Atasoy. Some injuries may be so severe that amputation revision may be the most sensible and functional solution.

Volar fingertip injuries also range from the simple to the more complex. These often involve multiple digits such as with lawnmower accidents. If bone is not exposed and the soft tissue defect is less than 1 cm in an adult, the wound is best left open and managed with soaks and dressings.[11] Such injuries heal with surprisingly good functional and cosmetic results. Larger soft tissue defects of the fingertip pulp may be more appropriately treated with a small split-thickness skin graft. On the other hand, if bone is exposed, one should consider either flap coverage or revision of amputation by trimming back exposed bone to obtain soft tissue coverage. If the loss is dorsally angulated, an advancement flap is indicated. A neurovascular V-Y advancement flap is classically described for this type of defect.[12] More extensive neurovascular island advancement flaps such as that represented by the step advancement flap described by Evans may be considered (Figure 39.13).[13] If the soft tissue loss is angulated in a more volar direction, a cross-finger flap (Figure 39.14),[14] or even an adjacent finger digital island flap or a homodigital flap, may be considered (Figures 39.15 and 39.16).[13,15] The latter requires microvascular tissue handling techniques.

If an amputated fingertip is retained, reimplantation may be considered. This will give an aesthetic nail reconstruction; however, more important, reimplantation of avulsed tissue containing either thumb pulp or index finger pulp should always be considered in view of the

FIGURE 39.13. **(A)** V-Y step advancement flap is reconstructed as an island based on the digital neurovascular structures. **(B)** This is advanced to the fingertip (as much as 2 cm advancement may be achieved) to cover a soft tissue defect that is dorsally angulated and so helps maintain the skeletal length of the finger.

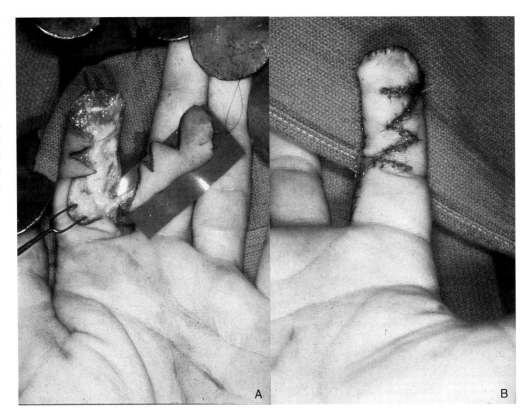

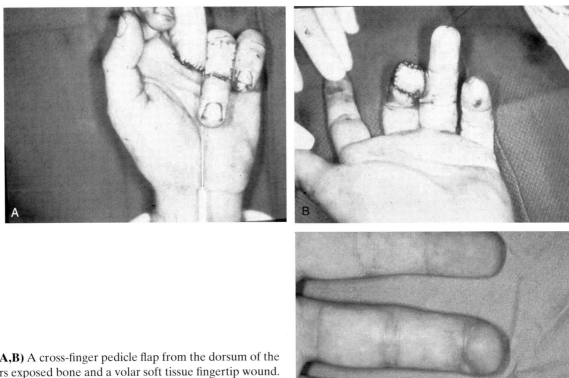

FIGURE 39.14. **(A,B)** A cross-finger pedicle flap from the dorsum of the ring finger covers exposed bone and a volar soft tissue fingertip wound. The dorsal donor site of the ring finger must be skin grafted, and the fingers must be kept joined together for 11 to 14 days before separating the two digits. **(C)** Long-term result shows a pleasing aesthetic reconstruction with preservation of digital length. Protective sensation at the fingertips is generally restored in time.

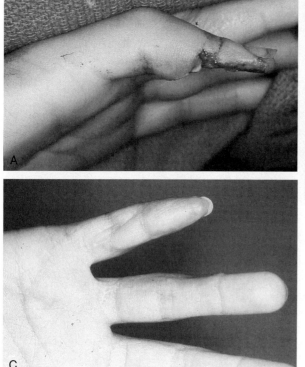

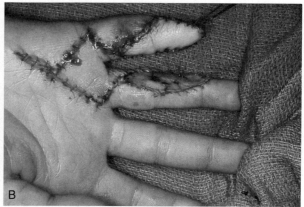

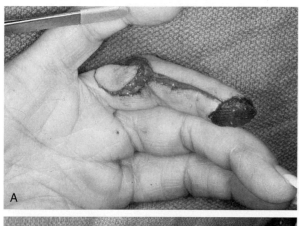

FIGURE 39.15. **(A)** A large volar avulsing wound has both bone and tendon sheath exposed on the little finger. **(B)** An arterialized flap based on the ulnar digital vessels of the ring finger (leaving the digital nerve intact to that ring finger) is transposed to the little finger soft tissue wound with skin grafting done to the donor defect. **(C)** Long-term functional recovery is seen.

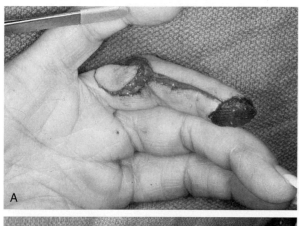

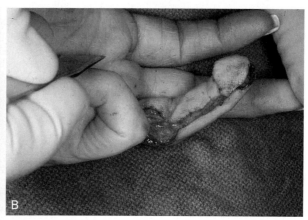

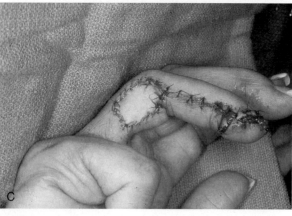

FIGURE 39.16. **(A)** A less extensive volar angulated pulp injury of the finger is seen. **(B,C)** A homodigital reverse pattern arterialized flap is transposed to the fingertip to avoid having to tether adjacent fingers together as would otherwise be the case with a cross-finger flap.

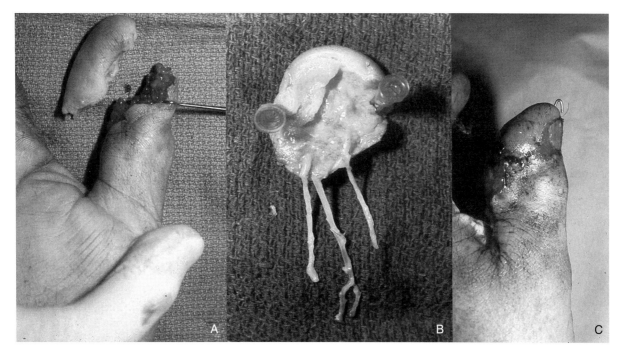

FIGURE 39.17. Microvascular reattachment of a traumatically avulsed thumb pulp.

functional importance of good sensation in these two digits (Figure 39.17).[11] When the amputated part has been too severely crushed, the thumb pulp may be reconstructed by a neurovascular island sensate flap ("kite flap") based on the vascular branches of the first dorsal metacarpal artery from the dorsoradial aspect of the proximal phalanx of the index finger and transposed to reconstruct the thumb pulp (Figure 39.18).[13]

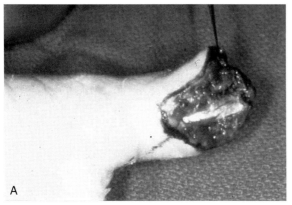

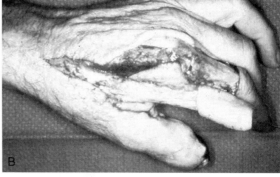

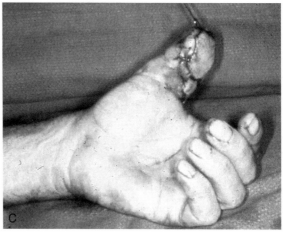

FIGURE 39.18. **(A)** Thumb pulp avulsion injury with the amputated part could not be salvaged. **(B,C)** A "kite" flap was used for reconstruction. This flap is subtended on the first dorsal metacarpal artery and is transposed from the dorsum of the index finger. Skin grafting is necessary for the donor site.

Open Soft Tissue Injuries and Complex Wounds

Before adequate tissue coverage can be safely provided, satisfactory wound debridement must be done.[16] Modern day debridement is much more aggressive than before, because in this era of microvascular tissue transfer we no longer fear being unable to cover exposed vital structures. Another basic tenet of wound management has in the past been the principle of delayed wound closure; however, with regard to upper extremity injuries, this concept is now being challenged. Functional outcome is of paramount importance in upper extremity injuries, and the more rapidly one can start hand therapy the better the chances of maximizing return of function. Treatment consisting of radical debridement, rigid fixation, immediate soft tissue resurfacing, and even immediate reconstruction of segmental bone defects and tendon loss, followed by early protective range of motion exercises, has been shown in some reports to result in excellent functional outcome.[16] All evidence is yet to be gathered to determine if the potentially increased risk of infection has outweighed improved function, decreased morbidity, and shortened hospital stay that might result from immediate soft tissue coverage and reconstruction. Adequate debridement and wound irrigation are key. Irrigation under a pressure of at least 7 psi has been shown to be effective but must be combined with the judicious use of parenteral antibiotics.

Once a wound has satisfied the requirements of closure, the reconstructive options must be considered. Each wound should be approached with the reconstructive ladder (Figure 39.19) in mind, and the simplest option that is best suited to both the general condition of the patient and the local requirements of the specific wound should be selected. Skin graft is suitable for wounds of large surface area that do not expose important structures, such as burn injuries; however, in the hand and upper extremity, a more durable wound coverage is often required. Skin grafts may be applied directly over tendons (if paratenon is intact), but they may not be very suitable because tendons adhere to overlying grafts, causing a deformity with tendon motion. More important, however, is the frequent secondary need for tenolysis and hence the requirement for coverage that is more durable than a skin graft. A skin graft may, on the other hand, provide useful temporary coverage when the severe nature of the patient's injuries precludes more elaborate immediate wound closure.

Our understanding of soft tissue coverage was clarified when McGregor popularized the concept of axial—and random—pattern flaps.[17] The former is a single pedicled flap with an anatomically recognized arteriovenous system running along its access. The groin flap, based on the superficial circumflex iliac artery, was one of the earliest axial pattern flaps described and is still frequently used for resurfacing of the upper extremity. A groin flap may be used for preliminary soft tissue coverage to conserve recipient vessels prior to needed further microvascular surgery such as a planned subsequent toe transfer. A groin flap may also have a role for soft tissue coverage of the hand where recipient arteries and veins are unavailable for free flap reconstruction. This occurs particularly in a patient with peripheral vascular disease, or one who has recovered from a significant soft tissue infection and cellulitis, or in a drug abuser or with extravasation injuries where recipient arteries, and in particular veins, may be unavailable (Figure 39.20). In contrast, a random pattern flap is one that lacks any significant bias in its vascular pattern. Such flaps were classically thought to need a length-base ratio of 1:1 to avoid distal tip necrosis; however, Milton showed that absolute flap length, not width, is crucial.

We now know that absolute survival flap length of random pattern flaps is determined by the axiality of the flap: that is, a longer flap can be obtained by orienting it along the longitudinal rather than the transverse axis of an extremity. This is because the predominant direction of the vessels is longitudinal, and so by random chance more vessels will run along the length of the flap. Increased flap length (that is, improved reliability) is also obtained by including fascia (so-called fasciocutaneous flaps) or by tissue expansion. The fascia carries with it its own inherent blood supply, while the capsule produced around the silicone tissue expander is also very vascular and so imparts viability to the overlying skin. Local and regional flaps are described by the way in which they are moved. There are two types: flaps that rotate about a pivot point (rotation and transposition flaps) and

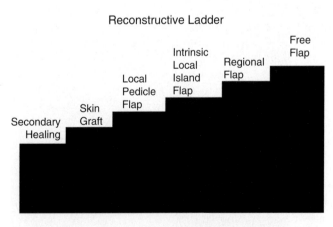

Reconstructive Ladder

FIGURE 39.19. The reconstructive ladder.

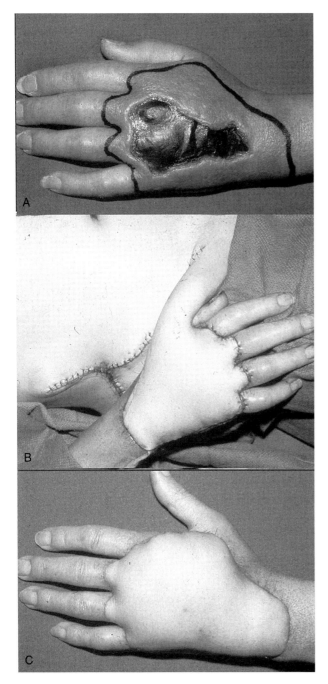

FIGURE 39.20. **(A)** An extravasation injury from a chemotherapy solution requires debridement. **(B,C)** Groin pedicle flap keeps the hand initially attached to the body, and the pedicle is separated after 3 weeks. (Courtesy of Melvin Spira, MD.)

advancement flaps.[17] Axial flaps may consist of skin only (e.g., groin flap), fascia and fasciocutaneous tissue (e.g., radial forearm, lateral arm, temporoparietal flaps), or muscle and musculocutaneous tissue (e.g., latissimus dorsi, rectus abdominis, and gracilis). Radial forearm flap

and posterior interosseus flap may be pedicled on the distal blood supply so that the venous flow is retrograde (Figure 39.21).[18]

Flaps offer a number of advantages over skin grafts.[17] They avoid contraction, fill dead space, cover important structures (vessels, bone, tendons, nerves), help clean up infection, enhance vascularity, and provide specific functions (e.g., latissimus muscle transfer to restore biceps function). Since Ger's use of muscle flaps for osteomyelitis in the 1960s, "antiinfection" has been attributed to muscle. Mathes has provided scientific data to support this premise. We believe it is the good blood supply of an axial pattern flap that provides the ability to "clean up" infection in a contaminated but nonetheless adequately debrided wound.

Reconstructive requirements of the upper extremity may be summarized as follows:

1. Replace the missing tissue type with a similar type. In the hand and fingers, thin and pliable soft tissue coverage is required.

2. There may be a subsequent or simultaneous need for secondary reconstruction of bone, tendon, and nerve in addition to the soft tissue requirements. Under these circumstances, skin grafts would be inadequate soft tissue coverage.

3. Flap reconstructions may need to be sensate, especially at the fingertips.[19]

4. The size of the defect needs to be reconstructed three dimensionally. A deep volume of soft tissue may be required as well as a large surface area in certain injuries.

5. Flap reconstruction may need to be functional and provide motion.

Injuries in the shoulder girdle region and upper arm can be covered by a wealth of potential pedicle muscle and cutaneous flaps. An example is a patient who had a gunshot wound to the lateral aspect of the deltoid region where a latissimus dorsi musculocutaneous flap not only helped provide soft tissue contour wound coverage but also augmented missing muscle function (Figure 39.22). Closure of elbow wounds has been described by a number of elaborate means; however, a large posterior arm rotation flap often readily covers the extensor aspect of the olecranon (Figure 39.23), and a transposition flap (with the donor site skin grafted) will cover vital exposed structures in the antecubital fossa. On the dorsum of the hand, a local random pattern flap provides thin and pliable soft tissue coverage. A transposition flap (Figure 39.24) shifted radially covered the exposed basilar thumb joint and allowed the metacarpal base and shattered trapezium to be reconstructed by soft tissue tendon interposition and immediate bone grafting.

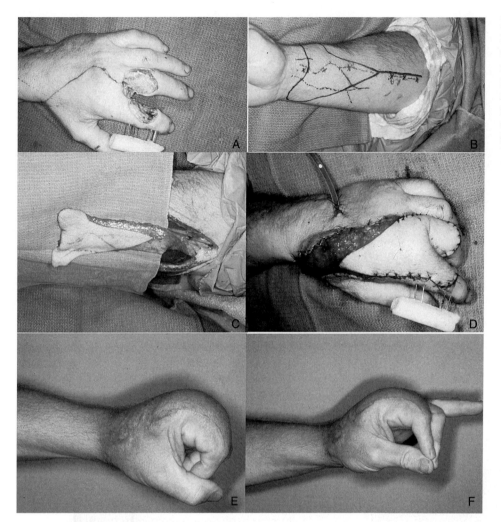

FIGURE 39.21. **(A)** A wound involving the web space and adjacent surfaces of the index and middle fingers. **(B–D)** A reverse flow radial forearm fasciocutaneous flap is transposed from the ipsilateral forearm distally to the traumatic defect. **(E,F)** Functional outcome.

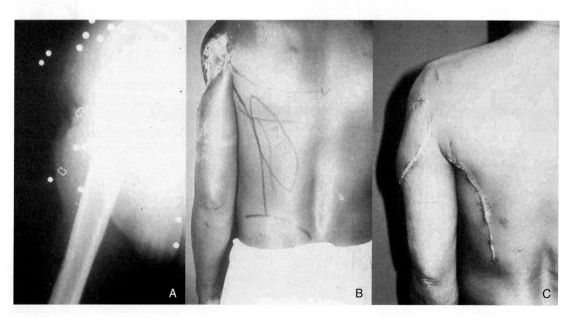

FIGURE 39.22. A wound of the deltoid area resulting from a shotgun blast is successfully covered with a latissimus dorsi musculocutaneous flap.

FIGURE 39.23. A rotation flap (arrow) designed on the posterior aspect of the upper arm readily covers an olecranon wound.

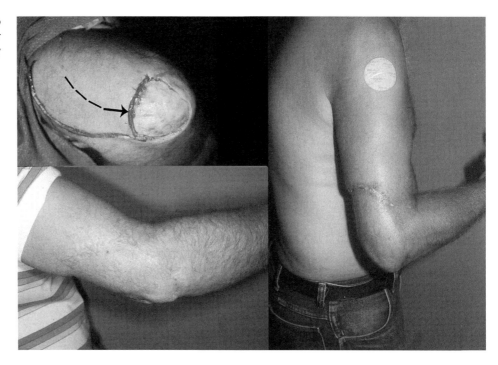

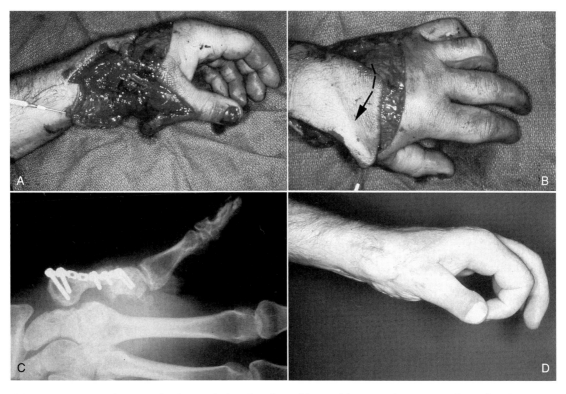

FIGURE 39.24. **(A)** A blast injury to the base of the thumb resulted in a shattered thumb metacarpal and trapezium and substantial soft tissue wound. **(B)** A transpositional flap pro-vides stable wound coverage (arrow). **(C)** Immediate bone reconstruction was undertaken. **(D)** Final reconstruction has restored thumb prehension.

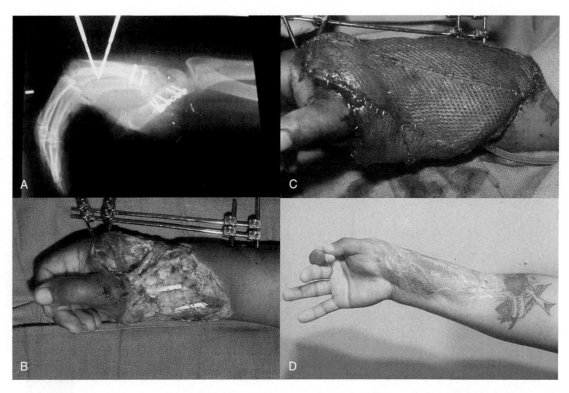

FIGURE 39.25. **(A,B)** A blast injury to the radial side of the distal forearm and hand. **(C)** Soft tissue coverage over the reconstructed bone with latissimus dorsi microvascular muscle transfer and a skin graft. **(D)** With time the muscle atrophies, and well-contoured reconstruction is restored.

Free vascularized tissue transfers are specifically indicated where there is a need to cover sites that ordinarily cannot be reached by pedicle flaps or to meet specific reconstructive requirements.[20] All areas of the upper extremity, unlike the distal third of the leg, can be reached by pedicle flaps. However, some defects may be so large as to make pedicle flaps impractical. A gunshot wound to the dorsoradial aspect of the wrist resulted in a very large soft tissue wound, tendon injuries, and comminuted fractures to the first metacarpal base and radial side of the wrist (Figure 39.25). Free bone graft reconstruction at the base of the thumb metacarpal with flexor carpi radialis tendon interposition and volar oblique ligament reconstruction to restore the anatomic configuration of the thumb basilar articulation with a traumatically destroyed trapezium was performed. This reconstruction was covered with well-vascularized soft tissue using latissimus dorsi muscle free flap covered by a skin graft. The transformed muscle will generally atrophy with time, and this will generally result in a good contour and

is preferred over the more bulky musculocutaneous flap.

A microvascular free flap is clearly required where certain reconstructive goals must be met, as in cases of segmental bone loss in the arm.[20] In this large soft tissue wound to the forearm from a shotgun injury with associated segmental bone defect, a reconstruction was performed with a composite myo-osseus flap using latissimus dorsi muscle and a serratus muscle with vascularized rib, all on a single thoracodorsal vascular pedicle (Figure 39.26). The muscle was covered with a split-thickness skin graft.

Finally, microvascular reconstruction enables single-stage reconstruction of bone and soft tissue and avoids hand dependency that would occur with a groin flap and enables motion at the earliest possible time when combined with rigid bone fixation. Early motion, well-vascularized soft tissue of adequate bulk, and extremity elevation reduce the risk of hand stiffness and contractures.

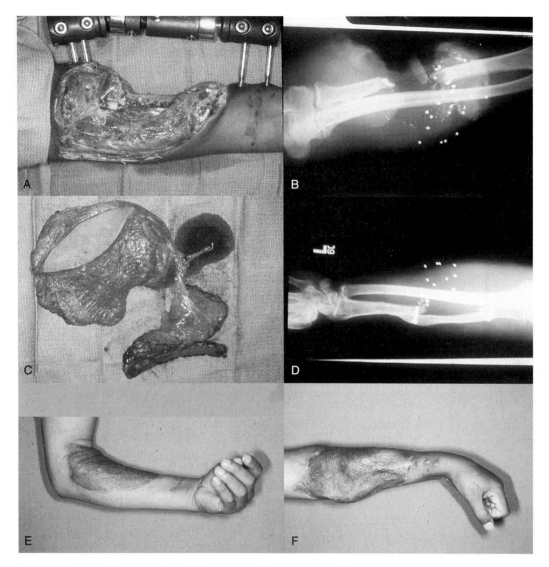

FIGURE 39.26. **(A,B)** Shotgun injury to the mid forearm with both significant soft tissue loss and segmental bone loss. **(C,D)** Composite microvascular transfer using the latissimus dorsi, ser-ratus anterior, and a rib all on a single thoracodorsal vascular pedicle enables a single-stage reconstruction of the soft tissue and bone defect. **(E,F)** Final outcome of the reconstruction.

Replantations and Amputations of the Upper Extremity

Replantation is the reattachment of a part that has been completely amputated. Revascularization requires reconstruction of vessels in a limb that has been severely injured or incompletely severed in such a way that vascular repair is necessary to prevent distal necrosis but some soft tissue (skin, tendon, nerves) is intact.[21] Revascularization generally has a better success rate than replantation, because venous and lymphatic drainage may be intact.

Minor replantation is a reattachment at the wrist, hand, or digital level, whereas major replantation is that performed proximal to the wrist.[21] This clinical distinction exists because, in the case of major replantations, ischemic time is crucial to viability of muscle and functional outcome. Ischemic muscle may result in myonecrosis, myoglobinemia, and infection that may threaten the patient's life as well as limb.

Amputations can be classified into three types[21]:

1. Guillotine amputation: This is used for tissue that is cut by a sharp object and is minimally damaged.

2. Crush amputations: A local crush injury can be converted into a guillotine injury simply by debriding back edges, but this may not be practically feasible for a more diffusely crushing injury.

3. Avulsion amputations: These are the most unfavorable type for replanting, because structures are injured at different levels. This may occur, for example, with a

so-called ring avulsion injury. Extensor tendons are shredded, flexor tendons are often avulsed at the musculotendinous junctions, and nerves are stretched and may be ripped from end organs.

Viability alone of a replantation is not construed as a measure of its success; useful function must be achieved. Replantation has both absolute and relative contraindications. It is strongly contraindicated at any level of amputation if there is significant concomitant life-threatening injury; severe chronic illness that precludes transportation or prolonged surgery; or extensive injury to the affected limb or amputated part. The following factors must also be considered when planning for potential replantation of amputated parts[22]:

1. Ischemia time: For amputated digits, more than 12 hours of warm ischemia is a relative contraindication. Promptly cooling the part to 4° to 10°C dramatically alters the ischemia factor, but even ischemia exceeding 24 hours does not preclude successful replantation. Ischemia time is more crucial for replants above the proximal forearm, and these should not be considered after more than 6 to 10 hours of warm ischemia time.

2. Affected parts: Good candidates for replantation are those who have amputations of the thumb or multiple digits or through the palm, wrist, and individual fingers distal to the insertion of the flexor digitorum superficialis tendon. Single digit injuries other than the thumb, in zone II, are generally not reattached because of the unfavorable functional outcome and the consequent adverse overall functional result on the hand with a single stiff finger. Because the function of the thumb accounts for 40% of total hand function, almost all amputated thumbs should be replanted with care taken to preserve the length of the thumb.

3. Patient considerations: A decision to replant a single digit proximal to the insertion of the flexor digitorum superficialis tendon is influenced by special circumstances, such as a patient who is a young woman or a professional musician or a child. Not only are sex, occupation, and age important considerations, but also mental health. For a child, an attempt should be made to replant almost any amputated part, because useful function can usually be anticipated and also because the child's eventual vocation is unknown. Old age is usually not a barrier to replantation provided that the vessels are not seen to be atherosclerotic when examined under the microscope. Mental stability is frequently difficult to assess in the limited time available for preoperative evaluation in the emergency room.

Amputation should not be considered an outmoded operation; rather, it is necessary when replantation might not be indicated.[22] When primary amputation is performed, the stump should be preserved with as much length as possible. An exception might be made if there is only a very short segment of proximal phalanx. If a ring or middle finger is involved, the short stump might have little value to the hand, in as much as small objects will fall through the gap. A short proximal phalangeal remnant at the index finger position may serve as an impediment to thumb to middle finger prehension. In all of these situations one might consider formal ray amputations to improve overall hand function.

The ends of the cut nerve should be allowed to retract or should be buried in muscle in order to minimize the occurrence of painful neuromas after amputation. Tendons should also be divided sharply and allowed to retract. The practice of suturing the flexor and extensor tendons over the end of the middle, ring, or small finger stump seriously impairs the motion of the uninjured fingers owing to the common origin of these flexors. There is an active flexion deficit in the uninjured digits, which nonetheless have a normal passive range. This is called the quadriga syndrome and is corrected by release of the flexor tendon remnant of the injured digit.

Operative Procedure for Replantation

Before transportation, the amputated part is placed in a clean, dry, plastic bag that is sealed and placed on top of ice in a Styrofoam container. This keeps the part sufficiently cool at 4° to 10°C without freezing.[21]

Bone shortening allows skin to be debrided back to where it is free of contusion and where direct tension-free closure can be achieved. In the thumb, bone shortening should be minimized to less than 10 mm. Bruner incisions may be used for exposure. The order of repair is usually bone, tendons, muscle units, arteries, nerves, and finally veins.[21]

In replanting the proximal portion of the digit, preplacing the sutures to the proximal and distal tendon ends enables the digit to be held in extension to expose microvascular structures on the volar surface. Once neurovascular repairs are completed, tendon ends are then simply coapted. Establishment of arterial flow before venous flow clears lactic acid from the replanted part. The functional veins can now also be detected by spurting bleeding. However, blood loss must be closely monitored.

For major replantations, reestablishing arterial circulation as rapidly as possible is crucial to limiting the ischemia time period.[21] A dialysis shunt or carotid shunt may be placed between the arterial ends. Intermittent clamping of the shunt may be necessary to restrict blood loss. In the upper extremity, bone shortening can be aggressive to achieve primary skin closure and primary nerve repair. Preparatory exploration of the distal amputated part under the microscope by an initial surgical team not only determines whether or not a replantation is technically feasible but also can be started while the patient is being prepared for the operating room. Judicious use of anticoagulants may enhance the success of the replantation. Topical application of 2% lidocaine or papaverine may help to relieve vasospasm.

Postoperative dressings consist of longitudinal strips of nonadherent mesh gauze, loose fluff gauze, and a plaster splint, and postoperative elevation minimizes edema and venous congestion. The patient's room must be kept warm, and smoking is forbidden postoperatively. Aside from antibiotics and analgesics, one aspirin tablet a day for its retarding effect on platelet aggregation is suggested. Postoperative monitoring is done hourly for color, pulp turgor, capillary refill, and digital temperature.

Tendon Injuries

Flexor Tendons

For better understanding and treatment of tendon injuries, the international agreement on anatomic nomenclature for the flexor and extensor zones of the hand was reached at the First Congress of the International Federation for Surgery of the Hand in Rotterdam in June 1980. Flexor tendon injuries are divided into five zones (Figure 39.27).[23] In zones I, II, and IV, each tendon is surrounded by a synovial sheath and is contained within a semirigid fibro-osseus canal. The synovial membrane has both parietal and visceral (epitenon) layers. In the other zones, the tendons are surrounded by loose areolar (paratenon) tissue. Healing in those parts devoid of a fibrous sheath is usually excellent because of the good blood supply from the paratenon. In addition, the profundus tendons in zone III have a segmental blood supply via the lumbrical muscles. Tendons in the carpal tunnel (zone IV) have a rich blood supply provided by the mesotenon; however, zone II and zone I have a precarious blood supply.[23] It is thought that complimentary

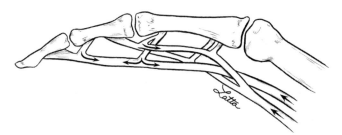

FIGURE 39.28. Vascular supply of flexor tendons in the digital flexor tendon sheath is derived through the vincula. Nutritional support of the synovium in this region is thus essential for tendon healing where blood supply is relatively tenuous.

nutritional support is provided by the synovial fluid. In order for tendon gliding to occur, the mesotenon has disappeared in the digital flexor sheaths except at the sites of the vincula that carry the vessels from the periosteum (Figure 39.28). They supply the longitudinal intrinsic vascular system, which runs through the tendons and is located chiefly in their dorsal and lateral aspects. The complimentary role of blood and synovial circulation can be extended to the understanding of tendon healing. Opposing but not mutually exclusive theories have been proposed to explain normal tendon healing. According to one theory, healing depends on blood supplied by adhesions formed from the sheath and surrounding tissues beginning a few days after injury. Tendon motion speeds regression of adhesions and strengthens the repair. A newer theory proposes that tendons completely devoid of blood supply will heal if bathed in synovial fluid.

A primary tendon repair is undertaken within a few hours of injury and is generally reserved for cleanly cut tendons.[24] Delayed primary repair may be performed from several hours up to 10 days after injury and is indicated for tidy but potentially contaminated wounds to allow for prophylaxis against infection before tendon repair. Relative contraindications to immediate tendon repair are (1) injuries more than 12 hours old; (2) crush wounds with poor skin coverage; (3) contaminated wounds, especially human bites; (4) tendon loss greater than 1 cm; (5) injury at multiple sites along with tendons; and (6) destruction of the pulley system. After 4 weeks, secondary repair is generally not possible because of retraction of the musculotendinous units so that reapproximation of the tendon ends produces undesirable joint flexion. Additionally, after 4 weeks the proximal tendon may coil and thicken, becoming too large to pass under the pulley into the flexor tendon sheath.

The surgeon's endeavors are directed to avoiding the four major complications that interfere with the smooth gliding and integrated action of tendons: adhesions, attenuation, rupture, and joint and soft tissue contractures.[23,24] Prerequisites for tendon repair are aseptic conditions in an operating room with good lighting, good instruments, adequate anesthesia (axillary block or general anesthesia), and loupe magnification.

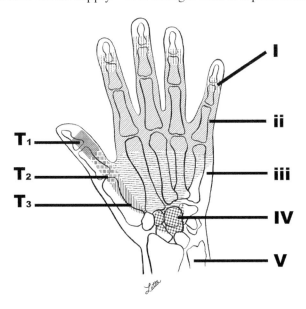

FIGURE 39.27. Flexor tendon zones of injury.

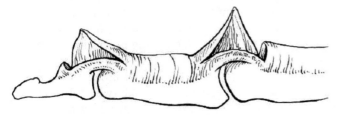

FIGURE 39.29. Access to lacerated tendons within the flexor tendon sheath is facilitated by enlarging the existing laceration in the sheath. However, avoid excising A2 or A4 pulleys.

Partial tendon injuries must be treated appropriately in order to produce a smooth juncture at the site of injury.[23] Prevention of complications rests with exploration of all wounds likely to cause partial flexor tendon lacerations. Partial lacerations of 50% or less are treated simply by trimming the lacerated portion and do not need to be sutured. Those partial injuries greater than 50% should be repaired. Nonrepaired, less than 50% partial lacerations have a significantly higher ultimate load and stiffness than those that are repaired. Failure to diagnosis a partial flexor tendon laceration at the time of primary repair may lead to delayed tendon rupture, entrapment between the tendon laceration and a laceration in the flexor sheath, or trigger finger.

Zone II tendon injuries merit special attention.[25] This zone is called the "no-man's land" of Bunnell. Three tendons (profundus and two slips of superficialis) traverse zone II, and they constantly interchange their mutual spatial relationships. Tendon injury in this region necessitates enlarging the sheath opening in order to gain access to sufficient tendon length for repair. The existing laceration in the sheath is used in making a longitudinal trap door incision so that a flap of sheath can be lifted up (Figure 39.29). Enough room is left for subsequent sheath closure if technically possible. Care should be taken to avoid excising the annular pulleys, especially A_2 and A_4, although it has been shown that as much as 50% of either of these two pulleys can be excised for on the flexor tendon sheath without any significant biomechanical consequences. Flaps can be raised on either side of these pulleys and repair performed by working on each side. It is difficult to repair both profundus and superficialis tendons if they are injured. Nonetheless, both should be repaired as resection of the superficialis reduces overall grip strength, predisposes to recurvatum and swan neck deformity at the PIP joint, and damages the vincula supply to the profundus.

Usually skin wounds have to be extended to display the divided tendon ends. The Bruner zigzag exposure is preferred. The tendons are handled with fine-toothed forceps only at their cut ends; their surface is never touched. The wrist is flexed, and a small Keith needle is passed transversely through the proximal tendon about

2 cm from its end, transfixing it to the skin and sheath but avoiding the neurovascular bundle. Immobilization of the tendon in this way facilitates tension-free repair. The ragged tendon ends may be squared off, but no more than a total of 1 cm should be resected, or some permanent contracture will result. The tendon ends are brought together by a single tension-holding "core suture." (A modified Kessler suture is preferred.) The transverse limb of the suture is placed volar to the longitudinal limbs and nearer to the tendon ends so as to "lasso" the lateral tendon fibers caught in the loops (Figure 39.30). Such locking loops increase by 10% to 50% the ultimate tensile strength of the repair. If this is not done, and a grasping loop rather than a locking loop is placed, tension on the suture line can open up the loop, increasing the propensity for gapping at the repair site. The ideal suture material for tendon repair has not been found. A 4-0 coated polyester or braided nylon is the best material for the core stitch.

Based on data from a number of studies and adjusting for friction, edema, and the effect of early repair stress,

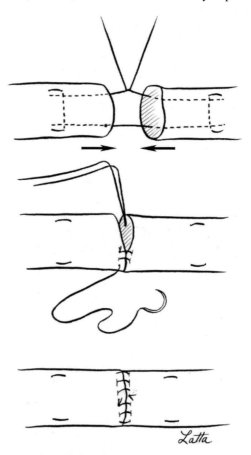

FIGURE 39.30. Locking core suture and running epitenon peripheral suture enable a strong, smoothly gliding flexor tendon repair to be achieved. Most would now add at least a second core suture or employ a double-stranded suture material because it has been shown that at least four strands crossing the repair site are optimum.

rough estimates allow for preparation of a strength versus force graph. The safety of any four-strand core suture repair can then be appreciated.[24] Some achieve a four-stranded core repair by using a double-stranded type of suture material. Others place a second core suture with a single-stranded material. Such a four-stranded core repair should permit light composite grip during the entire healing period.

Additionally, a running circumferential peripheral epitendon suture repair is also placed. This not only helps to smooth the surface of the repair site but adds to the ultimate tensile strength of the repair and reduces gap formation. A peripheral 6-0 nylon coapting suture serves the purpose. Thus, the characteristics of the ideal primary flexor tendon repair are (1) sutures easily placed in the tendon, (2) secure suture knots, (3) smooth junction of tendon ends, (4) minimal gapping at the repair site, (5) minimal interference with tendon vascularity, and (6) sufficient strength throughout healing to permit the application of early motion stress.

Zone I injury may be caused by a penetrating injury. However, closed traction injury may cause profundus tendon avulsion most frequently involving the ring or middle finger. For repair of zone I injuries a pull-out suture is necessary if distal tendon length is insufficient to repair the tendon securely (Figure 39.31), although suture bone anchors have now facilitated this mode of tendon repair into bone at the base of the distal phalanx.

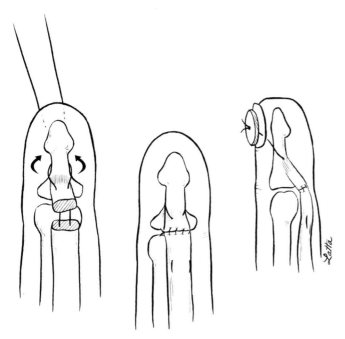

FIGURE 39.31. Method of performing a zone I tendon repair when there is inadequate distal tendon stump for a secure tendon-to-tendon junction repair. DIPJ, distal interphalangeal joint; PIPJ, proximal interphalangeal joint.

A 4-0 monofilament suture is placed transversely through the tendon 1 cm proximal to the cut end and is woven distally along each side of the tendon. A distally based periosteal flap is raised from the volar surface of the distal phalanx. The suture is passed under the flap and around the distal phalanx or through two drill holes and out through the nail over a button. The periosteal flap and distal tendon stump is secured over the repair. The pullout suture is retained for 6 weeks.

Postoperatively, hand elevation is important to reduce edema. The wrist is placed in about 20° of flexion and the metacarpophalangeal joints at about 40° to 60° of flexion. The splint is molded against the fingers with the interphalangeal joints fully extended. A system of rubberband dynamic traction may be used as described by Kleinert following repair of flexor tendons in zone II, with good results obtained in over 80% of cases.[25] An alternative regimen for postoperative care has been described by Duran in which a similar protective splint is used, but controlled passive mobilization is performed. Most recent hand surgery literature is replete with confirmation of the beneficial effects of applying early controlled forces to healing tissues.[26] Advocates of controlled active digital motion believe that this technique generates greater gliding of the healing tendon, fewer adhesions, and the ability to more rapidly achieve tendon strength than passive motion protocols.[25–27] Improved excursion of flexor tendons can be obtained by addition of a palmar bar to the Kleinert dynamic rubber-band protocol, and even greater excursion can be expected if wrist extension is added.

Differential excursion between the two digital flexors is dramatically increased by a synergistic splint that allows for wrist extension and finger flexion. This position of wrist extension and metacarpophalangeal joint flexion produces the least tension on a repaired flexor tendon during active digital flexion; thus, we have come to adapt the hinged brace technique advocated by Strickland and the so-called place and hold protocol.[23] A tenodesis splint with a wrist hinge is fabricated to allow for full wrist flexion, wrist extension of 30°, and maintenance of metacarpophalangeal flexion of at least 60°. Following composite passive digital flexion, the wrist is extended, and passive flexion is maintained. The patient actively maintains digital flexion and holds that position for approximately 5 seconds. The patient is instructed to use the lightest muscle power necessary to maintain digital flexion. This type of protected motion postoperative protocol extends for 6 weeks.

Extensor Tendons

Proper diagnosis and treatment of extensor tendon injuries requires quite a bit of knowledge of the relatively complex anatomy of the extensor mechanism of the

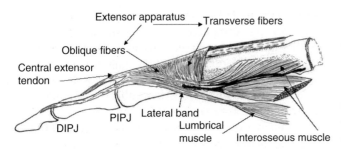

FIGURE 39.32. Anatomy of the extensor mechanism over the dorsum of the finger.

dorsum of the finger (Figure 39.32).[28,29] The common extensor tendon, through the sagittal bands, extends the metacarpophalangeal joint by lifting the volar plate at the base of the proximal phalanx (there is no bony attachment per se of the extensor tendon to the proximal phalanx itself). The central slip of the common extensor extends the PIP joint, and the conjoined tendon extends the DIP joint. Injuries to these structures can result from open lacerations or closed avulsions of the distal insertions.

All lacerations should be repaired if 50% or more of the width of the tendon is divided. Extensor tendon avulsions are most likely to occur at the DIP joint from a "jamming" type of injury that results in a mallet finger deformity (Figure 39.33).[30] If a bone fragment representing 50% or more of the articular surface is involved or if there is a volar subluxation of the DIP joint, an open reduction with internal fixation should be per-

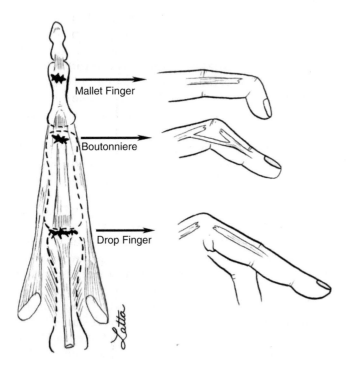

FIGURE 39.33. Depending on the location, extensor tendon injuries will result in mallet finger, boutonniere deformity, or a "dropped" fingertip.

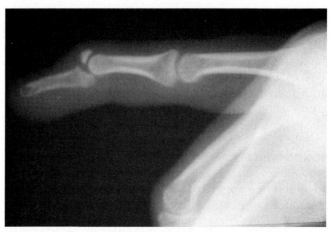

FIGURE 39.34. A mallet fracture from a closed injury requires open reduction and internal fixation such as this case with a large avulsion bone fragment and volar subluxation of the distal phalanx.

formed (Figure 39.34). If there is a tendon rupture or only a small piece of bone avulsed, good results can be obtained by 6 weeks of continuous splinting with the DIP joint in extension (Figure 39.35B). Subsequent to this splinting, the DIP joint should be further protected during sleeping hours for 2 more weeks.

Closed tears through the triangular ligament may be caused by joint subluxation or a jamming type of injury and result in a boutonniere deformity (see Figure 39.33).[31] The central slip attachment at the base of the middle phalanx is disrupted so that extension of that joint is altered. The lateral bands lose their support dorsal to the PIP joint axis and slip volar to it, becoming flexors of the PIP joint and extensors of the DIP joint. Within 6 weeks of injury these can be treated satisfactorily by extension splinting at the PIP joint but maintaining the DIP joint free for active flexion and extension (Figure 39.35A). If there is an open laceration to the central slip mechanism and adjacent triangular ligament, direct suture repair or reinsertion into bone by means of mini-bone anchor sutures should be performed followed by the same postoperative protocol as for a closed avulsion injury.

Extensor tendon injuries proximal to the PIP joint result in a drop finger (see Figure 39.33). They should be repaired and splinted for 4 weeks with the metacarpophalangeal joint at neutral. Common extensor tendon injuries over the dorsum of the hand and at the wrist must be repaired and then treated postoperatively by one of a number of different controlled motion protocols, one of which such schemes is a dynamic rubber-band extension outrigger brace or use of a relative motion splint as described by Merritt in which the affected digit is kept at a more dorsal pitch to the adjacent fingers, thus relaxing the repaired tendon.[28] This latter splint causes minimal interference with day-to-day activities during the rehabilitation period.

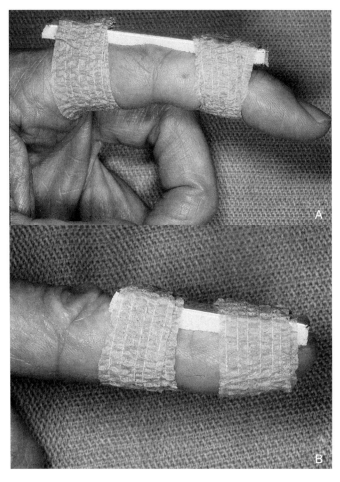

FIGURE 39.35. **(A)** Closed boutonniere proximal interphalangeal injury is treated by continuous finger splinting that immobilizes the joint but allows active flexion of the distal interphalangeal joint. **(B)** Closed mallet injury without a significant bone fracture is treated by continuous finger splinting for 6 weeks and immobilizes the distal interphalangeal joint.

Nerve Injuries

Severance of a peripheral nerve involves an acute loss of sensory, motor, and sympathetic functions. Knowledge of the motor and sensory distributions of the nerve allows for a clinical evaluation of the injury[32]; however, associated injuries such as fractures and muscle and tendon lacerations may complicate the evaluation. Loss of pseudomotor activity occurs within 30 minutes of the nerve injury; a loss of sweating can be demonstrated with a ninhydrin test. Nerve conduction studies, on the other hand, are not helpful immediately following the injury. They become useful 3 weeks after the injury. They demonstrate fibrillation and denervation potentials in muscles that are completely denervated so that in a closed injury they may differentiate between a neuropraxia and a neurotmeses. Later, nerve conduction studies may help monitor nerve regeneration after repair.[33]

From 25% to 75% of the nerve consists of connective tissue; thus, nerves heal by scarring, and the aim of surgical repair of a severed nerve is to minimize the degree of the scarring.[33,34] The epineurium completely surrounds the nerve and also binds groups of fascicles loosely together. Each fascicle is surrounded by a thin sheath of connective tissue called the perineurium that functions as a diffusion barrier. Rupture of the perineurial sheath results in loss of the conduction properties of the enclosed nerve fibers. Endoneurium provides the connective tissue packing between individual nerve fibers. During limb movement a peripheral nerve undergoes longitudinal excursion within its bed. The greatest excursion of peripheral nerves occurs at the wrist proximal to the carpal tunnel where the median nerve has 15.5 mm of gliding when the wrist ranges through a full arch of flexion and extension. Longitudinal excursion of the nerve during limb movement must be added to the normal retraction of the divided nerve when considering a repair.

Primary nerve repair is done within 72 hours of injury, delayed primary repair from 72 hours to 14 days, and secondary nerve repair in 14 or more days following injury. Factors that might influence the timing of nerve repair are the following:

1. Metabolic changes within the nerve: Peak metabolic activity in the nerve occurs within 4 to 20 days following injury, and it has been postulated that nerve repairs might optimally be performed in the second or third week postinjury. There are no clinical studies to support this hypothesis.

2. Muscle cell changes: Muscle spindles start to atrophy at 3 to 4 months. There is no hope of motor function return after 18 months.

3. Sensory end-organs: Sensory end-organs survive without nerve innervation, but the quality of sensation depends on the ability of the brain to decode messages received from the end-organs. Young patients accomplish better sensory recovery after a long delay (even more than a year) than can be achieved with adults. Fibrosis of the distal nerve channels may block axonal growth after a prolonged delay following injury, and this may also limit the degree of sensory recovery.

4. Wound condition: Treatment of skin loss, vascular insufficiency, and skeletal instability all take precedence over nerve repair. In the presence of a severely crushed or avulsed nerve or after a gunshot blast, secondary nerve repair is better at which time the proximal and distal extents of the nerve injury from the site of division can be better appreciated. Nonetheless, at the time of acute management of the wound, identification of cut ends and temporary approximation to maintain elastic length are helpful.

5. Patient condition: Nerve repair is an exacting operation and must be delayed until the patient's condition permits suitable circumstances.

Thus, primary neurorrhaphy is recommended when (1) the nerve is sharply incised, (2) there is minimal wound contamination, (3) there are no injuries that preclude obtaining skeletal stability or adequate skin cover, (4) the patient is sufficiently stable to undergo an operation, and (5) appropriate magnification and instrumentation are available.

Within a nerve, fascicles are not separate cables running in parallel throughout the length of the nerve. There are multiple interconnections between them resulting in an intraneural plexus.[32,34,35] This explains the difficulty of nerve reconstruction in cases of segmental loss and the often suboptimal clinical results following repair of even a sharply incised nerve laceration. Within hours of the nerve injury, the nerve cell body in the anterior horn of the spinal cord undergoes metabolic changes, and transected axons begin to sprout. Wallerian degeneration occurs in the entire segment distal to the injury and 1 to 2 cm proximal to it. The endoneurial tubes during this process are cleared of debris from axons and myelin, allowing a path for axonal regeneration. Subsequent axonal regeneration occurs at a maximum rate of 1 to 2 mm per day. In closed injuries, when the severity of a nerve injury is unknown, repeated clinical evaluations and electrical studies every 3 to 6 weeks will help distinguish between neuropraxia and axial axonal injury. In most cases, surgical exploration with repair is indicated after 3 months if no clinical recovery is detected.

Nerve repair is performed with magnification using microsurgical techniques and either epineurial or group fascicular suture placement. The repair should be tension free. Fibrin glue can be used in combination with a limited number of sutures. With sharp nerve lacerations, an epineurial repair provides as good a functional recovery as fascicular repair provided that anatomic landmarks such as vasa nervorum allow an accurate and precise matching of the cut nerve ends. Current investigation suggests that optimum nerve regeneration and matching of proximal and distal axons occur by a combination of neurotropism and contact guidance. A critical distance must exist between proximal and distal nerve segments to obtain the maximum benefit of neurotropism. With standard nerve grafting it is the surgeon who determines the topography of the proximal and distal fascicles. The fascicular alignment chosen may not always be appropriate. For small gaps, probably up to 3 cm in humans, experimental evidence suggests it might be more appropriate to place a polyglycolic acid tube to bridge the gap rather than to perform nerve grafting.

If a nerve gap exists, it may be overcome by proximal and distal mobilization or, in the case of the ulnar nerve, anterior nerve transposition; however, excessive mobilization of the nerve ends must be avoided as this impairs the vascularity of the nerve. If there is judged to be too much tension on the nerve repair (it cannot be held

together with 8-0 nylon sutures), nerve grafting (or in some instances placement of a nerve tube) must be done.[35] Donor sources are most frequently from the posterior interosseus nerve or the median antebrachial cutaneous nerve for small digital nerves and the sural nerve for nerve gaps of larger nerves.

Following repair, the affected part is splinted for 3 weeks to protect the anastomosis in a position of least tension. Secondary deformity for motor nerve injuries may be prevented by appropriate splinting (such as an anti-claw brace for ulnar palsy) until motor recovery occurs. After nerve repair, Tinel's sign is monitored as an index of progressive recovery.

Fractures and Dislocations

Pain, swelling, limited motion, and deformity suggest the presence of fracture or dislocation. Standard anteroposterior (AP) and lateral x-rays may miss some fractures and dislocations, and multiple x-ray views are frequently necessary to establish the exact diagnosis. Posteroanterior (PA), oblique, carpal tunnel, and stress views are often useful as are ancillary studies such as arthrography, bone scan, CT scan, and MRI.

Fractures may be rotated, angulated, telescoped, or displaced. Angulation is described by the direction in which the apex of the fracture points, and displacement is described by the direction of the distal fragment.[36,37] Fractures may be closed or open depending on whether or not a wound is involved; they may be complete, incomplete, or comminuted (more than two pieces); and they may be transverse, longitudinal, oblique, or spiral. Dislocation of joints may be complete or incomplete (subluxed) depending on the severity of the capsular injury. Displaced fractures or dislocations should be repositioned as soon as possible. This decreases soft tissue injury, decompresses nerves that might be stretched, and relieves kinking of blood vessels. Good bony contact and stability are essential for fractures to heal.

Some fractures are stable and require only external support in a splint or cast, whereas others are unstable and require internal support, which can be provided by Kirschner wires, internal wire sutures through drill holes in the fracture fragments, screws, or plates, or even external fixation devices. The more complicated the fixation, the more dissection is required to apply that fixation and therefore the greater is the potential for scarring about adjacent tendons and consequential stiffness; however, screws and plates can nonetheless establish a degree of rigid synostosis that will allow for early motion of the part and so potentially reduce the risk of cicatricial stiffness.

Intraarticular fractures require accurate reduction in order to preserve motion. Significant step-off on the articular surface may alter motion and lead to later development of arthrosis. Persistent rotational deformity and significant lateral angular deformity will generally not remodel with time, and this can be avoided by observing the alignment of the injured fingers as compared with adjacent digits while passively gently flexing them into a fist after reduction is obtained. If they do not fit comfortably adjacent to each other and do not point toward the distal pole of the scaphoid, a fresh attempt at reduction should be performed; thus, clinical observation of good anatomic alignment of fractures is important in assessing the final result. A thorough neurovascular examination should always be performed both before and after fracture reduction has been completed. Most common fractures and dislocations are discussed below.

Clavicle Fractures

Clavicle fractures represent one of the most common bone injuries (5% to 10% of all bone fractures). The mechanism of injury can be direct or indirect, such as falling on an outstretched hand. Clavicle fractures are classified into three groups: I (middle third), representing 80% of clavicle fractures; II (lateral third); and III (medial third). Diagnosis is usually easy, and complications are rare. However, high-velocity injuries may have multiple associated injuries such as a fracture to the ipsilateral scapula and upper ribs, pneumothorax, and neurovascular injuries.

Most middle third clavicular fractures heal uneventfully with nonoperative immobilization for 4 to 6 weeks, such as with the use of a sling.[38] A variety of slings, straps, and braces have not been shown to necessarily be superior to the others in the treatment of these fractures. Surgical treatment with open reduction and internal fixation is indicated in cases of open injury or pending skin disruption, neurovascular compromise, unstable floating shoulder (an associated fracture of the surgical neck of the scapula), or wide separation of the clavicular ends with soft tissue interposition. With lateral third fractures, the coracoclavicular ligament provides stability in most cases, allowing also for nonoperative treatment to be successful.

Proximal Humerus Fractures

Proximal humerus fractures make up 2% to 3% of upper extremity fractures and occur more frequently in elderly people, especially with associated osteoporosis. These are fractures proximal to the insertion of the pectoralis major and involve the proximal humeral shaft, head of the humerus, or anatomic neck or surgical neck of the humerus.[38] A fracture is considered nondisplaced, regardless of the number of fragments if translation is less than 1 cm and angulation is less than 45°. The blood supply of the humeral head is at risk in all fractures involving the anatomic neck.

Associated injuries are relatively frequent, including glenohumeral dislocation, injuries to the brachial plexus, axillary nerve, and also vascular injuries. Most cases result from indirect trauma (fall on the outstretched arm). Radiographic evaluation requires at least AP, lateral, and axillary views, and a CT scan may be helpful for the more complex cases. Most cases are only mildly displaced and can be treated nonoperatively with a comfort sling or splint. Early range of motion is essential and may be started as soon as the second week after injury.

With displaced fractures, closed or open reduction followed by percutaneous pinning or internal fixation is necessary. If the humeral head is devascularized, especially in elderly patients, the fracture may be more reliably treated with a hemiarthroplasty.

Humeral Shaft Fractures

Humeral shaft fractures extend from the insertion of the pectoralis major proximally to the supracondylar ridge distally. The level of the fracture relative to muscle insertions determines the deforming forces and angulation of the fracture. Above the deltoid insertion, the proximal fragment is pulled into adduction by the pectoralis major, and the distal fragment under the influence of the deltoid is displaced into adduction. Below the deltoid, the proximal fragment is abducted. The radial nerve is in close contact with the posterior aspect of the humerus, particularly in fractures involving the middle third of the shaft, and so it is potentially at risk for injury. Other potential associated injuries may include the brachial artery and the median and ulnar nerves. The mechanism of injury can be indirect by fall on an outstretched upper extremity but is more often through a direct injury.

The vast majority of these fractures can be treated nonoperatively such as using a hanging cast. Close follow up with x-rays every 4 to 6 weeks is necessary. Deformities of up to 20° to 30° of angulation or 2 to 3 cm of shortening are usually accepted. As soon as the fracture seems stable, functional bracing enables humerus immobilization so that shoulder and elbow rehabilitation can begin. Indications for surgery include open fractures, polytrauma, bilateral humerus fractures, floating elbow, segmental fracture, and vascular injuries, as well as obese and uncooperative patients. Radial nerve paralysis usually recovers spontaneously and in most cases therefore is usually not a surgical indication; however, if open reduction is indicated for other reasons, the radial nerve should be explored if the patient has a preexisting radial palsy. Open reduction and internal fixation is achieved by means of compression plate and screw fixation or by means of intramedullary nailing.

Fractures of the Distal Humerus

Fractures of the distal humerus may be intraarticular or extraarticular, and treatment is very challenging, often surgical, necessitating solid anatomic reduction that allows for early range of motion. Complications are frequent, including compartment syndrome, loss of fixation, nonunion, heterotopic calcification, and stiffness. The mechanism of injury is usually an indirect trauma, with the deforming forces transmitted with the elbow in either flexion or extension, or a varus or valgus deformity resulting in a variety of different fracture patterns. Neurovascular injuries may involve the brachial artery, median, ulna, or radial nerve around the elbow area.

Except for some nondisplaced stable fractures, there is generally no place for nonoperative treatment or percutaneous pinning of these fractures in adults. Surgical treatment in most cases requires anatomic reduction and fixation with lag screws or plates and screws, depending on the complexity of the fracture. Fixation should be solid enough to allow immediate range of motion to the elbow. Indomethacin may be helpful in reducing the incidence of subsequent heterotopic ossification. In children, supracondylar fractures are usually treated with closed reduction and percutaneous pinning.

Olecranon Fractures

If the fracture is thought to be nondisplaced, it should be checked radiographically with the elbow at 90° of flexion. If there is no separation with this increased flexion, immobilization for 3 weeks followed by sling and rehabilitation under supervision can then be undertaken. However, in all other cases open reduction and internal fixation are required for olecranon fractures. This is followed by early protected range of motion for these intraarticular fractures.[39]

Radial Head Fractures

Radial head fractures are usually caused by axial loading from a fall on an outstretched hand, and the radial head is impacted against the capitellum.[39] Mason classifies four types: type I, undisplaced fracture; type II, displaced fracture that involves only part of the radial head; type III, comminuted fracture; and type IV, fracture associated with elbow dislocation. Clinical examination should carefully rule out a distal radioulnar dissociation (Essex-Lopresti lesion).[40] Quality x-rays should rule out any other associated fractures such as to the coronoid, olecranon, and capitellum.

Nonoperative management is indicated for type I and type II fractures with less than 2 mm of displacement. Immobilization in a sling is necessary for 2 to 3 weeks followed by early active supervised range of motion. For all fractures with severe radial head displacement, surgical

treatment is indicated. Once surgical exposure has been achieved, evaluation of the degree of comminution and of elbow stability is required. The radial head can then be fixed or replaced. Radial head excision is not recommended, as it may result in instability.

Forearm Fractures

Forearm fractures might involve isolated fractures of the radius or ulna, or both bones may be fractured together. A Monteggia fracture is described as the association of an ulnar fracture and radial head dislocation. Galeazzi fractures are the association of a radius fracture and distal ulnar dislocation. More than for any other fractures, the radiographic examination should focus on the joints above and below the fractures. Examination evaluates the neurovascular integrity of the distal extremity. Compartment syndrome may also be associated.

For adults, isolated fractures of the ulna that are only mildly displaced can be treated with cast immobilization. All other fractures should generally be treated surgically. Bone fixation is achieved with either plate and screws or flexible intramedullary nails. In most cases, anatomic reduction of the forearm fracture will generally result in a spontaneous reduction of the radial head or the distal radioulnar joint when there is an associated proximal or distal dislocation. Finally, open fractures, especially when associated with a severe soft tissue injury, are often treated with external fixation.

Distal Radius Fractures

Fractures of the distal radius represent the most common that involve the upper extremity. Therapeutic modalities have evolved considerably over the past few years, but many controversies still persist. These injuries occur to different age population groups, elderly and young patients. In older patients these fractures are typically extraarticular and often follow a less severe trauma. Because the bone is osteoporotic, there is a relatively frequent need for supportive bone grafting. Immobilization should be as short as possible to prevent stiffness. In contrast, in young adult patients there is usually a high-energy trauma that results in intraarticular and comminuted distal radius fractures. Possible associated injuries include carpal or distal radioulnar instability and triangular fibrocartilage injury, and for these reasons the tendency is to more aggressively treat these patients surgically.

Colles and Smith fractures represent extraarticular fractures with, respectively, dorsal and volar displacement. A Barton's fracture is a marginal articular fracture involving the rim of the distal radius in a coronal plane. These fractures can be either anterior or posterior. Fractures in the sagittal plane may involve the radial styloid and are also known as "chauffeur's fractures." Fractures involving the lunate fossa of the distal radius are known as die-punch fractures. Scapholunate disassociations are often associated with fractures of the radial styloid. Rupture of the extensor pollicis longus tendon can occur as an early complication of even mildly displaced distal radius fractures.

Treatment may be closed for stable fractures that are not excessively displaced. For displaced fractures, a closed reduction may first be attempted. The criteria for an acceptable reduction include restoration of radial length, volar tilt, and radial inclination. Unstable fractures, or unacceptable reduction, need surgical management, and multiple described procedures include percutaneous pin fixation, open reduction with internal fixation, and external fixation.[41]

Scaphoid Fractures

Scaphoid is by far the most common carpal bone fracture. The scaphoid waste comes into contact in hyperextension with the dorsal rim of the radius when falling on an outstretched hand. Understanding blood supply to the scaphoid is important.[42] The proximal pole of the scaphoid is poorly vascularized, and all of its blood supply comes in a retrograde fashion from distal to proximal. For this reason, avascular necrosis and nonunion are frequent complications of proximal pole scaphoid fractures.

Fractures of the scaphoid are suspected in patients with pain and tenderness in the anatomic "snuffbox" or with tenderness elicited by pressure on the scaphoid tubercle.[43] Diagnosis is usually confirmed by AP, lateral, and oblique wrist x-rays, although an additional specific scaphoid radiographic view with the resting ulnar deviation may be helpful (Figure 39.36). If x-rays are negative with a strong clinical suspicion of a scaphoid fracture, a thumb spica cast should be applied with repeated x-rays performed within 10 to 15 days. An immediate bone scan or preferably a CT scan is another option when there is doubt about a potential scaphoid fracture. Early diagnosis is essential so that appropriate treatment can be instituted to reduce the risk of complications.

Closed treatment consists of 8 to 12 weeks of immobilization starting initially with a long arm and a thumb spica cast followed then with a short arm thumb spica cast. Unstable fractures with displacement more than 1 mm and an intrascaphoid angle of greater than 45° and associated ligamentous injuries and vertical pattern fractures that tend to be of a more unstable configuration should generally be treated surgically (see Figure 39.36). Modern cannulated screws or intraoperative fluoroscopy and arthroscopy may even allow a minimally invasive percutaneous fixation of some of these scaphoid fractures.

Metacarpal Fractures

Stable metacarpal fractures may be treated with splinting alone. Those with dorsal or volar angulation can be stabilized by percutaneous insertion of intramedullary fixation pins. If they are displaced or unstable, such as long oblique or spiral fractures, or multiple metacarpal fractures, open reduction and internal fixation should be performed.[36,37] The internal fixation can be achieved with Kirschner wires, lag screws, or plate and screws depending on the fracture pattern configuration.[44,45] Dorsally angulated fractures at the neck of the little finger metacarpal, the so-called boxer's fracture, do not require reduction if the dorsal angulation is less than 30°. Mobility of the carpometacarpal joint will compensate for this degree of angulation. If the angulation is greater than 30°,

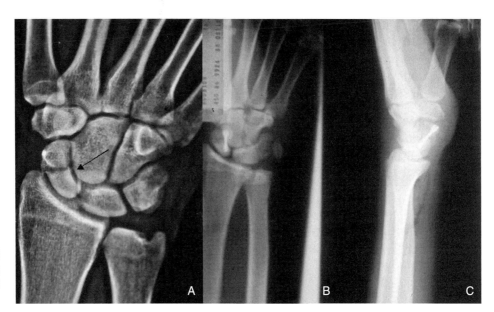

FIGURE 39.36. **(A)** Displaced scaphoid fracture (arrow). **(B,C)** This fracture has been treated with a cannulated screw.

the fracture should be reduced and if necessary maintained with internal fixation. Occasionally these fractures need to be opened in order to obtain satisfactory reduction and stability.

Oblique fractures at the base of the thumb metacarpal (Bennett's fracture) result in the small proximal fragment being held in position by the volar oblique ligament to the trapezium. The entire remaining portion of the thumb metacarpal is displaced dorsally and radially because of the pull of the abductor pollicis longus tendon. These structures should be properly reduced and secured with internal fixation. Comminuted fractures at the base of the thumb metacarpal (Rolando's fracture) are frequently treated by closed reduction. Accurate reduction is important to the ultimate function of the thumb, and, therefore, if the fragments are large and badly displaced, an open reduction is indicated. Fractures of the shaft of the thumb metacarpal tend to become displaced by the opposing muscle forces of the abductor and the adductor on the proximal and distal fragments, respectively; thus, even undisplaced fractures may with time become progressively more displaced and angulated, necessitating an internal fixation.

Phalangeal Fractures

In some cases, such as for irreducibility, malrotation, intraarticular fractures,[46] open fractures, segmental bone loss, and multiple fractures involving the hand, operative fixation is required (Figure 39.37). Overzealous treatment by open reduction and internal fixation can lead to excessive scarring, tendon adhesions, and stiffness.[44,45] In proximal phalangeal fractures, the interossei tend to flex the proximal fragment while the extensor mechanism extends the distal fragment, resulting in a volar angulation. In middle phalangeal fractures, the displacement depends on the level of the fracture relative to the insertion of the central slip. Displacement is dorsal in proximal fractures and volar in distal fractures. Stable fractures can be treated by initial immobilization followed by buddy taping and progressive mobilization. It is important to note that there is little correlation between clinical and radiographic bone healing. Mobilization is usually started after about 4 weeks based on clinical improvement. When operative treatment has secured solid rigid bony fixation, earlier range of motion may be instituted.

Fractures of the distal phalanx are very frequent. They represent half of all hand fractures. Most of them result from crush injuries with associated nailbed injuries. Precise reduction is generally not required; hence, treatment generally consists of splinting alone. Unstable shaft fractures, with overriding of the fragments, are indications for reduction and longitudinal Kirschner wire fixation.

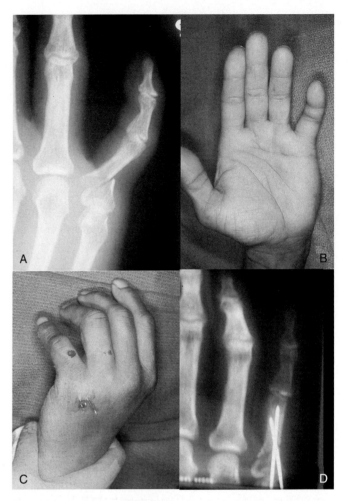

FIGURE 39.37. **(A,B)** A displaced proximal phalangeal fracture at the base of the little finger. **(C,D)** This was treated by closed manipulation of the fracture and percutaneous pinning to maintain stability.

Carpal Dislocations

The lunate and perilunate dislocations represent the most common form of wrist dislocation. They result from hyperextension of the wrist on an outstretched hand. The radiologic diagnosis may sometimes be difficult, and up to 25% of these injuries are still missed in the emergency room. They can be a pure lunate dislocation with rupture of the scapholunate (Figure 39.38) and lunotriquetral ligaments or a fracture-dislocation involving a transscaphoid perilunate dislocation or with a fracture involving the radial styloid, capitate, hemate, and triquetrum. Median nerve compression is frequently associated. Even though reduction can often be achieved by closed manipulation and distraction; surgical repair of the scapholunate and lunotriquetral ligaments are necessary with K-wire protection and splinting for 6 weeks.

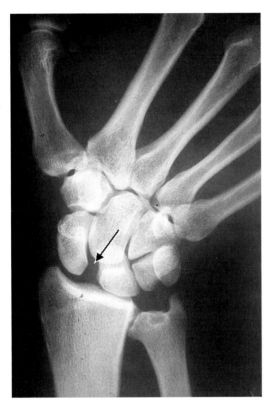

FIGURE 39.38. Scapholunate ligament disruption is indicated by a widened gap between the scaphoid and lunate bones (arrow).

Dislocations Involving the Hand

Closed dislocation of the PIP or DIP joints can frequently be managed by closed reduction and splinting. If the joint is unstable after reduction, it needs exploration for ligament repair.[46] A PIP joint volar dislocation is frequently associated with a tear in the triangular ligament of the extensor mechanism through which the head of the proximal phalanx protrudes and becomes trapped. Attempts at closed reduction fail, because they further tighten the fibers of the lateral bands and the central slip around each side of the protruding neck of the proximal phalanx. These injuries require open reduction with repair of the tear. Dorsal dislocations of the PIP joint involve the volar plate. Instability of the joint after reduction signifies that at least one collateral ligament is also involved, and open reduction and repair are required. If there is an avulsion from the volar base of the middle phalanx of a bone fragment representing one third or more of the articular surface, this may also require open reduction and internal fixation.

Palmar dislocations of the head of the index finger metacarpal often require metacarpal open reduction (Figure 39.39). The head of the metacarpal becomes trapped between the superficial, transverse palmar ligament, the flexor tendons and lumbrical muscles, and the natatory ligament, while the volar plate becomes trapped between the metacarpal head and the base of the proximal phalanx. Attempts at closed reduction are fruitless because of the entrapment phenomenon resulting from this arrangement. Open reduction may be approached through either the dorsum or the palm. In the latter approach, caution must be used to avoid injury to the digital nerves stretched over the metacarpal head. In either approach, the trapped volar plate must be released.

Metacarpophalangeal joint dislocation of the thumb often results from jamming it in a radial direction, thus tearing the ulnar collateral ligament. In about 75% of complete tears, the ulnar collateral ligament pulls proximally and comes to rest dorsal to the extensor hood (a Stener lesion) (Figure 39.40). These lesions cannot heal spontaneously, because the ulnar collateral ligament is prevented from reattaching to bone. They require operative repair. Radial deviation of the joint by 40° degrees or more or volar subluxation of the joint suggests a complete tear, and ligament repair should be performed. Stress radiographs (sometimes enabled only after the digit is anesthetized with a metacarpal block) may be required

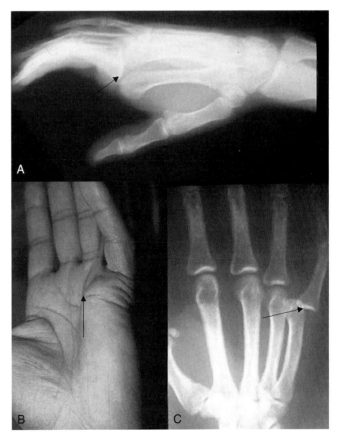

FIGURE 39.39. (A) Palmar dislocation at the head of the index finger metacarpal (arrow) was "irreducible" by closed technique. (B,C) A more unusual "irreducible" desiccation of the head of the little finger metacarpal is seen (arrows). The digital nerves are often stretched over the volar surface of the head of the metacarpal.

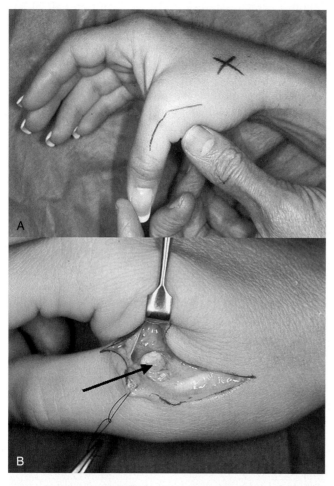

FIGURE 39.40. **(A)** Closed injury of the ulnar collateral ligament of the metacarpophalangeal joint of the thumb showing marked joint instability. **(B)** A classic Stener lesion is seen intraoperatively with a disrupted ulnar collateral ligament (arrow) tracking proximally and resting dorsal to the extensor hood.

to facilitate diagnosis of a complete ulnar collateral ligament injury of the thumb metacarpophalangeal joint.

Vascular Emergencies

Acute vascular injuries may follow closed or penetrating extremity trauma or may occur after iatrogenic injury. Fractures or dislocations may be causes of vascular injury. Onset of symptoms may be delayed, as the culmination of swelling, hypotension, and intimal injury all combine to result in late thrombosis and vascular insufficiency. Following the acute arterial injury, symptoms result from a combination of the adequacy of collateral circulation, posttraumatic sympathetic tone, and vasomotor control mechanisms. Patients with an upper extremity arterial injury who have adequate collateral circulation and normal vasomotor control may have minimal symptoms, and vascular reconstruction is not necessarily mandatory; however, adequate anatomic vasculature may be com-

promised by inappropriate distal functional control with consequent vasospasm and arteriovenous shunting.[47,48] For patients who have inadequate collateral circulation, the distal ischemia will further increase sympathetic tone and produce additional arterial spasm and induce more ischemia; thus, the effects of arterial injury in the upper extremity may be magnified by the additional presence of a concomitant nerve injury.[47,48]

If there is a noncritical arterial injury, reconstruction may be advocated to restore parallel flow in case of future injury, to enhance nerve recovery, to facilitate healing, and to prevent cold intolerance. However, reported patency rates even with microvascular techniques for single vessel repairs vary from 47% to 82%.[49] The following injuries, however, are optimally managed by vascular repair/reconstruction: axillary or brachial artery injury, combined radial and ulnar artery injury, and radial or ulnar artery injury associated with poor collateral circulation. The following are relative indications for repair: extensive distal soft tissue injury, technical ability to achieve repair without compromising patient well-being, and combined vascular and neural injury.[49] Need for arterial reconstruction requires assessment of adequacy of collateral circulation, and this is based primarily on initial clinical judgment to include assessment of color, capillary refill, turgor, and temperature; however, the final decision regarding arterial reconstruction is often made in the operating room after exploration. Once the injured structures have been isolated, potential bleeding sites controlled, and the hematoma evacuated, the distal extremity can be more adequately assessed.[47] At this time, the lacerated vessel ends are controlled by atraumatic vascular clamps, and the tourniquet is released. Capillary refill and turgor of the distal extremity is then assessed as is the backflow from the distal lacerated vessel ends. Digital blood pressure can be quantified with a sterile Doppler probe and cuff, and a digital brachial index of 0.7 or greater suggests adequate perfusion.[50] If there is poor collateral flow, then arterial reconstruction should be performed. At this time, the standard of care does not require arterial repair of isolated noncritical vessels. Brachial artery lacerations, particularly those injuries occurring above the origin of the profunda brachii, are reconstructed unless there are clinical contraindications. In combined radial and ulnar artery injuries, one or both vessels should be reconstructed. If possible, both vessels are repaired.

Preoperative evaluation, particularly for closed injuries, may be facilitated by special investigations; however, important details of the patient's history are also the presence of previous injury, particularly repetitive insults, blood dyscrasias, drug exposure, tobacco use, and factors that might be associated with connective tissue disorders. Physical examination for a vascular disorder of the upper extremity must include a thorough evaluation of the entire upper extremity, the neck, careful auscultation of the heart for heart murmurs, and auscultation for bruits in the neck or thoracic outlet region that might be supportive of embolic phenomena or might be an irregular rhythm from atrial fibrillation. A radial brachial index (RBI) and a digital brachial index (DBI) can be calculated. A DBI or RBI of less than 0.7 indicates inadequate arterial flow to a hand or digit and necessitates either medical or surgical intervention.[50] Differences of 15 mm Hg between fingers or a wrist-to-finger difference of 30 mm Hg is thought to indicate occlusion at the level of or distal to the palmar arch. A pressure difference greater than 20 mm Hg at the same level between the affected and contralateral extremity may also indicate arterial stenosis or occlusion.

Noninvasive vascular studies by pulse volume recordings and Doppler evaluations provide a wealth of information. Contrast arteriography provides the best anatomic structural information of the upper extremity vasculature but is nonetheless a static evaluation of the extremity. Information is optimized by using intraarterial vasodilators (such as Priscoline) to identify stenoses that might be secondary to vasospasm and substraction techniques that minimize background interference. The potential problems of arteriography include catheter-induced vasospasm with possible failure to observe distal arterial reconstitution because of vasospasm. Consider regional anesthetic block, such a stellate ganglion block, if vasospasm prevents adequate visualization.

Acute arterial occlusion can also occur from nonlacerating arterial injuries such as cannulation injuries, whereas acute occlusion in the upper extremity arteries may occur as the result of repetitive frequent trauma (hypothenar hammer syndrome), atherosclerosis, proximal embolic event, and systemic disease with or without a hypercoagulable state. Significant arterial occlusion produces ischemia and vasospasm. The prognosis may be related to etiology; for example, posttraumatic ulnar artery thrombosis has a much better prognosis than Buerger's disease. Repetitive trauma may produce localized thrombosis resulting from periadventitial scarring. The trauma may also potentially cause intima damage to the media, disruption of the internal elastic lamina, and exposure of endothelial collagen leading to aneurysmal dilatation and/or thrombosis. As with acute arterial lacerations, arterial thrombosis or embolism may have adverse distal deleterious effects based on the extent of the occlusion, the adequacy of the collateral flow, and the sympathetic tone.

Cannulation injuries most frequently involve the brachial or radial arteries such as following arterial blood studies, indwelling arterial catheters, and cardiac catheterization.[51] Surgical repair of the brachial artery is necessary in the presence of distal ischemia, active bleeding, or aneurysm. Surgical options may include resection and ligation, arterial reconstruction, and/or thrombectomy with embolectomy. The loss of a radial pulse

without ischemic symptoms distally is not an indication for acute care surgery. The extremity may be observed clinically in an awake and alert patient. In an unconscious patient, a Doppler probe and distal pressure measurements are helpful to evaluate the affected extremity.

Arterial injection injuries may occur during medical procedures or may be self-inflicted during drug abuse and occasionally a consequence of workplace exposure. Distal ischemia may occur following inadvertent or inappropriate injection of pharmaceutical products such as barbiturates, propoxyphene, and nonparenteral narcotics. Severe vascular events may occur following workplace injury involving solvents, paint products, and lubricants; however, intraarterial injection is infrequent in such workplace injuries. These injection injuries result in severe acute extremity ischemia on the basis of secondary vasospasm, chemical endarteritis, and arterial blockage with activation of the clotting cascade. There are generally acute symptoms of arterial insufficiency with diffuse hand swelling, numbness, and discoloration. The injection wounds often appear innocuous. There may be rapid development of skin and soft tissue necrosis. Diagnostic modalities are aimed at determining if there is segmental and reconstructible occlusive arterial disease. Unfortunately, end artery occlusion within the microvascular beds is common, and systemic anticoagulation with systemic support remains the only treatment option.

Management of ischemic symptoms secondary to a dialysis arteriovenous fistula includes ligation or banding.[52] Ligation may be required for recurrent thrombosis and resultant distal embolization. Documentation of a "steal" phenomenon requires recording of digital pressure before and after occlusion of the radial artery below the fistula. A DBI of less than 0.64 is significant. Banding or takedown of the shunt will then be required.

Acute arterial thrombosis that is secondary to either closed external posttraumatic occlusive disease or primary vascular occlusive disease is treated based on the severity of the distal ischemia, collateral circulation, and the vascular sympathetic tone. Treatment options are increased collateral blood flow through elimination of tobacco products, increased nutritional tissue blood flow with the use of calcium channel blockers, possibly a sympathectomy, either chemical or surgical (such as resection of the thrombosed segment and ligation as in the Leriche type sympathectomy), and surgical restoration of the circulation (through thrombectomy, resection and vein graft, arterial bypass), and/or thrombolytic therapy.[53,54]

High-Pressure Injuries

Pressure injection injuries to the hand are relatively uncommon, but the consequences of a missed diagnosis are very serious.[55,56] The severity of these injuries requires prompt response and urgent disposition. High-pressure injection guns are found in the industrial setting and are used for painting, lubricating, cleaning, and mass farm animal vaccinations. Materials that may be injected with these devices include paint, paint thinners, oil, grease, water, plastic, vaccines, and cement. A pressure of 100psi can penetrate through skin. These high-pressure injection guns generate pressures ranging between 3,000 and 12,000psi. Injection injuries can also be caused by other sources, such as defective lines and valves. Pneumatic hoses, grease boxes, and hydraulic lines can all cause a high-pressure injection injury.

Several factors affect the extent of tissue injury, including the type of material, amount of material, anatomic location of the injection, and velocity of the injected material, but the type of material injected is the most important prognostic factor. Oil-based paints and paint thinners can generate significant early inflammation leading to severe fibrosis. Because tendon sheaths of the index, middle, and ring fingers end at the level of the metacarpophalangeal joints, material injected at either the DIP or PIP flexion creases will remain within those digits; however, the tendon sheaths of the thumb and little finger extend all the way into the radial and ulnar bursae; thus, material injected at either the DIP or PIP of the little finger or at the interphalangeal flexion crease of the thumb has the potential for extension into the forearm and could even cause a compartment syndrome, carpal tunnel syndrome, or ulnar nerve compression in Guyon's canal.

Initial presentation of the patient with a high-pressure injection injury may be benign and subtle. This can result in mismanagement and in minimizing the patient's complaints. The break in the skin may be a very benign-looking pinhole-sized puncture site; however, several hours later the digit becomes increasingly more painful, swollen, and pale. Prompt recognition and realization of the severity of the injury is key. Antibiotic prophylaxis is started. Radiographs will help determine the extent of dispersion of the injected material. Nonlead-based paints may appear as subcutaneous emphysema, and grease may appear lucent on radiographs. On the other hand, lead-based paints may be seen as radiopaque soft tissue densities. Incisions are made to decompress the affected tissue and then perform an extensive exploration of all areas infiltrated by the injected material. Foreign material and all necrotic tissue must be debrided. Appropriate irrigation is performed to help reduce fibrosis and scarring. The wounds are then closed loosely over Penrose drains, left open to heal by secondary intention, or closed in a delayed manner. Despite prompt recognition and treatment, many can result in surgical amputation of the digits.

Frostbite and Chemical and Extravasation Injuries

Frostbite

Treatment of frostbite consists of restoring core body heat and rapidly rewarming the frozen extremity with a 44°C water bath until a digital flush appears. Active hand therapy must be instituted. The place of regional sympathectomy or possibly chemical sympathetic block in acute management of frostbite injuries is controversial; however, if disabling vasospastic syndrome persists as a chronic sequela to occult injury, digital sympathectomy is helpful.[57]

Avoidance of premature amputation is important. Demarcation and mummification of digits may take as long as 2 to 3 months.

Chemical Burns

Chemical burn injuries may affect the hands in industrial environments. Water lavage is the most important part of treatment and should be started at the scene of the accident. Its continuation for 1 to 2 hours for acid burns and longer for alkali burns is important. After lavage, treatment follows the same principles as those for thermal burns, although some chemicals require specific therapeutic antidotes.[58]

Reducing agents such as hydrochloric acid are merely diluted if only small amounts of water are available and therefore must be neutralized with soap or soda lime if massive water lavage is not available. Hydrofluoric acid is common in rust removers and degreasers. Hypocalcemia and hypomagnesemia have been reported with burns over more than 5% of the body surface area. Treatment requires immediate water lavage followed by subdermal injection of 10% calcium gluconate (painful if not combined with local or regional anesthesia). Calcium carbonate gel has more recently been used for topical application instead of the injection therapy. Injuries caused by phenol (not water soluble) require specific treatment with topical polyethylene glycol (PEG 400) followed by water lavage. Treatment of white phosphorous burns involves principally water lavage followed by identification and excision of the remaining phosphorous particles. Irrigation with dilute 1% copper sulfate solution helps identify the phosphorous particles. This is followed immediately by water lavage to avoid the toxic effects of the copper sulfate. Sterile debridement and delayed closure of phosphorous burns is then performed as necessary.

Extravasation Injuries

Injuries from extravasation of chemotherapeutic agents used to frequently affect the upper extremity; however, the use of more permanent subcutaneously tunneled central lines has reduced the incidence of these injuries. A number of specific antidotes have been recommended in the past. The treatment of these injuries has now been simplified. If extravasation is expected, the infusion must be stopped immediately. Cold packs are applied for 15 minutes four times a day for 58 hours and the extremity elevated. This regimen is effective for most injuries. If blistering, ulceration, and pain occur in the damaged tissue, however, progressive necrosis to the limits of the extravasation will then follow, and a surgical excision of all of the damaged tissue is necessary. The option for wound coverage following debridement will then depend on the extent of the debridement that was required and on the various tissues that might be exposed, but most such injuries can generally be treated with delayed split-thickness skin grafting.[59]

Compartment Syndrome

Compartment syndrome results in symptoms and signs occurring from increased pressure within a limited space that compromises the circulation and function of the tissues in that space.[60–62] High pressure in a closed space reduces capillary perfusion below a level necessary for tissue viability. Volkmann's ischemic contracture is the sequela of compartment syndrome. This results in fibrosed, contracted, and functionless muscle and in insensible nerves.

The relationship between local blood flow (LBF) and the arteriovenous (AV) gradient can be expressed by the following formula:

$$LBF = P_A - P_v$$

Local blood flow in a compartment equals local arterial pressure (P_A) minus local venous pressure (P_v) divided by the local vascular resistance (R). With the lowering of the local AV gradient, oxygen perfusion of the muscles and nerves decreases, function ceases, and muscle ischemia progresses to the death of that muscle and its subsequent replacement by fibrous tissue. Muscle ischemia that lasts for over 4 hours can also give rise to significant myoglobinuria, which may reach a maximum up to 3 hours after the circulation is restored. Significant myoglobinuria may produce renal failure, and, therefore, in the presence of myoglobinuria one must retain a high urinary output and an alkaline urine. A forced Mannitol-alkaline diuresis may be required.

A variety of injuries are known to cause compartment syndrome:

- Decreased compartment volume
  - Closure of fascial defects
  - Application of extensive traction to fractured limbs
  - Externally applied pressure (tight casts or dressings, lying on the limb)
- Increased compartment content
  - Bleeding
  - Increased capillary permeability (embolectomy, reperfusion after injury)
  - Trauma (fracture, contusion, wringer injuries)
  - Burns (thermal and especially electrical)
- Other injuries
  - Intraarterial drug injection
  - Cold exposure
  - Snake bite
  - Injection
  - High-pressure injection injuries
  - Increased capillary pressure
  - Venous obstruction or venous ligation
  - Diminished serum osmolarity such as nephrotic syndrome

The diagnosis of compartment syndrome must be based primarily on clinical evaluation of muscle and nerve ischemia (Figure 39.41). Although it is possible to measure intracompartment pressures, a decision to perform a fasciotomy must be based on a high degree of suspicion.[61,62] All too often attention is focused on the peripheral circulation, but compartment ischemia may be severe and still not affect color or temperature of the fingers, and distal pulses are rarely obliterated by compartment swelling; however, the circulation in the muscle and the nerve may be greatly reduced. Peripheral nerves will conduct impulses for 1 hour following ischemia and can survive for 4 hours with only neuropraxic damage. After 8 hours of total ischemia, irreversible nerve changes are complete. Ischemic skeletal muscle remains electrically responsive up to 3 hours following ischemia and may survive as long as 4 hours without irreversible damage, but at 8 hours complete irreversible damage has occurred.

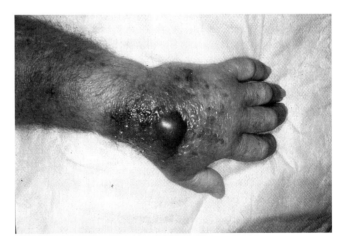

FIGURE 39.41. Patient with compartment syndrome has marked swelling of the hand and skin blistering. Clinical signs may not always be as florid as this.

The hallmark of muscle and nerve ischemia is pain. Pain is persistent, progressive, and unrelieved by immobilization. The pain is accentuated by passive muscle stretching, and this is the most reliable clinical test for making the diagnosis of compartment syndrome. The next most important clinical finding is diminished sensation, and this indicates ischemia of that nerve as it passes through the affected compartment. The third most important finding is weakness of the affected muscle. Finally, the closed compartments in the forearm and hand are palpated and are found to be tense and tender, confirming the diagnosis of compartment syndrome.

When performing a passive muscle stretch test, the examiner needs to keep in mind that there are 3 separate compartments in the forearm and 10 compartments in the hand. The muscles in the volar compartment of the forearm include the flexors of the finger, thumb, and wrist, and these muscles are tested by passive extension of the fingers, thumb, and wrist. The dorsal forearm compartment includes the finger, thumb, and ulnar wrist extensors and the long thumb abductor, and this compartment is therefore tested by passive finger and thumb and wrist flexion. The intrinsic compartments of the hand are tested by passively abducting and adducting the fingers while the metacarpophalangeal joints are maintained at full extension and the PIP joints in flexion. The adductor compartment of the thumb is tested by simply pulling the thumb into palmar abduction, and the thenar muscles can be tested by radial abduction of the thumb and the hypothenar muscles by extending and adducting the little finger.

Treated in the differential diagnosis of compartment syndrome are nerve injury and arterial injury. These diagnoses are differentiated as shown in Table 39.1.

When the clinical diagnosis is difficult because, either through inebriation or unconsciousness, the patient cannot cooperate, compartment pressure can be measured. The Whitesides technique[62] is simply performed by setting up an arterial line transducer system and connecting this to an 18-gauge needle. After the equipment is zeroed to atmospheric pressure, the needle is plunged into the compartment where pressure is to be measured. Such equipment is readily available in most acute care

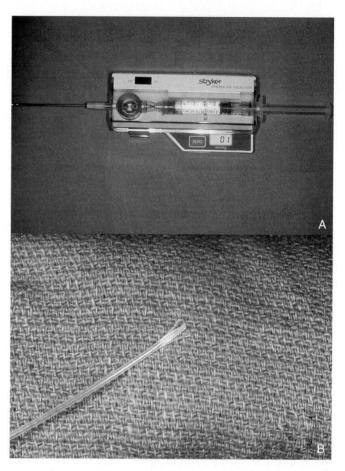

FIGURE 39.42. **(A)** A commercially available handheld device for measuring compartment pressure. (Courtesy of the Stryker Corporation.) **(B)** Tip of the indwelling slit catheter (enlarged).

settings in the intensive care unit, emergency room, and operating room. A commercially available intracompartment pressure monitoring system is made by the Stryker Corporation (Figure 39.42). This consists of a handheld monitor that is connected to a disposable indwelling slit catheter. The pressure threshold for fasciotomy remains controversial. However, Mubarak has recommended that fasciotomy be performed in patients with an intracompartment pressure greater than 30 mm Hg. Others have recommended that a pressure that is 20 mm Hg below diastolic should be the indicator.

If compartment syndrome is suspected, external compressive dressings and splints should be fully released immediately. If pain and clinical signs persist, then a fasciotomy is done.[60] Important principles with regard to performing a forearm fasciotomy are that damage to cutaneous nerves must be avoided; skin flaps are created to cover the median nerve at the wrist and flexor tendons in the distal forearm and the ulnar nerve at the elbow while awaiting secondary closure or skin grafting; the median or ulnar nerves can be released as they pass through the carpal tunnel and Guyon's canal; the brachial artery may be explored in conjunction with compartment

TABLE 39.1. Differential diagnoses of compartment syndrome as applied to nerve injury and arterial injury.

	Compartment syndrome	Arterial occlusion	Neuropraxia
Pressure increased in the compartment	+	−	−
Pain with stretch	+	+	−
Paresthesia or anesthesia	+	+	+
Paresis or paralysis	+	+	+
Pulses intact	+	−	+

+, Present; −, absent.

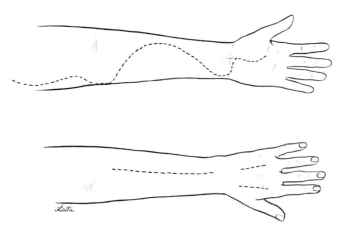

FIGURE 39.43. Proposed incisions for performing forearm and hand fasciotomies.

release; and straight line incisions across the wrist and elbow joint must be avoided to reduce the risk of subsequent contracture formation.

The palmar incision starts in the valley between the thenar and hypothenar muscles to release the carpal tunnel, and the incision then curves transversely across the flexion crease of the wrist to the ulnar border of the wrist (Figure 39.43). This incision thus avoids the palmar cutaneous branch of the median nerve and prevents flexion contracture across the wrist crease. It also provides an opportunity to release Guyon's canal as well. The incision then extends at least 5 cm in length proximally up the forearm before curving back in a radial direction so as to have a large skin flap that will cover the median nerve and distal forearm tendons. At the elbow the apex of the flap must be just radial to the medial epicondyle, and this flap then prevents linear contracture across the antecubital fossa and provides a cover for the brachial artery and the median nerve when the wound is left open. The incision can then readily be extended proximally up the arm without difficulty following the course of the brachial artery as necessary. The dorsal and "mobile wad" compartments of the forearm are readily released through a straight incision as needed. When performing a forearm fasciotomy, the decompression should be carried out along the entire volar compartment and always decompresses the carpal tunnel and is carried up proximally to the forearm to at least where the lacertus fibrosus (the bicipital aponeurosis) is released.

On the hand, the dorsal and volar interosseous muscle compartments and the adductor compartment to the thumb can be released through two parallel longitudinal incisions on the dorsum of the hand positioned over the second and fourth metacarpals. The thenar compartment and hypothenar compartments may be opened by longitudinal incisions along the radial side of the first metacarpal and the ulnar side of the fifth metacarpal, respectively. Fasciotomies to the digits are based on the degree of swelling present.

Postoperative splinting in an appropriate "safe" position and conforming dressings are essential. The wrist is kept in comfortable dorsiflexion, and the thumb is held in palmar abduction. Elevation of an extremity in a nondecompressed compartment problem does decrease tissue perfusion; however, once fasciotomy has been performed, postoperative elevation is recommended to promote venous drainage and reduce swelling. Most of the wounds can be partially closed at 5 days. If the skin cannot be closed secondarily within 10 days, a split-thickness skin graft can be applied to prevent excessive granulation tissue and lessen exposure of muscles and tendons to resulting fibrosis and scarring. Skin closure should not be done over questionably necrotic tissue or with excessive skin tension.

Acute Upper Extremity Infections

Kanavel[63] clarified the anatomy of the hand as it related to infection and applied this knowledge to the principles of surgical drainage. He injected the various spaces of the hand with plaster of Paris to delineate the anatomic boundaries and then by slowly increasing the injection pressure determined the manner of extension of simulated infectious processes when the spatial boundaries were breached. A hand infection may involve skin, subcutaneous tissue, tendon sheaths, joints, bone, and the deep spaces of the hand and forearm.[64] Acute infections are caused by a wide variety of pathogens but particularly the pyogenic bacteria and also on occasion by viruses.

Routes of Infection and Infecting Organisms

Septic thrombophlebitis affecting the hand or upper extremity is a complication related to the presence of an indwelling venous catheter. Such infections are managed by catheter removal and antibiotic therapy. Intravenous abscess may occasionally develop, extending along the venous system with systemic bacterial seeding, septicemia, and even death. Delaying vein excision can result in significant morbidity and death. A variety of microorganisms have been cultured, including *Streptococcus faecalis*, *Pseudomonas aeruginosa*, *Bacteroides fragilis*, other staphylococcal and streptococcal species, *Candida* species, and Enterobacteriaceae.

Toxic shock syndrome (TSS), a toxemia rather than a septicemia, has been reported following hand surgical procedures.[64] Although TSS usually presents with a benign-appearing local wound infection, the systemic symptoms include a desquamating rash, fever, hypotension, and multiple organ failure. Most surgical cases of TSS are associated with *Staphylococcus aureus* toxin-1 (TSST-1). The presence is confirmed in the patient's serum by a reverse passive latex agglutination test. A patient with TSS is transferred to intensive care monitoring. The wound is debrided, and any implants or drains are removed. The antibiotic choice is clindamycin, which is bacteriostatic and inhibits TSST-1 production.

The herpetic whitlow is caused by type I or II herpes simplex virus and may be confused with paronychia.[64] The infection begins with the appearance of small clear vesicles with localized swelling, erythema, and intense burning pain. The vesicles may appear turbid and then coalesce over the next 10 to 14 days before ulcerating. Tender lymphadenopathy and lymphangitis may be present. Diagnosis is confirmed by culturing the virus from the vesicular fluid, assessing immunofluorescent serum antibody titers, or performing a Tzanck smear. These measures are rarely required, because clinical diagnosis is usually sufficient. Treatment is nonoperative, because this infection is usually self-limiting. Vesicle unroofing for pain relief has been advocated. Antibiotic therapy and drainage may be indicated with bacterial superinfection. These infections occur particularly in patients whose fingers might be contaminated by oral flora, such as dental hygienists.

Despite these less usual routes of infection, most portals of entry to the hand by infecting microorganisms are by direct penetration, and most sites are involved by direct inoculation or by contiguous spread into adjacent sites; however, gonococcal infection may be a rare cause of tenosynovitis or septic joint by hematogenous spread. Infections may thus affect fingertips, tendon sheaths, and deep spaces of the hand, joints, and bone. Approximately 65% of hand infections are caused by aerobic organisms, with S. aureus isolated in about 35% of infections, the most common organism. Other commonly found aerobic organisms are alpha-hemolytic streptococci and group A beta-hemolytic streptococci. Gram-negative bacilli are uncommon but may occur from contaminated wounds or from wounds in patients who are drug abusers or have an altered immune status. The most striking difference in the microbial flora of human and animal bite wounds is the higher number of mean isolates per wound in human bites, the difference being mostly because of the presence of anaerobic bacteria.[65] Human bites can occasionally transmit other infectious diseases, such as hepatitis B, tuberculosis, syphilis, and actinomycosis. The incidence of *Eikenella corrodens* in human bite infections of the hand has been reported to vary between 7% and 29%. The most commonly isolated organisms from infected human bite wounds are, as in animal bites, alpha-hemolytic streptococci and *S. aureus*, beta-lactamase–producing strains of *S. aureus*, and *Bacteroides* species. Anaerobic bacteria are more prevalent in human bite infections than previously recognized and include *Bacteroides*, *Clostridium*, *Fusobacterium*, *Peptococcus*, and *Veillonella* species.

Most studies of animal bite wounds are focused on the isolation of *Pasteurella multocida*, disregarding the role of anaerobes. Recent studies, however, of gingival canine flora and of dog bite wounds point toward an oral flora of multiple organisms; *Pasteurella multocida* has been isolated from only 26% of dog bite wounds in adults. Most animal bites cause mixed infections of both aerobic and anaerobic bacteria.

Cat-scratch disease may follow a bite or a scratch from a cat, dog, or monkey and is caused by a recently named motile Gram-negative bacterium, *Afipia felis*. The cutaneous lesion develops into a red nodule; chills, fever, malaise, and tender regional axillary lymphadenopathy follow. The organism can be identified in both the primary lesion and in the draining nodes by the Warthin-Starry silver impregnation stain. A diagnostic skin test with a specific cat-scratch disease antigen is available. Cat-scratch disease has no specific treatment, but recovery is general complete in 2 to 5 months.

Anatomy of Hand Infections

Any hand infection, even on the volar surface, will include dorsal swelling because of the looser fascia on the dorsum of the hand and the paucity of fascial septa to the skin combined with the fact that the hand's lymphatic drainage runs palmar to dorsal. Dorsal swelling alone should not be mistaken for a dorsal hand infection. If a true dorsal infection is present, that aspect of the hand will be warm to the touch and painful to palpation.

A hand infection may include signs of lymphatic spread and ascending lymphangitis. The three primary lymph drainage sites for the hand are the epitrochlear nodes for the ring and little fingers, the axillary nodes for the thumb and index finger, and the deltopectoral nodes for the middle finger.

Figure 39.44 shows common sites of finger infections and depicts the route of spreading. Dorsal subcutaneous abscesses and peronychia occur commonly. A vesicle or pustule may be indicative of a felon beneath. Abscesses in the volar fat pad may point in a palmar direction or track to the dorsum before pointing; flexion creases often act as barriers to proximal or distal spread. An abscess in

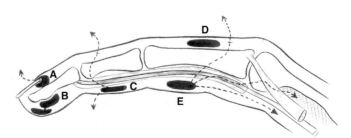

FIGURE 39.44. Common sites of hand infections and routes of spread of infections. (**A**) Paronychia. (**B**) Felon. (**C**) Volar middle phalangeal pulp abscess. (**D**) Dorsal finger abscess. (**E**) Volar infection may spread dorsally, proximally in subcutaneous layers, or through the lumbrical canal to deep palmar spaces.

the palmar (proximal) fat pad may spread either by tracking dorsally, passing the flexion crease barrier proximally, and entering the subcutaneous tissue of the palm or by the lumbrical canal to the deep palmar space. A collar-button abscess is an advanced lesion that usually arises at the metacarpophalangeal joint with abscess cavities on both the palmar and dorsal aspects of the hand. Such advanced lesions are rarely seen today with modern antibiotics and early surgical treatment of septic foci.

Types of Infections

Superficial Paronychial Infections

Paronychia is the most common infection of the hand and usually results from trauma to the eponychial or paronychial region.[66] Infection localizes around the nail base, advances around the nail fold, and burrows beneath the base of the nail. Swelling and erythema are present at the base of the nail and may extend up each paronychial side. If pus is trapped beneath the nail, pressure on the nail will evoke exquisite pain. Treatment incisions may not be necessary. A Freer elevator is used to lift approximately one fourth of the nail adjacent to the infected paronychium extending proximally to the edge of the nail. This portion of the nail is transected and gauze packing inserted beneath the nail fold. In runaround infections, an incision involving the junction of the eponychial fold with the paronychium may be required.

Infections at Intermediate Depths

Infections at intermediate depths are pulp space infections (felons) and also deep web space infections.[66] The former may involve the terminal pulp or the middle or proximal volar pulp spaces and may result from direct implantation or may represent spread from a more superficial subcutaneous infection. The pulp of the distal digital segment is a fascial space closed proximally by a septum joining the distal flexion crease to the periosteum where the long flexor tendon is inserted. This space is also partitioned by fibrous septa. Tension in the distal digital segment can become so great that the arteries to the bone are compressed, resulting in gangrene and necrosis of the distal three fourths of the terminal phalanx. The base of the terminal phalanx receives its blood supply from vessels that do not traverse this dense tissue. Spread from a pulp space infection may move into a joint space, to the underlying bone, or burst through the septum proximally to involve the rest of the finger. With infection of the distal digital pulp space, one must not wait for fluctuance before making the decision for surgery because of the danger of ischemic necrosis of the skin and bone. Clinical diagnosis is made by rapid onset of throbbing pain, swelling, and exquisite tenderness of the affected pulp space. Surgical draining is required. The two preferred possible incisions are either a single volar longitudinal incision or a unilateral longitudinal incision. The longitudinal incision must not cross the DIP joint flexion crease.

Web space abscesses result from either direct implantation or spread from a pulp space. A red and tender mass in the web space separates the fingers. Spread from this location may go proximally through the lumbrical canal to involve the deep spaces of the hand. Clinically there is loss of the normal palmar concavity with a widened space between the fingers. Dorsal swelling will be present, and it should not be mistaken for the infection site. A surgical incision is placed transversely across the web space. A counter longitudinal incision made be placed dorsally between the bases of the proximal phalanges, and generous communication is established between the two incisions (Figure 39.45).

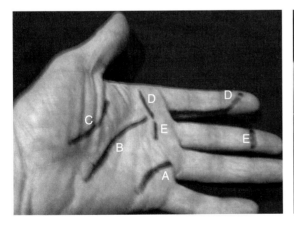 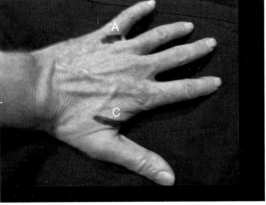

FIGURE 39.45. Surgical approaches to hand infections. **(A)** Web space (palmar and dorsal). **(B)** Midpalmar space. **(C)** Thenar space (palmar and dorsal). **(D)** Open drainage of finger (index). **(E)** Through-and-through irrigation of tendon sheath (middle finger).

Deep Infections

Deep Palmar Space Infections

Deep palmar space infections are localized to the deep spaces of the hand between the metacarpals and the palmar aponeurosis.[67] A transverse septum to the metacarpal of the middle finger divides the deep space into an ulnar midpalmar space and a radial thenar space. The transverse head of the adductor pollicis partitions the thenar space from the retroadductor space. Ballooning of the palm, thenar eminence, and posterior aspect of the web between the thumb and index finger is characteristic depending on which of the affected spaces is involved. The dorsal subaponeurotic space of the hand deep to the extensor tendons may also be affected by isolated infection, generally as a result of direct implantation. Dorsal hand swelling is accompanied by erythema and tenderness. Appropriate surgical incisions are illustrated in Figure 39.45.

For midpalmar space infections, a longitudinal curvilinear incision is the preferred approach. The preferred approach to surgical drainage of thenar space abscesses is a dual volar and dorsal incision. On the volar side the incision is made adjacent and parallel to the thenar crease. Great care is taken to avoid injury to the palmar cutaneous branch of the median nerve that is in the subcutaneous plane in the proximal part of the incision and to the motor branch of the median nerve that is in a deeper plane. The deeper dissection is carried bluntly toward the adductor pollicis and extended over the distal edge of the adductor. A second slightly curved longitudinal incision is made over the dorsum of the first web space. A Penrose drain is placed in each incision following thorough drainage of the respective spaces. A dorsal subaponeurotic space infection is sometimes difficult to differentiate from a simple cellulitis. A longitudinal incision is made directly over the abscess.[67]

Pyogenic Flexor Tenosynovitis

Kanavel's cardinal signs include the following: The finger is held flexed, as this position allows the synovial sheath its maximum volume and eases pain; symmetric swelling of the entire finger is present with edema of the back of the hand; the slightest attempt at passive extension of the affected digit produces exquisite pain; and the site of maximum tenderness is at the proximal cul-de-sac of the index, middle, and ring finger synovial sheaths in the distal palm or in the case of infection of the sheaths of the thumb and middle finger more proximally in the palm. The radial and ulnar bursae communicate in approximately 80% of cases and may simultaneously be infected. If they are both infected, the site of maximum tenderness is proximal to the flexor retinaculum at the wrist. Infections from the synovial spaces may spread into the deep palmar spaces by rupturing the proximal cul-de-sac in the palm. Bursal infections may spread into the forearm space of Parona, deep to the flexor tendons in the distal part of the forearm, and create a horseshoe-shaped abscess.

Pyogenic flexor tenosynovitis may be aborted with parenteral antibiotics, extremity elevation, and hand immobilization if the patient is seen within the first 24 to 48 hours of onset of infection. If the course is unsuccessful within 48 hours, or if the patient is seen more than 48 hours after onset of infection, surgical drainage must be undertaken. The preferred surgical approach is through two separate incisions.[68] A midaxial incision is made in the finger, usually on the ulnar side (on the radial side of the thumb and little finger). The digital artery and nerve remain with the volar flap, and the dissection proceeds to the tendon sheath. The synovium between A3 and A4 pulleys is incised. Cloudy fluid is encountered. A second incision is made in the palm over the tendon to drain the cul-de-sac. A 16-guage polyethylene catheter is inserted beneath the A1 pulley into the sheath. The sheath is flushed manually with sterile saline every 2 hours. After surgery, a bulky hand dressing absorbs the drainage.

Infections of the ulnar and radial bursae are the proximal extensions of the tendon sheath of, respectively, the flexor digitorum profundus of the little finger and the flexor pollicis longus of the thumb. Each may be opened and irrigated in a similar manner if involved.

Acute Fulminant Infections

Necrotizing Fasciitis

Necrotizing fasciitis is divided into two types based on bacteriology.[69] Type I consists of a combination of anaerobic bacteria and facultative aerobic bacteria, such as the Enterobacteriaceae, *Escherichia coli*, *Serratia marcescens*, *Klebsiella pneumoniae*, and streptococci other than group A. Type II consists of cases in which group A streptococci are isolated alone or in combination with *Staphylococcus aureus* or *Staphylococcus epidermidis*. *Vibrio vulnificus* from seawater may also result in a rapidly progressing necrotizing fasciitis. Predisposing factors, especially to the polymicrobial form of necrotizing fasciitis, are diabetes mellitus, alcoholism, vascular disease, and intravenous drug abuse.

Infection may first appear benign with a low-grade cellulitis; the progression is then rapid with development of moderate to severe pain. Lymphangitis is rare. Nonpitting edema, which can sometimes be massive, spreads beyond the erythematous area. Skin develops a patchy, dusky discoloration, and bullae are noted. Soft tissue crepitus is uncommon, but gas can often be demonstrated radiographically. Vascular thromboses in the subcutaneous plane result in skin necrosis. Infection dissects along fascial planes with necrosis of fascia and superficial fat. The fascia turns gray and liquefies, producing a watery exudate, "dishwater pus," in the fascial plane. Only radical surgical debridement can control the infection. All necrotic skin, fat, fascia, and muscle must be debrided, with fasciotomies extended well beyond the area of cellulitis, and even re-debridement performed within 24 hours should be considered.

Clostridial Myonecrosis (Gas Gangrene)

Clostridial myonecrosis is a rare anaerobic infection resulting from proliferation of Gram-positive rods. Gas gangrene infections may involve nonclostridial organisms. Exotoxins cause necrosis of muscle and subcutaneous tissue and in fact produce hydrogen sulfide and carbon monoxide and dissect along soft tissue planes. Early aggressive surgical debridement is essential, and intravenous penicillin is started immediately. The Gram stain reveals Gram-positive rods. Hyperbaric oxygen therapy is recommended as a treatment adjunct.

Diabetic Gangrene

Diabetic gangrene is usually seen in diabetic patients with peripheral vascular disease. Gram-negative and Gram-positive infections occur. Prompt aggressive debridement is important with use of broad-spectrum antibiotics.

Nondiabetic Gangrene

Nondiabetic gangrene is caused by mixed anaerobic and nonanaerobic organisms. Myonecrosis and soft tissue gas may be similar to those of clostridial infection. *Aeromonas hydrophila* from freshwater contamination can cause gangrene indistinguishable from a clostridial infection. Aggressive debridement and intravenous antibiotics are required.

Critique

Urgent intervention is needed for this upper extremity compartment syndrome. A complete fasciotomy is required, which necessitates opening three fascial compartments (volar, dorsal, and the mobile wad). The volar compartment encompasses the flexors of the wrist and fingers, along with the median and ulnar nerves. The posterior interosseous nerve and the extensors for the wrist and fingers are located in the dorsal compartment. The extensor carpi radialis longus and brevis, along with the brachioradialis, are found in the mobile wad. The incision for this fasciotomy starts proximal to the antecubital fossa and is extended distal to the midpalm, which will include releasing the carpal tunnel. The symptomatology and physical findings are too advanced for arm elevation. Also, a compartment syndrome can exist in the presence of palpable pulses.

Answer (C)

References

1. Green DP. General principles. In Green DP, Hotchkiss RN, Pederson WC, eds. Green's Operative Hand Surg, 4th ed. New York: Churchill Livingstone, 1999; 1–21.
2. Ramamurthy S, Hickey R. Anesthesia. In Green DP, Hotchkiss RN, Pederson WC, eds. Green's Operative Hand Surg, 4th ed. New York: Churchill Livingstone, 1999; 22–47.
3. Seiler JG. Anesthesia for hand surgery. In Essentials of Hand Surgery. Philadelphia: Lippincott Williams & Wilkins, 2002; 57–64.
4. Seiler JG. Casting and splinting. In Essentials of Hand Surgery. Philadelphia: Lippincott Williams & Wilkins, 2002; 57–64.
5. Seiler JG. Physical examination of the hand. In Essentials of Hand Surgery. Philadelphia: Lippincott Williams & Wilkins, 2002; 23–48.
6. Smith P. Injury. In Smith P, ed. Lister's The Hand: Diagnosis and Indications. 4th ed. London: Churchill Livingstone, 2002; 1–140.
7. Seiler JG. Anatomy. In Essentials of Hand Surgery. Philadelphia: Lippincott Williams & Wilkins, 2002; 4–22.
8. Metz VM, Wunderbaldinger P, Gilula LA. Update on imaging techniques of the wrist and hand. Clin Plast Surg 1996; 23:369–384.
9. Magid D, Thompson JS, Fishman EK. Computed tomography of the hand and wrist. Hand Clin 1991; 7:219–233.
10. Russell RC, Williamson DA, Sullivan JW, et al. Detection of foreign bodies in the hand. J Hand Surg 1991; 16A:2–11.
11. Brown RE. Fingertip and nailbed injuries in hand surgery. In Light TR, ed. Update II: American Society for Surgery of the Hand. Rosemont, IL: American Academy of Orthopedic Surgeons, 1999; 257–261.
12. Atasoy E, Loakimidis E, Kasdan ML, et al. Reconstruction of the amputated fingertip with a triangular volar flap. J Bone Joint Surg 1970; 52A:921–926.
13. Foucher G, Khouri RK. Digital reconstruction with island flaps. Clin Plast Surg 1997; 24:1–32.
14. Atasoy E. Reversed cross-finger subcutaneous flap. J Hand Surg 1982; 7:481–483.
15. Germann G, Rutschler S, Kania N, Raff T. The reverse pedicle heterodigital cross-finger flap. J Hand Surg 1997; 22B:25–29.
16. Breidenbach WC. Emergency free tissue transfer for reconstruction of acute upper extremity wounds. Clin Plast Surg 1989; 16:505–514.
17. Lister GD, Pederson WC. Skin flaps. In Green DP, Hotchkiss RN, Pederson WC, eds. Green's Operative Hand Surgery, 4th ed. New York: Churchill Livingstone, 1999; 1783.
18. Martin D, Dakhach J, Casoli V, Pellisier P, Ciria-Lorens G, Khouri RK, Beaudet J. Reconstruction of the hand with forearm island flaps. Clin Plast Surg 1997; 24:33–48.
19. Venkataswami R, Subramanian N. Oblique triangular flap: a new method of repair for oblique amputations of the fingertip and thumb. Plast Reconstr Surg 1980; 66:296–300.
20. Brown DN, Upton J, Khouri RK. Free flap coverage of the hand. Clin Plast Surg 1997; 24:57–62.

21. Scheker LR, Netscher DT. Replantations and amputations of the upper extremity. In Kasdan ML, ed. Occupational Hand and Upper Extremity Injuries and Diseases. Philadelphia: Hanley & Belfus, 1991; 215–231.

22. Zhong-Wei C, Meyer VE, Kleinert HE, et al. Present indications and contraindications for replantation as reflected by long-term functional results. Orthop Clin North Am 1981; 12:849–870.

23. Strickland JW. Development of flexor tendon surgery: twenty-five years of progress. J Hand Surg 2000; 25A:215–235.

24. Strickland JW. Flexor tendon injuries: II. Operative technique. J Am Acad Orthop Surg 1995; 3:55–62.

25. Lister GD, Kleinert HE, Kutz JE, Atasoy E. Primary flexor tendon repair followed by immediate controlled mobilization. J Hand Surg 1977; 2:441–451.

26. Gelberman RH, et al. Influences of the protected passive mobilization interval on flexor tendon healing. A prospective randomized clinical study. Clin Orthop 1991; 264:189–196.

27. Hung LK, Chan A, Chang J, Tsang A, Leung PC. Early controlled active mobilization with dynamic splintage for treatment of extensor tendon injuries. J Hand Surg 1990; 15A:251–257.

28. Aulicino DL. Extensor tendon injuries. In Light TR, ed. Hand Surgery Update II: American Society for Surgery of the Hand. Rosemont, IL: American Academy of Orthopedic Surgeons, 1999; 149–158.

29. Netscher DT. Extensor tendon injuries. In Goldwyn R, Cohen M, eds. The Unfavorable Result in Plastic Surgery: Avoidance and Treatment, 3rd ed. Philadelphia: Lippincott Williams & Wilkins, 2001; 751–770.

30. Brzezienski MA, Schneider LH. Extensor tendon injuries at the distal interphalangeal joint. Hand Clin 1995; 11:373–386.

31. Massengill JB. The boutonniere deformity. Hand Clin 1992; 8:787–801.

32. Sunderland S. The anatomic foundation of peripheral nerve repair techniques. Orthop Clin North Am 1981; 12:245–266.

33. Watchmaker GP, MacKinnon SE. Advances in peripheral nerve repair. Clin Plast Surg 1997; 24:63–73.

34. Jabaley ME, Wallace WH, Heckler FR. Internal topography of major nerves of the forearm and hand. J Hand Surg 1980; 5A:1–18.

35. Millesi H, Meissl G, Berger A. Interfascicular nerve grafting. Orthop Clin North Am 1981; 12:287–301.

36. Seiler JT. Fractures and dislocations of the metacarpals and phalanges. In Essentials of Hand Surgery. Philadelphia: Lippincott Williams & Wilkins, 2002; 91–113.

37. Stern PJ. Fractures of the metacarpals and phalanges. In Green DP, Hotchkiss RN, Pederson WC, ed. Green's Operative Hand Surgery, 4th ed. New York: Churchill Livingstone, 1999; 711–771.

38. Blake ER, Hoffman J. Emergency department evaluation and treatment of the shoulder and humerus. Emerg Med Clin North Am 1999; 17:859–876.

39. Ring D, Jupiter JB. Fracture-dislocation of the elbow. Hand Clin 2002; 18:55–63.

40. Stabile KJ, Pfaeffle HJ, Tomaino MM. The Essex-Lopresti fracture-dislocation factors in early management and salvage alternatives. Hand Clin 2002; 18:195–204.

41. Abboudi J, Kulp RW. Treating fractures of the distal radius with arthroscopic assistance. Orthop Clin North Am 2001; 32:307–315.

42. Amadio PC. Scaphoid fractures. Orthop Clin North Am 1992; 23:7–17.

43. Barton NJ. Twenty questions about scaphoid fractures. J Hand Surg 1992; 17B:289–310.

44. Kozin SH, Thoder JJ, Lieberman G. Operative treatment of metacarpal and phalangeal shaft fractures. J Am Acad Orthop Surg 2000; 8:111–121.

45. Stern PJ. Management of fractures of the hand over the last 25 years. J Hand Surg 2000; 25A:817–823.

46. Kiefhaver TR, Stern PJ. Fractures and dislocations of the proximal interphalangeal joint. J Hand Surg 1998; 23A: 368–380.

47. Koman LA, Ruch DS, Patterson-Smith B, et al. Vascular disorders. In Green DP, Hotchkiss RN, Pederson WC, eds. Green's Operative Hand Surgery, 4th ed. New York: Churchill Livingstone, 1999; 2254–2302.

48. Koman LA, Smith BP, Pollock FE Jr, et al. The microcirculatory effects of peripheral synthectomy. J Hand Surg 1995; 20A:709–717.

49. Gelberman RH, Nunley JA, Koman LA, et al. The results of radial and ulnar arterial repair in the forearm. Experience in three medical centers. J Bone Joint Surg 1982; 64A:383–387.

50. Sumner DS. Noninvasive assessment of the upper extremity and hand ischemia. J Vasc Surg 1986; 3:560–564.

51. Lee KL, Miller JG, Laitung P. Hand ischemia following radial artery cannulation. J Hand Surg 1995; 20B:493–495.

52. Redfern AV, Zimmerman NB. Neurologic and ischemic complications of upper extremity vascular access for dialysis. J Hand Surg 1995; 20A:199–204.

53. Freidman J, Fabre J, Netscher D, et al. Treatment of acute neonatal vascular injuries: the utility of multiple interventions. J Pediatr Surg 1999; 34:940–945.

54. Wheatley MJ, Marx MP. The use of the intra-arterial urokinase in the management of hand ischemia secondary to palmar and digital arterial occlusion. Ann Plast Surg 1996; 37:356–363.

55. Christodoulou L, Melikyan EY, Woodbridge S, et al. Functional outcome of high-pressure injection injuries of the hand. J Trauma 2001; 50:717–720.

56. Schnall SB, Mirzayan R. High-pressure injection injuries to the hand. Hand Clin 1999; 15:245–248.

57. Vogel JE, Dellon AL. Frost bite injuries of the hand. Clin Plast Surg 1989; 16:565–576.

58. Bentvdena PE, Deane LM. Chemical burns of the upper extremity. Hand Clin 1990; 6:253–259.

59. Larson DL. What is the appropriate management of tissue extravasation by anti-tumor agents? Plast Reconstr Surg 1985; 75:397–405.

60. Gelberman RH, Zikaib GS, Mubarak SJ, et al. Decompression of forearm compartment syndromes. Clin Orthop 1978; 134:225–229.

61. Mubarak SJ, Hargens AR. Acute compartment syndromes. Surg Clin North Am 1983; 63:539–565.

62. Whitesides TE, Haney TC, Morimoto K, et al. Tissue pressure measurements as a determinant for the need of fasciotomy. Clin Orthop 1975; 113:43–51.

63. Kanavel AB. An anatomical, experimental, and clinical study of acute phlegmons of the hand. Surg Gynecol Obstet 1905; 1:221–260.

64. Ouellett EA. Infections. In Light TR, ed. Hand Surgery Update II: American Society for Surgery of the Hand. Rosemont, IL: American Academy of Orthopedic Surgeons, 1999; 411–421.

65. Mennen U, Howells CJ. Human fight-bite injuries to the hand: a study of 100 cases within 18 months. J Hand Surg 1991; 16A:431–435.

66. Jebson PJL. Infections of the fingertip: paronychias and felons. Hand Clin 1998; 14:547–555.

67. Jebson PJL. Deep subfascial space infections. Hand Clin 1998; 14:557–566.

68. Neviaser RJ. Closed tendon sheath irrigation for pyogenic flexor tenosynovitis. J Hand Surg 1978; 3:462–466.

69. Gonzalez MH, Kay T, Weinzweig N, Brown A, et al. Necrotizing fasciitis of the upper extremity. J Hand Surg 1996; 21A:689–692.

40
Peripheral Vasculature

David V. Feliciano

Case Scenario

A high school cheerleader sustains a right supra-condylar fracture (radiographic confirmation) after tripping and falling on her outstretched arm. There is evidence of a slight neurologic deficit and vascular insufficiency with diminished distal pulses. The patient has no other injuries and is hemodynamically stable. Which of the following is the most appropriate definitive management approach for the injury?

(A) Immobilization of the elbow flexed to 90°
(B) Immobilization of the elbow flexed at 45°
(C) Traction of the forearm, with countertraction proximally
(C) Open exploration and reduction
(E) Traction applied to the hyperextended elbow

Upper Extremity

Upper Extremity Highlights

1. At least 10% of arterial emboli from cardiac or proximal arterial sources occur in the upper extremities.
2. The rare patient with ischemia in the hand after removal of an arterial line should first receive an intraarterial infusion of a thrombolytic agent.
3. Recently occluded prosthetic grafts used for angioaccess should have the venous end opened to allow for thrombectomy and verification of patency of the arterial and venous anastomoses.
4. Actively bleeding injuries in the second portion of the axillary artery are best exposed by division of the tendon of the pectoralis minor muscle at the coracoid process.

5. Extraanatomic bypass grafts are indicated when there is loss of soft tissue over an extensive arterial injury *or* when there is simultaneous infection in soft tissue and underlying artery or arterial repair.
6. The three musculofascial compartments of the forearm are the volar, dorsal, and "mobile wad."

Embolic Occlusion of the Brachial Artery

Although arterial emboli from a cardiac or proximal arterial source most commonly lodge at or below the bifurcation of the abdominal aorta, at least 10% occur in the upper extremities.

Diagnosis

Arterial emboli from a cardiac source such as atrial fibrillation, atherosclerotic cardiac disease, or a cardiomyopathy may lodge in the proximal brachial artery at the origin of the profunda brachii (deep brachial) artery. Because of the extensive collateral flow to the forearm through the profunda brachii artery, there may be a delay in presentation of the patient if the embolus lodges distal to its origin. The patient will complain of paresthesias in the fingers and pain in the forearm. Physical examination will confirm pale fingers, the absence of palpable radial and ulnar pulses, and a brachial–brachial index less than 0.4 to 0.5.

When the diagnosis is strongly suspected and there is no obvious contraindication (i.e., recent cerebrovascular accident), a bolus of intravenous heparin sodium at a dose of 10,000 U should be administered. As further workup proceeds, heparin is administered at 500 to 1,500 U/hr to maintain the partial thromboplastin time at 2 to 2.5 times normal. In thin patients with an acute presentation, it may be possible to localize the site of the embolic occlusion by careful palpation of brachial pulsations on the medial arm. When the patient has presented in a delayed fashion or the size of the arm precludes palpation of brachial pulsations, a diagnostic arteriogram is indicated to localize the embolus. This study can be helpful for all patients, however, to document a high bifurcation of the brachial artery and the presence of further clot at the origin of either the radial or the ulnar artery.

Treatment

Because the operative approach is simple, direct thrombolytic therapy is not indicated. A preoperative partial thromboplastin time should be measured as the patient has been heparinized as noted above, and a dose of an intravenous cephalosporin antibiotic should be administered. Before operation, the patient is positioned with the trunk on the side of the occlusion at the very side edge of the operating table and the upper extremity abducted 90° on an armboard. Some surgeons choose to place a 2-inch diameter rolled sheet longitudinally under the ipsilateral trunk and shoulder to further elevate the axilla for ease of proximal exposure, should this be needed. Skin preparation includes the ipsilateral neck, chest, axilla, and entire upper extremity to the fingertips. A sterile plastic bag can be used to cover the hand in light-skinned patients to allow for visualization of color changes after the embolectomy has been completed. Another option is to cover the hand, forearm, and distal arm in an orthopedic stockinette.

A 7- to 8-cm longitudinal incision overlying the area of the embolus is made on the medial arm in the biceps–triceps groove, the deep fascia is incised over the neurovascular bundle, and its surrounding sheath is incised. It is often possible to expose the proximal brachial artery with only minimal dissection of the medially placed median nerve. The two brachial veins surrounding the artery will have to be dissected away before proximal and distal control of the brachial artery can be obtained with 360° vascular loops (Dev-O-Loops, The Ludlow Co., Chicopee, MA). The area of isolation is ideally at the site of the embolus where distal arterial pulsations disappear.

A transverse arteriotomy is made at the site of occlusion using a No. 11 or 15 blade, and the embolus is extracted by manual compression of the now-collapsed arterial segment. A No. 4 balloon embolectomy catheter is then passed retrograde for 15 to 20 cm under proximal vascular control. The inflated balloon is withdrawn and, if no proximal embolus is retrieved after two passes, 10 to 15 mL of a solution of 50 U heparin/mL of saline is injected before the proximal vessel loop is tightened. A No. 3 balloon embolectomy catheter is then passed distally for 30 to 40 cm. To clear the orifices of both the radial and ulnar arteries distally, it is worthwhile to rotate the balloon catheter on second and third passes as it approaches the presumed or known site of the bifurcation of the brachial artery. Vigorous backbleeding without clot is reassuring, and 10 to 15 mL of heparinized saline solution is injected distally before the distal vessel loop is tightened.

The arteriotomy is closed with interrupted sutures of 6–0 polypropylene. Proximal and distal flushing is completed before the last three sutures are tied down. The distal vessel loop is removed to allow for evacuation of intraluminal air as the last sutures are tied down. After removal of the proximal vessel loop, the return of palpable radial and ulnar pulses at the wrist obviates the need for a completion arteriogram.

Postoperative screening to determine the source of the embolus is mandatory. The primary diagnostic test is transesophageal echocardiography, as 75% to 80% of peripheral emboli have a cardiac source (atrial or ventricular thrombus, subacute bacterial endocarditis, Libman-Sacks endocarditis, atrial myxoma, paradoxical embolus). Screening for a proximal source in the ascending or transverse thoracic aorta or proximal innominate or subclavian artery is accomplished using thoracic computed tomography (CT), CT arteriography, or a standard arch aortogram.

Even when the source of the embolus cannot be detected by the screening methods listed, long-term anticoagulation with daily warfarin sodium is mandatory.

Arterial Thrombosis Secondary to a Monitoring Device

Short- or long-term cannulation of either the radial or brachial artery is commonly used in critically ill patients. Before insertion of a cannula in either artery, it is appropriate to perform the modified Allen test described in 1966.[1,2] Although the sensitivity of this test is not 100%, a positive result should preclude cannulation of the artery in question. Once an arterial cannula is inserted in any extremity, continuous or intermittent flushing with heparinized saline solution is routine and should lower the incidence of thrombosis. Unfortunately, partial or complete thrombosis, particularly after the insertion of a radial artery line, occurs in up to 20% to 30% of patients if the cannula is left in place for more than 3 days.[3,4] Ischemic complications in the hand or fingers remain rare, however, in the absence of hypotension or need for drugs that cause vasoconstriction.[5]

Diagnosis

The ipsilateral hand and fingers should be inspected on a regular basis by the surgical team and nursing personnel once an arterial cannula has been inserted in an intubated patient. Evaluation on an hourly basis as part of the assessment of vital signs is appropriate when the patient is septic, hypotensive, and/or being administered drugs that cause vasoconstriction. Should the fingers or hand become cool, blanched, or mottled, the cannula is removed immediately. Failure of the local circulation to improve is strongly suggestive that local thrombosis or distal embolization has occurred.

Treatment

It has long been recognized that the three options for treatment of these patients include a cervicothoracic sympathetic block (stellate ganglion block) by an anesthesiologist, infusion of a thrombolytic agent, or a direct surgical approach. These can obviously be used in combination, but it is appropriate to obtain consultation from anesthesiology for the stellate ganglion block as a decision on a thrombolytic agent versus surgery is being considered.

In most situations, definitive therapy is best accomplished using an intraarterial infusion of a thrombolytic agent such as urokinase or tissue plasminogen activator (tPA). With either agent the infusion catheter should be placed within the thrombus by the interventional radiologist and periodic arteriograms performed to assess the therapeutic response. With successful resolution of the thrombus, the catheter is removed when the fibrinogen level is more than 100 mg/dl.[6]

Failure of infusion of a thrombolytic agent or early rethrombosis after cessation of a thrombolytic agent and administration of an anticoagulant should prompt a surgical attempt at salvage if the fingers or hand remain ischemic after cannulation of the radial artery. After preparation of the arm and forearm in the operating room, a 2.5-cm longitudinal incision is made in the distal volar forearm directly over the radial artery. Once proximal and distal arterial control has been obtained with vessel loops, a transverse arteriotomy is performed. Local thrombus is extracted; a No. 3 Fogarty balloon catheter is then passed into the distal radial artery and deep palmar arch and retrieved in a gentle fashion. After the infusion of 10 to 15 mL of heparinized saline distally, the transverse arteriotomy is closed with interrupted 7–0 polypropylene sutures using the flushing sequence described previously. Early rethrombosis suggests the need for a segmental resection of the area of the radial artery injured by the catheter and insertion of a cephalic vein interposition graft. Postoperative infusion of a low dose of thrombolytic agent may be a useful adjunct.

Occlusion or Infection of an Angioaccess Graft

Early occlusion of a prosthetic looped graft in the volar forearm or straight graft in the arm is caused by one of the following: (1) technical problems with one of the

anastomoses; (2) kinking or twisting of the prosthetic graft; (3) inadequate flushing of the graft before releasing vascular clamps; or (4) failure to recognize upstream venous narrowing or occlusion. After the administration of intravenous heparin at a dose of 1 mg/kg and a cephalosporin antibiotic, proximal and distal vascular control of the recipient vein and the prosthetic graft is obtained. The prosthetic graft proximal to the venous anastomosis is opened in a transverse manner.

Retrograde passage of a No. 4 or 5 Fogarty balloon catheter should remove any thrombus, verify patency of the proximal (arterial) anastomosis, and rule out kinking or twisting of the prosthetic graft. Successful prograde passage of a No. 6 or 7 Fogarty balloon catheter should rule out narrowing of the distal (venous) anastomosis or upstream venous narrowing or occlusion. If there is still concern about the latter problem because of "catching" of the balloon catheter as it is withdrawn, an intraoperative venogram is performed through the graftotomy. A tapered infusion catheter is first inserted through the graftotomy and held in place by a tight vessel loop. Either a fluoroscopic image or a hard-copy upstream venogram is obtained after injecting 35 mL of a 60% iodine-based contrast agent. Upstream venous narrowing will mandate extension of the angioaccess graft above this point or an attempt at balloon dilatation. A marked narrowing in a more proximal vein will need to be treated by balloon dilatation and insertion of an endovascular stent in an interventional radiology suite.

Infection of a prosthetic angioaccess graft may present as a false aneurysm along the body of the graft, erosion of the graft through the patient's skin with or without hemorrhage, or pus draining from one or both anastomotic sites (Figure 40.1). As with other infected prostheses, the graft will almost always have to be removed to

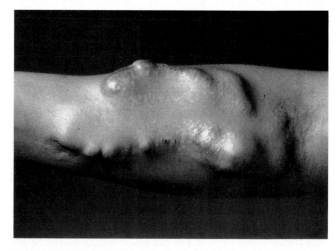

FIGURE 40.1. Infected forearm prosthetic angioaccess graft with multiple pseudoaneurysms.

clear the infection. Also, removal of a thrombosed graft is significantly easier than one that is still patent. In the hands of the occasional angioaccess surgeon, it is best to obtain control of the brachial artery with a vessel loop proximal to the old arterial anastomosis before it is exposed. After the administration of 1 mg/kg of intravenous heparin, the proximal (arterial) anastomosis is exposed and the presence of infection verified. The proximal brachial artery is occluded, and a decision is reached on whether a 1.5 to 2.0 mm cuff of graft can be left to allow for easy closure of the arterial end with a continuous 6–0 polypropylene suture after removal of the remainder of the graft. The absence of pus at this location makes this an acceptable option, whereas the presence of pus around the proximal anastomosis would generally rule out this option. In the latter instance, complete removal of the arterial end of the graft will force the use of one of several unpleasant options. These would include primary closure of a rigid arteriotomy site, the insertion of a small cephalic vein patch as an arterioplasty, or segmental resection of the brachial artery with an end-to-end anastomosis. The same principles can be applied to the venous anastomotic site, although the risk of a postoperative blowout of the repair caused by residual infection is significantly less.

Traumatic Injuries to Arteries

Injuries to the axillary, brachial, radial, or ulnar arteries account for approximately 45% to 52% of peripheral arterial injuries treated in civilian trauma centers.[7,8] Because of its length and exposed position in the upper extremity, injuries to the brachial artery are 3 to 3.5 times more common than those to the axillary artery.

Diagnosis

Traumatic occlusion or transection of the axillary or brachial artery without a subsequent repair does not always result in loss of the upper extremity because of the extensive collateral flow in this area. In DeBakey and Simeone's review of 2,471 arterial injuries in American military personnel in World War II, injuries to the axillary artery (n = 74), most of which were treated by ligation, resulted in an amputation rate of 43.2%.[9] In similar fashion, injuries to the brachial artery below the origin of the profunda brachii artery (n = 209) that were treated by ligation resulted in an amputation rate of 25.8%.[9] Therefore, a major injury to the axillary or brachial artery may be more subtle than one to the superficial femoral artery; that is, a wavering pulse (intermittently palpable) or audible Doppler pulse may be present, even with a proximal occlusion or major injury.

A patient with "hard" signs of an arterial injury (external hemorrhage, pulsatile hematoma, decrease in or loss of pulse and distal ischemic signs, or palpable thrill/audible bruit) after a penetrating injury should be moved to the operating room immediately with few exceptions. Diagnostic studies as previously described are not indicated, although an on-table surgeon-performed preoperative retrograde or antegrade brachial arteriogram may help determine the extent of injuries after a shotgun wound from a distance. For the patient with "hard" signs of an arterial injury after blunt trauma, there is often a need to rule out life-threatening injuries to the brain, thorax, or abdomen using CT before moving the patient to the operating room. It is appropriate, however, to realign any displaced fracture with traction or a splint or to reduce any dislocated joint as soon as possible to see if distal pulses return.

A patient with "soft" signs of an arterial injury (history of arterial bleeding, proximity of extremity injury to artery, nonpulsatile hematoma, or injury to adjacent nerve) needs further diagnostic evaluation. Diagnostic options include formal arteriography in an interventional radiology suite, surgeon-performed arteriography in the emergency center or operating room, or observation only. There are not enough data to justify the use of CT arteriography or magnetic resonance imaging (MRI) arteriography in evaluating possible peripheral vascular injuries at this time. The major disadvantage to formal arteriography in an interventional radiology suite is the associated time delay. Even during daylight hours, a minimum delay of 60 minutes is expected by the time the study is scheduled, the patient is transferred to the radiology suite, and the study is completed.

When the delay is likely to be even longer, a surgeon-performed arteriogram in the emergency center is appropriate.[10] Possible injuries to the proximal brachial and axillary arteries are evaluated by a retrograde brachial–axillary technique. An 18-gauge, 5.23-cm disposable catheter over needle is inserted into the distal brachial artery toward the shoulder by immobilizing the vessel against the humerus. A blood pressure cuff is then placed on the distal arm below the catheter in the brachial artery, and the arm is abducted to 90% and externally rotated. As the patient's head is turned away from the side of the injection, the blood pressure cuff is inflated to 300 mm Hg, and 50 mL of 60% meglumine diatrizoate dye is rapidly injected. A properly performed retrograde one-shot arteriogram will visualize the ipsilateral brachial, axillary, subclavian, and carotid arteries (Figure 40.2). With a possible injury to the distal brachial artery, the catheter over needle is inserted into the proximal brachial artery toward the hand. The distal arteriogram is performed with the arm once again abducted on an armboard. When the "one-shot" hard-copy arteriogram does not clearly visualize the area in question, a repeat injection can be performed depending on the patient's renal status.

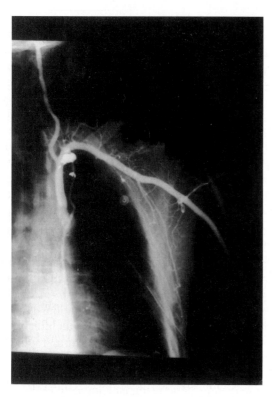

FIGURE 40.2. Retrograde brachial-axillary-subclavian arteriogram performed in the emergency center.

Treatment

When an arteriogram documents an abnormality in the wall of the vessel (intimal flap or irregularity, subintimal hematoma, spasm, or small pseudoaneurysm) but intact flow to the hand, there are three options. These include continued observation ("nonoperative management") with a repeated arteriogram in 3 to 7 days; insertion of an endovascular stent or stent graft; or operation. Nonoperative management is 87% to 95% successful when chosen for the appropriate lesions listed earlier.[11,12] If the patient refuses a follow-up arteriogram, careful education regarding acute and chronic signs of arterial occlusion is imperative. Also, the patient should have scheduled follow-up visits to the office or clinic for the next 2 months to detect signs of ischemia, expansion of a pseudoaneurysm, or delayed development of an arteriovenous fistula. Endovascular stenting is rarely considered for modest injuries to the axillary, brachial, or forearm arteries, as operation is so easily performed and does not usually threaten the life of even the multiply-injured patient. Operation, of course, is difficult to justify when there is not a significant pseudoaneurysm or arteriovenous fistula, and pulses at the wrist are still present despite a proximal arteriographic abnormality.

For the patient who presents with hard signs of an injury to the axillary or brachial artery, immediate operation is indicated as previously mentioned. Because

occlusion of the radial or ulnar artery leads to loss of the hand only 1% to 5% of the time, this particular lesion may be treated nonoperatively. In the operating room, skin preparation includes the entire anterior and lateral neck and chest and entire upper extremity to the fingertips as previously described. One lower extremity from the umbilicus to the toenails should be prepped, as well, to allow for retrieval of the greater saphenous vein from the groin or ankle area. It is helpful to cover the entire upper extremity in an orthopedic stockinette and place it at the side of the patient if an injury to the first or second portion of the axillary artery is suspected. This will allow more room for the operating team as well as relax the muscles around the shoulder girdle as dissection proceeds. With a suspected injury to the third portion of the axillary artery, the upper extremity is abducted at 90° and placed on an armboard.

The axillary artery starts at the lateral border of the first rib and becomes the brachial artery at the lateral border of the teres major muscle.[12] The operative approach varies depending on whether the arterial injury is located in the first portion (lateral border of the first rib to medial border of the pectoralis minor muscle), second portion (behind the pectoralis minor muscle), or third portion (lateral border of the pectoralis minor muscle to lateral border of teres major muscle). Injuries to the first or second portions that are not actively hemorrhaging are most commonly approached through an infraclavicular incision centered on the midclavicle.[14] After splitting the upper fibers of the pectoralis major muscle in a transverse fashion, the clavipectoral fascia is divided. Proximal arterial control is obtained by retracting the anteriorly positioned axillary vein in an inferior fashion and placing a vessel loop around the axillary artery just inferior to the clavicle. Distal control is obtained, as needed, by extending the infraclavicular incision into an incision in the deltopectoral groove (Figure 40.3). Should active hemorrhage from the second portion of the artery occur during dissection or the tamponaded injury is in the second portion, lateral retraction of the tendon of the pectoralis minor tendon is necessary. Persistent inadequate exposure of this arterial location mandates division of the tendon of the pectoralis minor muscle near the coracoid process to preserve the medial pectoral nerve. An injury in the third portion can be approached through the aforementioned incision in the deltopectoral groove. An alternate, but uncommonly utilized, approach involves a lateral pectoral incision along the edge of the pectoralis major muscle.

Injuries to the axillary artery, particularly those that are bleeding actively, are challenging because of the adjacent cords of the brachial plexus. The blind application of angled vascular clamps often entraps portions of the cords, leading to a partial brachial plexopathy for 12 to 24 months. Therefore, elevation of the injured artery

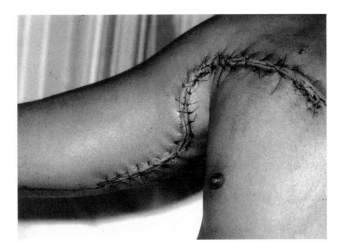

FIGURE 40.3. Standard incision for exposure of entire axillary and proximal brachial arteries.

proximally and distally with vessel loops is mandatory before vascular clamps are applied. The second problem in dealing with injuries at this location is the somewhat fragile nature of the axillary artery. This artery is rarely involved with significant atherosclerosis and is extraordinarily soft with a consistency that sometimes approaches that of the subclavian artery. Lateral repairs performed with suture bites that are too thin or end-to-end repairs performed under tension will lead to sutures tearing through when vascular clamps are released.

The brachial artery starts at the lateral border of the teres major muscle, courses through the medial arm, and bifurcates at the radial tuberosity of the forearm. The operative approach in the arm has been described previously. When an injury occurs near the elbow, the standard S-shaped incision extending from the medial biceps–triceps groove is used. This incision crosses the antecubital fossa and then turns longitudinally beyond the midaspect of the volar side of the forearm. The fascia overlying the neurovascular bundle medially and the bicipital aponeurosis beneath the antecubital fossa are divided to allow for complete exposure of the brachial artery proximal to its bifurcation.

There is a logical sequence for performing a complex repair (end-to-end anastomosis or insertion of a graft) of the axillary or brachial artery after proximal and distal arterial control has been obtained with vessel loops. When an end-to-end anastomosis is to be performed, a posterior knot is usually placed at 6 o'clock. If exposure is limited, as in an end-to-end anastomosis performed near the clavicle, it is helpful to perform the first one third of the posterior anastomosis in an open fashion (no posterior knot) in both directions to allow for complete visualization of all suture bites.[15] After this portion of the anastomosis is complete, the ends of the artery are pushed together as both sutures are pulled tight. Because both ends of the artery are now stabilized, a No. 5 or 6 Fogarty embolectomy catheter is passed proximally and distally to remove any thrombolic or embolic material. Approximately 10 to 15 mL of heparinized saline solution (50 U/mL of solution) is then injected into each end of the artery, and the vascular clamps are reapplied. The remaining two thirds of the anastomosis is completed by running one end of the continuous suture along one side and the other end along the other side. The last few loops of suture, however, are left loose to allow for flushing before the anterior knot is tied. The proximal vascular clamp is removed for flushing and then reapplied. The distal vascular clamp is removed to allow for flushing, as well. As air is evacuated by the distal flushing, the two suture ends are pulled up tight and tied. Once the first knot has been tied, the proximal arterial clamp is released. Bleeding from suture holes is controlled by the application of oxidized regenerated cellulose (Surgicel, Johnson & Johnson Medical, Inc., Arlington, TX) or Avitene (Med Chem Products, Inc., Woburn, MA). Because distal in situ thrombosis is very unusual during proximal arterial repairs in the upper extremity, the return of palpable pulses at the ipsilateral wrist obviates the need for a completion arteriogram. When distal pulsations are diminished or absent after removal of the vascular clamps, a completion arteriogram is mandatory.

When an interposition graft will be necessary to restore arterial continuity in the upper extremity, a reversed autogenous saphenous vein graft from the thigh of an uninjured lower extremity is the first choice. In the 15% to 20% of young male patients with saphenous veins that are too small for replacement of a major vessel such as the axillary artery, a ringed polytetrafluoroethylene synthetic graft is an acceptable alternative. The operative technique for each anastomosis may be as described above, or a more traditional approach may be used. The triangulation approach described by Carrel[16] involves placing stay sutures at 120° intervals on the circumference of the graft and on the recipient vessel. After these are tied and the ends of the graft and recipient vessel are in apposition, each 120° segment of the anastomosis may be readily approximated by a continuous suture technique. A related approach that is pertinent to the use of a rigid polytetrafluoroethylene interposition graft is to place only two stay sutures 180° apart to appose the ends of the graft and recipient vessel. When an interposition graft has been inserted, the terminal flushing maneuvers and evacuation of air are performed as described previously as the second anastomosis is completed.

When an interposition graft has been inserted to complete an arterial repair in the upper extremity, it is the practice of the author to place all adult patients on an intravenous drip of 10% dextran 40 in 5% dextrose (10% Gentran 40, Baxter Healthcare Corp., Deerfield, IL) at a dose of 40 mL/hr × 3 days. This agent can prevent or reverse cellular aggregation and will prolong the bleeding time. In addition, adult patients are started on 81-gr aspirin tablets once a day by rectal suppository or orally starting in the recovery room and maintained on this medication for the next 3 months.[17]

There are two other innovative operative techniques that may be helpful in trauma and infection problems involving the arteries of the upper extremity. The first is the use of extraanatomic bypass grafting. The indications for this technique include (1) loss of soft tissue over injured artery or vein; (2) postoperative wound infection with blowout of underlying arterial repair; or (3) simultaneous infections in soft tissue and underlying artery secondary to injection of illicit drugs.[18] In each of these situations, the arterial bypass graft is placed in a separate subcutaneous tunnel from the area of missing or infected soft tissue. The operative technique involves longitudinal extension of the operative incision or soft tissue defect to expose healthy proximal and distal artery. The extensions are usually 4 to 6 cm long to allow for transection of the healthy portion of the proximal artery followed by the performance of an end-to-end anastomosis to a reversed saphenous vein graft from an uninjured lower extremity. The proximal graft is then tunneled at an angle away from the soft tissue defect or infection through healthy soft tissue. The anastomosis of the extraanatomic bypass graft to distal healthy artery is once again performed beyond the soft tissue defect or infection. As a final step, both proximal and distal anastomoses and the ends of the extraanatomic bypass graft are covered by suture closure of the healthy soft tissue at the previously described extensions (Figure 40.4).

The other innovative operative technique is the use of temporary intraluminal shunts in arteries and/or veins of both the upper and lower extremities. The indications for this technique include (1) Gustilo IIIC combined orthopedic-vascular injuries, including mangled extremities or near amputations; (2) preservation of an amputated upper extremity at the arm, forearm, or wrist level before replantation; or (3) rapid restoration of arterial inflow or venous outflow, or both, as part of a peripheral vascular damage-control operation in the patient near death.[19] With the Gustilo IIIC fractures or partial/complete amputations of the upper extremity, the first operative priority is insertion of a temporary intraarterial plastic shunt by the general/trauma/vascular surgeon. This allows for appropriate orthopedic stabilization, reconstruction, or debridement before formal revascularization with interposition grafts. Of course, definitive repair

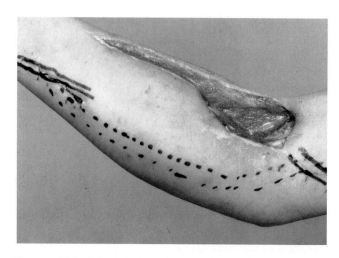

FIGURE 40.4. Infected pseudoaneurysm of the distal right brachial and proximal radial and ulnar arteries underlying severe cellulitis was replaced by an extraanatomic saphenous vein bypass graft from the distal brachial artery (end-to-end) to the midulnar artery (end-to-side). The path of the graft is marked on the skin. (Reprinted from Feliciano DV. Heroic procedures in vascular injury managment. The role of extraanatomic bypasses. Surg Clin North Am 2002; 82:115–124, with permission from Elsevier.)

with such grafts may be performed at a second operation depending on the patient's other injuries and metabolic state. For patients with prehospital near-exsanguination and a need for a damage-control operation, the rapid insertion of a temporary intraarterial plastic shunt preserves the injured extremity in the patient with "metabolic failure" from hemorrhage. Such patients have a body temperature less than 35°C, an arterial base deficit less than −10 to −15, and/or an intraoperative coagulopathy.[20] A prolonged arterial repair under these circumstances will endanger the patient's life, and damage-control principles mandate a short first operation to control hemorrhage and restore arterial inflow (or venous outflow).

The operative technique involves obtaining proximal and distal control around the injured portion of the artery (or vein). After debridement of the injured section, a Fogarty balloon catheter is passed into the proximal and distal artery. The usual injection of 10 to 15 mL of heparinized saline (50 U/mL) into each end is deferred for coagulopathic patients. The largest plastic shunt that will fit into both ends of the transected artery is chosen. The most commonly utilized shunt is an Argyle Carotid Artery Shunt (Sherwood Medical, St. Louis, MO) ranging in size from 8 to 14 Fr. A hemostat is placed at the midaspect of the shunt, and the shunt is inserted into the proximal artery for 8 to 10 mm. A 2–0 silk tie is tightened down near the end of the artery to hold the shunt in place. The hemostat is removed to verify flow through the shunt and then reapplied. The distal end of the shunt is then inserted into the distal end of the artery for 8 to 10 mm and fixed in place with another 2–0 silk tie, and the hemostat is removed to restore arterial flow. With larger intraluminal shunts and adequate venous outflow from the upper extremity, anticoagulation will not be necessary. After orthopedic procedures have been completed or when the patient undergoing damage-control shunting has been stabilized in the intensive care unit, the shunts can be removed. Before removal, however, an assessment is made of the distance between the two ends of the shunted artery. As the injured artery has already been debrided and further debridement at the sites of the 2–0 silk sutures will be necessary, most patients will require insertion of a saphenous vein interposition graft. The graft is retrieved from the thigh of an uninjured lower extremity in the usual fashion.

A decision on anticoagulation is made depending on the extent of the patient's injuries and current coagulation tests. In the absence of injuries to the brain, intraabdominal solid organs, or soft tissues of the injured extremity, a 1 mg/kg loading dose of intravenous heparin is administered before the ends of the artery around the intraluminal shunt are clamped. The 2–0 silk sutures are cut, the crushed ends of the artery are removed, a Fogarty balloon catheter is passed proximally and distally, and the saphenous vein interposition graft is sewn in place as described earlier.

Traumatic Injuries to Veins

Diagnosis

Injuries to veins in the upper extremities are infrequently discussed. Diagnostic tests such as venograms are not employed to document the presence of a peripheral venous injury as the consequences of missing such an injury are so modest; that is, pressure dressings usually control venous hemorrhage from small injuries, and late venous pseudoaneurysms are extraordinarily rare. The only indications for operation are venous bleeding not controlled by a pressure dressing or the suspected or known presence of an associated arterial injury.

Treatment

The incisions previously described for arterial injuries in the upper extremities are the same ones used for possible venous injuries. Proximal and distal control around a major venous injury, however, can be awkward because of multiple venous branches. As the venous system is characterized by low pressure, the use of small, medium, and large metal clips for ligation followed by division of venous branches is appropriate as exposure and control are obtained. Proximal and distal control around an area of injury can usually be maintained with use of vessel loops under tension rather than with angled vascular clamps.

Because of the presence of valves in the venous system, injection of heparinized saline toward the hand after distal venous control has been obtained is not performed. For the same reason, passage of a Fogarty balloon catheter toward the hand or toward the heart is inappropriate.

Essentially all major injuries to the brachial or axillary venae comitantes or veins can be ligated as there are extensive venous collaterals throughout the upper extremity. On rare occasions in stable patients with an isolated major injury to the axillary vein, resection and an end-to-end anastomosis or insertion of a saphenous vein interposition graft has been performed. Lateral venorrhaphies for lesser injuries are performed with interrupted or continuous sutures of 7–0 polypropylene. With a meticulous suture technique, peripheral venous repairs (most studied in the lower extremities) have been documented to have short-term patencies exceeding 75% in several reports.[21,22]

Compartment Syndromes and Fasciotomies

Diagnosis

A compartment syndrome is defined as increased pressure within a closed fascial space that reduces capillary perfusion to a level less than that required for the viability of tissues.[23] Most compartment syndromes result from an increase in content of the compartment as caused by edema or hemorrhage or, on rare occasions, by chronic overexertion of muscles. Trauma and/or ischemia to the extremity remain the most common causes.

A history of a delay in presentation when ischemia in an extremity is present should make the attending physician suspicious that a compartment syndrome is present or is likely to develop. The patient will often complain of pain out of proportion to the extent of an injury, as well. General findings on physical examination that increase the likelihood of a compartment syndrome occurring include systemic shock in combination with an ischemic extremity, evidence of a crush injury, and marked swelling of the extremity. The presence of a tender or tight musculofascial compartment does not, however, precisely correlate with the presence of a compartment syndrome. Rather, pain on passive stretch of muscles in the compartment is strongly suggestive. Other neurologic findings that often suggest the presence of an established compartment syndrome include hypesthesia in the sensory distribution of a nerve that courses through the compartment in question or weakness of the involved muscles. Finally, restoration of arterial inflow after a greater than 4- to 6-hour delay, the need to clamp arterial inflow and venous outflow vessels at the time of vascular repair, and ligation of a major outflow vein are procedures at operation that make a compartment syndrome more likely to develop. Also, it is important to note that distal pulses in an extremity are often still palpable or audible by a Doppler device after a revascularization procedure even though a compartment syndrome is present.

One approach in vascular or trauma surgery services has been to perform a fasciotomy to relieve a suspected compartment syndrome whenever any of the historical, physical, or operative factors described earlier are present. An aggressive approach such as this will avoid missing a compartment syndrome, but will surely result in some unnecessary or "prophylactic" fasciotomies. Another approach is to measure the intracompartmental pressure (normal, 4 to 8 mm Hg) and only perform fasciotomy when a certain elevated pressure has been reached. A large number of techniques for measurement of intracompartmental pressure have been described. including (1) needle injection, (2) wick catheter, (3) slit catheter, (4) arterial transducer, and (5) the STIC device (Solid-State Transducer IntraCompartmental Monitor System, Stryker Surgical, Kalamazoo, MI).[23–25] Unfortunately, there is little consensus in the literature about the absolute intracompartmental pressure that mandates a fasciotomy to avoid permanent muscular or neural damage. A rising pressure more than 30 mm Hg,[24,26] a pressure more than 45 mm Hg[23] or a less than 20 mm,[27] or a 30 mm Hg[28] difference between diastolic blood pressure and the intracompartmental pressure have all been suggested over the past 25 years. In a somewhat ecumenical approach, the American College of Surgeons Committee on Trauma poster entitled "Management of Peripheral Vascular Trauma" (2002) suggests that fasciotomy be performed for pressures ">30–35 mm Hg."[29]

Treatment

Fasciotomies to relieve compartment syndromes in the upper extremities account for only 20% of all fasciotomies performed after trauma and even less after nontrauma vascular occlusions. Therefore, many surgeons are not familiar with the operative techniques that are utilized.

The forearm is divided into three musculofascial compartments, including volar, dorsal, and the "mobile wad."[27] Other authors describe superficial flexor, deep flexor, and extensor compartments.[24] The volar compartment (flexion, pronation, supination) is opened first using the "ulnar approach." The incision begins on the lateral (radial side) of the forearm distal to the antecubital fossa, proceeds transversely across the forearm parallel to the arm–forearm fold, and then makes a right angle turn down the ulnar volar aspect of the forearm. At the wrist, the ulnar incision curves toward the radial side until it crosses the carpal tunnel along the thenar crease of the palm. The fascia overlying the flexor digitorum sublimis

and flexor carpi ulnaris muscles is divided from the aponeurosis of the elbow down to the carpal tunnel at the wrist (decompression of superficial flexor compartment). These two muscles are separated with retractors, the ulnar nerve and artery are identified overlying the flexor digitorum profundus, and the fascia overlying this muscle and the flexor pollicis longus is divided as well (decompression of deep flexor compartment). After complete decompression of the volar compartment, it is worthwhile to remeasure the intracompartmental pressure in the dorsal (extensor) and mobile wad compartments. Should these pressures still be elevated, the dorsal compartment is approached through a skin incision in the pronated forearm from the lateral epicondyle of the humerus to the midline of the wrist. The fasciotomy is performed in the interval between the extensor digitorum communis and extensor carpi radialis brevis muscles toward the radial side of the forearm. The role of epimysiotomy of decompressed muscles is unclear, and a carpal tunnel release at the wrist is often added if the wrist and hand are swollen.

Any pale forearm muscle that still contracts with stimulation from the electrocautery device should be left in place at the first operation. The entire forearm is then covered with a bulky dressing and elevated by attaching a forearm stockinette to an intravenous pole. After 3 to 7 days of elevation in patients with obviously viable forearm muscles, the patient is returned to the operating room. Closure of the skin incision is best accomplished by undermining the subcutaneous tissues and placing multiple interrupted vertical mattress skin-only sutures of 2–0 nylon. When the tension is too great to complete the skin closure with sutures, a split-thickness skin graft harvested from the anterolateral thigh is applied.

Lower Extremity

Lower Extremity Highlights

1. Catheterization injuries to the femoral artery include retroperitoneal and intraperitoneal hemorrhage, acute thrombosis, and acute pulsatile hematomas in the groin.
2. Approximately 45% of arterial emboli from cardiac or proximal arterial sources lodge at the bifurcation of the common femoral artery.
3. Failure of a transfemoral balloon catheter embolectomy is usually the result of simultaneous embolism to the popliteal or trifurcation vessels *or* to atherosclerotic disease locally or at Hunter's canal.
4. An infected femoral artery pseudoaneurysm in the drug addict must be completely excised; fortunately, the need for revascularization is uncommon.

5. Embolic occlusion of the "trifurcation" vessels mandates below-knee exposure of the anterior tibial, posterior tibial, and peroneal arteries, which usually requires division of the anterior tibial vein.

6. Temporary intraluminal plastic arterial (and venous) shunts in the extremities are indicated for patients with Gustilo IIIC combined orthopedic–vascular injuries or as part of peripheral vascular damage control for patients with near exsanguination.

7. A below-knee two-incision four-compartment fasciotomy is advised when the measured intracompartmental pressure is more than 30 to 35 mm Hg.

Catheterization Injuries of the Femoral Artery

Diagnosis

Catheterization of the common femoral artery is generally utilized for truncal or peripheral angiography or angioplasty, cardiac catheterization, coronary angioplasty or insertion of stents, and insertion of intraaortic balloons. Complications that occur include intraperitoneal and retroperitoneal hemorrhage, thrombosis of the common femoral or external iliac artery, and the development of a pseudoaneurysm or arteriovenous fistula in the groin.[30,31] In one review, the need for surgical intervention ranged from 0.6% after diagnostic cardiac catheterization to 11.5% after insertion of an intraaortic balloon.[30]

Intraperitoneal hemorrhage from perforation of the distal external iliac artery will often lead to an initial episode of hypotension during the catheterization procedure. Changes on the cardiac monitor suggestive of ischemia are usually absent at this point. After a response to the infusion of fluids, hypotension will recur, and the catheterization procedure may have to be terminated. The general or vascular surgeon notified at this point should confirm the diagnosis by physical examination of the abdomen supplemented by a surgeon-performed ultrasound. Using a 3.5 MHz probe (3.5×10^6 cycles/sec), the presence of anechoic (black) fluid in Morison's pouch, the splenorenal area, or the pelvis on the abdominopelvic ultrasound confirms the diagnosis of intraabdominal hemorrhage.

The patient with retroperitoneal hemorrhage may develop hypotension hours after the catheterization procedure has been completed. The hypotension that develops will usually respond to the infusion of fluids, and emergency laboratory studies will confirm new-onset anemia. An abdominopelvic CT is often performed before the surgeon is called if the patient is reasonably stable. A CT performed with intravenous contrast that does not demonstrate extravasation into the distal retroperitoneum suggests that the injury has been tamponaded by surrounding clot. Extravasation of contrast into the retroperitoneal hematoma confirms continued bleeding and mandates operation if coagulation studies are normal.

Acute thrombosis of the common femoral or external iliac artery secondary to dissection during the catheterization procedure or compression of the arterial entrance site at the completion of the procedure will cause immediate symptoms. The patient will complain of pain or numbness in the ipsilateral foot. The femoral artery pulse in the groin may be diminished or absent along with popliteal and pedal pulses. A temperature change in the skin will be present in the distal thigh and below. In the absence of preexisting symptoms, such as ipsilateral decreased pedal pulses, claudication, rest pain, or distal arterial ulcers, the diagnosis of thrombosis secondary to the catheterization procedure is most likely.

A palpable pulsatile mass that develops in the groin after a catheterization procedure is an acute pulsatile hematoma. Such lesions are commonly, but incorrectly, described as "pseudoaneurysms." The diagnosis is made on physical examination and confirmed with a surgeon-performed ultrasound using a 7.5 MHz linear probe.

The rare arteriovenous fistula that develops after a catheterization procedure is detected by the presence of a palpable thrill/audible bruit on physical examination. The diagnosis is confirmed using duplex ultrasonography, a combination of real-time B-mode imaging and pulsed-wave Doppler, or color duplex imaging ("triple imaging") in a vascular laboratory.

Treatment

The operative approach to intraperitoneal or retroperitoneal hemorrhage from a catheterization injury may vary according to the training of the surgeon. A general surgeon consulted for such a patient may feel more comfortable approaching a distal injury to the external iliac artery through a lower midline laparotomy. This is especially true with hypotensive or obese patients or with those who have had previous surgery in the same groin.[32] After evacuation of intraperitoneal blood, the small bowel is eviscerated to the right and the sigmoid colon to the left. In the profoundly hypotensive patient, the midline retroperitoneum is opened and a DeBakey aortic clamp is used to cross-clamp the infrarenal abdominal aorta. As the patient is resuscitated, the distal retroperitoneum 2 to 3 inches proximal to the inguinal ligament is opened over the external iliac vessels as they come out of the pelvis. The external iliac artery is encircled with a vessel loop that allows for the vessel to be pulled proximally and elevated away from the adjacent external iliac vein. Further sharp dissection directly on the artery should demonstrate the area of perforation, which is then oversewn with interrupted 6–0 polypropylene sutures. Should the distal external iliac artery not be injured, the adjacent vein is dissected toward the inguinal ligament. A vessel loop that encircles the external iliac vein will increase hemorrhage from a more distal perforation and should be avoided. Other general or vascular surgeons will approach presumed distal injuries to the external iliac artery (or vein) by dividing several centimeters of the inguinal ligament over the vessels. Another approach is to perform release of the inguinal ligament.[33] When the vascular injury is approached through the groin, a small Cooley C-shaped vascular clamp may be used to obtain proximal arterial control in the retroperitoneum. A vascular clamp applied to the common femoral vein in the groin may cause a modest decrease in hemorrhage from the distal external iliac vein as dissection proceeds superiorly to the area of the perforation.

Acute thrombosis of the common femoral or external iliac artery is approached through a longitudinal incision overlying the femoral vessels in the groin. The longitudinal incision allows for complete exposure of the distal external iliac artery by partial division of the inguinal ligament. Also, as many patients undergoing catheterization of the femoral artery have underlying atherosclerosis, complete dissection of the origins of the superficial femoral and profunda femoris arteries can be accomplished as well. After the administration of a 1-mg/kg loading dose of intravenous heparin and with vessel loops placed around the distal external iliac artery or the proximal common femoral artery, the superficial femoral artery, and the profunda femoris artery, an angled vascular clamp is applied to the external iliac or common femoral artery. Distal control on the branch vessels can often be accomplished by placing the vessel loops on traction. A 12-mm longitudinal arteriotomy is made over the site where the arterial pulse was noted to disappear prior to placing the proximal vascular clamp. After 6–0 polypropylene stay sutures are placed on either side of the arteriotomy to enhance exposure, local thrombus is manually extracted. The lumen is washed clean with heparinized saline solution and inspected carefully for size, presence of an elevated plaque, or an injury to the posterior wall. When none of these is present, a No. 5 to No. 7 Fogarty embolectomy catheter is passed retrograde through the arteriotomy under manual or vessel loop control for a distance of 10 to 15 cm. The balloon on the catheter is inflated to the listed size using a tuberculin syringe and withdrawn gently. When two consecutive passes of the balloon catheter proximally yield no thrombus and free flow of pulsatile arterial blood is noted, 10 to 15 mL of heparinized saline (50 U/mL) are injected before the proximal arterial clamp is reapplied. The vessel loops on the superficial femoral and profunda femoris arteries are released one at a time to confirm that

vigorous backbleeding is present. If this does not occur, No. 3 to No. 5 Fogarty embolectomy catheters are passed distally as described above. Should severe local atherosclerosis be present when the arteriotomy is first made and the thrombus has been extracted, an endarterectomy through the media of the common femoral artery may be necessary. The arteriotomy is then closed with a saphenous vein or thin-walled polytetrafluoroethylene patch angioplasty.

For the past 10 to 15 years, ultrasound-guided compression of postcatheterization "pseudoaneurysms" in the groin has been the standard of care.[34] In general, 15-minute periods of compression are followed by ultrasound examination using a 7.5 MHz linear probe of the pseudoaneurysm to confirm thrombosis of the extraluminal blood. The technique is successful because of the small perforations that standard catheterizations create.

In most patients, an acute arteriovenous fistula in the common or superficial femoral artery is approached through the longitudinal groin incision described above. Proximal and distal arterial control is obtained using vascular clamps or vessel loops. The area of adherence is separated, a finger is used to control hemorrhage from the small venotomy, and the arterial and venous perforations are closed with interrupted 6–0 polypropylene sutures.

Embolic or Thrombotic Occlusion of the Femoral Artery

Diagnosis

In patients with peripheral arterial emboli originating from atrial fibrillation, atherosclerotic cardiac disease, cardiomyopathy, or proximal atherosclerosis (rare), approximately 45% lodge at the bifurcation of the common femoral artery.[35] The sudden signs of acute femoral artery embolic occlusion are well known and have been described previously for patients with catheterization-induced thrombosis of the common femoral artery.

In the absence of atrial fibrillation, atherosclerotic cardiac disease, or a cardiomyopathy, an acute thrombotic occlusion of the common femoral artery may be present. As noted previously, this is more likely to be present when there is a history of ipsilateral decreased pedal pulses, claudication, rest pain, or distal arterial ulcers.

Treatment

Some elderly patients will present in a delayed fashion after an embolism to or thrombosis of the femoral artery and have advanced ischemic changes of the foot or leg. Such changes include a cold insensate foot or leg without movement or even early manifestations of gangrene. As resuscitation is initiated, it is important to measure serum potassium, creatinine, arterial blood gases, and urine myogloblin in these patients even if revascularization is not planned. The presence of hyperkalemia, an elevated creatinine level, metabolic acidosis, and myoglobinuria are strongly suggestive of rhabdomyolysis.[36] Although an early amputation would theoretically correct these metabolic problems, they already increase the risk of any type of anesthesia in the elderly patient. The hyperkalemia and metabolic acidosis are treated in the standard fashion, and a Swan-Ganz catheter is used to direct needed fluid resuscitation to correct the elevated creatinine level and clear myoglobin from the urine. In addition, the urine is alkalinized by the administration of intravenous bicarbonate. When the patient's hyperkalemia and acidosis are corrected and clearing of urine is noted, the patient is taken to the operating room. The level of amputation, the management of the stump, and the need for a femoral embolectomy or thrombectomy to aid healing of the stump are based on the patient's condition and on the local physical findings at the time of amputation.

There are patients in whom the viability of the extremity is unclear at the time of presentation or even after resuscitation. In some there may be a concern that a compartment syndrome secondary to prolonged ischemia followed by vigorous resuscitation may be compromising the physical examination of the leg and foot. It is appropriate for such patients to initiate the operative procedure with a short incision in the position of a normal below-knee anterior/peroneal compartment fasciotomy at the mid-leg (to be described). A 3- to 4-inch fasciotomy over the anterior compartment of the leg will allow for confirmation of dead versus viable muscle that bulges through the incision. Amputation followed by an embolectomy or thrombectomy in the common femoral artery is appropriate in the first instance. With bulging viable muscle, a below-knee four-compartment fasciotomy (to be described) is performed followed by the embolectomy or thrombectomy.

Based on the paper by Blaisdell et al.[37] in 1978, some surgeons choose to treat patients with a viable extremity and a period of ischemia in the lower extremity exceeding 10 to 12 hours with high-dose heparin rather than an acute care embolectomy or thrombectomy. The 20,000 units of heparin recommended as an initial bolus is followed by a continuous infusion of 2,000 to 4,000 units per hour.[37]

The preferred approach for other patients with acute embolic occlusion of the common femoral artery is to administer a 10,000-unit intravenous bolus of heparin as the patient is prepared for an acute care operation. When thrombotic occlusion is strongly suspected, an abdominal aortogram with bilateral femoral arterial runoff studies is often performed before heparin is administered. After a partial thromboplastin time is checked and a dose of an intravenous cephalosporin antibiotic is administered, a longitudinal incision is made over the common femoral artery. Once the common femoral, superficial femoral, and profunda femoris arteries have been encircled with vessel loops, the common femoral artery is clamped and traction or bulldog vascular clamps are applied to the branch vessels. A transverse arteriotomy just proximal to the bifurcation is made in patients with a probable diagnosis of embolic occlusion. If the common femoral artery has an extensive amount of plaque on palpation and the history is supportive of thrombotic occlusion, some surgeons choose to make a longitudinal arteriotomy just proximal to the bifurcation.

The embolus is extracted from the common femoral artery by manual compression of the now-collapsed arterial segment. Much as with embolic occlusion of the proximal brachial artery, a No. 4 or No. 5 balloon embolectomy catheter is passed retrograde for 15 to 20 cm under proximal vascular control. If no proximal embolus is retrieved after two passes, 10 to 15 mL of a solution of 50 units of heparin/mL of saline is injected. A No. 4 balloon embolectomy catheter is then passed distally for its entire length down the superficial femoral artery. Very gentle traction is placed on the inflated balloon as it is withdrawn, and the balloon is partially deflated each time resistance is encountered. This is necessary to avoid stripping diseased intima from such a commonly diseased artery in adults. It is unlikely that all infrapopliteal "trifurcation" vessels will be cleared of embolic material, if present, by distal passage of a balloon catheter from the common femoral artery. In one study performed in cadavers, embolectomy catheters passed from the groin entered the peroneal artery in 90% of instances.[38] After the injection of 10 to 15 mL of heparinized saline into the superficial femoral artery, a No. 3 balloon embolectomy catheter is passed for 15 cm into the profunda femoris artery. It may be useful to dissect out the first bifurcation of this vessel if extensive embolic material is present to allow for passage of the catheter into separate branches. Once again, great care is taken not to disrupt atherosclerotic plaque as the balloon catheter is withdrawn from this often fragile vessel. After the injection of heparinized saline, the common femoral arteriotomy is closed with interrupted 6–0 polypropylene sutures and terminal flushing as previously described. As a completion arteriogram is mandatory after embolectomies performed in the lower extremity, one option is to pass a 20-gauge short plastic catheter over metal needle through the last gap in the arteriotomy site before the final one or two 6–0 polypropylene sutures are placed. A completion femoropopliteal–tibioperoneal arteriogram can be performed by injecting 35 mL of 60% meglumine diatrizoate dye and counting "1,000, 2,000," up to "5,000" before the hard-copy x-ray film is shot. The x-ray cassette

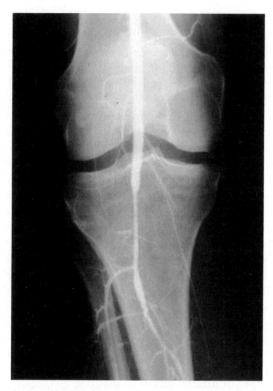

FIGURE 40.5. An intraoperative transfemoral postembolectomy arteriogram-documented spasm in the distal popliteal artery as the cause of diminished pedal pulses.

is placed to encompass the distal superficial femoral artery, popliteal artery, and the proximal one third to one half of the shank vessels (Figure 40.5). Another approach is to visualize the same area using fluoroscopic imaging.

The management of thrombotic occlusion of the common femoral artery is somewhat beyond the focus of this chapter. After removal of local thrombus, attempted passage of a balloon catheter will document whether proximal, local, and/or distal atherosclerotic narrowing or occlusive disease is present. Therapeutic options vary depending on the location and extent of disease. They include local endarterectomy/patch angioplasty, insertion of a crossover femorofemoral bypass graft, or, on occasion, the insertion of an aortobifemoral bypass graft. When associated occlusion of the superficial femoral artery at Hunter's canal is present, an acute care femoropopliteal bypass may have to be performed.

Ruptured Femoral Artery Pseudoaneurysm Secondary to Inadvertent Injection of Illicit Drugs

Diagnosis

There are few peripheral vascular surgical emergencies more dramatic than the rupture of an infected femoral artery pseudoaneurysm. These may occur rarely in patients with infected limbs of aortobifemoral bypass grafts. Others occur in drug addicts who have inadvertently injected contaminated material into the wall of an artery adjacent to the intended vein. The "traumatic infected pseudoaneurysm" that results can present as a pulsatile mass in the groin or as an arterial hemorrhage from the apex of the mass.[39] In the former instance, a surgeon-performed ultrasound using a 7.5 MHz linear probe will confirm the presence of a fluid-filled cavity outside the common femoral artery. When bleeding is present, a presumptive diagnosis is made based on the patient's history of self-administered needle injections into vessels in the groin.

Treatment

For the bleeding patient, immediate pressure is applied as standard resuscitation is performed. Aspiration of the infected pseudoaneurysm with a small needle at another site will allow for appropriate culture and sensitivity studies. Once hemorrhage has stopped, a bulky pressure dressing similar to that used after arteriograms performed through the common femoral artery is applied. Intravenous antibiotics, particularly those with antistaphylococcal coverage, are started immediately. The presence of methicillin-resistant *Staphylococcus aureus* in community-acquired infections is now well documented and should be considered when choosing an antibiotic.

After 18 to 24 hours of intravenous antibiotics, the patient is taken to the operating room for complete excision of all infected segments of the femoral artery. When a large infected pseudoaneurysm of the common femoral artery is present, proximal arterial control is obtained via a lower abdominal quadrant extraperitoneal approach (to be described). Also, the longitudinal groin incision may have to be extended distally in order to allow for complete excision of infection in the proximal superficial femoral artery. All infected arterial segments are excised, including the proximal profunda femoris artery, if necessary. The arterial ends are suture ligated with polypropylene suture, covered with a transposition muscle flap if soft tissue coverage is inadequate, and the remainder of the infected area is packed open.[40]

It is common knowledge in public hospitals that a surprising number of patients with excision of the common femoral artery and its bifurcation vessels continue to have a viable lower extremity. This has been confirmed in a large published series.[41] A lower extremity that is ischemic preoperatively or in the early postoperative period will have to be revascularized. One option is the insertion of an extraanatomic prosthetic graft from the ipsilateral external iliac artery through the obturator foramen to a segment of the superficial femoral artery distal to the infected cavity in the groin.[42,43] Another is the insertion of an interposition autogenous superficial femoral vein graft retrieved from the contralateral thigh.[44]

Embolic Occlusion of the Popliteal "Trifurcation" Vessels

Diagnosis

In patients with arterial emboli in the lower extremity originating from the previously described sources, transfemoral embolectomy may fail to reestablish blood flow to the foot. One reason may be associated atherosclerotic disease in the superficial femoral artery at Hunter's canal that is noted on a completion arteriogram. Another may be an embolus to the popliteal artery or to the "trifurcation" vessels of the shank, the particular focus of this section.

Treatment

The appearance of an embolus in the popliteal artery on a postfemoral embolectomy arteriogram mandates reopening of this vessel. Repeated distal passage of the No. 4 balloon embolectomy catheter is performed until the embolus is retrieved. Failure of retrieval suggests that a chronic thrombus or underlying atherosclerosis is present. One option is to perform a distal medial thigh incision along the anterior border of the sartorius muscle. After the fascia is incised, the sartorius muscle is retracted posteriorly and the vastus medialis muscle anteriorly. The popliteal vessels are exposed, and chronic disease is confirmed by palpation. If a softer segment of popliteal artery can be palpated beyond this point, a popliteal-shank intraoperative arteriogram can be performed. This will allow for proper selection of a site for distal anastomosis of a salvage femoropopliteal or femorotibial bypass graft.

Should the completion arteriogram document likely embolic occlusion of two or more "trifurcation" vessels, a local embolectomy is indicated. An 8-cm longitudinal incision beginning at the posterior edge of the condyle of the tibia is made in the medial infrapopliteal area, approximately 1 cm below the posterior edge of the tibia. It is imperative to avoid injury to the greater saphenous vein, which usually lies posterior to the incision described. After the fascia is incised posterior to the edge of the tibia and inferior to the overlying tendons of the sartorius, gracilis, and semitendinosus muscles, the medial head of the gastrocnemius muscle is retracted posteriorly. To obtain appropriate exposure in large patients, the electrocautery may be used to separate the medial attachments of the soleus muscle to the tibia as well. A proper "trifurcation" embolectomy mandates the placing of vessel loops around the distal popliteal, anterior tibial,

posterior tibial, and peroneal arteries. This dissection is somewhat tedious, especially if there is associated atherosclerosis at this location. Proper exposure of all vessels will usually involve careful ligation and division of the anterior tibial vein and separation of the posterior tibial and peroneal arteries from their associated veins. Once complete exposure and arterial control have been obtained, a 1-mg/kg loading dose of intravenous heparin is administered. The direction of incision in the distal popliteal artery is the surgeon's choice. Using both hands, a No. 3 balloon embolectomy catheter is first directed down the oblique course of the anterior tibial artery to the ankle. If no distal embolus is retrieved after two passes, 10 to 15 mL of a solution of 50 U heparin/mL of saline is injected before tightening the loop on this vessel is tightened. Subsequent passes of the balloon embolectomy catheter down the posterior tibial and peroneal arteries are performed, as well, followed by the injection of regional heparinized saline as described. A diseased distal popliteal artery at the site of the arteriotomy is managed with a small vein patch angioplasty using a continuous 6–0 or 7–0 polypropylene suture. Once again, a completion arteriogram is appropriate to confirm the restoration of arterial inflow to the foot.

Traumatic Injuries to Arteries

Injuries to the femoral, popliteal, or shank arteries account for approximately 48% to 55% of peripheral arterial injuries treated in civilian trauma centers.[7,8] Because of its length and exposed position in the lower extremity, injuries to the common or superficial femoral artery are 2 to 2.5 times more common than those to the popliteal and shank arteries.

Diagnosis

Traumatic occlusion or transection of the common or superficial femoral or the popliteal artery without a subsequent repair results in a much higher loss of the lower extremity as compared to analogous injuries in the upper extremity as previously described. The lack of collateral vessels in otherwise healthy young injured patients mandates early diagnosis and treatment for the main "end" arteries listed. In DeBakey and Simeone's review[9] of 2,471 arterial injuries in American military personnel in World War II, injuries to the common femoral or superficial arteries, most of which were treated by ligation, resulted in amputation rates of 81.1% and 54.8%, respectively. In similar fashion, injuries to the popliteal artery treated by ligation resulted in an amputation rate of 72.5%.[9]

Much as with arterial injuries in the upper extremity, patients with injuries in the lower extremity are separated into those with "hard" or "soft" signs of an arterial injury. Once again, the only patient with hard signs who may benefit from an on-table surgeon-performed preoperative femoral arteriogram is one with a shotgun wound and pellets covering a wide area of the thigh. For the patient with soft signs and likely delays before a formal arteriogram can be performed, a surgeon-performed femoral arteriogram in the emergency center is appropriate if the surgeon is uncomfortable with observation.[10] The 18-gauge, 5.23-cm disposable catheter over needle is inserted into the common femoral artery toward the head just inferior to the inguinal ligament. To evaluate the common or superficial femoral artery, 25 to 30 mL of 60% meglumine diatrizoate dye is injected rapidly. As the injection is completed, a one-shot hard-copy arteriogram or a fluoroscopic image is obtained of the common and superficial femoral arteries.[10] Excellent images of the popliteal and shank arteries can be obtained by injecting 35 mL of contrast, counting "1,000, 2,000, 3,000, 4,000, 5000," and then performing the one-shot exposure or the fluoroscopy.[10] When the area of the vessel in question is not visualized, the timing of a second shot or fluoroscopic image is adjusted, as needed.

Treatment

Arterial wall abnormalities documented on formal or surgeon-performed arteriograms associated with intact pedal pulses are managed with observation, insertion of an endovascular stent or stent graft, or operation. Much as with such limited injuries documented in the major arteries of the upper extremity, careful follow-up of nonoperated patients is necessary to document progression rather than healing of the lesion.

Skin preparation of patients with hard signs should extend from the nipples to the toenails bilaterally and encompass the entire circumference of both lower extremities. Once again, a sterile plastic bag can be used to cover the foot of light-skinned patients. Another option is to cover the foot, leg, and thigh in an orthopedic stockinette. Injuries to the common femoral, proximal superficial femoral, or profunda femoris arteries are approached through the previously described longitudinal groin incision inferior to the inguinal ligament. An injury right at the inguinal ligament or the presence of a large pulsatile hematoma overlying the groin and inguinal ligament will mandate obtaining more proximal arterial control. An ipsilateral oblique anterior flank incision is made 3 cm above the inguinal ligament. Successive muscle and aponeurotic layers including the transversus abdominis muscle and transversalis fascia laterally are divided. The peritoneum is pushed medially using spongesticks to enter the retroperitoneal space and expose the psoas muscle. After the ureter is elevated with the peritoneum, the external iliac artery is encircled with a vessel loop and clamped for proximal arterial control.

Once proximal and distal control has been obtained around arterial injuries in the groin, certain principles should be kept in mind. One is that the profunda femoris artery should not be sacrificed for reasons of exposure. Even if an end-to-end anastomosis or insertion of an interposition graft into the common femoral artery has been necessary, it is not difficult to reimplant the end of the profunda femoris artery into this reconstructed segment. This involves rotating the vascular clamps on the common femoral artery 90° toward the midline. A small posterolateral arteriotomy in the common femoral artery or graft replacement will then allow for an end-to-side anastomosis to the profunda femoris artery using 6–0 polypropylene suture.

Another principle is that the greater saphenous vein from an uninjured thigh remains the interposition arterial conduit of choice. Therefore, one should always avoid the temptation to retrieve the adjacent greater saphenous vein as an interposition conduit to replace an injured common or superficial femoral artery in the groin or thigh. This is inappropriate, especially in a patient with an associated injury to the ipsilateral common or superficial femoral vein that may thrombose after even a meticulous repair.

Two of the operative techniques mentioned previously have particular applicability with arterial injuries in the lower extremities. An extraanatomic bypass graft should always be considered when a close-range shotgun blast causes an extensive arterial injury associated with a large defect in soft tissue of the groin or thigh. Because such a wound will require extensive debridement and repeated open packing for weeks, any arterial repair with a saphenous vein graft should be routed well around the defect through healthy soft tissue. Also, the use of a temporary intraarterial luminal shunt should always be considered in near-exsanguinated patients with the sequelae of shock (Figure 40.6). This approach obviates the need for a deci-

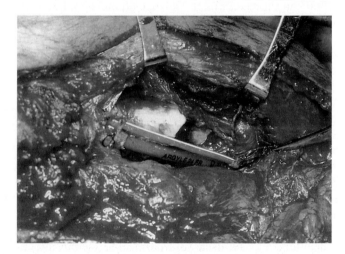

FIGURE 40.6. A 14-F "carotid artery" shunt in the popliteal artery and a 24-F thoracostomy tube shunt in the popliteal vein in a railroad worker with a crush injury to the distal thigh.

sion on life versus limb as it allows for salvage of both in properly selected patients.

Injuries to arteries below the groin are approached through longitudinal incisions as well. The superficial femoral artery in the proximal three fourths of the thigh lies posterior to the inferior edge of the sartorius muscle. With anterior mobilization of this muscle and division of the surrounding sheath, the superficial femoral artery (and vein) are easily exposed. In the distal one fourth of the thigh, exposure of the proximal popliteal artery involves mobilizing the sartorius muscle posteriorly and the vastus medialis muscle anteriorly. Occasionally, the adductor magnus tendon comprising the edge of the adductor hiatus may have to be divided as well.[45] The entire popliteal artery system is exposed by extending the medial distal thigh incision into an incision 1 cm posterior to the edge of the tibia. The tendons of the sartorius, gracilis, and semitendinosus muscles will often require division 1 to 2 cm away from their insertions on the tibia for complete exposure. Each tendon should be divided between two colored sutures, with different colors used for each of the three tendons. This will allow for accurate reapproximation of the tendons following the arterial repair.

The principles of arterial repair are the same in the lower extremity as previously described for the upper extremity (Figure 40.7). In medical centers that care for large numbers of penetrating arterial wounds in the lower extremities, only one third can be repaired with simple lateral sutures. Over two thirds will require segmental resection, and the majority of these (55% to 60%) will have an interposition graft inserted.[46]

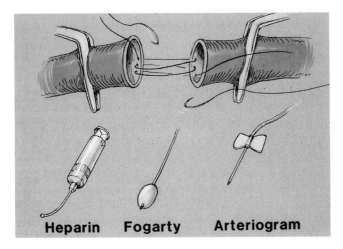

FIGURE 40.7. Fine points in peripheral arterial repair include use of small vascular clamps or Silastic vessel loops, open anastomosis technique, regional heparinization, passage of a Fogarty catheter proximally and distally, and arteriography on completion. (Courtesy of Baylor College of Medicine, Houston, Texas, ©1981.)

One area in which the repair of arteries in the lower extremity differs from that in the upper extremity is in the management of extensive distal injuries. Although loss or ligation of the radial or ulnar artery will rarely result in loss of the hand, the loss of two shank arteries from an extensive blunt injury will often lead to a below- or above-knee amputation. Certain patients with these injuries have true mangled extremities and will be served best by an immediate amputation. Others will have disruption or thrombosis of the tibioperoneal trunk or of the anterior tibial artery and one of the branches of the tibioperoneal trunk. The combination of a crushing or shearing injury and loss of two main arteries will often leave one or more muscle compartments of the leg and/or the foot ischemic. In such patients innovative bypasses originating in the distal popliteal artery and crossing over a fracture site may be necessary to restore adequate arterial flow to the leg and foot.

Traumatic Injuries to Veins

Diagnosis

As with venous injuries in the upper extremities, the only indications for operation are venous bleeding not controlled by a pressure dressing or the suspected or known presence of an arterial injury.

Treatment

Venous injuries in the lower extremities are approached through the usual longitudinal incisions and managed as previously described. The one unique aspect of management is the much stronger emphasis on repair rather than ligation. The popliteal vein and superficial femoral vein inferior to its junction with the profunda femoris vein are true end veins draining the leg. Ligation of either of these veins has some theoretical disadvantages. There is always the concern that a below-knee compartment syndrome will develop in the early postoperative period, that there will be an acute adverse impact on arterial inflow into the shank, and that chronic edema of the leg will occur.[46–50] Several civilian series have documented that venous ligation in the popliteal and superficial femoral veins is surprisingly well-tolerated in young trauma patients.[46–49] This is particularly true if absolute bed rest and elevation of the injured lower extremity for the first 5 to 7 days after ligation are mandatory.[50] There is not a clear-cut increase in the need for postligation fasciotomy, amputations are rare, and edema of the leg often resolves over time.[46–49] This is in marked contrast to the 50% edema reported after ligation of the popliteal vein during the Vietnam War.[51]

Nonetheless, in the absence of near exsanguination and sequelae of shock such as severe hypothermia, profound metabolic acidosis, and an intraoperative coagulopathy,

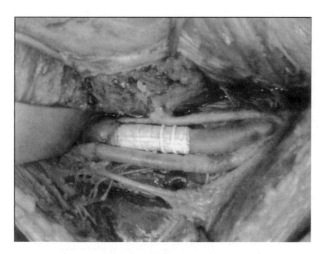

FIGURE 40.8. A 10-mm ringed polytetrafluoroethylene graft in the distal superficial femoral vein.

the superficial femoral and popliteal veins should be repaired. Options for repair include lateral venorrhaphy with 6–0 polypropylene suture, vein patch venoplasty using the greater saphenous vein from the contralateral ankle, or insertion of an autogenous saphenous vein graft or externally supported polytetrafluoroethylene graft (Figure 40.8)[22,46–49,52,53] Because of the time needed to make spiral and panel vein grafts and the mixed patency rates reported, these are rarely performed in American trauma centers.[53,54]

When damage-control venous surgery is necessary because of near exsanguination, thoracostomy tubes in sizes of No. 20 to No. 24 French are used as intraluminal shunts. These large tubes fit the veins of the thigh and groin and rarely thrombose in the absence of postoperative hypotension.

After any type of complex venous repair in the lower extremity, it is the practice of the author to wrap the entire lower extremity with an elastic bandage at modest tension to avoid causing a compartment syndrome. The lower extremity is elevated on three to four pillows for 5 to 7 days, and strict bed rest is mandatory as previously described. Dextran 40 is administered intravenously at 40 mL/hr × 3 days, and an 81-gr aspirin tablet is administered once a day by rectal suppository or orally starting in the recovery room. The aspirin is continued for 3 months. A duplex venous study is performed before discharge.

Compartment Syndromes and Fasciotomies

Diagnosis

Palpation of the muscle compartments of the leg is very inaccurate in diagnosing a compartment syndrome. Therefore, compartment pressures are measured using one of the devices previously described. Because the anterior compartment of the leg is prone to developing a compartment syndrome in high-risk patients, the pressure is always measured first in this compartment. If the pressures in this compartment and in the deep posterior compartment immediately posterior to the tibia are greater than 30 to 35 mm Hg, a below-knee two-incision four-compartment fasciotomy is performed.

A compartment syndrome of the thigh is uncommon, but it has occurred in patients with severe pelvic fractures, ligation of the common or external iliac vein or common femoral vein, or, on rare occasions, with severe fractures of the femur. This entity will be present in many patients with the secondary extremity compartment syndrome following resuscitation from near exsanguination as well.[55] A compartment pressure greater than 30 to 35 mm Hg in either the anterior or posterior compartment is an indication to perform a thigh two-incision three-compartment fasciotomy.

Treatment

The leg is divided into four musculofascial compartments, including anterior, peroneal, superficial posterior, and deep posterior. The anterior and peroneal compartments are approached through a 25- to 30-cm longitudinal incision 2 cm anterior to the upper edge of the fibula. The subcutaneous tissue and skin of both flaps are mobilized using traction with rake retractors and manual pressure with a laparotomy pad over fingers. Perforating vessels are divided and ligated with 3–0 silk ties to eliminate postoperative oozing in coagulopathic patients. When the intermuscular septum is clearly visualized or palpated, separate longitudinal fasciotomies approximately 4 cm apart are made over the entire anterior and peroneal compartments. The superficial and deep posterior compartments are approached through a 25- to 30-cm longitudinal incision 2 cm posterior to the lower edge of the tibia. Care should be taken to avoid injury to the greater saphenous vein and nerve. The subcutaneous tissue and skin of both flaps are mobilized as above. The superficial posterior compartment is visualized by further traction on the posterior skin flap and opened over its entire length with a longitudinal incision. The deep posterior compartment may often be visualized in the distal aspect of the calf through the standard skin incision. Complete decompression of this musculofascial compartment posterior to the tibia and medial to the fibula will, however, require detachment of the soleus muscle from the back of the tibia.[56]

The thigh is divided into three musculofascial compartments, including the quadriceps (anterior), hamstrings (posterior), and adductors (medial). The quadriceps compartment is approached through a 30-cm longitudinal anterolateral incision along the iliotibial tract from the intertrochanteric space to the lateral epicondyle of the distal femur. A longitudinal fasciotomy is made, and the fascia can be lifted off the rectus femoris muscle anteriorly as well. Access to the hamstrings compartment is obtained by mobilizing the vastus lateralis muscle anteriorly. The thick intermuscular septum medial to this muscle is then opened with a longitudinal incision to decompress the hamstrings compartment. If pressure in the adductor compartment is still elevated after the other two compartments of the thigh have been opened, the adductor compartment is approached through a 30-cm medial and longitudinal skin incision posterior to the sartorius muscle. After minimal mobilization of the skin and subcutaneous flaps, a longitudinal fasciotomy incision is made over the adductor muscles.

Critique

A supracondylar fracture with an associated neurologic deficit or vascular insufficiency dictates an open reduction that will allow exploration of the involved structures. Traction applied to the hyperextended elbow is contraindicated, for such a maneuver could cause further compression and injury of the neurovascular structure. Unfortunately, this injury could lead to a Volkmann's ischemic contracture.

Answer (D)

References

1. Allen EV. Thromboangiitis obliterans: methods of diagnosis of chronic occlusive arterial lesions distal to the wrist with illustrative cases. Am J Medical Sci 1929; 1–78:234–244.
2. Ejrup B, Fischer B, Wright IS. Clinical evaluation of blood flow to the hand: the false-positive Allen test. Circulation 1966; 33:778–780.
3. Gardner RM, Schwartz R, Wong HC, et al. Percutaneous indwelling radial-artery catheters for monitoring cardiovascular function. Prospective study of the risk of thrombosis and infection. N Engl J Med 1974; 290:1227–1231.
4. Bedford RF. Long-term radial artery cannulation: effects on subsequent vessel function. Crit Care Med 1978; 6:64–67.
5. Johnson FE, Sumner DS, Strandness DE Jr. Extremity necrosis caused by indwelling arterial catheters. Am J Surg 1976; 131:375–379.
6. Comerota AJ, Malone MD. Simplified approach to thrombolytic therapy of arterial and graft occlusion. In Yao JST, Pearce WH, eds. Practical Vascular Surgery. Stamford, CT: Appleton & Lange, 1999: 321–334.
7. Mattox KL, Feliciano DV, Burch J, et al. Five thousand seven hundred sixty cardiovascular injuries in 4459 patients. Epidemiologic evolution 1958 to 1987. Ann Surg 1989; 209:698–707.
8. Frykberg ER, Schinco MA. Peripheral vascular injury. In Moore EE, Feliciano DV, Mattox KL, eds. Trauma, 5th ed. New York: McGraw-Hill, 2004: 969–1003.
9. DeBakey ME, Simeone FA. Battle injuries of the arteries in World War II. An analysis of 2,471 cases. Ann Surg 1946; 123:534–579.
10. O'Gorman RB, Feliciano DV. Arteriography performed in the emergency center. Am J Surg 1986; 152:323–325.
11. Frykberg ER, Vines FS, Alexander RH. The natural history of clinically occult arterial injuries: a prospective evaluation. J Trauma 1989; 29:577–583.
12. Stain SC, Yellin AE, Weaver FA, et al. Selective management of nonocclusive arterial injuries. Arch Surg 1989; 124:1136–1141.
13. Wind GG, Valentine RJ. Axillary artery. In Wind GG, Valentine RJ, eds. Anatomic Exposures in Vascular Surgery. Baltimore: William & Wilkins, 1991: 138–157.
14. Graham JM, Mattox KL, Feliciano DV, et al. Vascular injuries of the axilla. Ann Surg 1982; 195:232–238.
15. Feliciano DV. Managing peripheral vascular trauma. Infect Surg 1986; 5:659–669, 682.
16. Carrell A. The surgery of blood vessels. Johns Hopkins Hosp Bull 1907; 18:18–28.
17. The Dutch Bypass Oral Anticoagulants or Aspirin Study Group. Efficacy of oral anticoagulants compared with aspirin after infrainguinal bypass surgery. The Dutch Bypass Oral Anticoagulants or Aspirin (BOA) Study: a randomized trial. Lancet 2000; 355:346–351.
18. Feliciano DV. Heroic procedures in vascular injury management. The role of extra-anatomic bypasses. Surg Clin North Am 2002; 82:115–124.
19. Feliciano DV. Evaluation and treatment of vascular injuries. In Browner BD, Jupiter JB, Levine AM, Trafton PG, eds. Skeletal Trauma: Basic Science, Management, and Reconstruction. Philadelphia: W.B. Saunders, 2003: 250–267.
20. Feliciano DV, Moore EE, Mattox KL. Trauma damage control. In Moore EE, Feliciano DV, Mattox KL, eds. Trauma, 5th ed. New York: McGraw-Hill, 2004: 877–900.
21. Sharma PVP, Shah PM, Vinzons AT, et al. Meticulously restored lumina of injured veins remain patent. Surgery 1992; 112:928–932.
22. Parry NG, Feliciano DV, Burke RM, et al. Management and short-term patency of lower extremity venous injuries with various repairs. Am J Surg 2003; 186:631–635.
23. Matsen FA III. Compartmental Syndromes. New York: Grune & Stratton, 1980.
24. Amendola A, Twaddle BC. Compartment syndromes. In Browner BD, Jupiter JB, Levine AM, Trafton PG, eds. Skeletal Trauma: Basic Science, Management, and Reconstruction. Philadelphia: W.B. Saunders, 2003: 268–292.
25. Feliciano DV, Cruse PA, Spjut-Patrinely V, et al. Fasciotomy after trauma to the extremities. Am J Surg 1988; 156:533–536.
26. Mubarak SJ, Hargens AR. Compartment syndromes and Volkmann's contracture. Philadelphia: W.B. Saunders, 1981: 117.
27. Whitesides TE Jr, Heckman MM. Acute compartment syndrome: update on diagnosis and treatment. J Am Acad Orthop Surg 1996; 4:209–218.
28. McQueen MM, Court-Brown CM. Compartment monitoring in tibial fractures. The pressure threshold for decompression. J Bone Joint Surg Br 1996; 78:99–104.

29. Feliciano DV. Management of peripheral vascular trauma (Poster). American College of Surgeons Committee on Trauma/Subcommittee on Publications. Chicago: American College of Surgeons, 2002.

30. Skillman JJ, Kim D, Baim DS. Vascular complications of percutaneous femoral cardiac interventions. Incidence and operative repair. Arch Surg 1988; 123:1207–1212.

31. Cutler BS, Okike ON, Vander Salm TJ. Surgical versus percutaneous removal of the intra-aortic balloon. J Thorac Cardiovasc Surg 1983; 86:907–911.

32. Franco CD, Goldsmith J, Ohki T, et al. Iatrogenic vascular injury. In Hobson RW II, Wilson SE, Veith FJ, eds. Vascular Surgery: Principles and Practice, 3rd ed, revised and expanded. New York: Marcel Dekker, 2004: 1098.

33. Franco CD, Goldsmith J, Veith FJ, et al. Management of arterial injury produced by percutaneous femoral procedures. Surgery 1993; 113:419–425.

34. Hajarizadeh H, LaRosa CR, Cardullo P, et al. Ultrasound-guided compression of iatrogenic femoral pseudoaneurysm. Failure, recurrence, and long-term results. J Vasc Surg 1995; 22:425–433.

35. Mills JL, Porter JM. Basic data related to clinical decision-making in acute limb ischemia. Ann Vasc Surg 1991; 5:96–98.

36. Sharp LS, Rozycki GS, Feliciano DV. Rhabdomyolysis and secondary renal failure in critically ill surgical patients. Am J Surg 2004; 188:801–806.

37. Blaisdell FW, Steele M, Allen RE. Management of acute lower extremity arterial ischemia due to embolism and thrombosis. Surgery 1978; 84:822–831.

38. Short D, Vaughn GD III, Jachimczyk J, et al. The anatomic basis for the occasional failure of transfemoral balloon catheter thromboembolectomy. Ann Surg 1979; 190:555–556.

39. Wilson SE, Van Wagenen P, Passaro E Jr. Arterial infection. Curr Probl Surg 1978; 15:1–89.

40. Strinden WD, Dibbell DG Sr, Turnipseed WD, et al. Coverage of acute vascular injuries of the axilla and groin with transposition muscle flaps: case reports. J Trauma 1989; 29:512–516.

41. Ting AC, Cheng SW. Femoral pseudoaneurysms in drug addicts. World J Surg 1997; 21:783–787.

42. DePalma RG, Hubay CA. Arterial bypass via the obturator foramen. An alternative in complicated vascular problems. Am J Surg 1968; 115:323–328.

43. Fromm SH, Lucas CE. Obturator bypass for mycotic aneurysm in the drug addict. Arch Surg 1970; 100:82–83.

44. Valentine RJ, Clagett GP. Aortic graft infections: replacement with autogenous vein. Cardiovasc Surg 2001; 9:419–425.

45. Wind GG, Valentine RJ. Axillary artery. In Wind GG, Valentine RJ, eds. Anatomic Exposures in Vascular Surgery. Baltimore: William & Wilkins, 1991: 384–388.

46. Feliciano DV, Herskowitz K, O'Gorman RB, et al. Management of vascular injuries in the lower extremities. J Trauma 1988; 28:319–328.

47. Bermudez KM, Knudson MM, Nelken NA, et al. Long-term results of lower-extremity venous injuries. Arch Surg 1997; 132:963–968.

48. Yelon JA, Scalea TM. Venous injuries of the lower extremities and pelvis: repair versus ligation. J Trauma 1992; 33:532–536.

49. Timberlake GA, O'Connell RC, Kerstein MD. Venous injury: to repair or ligate—the dilemma. J Vasc Surg 1986; 4:553–558.

50. Mullins RJ, Lucas CE, Ledgerwood AM. The natural history following venous ligation for civilian injuries. J Trauma 1980; 20:737–743.

51. Rich NM, Hobson RW, Collins GJ Jr, et al. The effect of acute popliteal venous interruption. Ann Surg 1976; 183:365–368.

52. Feliciano DV, Mattox KL, Graham JM, et al. Five-year experience with PTFE grafts in vascular wounds. J Trauma 1985; 25:71–82.

53. Pappas PJ, Haser PB, Teehan EP, et al. Outcome of complex venous reconstructions in patients with trauma. J Vasc Surg 1997; 25:398–404.

54. Zamir G, Berlatzky Y, Rivkind A, et al. Results of reconstruction in major pelvic and extremity venous injuries. J Vasc Surg 1998; 28:901–908.

55. Tremblay LN, Feliciano DV, Rozycki GS. Secondary extremity compartment syndrome. J Trauma 2002; 53:833–837.

56. Amendola A, Twaddle BC. Compartment syndromes. In Browner BD, Jupiter JB, Levine AM, Trafton PG, eds. Skeletal Trauma: Basic Science, Management and Reconstruction. Philadelphia: W.B. Saunders, 2003: 268–292.

Part III
Administration, Ethics, and Law

41
Understanding the Latest Changes in EMTALA: Our Country's Emergency Care Safety Net

Thomas R. Russell

On April 7, 1986, President Ronald Reagan signed into law the Consolidated Omnibus Budget Reconciliation Act of 1985, which incorporated legislation known as the Emergency Medical Treatment and Labor Act (EMTALA) to address the problem of "patient dumping" by hospital emergency departments. Although originally designed to serve as a safety net for emergency patients, the statute grew in both scope and complexity during the following two decades, wreaking widespread confusion within the physician and hospital communities regarding their respective responsibilities under the law.

During the 1990s, this confusion, particularly over physician on-call requirements, grew to such mammoth proportions that the involved players in the health care delivery system began petitioning Congress and the Health Care Financing Administration (now known as the Centers for Medicare and Medicaid Services [CMS]) in earnest for clear and understandable guidance about EMTALA mandates. As part of this effort, physician and hospital groups also urged Congress and the agency to revise the regulations to better reflect the original intent of the statute.

Thankfully, these efforts paid off when CMS finally issued new EMTALA regulations that went into effect November 10, 2003, providing guidance that better clarifies physician and Medicare-participating hospital responsibilities under the law. This chapter examines the main tenets of the revised EMTALA regulations and their positive impact on the future of surgical practice and emergency surgical care, as well as highlight lingering issues that need to be addressed. Finally, new trends in the delivery of care that are influencing acute care are discussed.

Understanding the Basics for Hospitals: Obligation to Examine, Treat, and Stabilize

In January 1985, San Francisco General Hospital became the final destination for the triage and treatment of Eugene "Red" Barnes, a 32-year-old unemployed mechanic who had been fatally wounded when he was stabbed in an altercation outside an abandoned hotel in Richmond, California. An investigation into the emergency care that Mr. Barnes received before arriving at San Francisco General revealed a number of weaknesses in our country's emergency care safety net for the uninsured, primarily the lack of a federally mandated obligation for hospitals to examine, treat, and stabilize all patients with an emergency condition regardless of the patient's insurance coverage.

Under EMTALA, this obligation is triggered when an individual comes to a hospital's dedicated emergency department or presents on hospital property *and* requests an examination or treatment of a medical condition or a request is made on the individual's behalf. In the absence of such a request, EMTALA would also apply if a prudent layperson observer believes that an individual needs examination or treatment for a medical condition.

This main tenet of EMTALA has expanded and contracted over the years based on the interpretation of what constitutes a "hospital emergency department." The current regulations state that a dedicated emergency department is defined as any department of the hospital (located on or off the main hospital campus) that is licensed by the state as an emergency department; held out to the public as providing emergency services; or has provided at least one-third of its outpatient visits for treatment on an urgent basis during the previous year.[1] Exceptions to this rule are individuals who come to off-campus outpatient clinics that do not routinely provide emergency services or patients who have begun to receive scheduled, nonemergency outpatient services at the main campus of the hospital.

Once the hospital determines that the individual does indeed have an emergency medical condition, that hospital must stabilize the emergency condition or, if it is unable to stabilize the patient, must transfer the patient to a hospital that is capable of providing such treatment.

The latter aspect of this requirement was included to ensure that patients with severe injuries or very complex medical conditions are examined and triaged to the appropriate acute care facility as quickly as possible.

Penalties, Enforcement, and Resolution of EMTALA Violations

When CMS receives a report of an alleged EMTALA violation, the agency's regional office sends state surveyors to conduct an investigation. Generally, in determining ETMALA compliance, CMS will consider all relevant factors and look for specific patterns of care that could point to EMTALA infractions.

Hospitals that fail to comply with EMTALA-mandated responsibilities can have their Medicare participation terminated and can be subject to civil monetary penalties of up to $50,000 per violation. If a physician serving as "an agent of the hospital" on its on-call panel is called by the hospital to provide acute care screening or treatment and either fails or refuses to appear within a reasonable period of time, that physician may be in violation of EMTALA and could also face fines of up to $50,000 per violation. Patients who have suffered physical harm and hospitals that believe they have incurred a financial loss as a result of an inappropriate transfer also have a private right of action against hospitals that violate EMTALA.

In its January 2001 report entitled "The Emergency Medical Treatment and Labor Act: The Enforcement Process," the Department of Health and Human Services' Office of Inspector General recommended that CMS make certain that providers will not be terminated from the Medicare program for an EMTALA violation without peer review. Congress implemented that recommendation in the Medicare Prescription Drug, Improvement, and Modernization Act by requiring HHS to request a quality improvement organization review before making a compliance determination that would terminate a hospital's Medicare privileges. An exception to this rule would be in the case when a delay would jeopardize the health and safety of the individual. Also, in response to complaints from hospitals and physicians that they are kept in the dark as to whether an EMTALA investigation, once opened, is ongoing or has been resolved, the act also requires that a procedure be established to notify hospitals and physicians when an EMTALA investigation is closed.

Physician Obligations Under EMTALA

Many surgeons complain about the numerous EMTALA obligations that the federal government has imposed on the physician community. In truth, the statute does not place any direct obligations or liabilities on physicians. EMTALA focuses its mandates on hospitals or "agents of the hospital," for example, hospital medical staff or on-call physicians. It is when they fall into the latter group that physicians come under the scrutiny of the law.

If one examines EMTALA, he or she will realize that the statute maintains that the hospital, and not its medical staff or individual physicians, is responsible for maintaining an on-call roster for the emergency department. However, when physicians join the medical staff of a hospital or agree to take a call, they become a "responsible physician" under EMTALA by virtue of entering into a contract with the hospital to examine, treat, and/or transfer individuals who are covered by the law.[2] In doing so, they are now acting as agents of the hospital and therefore share responsibility and liability with the hospital for providing EMTALA-related services. This is true regardless of whether or not the contract references EMTALA responsibilities.

Because the final responsibility for maintaining on-call coverage falls on the hospitals, the medical staff bylaws for these institutions usually include language that requires physicians to comply with hospital policies and procedures as a condition of maintaining their clinical privileges at the hospital. This language, which is congruent with standards issued in the Joint Commission on Accreditation of Healthcare Organizations' manual, encompasses the hospital's policy for on-call coverage.

Although surgeons "voluntarily" accept their role as agents of the hospital when they secure privileges, many of them receive little training regarding the EMTALA guidelines and, thus, are often unsure of their responsibilities under the statute. This fact was illustrated in a past survey of hospital emergency departments conducted by the Department of Health and Human Services (DHHS) Office of Inspector General (OIG). In a 2001 report, OIG found that "training increases EMTALA awareness, and nearly two-thirds of emergency physicians, nurses, and registration staff receive training. However, only one-quarter of on-call specialists are trained on EMTALA guidelines."[4]

Since the inception of EMTALA, surgeons have found it difficult to distinguish between their responsibilities under the law versus "policy" developed by hospitals to comply with EMTALA. The following sections of this chapter examine the various issues that surgeons should be aware of when serving as an agent of the hospital, either on its medical staff or on an on-call panel.

EMTALA On-Call Requirements

Continuous Call

EMTALA requires that Medicare-participating hospitals maintain an on-call list of physicians to provide services to patients who seek care in hospital emergency departments. The CMS has provided several memoranda and guidance documents since the original EMTALA regulations were released to help clarify various provisions of the act, including the on-call provisions. Despite the agency's attempts to clear up ambiguity, it has remained a challenge for physicians to know what EMTALA mandates; whether hospital bylaws relating to emergency care are actually required by EMTALA; and how the law should be interpreted in specific circumstances.

The most onerous, and perhaps most confusing, aspect of EMTALA for surgeons and other physicians is the on-call requirements. Hospitals, often out of fear of EMTALA violations, impose unrealistic on-call requirements on their physicians. It is not uncommon for a single specialist who covers multiple hospitals to be required, as a condition for joining a hospital's staff, to be on-call 24 hours a day, 7 days a week. In some cases, surgeons have been expected to leave their office practice activities, or even an operation, in order to respond to emergency department calls at the hospitals for which they have privileges. A "24–7" demand for on-call services creates such unrealistic schedules and unreasonable demands for surgeons and other specialists that a number of these practitioners have altered their practices, often dropping privileges at a number of hospitals, in an effort to maintain viable practices and some semblance of quality of life.

Many areas of the country have an insufficient population base to support a large number of specialists in certain fields, such as neurosurgery, cardiovascular services, pediatric surgery, obstetrics/gynecology, and orthopedics. This situation is especially true in rural areas and in areas that have small hospitals providing care to populations spread out over a great distance. Being selective about the day or circumstance for providing on-call services in these areas is usually not an option for these high-risk specialties.

Recognizing this burden, CMS revised the on-call language to state that a hospital's on-call list must be maintained in a manner that best meets the needs of the hospital's patients who are receiving services required under EMTALA *in accordance with the capability of the hospital, including the availability of on-call physicians.* The CMS intended this modification to provide more flexibility for hospitals and their medical staffs to determine how best to provide emergency medical care and respond to on-call needs. The agency states that these decisions can be made reasonably only at the individual hospital level through coordination between the hospitals and their staff of physicians.[4]

The CMS issued this clarification in the latest regulations because of confusion over one of the most perpetuated myths of EMTALA—the existence of the "rule of three," which states that if a hospital has more than three physicians within a specialty, it must provide continuous emergency department coverage for that specialty. The CMS makes it clear that no such rule exists; however, many hospitals have developed policies based on this principle, and physicians historically have been led to believe that it is mandated by EMTALA.

Some people have argued that EMTALA should require a minimum number of hours for individual physicians to be on call, the times for which physicians should be on call, or the number of physicians needed to fulfill on-call responsibilities at particular hospitals. The CMS has rejected these proposals from a practical standpoint. The agency maintains that the wide variations with regard to medical staff size, specialty mix, and general capabilities that exist among institutions that participate in the Medicare program make it infeasible to mandate a particular minimum level of on-call coverage that must be maintained by all hospitals.

The latest changes to EMTALA provide other specific clarifications regarding on-call requirements that are aimed at allowing hospitals and their medical staffs to develop more realistic policies and procedures to achieve the goals of EMTALA and to address critical issues that have long concerned surgeons and other physicians with regard to the regulations.

Simultaneous Call

Many surgeons hold privileges at several hospitals, particularly in areas where shortages of certain specialties exist. The CMS has only recently established that it is critically important for the interests of patients and hospital emergency departments that physicians be permitted to be on-call at more than one hospital simultaneously.[6] In updating its policy, the agency recommends to hospitals that they notify each other when a physician is on-call at more than one hospital simultaneously and that each hospital involved be made aware of the physician's on-call schedule. Furthermore, hospitals are required to have in place written policies and procedures to follow in situations when a physician is on-call at another hospital and is unable to respond. Such policies and procedures could include arranging for a back-up on-call physician or executing an appropriate transfer.[7]

Scheduling Elective Surgery While On-Call

Performing elective surgery while on call has become an issue that surgeons struggle with in an effort to maintain their regular busy practice while fulfilling EMTALA requirements. In the past, the CMS has made conflicting statements in guidelines regarding whether physicians who cannot respond to an emergency call because they are performing elective surgery have violated EMTALA. To clarify this issue, the agency now emphatically states in the current regulations that EMTALA does not prohibit surgeons from performing elective surgery while on call. This is welcome news to many surgeons who are on call for days or weeks at a time.

Scope of Privileges

"Many physicians limit their scope of practice to well-defined subspecialty areas, even though they are often credentialed by their hospitals to perform all surgery for the broader specialty for which they are board-certified." For example, a neurosurgeon, with limited privileges for spine surgery, would argue that he or she is not required to take call for head trauma. Surgeons should be aware that the CMS addresses this issue in the current regulations, and hospitals may soon begin to move toward defining core privileges for a number of specialties.

The CMS states that "a physician who is in a narrow specialty may, in fact, be medically competent in his or her general specialty and in particular may be able to promptly contribute to the individual's care by bringing to bear skills and expertise that are not available to the emergency physician or other qualified medical personnel at the hospital." CMS also stresses that although the emergency physician and the on-call specialist may need to discuss the best way to meet the individual's medical needs, the agency believes any disagreement between the two regarding the need for the on-call physician to come to the hospital and examine the individual must be resolved by deferring to the medical judgment of the emergency physician or other practitioner who has personally examined the individual.[8]

Although the new EMTALA regulations clarify that on-call coverage determinations are to be made jointly by the hospital and the physicians on its on-call roster, it is the hospitals that are put in the position of ensuring that policies and procedures are in place to provide coverage of emergency department services. In turn, physicians practice at hospitals under privileges extended to them by those hospitals. If a physician refuses to assume on-call responsibilities or to carry out the responsibilities he or she has assumed, the hospital could suspend, curtail, or even revoke the offending physician's privileges.

Thus, hospitals will still maintain a tremendous amount of leverage in the development of on-call policies and schedules. Despite this fact, surgeons should take solace in knowing that they now have more concrete knowledge of what EMTALA requires, an invaluable asset when negotiating privileges with hospitals, working to maintain a viable practice, and striving to provide comprehensive emergency care in their communities.

Some individuals may argue that the CMS's most recent actions "relax" EMTALA standards and will endanger the safety net established by the law. Physicians believe that the clarifications made to EMTALA hold promise to have a positive impact on a situation that has been, up to the present time, increasingly unsustainable.

EMTALA Reforms Included in Medicare Prescription Drug Law

Managed Care Reimbursement for EMTALA-Related Services

Managed care plans often require preauthorization for services delivered in the emergency room. Under EMTALA, though, Medicare-participating hospitals or physicians are barred from seeking preauthorization before providing medical treatment unless such activities do not delay required screening and stabilization services. Thus, hospitals and physicians often wind up in a financial quandary when treating managed care patients in the emergency room—either foregoing payment or risking the imposition of EMTALA fines.

A key provision in the new Medicare Prescription Drug, Improvement, and Modernization Act (MPDIMA), which was signed into law December 8, 2003, addresses the issue of managed care plans making retrospective denials for emergency screening and stabilization services. Under MPDIMA, medical necessity determinations for EMTALA services must be made "on the basis of the information available to the treating physician or practitioner (including the patient's presenting symptoms or complaint) at the time the item or service was ordered or furnished by the physician or practitioner (and not on the patient's principal diagnosis)."

Many experts in the medical community and in Congress have long advocated that managed care plans be required to pay for justifiable screening and treatment services provided under EMTALA. Hopefully, this key reform in the Medicare prescription drug law will resolve many of the disputes that hospitals and physicians often encounter with the managed care community's approach to reimbursement for emergency care services.

EMTALA Technical Advisory Group

Another key provision of MPDIMA establishes a new EMTALA Technical Advisory Group "to review issues related to EMTALA and its implementation." Table 41.1 lists its responsibilities. Membership in the advisory group will consist of 19 individuals, including the administrator of the CMS and the OIG of the Department of Health and Human Services. Seven slots on the advisory group are reserved for representatives from the

TABLE 41.1. General responsibilities of the EMTALA technical advisory group.

1. Shall review EMTALA regulations
2. May provide advice and recommendations to the Secretary of DHHS with respect to those regulations and their application to hospitals and physicians
3. Shall solicit comments and recommendations from hospitals, physicians, and the public regarding the implementation of such regulations
4. May disseminate information on the application of such regulations to hospitals, physicians, and the public.

physician's community in the areas of emergency medicine, cardiology or cardiothoracic surgery, orthopedic surgery, neurosurgery, pediatrics or a pediatric subspecialty, obstetrics/gynecology, and psychiatry. The physician and hospital communities are optimistic that this new group will help CMS in its future deliberations on implementing changes in EMTALA regulations.

Issues Remaining

Although the federal government has come a long way in addressing the concerns of the medical community regarding the scope of EMTALA, a number of issues remain that will continue to impact access to emergency surgical care. These issues include managed care reimbursement policies and emergency room overcrowding; proliferation of single-specialty hospitals; lack of liability protections for EMTALA-related services; and growing burdens on trauma centers and community hospitals.

Managed Care Pressures

I have discussed how Congress has now addressed the issue of managed care reimbursement for EMTALA-related services, but there are a number of other practices used by this industry that continue to place stress on the emergency care safety net. One such pressure revolves around patients' inability to receive timely access to specialty care in the nonhospital setting. More often than not, managed care plan enrollees, some knowledgeable about EMTALA requirements, may use the emergency room when they cannot get an appointment with their regular specialist or primary care physician. Add to this number the more than 40 million uninsured who view the emergency room as their primary source of health care and the result is massive overcrowding. This kind of non-emergent saturation of emergency room departments across the country, particularly in urban areas, is resulting in numerous injured patients being unnecessarily diverted—causing critical delays for individuals requiring acute care.

Impact on Trauma Centers and Community Hospitals

Although many physicians are heralding the recent changes in EMTALA's on-call requirements, others, particularly in the trauma community, are worried that these changes will further exacerbate the financial difficulties facing trauma centers and community hospitals. Under EMTALA, hospitals are now only required to maintain an on-call list "in a manner that best meets the needs of the hospital's patients in accordance with the capability of the hospital, including the availability of on-call physicians."[9]

Many trauma professionals believe that this change in the regulation will provide hospitals, particularly for-profit entities, with the ability to shield themselves from caring for severely injured patients by limiting on-call schedules. For example, some hospitals may only provide on-call coverage until 9:00 p.m. every night, leaving the local trauma center as the provider of last resort.

One trend that will likely grow as a result of this change will be increased demands by specialists for hospitals to provide on-call compensation or stipends for emergency room coverage. The trauma community views this as yet another financial burden that trauma centers and community hospitals will have to bear in order to maintain their trauma designation or to keep the doors of their emergency room open.

Some other old and new factors that will likely influence the viability of trauma centers in the future include lack of medical liability protections for EMTALA-related services and the exploding growth of specialty hospitals in areas such as cardiac and orthopedic care. At the federal level, Congress is examining both of these issues. In terms of medical liability protection, some legislators are calling for a narrow approach to medical liability reform that would focus solely on providing caps on noneconomic damages for EMTALA and OB-GYN services. With regard to the growth of specialty hospitals, Congress has imposed an 18-month moratorium on physician investments in specialty hospitals through mid 2005 in order to study the impact of this growing trend in care delivery on patient access to specialty services, particularly in the emergency room environment.

Suggestions from the Surgical Community for Solidifying the Safety Net over the Next Decade

In pulling together this chapter, I reached out to a broad array of surgeons from all parts of the country, physicians who are on the front lines of providing emergency surgical care. Without exception, all of these individuals applauded the recent changes in EMTALA. Some of them also had very good suggestions regarding aspects of the law that should be addressed to better enhance timely patient access to specialized emergency care. These suggestions include better hospital triage and transfer policies; more flexibility regarding on-call response time; and evaluation of hospital staff cutbacks and recent implementation of the 80-hour resident work week on hospital capacity.

Although greatly abbreviated here, the preceding comments were all presented to me with one goal in mind—improving care for the emergency patient. Surgical schedules and caseloads are increasing, reimbursement is declining, and liability insurance premiums are skyrocketing. In the twenty-first century, these trends have led many surgeons to alter their practices in ways that would have seemed unimaginable a decade ago: limiting scope of privileges, dropping participation in hospital medical staffs, and requesting stipends for providing on-call coverage.

Many individuals outside the profession mistakenly view these changes in surgical practice as selfish and self-serving, but surgeons know that these modifications have often become necessary in order to maintain a viable practice so that they may continue treating patients, albeit for a reduced range of services. Despite this fact, surgeons whom I have spoken to about the EMTALA issue tell me that they still view the ability to provide charity care as an integral part of why they became a physician and that hopefully they will be able to continue to provide services to the local community in this regard.

It is a shame that the last 20 years of government involvement in strengthening the emergency care safety net may have inadvertently weakened it to the breaking point. Surgeons, in general, state that, to mend this safety net, our country and government must recognize the public good that emergency medical and trauma systems provide to Americans every day. As such, legitimate EMTALA services would then become a mandated covered benefit under both Medicare *and* private health insurance plans; hospitals and physicians would receive reasonable liability protections for treating emergency and severely injured patients; and funding would be increased to help properly staff emergency rooms so that patients are evaluated and triaged quickly and *appropriately*.

References

1. Federal Register, Vol. 68, No. 174, Part II. Medicare Program; Clarifying Policies Related to the Responsibilities of Medicare-Participating Hospitals in Treating Emergency Medical Conditions; Final Rule. DHHS, CMS. September 9, 2003: 53263.
2. Bitterman R. Overview of Hospital and Physician Responsibilities Mandated by EMTALA. Foster. Providing Emergency Care under Federal Law: EMTALA. Dallas: The American College of Emergency Physicians, 2000: 21.
3. Joint Commission on Accreditation of Healthcare Organizations. Manual, 1999, Medical Staff Standard 1.1.3.
4. DHHS Office of Inspector General Report OEI-090-98-00220. The Emergency Medical Treatment and Labor Act: Survey of Hospital Emergency. January 2001: 2.
5. 68 Federal Register. September 9, 2003: 53264.
6. Department of Health and Human Services, Centers for Medicare and Medicaid Services Survey and Certification Letter No. S&C-02-34, June 13, 2003.
7. 68 Federal Register. September 9, 2003: 53254.
8. 68 Federal Register. September 9, 2003: 53255.
9. 68 Federal Register. September 9, 2003: 53264.

42
Informed Surgical Consent

Linda S. Laibstain and Robert C. Nusbaum

General Rule

Informed surgical consent is a legal doctrine in force throughout each of the 50 United States, and it is governed by statute or by case law, or both, in every state. There is uniformity in principle, but sufficient variation exists to require the surgeon to be familiar with the specific statutes, where they exist, and the applicable case law, of the state in which he or she practices.

The basic rationale for informed consent was stated by Justice Cardozo in a 1914 decision in the Superior Court of New York: "Every human being of adult years and sound mind has a right to determine what shall be done with his own body; and a surgeon who performs an operation without his patient's consent commits an assault, for which he is liable in damages."[1] Subsequent case law makes clear that a patient's agreement to a proposed course of treatment is legally effective only to the extent that he or she has been informed as to (1) what the diagnosis or problem is, (2) what is to be done, (3) the risks involved, and (4) the alternatives to the contemplated treatment—hence the term "informed consent."

Failure to obtain informed surgical consent can expose the surgeon to liability for damages for assault and battery, or negligence, or both, unless the failure is excused by justifiable exceptions, such as medical emergency or other situations discussed in this chapter.

Evidence of Consent

Informed surgical consent is best evidenced by a document signed by the patient and covering, among other desirable subjects, the elements set forth above, namely, a description of the diagnosis and proposed treatment, the risks, and the alternatives. It is important that the contents of the document be understandable by people of ordinary intelligence. The surgeon should make certain that the patient has read and understood the document

and cannot safely rely upon a recitation to that effect at the foot of the signed document. Supplementary oral explanation by the surgeon or a qualified assistant is good practice and should be the rule rather than the exception. Such explanations should be documented at the time in the patient's record. In the case of a language barrier, an interpreter may be needed to ensure that the patient understands what is being explained and what consent is being given. If the patient cannot read, the medical record should contain a notation that the document has been read or explained to the patient.

Most hospitals will supply one or more required forms designed to obtain informed consent for surgery and related procedures, including such matters as administration of anesthesia, consent for students to be present to observe, and consent for preservation of removed organs and tissue for use in the advancement of medical science and education. In most situations, patients have the right to cross out provisions of the consent form to which they object, for example, use of their organs or tissue for research or education or the presence of student observers. The surgeon should become familiar with these forms, and keep them readily available. In the final analysis, it is the surgeon's responsibility to see that the consent form used in a given case adequately describes the contemplated treatment, the risks, and the alternatives. The Hospital Law Manual published by Aspen Publishers, Inc., contains an excellent chapter on consents and a comprehensive appendix of useful forms.[2]

What Constitutes a Medical Emergency

It is well settled in the law and the practice of medicine that there is an exception to the informed consent doctrine for cases of medical emergency. Many states have enacted laws and many courts have rendered decisions as to what elements are necessary to constitute an emergency, justifying the performing of medical or surgical procedures in the absence of informed consent. Surgeons should rely on the "medical emergency" exception only when a real medical emergency exists, "requiring immediate action for the preservation of the life or health of the patient under circumstances in which it is impossible or impracticable to obtain the patient's consent or consent by anyone authorized to assume such responsibility."[3] A "medical emergency" is a condition that endangers the life or health of a patient.[4] It must be a condition for which immediate surgery is required to save the life of a patient, to preserve a patient's organs or limbs, or to alleviate a patient's suffering and pain.[5]

One state statute defines a medical emergency as a situation in which (1) in competent medical judgment, the proposed surgical or medical treatment or procedures are reasonably necessary; and (2) a person authorized to consent (for the patient) is not readily available and any delay in treatment could reasonably be expected to jeopardize the life or health of the person affected or could reasonably result in disfigurement or impaired faculties.[6]

Exceptions to Informed Consent

It is generally recognized that "a patient's consent is limited to those procedures made known and contemplated at the time consent is given."[7] Some courts have carved out limited exceptions for situations in which unexpected or acute care conditions or problems arise during the course of an authorized procedure. While performing surgery for which there is an authorized consent, a surgeon may face an unanticipated emergency. Courts have permitted exceptions to the informed consent requirement in situations where it could be shown that there was an immediate threat to the patient's life or health without time to awaken the patient from anesthesia or obtain a family member's consent. In the absence of consent, courts are particularly hesitant to sanction the removal of a patient's organs or limbs without compelling reasons, especially so in situations involving the removal of reproductive organs.

The case of *Barnett v. Bacharch* provides guidance for the surgeon who encounters an unanticipated emergency during the course of surgery. In *Barnett*, the patient, who was pregnant and complaining of pain in her lower abdomen, was diagnosed as having a tubal pregnancy. While the patient was under anesthesia, the surgeon found she had an acute appendix and, without consulting the patient's husband, removed the appendix. The court held that an acute appendix, with potentially dangerous consequences if not removed immediately, created a medical emergency sufficient to justify its removal without additional consent.[8]

In the Louisiana case of *Douget v. Touro Infirmary*, a patient with a lengthy history of surgeries and extensive adhesions underwent an anterior lumbar fusion operation by a physician experienced in this type of procedure.

During the surgery, the physician encountered hundreds of adhesions and other unanticipated complications, including serious hemorrhaging. As a result of these complications, the surgeon determined that one of the patient's kidneys had only a slight chance of survival and, if not removed, might result in severe sepsis. In addition, the surgeon removed the patient's spleen, believing it was impossible to save. The court, in the *Douget* case, affirmed the jury's decision that an acute care situation existed, requiring immediate action by the surgeon. The court held that prolonging the anterior fusion operation for the surgeon to leave the operating room to explain the situation to the patient's husband and request his informed consent could have resulted in jeopardizing the life or health of the patient's wife.[9]

An example of a court reaching a different decision is *Tabor v. Scobee*, a case in which a 20-year-old patient consented to an operation for appendicitis. During the procedure, the surgeon determined that the patient's fallopian tubes were infected, swollen, and sealed off at both ends. The surgeon proceeded to remove them, believing that failure to do so within the next several months could result in serious harm or death. He was unable to obtain the patient's consent because she was under anesthesia and did not attempt to obtain the consent of the patient's stepmother, apparently in the hospital at the time. The court held that the patient's medical condition did not constitute a "medical emergency," because there would be an opportunity for the patient to make an informed decision without immediate jeopardy to her life or health.[10]

A similar situation occurred in the Louisiana case of *Rogers v. Lumbermens*, in which the surgeon, engaged to perform a simple appendectomy, also performed a hysterectomy as a precautionary measure, without the knowledge or consent of the patient or her husband. The court found that no emergency existed to justify the surgery under the circumstances.[3]

Surgeons must recognize that procedures otherwise considered emergencies may not justify surgery without consent if there is a reasonable opportunity to obtain consent.

The Unconscious Patient

An exception to the informed consent doctrine is generally recognized for treatment of an unconscious patient in need of acute care surgery. This is based on the proposition that "when the patient is unconscious and in immediate need of acute care medical attention, the duties of disclosure imposed by the doctrine of informed consent are excused because irreparable harm and even death may result from the physician's hesitation to provide treatment.[11]

This proposition is illustrated by the often-cited case of *Jackovach v. Yocom*, decided by the Supreme Court of Iowa in 1931. Albert Jackovach, a 17-year-old boy, was injured while trying to jump off a moving train. After being dragged along the tracks, he was taken to the local hospital, where he was found to have a serious scalp wound, which was bleeding profusely, and a severely mangled and crushed elbow joint and arm. Before taking the patient to the operating room, efforts were made to reach his parents, who lived in a town approximately 8 miles away and who did not have a telephone. Neither of his parents was located until some time after the operation was completed.

Evidence at trial showed that the patient initially was taken to the operating room, where he was put under anesthesia for treatment of his head wound to stop the flow of blood and to save his life. The surgeon, assisted by two other physicians, determined that the crushed and mangled condition of the patient's arm was a "menace" to his life and that it was necessary to amputate the arm. Despite the subsequent argument of the patient and his parents that x-rays should have been taken and consent obtained before the patient's arm was amputated, the court held that consent was implied by the circumstances of the situation. The court made a key finding, in the ensuing 70 years frequently referred to by those in the medical and legal professions: "If a surgeon is confronted with an emergency which endangers the life or health of the patient, it is his duty to do that which the occasion demands within the usual and customary practice among physicians and surgeons in the same or similar localities, without consent of the patient."[12]

The Iowa court also noted the futility and potential dangers to the patient if his physicians were to release him from the anesthesia for the sole purpose of ascertaining whether the patient and his parents would consent to the amputation.

Capacity to Consent

In addition to making a medical diagnosis, a surgeon may need to make a determination of a patient's capacity to provide informed consent. This determination is to establish whether the patient is capable of understanding his or her medical condition, the nature and effect of the proposed treatment, and the risks involved in proceeding both with and without such treatment, including alternatives, if any.[13] Although it is clear that a patient who is unconscious does not have the capacity to consent, the issue is not always clear in situations involving patients with diminished capacity resulting from trauma, head injuries, intoxication, or other impairments that can affect the patient's ability to understand the elements described above.

When a physician determines that a patient is incapable of providing consent for an acute care procedure, the physician should attempt to locate and obtain the consent of a family member, if at all practicable.[13] If a family member cannot be located and if in the physician's judgment the patient will suffer harm as a result of the delay, the surgeon should proceed with appropriate treatment or surgery.[14]*

Intoxicated Patients

The issue of capacity frequently arises in the treatment of intoxicated patients who refuse to authorize recommended procedures. Although each patient must be evaluated individually for ability to give informed consent, courts generally give deference to the practice of good medicine. Illustrative of this proposition is the case of *Miller v. Rhode Island Hospital*, in which a patient was admitted to the hospital's trauma service following a vehicular accident, resulting in injuries to his head, face, and ribs. He was evaluated by three trauma team physicians and underwent a number of diagnostic tests. The patient, found to have the equivalent of 16 alcoholic drinks in his blood, objected to the physician's plan to perform a diagnostic peritoneal lavage, which was established hospital protocol for a patient with his injuries. The patient later sued the hospital, complaining that anesthesia was administered and the procedure performed over his vehement objection. The Supreme Court of Rhode Island, in a detailed analysis, agreed with the surgeon's decision and the hospital's policy to perform a nonconsensual peritoneal lavage if the patient suffered an injury likely to cause internal injuries and if the "patient's mental status was impaired by drugs, alcohol or an injury to the head, such that the patient cannot sense or report symptoms of internal bleeding."[15] The court noted that the treatment was consistent with the standards established by the American College of Surgeons and that the surgeon's decision to perform the procedure was supported by his findings and by other physicians present at the time.

Minors

As a general rule, the medical emergency exception to the informed consent doctrine also applies to minors.

---

* As technology advances and methods and speed of electronic communication (cellular telephones, fax machines, etc.) evolve, there are more options available to reach family members, if they can be identified and located. The practicality of using these communications should be balanced against the patient's medical needs, based on the best judgment of the surgeon.

Although a parent or guardian's consent is normally required to treat a minor, it is generally not required if the delay would likely result in immediate injury or death.[16]

Most states have statutes that deal with consent for acute care medical treatment of minors. For example, Massachusetts statute law provides:

No physician, dentist or hospital shall be held liable for damages for failure to obtain consent of a parent, legal guardian or other person having custody or control of a minor child . . . to emergency examination or treatment, including blood transfusions, when delay in treatment will endanger the life, limb or mental well-being of the patient.[17]

Surgeons should be familiar with their hospitals' procedures for providing emergency medical care to minors when parents cannot be located, including how to get in touch with designated hospital administrators/personnel to implement the procedures. This is especially important in situations involving life-threatening conditions that, although serious, allow time for obtaining a court order in the absence of consent of a parent or legal guardian. Courts are inconsistent in their application of the emergency exception with respect to minors in cases where neither consent nor a court order was obtained before acute care surgery.[16] Hospital attorneys often have standing arrangements to obtain an expedited hearing for court approval of acute care surgery or related treatment in cases where voluntary consent is unavailable and dire consequences may result if surgery is too long delayed.

Some courts recognize an exception for the mature minor. This exception allows a minor to give informed consent "if it is determined that the patient has the ability and maturity to understand and comprehend the nature of his or her condition, proposed treatment, the associated risks and potential results in view of the surrounding circumstances."[16]

Although court decisions vary depending on the specific facts, the *Jackovach* case described above, in which physicians amputated the patient's arm, while the patient was under anesthesia for life-threatening head injury, and the *Luka* case that follows, are examples of judicial deference to the decisions of surgeons practicing good medicine with respect to minors in acute care situations. In *Luka v. Lowrie*, a 15-year-old boy was brought to the hospital with a mangled and crushed foot. Shortly after giving his name and the street where he lived, he lapsed into unconsciousness. The surgeon, after learning that the patient's parents were not in the hospital and upon consultation with four other physicians, agreed that an immediate amputation of the patient's foot was necessary to save the patient's life. The court ruled that the surgeon's decision to operate, in the absence of consent, was appropriate given the condition of the patient and the potential consequences if surgery was not performed.[18]

Patient's Refusal to Consent

It is a well-established principle in law and medicine that a competent person may refuse to consent to medical treatment and that a physician must respect a competent person's refusal of treatment, even in an emergency. The right to refuse medical treatment applies to all forms of medical treatment, including life-saving and life-sustaining procedures. It also includes refusal of blood transfusions, an issue that frequently arises in the context of an emergency as well as during the course of non-emergency medical treatment.[19]

Because issues involving patients' refusal of treatment, including refusal of blood transfusions, frequently arise in life-threatening situations, physicians and hospitals are sometimes unwilling to proceed with what they consider unsound medical practice—hence the large number of these types of cases that are brought before the courts for resolution.[20] Courts often reach different decisions on these issues, based in large part on the specific factual situations and the level of the patient's competency to make an informed decision.

A Florida court has held that a patient with kidney disease, who was likely to die within a few hours without a blood transfusion, had the right to refuse the transfusion. The court found that the patient was competent and mentally alert, and there was no overriding reason to require a transfusion that would violate the patient's religious beliefs. The court made it clear that the patient had the right to refuse a transfusion for himself as a matter of self-determination but stated that its conclusion was limited to the facts before it and that the outcome might be different for a parent or guardian refusing treatment for another person.[21]

In re Quackenbush deals with a 72-year-old competent patient who refused to consent to amputation of his legs, despite likely death from gangrene in a matter of weeks without the surgery. The patient had declined medical treatment for 40 years and described himself as a "conscientious objector" to medical care. The New Jersey court upheld the patient's right to refuse treatment and declined a petition by the hospital to order surgery.[22]

An unusual case from the Supreme Judicial Court of Massachusetts illustrates the type of dilemma that can be faced by emergency personnel. This case was brought by the parents of a young woman, Catherine Shine, an asthmatic, who presented to the emergency room with a severe asthma attack. Having suffered from this condition all her life, and knowledgeable about various treatments, she made it known to hospital personnel (and they agreed) that only oxygen would be administered. After the patient removed the oxygen mask because it gave her a headache, the emergency room attending physician determined that she required intubation. The patient was restrained and intubated, contrary to her stated instructions. The patient, having been traumatized by these events, vowed never to go to a hospital again. Two years later, while suffering an asthma attack, she adamantly refused to go to a hospital. She was finally taken by ambulance to a hospital, where she died 2 days later, despite medical treatment. The court declined to dismiss the case, ruling that a jury could consider whether the treating physician took all steps necessary to obtain the patient's consent or the consent of a family member for treatment.[23]

Issues involving refusal to give consent, particularly for blood transfusions, can be problematic with an unconscious patient, a patient with limited capacity, or a minor. They sometimes arise when family members voice the patient's objection, religious or otherwise, contrary to the physician's recommendation. When confronted with a parent's or representative's refusal to consent to treatment, the physician should seek the assistance of designated hospital personnel (on-call administrator, legal counsel, etc.) to obtain guidance or to petition the courts, if necessary. Courts generally analyze these matters on a case by case basis, depending, in part, on whether the patient has previously expressed instructions, the patient's condition, and, in some circumstances, whether there is a compelling state interest in the preservation of life that outweighs the patient's religious tenets expressed by family members.[20]

Documentation

When treating a patient over his or her objection, or when there are issues as to the patient's capacity to give informed consent, the physician should (1) document objective findings, for example, blood alcohol levels and Glasgow Coma Scores; (2) document in the patient's record the subjective findings forming the basis for the decision; (3) consult with other physicians or health care providers, if feasible; (4) document efforts to reach family members or otherwise obtain consent; and (5) document the need for the immediacy of the procedure.

It is obligatory that surgeons be familiar with their own state statutes, leading cases, and hospital policies and regulations concerning informed consent in order to make sound decisions. Some states provide detailed requirements for informed consent and specific exemptions for acute care procedures, but others provide little or no guidance. Most hospitals have regulations for performing surgery when the patient's consent is not available, including protocols for notification of "on-call administrators." These individuals are usually well informed and very helpful. Adhering to hospital guidelines, as well as thorough documentation of the physician's reasons for performing acute care surgical procedures without the

consent of the patient or a representative are essential for all concerned.

In conclusion, it is impossible to anticipate the variety of situations that may present themselves to the emergency physicians, often requiring quick decisions. However, there are certain steps the surgeon and other medical personnel can and should take to ensure good medicine while limiting exposure to liability for performing medical procedures to which the patient or his family express objections or may object in the future.

The following guidelines are suggested:

1. Be familiar with the laws in the state where you operate with respect to informed consent, refusal of treatment, treatment of incapacitated patients, minors, and so forth.

2. Know your hospital's policies for treatment in emergency situations—know the hospital administrator or designated person to contact when emergency/consent issues arise and know how to get in touch with that person.

3. Have available informed consent forms for surgical procedures, ancillary procedures (e.g., anesthesia), and other treatment. Use the forms!

4. Consult with other physicians and health care providers on difficult issues, time permitting. This includes involvement of others in decisions to operate, administer anesthesia, and order transfusions.

5. Discuss with the patient, and/or his or her designated representative, the diagnosis and nature of the patient's condition, the proposed treatment and material risks, and alternatives to that treatment.

6. Document your findings, diagnosis, and treatment.

7. Document discussions with patient and representative concerning consent issues.

8. Practice good medicine!

References

1. *Schloendorff v. Society of New York Hospital*, 211 N.Y. 125, 129–130, 105 N.E. 92, 93 (1914).
2. Hospital Law Manual. New York: Aspen Publishers, Inc., 2006.
3. *Rogers v. Lumbermen's Mutual Casualty Company*, 119 So. 2d 649, 650 (1960).
4. *Jackovach v. Yocom*, 212 Iowa 914, 237 N.W. 444, 449 (1931).
5. *Sullivan v. Montgomery*, 155 Misc. 448, 279 N.Y.S. 575 (1935).
6. Louisiana Revised Statutes 40:1299.54 (2006).
7. Consent to medical and surgical procedures by Arnold J. Rosoff. In Hospital Law Manual. New York: Aspen Publishers, Inc., 2006: 1–252.
8. *Barnett v. Bacharch*, 34 A. 2d 626 (1943).
9. *Douget v. Touro Infirmary*, 537 So. 2d 251, 260 (1988).
10. *Tabor v. Scobee*, 254 S.W. 2d 474 (1951).
11. Hartman K, Liang B: Exceptions to informed consent in emergency medicine. Hosp Physician 1999; 35:53–59.
12. *Jackovach v. Yocom*, 212 Iowa 914, 237 N.W. 444, 449 (1931).

13. *Miller v. Rhode Island Hospital*, 625 A. 2d 778, 785 (1993).
14. *Canterbury v. Spence*, 464 F. 2d 772, 788, 789 (1972).
15. *Miller v. Rhode Island Hospital*, 625 A. 2d 778, 781 (1993).
16. Veilleux D. Medical practitioner's liability for treatment given child without parent's consent, 67 A.L.R. 4th 511, The Lawyers Co-operative Publishing Company, 2004.
17. Mass. Gen. Laws Ann. Ch. 12 §12F (2006).
18. *Luka v. Lowrie*, 171 Mich. 122, 136 N. W. 1106 (1912).
19. *In re Brown*, 294 Ill. App. 3d 159, 689 N. E. 2d 397, 228 Ill. Dec. 525 (1997); appeal denied, 177 Ill. 2d 570, 698 N. E. 2d 543 232 Ill. Dec. 452 (1998).
20. Karnezis K. Patient's right to refuse treatment allegedly necessary to sustain life, 93 A.L.R. 3d 67, The Lawyers Co-operative Publishing Company, 2004.
21. *St. Mary's Hosp. v. Ramsey*, 465 So. 2d 666 (Fla. Dist. Ct. App. 4th Dist. 1985).
22. *In re Quackenbush*, 156 N. J. Super. 382, 283 A. 2d 785 (1978).
23. *Shine v. Vega*, 429 Mass. 456, 709 N. E. 2d 58 (1999).

43
Advance Directives

David G. Jacobs

These are the duties of a physician—to cure sometimes, to relieve often, to comfort always

Anonymous[1]

This chapter discusses the issues surrounding advance directives, focusing specifically on the impact these documents may have on the care of the acute care surgical patient. At first, it may seem somewhat unusual to include a chapter on this topic in a text devoted to the care of the acute care surgical patient. However, it is important to remember that acute surgical illness, whether from injury, sepsis, or shock, may render the patient incapable of participating in decision making at the time of presentation. Furthermore, the nature of acute surgical illness not infrequently results in postoperative complications, organ failure, and prolonged intensive care unit stays, requiring invasive and expensive treatment modalities that, for some patients, may be life saving but, for others, may simply be death delaying. Thus, some understanding of the history of advance directives, the types of documents that currently exist, and their relative advantages and disadvantages is necessary to ensure optimal outcomes for this patient population.

In this regard, the word "outcomes" is used in its broadest sense, as the treatment goals from the patient's perspective may be radically different from those of the treating surgeon. Advance care planning in general, and advance directives in particular, refers to a process whereby a patient rendered temporarily or permanently incapable of participating in treatment decisions can exert his or her right to autonomy, thus ensuring a favorable outcome from the patient's perspective.

History of the Development of Advance Directives

Ethical Foundation

The principle of autonomy, the right of each person to determine what will or will not be done to his or her body, is one of the guiding bioethical principles of our time. So basic and fundamental is this right that most courts now appear to recognize it as the first principle of medical ethics.[2] This principle provides the ethical foundation for the "Patient's Bill of Rights" approved by the American Hospital Association in 1973, in which the express right of a competent patient to refuse treatment was supported.[3] In the same year, the American Medical Association recognized the reciprocal rights of both patient and physician to determine appropriate end-of-life treatments.[4] Current opinion suggests that patient autonomy is so fundamental to medical decision making that it should be extended even to individuals who, because of acute or chronic illness, are no longer able to direct their own medical care. This, in turn, mandates the creation of some means of exerting this autonomy after medical decision-making capacity has been lost, that is, advance directives.

Two other principles of modern medical ethics are important to consider when discussing advance care planning—beneficence and social justice. Beneficence declares that whatever is best for each person should be accomplished, whereas social justice holds that resources, particularly scarce ones, should be allocated fairly. As will be discussed later, both of these principles, along with autonomy, strongly influence end-of-life care and thus impact advance care planning as well. In most cases, medical care can delivered in such a way as to be consistent with all three of these principles. However, under certain circumstances, particularly in end-of-life situations, it may not be possible to satisfy all principles simultaneously. When this occurs, the relative primacy of autonomy as an ethical principle will generally direct the decision making.

Legal Foundation

Advance directives have existed, in one fashion or another, for more than 30 years, as evidenced by Kutner's proposal of a "living will" in 1969 as a way for a patient with terminal illness to specify the nature of future medical care.[5] However, it was not until the well-publicized case of Karen Ann Quinlan in 1976 that a patient's right to refuse medical care in certain "terminal" situations gained the public's attention and support. In this case, the State Supreme Court of New Jersey authorized the discontinuance of ventilatory support from Ms. Quinlan (thus effectively allowing her death) on the basis of a patient's right to privacy. Just as important, however, was the Court's recognition that this authority extended to Ms. Quinlan's parents, without whom the patient's right to privacy would have been lost.[6]

Advance care planning, however, was still virtually nonexistent until two significant developments, both of which occurred in the early 1990s. The first was the case of *Cruzan vs. Director, Missouri Department of Health*.[7] This case involved a young woman who was rendered severely and permanently mentally incapacitated as a result of a motor vehicle crash. There was universal agreement among her physicians that she was indeed in a "persistent vegetative state" from which she would not recover. She was successfully weaned from mechanical ventilation, but continued to receive enteral nutrition via a surgically placed gastrostomy tube. Her parents petitioned the Court to force termination of her nutritional support, citing their daughter's statement that she would not want to continue to live if she could not be "at least halfway normal." Their request was granted, only to be overturned on appeal by the Missouri State Supreme Court on the grounds that the parents had not supplied "clear and convincing" evidence that Ms. Cruzan would have rejected such treatment. This decision was then further appealed to the United States Supreme Court that, in a split decision (5–4), upheld the State Supreme Court's decision to refuse termination of nutritional support. Although the majority opinion of the Supreme Court recognized the patient's right to autonomy, it also recognized the right of every state to determine criteria by which the authenticity of the patient's end-of-life wishes could be deduced. Despite siding with the majority, Justice O'Connor appeared to strongly support the right of a previously competent, now incompetent patient to direct his or her own end-of-life care when she wrote the following:

Few individuals provide explicit oral or written instructions regarding their intent to refuse medical treatment should they become incompetent. States which decline to consider any evidence other than such instructions may frequently fail to honor a patient's intent. Such failures might be avoided if the State considered an equally probative source of evidence: the patient's appointment of a proxy to make health care decisions on her behalf. . . . Today's decision, holding only that the Constitution permits a State to require clear and convincing evidence of Nancy Cruzan's desire to have artificial hydration and nutrition withdrawn, does not preclude a future determination

that the Constitution requires the States to implement the decisions of a patient's duly appointed surrogate.[8]

This statement by Justice O'Connor, suggesting a possible role of the federal government in mandating compliance with a surrogate's medical decisions, provided significant impetus to the adoption of advance directive legislation. Two additional lessons from the Cruzan decision are germane to this discussion. First, there is no distinction made among the various forms of life-sustaining treatment; nutrition and hydration are no different from mechanical ventilation and other more invasive therapies when considering "life-support" strategies. Second, there is no ethical or legal difference between withholding and withdrawing treatment from a patient. Thus, the physician need not be concerned that initiating a particular "life-support" therapy will preclude him or her from withdrawing that therapy on the patient's behalf in the future.[9]

The Patient Self-Determination Act

The second event that was critical in fostering the development of advance directives was the Patient Self-Determination Act (PSDA) of 1990.[10] This federal legislation required that all health care institutions (hospitals, nursing homes, health maintenance organizations, etc.) that received federal funding provide written information to each adult patient regarding that patient's legal right to make decisions concerning medical care, to refuse treatment, and to formulate advance directives. In addition, the institution was required to document advance directives in the patient's medical record, ensure compliance with state law regarding advance directives, and avoid making care conditional on completion of such directives. The purpose of the PSDA was a good one—to encourage discussions between patients and physicians regarding end-of-life care preferences, thus facilitating patient autonomy.

Some, however, have suggested a more jaded and sinister rationale behind this legislation, a financial motive. The PSDA as passed was a part of the Omnibus Reconciliation Act of 1990 that, among other things, provided for an overall net reduction in Medicare payments to health care institutions. This raises an intriguing question: Does more widespread use of advance directives have any impact on health care expenditures? Chambers et al.,[11] in a study of nearly 500 Medicare patient deaths, documented a mean inpatient charge of $30,478 for patients with advance directives compared with $95,305 for those without directives, even after controlling for severity of disease, use of an intensive care unit, and number of procedures. Similar findings have been noted by Weeks et al.[12] Thus, the use of advance directives, by limiting presumably unwanted expensive end-of-life care, resulted in the potential of significant cost savings.

Other authors have examined this issue and have found no decrease in health care expenditures for patients with advance directives.[13,14] Some of the discrepancy between these findings may be due to the relatively large number of patients in some of these studies whose advance directives were not followed, resulting in comparable charges for both groups. Future studies comparing patients whose directives were actually followed with those whose directives were ignored will be necessary to determine whether advance directive use reduces health care costs.

The larger ethical issues raised here—the societal value of end-of-life care and who should pay for it—relate directly to the third ethical principle described earlier—social justice, the equitable allocation of scarce resources. Whether the impetus for creation of the PSDA was autonomy, beneficence, social justice, or some combination of these principles, will probably never be known.

The immediate impact of the Cruzan decision and the PSDA was the rapid development and dissemination of legislation regarding advance directives. All 50 states have enacted advance directive legislation of one type or another, and all of these laws provide immunity to physicians and other health professionals who follow the patient's wishes as expressed in a living will. However, there is a great deal of variability from state to state regarding the form, function, and authority ascribed to these documents.[15] This lack of uniformity has weakened the overall effectiveness of advance directive legislation and has created obstacles to both patients and physicians in terms of completing these documents. Advance directive laws vary significantly among states in such areas as who can be designated as a proxy, the conditions under which these directives can be activated, and even the process by which these documents can be revoked. Some states restrict their living will laws to directives that *limit* resuscitative efforts in end-of-life care, whereas others allow their documents to specify "aggressive" care.

Most states authorize both living wills and the appointment of a health care power of attorney. However, three states, Massachusetts, Michigan, and New York, authorize only the appointment of a health care agent, while one state, Alaska, authorizes only the use of living wills.[16] Therefore, it is incumbent on the patient and physician to be familiar with the limitations and restrictions set forth by their particular state as well as to recognize that an advance directive drawn up in accordance with one state's regulations may not be recognized in a different state. It has been recommended that patients have advance directives drawn up for each state in which they may find themselves requiring this sort of "protection." In an attempt to reduce confusion and to provide for some consistency across the states regarding advance directives, the National Conference of Commissioners on Uniform State Laws proposed the Uniform Health-Care Decisions Act in 1993 that provides for a uniform, consistent approach to advance directive implementation, management, and enforcement within and between state jurisdictions.[17] Unfortunately, to date this legislation has been adopted by less than 10 states.

Sadly, the PSDA does not seem to have had much impact on advance care planning in the United States. Today it is estimated that only 10% to 15% of patients have actually signed advance health care directives.[18–23] The reasons behind this apparent lack of interest in completing advance directives are many, varied, and not well understood.[24,25] Perhaps the most comprehensive study to examine the impact of advance health care decision making in the post-PSDA era is the SUPPORT study, in which 9,105 seriously ill patients in five teaching hospitals participated in an intervention in which a nurse facilitated communication among the patient, family, physicians, and hospital staff to improve understanding of outcomes and promote advance care planning. Only 20% of these patients had an advance directive prior to the study, and the intervention did nothing to improve this rate. The study also documented poor physician–patient communication regarding cardiopulmonary resuscitation preferences and other end-of-life issues, even for those few patients who had completed advance directives.[26–28] Despite the fact that the PSDA mandates that patients admitted to health care institutions be given the opportunity to complete these documents, there is essentially uniform agreement that this is not the optimal time, from either a patient or physician perspective, to enter into these types of discussions.[29–31] Many patients, because of the illnesses that have prompted hospital admission, may not be in a position to discuss advance directives. Furthermore, it seems intuitive that many of the patients who are *able* to discuss advance directives may not be *willing* to do so, as these discussions may perhaps heighten fears and suspicions.

This perception is corroborated in the SUPPORT study, in which more than 50% of patients refused to discuss end-of-life management when they were seriously ill.[26] Other authors have reached similar conclusions,[32,33] but work by Reilly et al.[34] suggests that in excess of 80% of hospitalized patients are willing to undertake such discussions with their physicians. Importantly, only 47% of patients actually had these discussions, highlighting the reluctance that physicians have in initiating these conversations. The health care facility, therefore, caught between legislation requiring them to provide patients with this opportunity and physicians reluctant if not unwilling to engage patients in these discussions, has relegated the responsibility of providing information regarding advance directives to hospital admissions personnel who, in many cases, distribute this information in a perfunctory fashion along with a myriad of other required patient notifications, including forms for authorization for treatment, release of information, and authorization for assignment of benefits. Thus the potential impact of the PSDA has been significantly hampered.[20,35]

One potential solution would be to distribute advance directive information to patients prior to hospital admission. Cugliari et al.[36] documented a significantly higher rate of advance directive completion (40% vs. 4%) by simply distributing information about directives one day before admission as opposed to at the time of admission. Although this represents a marked improvement in document execution, it does not provide for physician involvement, nor does it address the needs of patients admitted under nonelective circumstances.

For these and other reasons, it is generally acknowledged that discussions regarding advance directives should occur between a patient and his or her primary care physician in the outpatient setting, well in advance of the need for implementation of such directives.[18,29] Evidence, however, suggests that these outpatient discussions are not occurring.[37,38] Why not? When polled, the majority of patients favor hearing about their illnesses and their health care options but believe that these discussion should be initiated by the physician.[19,39–42] Multiple studies have documented the extent of, and reasons for, physician reluctance to initiate discussion about advance directives.[18,39,43,44]

Some physicians perceive that their patients will respond negatively to a discussion on advance directives, particularly at the time of hospital admission. However, this concern is not born out in the published literature.[18,19,45] Furthermore, many physicians have not been provided the training necessary to undertake these types of discussions,[46,47] nor are they compensated for the time that would be required to adequately discuss the issues.[38] For example, advocates of the Values History, one particular directive, estimate that it might take five patient visits or 1 year to complete this document. Another recent study noted that physicians with expertise in the area of advance directives spend, on average, 15 minutes per office visit in discussions about these issues with their patients.[48] Given the time and financial constraints imposed upon modern-day medical practices, extensive patient–physician discussions about advance directives may not be an option.[49] Some have recommended the use of financial incentives to hospitals or physicians to encourage patient–physician discussion,[50,51] but, to date, no legislative provisions have been made to support this. Finally, for both the physician and the patient, ethnicity and sociocultural norms seem to play a role in advance directive discussions and decision making.[52–56] Clearly, greater effort needs to be expended in identifying the causes for the underutilization of these documents and in finding solutions for them.

Types of Advance Directives

Advance directives may be classified in several ways and, as a result, describing the various types of documents can be confusing. Most commonly, *advance directives* refers to any document in which a competent patient makes known his or her wishes regarding the nature and extent of medical care desired should he or she lose decisional capacity in the future. Others use the term to specifically refer to those directives that are "advisory" in nature. The American Medical Association describes two categories of advance directives, advisory and statutory.[57]

Advisory documents attempt to accurately represent a patient's wishes and might include such things as a worksheet containing potential end-of-life scenarios with choices indicating the patient's preferred mode of treatment. Alternatively, they might include a statement of values that could provide a framework on which the physician and the family could base their subsequent decisions. Other examples include notes written by a physician in the medical record reflecting discussions that he or she has had with the patient, as well as written documentation of conversations between the patient and family members. Regardless of their form, these documents are legally binding under the law.

Statutory documents give physicians immunity from malpractice for following a patient's wishes. Examples of these documents include living wills and durable power of attorney for health care designations. Importantly, the degree of flexibility and options accorded the patient by these documents varies significantly from state to state and, as a result, may not provide the desired amount of "protection" required by the patient, as one state's document may not be recognized as valid in another state. Regardless of how these documents are classified, the two documents with which both patients and physicians should be most familiar are the living will and the durable health care power of attorney.

Living Wills

Living wills represent the earliest form of advance directive, dating back to 1969.[5] In general, living wills are documents that instruct physicians on the type of medical care the patient would like to receive in the event he or she loses decision-making capacity. The language in these documents is generally broad and conceptual rather than specific, although many living will forms do enable patients to add specific requests. Advantages of the living will include the fact that these documents allow the patient the opportunity to specify both the conditions under which certain treatments should be provided or withheld (qualifying statements) as well as the nature of those treatments (directive statements). Thus, for example, a patient may specify that endotracheal intubation may be carried out as part of an operative procedure but not in the event of cardiopulmonary arrest.

Living wills have generally been used to *limit* interventions provided to the patient at the end of life, but this is by no means the only type of medical directive provided for by living wills. Some patients have used living wills to indicate their desire to have all treatment options and resuscitative measures provided to them, irrespective of clinical circumstances.[58] Others have used living wills to designate that medical care be carried out according to specific religious customs or traditions,[59–61] whereas others have used these documents to indicate their desire to donate their organs upon their deaths.[49,50] Clearly, however, the most common purpose for the completion of living wills is to limit the use of certain medical interventions perceived by the patient to be unnecessary or unwarranted in end-of-life situations.

Unfortunately, the language used in most living wills is sufficiently vague and ambiguous so as to render their interpretation meaningless in many clinical situations. Use of words such as "terminal condition," "extraordinary means," "imminent death," and others have introduced an unwanted degree of subjectivity into the interpretation of these documents by both physicians and family members.[62] Some authors (and states) have attempted to reduce this ambiguity by attaching either to the living will itself or to another form of advisory document either a scenario-based or value-based assessment to give the patient the opportunity to make clear under what specific conditions and circumstances "aggressive" end-of-life care would be provided.[49,50] Others have argued, however, that inclusion of these additional documents does nothing to ensure that the intent of the patient will be sustained when required and that these "enhancements" may actually restrict patient autonomy.[63,64]

Ethical arguments have, as well, been raised against the use of living wills on the basis of the concept of "personhood."[65] This point of view holds that it is inappropriate to bind individuals to a decision that they made when they possessed perhaps a completely different set of values and interests. For example, should a pleasantly demented, but functional, individual be denied "aggressive" end-of-life care simply because he or she, 20 years previously, believed that "dementia" would represent an unacceptable quality of life? Despite these concerns, living wills have been demonstrated to increase the accuracy of substituted judgments by hospital-based physicians in contrast to primary care physicians or family surrogates.[66] Thus, determining the presence of completed advance directives may be of value to the "emergency" physician or surgeon, where prior knowledge of the patient's wishes may influence care.

Durable Health Care Power of Attorney

The other common form of advance directive is the durable health care power of attorney (DHPA) in which a competent patient identifies an individual who will act as that patient's surrogate under those circumstances in which the patient loses decision-making capacity. This individual could be a family member, friend, or even physician, and, in most states, the DHPA requires the signature of the named surrogate or "proxy." This form of advance directive has the advantage of preserving the patient's right to informed consent in that, under conditions of lost decision-making capacity, the surrogate would be informed of the risks and benefits of proposed treatment strategies and then would make decisions on behalf of the patient using the "substituted judgment" standard—that is, making the decision that the patient would make were the patient capable. When a proxy does not possess sufficient information to use the substituted judgment standard, a decision would be made using the "best interests" standard in which the proxy makes decisions that maximize patient benefit, consistent with the ethical principle of beneficence.

The DHPA, unlike the living will, therefore, provides the patient with an opportunity for decision-making under conditions that may not have been anticipated at the time that the directive was executed and therefore not specifically addressed within the living will. In this fashion, a DHPA adheres more faithfully to the doctrine of informed consent, which requires that a decision be made *after* the diagnosis has been established and all available treatment options with the attendant risks and benefits have been considered. For these reasons, most authorities recommend completion of a DHPA at a minimum, along with a living will if desired.[64] So important is the presence of a proxy under these circumstances that some states have enacted legislation providing for designation of a surrogate decision maker (in order of priority: guardian, spouse, adult children, parent, sibling, adult grandchild, friend, estate guardian) who would be empowered to make health care decisions for the incompetent patient based on the "substituted judgment" or "best interests" principle in the event that an advance directive has not been completed.[67]

A brief discussion of the concepts of "competence" and "capacity" is necessary here as DHPAs only become effective when the patient loses decision-making capacity or competence. Hence, the assessment of capacity is integral to establishing and preserving patient autonomy. The task of determining who is competent and who has lost medical decision-making capacity can be challenging at times, but typically the process is straightforward and can (and should) be completed by the physician primarily responsible for the patient's care. It should not usually be necessary to involve psychiatrists in these

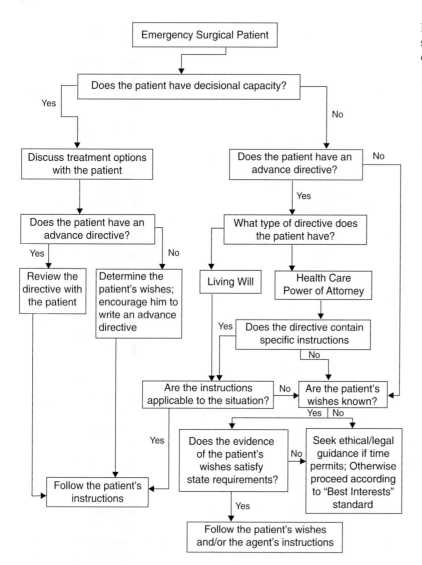

FIGURE 43.1. Decision making in emergency surgery. (Reprinted with permission from Yamani et al.[74])

determinations. Also, it should be emphasized that, although the terms "capacity" and "competence" are frequently used interchangeably, there are some important differences. "Competence" is a *legal* term and refers to an individual's ability to make rational, informed decisions about one's life and property.[68] Individuals over the age of 18 years are presumed to be competent unless declared otherwise by a court of law. Capacity is a *medical* term, is very much related to the concept of autonomy and informed consent, and can be defined as the "ability to understand the significant benefits, risks, and alternatives to proposed health care, and to make and communicate a health care decision."[17]

Unlike competence, capacity is not absolute and must always be interpreted in a temporal and situational context. Therefore, a particular patient may possess the capacity for certain medical decisions, but not others, or at one point in time, but not another. For example, a postoperative acute care surgical patient may lack the capacity to make decisions regarding the appropriateness of

instituting dialysis or mechanical ventilation, but the capacity to choose an appropriate DHPA may well be preserved. Similarly, this patient's capacity for medical decision making may fluctuate over time, depending upon clinical status, medications administered, and the nature and extent of medical procedures to which the patient has been subjected.

The approach to determining loss of decisional capacity should be orderly and systematic. A standard mini-mental status examination involving an assessment of alertness, attention, memory, and reasoning will identify the majority of patients lacking decisional capacity. On occasion, these more basic functions will be preserved, necessitating a specific assessment of the patient's capacity relative to the specific medical issue in question. Although many criteria have been proposed, and several evaluation tools exist to aid in the determination of decisional capacity, none has been proven to be superior to another.[69–72] In its simplest terms, the capacity assessment need only address the two questions contained in the earlier definition of capacity: (1) Does the patient understand the significant benefits, risks and alternatives to the proposed plan of care? (2) Can the patient make and communicate a health care decision? In order to give patients the very best chance to establish their decisional capacity (and thereby retain their autonomy), they must be provided with a thorough explanation of the risks and benefits of, and alternatives to, the proposed intervention. This is why the physician responsible for the patient's care is likely to be in a better position to judge the patient's decisional capacity than is the psychiatric specialist. Once the question of decisional capacity has been determined, medical decision making can then proceed, guided by the physician, the patient (if not incapacitated), the advance directive (if present), and other patient advocates (decisionally incapacitated patient, no advance directive). The American Medical Association's Policy Statement E-2.20, *Withholding or Withdrawing Life-Sustaining Medical Treatment*, nicely summarizes this approach to decision making.[73] An algorithm showing how this process might occur is given in Figure 43.1.[74]

Advance Directives: Unfulfilled Potential

The potential of advance directives to significantly alter end-of-life care in the United States has never been realized for two major reasons. The first, the overall small percentage of Americans who have actually completed advance directives, was discussed earlier. Second, even for patients who have completed these directives, there is little evidence that they actually alter end-of-life care.[75,76] In one study of the impact of advance directives on hospital and skilled nursing facility care, care was consistent with the directive in only 75% of cases. Interestingly, of those cases when care was *inconsistent* with the directive, 75% actually received *less* aggressive care than specified in the directive.[76] It is obvious that possession of an advance directive does not guarantee that the patient's *intent* will be achieved. Why are these documents not effective? There appear to be several reasons.

First, it is important to recognize that the advance directive may not actually reflect the patient's wishes or intent. There may be several reasons for this, including limitations placed on these documents by the states in which they are drafted. For example, some states have no provisions in their living wills for a patient to refuse artificial nutrition and water should they desire. Furthermore, many patients are not receiving any education about, or help with completion of, these documents, including guidance from physicians. Although the intent of the PSDA was to encourage patient–physician interaction regarding this issue, there is little evidence that

meaningful discussion is occurring from either a quantitative standpoint (percentage of patients who have had *any* discussion about the content of their advance directives with their physicians)[77] or a qualitative one (percentage of patients who have a *good* understanding of the content of their advance directives).[78]

Not infrequently, the physician is unaware of the existence of advance directives.[28,79] In one recent study of seriously ill intensive care unit patients, only 5% of patients had completed advance directives at the time of admission. Of those with advance directives who subsequently died, 11% underwent "unwanted" cardiopulmonary resuscitation because of lack of awareness of the advance directive on the part of the physician.[80] Many patients have completed advance directives and have not informed either their physician or their family.[81] The Internet has provided easy access to a myriad of advance directive products, and many patients are completing these without the knowledge or assistance of their physicians. Hence, when the patient loses decisional capacity, no one is aware of the existence of directives that might aid in decision making.

One possible solution would be a requirement that these documents be co-signed by both the physician and the proxy, if one has been selected.[81] Even if an advance directive is known to exist, it may not be readily available to the health care team at the time of presentation. These documents may be in the possession of family members, surrogates, or in the office chart of the primary care physician. Morrison et al.,[82] in a study of 114 geriatric patients with previously executed advance directives, noted that only 26% of patients had these directives recognized during their hospitalizations. More importantly, of the subgroup of patients judged not to have decisional capacity during these hospitalizations, only 26% had their directives recognized.[82] Some have recommended the actual appending of the advance directive to the Medicare card such that its contents would be immediately available to health care providers.[83] Others have called for the creation of a central repository that would contain not only a patient's advance directive but also the names and contact information of the primary care physician and any surrogates named by the patient.[57]

An additional shortcoming of advance directives, already alluded to, is the vague and imprecise language employed in many of these documents, found both in the *qualifying* statements within the document ("*if* my condition is __"), as well as in the *directive* statements ("then I do not wish __"). This, in turn, allows for significant differences in interpretation of the patient's actual intent among the various health care providers and patient surrogates. Many qualifying statements specify conditions such as "terminal," "incurable," and "no reasonable expectation of recovery" that defy strict definition, thus potentially allowing unwanted aggressive care to proceed on purely subjective grounds. It has been well documented that many physicians choose not to adhere to advance directives because they believe that the patient's condition does not meet the criteria outlined in the qualifying statements.[24,64,65,75]

Even when there is universal agreement that the criteria set forth in the qualifying statement have been met, the intent of the advance directive may be subverted, intentionally or unintentionally, through the physician's interpretation of the terms "extraordinary means," "heroic measures," or "life-prolonging procedures" employed in the directive statements. For example, a blood transfusion and therapeutic endoscopy for a bleeding duodenal ulcer may seem extraordinary to the patient, but may be entirely reasonable in the physician's mind, given the high likelihood of short-term "cure." This highlights the shortcomings of the living will compared with the DHPA in that, under this specific scenario, the risks and benefits of blood transfusion and endoscopy could be discussed with the patient's proxy, allowing authentic decision-making consistent with the patient's values and beliefs to occur in real time.

The DHPA, however, may not be the ultimate answer either. Not infrequently, the DHPA is unaware that he or she has been chosen to serve in this capacity and, when presented with this information, may be unwilling or unable to serve. Furthermore, the chosen proxy, even if willing to serve, may have ideological differences with the course of action dictated by the advance directive and therefore is unable to carry out the directive. Under these circumstances, a family member or some other surrogate will need to be identified who can fulfill this role. Finally, it is not at all clear that proxies can reliably make health care decisions for the patient using the "substituted judgment" standard.[84–90] This once again highlights the need for thorough discussion among the patient, surrogate, and physician in order that the patient's preferences and wishes be carried out.

Advance Directives: Relevance to the Acute Care Surgeon

The principle of patient autonomy, although difficult to achieve, must still be preserved in the acute care setting. Thus, informed consent, either implicit or explicit, is necessary for all procedures, diagnostic tests, or treatments to be instituted. Frequently, however, the patient requiring acute care surgery lacks the requisite decision-making capacity to provide informed consent. Under these circumstances, a physician may render treatment without the patient's informed consent. The underlying legal principle for this is termed *implied* or *presumed* consent, and it applies when the patient is deemed to be "incompetent."[91]

Ethically speaking, the principle of patient autonomy no longer prevails because preservation of autonomy under these circumstances would require the identification of a surrogate decision maker, thus delaying potentially life-saving medical therapy. Instead, beneficence becomes the dominant ethical principle, directing that treatment be provided according to what a "reasonable" person would want, for example, resuscitation. If, however, an *authentic and relevant* advance directive is immediately available, an unlikely event, then autonomy once again prevails, and care consistent with the directive should be provided.

Here, the determination of "authenticity" and "relevance" is critical. In order to be judged to be authentic, the directive must have been appropriately and officially executed, with the necessary signatures and co-signatures. Advance directive identification bracelets and wallet cards present greater challenges in establishing authenticity, not to mention patient intent, and these should probably be ignored in the acute care setting unless their intent is clearly unambiguous.[91] "Relevance" is the second test to which the advance directive must be subjected. The responsible physician must ensure that the qualifying and directive statements set forth in the patient's advance directive apply to the clinical scenario at hand. Thus, the elderly patient with acute cholecystitis should not be denied cholecystectomy when the directive specifies "no heroic measures in the event of terminal illness." Certainly the ambiguity of this statement precludes an unambiguous interpretation of the patient's intent, but it is probably wiser to proceed with cholecystectomy, and then reevaluate, with any available surrogates, the intent of the directive in the early postoperative period, remembering that there is no difference, from an ethical standpoint, between withholding an intervention, and withdrawing it.

An advance directive may also lead to a situation wherein the surgeon finds himself or herself ethically in disagreement with the care parameters outlined in the directive. This may be due to a directive that specifies aggressive care in circumstances that the surgeon believes represent medical futility, or, conversely, where the surgeon believes that care prohibited by the directive will be of benefit to the patient. Under this circumstance, the physician is under no obligation to passively adhere to the dictates of the directive. The physician, however, does have a responsibility to not abandon the patient and therefore is charged with the responsibility of finding a physician who can, in good conscience, carry out the dictates of the patient's advance directive. Occasionally, input from an institutional ethics committee can help to resolve differences between the health care team and the advance directive (or the proxy) and thereby avoid the necessity of identifying alternate health care providers. As a last resort, some states have enacted binding legislation that provides for a legal solution to these conflicts.[92] All other reasonable efforts should be exhausted before resorting to this form of "mediation."

One circumstance that is perhaps unique to the emergency surgeon is that of the patient with a do-not-resuscitate (DNR) type of advance directive that sustains cardiopulmonary arrest in the course of an operative procedure. Ideally, this eventuality will have been discussed with the competent patient (or the proxy) prior to undertaking the operative procedure and clear agreement reached on the course of action to be followed under this circumstance.[93] The emergent nature of the procedure does not release the surgeon from the obligation of exploring these difficult types of issues with the patient and/or proxy and documenting the results of these discussions in the medical record. In the event that intraoperative cardiac arrest does occur without some mutual understanding having been reached regarding the role of cardiopulmonary resuscitation, arguments have been made for both suspension of and adherence to the DNR order.

Proponents of withholding cardiopulmonary resuscitation emphasize the right of the patient to expire peacefully while under anesthesia and, just as importantly, avoiding the possibility of condemning the patient to continuing to endure the unacceptable existence that prompted the DNR order in the first place.[94] Reasons cited for utilizing cardiopulmonary resuscitation include the view that resuscitation is, in fact, part of, indeed inseparable from, the operative procedure itself and that the decision to proceed with surgery carries with it an obligation to employ all available methods to achieve patient survival. Furthermore, given the readily available resources in the operating room and the many potentially reversible causes of intraoperative cardiac arrest that occur there, the outcomes following intraoperative cardiac arrest are far better than cardiac arrest that occurs anywhere else. Thus, the overall poor postcardiac arrest outcomes that may have prompted the DNR order may not pertain under these circumstances.[95]

A middle-of-the-road approach takes into consideration the cause of the cardiac arrest, recommending cardiopulmonary resuscitation if the etiology of the arrest is easily correctable or iatrogenic in nature and withholding cardiopulmonary resuscitation if the patient's underlying process has precipitated the arrest. Such distinctions are not always possible, and so, if there is any doubt about the exact etiology of the arrest, resuscitative efforts should be undertaken, recognizing that support can always be withdrawn at some future point should the patient's clinical condition so warrant. The American College of Surgeons' Statement on Advance Directives by Patients: "Do Not Resuscitate in the Operating Room" discourages both the automatic enforcement or cancellation of DNR orders and instead advocates a policy of "required reconsideration" of previous advance directives whereby the patient (or proxy) and responsible physician reach consensus regarding the approach to be taken in the event of intraoperative cardiac arrest based on perceived risks and benefits.[96]

Recommendations

Although advance care planning offers patients the opportunity to preserve autonomy in end-of-life decision making, many are not taking advantage of the benefits these documents provide. Furthermore, the potential impact of advance directives on end-of-life care is substantially reduced by the vague and ambiguous language contained in these documents, the lack of uniformity and portability across state lines, and the physician's lack of awareness of, and access to, these directives in critical situations. If advance care planning is ever to achieve the potential that was intended for it, then change, both legislative and behavioral, is needed. Some potential solutions include the following:

- Institute widespread educational programs for patients regarding the importance of advance care planning.
- Create educational and financial incentives for physicians to initiate and maintain end-of-life discussions with patients.
- Mandate that all advance directives be discussed with and co-signed by the patient's physician.
- Create federal legislation that mandates the use of uniform language and medical care options in advance directives and that provides for reciprocity in directive recognition across all 50 states. The Uniform Health Care Decisions Act of 1993 represents a good example of such legislation and should be widely adopted.[17]
- Establish a central repository for advance directives. This would provide for consistent access to these documents when the primary care physician or surrogate is not available to guide treatment.

Finally, it must be reemphasized that advance care planning involves much more than completion of an advance directive. Rather, it is the patient–physician communication that occurs in the process of completing the directives that is critical. Through these discussions, both patient and physician gain greater insight into those values that will guide end-of-life care, the patient understands and appreciates more fully what medical options exist for end-of-life care, the development of patient–physician trust is enhanced, and patient autonomy is reinforced. In the acute care setting, it is the surgeon's responsibility to seek the presence of these directives, verify their authenticity, and honor them unless doing so would create an ethical conflict for the surgeon. Furthermore, the emergency surgeon, when clinical circumstances permit, should take advantage of any and all opportunities to initiate thoughtful and careful discussions with patients and/or their surrogates regarding end-of-life treatment preferences. This in turn ensures that autonomy is preserved, beneficence is maximized, and social justice is facilitated.

References

1. Strauss M, ed. Familiar Medical Quotations. Boston: Little, Brown and Company, 1968.
2. Furrow BR GT, Johnson SH, et al. Bioethics: Health Care Law and Ethics, 3rd ed. St. Paul: West Group, 1997.
3. American Hospital Association: A Patient's Bill of Rights. Chicago: AHA, 1973.
4. Judicial Council of the American Medical Association: Report on Physician and the Dying Patient. Chicago: AMA, 1973.
5. Kutner L. Due process of euthanasia: The living will, a proposal. Ind Law J 1969; 44:539–554.
6. *In re Quinlan.* Vol 10: 70 NJ; 1976:355 A.352d647.
7. *Cruzan v Director, Missouri Department of Health*: 497 U.S. 261, 110 S. Ct. 2841, 111 L.Ed.2d 224; 1990.
8. O'Connor S. 881503 Concur v. Director, Missouri Dept. of Health. 497 US 261 1990. Available at: http://supct. law.cornell.edu/supct/html/88-1503.ZC1.html. Accessed January 9, 2004.
9. Fairman RP. Withdrawing life-sustaining treatment. Lessons from Nancy Cruzan. Arch Intern Med 1992; 152(1):25–27.
10. Omnibus Reconciliation Act of 1990. Public Law No. 101–508. 1990; Sec. 4206.
11. Chambers CV, Diamond JJ, Perkel RL, Lasch LA. Relationship of advance directives to hospital charges in a Medicare population. Arch Intern Med 1994; 154(5):541–547.
12. Weeks WB, Kofoed LL, Wallace AE, Welch HG. Advance directives and the cost of terminal hospitalization. Arch Intern Med 1994; 154(18):2077–2083.
13. Schneiderman LJ, Kronick R, Kaplan RM, Anderson JP, Langer RD. Effects of offering advance directives on medical treatments and costs. Ann Intern Med 1992; 117(7):599–606.
14. Teno J, Lynn J, Connors AF Jr, et al. The illusion of end-of-life resource savings with advance directives. SUPPORT Investigators. Study to Understand Prognoses and Preferences for Outcomes and Risks of Treatment. J Am Geriatr Soc 1997; 45(4):513–518.
15. Gillick MR. Advance care planning. N Engl J Med 2004; 350(1):7–8.
16. Source: Partnership for Caring, Inc; March 2000 Data. Available at: http://www.partnershipforcaring.org/Resources/developments_set.html. Accessed January 26, 2004.
17. National Conference of Commissioners on Uniform State Laws. Uniform Health-Care Decisions Act. Available at: www.law.upenn.edu/bll/ulc/fnact99/1990s/uhcda93.pdf. Accessed January 26, 2004.
18. Gamble ER, McDonald PJ, Lichstein PR. Knowledge, attitudes, and behavior of elderly persons regarding living wills. Arch Intern Med 1991; 151(2):277–280.
19. Emanuel LL, Barry MJ, Stoeckle JD, Ettelson LM, Emanuel EJ. Advance directives for medical care—a case for greater use. N Engl J Med 1991; 324(13):889–895.
20. La Puma J, Orentlicher D, Moss RJ. Advance directives on admission. Clinical implications and analysis of the Patient Self-Determination Act of 1990. JAMA 1991; 266(3):402–405.
21. Johnson RF Jr, Baranowski-Birkmeier T, O'Donnell JB. Advance directives in the medical intensive care unit of a community teaching hospital. Chest 1995; 107(3):752–756.
22. Gross MD. What do patients express as their preferences in advance directives? Arch Intern Med 1998; 158(4):363–365.
23. Hanson LC, Rodgman E. The use of living wills at the end of life. A national study. Arch Intern Med 1996; 156(9):1018–1022.
24. Wolf SM, Boyle P, Callahan D, et al. Sources of concern about the Patient Self-Determination Act. N Engl J Med 1991; 325(23):1666–1671.
25. Llovera I, Ward MF, Ryan JG, et al. Why don't emergency department patients have advance directives? Acad Emerg Med 1999; 6(10):1054–1060.
26. Teno J, Lynn J, Wenger N, et al. Advance directives for seriously ill hospitalized patients: effectiveness with the patient self-determination act and the SUPPORT intervention. SUPPORT Investigators. Study to Understand Prognoses and Preferences for Outcomes and Risks of Treatment. J Am Geriatr Soc 1997; 45(4):500–507.
27. Teno JM, Licks S, Lynn J, et al. Do advance directives provide instructions that direct care? SUPPORT Investigators. Study to Understand Prognoses and Preferences for Outcomes and Risks of Treatment. J Am Geriatr Soc 1997; 45(4):508–512.
28. The SUPPORT Principal Investigators. A controlled trial to improve care for seriously ill hospitalized patients. The study to understand prognoses and preferences for outcomes and risks of treatments (SUPPORT). JAMA 1995; 274(20):1591–1598.
29. Loewy EH, Carlson RW. Talking, advance directives, and medical practice. Arch Intern Med 1994; 154(20):2265–2267.
30. White ML, Fletcher JC. The Patient Self-Determination Act. On balance, more help than hindrance. JAMA 1991; 266(3):410–412.
31. Doukas DJ. Competency and the routine discussion of advance directives. Am Fam Physician 1992; 45(2):473–474.
32. Frankl D, Oye RK, Bellamy PE. Attitudes of hospitalized patients toward life support: a survey of 200 medical inpatients. Am J Med 1989; 86(6):645–648.
33. Singer PA, Martin DK, Lavery JV, Thiel EC, Kelner M, Mendelssohn DC. Reconceptualizing advance care planning from the patient's perspective. Arch Intern Med 1998; 158(8):879–884.
34. Reilly BM, Magnussen CR, Ross J, Ash J, Papa L, Wagner M. Can we talk? Inpatient discussions about advance directives in a community hospital. Attending physicians' attitudes, their inpatients' wishes, and reported experience. Arch Intern Med 1994; 154(20):2299–2308.
35. Annas GJ. The health care proxy and the living will. N Engl J Med 1991; 324(17):1210–1213.

36. Cugliari AM, Miller T, Sobal J. Factors promoting completion of advance directives in the hospital. Arch Intern Med 1995; 155(17):1893–1898.

37. Markson LJ, Fanale J, Steel K, Kern D, Annas G. Implementing advance directives in the primary care setting. Arch Intern Med 1994; 154(20):2321–2327.

38. Morrison RS, Morrison EW, Glickman DF. Physician reluctance to discuss advance directives. An empiric investigation of potential barriers. Arch Intern Med 1994; 154(20): 2311–2318.

39. Shmerling RH, Bedell SE, Lilienfeld A, Delbanco TL. Discussing cardiopulmonary resuscitation: a study of elderly outpatients. J Gen Intern Med 1988; 3(4):317–321.

40. Havlir D, Brown L, Rousseau GK. Do not resuscitate discussions in a hospital-based home care program. J Am Geriatr Soc 1989; 37(1):52–54.

41. Joos SK, Reuler JB, Powell JL, Hickam DH. Outpatients' attitudes and understanding regarding living wills. J Gen Intern Med 1993; 8(5):259–263.

42. Johnston SC, Pfeifer MP, McNutt R. The discussion about advance directives. Patient and physician opinions regarding when and how it should be conducted. End of Life Study Group. Arch Intern Med 1995; 155(10):1025–1030.

43. Kohn M, Menon G. Life prolongation: views of elderly outpatients and health care professionals. J Am Geriatr Soc 1988; 36(9):840–844.

44. McCrary SV, Botkin JR. Hospital policy on advance directives. Do institutions ask patients about living wills? JAMA 1989; 262(17):2411–2414.

45. Lo B, McLeod GA, Saika G. Patient attitudes to discussing life-sustaining treatment. Arch Intern Med 1986; 146(8): 1613–1615.

46. Tulsky JA, Fischer GS, Rose MR, Arnold RM. Opening the black box: how do physicians communicate about advance directives? Ann Intern Med 1998; 129(6):441–449.

47. Tulsky JA, Chesney MA, Lo B. How do medical residents discuss resuscitation with patients? J Gen Intern Med 1995; 10(8):436–442.

48. Roter DL, Larson S, Fischer GS, Arnold RM, Tulsky JA. Experts practice what they preach: a descriptive study of best and normative practices in end-of-life discussions. Arch Intern Med 2000; 160(22):3477–3485.

49. Doukas DJ, McCullough LB. The values history. The evaluation of the patient's values and advance directives. J Fam Pract 1991; 32(2):145–153.

50. Emanuel LL, Emanuel EJ. The Medical Directive. A new comprehensive advance care document. JAMA 1989; 261(22):3288–3293.

51. Hickey DP. The disutility of advance directives: we know the problems, but are there solutions? J Health Law 2003; 36(3):455–473.

52. Romero LJ, Lindeman RD, Koehler KM, Allen A. Influence of ethnicity on advance directives and end-of-life decisions. JAMA 1997; 277(4):298–299.

53. Blackhall LJ, Murphy ST, Frank G, Michel V, Azen S. Ethnicity and attitudes toward patient autonomy. JAMA 1995; 274(10):820–825.

54. Caralis PV, Davis B, Wright K, Marcial E. The influence of ethnicity and race on attitudes toward advance directives, life-prolonging treatments, and euthanasia. J Clin Ethics 1993; 4(2):155–165.

55. Eleazer GP, Hornung CA, Egbert CB, et al. The relationship between ethnicity and advance directives in a frail older population. J Am Geriatr Soc 1996; 44(8):938–943.

56. Mebane EW, Oman RF, Kroonen LT, Goldstein MK. The influence of physician race, age, and gender on physician attitudes toward advance care directives and preferences for end-of-life decision-making. J Am Geriatr Soc 1999; 47(5):579–591.

57. American Medical Association. E-2.225: Optimal Use of Orders—Not-To-Intervene and Advance Directives. April 17, 2003. Available at: http://www.ama-assn.org/ama/pub/category/print/8462.html. Accessed January 22, 2004.

58. Kapp MB. Response to the living will furor: directives for maximum care. Am J Med 1982; 72(6):855–859.

59. Grodin MA. Religious advance directives: the convergence of law, religion, medicine, and public health. Am J Public Health 1993; 83(6):899–903.

60. Ridley DT. Honoring Jehovah's Witnesses' advance directives in emergencies: a response to Drs. Migden and Braen. Acad Emerg Med 1998; 5(8):824–835.

61. Kleinman I. Written advance directives refusing blood transfusion: ethical and legal considerations. Am J Med 1994; 96(6):563–567.

62. Thompson T, Barbour R, Schwartz L. Adherence to advance directives in critical care decision making: vignette study. BMJ 2003; 327(7422):1011.

63. Brett AS. Limitations of listing specific medical interventions in advance directives. JAMA 1991; 266(6):825–828.

64. Silverman HJ, Vinicky JK, Gasner MR. Advance directives: implications for critical care. Crit Care Med 1992; 20(7): 1027–1031.

65. Tonelli MR. Pulling the plug on living wills. A critical analysis of advance directives. Chest 1996; 110(3):816–822.

66. Coppola KM, Ditto PH, Danks JH, Smucker WD. Accuracy of primary care and hospital-based physicians' predictions of elderly outpatients' treatment preferences with and without advance directives. Arch Intern Med 2001; 161(3): 431–440.

67. Menikoff JA, Sachs GA, Siegler M. Beyond advance directives–health care surrogate laws. N Engl J Med 1992; 327(16):1165–1169.

68. Grisso T. Evaluating Competence. New York: Plenium Press, 1986.

69. Appelbaum PS, Grisso T. Assessing patients' capacities to consent to treatment. N Engl J Med 1988; 319(25):1635–1638.

70. Drane JF. Competency to give an informed consent. A model for making clinical assessments. JAMA 1984; 252(7): 925–927.

71. Grisso T, Appelbaum PS, Hill-Fotouhi C. The MacCAT-T: a clinical tool to assess patients' capacities to make treatment decisions. Psychiatr Serv 1997; 48(11):1415–1419.

72. Tunzi M. Can the patient decide? Evaluating patient capacity in practice. Am Fam Physician 2001; 64(2):299–306.

73. American Medical Association. E-2.20: Withholding or Withdrawing Life-Sustaining Medical Treatment. July 22,

2002. Available at: http://www.ama-assn.org/ama/pub/category/print/8457.html. Accessed January 9, 2004.

74. Yamani M, Fleming C, Brensilver JM, Brandstetter RD. Using advance directives effectively in the intensive care unit. Terminating care in the presence—or absence—of directives. J Crit Illn 1995; 10(7):465–467, 471–473.

75. Teno JM, Stevens M, Spernak S, Lynn J. Role of written advance directives in decision making: insights from qualitative and quantitative data. J Gen Intern Med 1998; 13(7):439–446.

76. Danis M, Southerland LI, Garrett JM, et al. A prospective study of advance directives for life-sustaining care. N Engl J Med 1991; 324(13):882–888.

77. Virmani J, Schneiderman LJ, Kaplan RM. Relationship of advance directives to physician-patient communication. Arch Intern Med 1994; 154(8):909–913.

78. Fischer GS, Tulsky JA, Rose MR, Siminoff LA, Arnold RM. Patient knowledge and physician predictions of treatment preferences after discussion of advance directives. J Gen Intern Med 1998; 13(7):447–454.

79. Teno JM, Lynn J, Phillips RS, et al. Do formal advance directives affect resuscitation decisions and the use of resources for seriously ill patients? SUPPORT Investigators. Study to Understand Prognoses and Preferences for Outcomes and Risks of Treatments. J Clin Ethics 1994; 5(1):23–30.

80. Goodman MD, Tarnoff M, Slotman GJ. Effect of advance directives on the management of elderly critically ill patients. Crit Care Med 1998; 26(4):701–704.

81. Emanuel EJ, Emanuel LL, Orentlicher D. Advance directives. JAMA 1991; 266(18):2563.

82. Morrison RS, Olson E, Mertz KR, Meier DE. The inaccessibility of advance directives on transfer from ambulatory to acute care settings. JAMA 1995; 274(6):478–482.

83. Pollack S. A new approach to advance directives. Crit Care Med 2000; 28(9):3146–3148.

84. Seckler AB, Meier DE, Mulvihill M, Paris BE. Substituted judgment: how accurate are proxy predictions? Ann Intern Med 1991; 115(2):92–98.

85. Suhl J, Simons P, Reedy T, Garrick T. Myth of substituted judgment. Surrogate decision making regarding life support is unreliable. Arch Intern Med 1994; 154(1):90–96.

86. Hare J, Pratt C, Nelson C. Agreement between patients and their self-selected surrogates on difficult medical decisions. Arch Intern Med 1992; 152(5):1049–1054.

87. Ouslander JG, Tymchuk AJ, Rahbar B. Health care decisions among elderly long-term care residents and their potential proxies. Arch Intern Med 1989; 149(6):1367–1372.

88. Zweibel NR, Cassel CK. Treatment choices at the end of life: a comparison of decisions by older patients and their physician-selected proxies. Gerontologist 1989; 29(5):615–621.

89. Tomlinson T, Howe K, Notman M, Rossmiller D. An empirical study of proxy consent for elderly persons. Gerontologist 1990; 30(1):54–64.

90. Uhlmann RF, Pearlman RA, Cain KC. Physicians' and spouses' predictions of elderly patients' resuscitation preferences. J Gerontol 1988; 43(5):M115–121.

91. Iserson KV. Nonstandard advance directives: a pseudoethical dilemma. J Trauma 1998; 44(1):139–142.

92. Fine RL, Mayo TW. Resolution of futility by due process: early experience with the Texas Advance Directives Act. Ann Intern Med 2003; 138(9):743–746.

93. Peterson LM. Advance directives, proxies, and the practice of surgery. Am J Surg 1992; 163(3):277–282.

94. Walker RM. DNR in the OR. Resuscitation as an operative risk. JAMA 1991; 266(17):2407–2412.

95. Cohen CB, Cohen PJ. Do-not-resuscitate orders in the operating room. N Engl J Med 1991; 325(26):1879–1882.

96. Statement of the American College of Surgeons on Advance Directives by Patients. "Do Not Resuscitate" in the operating room. Bull Am Coll Surg 1994; 79(9):29.

44
The Nonviable Patient and Organ Procurement

Frederic J. Cole, Jr., Jay N. Collins, and Leonard J. Weireter, Jr.

The current state of medical technology and critical care support is such that people who never had a chance of survival a generation ago routinely leave the hospital and return to productive lives. The unfortunate side effect of this remarkable advance is that not all patients fare so well. The patient rapidly delivered to tertiary care for resuscitation only to be found to have a lethal central nervous system disease is a common occurrence on trauma and critical care services. The concept of the non-salvageable patient and the role of futile care has become a regular part of conversations among medical staff at all levels—physician, nursing, resident, medical student, and allied health professional. Recognition of this patient is not always simple. We will argue these issues among ourselves. Who is nonsalvageable? What care is futile? How do we broach this with the families of these patients?

The evolution of solid organ transplantation needed the recognition of cerebral death criteria as a method to identify potential viable organ donors. How one determines cerebral death is unfortunately not uniform as it exists at the law—medicine interface. Criteria are agreed on, but application of the criteria is variable. Then there is the issue of how does one care for the potential donor in the workup phase of transplantation. This requires as much if not more critical care resources than the care of the original insult that culminated in cerebral death in the first place. This chapter attempts to put these issues into perspective and to offer a methodology to deal with the questions raised.

Defining the Problem

Consider two cases, which are common in the practice of emergency surgery:

1. A previously vigorous 74-year-old woman in the intensive care unit following sigmoid colectomy, end colostomy, and Hartmann's pouch for perforated diverti-culitis with peritonitis is receiving aggressive ventilator therapy for respiratory insufficiency, fluids, and low-dose vasoactive agents for distributive shock. She has mild renal insufficiency but is not requiring dialysis. She is receiving enteral nutritional support and broad-spectrum antibiotics for generalized peritonitis and returns to the operating room several times for repeated peritoneal irrigation and debridements and drainage of interloop abscesses. Gradually her sepsis resolves, the vasopressors are weaned off, her renal function improves, her respiratory function improves, and she is weaned successfully from the ventilator. She transfers to the floor and eventually goes to the acute rehabilitation unit.

2. A 68-year-old man sustains a fall from a ladder while cleaning out the gutters. He suffers a right flail chest with fractures of ribs 3 to 8, right hemopneumothorax treated by right tube thoracostomy, and a closed midshaft tibia fracture. He undergoes intramedullary nailing of the tibia fracture the day of injury and is admitted to the intensive care unit postoperatively for monitoring. He has a history significant only for mild hypertension and diabetes. Despite aggressive pain control measures, his pulmonary toilet is poor. He develops progressive respiratory dysfunction, culminating in intubation and mechanical ventilation. He develops a Gram-negative ventilator-associated pneumonia requiring broad-spectrum antibiotic therapy. Despite appropriate stress ulcer prophylaxis, he suffers a hemodynamically significant upper gastrointestinal bleed requiring endoscopic intervention. He develops acute renal failure related to his hemorrhage and requires dialysis. Over the ensuing weeks, his condition waxes and wanes with rallying periods during which he seems to clear his infections and begins to make progress in being weaned from the ventilator. Such a rally is then followed by another fever spike, leukocytosis, positive culture, drop in blood pressure, and intolerance of work of breathing and enteral feeding. Support is increased; another rally ensues, followed by deterioration.

Surgeons are trained and comfortable with the first scenario. They expect to intervene surgically in the diseases of critically ill patients and then support them as they recover. They are comfortable employing the variety of advanced technologies, therapies, medicines, and surgical techniques common in the modern intensive care unit to return their critically ill patients to their previous state of health. This is, after all, why we admit our patients to intensive care units: to employ technology in the form of monitoring devices, ventilators and respiratory care, dialysis machines, and medicines such as antibiotics, sedatives, analgesics and vasoactive agents to support their vital functions and physiology as they recover from their primary disease processes.

Surgeons are much less comfortable with the second scenario, which is all too familiar despite all of the advanced technologies and therapies available in the modern intensive care unit. Up to 40% of intensive care unit patients do not survive to leave the hospital.[1-3] As the scenario implies, the physiology and vital functions of such patients can be maintained for quite some time before an irreversible terminal event occurs. Such maintenance does not come without cost. There is an obvious monetary cost to continuing to provide aggressive intensive care. The rising percentage of the Gross Domestic Product that the cost of medical care represents in our country has led to pressure from employers, the federal government, and third-party payers on doctors and hospitals to keep costs down. A significant portion of this money is spent in the last weeks of life in intensive care units.[4]

There is also a cost in terms of resources. Hospital beds in general and intensive care beds in particular are at a premium as hospitals struggle with staffing shortages and need for efficiency. It is all too common for the emergency departments of our hospitals to be boarding a number of critically ill patients waiting for an intensive care unit bed. There are human costs to providing this support as well. The patient is frequently in pain and fearful or anxious.[1] There is an emotional toll on families and caregivers as repeated efforts fail to restore health.[5] Inevitably, someone begins to question whether aggressive care with curative intent should continue. This may be a family member or one of the critical care team.

The Problem with Futility

There has been a change in the last 40 years in how such issues are addressed and managed.[6] This change parallels a shift in the ethical imperative in the doctor–patient relationship from the historical norm of benign paternalism to one of primacy of patient autonomy.[6-8] Whereas there was little room for discussion in the past when the physician, the subject matter expert, recommended a course of

treatment, today we place a great deal of emphasis on the need for the patient (or the patient's surrogate) to actively participate in selecting the appropriate course of action. Thus any unilateral decision on the part of the physician to continue curative care or to withdraw life-sustaining therapies is today viewed with disdain.[9]

Interestingly, this emphasis on patient autonomy has emerged even as physicians have become more willing to limit and/or withdraw aggressive life-sustaining therapy. In contrast to the Karen Quinlan case in which conflict between Ms. Quinlan's physicians and family arose over the wish of the family to have potentially life-sustaining therapy (the ventilator) discontinued and the doctors' refusal, today the conflict is more likely to be over the insistence of the family that some life-sustaining therapy be continued after the critical care team believes that there is no hope of any long-term benefit from continuation of the therapy.[8,10]

This leads inevitably to a discussion of medical futility. There are legal and ethical precedents that physicians need not provide futile care.[6,8,11,12] From a physician's perspective, this concept is at first deceivingly simple. The historical goal after all is to return the patient to his or her premorbid state of health, and, failing that, returning them to an acceptable state of health with minimal morbidity. Being able to function independently, or with some assistance, but, at a minimum, being able to interact with one's environment in a meaningful manner are laudable goals, and physicians quickly point them out. Some have advocated that determination of futility is purely a function of the medical staff assessing the patient, determining that there is no realistic hope for meaningful recovery, and making the "diagnosis" of futility.[8-11]

There are a number of problems with physician-defined futility. First, determining which patients cannot achieve meaningful survival is less than an exact science. Physicians are certainly subject matter experts with respect to disease, options for treatment, and prognosis, but they are not able to accurately predict who will survive and who will not.[1] There are a number of severity of illness scores: Simplified Acute Physiology Score (SAPS), Injury Severity Score (ISS), Mortality Prediction Model (MPM), Therapeutic Intervention Scoring System (TISS), and the various versions of Acute Physiology and Chronic Health Evaluation (APACHE), among others. None has reliably been demonstrated to accurately predict mortality for individual patients[10,13] Any physician who has cared for critically ill patients for any length of time can relate stories of patients who all thought were hopeless only to see them walk back into the unit months later to thank the staff.

Second is the matter of defining meaningful survival. Differing life experiences, religious traditions, and education will lead to different definitions. For some, any life is God-given and therefore inviolable. For others, the absence of higher cortical function (persistent vegetative state) is synonymous with an unacceptable existence, making efforts to maintain vital functions futile. In the final analysis, determination of futility always involves a value judgment. Physicians are not subject matter experts in this arena. A third problem with physician-determined futility has already been suggested. The rising cost of medical care has put pressure on hospitals and doctors to be cost effective. Thus there is an implicit conflict of interest for the physician who is tasked with managing hospital and societal resources at the same time that one is providing optimum care for individual patients.

The patient then is left with the task of determining what futility is.[10] The physician serves to inform the patient regarding reasonable expectations for what may transpire with various courses of action.[14] Unlike the situation of a patient with a progressing malignancy, patients in the intensive care unit for whom these discussions become pertinent are rarely able to participate in them at the time that they become pertinent.[1] The decision then falls to the patient's surrogate, usually the next of kin, but potentially a court-appointed guardian when there is no next of kin.[8,10,14]

Communication Is the Key

One result of the shift to an emphasis on patient autonomy in the patient—physician relationship is that many patients will have executed "living wills," or medical powers of attorney, which may provide insight into what the patient's wishes might be in the event of catastrophic illness. Hospitals are now required to inquire and document patients' preferences with respect to resuscitation.[15] There is an increased awareness of these issues by the lay public through television programs and other media, and families are more likely to have discussed these issues than in the past.

Nevertheless, there is some reluctance to engage patients or their families in discussion of these issues. Some providers fear that they will unnecessarily alarm the patient and family or that such conversation will give a false sense that the team is abandoning the patient.[1,13,16,17] Indeed, abruptly engaging in a discussion regarding withdrawal of care after weeks of aggressive curative care can be confusing to the family as well as the critical care team. A better approach is one of continuing conversations in which current condition, planned interventions, and expectations are honestly discussed.[1,13,17–19] Such discussions should involve all available stakeholders: patient/family/surrogate, physicians, nurses, therapists, clergy, and social workers. There has been little formal training in how to conduct such conversations in the past. Inadequate training can also lead to inhibition in addressing end of life issues.

There are a number of models for these discussions. The most familiar is the "family conference" in which a formal meeting is arranged involving all of the parties mentioned above. Frequently such meetings are called to ask "the question" of the family when the physicians believe that further curative efforts are not of benefit. These then become high-stakes discussions with a significant amount of tension. There are less formal "daily updates," which generally involve physicians, nurses, or other members of the critical care team transmitting information regarding the patient's condition to the family in a more informal setting, often at the bedside. Unfortunately, these conversations do not always address what the patient's wishes may or may not have been. They tend to be focused on where the patient is on the road to recovery and what the next therapeutic or diagnostic steps may be. A new innovation in transmitting information to families is the practice in many intensive care units of having family members attend and participate in daily rounds. This provides the family with medical information and with an opportunity for discussions regarding the patient's previously stated goals and wishes.

Whatever method is utilized, the crucial element is that there is an ongoing dialogue between the critical care team and the decision makers. Early discussion of what the patient's values and goals are regarding their health and life combined with realistic assessment of the patient's risk of death and impairment are critical to forging a mutually supportive relationship between the family and the health care team. Such a relationship allows the family and the providers to work together continuously to meet the patient's goals rather than coming together for high-stakes decision making regarding discontinuation of life-sustaining therapy at the end of the patient's illness without a solid basis for working together.

There can be a continuum from curative to palliative care using this approach.[20] There is emphasis on relief of symptoms and patient autonomy throughout the episode of care. When possible, conversations before illness or surgery among family, patient, and physician can lay the groundwork by establishing the patient's values, goals, and expectations for treatment. Decisions can be made regarding limitations and end points of therapy that the patient finds appropriate. In the world of acute care surgery, such discussions can rarely occur as the acute treatment plan is developed and implemented. Early and ongoing discussions with the family can be utilized to learn what may have been discussed earlier in the nonacute setting among the patient, the family, and/or the primary care physician. There may be a living will, which should be sought for inclusion in the medical record.

As treatment proceeds and milestones are either met or missed, reassessment of the consistency of the current plan with the patient's goals can be determined. Each therapy can be evaluated with respect to its ability to help the patient achieve the goal of therapy. Treatments that do not further the patient's goals may be withdrawn.[1,4,13,18] As "cure" is increasingly recognized to not be a realistic goal, the focus changes and palliative therapies, instituted at the outset, are the only ones left in place. The importance of involvement of the entire health care team cannot be overemphasized. All stakeholders must possess the same objective data and subjective evaluations of those data to formulate a coherent and cohesive plan of care.

Once the decision is made to change the focus of care from cure to palliation, it is important to understand how such care is most effectively delivered. There is an abundance of evidence that patients and their families have not been satisfied with the end-of-life care being provided in intensive care units.[1,19,21] Consistent areas of concern are communication and symptom relief. Both of these components must be adequately addressed for effective end-of-life care to be rendered.[1,18,19,21,22]

End-of-Life Care

The importance of effective communication has already been emphasized with respect to including all stakeholders in the conversation and sharing all relevant data, opinions, and thoughts. How the communication occurs is at least as important as the information being exchanged. Surgeons, physicians, and nurses are busy people. There is never enough time in the day to accomplish all that lies before us. Nevertheless, it is imperative that the health care workers be invested in these conversations leading to and following a decision to cease seeking cure. It is important that the family know that the surgeon is committed to the process and is not "squeezing them in" between cases.[22] These discussions must not be rushed. The family needs the opportunity to work through the issues and to express their opinions, beliefs, and concerns. This cannot be done effectively on the fly in the hallway. A comfortable room apart from the intensive care unit needs to be available for such conversations to occur in private without interruption.[19,22]

Although autonomy dictates that the ultimate decision regarding cessation of curative care lies with the family, the primary physician must take an active role in the decision to pursue palliative end-of-life care. The physician must lend medical expertise to the process as well as shepherding the family through its steps: not deciding for them, but facilitating their decision. This may involve sharing their opinions, feelings, and doubts in a genuine and honest manner. Such interactions may require clinicians to expose their own vulnerabilities and preclude them from maintaining a safe emotional distance. Thus clinicians must have come to terms with their own thoughts about death and dying and be comfortable sharing them.[22]

There are a number of issues to be addressed in providing effective end-of-life care. Communication has been emphasized and cannot be overemphasized. The surgeon, nurses, and other professionals who were involved in the process of shifting focus to palliation must continue to be attentive to the patient and the family.[1,18,19,22] Assurances to this effect must be given and realized. Some of the dissatisfaction families have reported in recent years has to do with the sense of abandonment caused by infrequent assessments by and interactions with the staff once the decision to abandon seeking cure is made. Effective care mandates frequent assessments of the efficacy of prescribed therapies and emergence of new symptoms.[1] Realistic information regarding the anticipated course needs to be communicated to the family, updated, and changed as the clinical situation changes.[22]

The focus of end-of-life care is symptom relief for the patient. Further details regarding specific strategies are outlined below. Frequent assessment of symptoms and therapies should be undertaken as noted earlier. The family should be involved in this evaluation as well. Pain relief tends to be the primary end point. Evidence of pain may include restlessness, agitation, tachycardia, hypertension, and tachypnea. Other concerns may include anxiety, dyspnea, abdominal distension or pain, and nausea. There may be a trade-off between alertness and symptom relief. Which gets preference is determined through ongoing discussions with the family and patient if he or she are able to participate.

The family must also be included in the care. It is a tremendously stressful time as they anticipate the loss of their loved one. Ideally they should have access to a waiting room in proximity to the intensive care unit. It should be comfortable with telephone access to an outside line and a television. Some intensive care units make Internet access available to patients' families, and post updates on patient condition to the unit Web page. The family should have ready if not immediate access to nourishment and refreshments. There should be nearby accommodations (within the hospital) for them to sleep as well.[23]

Access to the patient should be liberal. If the intensive care unit has restricted visiting hours, they should be opened up for the family, allowing them to spend as much time as possible and desired with their loved one. Restrictions on personal items should be liberalized as well as restrictions on the number of visitors to the extent possible. The family may also be allowed and encouraged to participate in personal care of the patient if desired.[1,17,23] To some extent this re-creates the situation in the past when people died at home with their families attending to them. Being able to provide hands-on comfort care to their loved one can greatly assist some family members in coming to acceptance and work through their grief.

All therapies must be evaluated for their contribution to the goal of symptom relief. Many routine interventions such as daily laboratory tests will be discontinued on this basis to prevent the pain of venipuncture. Agents for oral thrush may be continued as providing treatment for the symptoms related to the infection, whereas systemic antibiotics for other infections may be discontinued, especially if the agents require intravenous access. Fevers are treated with antipyretics, but ice packs and other topical coolants are avoided as being productive of discomfort.[18]

Symptoms of pain and distress are well treated with narcotics, such as morphine, and benzodiazepines. Transdermal narcotic administration systems are particularly useful if intravenous access is a problem. Respiratory depression is rarely observed in this patient population despite significant doses. One series demonstrated no difference in time to death for patients who received narcotics and those who did not. The implication is that it is the disease process that determines time of death.[18,24] Haloperidol can be of use if there is also delirium present. Doses of all agents must be titrated to effect. Use of pain and sedation scales may be very useful.

Withdrawal of Life-Sustaining Treatment

All of the foregoing processes described as being optimal palliation are appropriate for both curative care and end-of-life care. The area of removing therapies that are deemed inconsistent with the goals of palliation when the decision has been made that cure is no longer a reasonable end point is a frequent concern for many practitioners. While no provider is interested in continuing modalities that are frequently painful or at least uncomfortable, may interfere with interaction with family members, or create other problems when they are no longer deemed capable of returning the patient to health, neither are they interested in causing pain, distress, or being accused of assisting suicide or killing the patient.

With respect to the last point first, it is appropriate to recall that discontinuation of an unwanted therapy is equivalent ethically and legally to withholding the therapy in the first place. The principle of autonomy allows patients to choose what therapies they will and will not accept. This is different from the situation in which a patient requests an intervention that has no purpose other than to hasten or cause death—so-called physician-assisted suicide. This last remains illegal in most places in the United States. Legitimate therapies or treatments have as their goal restoration of health. When this is no longer possible, or when the burden of the treatment is too great in the opinion of the patient or the surrogate, the treatment may be foregone.

The interventions most likely to be considered for withdrawal in the intensive care environment are mechanical ventilation, administration of vasopressors and inotropes, hemodialysis, antibiotics, enteral/parenteral nutrition, and intravenous fluids.[18] The last to be withdrawn is likely to be mechanical ventilation because of concerns regarding airway maintenance and symptoms of respiratory insufficiency. Some practitioners will remove the interventions sequentially, saving ventilation for last in the hope that the patient will expire without needing to have the ventilator removed.[13,18] The areas of nutrition and hydration are the others most likely to be problematic for clinicians and families to remove.[18,23] Concerns regarding both of these actions can be addressed through consideration of symptoms likely to result and how to treat those symptoms.

Removal of vasopressors and inotropes will likely result in hypotension, and frequently death rapidly ensues. There may rarely be agitation, but this is well treated with sequential doses of a benzodiazepine.[23] The consequences of discontinuing hemodialysis—acidosis, fluid overload, uremia, and electrolyte imbalance—for the most part require no intervention.[18] Uremia may result in gastritis that can be managed with antacids or acid-secretion suppression. Dyspnea from hypervolemia or uremic pericardial or pleural effusions may be relieved by administration of oxygen, morphine, benzodiazepines, and fluid restriction.[18] Discontinuation of antibiotics rarely causes symptoms. If fever is present and causing the patient discomfort, it can be treated with antipyretics, alternating acetaminophen with nonsteroidal antiinflammatory agents.[18]

Those who are dying typically do not experience hunger. In fact, administration of feedings may cause abdominal distention and distress.[18,23] Knowledge of these facts goes a long way in eliminating concern about "withholding food" from the patient and allowing them to "starve." The dying similarly do not often complain of thirst but do commonly complain of dry mouth. Sips of liquids, ice chips, and use of glycerin swabs, lip balm, and petroleum jelly can all be useful in relieving this symptom. Continued provision of adequate oral hygiene is also important. Thrush should be treated with antimonilial agents. Nausea when it occurs can be treated with a number of antiemetics.

There are different approaches to discontinuation of mechanical ventilation: immediate extubation, terminal weaning with or without extubation, discontinuation of the ventilator without weaning, and continuation of intubation. There are proponents of each method who typically justify their approach as being more comfortable for the patient. Regardless of which approach is selected, appropriate preparation is necessary. The degree of respiratory insufficiency should be assessed so that the family can be properly counseled as to what to expect:

rapid demise or independent ventilation for some time. The family must also understand that independent ventilation may continue for days or weeks or even become permanent (e.g., in the case of the persistently vegetative patient with no other significant organ dysfunction). The family and the caregivers should all understand what symptoms are likely to occur and what treatments to relieve the symptoms will be administered.[1,13,18,22,23]

Before mechanical ventilation is discontinued, administration of an anxiolytic such as midazolam is appropriate. If the ventilator support is to be gradually decreased to off (terminal wean), distress in the form of tachypnea, tachycardia, and restlessness may occur. These symptoms may be effectively treated with bolus doses of morphine, additional doses of midazolam, and/or a morphine infusion. Titration of the medications may be necessary to keep symptoms in check. Good tracheal toilet before extubation and an antisecretory agent (glycopyrrolate) may reduce problems with secretions (although creating dry mouth).

In contrast to the controlled discontinuation of life support that follows discussions about the futility of further care and what the patient would desire, families are often thrown into chaos when their loved one has suffered a rapid-onset devastating cerebral event. Subarachnoid hemorrhage from a ruptured aneurysm, blunt cerebral injury from a motor vehicle crash or assault, or a gunshot wound to the head renders the victim almost but not quite dead. Worse yet, while the brain has been devastated the remainder of cardiopulmonary function continues almost as if nothing has happened. The deterioration of cerebral function can be tracked as the brain stem reflexes are lost from cephalad to caudad. Eventually the lowest lying reflexes, those controlling spontaneous respiratory drive and heart rate control, are lost. Unfortunately, the patient still exhibits a blood pressure, heart rate, and body temperature because of our intensive interventions. We tell families that their loved one is dead. They ask how, the monitor shows a blood pressure and heart rate. Now begins a potentially tedious and uncomfortable discussion about how people can die because their brain is dead.

Lifenet, our organ procurement organization, has developed a program utilizing specially trained chaplains to facilitate this discussion with families of a potential organ donor. After the family has been informed that cerebral death criteria have been met, this chaplain approaches the family regarding organ donation. It is clear that this chaplain is separate from the team caring for the patient before the declaration of cerebral death. They are there to discuss organ donation, inquire as to the wishes of the patient regarding donation, if known, and answer questions that guide the family through the process of considering donation.

The Determination of Brain Death

The brain is the organ most sensitive to loss of oxygen and perfusion. Its function may be irreversibly lost despite preservation of other organ functions. However, the advances in intensive care units over the years have allowed many patients who would have died to now survive for days or weeks without evidence of neurologic activity or hope for recovery. This progress in health care identified a major problem: What should be done for patients with no chance of recovery of neurologic function? In 1968, an ad hoc committee at Harvard University defined irreversible coma, or brain death, as a persistent comatose state of a known etiology with the absence of movement, brain stem reflexes, and breathing.[25] Based on this information, the American Bar Association, American Medical Association, and the National Conference of Commissioners on Uniform State Laws developed the Uniform Determination of Death Act in 1980.[26] In it, death has occurred in "an individual who has sustained either (1) irreversible cessation of circulatory and respiratory functions, or (2) irreversible cessation of all functions of the entire brain, including the brain stem. A determination of death must be in accordance with accepted medical standards." This declaration is accepted as law in all 50 states.

However, there is no one defined method to determine brain death. The criteria for the declaration of brain death are established by the individual states and vary from state to state. In some states, state law outlines the procedure for the determination of brain death. In others, the individual hospital facilities have the authority to enact a policy that describes the procedure for the determination of brain death. Written documentation of loss of all neurologic activity by either one or two licensed physicians is usually all that is required. In some states, one of the physicians is required to be a neurospecialist, but this may not always be possible, especially in smaller hospitals. In some states there must be an interval of 6 hours between the times of examinations, whereas in others no time interval is required.[27] The determination of brain death does need to be in accordance with acceptable medical standards. In general, brain death is demonstrated by the complete loss of activity of the cerebral cortex with the absence of function of the midbrain, pons, and medulla. This is clinically demonstrated by the persistence of a comatose state, loss of all brain stem reflexes, and loss of spontaneous respirations. These guidelines were published by the American Academy of Neurology in 1995.[27]

The declaration of brain death requires a thorough neurologic examination, certainty about the etiology of the patient's comatose state, and exclusion of contributing factors.[28] Severe hypothermia, locked-in syndrome, drug intoxication, and Guillan-Barre syndrome with cranial nerve involvement are all examples of conditions that may mimic a state of persistent coma.[29] The certainty of irreversibility of the comatose state must be established as well as the etiology. In adults brain death is most often a result of cerebrovascular disease or traumatic brain injury.[29] A computed tomographic (CT) scan of the brain is essential in determining the etiology of coma. This may reveal a mass effect, herniation of the brain stem, infarction, hemorrhage, or edema. At times the early CT findings after cardiopulmonary arrest, hypoperfusion, or central nervous system (CNS) infections may be normal, and follow-up CT scans are warranted. If the head CT is normal and suspicion of CNS infections is high, a diagnostic lumbar puncture is indicated.

Before brain death is considered, the individual must be as physiologically normal as possible. Severe electrolyte, acid–base, or endocrine abnormalities must be corrected and excluded as causes of the coma. Patients must be free of all toxins, sedatives, narcotics, neuromuscular blockers, and other mind-altering drugs. This may require a period of observation to ensure that all drugs have been metabolized and eliminated. Patients must be normotensive and normothermic. Patients may be receiving vasopressors as needed to maintain a normal blood pressure (a mean arterial pressure of 60 mm Hg or greater). Coma from hypothermia must be excluded. Rewarming measures may be required until the core temperature is at least 32°C.[27]

Once a patient is thought to have sustained an irreversible brain injury and is metabolically normal, a thorough neurologic examination needs to be performed. The diagnosis of brain death requires documentation of a coma, absence of brain stem reflexes, and apnea. A persistent comatose state is one in which there is no response to any type of external stimuli. Patients do not spontaneously open their eyes or respond to verbal commands. Painful stimulation such as supraorbital or nail bed pressure does not result in movement or withdrawal of any extremity. However, spinal reflexes remain intact in a brain dead patient. This may result in spontaneous movements of the arms and legs or flexion at the waist. Although these movements can be shocking, this does not contradict the diagnosis of brain death if all other criteria are met. Decorticate or decerebrate posturing and seizure activity imply cortical activity and are not consistent with brain death.

An examination of brain stem reflexes reflective of cranial nerve (CN) function needs to be completed next.[27] Pupillary response to light measures the activity of CNs II and III. Fixed and dilated pupils unresponsive to light suggest loss of midbrain function. Gentle touching of the cornea with a cotton tip swab normally results in blinking of the eye. Loss of this corneal reflex (CNs V and VII) suggests loss of mid pons activity. If the eyes remain fixed forward with rapid rotation of the head, loss of the oculocephalic reflex (CNs VIII, III, and VI) has occurred. Loss of the oculovestibular reflex (CNs VIII, III, and VI) implies loss of lower pons activity. This occurs when ice-cold water is instilled in the ear canal and the eyes do not move. Pharyngeal (gag) and tracheal (cough) reflexes (CNs IX and X) are best tested by irritating the hypopharynx with a tongue depressor or the trachea with a suction catheter through the endotracheal tube. Absence of all of these central reflexes demonstrates loss of function of the midbrain and pons.

After the loss of brain stem reflexes has been documented, the presence of apnea must be demonstrated. While keeping the patient well oxygenated, one looks for the absence of respirations in response to an elevated partial pressure of carbon dioxide (pCO_2). The patient is initially preoxygenated with 100% oxygen.[29] Arterial blood gas (ABG) is then measured to document a normal pCO_2 (38 to 42 mm Hg). The ventilator is turned off and a catheter is placed through the endotracheal tube to the level of the carina. Oxygen is delivered at 6 to 10 L/min. Oxygen saturation is continuously measured by a pulse oximeter. During the apnea test the physician must remain at the bedside for the entire test period to watch for the absence of respiratory efforts. Any attempt at respiration shows the patient to have some function of the medulla oblongata, and the test is negative. Without respirations, the pCO_2 usually rises 3 to 5 mm Hg/min. After 5 to 8 minutes an ABG sample is drawn. If the pCO_2 is greater than 60 mm Hg or has risen more than 20 mm Hg from baseline and the patient has demonstrated no efforts at respiration, the apnea test is positive and supports the diagnosis of brain death.

If these tests cannot be reliably performed or are indeterminate, other confirmatory tests may need to be performed. It may be difficult to do cranial nerve testing in patients with facial trauma or previous ocular abnormalities. Patients with severe drug intoxication may require an extended period of time to clear their system of the drugs. It may not be possible to do an apnea test on a patient with chronic obstructive pulmonary disease, severe retention of CO_2, or severe hypoxemia. These confirmatory tests are also recommended for children under 1 year of age.[30]

The absence of blood flow to the brain is diagnostic of brain death. No visualization of the intracranial arteries on cerebral angiography results when intracranial pressure is greater than systemic arterial pressure. The external carotid artery may fill, but there is no visualization of flow at the circle of Willis or at the base of the skull. A nuclear brain scan with technetium has good correlation with angiography and will show no intracranial uptake of the radionucleotide. This results in the "hollow skull" sign and is diagnostic of brain death. Transcranial Doppler ultrasonography can also demonstrate lack of blood flow to the brain. Small systolic peaks in early systole without diastolic flow or reverberating flow indicate a very high vascular resistance and elevated intracranial pressure.[31] Finally, absent electrical activity for at least 30 minutes on electroencephalography supports the diagnosis of brain death.

Once an individual has been declared brain dead, that person is legally dead and all artificial means of support, including the ventilator, may be discontinued. However, it is appropriate to discuss this diagnosis with the family before removing support. Ideally the family is aware of the severity of the situation and the diagnosis of brain death is not a surprise. The option of organ donation may be considered at this time but is best approached from someone outside the primary health care team.

Care of the Potential Organ Donor

Once patients are determined to be brain dead and potential organ donors, they are at risk for a number of adverse events unless fastidious attention is directed to their care. Complicating factors include the disease processes that lead to cerebral death and the subsequent deterioration as CNS regulation of vital physiologic functions is lost. Trauma with its soft tissue injury, hemorrhage-related shock, and preexisting coronary artery disease become important contributors to the physiologic demise of the potential donor. The time constraints imposed are variable, ranging from very short for a hemodynamically unstable patient to almost as long as 18 to 24 hours.

Adequate tissue perfusion is essential to maintaining satisfactory end-organ function for transplantation. The end points of resuscitation include normalizing hemodynamics and maintaining acid–base balance, normal coagulation function, and temperature control. A urine output of 0.5 to 1.0 mL/kg/hr is a common surrogate of adequate perfusion. Care of the potential donor can be a challenge as the mechanisms of dying clash with the need to maintain physiologic viability. This section addresses care of the potential donor in the time interval during which tissue typing and donor evaluation occurs before harvesting and transplantation. The focus is on common conditions encountered and their treatment.

Cardiovascular System Issues

Cardiovascular integrity is required to maintain an adequate donor for organ transplantation. A minimum mean arterial pressure of 60 to 70 mm Hg should be the goal as this will ensure adequate organ perfusion. Pressure measurement devices include automated cuff measurements, depending on auscultatory technology and arterial lines. Although both methodologies have advantages and disadvantages, the ability to sample blood via the arterial line makes that the preferable method for measuring blood pressure. Location of the arterial line is at the discretion of the practitioner, and common practice favors the radial or brachial position. Femoral arterial catheterization for pressure monitoring carries an increased infection risk and is discouraged, although there are circumstances in which that route should be used. Fastidious attention to detail to minimize infection and other risks is necessary to preserve optimal end-organ function.

Shock, the inability to meet the oxygen needs of the tissue beds, is a common problem and will interfere with transplantation success unless dealt with rapidly and correctly. Shock can be the result of the injury or disease state that preceded cerebral death but can also arise from the treatment of that injury or disease. Hypotension, usually as a manifestation of hypovolemic shock, is common. This may occur when hemorrhage has been inadequately treated. Overly aggressive diuretic therapy directed at intracranial pressure may also decrease blood pressure. Diabetes insipidus with inadequate fluid replacement will also decrease blood pressure. Alternatively, hypotension may result from vasodilation as occurs in severe infection. The intrinsic pumping function of the heart may be so compromised that the cardiac output fails to increase blood pressure appropriately to meet end-organ needs. Regardless of etiology, rapid determination of cause and institution of treatment are essential if organ function suitable for transplantation is to be achieved.

The parties responsible for maintaining the potential donor need a thorough understanding of the events leading to cerebral death determination. Detailed conversation with the team treating the patient before cerebral death declaration will help clarify many of these details. Not uncommonly, the Organ Procurement Agency has a long-standing relationship with the intensive care practitioners and is in close communication with them leading up to the declaration of cerebral death. The family, once consent for donation has occurred, may be a good source for background medical information that might not be related to the events leading to cerebral death. A thorough medical history is part of the Organ Procurement Agency representatives' requirements, but instability in the potential donor and the urgency to treat may preclude that discussion from occurring in a timely fashion.

The etiology of hypotension may be multifactorial. Hemorrhage control needs to be ensured. Replacement of intravascular volume should readily correct the pressure if hypovolemia is the issue. Central venous pressure determination is an adjunct to shock therapy in that determination of the filling pressures of the right heart can be used as a surrogate for left ventricular end diastolic volume determination. Ideally, central venous pressure should be maintained in the range of 8 to 12 mm Hg.

More specific information can be determined with a flow-directed pulmonary artery catheter. This allows measurement of the pulmonary artery pressure at occlusion of the pulmonary artery, the "wedge" pressure, which in the absence of mitral valve pathology looks directly into the left atrium and ventricle during diastole. Normal pressures range from 12 to 15 mm Hg. Cardiac output can be determined with a pulmonary artery catheter and a variety of physiologic variables calculated from the data determined. Central venous oxygen saturation measured from the pulmonary artery is available and is used to determine if whole-body oxygen utilization is appropriate.

The decision to use one device versus another is dictated by the stability of the patient, the preceding clinical course, and the need for greater information to help elucidate the reasons for ongoing hemodynamic instability. The risks of both devices are low in experienced hands. Pneumothorax with subsequent pulmonary complications occurs in approximately 2% of central venous line placements. The pulmonary artery catheter has a risk of cardiac valvular damage or of inciting arrhythmias in certain populations. As with any invasive device, it is the responsibility of the health care professional to balance the risk of the device with the benefit derived from the information the device provides.

Once the type of central pressure monitoring has been decided, the practitioner needs to be attentive to the data derived. Fluid administration may take the form of crystalloid or colloid. The argument here is beyond the scope of this discussion and is frequently left to a given protocol employed by the treating institution. It is important to realize that dogmatic adherence to any given position may be detrimental, and fluid administered should reflect the needs of the patient. Packed red blood cell transfusion for ongoing hemorrhage or significant anemia, fresh-frozen plasma or platelets for specific coagulopathy defects, and crystalloid fluids for dehydration replacement as commonly seen with the development of diabetes insipidus represent appropriate utilization of these substances.

The balance between over- and underhydration underscores the crystalloid colloid controversy. Ideally, one would like to construct a Starling curve with optimal cardiac output response to ensure end-organ perfusion. Failing that, one needs to be suspicious that specific diseases such as pneumothorax, tension pneumothorax, cardiac tamponade, or cardiogenic shock may be present. Identification and treatment of a specific condition should lead to resolution and return to stable, normal hemodynamics.

Associated with brain injury is a release of catecholamines, epinephrine, norepinephrine, and dopamine. Cerebral herniation is accompanied by a profound coronary vasospasm that may induce significant myocardial ischemia with decreases in cardiac contractility that occur over minutes to hours. As cerebral death is completed and neural control lost, there will be a profound vasodilation with further drop in blood pressure as a relative hypovolemia is induced.[32-35] Aggressive use of echocardiography to evaluate contractile function and measure ejection fraction may be the best way to track this development and monitor therapy. Pharmacologic support of the failing heart and circulation requires judicious use of alpha- and beta-agonists to provide inotropic support for contractility while controlling heart rate so as not to further exacerbate myocardial ischemia.[36] If adequate preload has been obtained, as measured by central filling pressures, and mean arterial pressure is still less than 60 mm Hg, cardiac contractility may be augmented with inotropic agents such as dopamine. Dosing can begin between 5 and 10 mg/kg/min. The point is that hypotension with mean arterial pressure less than 60 mm Hg needs rapid treatment. Fluids plus inotropic agents to increase the mean arterial pressure are essential. Maintaining this pressure between 80 and 90 mm Hg is a reasonable goal. Alternatively, the systolic blood pressure needs to be maintained greater than 100 mm Hg. A more aggressive inotropic agent use should be discussed with the transplant surgeons. Use of such agents may be part of a predetermined resuscitation protocol. The inability to keep the mean arterial pressure above 60 mm Hg will compromise donor organ function and threaten the viability of the donor.

The role of thyroid hormone replacement therapy in this situation is controversial. Triiodothyronine infusion is associated with increased myocardial contractility independent of beta-receptors, possibly because of calcium-dependent cardiac contractile proteins.[37-39] The decision to use or not to use such replacement should be the result of specific protocol development by the treating team. A typical dosing regimen is levothyroxine 200 μg/250 mL normal saline (NS) and begun at 20 μg/hr and 25 mL/hr, with a maximum dose of 30 μg/hour to keep systolic blood pressure above 100 mm Hg.

Alternative etiologies of hypotension include specific medication effects during support of the patient in the time leading up to cerebral death declaration. Aggressive diuretic therapy leading to hypovolemia should be detected and volume status restored. The use of barbiturate coma can result in a negative inotropic effect on the heart. This should be resolved before the declaration of cerebral death but may have residual effects that need to be addressed independently.

A specific cause of hypovolemia with cardiac consequences is the development of diabetes insipidus. The loss of hypothalamic–pituitary function with decreased release of posterior pituitary hormones, especially vasopressin, results in an unchecked urinary output as the antidiuretic effect is lost. Volume-for-volume fluid replacement is necessary, and intravenous vasopressin may be needed to ameliorate the condition. The diagnosis of diabetes insipidus is made by the production of large volumes, often several hundred milliliters per hour, of dilute urine as characterized by a specific gravity less than 1.005.

Hypertension, a mean arterial pressure consistently above 100 mm Hg, can cause adverse cardiac effects if left untreated. Hypertension and bradycardia are the cardiovascular hallmarks that accompany brain stem herniation and require no particular treatment other than that directed at the CNS pathology. Long-standing hypertension increases the stress on the myocardium, and the degree of injury is a function of the degree and duration of the hypertension. Short-acting beta-blockers or carefully titrated vasodilating agents can be used intravenously to obtain the blood pressure control necessary. Sodium nitroprusside in doses of 0.3 μg/kg/min up to 10 μg/kg/min may be used to control severe hypertension. Rapid vasodilatation with sudden drops in mean arterial pressure can occur with nitroprusside use, so fastidious titration is essential. Frequently, hypertension requires no specific therapy other than awareness of its presence.

Fluid and Electrolyte Issues

Fluid and electrolyte disturbances are commonly seen in the potential organ donor. They, like the cardiovascular abnormalities, result from the disease process leading to cerebral death or from the therapy preceding cerebral death declaration, or they are sequelae of the loss of neurologic control that accompanies death. Vasopressin is elaborated by the posterior pituitary and acts as a potent antidiuretic agent under normal conditions. With the development of cerebral demise the pituitary no longer elaborates vasopressin with the resultant loss of regulation of renal tubule function.[40–42] Urine output consists of dramatic volumes of dilute urine, as no concentrating or resorptive ability exists. A urine specific gravity less than or equal to 1.005 in the face of no diuretic therapy and urine output frequently in excess of hundreds of milliliters hourly supports the diagnosis. Therapy is directed at reestablishing the hormonal control of fluid resorption in the kidney. Vasopressin administered as an intravenous bolus dose of 5–10 units followed by a titratable infusion in conjunction with volume-for-volume replacement of urinary loss with 0.25 NS can readily correct the problem. Alternatively, intermittent doses of intravenous desmopressin, 1–2 μg every 2 hours, until urine output is in the range of 200 mL/hr, can be used. Pros and cons of vasopressin and desmopressin center on the vasoconstrictive effects of vasopressin on donor organs and potential detrimental effects of desmopressin on the transplanted kidney.[43–45]

The free water deficit induced by such diuresis can be substantial and requires aggressive correction. The hypernatremia that accompanies diabetes insipidus is a reflection of water loss far in excess of any sodium loss and can be used to determine the volume deficit in liters that results. The free water deficit is calculated as follows:

Free water deficit (liters)
= 140 (0.6 × weight in kg)/measured Na⁺

Replacement should proceed with 0.25 NS administered to meet 50% of the deficit over 3 to 4 hours and the remainder as reassessment of the sodium and fluid status dictates.[46]

Inadequate glucose control can produce an osmotic diuresis. Serum glucose in excess of 300 mg/dL in conjunction with marked glucosuria should prompt aggressive glycemic control with intravenous insulin and water replacement as outlined above. Glycemic control with blood glucose less than or equal to 250 mg/dL with normalization of intravascular volume should be rapidly obtained.

Hyponatremia is far less common. It is of little concern until sodium drops below 125 mg/dL. One confounding variable is the fact that pseudohyponatremia results from elevation of serum glucose that artificially lowers measured sodium. To correct for the sodium, 3 mg/dL should be added to the measured sodium for every 100 g/dL of glucose elevation over 300 mg/dL.

Abnormalities of potassium and magnesium require correction as the potential for cardiac arrhythmia increases with marked increased or decreased levels of these electrolytes. Most intensive care units have potassium replacement protocols to maintain potassium levels in the normal range. Hyperkalemia may require more aggressive methods to bring the levels into the normal range. Glucose and insulin shift potassium into the intracellular space and allow rapid albeit short-term control. Binding resins and dialysis, although commonly used in critical care, may not be appropriate for the donor population. Specific protocols for replacement and control of potassium, magnesium, and calcium should be developed and utilized by the care team in conjunction with the transplant surgeons.

Acid–Base Balance Issues

Acid–base disturbances reflect underlying pathophysiology and need to be addressed quickly. Acidosis, pH < 7.20, carries a risk of decreasing cardiac contractility and inducing cardiac arrhythmia. Renal blood flow decreases and serum potassium level increases as acidosis worsens. There is also a diminished responsiveness to catecholamines. Alkalosis induces coronary vasospasm and is also associated with arrhythmia risk. Potassium and magnesium are shifted intracellularly, which may have a role in cardiac irritability. Hemoglobin–oxygen binding intensifies in alkalosis making peripheral offloading at the tissue interface more difficult, leading to microcirculatory hypoxia.

Acidosis is probably a more commonly encountered problem. Respiratory causes are amenable to correction of minute ventilation. Respiratory alkalosis is seen if hyperventilation has been utilized to control intracranial hypertension before cerebral death declaration or if severe volume contraction has been protracted and untreated.

Metabolic acidosis can arise for a number of reasons many of which should have been clarified before declaration of death. The anion gap is an easy method to stratify etiologies. The anion gap represents the difference between the cation and anion species present in plasma:

$$AG = (Na^+ + K^+) - (Cl^- - HCO_3^-)$$

A normal anion gap is 8 to 12. A normal anion gap acidosis results from early renal failure, prolonged total parenteral nutrition use, prolonged hyperventilation, or the use of acetazolamide as a diuretic.[47–49]

An increased anion gap acidosis commonly reflects inadequately resuscitated shock. Elevation of the base deficit and serum lactate level will corroborate shock as the likely etiology. Alternatively, established renal failure may be an etiology. Other common causes such as diabetic ketoacidosis, toxin ingestion, and hyperosmolar nonketotic states should have been identified and rectified before the declaration of cerebral death. Correction of the acidosis is directed at the primary cause. Shock needs to be resuscitated and ketoacidosis corrected with insulin and intravenous fluid. Occasionally bicarbonate will need to be administered to mitigate the effects of the acidosis before correction of the underlying pathology is complete. The HCO_3 deficit can be calculated as follows:

$$mEq\ HCO_3 = 24 - [measured\ HCO_3 \times 0.4$$
$$(patient\ weight\ in\ kg)]$$

This will determine the HCO_3 quantity to be replaced and avoid overzealous administration with overshooting the target pH and subsequently inducing alkalosis.

Coagulation System Issues

Coagulation defects may arise as a consequence of medications used by the patient before the events leading to cerebral death or as part of the recent disease and treatment. Coagulation is a temperature-dependent series of reactions. Body temperatures less that 92°F are associated with shutdown of the coagulation cascade as platelet function virtually stops. Temperature control becomes essential to minimize this risk.

Coumadin, aspirin, clopidogrel, and ticlopidine are commonly used outpatient anticoagulants. Heparin is routinely used in the hospital therapeutically or to help maintain indwelling arterial lines as a flush solution. The use of these agents needs to be specifically sought and appropriate measures taken to counter their effects as necessary.

Consumptive coagulopathy frequently accompanies severe trauma with massive hemorrhage. Replacement of lost blood with component therapy from the blood bank frequently underestimates the need for specific coagulation components. Replacement of platelets and use of fresh-frozen plasma or cryoprecipitate, alone or in combination, will be dictated by the clinical situation and the laboratory data obtained. A specific coagulation defect known as disseminated intravascular coagulation represents a breakdown in the balance between clot formation and lysis, with the scales tilted in favor of clot lysis. In the scenario of the cerebral death patient, overwhelming sepsis can be an etiology of disseminated intravascular coagulation, but more commonly it is severe cerebral injury. The brain is a tremendous tissue thromboplastin reservoir. The injured brain releases large quantities of tissue thromboplastin. The result is an augmented coagulation system. The response to this abnormal clot formation is an upregulation of plasmin activity and increased clot lysis. The key to the diagnosis of disseminated intravascular coagulation is the knowledge of the pathophysiology. Prolongation of the protime (PT) and partial thromboplastin time (aPTT) and a decrease in the platelet count and fibrinogen levels demonstrate consumption of the coagulation cascade elements. Detection of fibrin degradation products and D-dimer species reflect the increased lytic activity. Classically therapy is directed at the inciting cause with support of the coagulation system with factor replacement as indicated. Systemic heparization as a way to stop the coagulation and thus interrupt the process is advocated as an adjunct. Unfortunately in the cerebral death patient the head injury is not treatable. Heparin probably has no role here either. Therapy is directed at specific factor replacement to help control the coagulation abnormality in the short term. Regular determination of the hospital disseminated intravascular coagulation screening panel will detect all the components of the coagulation system and allow appropriate correction. Overwhelming infection, a common disseminated intravascular coagulation initiator and usually precluded organ donation, is not usually a consideration in care of the donor. Obstetric causes of disseminated intravascular coagulation, such as amniotic fluid embolus, are distinctly unusual in this situation.[50]

Temperature Regulation Issues

The center of temperature regulation resides in the hypothalamus. With cerebral death, temperature regulatory function is lost. Patients may demonstrate hyper- or hypothermia. Hyperthermia reflects inflammatory drivers from the cytokine cascade as a response to injury or infection. The increased cellular metabolic rate with increased oxygen consumption can be detrimental to end-organ function. The possible role of infection driving such fever response needs to be considered and sources of infection sought.

The inability to respond to environmental cooling commonly accompanies cerebral death. Therapy of the injury or disease preceding death uses medications and fluid administration none of which is at body temperature. Intensive care unit rooms are kept at temperatures comfortable for the medical staff rather than the patients' needs. As in the discussion of coagulation, temperature protection is a critical factor to be concerned about, as it is far easier to maintain body temperature that it is to recoup it. The goal should be as normal a body temperature as possible, with temperatures <34°F not acceptable. This will avoid the coagulopathy effects and minimize the cardiac irritability cold induces. Easy ways to maintain body temperature include heater circuits on ventilators, forced air warmer blankets, keeping environmental temperature above 80° to 85°F, or using specific warming lights on the patient. More aggressive maneuvers to regain lost temperature include lavage with warm saline via nasogastric tubes, urinary catheters, tube thoracostomies, or peritoneal lavage. Cardiopulmonary bypass allows excellent temperature control and is a specific hypothermia treatment. Its use for the potential organ donor would need to be discussed with the transplant surgeons before proceeding.

Ventilator Management Issues

The medical staff caring for the potential organ donor needs to be aware of the type of ventilator support employed.[51] Frequently, the ventilator management will have been set by the treating team before the declaration of cerebral death. The lung pathology will determine the ventilator mode used, but the goal remains to minimize further lung injury while providing maximum support for oxygenation and ventilation functions. There are a number of ventilator modes utilizing pressure or volume as the driving force behind gas exchange. The treatment team needs to be cognizant of the concepts of positive end-expiratory pressure, airway pressures, peak, mean, and plateau and how these can be interpreted and manipulated. Current ventilator management tries to minimize FIO_2 and keep peak airway pressure less than $35\,cm\ H_2O$. FIO_2 in excess of 60% is detrimental to the alveolar capillary architecture and gas exchange. Peak airway pressure less than $35\,cm\ H_2O$ pressure minimizes barotrauma and the risk of pneumothorax. The ARDS net study[52] advocates a lower tidal volume of $6\,mL/kg$ and a plateau pressure less than $30\,cm\ H_2O$ as a method to decrease morbidity and mortality in acute lung injury. As many of these potential donors have suffered trauma, this can be a prudent plan of respiratory care. Specific consultation with the transplant surgeons or the pulmonary consultants involved in the donor screening program is essential to minimize pulmonary injury, especially if lung transplantation is being considered.

In summary, death in modern intensive care units remains an all too common occurrence. A transition in approach has occurred from maintaining life at all costs to recognizing that a point may be reached beyond which life may be maintained temporarily, but the efforts truly represent a prolongation of dying. Thus many of the patients dying in intensive care units today have undergone some withdrawal of therapy. There is abundant evidence that the process of moving from curative to palliative care has historically been poorly managed. A common avenue into end-of-life discussions involves cerebral death. The recognition of cerebral death set the stage for the progression of organ donation and transplantation. How to determine cerebral death and then to care for the patient and the patient's family are important issues. Regardless of the factors leading to the discussion, the characteristics of good end-of-life care can be identified: communication, attentiveness to symptoms, care of the family, and access. Specific skill sets that enable clinicians to be more effective in this setting can similarly be identified and taught.[20,22] Increased attention to these matters in formal training programs can only help improve care of surgical patients dying in the intensive care unit.

References

1. Nelson JE, Danis M. End-of-life care in the intensive care unit: where are we now? Crit Care Med 2001; 29(Suppl): N2–N9.
2. Knaus WA. Prognosis with mechanical ventilation: the influence of disease, severity of disease, age, and chronic health status on survival from an acute illness. Am Rev Repir Dis 1989; 140:S8–S13.
3. Cohen IL, Lambrinos J. Investigating the impact of age on outcome of mechanical ventilation using a population of 41,848 patients from a statewide database. Chest 1995; 107:1673–1680.
4. Rivera S, Dong K, Garone S, et al. Motivating factors in futile clinical interventions. Chest 2001; 119:1944–1947.
5. Cohen NH. Assessing futility of medical interventions—is it futile? Crit Care Med, 2003; 31(2):646–648.
6. Fetters MD, Churchill L, Danis M. Conflict resolution at the end of life. Crit Care Med 2001; 29(5):921–925.
7. Burt RA. The Medical futility debate: patient choice, physician obligation, and end-of-life care. J Palliative Med 2002; 5(2):249–254.
8. Veatch RM, Spicer CM. Medically futile care: the role of the physician in setting limits. Am J Law Med 1992; 18(1–2): 15–36.

9. Brennan TA. Physicians and futile care: using ethics committees to slow the momentum. Law Medicine Health Care 1992; 20(4):336–339.

10. Ayres SM. Who decides when care is futile? Hosp Pract 1991; 26(9A):41–53.

11. Miles SH. Medical futility. Law Medicine Health Care 1992; 20(4):310–315.

12. Loefmark R, Nilstun T. Conditions and consequences of medical futility—from a literature review to a clinical mode. J Med Ethics 2002; 28:115–119.

13. Stroud R. The withdrawal of life support in adult intensive care: an evaluative review of the literature. Nursing Crit Care 2002; 7(4):176–184.

14. Blake DC. Bioethics and the law: the case of Helga Wanglie: a clash at the bedside—medically futile treatment v. patient autonomy. Whittier Law Rev1993; 14:119–128.

15. Joint Commission on Accreditation of Healthcare Organizations. Comprehensive Accreditation Manual for Hospitals, 2004; Ethics, Rights and Responsibilities Standards. Washington, DC: JCAHO, 2004.

16. Levy MM. Conflict resolution at the end of life. Crit Care Med 2001; 29(2S):N56–N61.

17. Levy MM. Compassionate end-of-life care in the intensive care unit. Crit Care Med 2001; 29(2S):N1–N2.

18. Brody H, Campbell ML, Faber-Langendoen K. Withdrawing intensive life-sustaining treatment—recommendations for compassionate clinical management. N Engl J Med 1997; 336(9):652–657.

19. Clarke EB, Curtis JR, Luce JM, et al. Quality indicators for end-of-life care in the intensive care unit. Crit Care Med 2003; 31(9):2255–2262.

20. Nelson JE. Saving lives and saving deaths. Ann Intern Med 1999; 130:776–777.

21. SUPPORT Principal Investigators. A controlled trial to improve care fro seriously ill hospitalized patients. The study to understand prognoses and preferences for outcomes and risks of treatments (SUPPORT). JAMA 1995; 274(20):1591–1598.

22. Levy MM. End-of-life care in the intensive care unit: can we do better? Crit Care Med 2001; 29(2S):N56–N61.

23. Truog RD, Cist AFM, Brackett SE, et al. Recommendations for end-or-life care in the intensive care unit: The Ethics Committee of the Society of Critical Care Medicine. Crit Care Med 2001; 29(12):2332–2348.

24. Wilson WC, Smedira NG, Fink C, et al. Ordering and administration of sedatives and analgesics during the withholding and withdrawal of life support from critically ill patients. JAMA 1992; 267:949–953.

25. A definition of irreversible coma: report of the Ad Hoc Committee of the Harvard Medical School to Examine the Definition of Brain Death. JAMA 1968; 205:337–340.

26. Uniform Determination of Death Act, 12 Uniform Laws Annotated (U.L.A.) 589 (West 1993 and West Supp. 1997).

27. The Quality Standards Subcommittees of the American Academy of Neurology. Practice parameters for determining brain death in adults. Neurology 1995; 45:1012–1014.

28. Wijdicks EF. Determining brain death in adults. Neurology 1995; 45:1003–1011.

29. Wijdicks EF. The diagnosis of brain death. N Engl J Med 2001; 344:16:1215–1221.

30. American Academy of Pediatrics Task Force on Brain Death in Children. Report of special task force: guidelines for the determination of brain death in children. Pediatrics 1987; 80:298–300.

31. Petty GW, Mohr JP, Pedley TA, et al. The role of transcranial Doppler in confirming brain death: sensitivity, specificity and suggestions for performance and interpretation. Neurology 1990; 40:300–303.

32. Novitzky D, Hicomb WN, Cooper DKC, et al. Electrocardiographic, hemodynamic and endocrine changes occurring during experimental brain death in the Chacma baboon. J Heart Transplant 1984; 4:63–69.

33. Bittner HB, Chen EP, Kendall SWH, et al. Brain death alters cardiopulmonary hemodynamics and impairs right ventricular power reserve against an elevation of pulmonary vascular resistance. Chest 1997; 111:706–711.

34. Darracott-Cankovic S, Stoven PGI, Wheeldon D, et al. Effect of donor heart damage on survival after transplantation. Eur J Cardiothorac Surg 1989; 3:525–532.

35. Owen VJ, Buston PBJ, Michel MC, et al. Myocardial dysfunction in donor hearts. Circulation 1999; 99:2565–2570.

36. Novitzky D. Donor management: state of the art. Transplant Proc 1997; 29:3773–3775.

37. Ririe DG, Butterworth JF, Royster RL, et al. Triiodothyronine increases contractility independent of beta-adrenergic receptor or stimulation of cyclic 3–5-adenosine monophosphate. Anesthesiology 1995; 82:1004–1012.

38. Timek T, Bonz A, Dillman R, et al. The effect of triiodothyronine on myocardial contractile performance after epinephrine exposure: implications for donor heart management. J Heart Lung Transplant 1998; 17:931–940.

39. Novitzky D. Selection and management of cardiac allograft donors. Curr Opin Cardiol 1996; 11:174–182.

40. Gramm HJ, Meinhold H, Bicket U, et al. Acute endocrine failure after brain death. Transplantation 1992; 54:851–857.

41. Howlett TA, Keogh AM, Perry L, et al. Anterior and posterior pituitary function in brain-stem–dead donors. Transplantation 1989; 47:828–834.

42. Powner DJ, Hendrich A, Lagler RG, et al. Hormonal changes in brain dead patients. Crit Care Med 1990; 18:702–708.

43. Debelak L, Pollak R, Ruland C. Arginine vasopressin versus desmopressin for the treatment of diabetes insipidus in the brain dead organ donor. Transplant Proc 1990; 22:351–352.

44. Hirsch L, Matzner MP, Huber WO, et al. Effect of desmopressin substitution during organ procurement on early renal allograft function. Nephrol Dial Transplant 1996; 11:173–176.

45. Guesde R, Barrou B, Leblanc I, et al. Administration of desmopressin in brain dead donors and renal function in kidney recipients. Lancet 1998; 352:1178–1181.

46. Powner DJ, Kellum JA, Darby JM. Abnormalities in fluid, electrolyte and metabolism of organ donors. Prog Transplant 2000; 10:88–96.

47. Androgue HJ, Madias NE. Management of life threatening acid–base disorders First of two parts. N Engl J Med 1998; 338:26–34.

48. Androgue HJ, Madias NE. Management of life threatening acid–base disorders second of two parts. N Engl J Med 1998; 338:107–111.

49. Powner DJ, Kellum JA. Maintaining acid–base balance in organ donors. Prog Transplant 2000; 10:98–105.

50. Powner DJ, Reich HS. Regulation of coagulation abnormalities and temperature in organ donors. Prog Transplant 2000; 10:146–153.

51. Powner DJ, Darby JM, Stuart SA. Recommendations for mechanical ventilation during donor care. Prog Transplant 2000; 10:33–40.

52. Brower RG, Morris A, Schoenfeld D, et al. for the ARDS network. Ventilation with lower tidal volumes as compared with traditional tidal volumes for acute lung injury and the acute respiratory distress syndrome. N Engl J Med 2000; 342:1301–1308.

45
Ethical Dilemmas and the Law

Ira J. Kodner, Daniel M. Freeman, Robb R. Whinney, and Douglas J. E. Schuerer

Considerations for Surgeons

General Concepts

Defining the Problem

Professional responsibilities have been a concern of surgeons since antiquity; however, the last 25 years have displayed a dramatic growth of both professional and societal attention to moral and ethical issues involved in the delivery of health care. This increased interest in medical ethics has occurred because of such factors as the greater technological power of modern medicine, the assigning of social ills to the responsibility of medicine, the growing sophistication of patients and the information available to them, the efforts to protect the civil rights of the increasing disadvantaged groups in our society, and the continued rapidly escalating costs of health care, including medical malpractice costs. All of these factors contribute to the urgency of dealing with ethical and moral issues involved in the delivery of modern emergency surgical care.[1]

The terms *ethics* and *morals* are often used interchangeably to refer to standards regarding right and wrong behavior. *Morals* refer to conduct that conforms to the accepted customs or standards of a people. They vary with time and with the nature of society at that time. *Ethics* is the branch of philosophy that deals with human conduct and can be described as applied morals. *Medical ethics* refers to the ethics of the practice of medicine. *Clinical ethics* refers to the ethics of delivering patient care. The term *bioethics* includes the ethics of all biomedical endeavors and encompasses both medical and clinical ethics.[2] The law serves to delineate the formal rules of society. It expresses a kind of minimal societal ethical consensus, which society is willing to enforce through civil judgments or criminal sanctions. The law does not always prohibit behavior deemed unethical; however, it will usually set a minimal standard for conduct. Those of us who practice clinical surgery, especially acute care surgery, often have trouble differentiating ethical issues from legal issues. It is the purpose of this chapter to clarify this dichotomy. It should be stated from the outset that it is more important to understand the process of dealing with these issues than to assume that anyone can clearly state what is ethically right or wrong in a complex medical/surgical dilemma. The law, on the other hand, can be very explicit and can vary from state to state.

Surgeons live and practice an intense form of applied ethics. We deliver bad news; we guide patients and their families through complicated decisions to arrive at appropriate informed consent; we live a code of truth and trust among ourselves, our patients, and our trainees; we must deal with the end-of-life issues; and we make plans for extended, palliative, and hospice care. Finally, as only we surgeons know, we must go to bed at night knowing that in the morning we will spend hours with someone's life literally in our hands.

In recent decades, although we can technically and scientifically do more for our patients than ever before, our personal, trusting relationship with them has deteriorated to the point where it is sometimes adversarial. We have allowed medicine to become a business, guided in many cases by the financial bottom line rather than by the uncompromising concern for a sick person. Within this fast-moving corporate system, we see too many patients, do too much surgery, and do not have time to develop a close mentoring relationship with our chosen role models or with our trainees.[3]

Just as with medicine and science, bioethics and legal underpinnings of bioethical decision making are evolving all the time. In this chapter, we will not discuss all possible bioethical issues but will limit ourselves to those that may be of concern to acute care surgery and to surgery in general. Other important issues relating to such matters as property rights, genetics, and assisted reproduction, which do not present themselves to the acute care surgeon's practice, are not discussed.

What Makes the Surgeon Special?

Undergoing major surgery is an extreme experience that changes people's lives. Surgeons are repeatedly involved in these extreme experiences of others. This makes surgeons uniquely placed among health care professionals to understand the experiences of their patients.

Miles Little explains that there are special ethical considerations for surgeons.[4] These include rescue, proximity, ordeal, aftermath, and presence. These terms help to define the ethical relationship between the surgeon and his or her patients.

Rescue, he describes as the first pillar of surgical ethics. It deals with the fact that surgery conveys power and that power is socially endorsed and may be reinforced by the surgeon's individual charisma; but, as with all power, it must be constantly renewed and revalidated. Patients have no choice but to acknowledge surgical power when they consult a surgeon. There is always an element of surrender in the surgical relationship, but it is a surrender that presupposes rescue. Accepting rescue as a legitimate principle justifies respect for dependence in the surgical relationship. Surgeons, themselves, sometimes need help and rescue from colleagues when they have trouble with complicated diagnostic, management, or operative procedures.

Proximity occurs in surgery as in no other act. To operate on people involves entering their bodies and becoming privy to secrets denied even to the owner of the body. Little states: "To get to my body, my doctor has to get to my character. He has to go to my soul. He doesn't only have to go through my anus."[4] This proximity to the patient can make special ethical demands on the surgeon. This proximity carries with it the penalties of closeness and particularly the pains of failure. Some surgeons find that distancing themselves from their patients makes failure easier to bear. Understanding the privileges and risks of proximity is critical for the compassionate surgeon.

Ordeals are periods of extreme experience, capable of disrupting our lives. Little explains that all medical encounters are ordeals. Patients yield autonomy, acknowledge dependence, place trust, face risk, confront embodiment and mortality, lose control over time and space, and experience alienation, pain, fear, discomfort, suffering, and boredom. Surgeons, especially those providing emergency care, observe and participate in the lives of patients with serious illnesses. A surgeon who understands the ordeal of the surgical episode can better help his or her patient through such extreme experiences.

Aftermath deals with the reality that surgery leaves physical and psychological scars that may persist for life. It is very difficult to communicate the concept of suffering to someone who has not suffered. Little describes surgeons as being in a unique position to understand the existential threats that their patients experience, the sense of mortality and bodily frailty they live with, and the difficulty of explaining extreme experience to others. When death approaches our patients, we must remember, not deny, our own mortality. Such an approach takes courage and a sense of personal security, and this does not suit everyone, whether patient or surgeon.

Presence, as a virtue and a duty, is what the patient desires of the surgeon during all phases of the surgical encounter. Most surgeons have the stamina and cognitive ability to be present for their patients, but not all of us process the personal attributes of charisma, confidence, energy, and empathy, which are necessary to engender trust from our patients and our staff. Sometimes, amazingly, our mere presence means more to our patients than defects in the manner with which we deal with them. Even if we cannot teach sensitivity, we can emphasize the importance of surgical presence.

Thus, surgeons are privileged to lead lives of great complexity and moral richness. We can acquire a profound understanding and recognition of patient experience and suffering. Our proximity to patients seeking rescue, facing ordeals, and experiencing the aftermath of surgery presents us with a great challenge.

Special Problems of Acute Care Surgery

Surgeons, unlike other members of the emergency health care team, take on a different level of responsibility as they encounter patients in the acute care facility. The difference is that the surgeon is not going to just treat the patient in the acute care facility. For the surgeon, the initial contact in the emergency room may be just the beginning of a longer term relationship. With no previously established doctor–patient relationship, the surgeon and the patient may well be heading to the operating room for sometimes massive and sometimes potentially "futile" surgery. The surgeon and the surgical team take on the continued responsibility of the operative procedure itself, the postoperative care, and usually the long-term follow up and management of any complications and dilemmas that may result from the initial encounter. This intense relationship is often established very quickly and under frequently adverse circumstances. The family and religion may not be known, the patient may be unconscious and certainly will be once the procedure starts, and he may even be on death's door because he was shot by a policeman who had the intention of killing him but was not successful.

Arthur R. Derse nicely delineates the array of ethical issues that arise in delivering acute surgical care.[2] These include informed consent, refusal of treatment, determination of decision-making capacity, treating patients despite their refusal, maintaining confidentiality while respecting the duty to warn others, limiting treatment over issues of "futility," treating pain at the end of life, and acting as a Good Samaritan. He goes on to describe the unique ethical issues that can arise because of the acute care environment in which care must be delivered. Among these are (1) the need for rapid decision making, often based on incomplete information; (2) the fact that the patient has had a sudden change in health and has no choice of physician; (3) the lack of a prior physician–patient relationship, resulting in difficulty establishing trust; (4) the fact that the patient may be hostile, non-compliant, or impaired because of alcohol or drugs, may be in police custody, or may have injuries or illnesses related to illegal or socially unacceptable activities; (5) the unique ethical issues associated with the initiation and discontinuation of resuscitation; and (6) the fact that acute care facilities are often the health care providers of last resort for much of the indigent in the United States. Obviously, many of these ethical issues have legal components as well.[2]

Unlike surgeons caring for acute care patients, people in most professions have the luxury of time and the opportunity to redo their work in order to remedy any mistakes. Attorneys can appeal their cases. Accountants can file an amended return. Movie directors can yell: "Cut! Take two!" and reshoot the scene. All doctors understand that they will probably be second guessed. As everyone who has ever watched a television police drama knows, the first thing a police officer must say to an arrested person is the famous *Miranda* warning. What most people do not remember is the requirement that those warnings be given is the result of a Supreme Court decision rendered in June 1966. As a practical matter, the court was telling the arresting police officer, in the heat of making an arrest, that he should have known something that took the court system 3 years to contemplate and research. The bottom line for surgeons who work under the same kinds of time pressures is to do what you think is best. You must use your judgment, based on your medical knowledge and your experience. You are on the front line, and you do not have the luxury of waiting 3 years for the Supreme Court to tell you how to handle a potential situation. However, you also want to be as scrupulous as possible in making sure that bioethical and legal guidelines are followed for both the benefit of the patient and, frankly, as protection for yourself.

Although it is crucial for the practice of medicine in all fields that practitioners be familiar with bioethical concepts, it is unrealistic for acute care surgeons to be expected to be knowledgeable about the nuances requiring detailed understanding of controversial bioethical dilemmas. However, it is important for surgeons to have a working knowledge of general medical ethical principles and of how these principles affect decisions involved with treating patients. Our goal is to distill the general bioethical concepts and their underlying applications to specific situations that acute care surgeons may face into a cogent and concise tool for routine use, for inclusion in training, and as a reference resource. For specific dilemmas, time permitting, surgeons should obtain an opinion from the hospital ethics consultation service and/or from hospital counsel. By doing so, one can gain the experience and imprimatur of opinions from those who have dealt with such issues and whose training gives them the experience to deal with them in a knowledgeable way. It also serves as a cushion of knowledge for the physician when discussing the matter with a patient or the family. Surgeons should do all they can for the patient while at the same time doing what they need to do to protect themselves from personal risk and possibly from negative legal ramifications.

Similarly, doctors have a positive duty to themselves not to get into situations that violate their own personal beliefs, whether religious or medical. This includes thinking a step or two ahead of the current situation to know what the ramifications of a course of treatment may be. If the anticipated actions may violate a doctor's own personal tenants, he or she should refer the patient to another physician. The most obvious of these situations comes up with regard to religious beliefs. If, for example, a doctor has religious beliefs that would preclude *withdrawal of life support*, the doctor should be very careful about getting into a situation with a patient that might later dictate putting someone on life support. It may, down the line, become bioethically or medically appropriate to withdraw life support. If a physician cannot do that, he or she needs to know that up front and be prepared to withdraw from the case. A similar situation involves doctors who do not believe in *abortion*. They should not get themselves into medical situations where an acute care termination of a pregnancy may become the best medically viable option. Surgeons must always be prepared to protect themselves *and* their patients and must recognize their duties, both legal and ethical. Surgeons need to be aware of these duties and avoid situations where they may come into conflict. This can be very difficult at times.

Principles of Bioethics

Philosophical Principles

Two fundamental theoretical philosophical concepts exist for constructing a theory of ethics: deontologic and consequentialist. A deontologic theory relies on *rules*, and a consequentialist theory relies on *outcomes*.[2] From these theories are derived *principles of ethics*, such as those delineated by Beauchamp and Childress[5]: respect for autonomy (patient self-determination), beneficence ("doing good"), nonmaleficence ("do no harm"), and justice (fairness).

Respect for Autonomy

Adult patients with decision-making capacity have a right to their preferences regarding their own health care. This right is grounded in the legal doctrine of informed consent. Informed consent means that patients must give their voluntary consent to treatment after receiving all appropriate and relevant information about the nature of their problem, the expected consequences of the recommended treatment, and the treatment alternatives.

This is probably the most crucial legal concept in bioethics. It simply means that a physician cannot touch a person without first getting permission and without telling the individual of the possible ramifications of that "touching." Touching someone without his or her consent is, in legal terms, a "battery," which could result in a lawsuit for damages. Therefore, the principle is, *medical treatment without consent is a battery*. The first major case in this area concluded that

Every human being of adult years and sound mind has a right to determine what shall be done with his own body; and a surgeon who performs an operation without his patient's consent commits an assault, for which he is liable in damages. . . . This is true except in cases of emergency where the patient is unconscious and where it is necessary to operate before consent can be obtained.[6]

This case was decided before the concepts of "living wills" and "durable powers of attorney" came into being. These concepts both facilitate and complicate the consent process because consent must be obtained, if time permits, through documents or via surrogate decision making. Subsequent cases refined the requirements of consent to add to the concept of "informed" consent. The courts now require not only that the patient consent to the procedure, either themselves or through a proper surrogate, but also that the patient be given sufficient information to make an informed decision. The courts have held that the quality and quantity of information given to the patient must be sufficient for the reasonable patient to understand, not the doctor. The law has established the doctrine of the "reasonable man" to be used in deciding what is acceptable in many areas of delivering acute surgical care.

Doctors are duty bound to respect the autonomy of each competent patient. The patient is the ultimate decision maker about what he or she wants. The doctor may differ, even vehemently, with the patient's decision; however, the patient has the final say. There are exceptions to this rule also, such as the patient who demands a certain kind of treatment that the doctor knows will not be efficacious. Permitting autonomy to trump nonmaleficence poses a serious problem. A simple example of this is a patient who demands antibiotics to treat a viral infection. Giving the requested antibiotic complies with the autonomy principle; however, in the long run, it is con-ceivable that giving an antibiotic in such a case would violate the principle of nonmaleficence, would impose the concept of futility, and in the long run might enhance the capacity of bacteria to become resistant to certain antibiotics, thus even bringing into play the concept of justice. Even this simple example illustrates how medical ethical conundrums are frequently the result of conflicting duties. If the patient is unable to make his or her own decision, the treating surgeon must respect the decision made by a surrogate decision maker, such as one designated in a health care *durable power of attorney*.

Beneficence

The principle of beneficence, simply stated, is that the physician has a duty to act in the best interest of his or her patients. Beneficence is doing good and is the reason most of us chose to become doctors. Beneficence, or doing good, is probably the universal tenet of the medical profession.

Nonmaleficence

Nonmaleficence is essentially the philosophical principle "first do no harm." It derives from knowing that patient encounters with surgeons can prove harmful as well as helpful. This principle includes not doing harm, preventing harm, and removing harmful conditions. For those physicians caring for patients in an acute care environment, it also includes the concept of security, protecting oneself and one's team, as well as the patient, from harm.[7]

This concept also incorporates the principle of *avoiding killing*. This seems obvious on its face value; however, what is a doctor to do when confronted with a situation where the administration of sufficient medication to alleviate the pain of a patient might have the *secondary effect* of diminishing respiration and actually hastening the patient's death? This is, of course, the crux of the major debate that is ongoing over "physician-assisted suicide." There are other situations where avoiding killing must be taken into account. *Abortion*, depending on one's personal beliefs, might fall into this category. This could create a conflict between the duty to respect the autonomy of the patient and the personal religious beliefs of the treating physician.

Justice

Justice is *fairness*. It is required to ensure that medical decisions are made with reason and honesty. Selfish or biased influences must be recognized and avoided.[8] For many the term *justice* includes the concept of "distributive justice." This form of justice includes not only the surgeon's obligation to an individual patient but also fairness in the allocation of resources for the good of the broader society. It is this concept of justice that becomes the basis for society-wide health care policy determination. "Distributive justice" implies that all individuals and groups should share in society's benefits and burdens. This presents an ethical challenge for the surgeon dealing with an individual patient who mistakenly believes that he or she should limit or terminate care based on a need to limit health care resource expenditures for the good of society.[7] It was this temptation to place the good of society before the good of an individual that led the physicians of Europe to fall prey to the fallacious doctrines being promulgated by the Nazi government.[9]

Surgeons providing emergency care should be prepared to respect and seek to understand people from many cultures and from diverse socioeconomic groups. In the United States, acute care facilities are obligated to provide necessary care to all patients, regardless of ability to pay. Our current business-based medical delivery system makes it difficult to abide by the principle of having access to appropriate inpatient and follow-up medical care dictated by the patient's financial situation. Provision of acute care surgical treatment should not be based on gender, age, race, socioeconomic status, or cultural background. No patient should ever be abused, demeaned, or given substandard care.[1]

Religion and Medical Ethics

In many societies, religion has been looked upon as the determinant of ethical norms. In American society, we are multicultural with no single religion holding dominance over the entire population. Therefore, a value-based approach to ethical issues depends on the individual patient's values. However, religion still influences bioethical concepts and decisions. Clinical bioethics, in fact, uses many decision-making methods, arguments, and ideals that originated from religion. It is also important for the individual clinician to understand his or her own personal spirituality in order to relate better to patients and families seen in the crisis of the emergency center, who will represent a broad range of religious an ethnic backgrounds. Although religions may appear dissimilar, most are based on some form of the Golden Rule, which holds, "do unto others as you would have them do unto you." Problems frequently arise when trying to apply religion-based rules to specific clinical, ethical situations.

In so-called modern times, the United States began turning away from a reliance on religious principles, relying instead on more generic secular principles; and the medical/surgical community was no exception. As previously described, we have come to rely instead on the four ethical principles of autonomy, beneficence, nonmaleficence, and fairness. These are the principles that have guided ethical thinking and have been instrumental in forming health care policies in the United States and other western countries over the past three decades.[7]

In a recent survey of physicians' attitudes toward spirituality in clinical practice, 85% said physicians should be aware of the patient's religious and spiritual beliefs. The survey went on to show that, although many physicians believe that they should inquire about their patients' beliefs, fewer than 10% of doctors actually do so, even among dying patients. There are no hard data to support the benefits of taking a spiritual history, but there is some indirect evidence in support of the practice. Religion is one of the most common ways by which patients cope with medical illness. Religious beliefs are known to be significant influences and medical decisions, especially those made by patients with serious illnesses. In addition, the faith community is a primary source of support for many medically ill patients; and such social support is associated with better adherence to therapy and improved medical outcomes. Several surveys have revealed that, from the patient's point of view, satisfaction with the emotional and spiritual aspects of care was at one of the lowest ratings among all clinical care indicators and was one of the highest areas in need of quality improvement.[10]

The purpose of taking even a brief spiritual or religious history is to learn how patients cope with their illnesses, the kinds of support systems available to them in the community, and any strongly held beliefs that might influence delivery of emergency medical care. Venturing into this delicate area is obviously fraught with some hazards. Surgeons must be extremely cautious about prescribing religion to nonreligious patients, forcing a spiritual history on patients who are not religious, encouraging a patient to believe their practices and specific ways, attempting to provide spiritual counsel to patients, and arguing with patients over religious matters.[10] It is also imperative for surgeons to be comfortable enough with their own beliefs to allow patients to pray for us, according to the faith of their own religion. No comment more than a simple and sincere "thank you" is usually indicated.

Legal Principles

In the United States, law is created in one of two systems—federal or state—and is made by judges (common law), legislatures (statutory law), and executive agencies empowered by legislatures (regulatory law). The fundamental document that creates and delineates these powers is the U.S. Constitution. *Civil law*, including malpractice, is usually enforced by monetary judgments. *Criminal law*, including physician-assisted suicide, is usually enforced by fines and/or imprisonment.[2]

There are three kinds of law that affect the practice of surgery: *statutes, regulations* promulgated by an administrative agency pursuant to a statute, and *case law*. The legislatures are the designated policy-making entities in our system; regulations are written to comply with legislative directives; and the courts are charged with resolving disputes between parties, usually as directed by statute, if there is a relevant one. Courts issue written opinions when there is a conflict that results in a lawsuit, especially when the interpretation of a statute or a regulation is in question. The most difficult situations are those where the court is faced with a matter of "first impression," one that the legislature has not specifically addressed. The courts, and their written opinions, on this type of case frequently ask the legislature for guidance in future situations. Until the legislature acts, the written opinion of the court is the only guidance physicians have, and hospital counsel sometimes must interpret this.

Doctors should be generally familiar with state law. There are different state laws about many bioethical matters, such as definition of death, competency, and organ donation. Many doctors move from state to state during their careers, and having a general understanding of the state laws governing situations that may arise in their acute care surgical practice is crucial. However, most important legal principles that apply to ethical dilemmas in delivering emergency surgical care are widely accepted among several states. There are some glaring discrepancies in these commonalities, including the neurologic criteria for death—a person may be legally dead in one state but not in another—and the legality of physician-assisted suicide (punishable as a crime in all states except Oregon).

Malpractice

Judges, not the legislature, establish the standards that constitute medical malpractice. The familiar elements of medical malpractice include *duty, breach, causation,* and *damages.* Decisions are based on the standard of care, and judges have developed the methods of determining the standards over many years, after the review of many cases. Thus, the courts rule on a specific set of facts that have already occurred. This is extremely frustrating for those practitioners of acute care surgery who need to know what the law would say any particular situation, as it is occurring, not in retrospect.

Unfortunately, resolution of controversy over medical and surgical ethical issues has been the domain of law, not philosophy or medicine. So far, perhaps because of legal constraints, medicine has been unable to "police itself." Because the law has come to champion individual rights and to hold physicians liable for malpractice, it has served to erode medical paternalism as it has elevated patients' rights. This has had the damaging effect of encouraging many physicians to be more concerned with avoiding litigation than with "doing the right thing." The law has had understandable difficulty in sorting out the complicated physician–patient relationship, and thus law does not mandate the ethical behavior in these relationships.

Statutory Law

Statutory law is made by legislatures and includes such issues as "the statute of limitations," which defines how long after an adverse event a patient is able to sue a physician for malpractice, and, in some states, statutes on "informed consent."

The Emergency Medical Treatment and Labor Act (EMTALA) is another example of a federal statutory law. It was originally enacted as part of the Consolidated Omnibus Budget Reconciliation Act of 1986. Congress enacted EMTALA as a remedy for "patient dumping." The legislature was particularly concerned about hospitals refusing to render acute care because of lack of insurance or the economic ability to pay, but soon came to realize that care was also being refused on the basis of race or other discriminatory criteria. The Act requires that a basic screening examination be provided to all patients seeking care. It therefore became illegal, as well as unethical, to withhold therapy from the poor just because they do not have the ability to pay.[11]

Compilations of statistics from major county hospitals across the country conclude that as many as 650,000 patients were "dumped" annually, and the resulting transfer led to substandard care and or life-threatening situations in 25% to 33% of them. The economic impact of EMTALA on hospitals and acute care physicians has been enormous. Patients without the means to pay for medical care know that they cannot be turned away from the emergency room. Therefore, they use it as their primary care facility. As a result, the hospitals and acute care physicians and surgeons now carry the burden of the nation's uninsured without compensation. For many health care facilities, this money lost in the emergency room can mean the difference between bankruptcy and solvency.[12]

Regulatory Law

Administrative laws are created by regulatory agencies, including state medical boards. Recent examples of regulatory law include not only EMTALA but also the Health Insurance Portability and Accountability Act of 1996 (HIPAA). HIPAA, like EMTALA, was intended to protect patients' right of privacy and guarantee them continuation of health insurance coverage should they change employers. Also like EMTALA, HIPAA has many ramifications leading to a huge economic impact on the precarious costs of delivering medical care. Although the good aspects of it are necessary and noble, the burdens of increased costs will be crippling to some health care facilities and will probably significantly curtail many clinical research endeavors.

Physician-Based Ethics

General Principles

Mark Siegler, a physician, and his co-authors of *Clinical Ethics*, fifth edition, present a technique for using case analysis as a practical approach to solving ethical dilemmas in clinical medicine. Contrary to most texts on health care ethics that are organized around the ethical *principles* of respect for autonomy, beneficence, nonmaleficence, and fairness, their publication provides a straightforward *method* for clinicians to use in sorting out the pertinent facts and values of any case into an orderly pattern that facilitates the discussion and resolution of ethical problems.[13] Their technique corresponds to the way in which clinicians usually analyze actual cases. It assimilates the ethical principles and circumstances that comprise a method to facilitate the analysis of cases involving ethical issues.

The "Clinical Ethics" System

Siegler and his colleagues suggest that all clinical cases, especially those raising an ethical dilemma, should be analyzed by the topics of (1) medical indications, (2) patient preferences, (3) quality of life, and (4) contextual features (the social, economic, legal, and administrative context in which the case occurs). The authors emphasize that, although the facts of each case can differ, these four topics are always relevant. The topics organize the facts of the particular case and, at the same time, call attention to the ethical principles appropriate for each case. The intent is to show clinicians that these four topics provide a systematic method of identifying and analyzing the ethical problems occurring in clinical medicine (Figure 45.1).[13]

We find it extremely helpful to utilize this case management system, which is very similar to our usual approach of managing a patient and his or her problem by taking a history in an organized fashion and proceeding to do a physical examination, analyze the laboratory data, and come to a plan for managing the case. Examination of the Figure 45.1 shows that the authors have clearly related to clinical situations the basic ethical principles previously described. They go on to emphasize that most ethical conflicts can be resolved by falling back on the "medical indications" that represent the medical facts of the case. This information plus the second category of "patient preferences" almost always will lead the clinical surgeon to a resolution of the ethical problem. If the ethical dilemma results from conflict among the patient,

■ MEDICAL INDICATIONS	■ PATIENT PREFERENCES
The Principles of Beneficence and Nonmaleficence	The Principle of Respect for Autonomy
1. What is the patient's medical problem? history? diagnosis? prognosis? 2. Is the problem acute? chronic? critical? emergent? reversible? 3. What are the goals of treatment? 4. What are the probabilities of success? 5. What are the plans in case of therapeutic failure? 6. In sum, how can this patient be benefited by medical and nursing care, and how can harm be avoided?	1. Is the patient mentally capable and legally competent? Is there evidence of incapacity? 2. If competent, what is the patient stating about preferences for treatment? 3. Has the patient been informed of benefits and risks, understood this information, and given consent? 4. If incapacitated, who is the appropriate surrogate? Is the surrogate using appropriate standards for decision making? 5. Has the patient expressed prior preferences, e.g., Advance Directives? 6. Is the patient unwilling or unable to cooperate with medical treatment? If so, why? 7. In sum, is the patient's right to choose being respected to the extent possible in ethics and law?
■ QUALITY OF LIFE	■ CONTEXTUAL FEATURES
The Principles of Beneficence and Nonmaleficence and Respect for Autonomy	The Principles of Loyalty and Fairness
1. What are the prospects, with or without treatment, for a return to normal life? 2. What physical, mental, and social deficits is the patient likely to experience if treatment succeeds? 3. Are there biases that might prejudice the provider's evaluation of the patient's quality of life? 4. Is the patient's present or future condition such that his or her continued life might be judged undersirable? 5. Is there any plan and rationale to forgo treatment? 6. Are there plans for comfort and palliative care?	1. Are there family issues that might influence treatment decisions? 2. Are there provider (physicians and nurses) issues that might influence treatment decisions? 3. Are there financial and economic factors? 4. Are there religious or cultural factors? 5. Are there limits on confidentiality? 6. Are there problems of allocation of resources? 7. How does the law affect treatment decisions? 8. Is clinical research or teaching involved? 9. Is there any conflict of interest on the part of the providers or the institution?

FIGURE 45.1. The four topics: case analysis in clinical ethics. (Reprinted by permission of The McGraw Hill Companies from Jonsen et al.[13])

the family, the health care team, or institutional policy, then adequate resolution may depend on applying analysis of the additional categories of "quality of life" and the array of "contextual features." It is amazing how often reviewing and relying on what the medical facts of the situation actually are can clarify the intensity and emotion of even the most complex situation.

Specific Dilemmas of Acute Care Surgery

Categories of Patient Encounters

Severe Emergency: Life in Immediate Jeopardy

An example of a severe emergency is when a critically ill person is brought in after a severe motor vehicle accident or after suffering a serious gunshot wound to the chest. Certainly, there is no preestablished doctor–patient relationship, there is little chance that there will be a reliable surrogate, and many ethicists have questioned if a patient in such dire straits ever has a decision-making capacity.

Urgent: Serious Problem needing Surgery

An example of an urgent emergency is when a patient is brought in with a ruptured abdominal aortic aneurysm. The individual is in hypovolemic shock, is terrified, but is still cognizant of the situation and what is happening. There certainly is no preexisting doctor–patient relationship, and no one is absolutely sure of the patient's decisional capacity, especially if the patient disagrees with the recommendation of the surgical team. In such a case, when there is some but not much time, the presence of a surrogate and clearly described advance directives would be extremely helpful.

Semi-Elective: Will Probably Need Surgery

An example of a semi-elective emergency is when an elderly patient with known extensive intraabdominal cancer presents with a significant, unresolving intestinal obstruction. It is clear that the obstruction can be relieved only by surgery, but it is not clear that this will be beneficial to the patient. In this case, the patient's decisional capacity, the existence of advance directives, or the presence of a reliable surrogate is very important, and there is enough time to pursue the intended desires of this patient.

Informed Consent

General Concepts

Studies have revealed that doctors may not adequately inform patients, patients may not understand the information, and such information rarely affects the patient's decision to follow the physician's recommendations. Despite these facts, American courts have long held that a patient's informed consent to a medical or surgical pro-

cedure or test is essential. The physician must give the patient sufficient information to make an intelligent decision before any action is performed. The laws dealing with informed consent require the surgeon to describe to the patient the nature of the procedure and the risks, benefits, and alternatives, including no treatment at all. Ethical consensus on just how much disclosure is adequate is still very controversial. What is clear is that permission must be given *voluntarily,* that is, without coercion from the physician or anyone else involved in rendering health care and, especially, those participating in the implementation of a research project.

The current interpretation of the law requires several elements to constitute "informed consent." The physician must disseminate the following information to the patient or acting surrogate to meet that standard:

1. A full explanation of the treatment procedure that the doctor wishes to pursue and what it involves, including the necessity for anesthesia and other support functions.
2. The reason the doctor selected this particular treatment, including the doctor's judgment as to why this procedure is chosen to alleviate, cure, or minimize the medical/surgical problem.
3. The risks of the recommended treatment, including the risks of both the treatment itself and any corollary threats to the patient. Doctors should, in satisfying this requirement, include discussion of their own particular experience with the procedure as well as that of the hospital and the medical/surgical colleagues who will be assisting.
4. The benefits the patient will receive from the proposed treatment. This is similar to the choice of treatment information previously described in that it requires the doctor to explain what the potential benefits will be from the procedure.
5. The chances that the proposed treatment will remedy the problem. This is similar to the information included when describing "benefits and risks" and should also include a description of the past experience of the surgeon in performing this specific procedure, as well as the outcomes that the surgeon has obtained.
6. The alternative treatment options for the given problem. This is similar to explaining the choice of treatment but emphasizes what other treatment options are available and why this surgeon has chosen this particular procedure.
7. The effects that refusal to accept the proposed treatment will have on the patient. This must entail a frank discussion of the ramifications of failure to receive the suggested treatment and whether it is life threatening or of a lesser degree of medical difficulty. This is when the surgeon must be most sensitive to the patient's religious, cultural, and ethnic background.

Here the law states that the sufficiency of the level of information will be judged from the *patient's* point of view, not the doctor's. If a surgeon explains a proposed treatment to the patient in terms that only another surgeon can understand, then the patient is not truly "informed." This requires communication skills. Every profession has its own jargon. Physicians must strive to ensure that the language they use is clearly understandable. Achieving acceptable levels of communication may be complicated by language, cultural, and socioeconomic factors. A manager responsible for building a new jetliner was credited with saying: "The main problem with communication is the illusion that it has actually occurred." All too frequently, patients and families come away from discussions where the surgeon thinks he or she has effectively communicated and the patient and family seemed to understand, but they did not. Sometimes it just comes down to faith in the doctor or an individual's unwillingness to reveal his or her lack of comprehension. The physician must use "common sense" in determining whether fully informed consent has truly been granted, taking into account that some cynics claim: "The problem about common sense is that it is not common."

As with every rule of law, there are certain exceptions to the requirement for informed consent. When there is an acute care situation that could result in the death of the patient, time is of the essence, and there is no surrogate decision maker present, the *consent requirement* is waived. Similarly, when the situation is not an emergency, but the patient is for one reason or another not able to give consent due to unconsciousness, coma, mental disability, or other cause of inadequate decision-making capacity, and there is no advance directive nor surrogate, informed consent is not necessary. There is also a therapeutic exception to the rule. If the physician believes that revelation of the normally required information would have a negative effect on the patient's health, fully informed consent is not necessary. This usually arises in the context of a psychiatric patient. Also, when a competent patient *refuses* to receive information upon which to base a decision, this requirement is waived. There can also be a waiver of the necessity for informed consent when the *government* requires certain medical tests or treatment in the face of possible medical or national security emergencies.

A common misconception among those rendering emergency care is that anyone who presents to an acute care facility falls into the "emergency exception" to informed consent. The emergency exception allows a physician to treat a patient without obtaining informed consent. This exception requires the following: the patient must be unconscious or without the capacity to make a decision, and no one else legally authorized to make such a decision is available; time must be of the essence in avoiding risk of serious bodily injury or death; and, under the circumstances the action proposed would be that to which a "reasonable person" would consent. The emergency exception does not apply if the patient has decision-making capacity and is able to communicate a decision about medical care.[2]

Using Newly Deceased Patients for Teaching Purposes

A unique problem exists for the medical/surgical team caring for patients in the emergency department of a teaching hospital. It involves using the newly dead for teaching purposes. This most commonly involves teaching medical students and residents the techniques of endotracheal intubation. The issue is, do surgeons have the right to perform procedures on a newly deceased person without obtaining permission (informed consent) from the surviving family? The dilemma is complicated by the fact that no better teaching opportunity exists for the trainees, who can then go forward, when adequately trained, to save lives and relieve suffering in the future. Clearly, no harm can be done to one who is dead. Furthermore, to our knowledge, there are no state statutes that specifically prohibit the teaching of procedures using newly dead patients; and no court has considered this issue. Although before death a patient has constitutional protection against nonconsensual invasion of his or her body, it has been established by various state courts that constitutional rights do terminate at the time of death.

Although the law in this situation is very forgiving, compassionate and ethical considerations should supervene. Policies have been proposed to deal harmoniously with these situations. Institutions should determine which trainees have a legitimate need to master the techniques afforded by practicing on the newly deceased patient. Only nonmutilating procedures should be permitted. The teaching of resuscitation skills on the newly deceased must be part of a structured learning sequence rather than an opportunistic and sporadic event.

Many ethicists now agree that permission must be obtained. They reject the arguments of those who wish to make this practice an exception to widely recognized standards of consent. Most believe that this can be compassionately expedited by a physician explaining to the family the importance and benefits that derive from their granting of permission to perform these teaching procedures.[14] Several medical studies have found that patients and families are likely to consent to such procedures but prefer to be asked permission first. Even the law advises that in this day of increasing recognition of personal autonomy, it is probably prudent to approach the next of kin for permission before performing procedures on the newly deceased.[15]

Participation in Research

Good research is described as that which enhances our ability to prevent illness or injury, to improve the quality or decrease the cost of care, or to improve the lives of our patients. Such research also must protect subjects and patients from harm, preserve their confidentiality, and allow them to enter freely as participants. Subjects and patients must be allowed to make an informed choice to participate, or not, without fear that their treatment might be compromised if they decline the request of the investigator. For a research project to be ethical, it must also be well designed and must investigate an issue of importance for which the answer does not yet exist. Protocols must be scientifically sound and likely to yield meaningful conclusions. Good research is therefore ethical, and bad research is unethical.[16]

In June 1966, Henry Beecher published an analysis of ethics and clinical research.[17] His benchmark article accelerated the movement that brought human experimentation under rigorous federal and institutional control. Although Beecher was not the first to direct attention to abuses in human experimentation, his presentation of 22 examples of investigators who endangered "the health or the life of their subjects" without informing them of the risks or obtaining their permission was a critical element in reshaping the ideas and practices governing human experimentation.[18]

Special issues for informed consent arise when the acute care patient is asked to participate in a research project. The time for decision making is usually short, and the principle investigator of the project may also be the one administering care. This raises issues of both adequate informed consent and the risk for coercion of the patient to participate in the study. The acute care surgeon researcher should abide by basic principles as outlined by the National Commission for the Protection of Human Subjects of Biomedical and Behavioral Research and by the Declaration of Helsinki. There are also prevailing federal, institutional, and professional guidelines that govern human and animal research. To be ethical, studies must be well designed and worth the risk to patient and society. The institution's review board should approve the study, and the investigator should take the responsibility to ensure adequate informed consent, confidentiality, and appropriate protection of the patient's well being.[1]

Acute care physicians must ensure that trials involving human subjects address issues of potentially significant value and are conducted ethically. The Nuremberg Code obligates researchers to prepare descriptions of the probability and magnitude of all physical, psychological, social, and economic risks and to minimize unnecessary pain and suffering. Consent must be voluntary and without any element of force, coercion, or deceit.[11] When discussing the potential risks of a proposed procedure, the investigator must quantify minimal, low, or high risk using examples from everyday life. Potential benefits from a research project may apply to the individual, to society, or to both. When discussing the benefits of a proposed study, one must distinguish clearly between therapeutic and nontherapeutic research. Researchers must clearly differentiate, for the patient, the balance between potential benefit to the patient and any potential risks associated with the protocol. No matter how great the benefit to society, it would not be ethical to expose a subject to anything greater than minimal risk if there is little direct benefit to the patient.[16]

Consent must never be assumed. This concept is especially confusing for research studies conducted in the acute care setting. Many would question the validity of truly "informed" consent rendered by someone who is acutely ill or severely injured. Especially for research, the principle still holds that consent must be valid; it must be informed, understood, and voluntarily given. Subjects, or their surrogates, must have enough information in a comprehensible form to enable them to make a proper judgment as to whether or not to participate in the requested study. Normally, this requires time for reflection before a decision to enroll. This concept is frequently stressed in the acute care situation. Here, the acute care surgeon may be forced to act in the patient's best interests and to presume consent on the basis of necessity. Clearly, this is only appropriate for interventions that will benefit the patient directly, and actual consent should be obtained as soon as possible afterwards. In a research context, the intervention must be part of a protocol approved by an independent institutional committee, such as an internal review board, and should present no more than minimal risk to the patient.[16]

Conflict of Interest: Industry and Drug Money

Many acute care surgeons interested in research have difficulty obtaining extramural support for their projects and thus turn to private sources, namely, the biomedical and pharmaceutical industry. Industry support for biomedical research now exceeds the support from all federal funding sources. The liaison between academic surgery and industry introduces the possibility of remarkable benefits especially to patients; however, differences between the fundamental goals of physicians and industry can create serious conflicts. Industry strives to complete clinical trials expeditiously and to publish positive results. Conversely, the primary goal of the surgical investigator is to advance and disseminate knowledge by the unimpeded exchange of ideas, despite secondary professional, financial, institutional, and sociopolitical objectives.

Critics maintain that the physician–industry relationship will only serve to potentiate bias; and loss of objectivity will fundamentally poison the way research is conducted. Currently, however, the lifeblood of clinical research is external support requiring a productive relationship with the biomedical industry. This potential conflict of interest can be resolved only by scrupulously implementing the principles of integrity, honesty, respect, and equity. Even the mere appearance of a conflict of interest could jeopardize the investigator's integrity and undermine public trust. Surgeon investigators involved with industry-sponsored research should meticulously divorce themselves from any personal or commercial conflict that could compromise patient loyalty or well-being.[11] Ethical recruitment of patients into research protocols is especially challenging for surgeons who, under the current system of financial remuneration, may receive more money by having the patient participate in a study than he or she would receive for doing the surgical procedure indicated for the patient.

A common challenge involves investigators who received industry-funded materials, discretionary funds, research equipment, and trips to meetings. Investigators must be aware that subsequent restrictions and expectations can create conflicts of interest. These seemingly innocent economic factors become a conflict any time they influence study design, interpretation of results, or the timing and method by which results are reported. The personal gain of the investigator such as ownership of stock or receipt of funds for testing drugs or devices can introduce bias and compromise objectivity. On the other hand, is not inappropriate for an investigator to receive economic rewards from a drug or device that is commensurate with his or her efforts involved in the development of the product. It is also acceptable for investigators to receive consultant and lecture fees from companies whose product they are testing, provided that the remuneration is proportionate with his or her efforts and that it is clearly reported, in advance, of all presentations and is clearly stipulated in any publications. It is unethical, however, to sell or purchase stock or to have a direct financial interest in the product under investigation until the relationship between the investigator and the company has been terminated and the results of the research have been published or made public. Although opponents argue that disclosure cannot heal the financial conflicts of interest, it does recognize public concerns, protect the credibility and reputation of investigators, and alert readers as they analyze the published report.[11]

The practice of pharmaceutical companies bestowing gifts on physicians is well documented. These gifts, however, cost money; and that cost is ultimately passed on to the patients without their explicit knowledge. The biomedical industry has clearly made outstanding contributions toward the advancement of modern scientific medicine; however, obvious conflict of interest occurs when physicians accept personal gifts that have no benefit to their patients. Acceptance of individual gifts that did not benefit patients, such as trips and subsidies for medical educational conferences at which physicians are not speakers, is strongly discouraged. The acceptance of even small gifts has been shown to affect clinical judgment and to heighten the perception (or reality) of a conflict of interest. Until specific guidelines are established, common sense should always prevail: no gifts should be accepted if suspected strings are attached.[11]

Autonomy, Decision-Making Capacity, and Competency

General Concepts

Individual freedom is one of the basic tenets of modern bioethics. This freedom is usually referred to as *autonomy*. This principle implies that a person should be free to make his or her own decisions. It is somewhat the antithesis of the medical profession's long practiced *paternalism* whereby the physician acted on what he or she thought was "good" for the patient, whether or not the patient agreed. The concept of autonomy applies to many interpersonal relationships and is essentially a respect for each person as an individual.

It has been difficult for many physicians, perhaps especially surgeons, and even more so for acute care surgeons, to accept the principle of patient autonomy. This is not difficult to understand, because accepting this principle implies a change in the physician's relationship with the patient. The physician must now be a partner in his or her patients' care; must become an educator, teaching uninformed patients enough about their diseases to make rational decisions; and, most distressing, must allow autonomous patients to make foolish choices. For physicians dedicated to helping their patients, allowing them to select what the physician considers a terrible treatment option, or even refusing treatment altogether, is a very frustrating change.[7]

On the other hand, experienced surgeons, especially those involved in rendering emergency care, know that their patients significantly rely on them for guidance through complicated choices, often when life itself is on the line. This is, of course, a form of paternalism that patients request and to which they are entitled. The key to accomplishing this ethically and successfully is based on the principle of *trust*. For surgeons, the establishing of this trust must begin at the inception of the relationship and sometimes must be very quickly accomplished. It can be very difficult for nonsurgical colleagues in medicine to understand and accept this element of paternalism required in the surgeon–patient relationship.

The crucial issue for the surgeon seeking autonomous informed consent is the *decision-making capacity* or *competence* of the patient involved. Understanding the differences between these terms is important, especially if the patient disagrees with the advice of the surgeon or refuses potentially life-sustaining treatment.

The determination of decision-making capacity involves more than just completing a mental status examination and includes the ability of the patient to take in information, to evaluate a decision based on personal values, to make a decision, and to communicate the choice of decision to the physician. The concept of medical decision-making capacity is one based on the ethical and practical evaluation of the team providing medical and surgical care. This is distinguishable from a legal determination of *incompetence*. A patient is always assumed to be legally *competent* unless a court has declared otherwise. For example, patients may not have been declared incompetent by a court but may have lost the capacity to make decisions about their medical care because of their current medical conditions, including intoxication, stroke, hypoxia, blood loss, dementia, and severe trauma. The determination of decision-making capacity varies in stringency with the seriousness of the impact of the decision. For example, the more severe the risk posed by the patient's decision, the more stringent should be the standard of determining capacity. This provides an increased protection for patients of questionable capacity when the potential harm from their decision is greater. This reaches the pinnacle of importance when a patient refuses treatment for a potentially life-threatening condition. These decisions are often difficult to make in the acute care environment, and the treating surgeon must sometimes make practical ethical decisions that go beyond the basic law of informed consent.

Refusal of Treatment

Ethical dilemmas usually occur when there is disagreement among the patient, the family, and the health care team. The clearest example is a patient's refusal to accept the recommended treatment. This is especially critical for the patient who has decision-making capacity and refuses potentially life-sustaining treatment. The United States Supreme Court, in the Cruzan case, upheld the right of persons to refuse life-saving medical treatment, including resuscitation, ventilators, artificial nutrition and hydration, and blood transfusions. The court based its decision on "the right of every individual to the possession and control of his own person, free from all restraint or interference of others, unless by clear and unquestionable authority of law under the liberty interest protected by the Due Process clause of the Fourteenth Amendment of the Constitution." The courts have, however, identified four *state interests* that override the refusal or termination of medical treatment on behalf of competent and incompetent persons, including the preservation of human life, the protection of the interests of innocent third persons, the prevention of suicide, and the maintenance of the integrity of the medical profession.

In exercising rights under the autonomy principle, each competent patient can refuse treatment, even if the results of such refusal will be death. This situation comes up most often in the case of religious or cultural beliefs. Jehovah's Witnesses are probably the most familiar example of this dilemma. They refuse to accept blood transfusions, based on their religious beliefs. Such refusal, especially when major surgery is indicated, clearly poses the likelihood of avoidable death. Still, the competent patient's autonomy must rule. There may be times when the treating surgeon doubts the competency of the patient refusing treatment. In such a case, if time permits, in order to protect the doctor and the hospital, it may be appropriate to seek a court order permitting the indicated procedure or blood transfusion. The courts will weigh the possible benefits of the treatment against the potential negative effects, risks, and the potential burdens on the patient; and they will issue a ruling. This ruling will insulate the treating physician and the institution from legal liability.

There are situations when parents or guardians are involved in refusal to accept and allow treatment on behalf of minors. These are the most common instances when court intervention is sought. To resolve the problem, the courts must balance the best interests of the child against the desires of the parents.

Certainly, refusal of a life-sustaining medical treatment should be accompanied by a full assessment of decision-making capacity and by an understanding from the patient of the consequences of refusal. If uncertainty prevails, the surgeon on the firing line should still "err on the side of life."

Telling the Truth/Disclosing Errors

Physicians have a duty to tell their patients the truth. This seems so obvious that it merits no further discussion. However, there may be circumstances when telling the "whole truth" to a patient will have a negative impact on his or her overall well-being. If the physician believes that telling the patient everything about the condition in question, which is a duty, will have a dramatic negative effect on the patient's well-being, the physician must decide which duty is more important.

"Truth telling" also would apply in situations involving medical mistakes, even those mistakes that are minor and arguably have no detrimental effect on the patient. To illustrate this point, consider a doctor awakened in the middle of the night who orders 1 mg of a drug but the appropriate dose is 0.1 mg. The overdose has no detrimental effect on the patient, so, does the doctor still have a duty to reveal the error that he or she made? Ostensibly, this question would seem to be easy to answer: Just tell the truth! However, if informing a patient whose confidence in the medical profession is very low and whose mental stability might be diminished by finding out about a medical error, notwithstanding the fact that the error had no detrimental effect, do doctors still have a duty to tell the truth? In this situation, it might violate the duty of nonmaleficence by doing something that will hurt the patient.

Impaired Decision-Making Capacity

Examples of patients having impaired decision-making capacity include minors, mentally handicapped persons, those with organic brain disease or in toxic states, and those with psychiatric conditions, including suicidal risk. Determining the point at which a minor has the capacity to make medical decisions is often very complicated, and the relevant laws vary among states.[19] For example, an "emancipated" minor can make his or her own medical decisions. This includes individuals younger than the age of majority who are living on their own, are married, or are in the military.

Even patients with Alzheimer's disease cannot all be regarded as having lost their decision-making capacity. Depending on the severity of their disease, they may well be able to participate in much of the decision-making process. This of course depends on the status of their disease and on the complexity and implications of the decision to be made.

Suicidal Patients

Respect for autonomy has always had its limits. When treating a suicidal patient in the emergency department, the surgeon is faced with a conflict between the ethical principles of *beneficence* and *respect for autonomy*. Sorting out this dilemma is usually based on whether the suicidal patient is currently capable of making a rational, autonomous decision. It also raises the perplexing question: can suicide sometimes be a rational choice? Generally, surgeons intervene with the suicidal patient based on the assumption that the person is suffering from mental illness and impaired judgment. This assumption is usually correct, with 90% of suicides being found to be associated with a mental illness such as depression, substance abuse, or psychosis.[20]

Therefore, relying on the principle of beneficence, surgeons almost always treat the injuries inflicted by suicidal patients despite their expressed intention to die. The conflict arises when the reasons for suicide appear "good," such as in the case of the terminally ill cancer patient with severe, uncontrollable pain. Is the application of life-saving intervention truly a beneficent act in the patient's best interest? Several studies have shown that physicians rendering care in the emergency department are not likely to recognize treatable depression in

their patients. These studies also confirm that 80% of patients who attempted suicide do not continue to wish to die. Thus, although some patients might make a rational decision to commit suicide, in most cases the surgeon delivering emergency care must assume that the person's judgment is impaired and proceed with life-saving measures.[20]

Advance Directives

General Principles

When a patient does not have the decision-making capacity to give informed consent, or there is no time to ask the patient or his or her surrogate about treatment preferences, *advance directives* express in writing what the patient's choices would be if he or she had decision-making capacity. Advance directives include living wills, durable powers of attorneys, and other written documents. In 1991, the federal government passed the Patient Self-Determination Act (PSDA), which required that health care institutions advise and educate patients regarding advance directives. This affected all institutions participating in the Medicare and Medicaid programs. This law was supposed to increase the use of advanced directives and thus prevent unwanted care. In fact, a major study of advanced directives and seriously ill patients revealed that the PSDA had little impact on health care in the United States. This was the Study to Understand Prognoses and Preferences for Outcomes and Risks of Treatments (SUPPORT), which showed that only 20% of seriously ill patients had advance directives even after the SUPPORT intervention and the PSDA.[21]

Despite these studies, it is still imperative for surgeons rendering acute care to understand the principles involved and the advantages of advocating for appropriate advance directives for patients and their families. An advance directive is any proactive document stating the patients' wishes in various situations should they be unable to state their own wishes.

Some states have specific language for each type of document and provide reciprocity for other states. Both the living will and a durable power of attorney can be prepared without the benefit of state-approved language as long as the intention of the person executing the document is clear. Such directives provide advanced informed consent for a myriad of courses of treatment, including issues of pain medication, "do not resuscitate" orders, or management should the individual enter some level of persistent vegetative state. In a complete set of these documents, the patient has given full thought to all of the possibilities that might occur and has decided what course of treatment he or she wants. Unfortunately, most patients have not executed these documents, or they have not given sufficient thought to what their wishes are.

Furthermore, many times when a power of attorney is granted to a surrogate decision maker, the surrogate has not had a full discussion of the wishes of the signatory.

Living Will

The living will, which was adopted by many states in 1990, is a document suitable for *terminally ill patients* and the treating physician accepts the patient's wishes regarding withholding of care, including requests restricting heroic resuscitative efforts, in advance. Many state that no life support be used when meaningful recovery will not occur. In a living will, the signatory indicates what his or her choices would be for medical treatment when death is imminent and the individual's wishes are unable to be communicated to the treating physician. Under most state laws, living wills indicate the signatory's desire to die a natural death and indicate unwillingness to be kept alive by so-called heroic measures. This usually amounts to a "do not resuscitate" order. In some states, it also indicates the patient's wishes concerning the level of pain medication, hydration, and nutrition to be administered if he or she lapses into a nondecisional condition. In most states the activation of the terms of a living will require an imminent demise and a second physician's opinion corroborating that determination. Unfortunately, many people believe that the living will is the best form of advanced directive and do not realize that it is only intended for the terminally ill.

Durable Power of Attorney

A durable power of attorney for health care specifies a surrogate decision maker in the event that the patient no longer has the capacity to make medical decisions. The durable power of attorney is a written document that gives the authority to another person, usually a spouse or relative, to make decisions regarding health care if the patient is incapacitated and unable to make decisions for himself or herself. The reason it is called "durable" is to ensure that the signatory knows that it can be revoked and or changed at any time. This provides the freedom to change both who the surrogate is and what the patient's stated wishes, if any, are. This is important in situations such as divorce, when the person executing the power of attorney may want to change the surrogate before the divorce becomes final, or when family dynamics create a desire to change the surrogate.

Thus, the patient designates a surrogate decision maker to participate in all significant treatment decisions and to be kept up to date regarding the patient's health care. The durable power of attorney works best when the patient has discussed with the surrogate his or her values and beliefs, as these would apply when complex decisions regarding health care issues are made. If there is no durable power of attorney, surrogate decision makers may be sought based on state laws. There is usually a defined hierarchy regarding surrogate decision makers: spouses, adult children, siblings, and so forth. Such a surrogate decision maker must be acting in the best interest of and according to the wishes and values of the patient. The durable power of attorney is a better form of advanced directive than the living will because; in the former, a surrogate can be educated about the nuances and options regarding each stage of treatment or non-treatment.[21]

Problems

In many situations the surrogate has the legal authority to make a decision but is not aware of what the patient would want. This is the fault of the patient, and all persons, when naming a surrogate decision maker, have a responsibility to fully explain what they would want in certain medical treatment situations. Failure to do so puts the burden on the surrogate to speculate what the patient would do were he or she able to make the decision.

There are two standards that apply when the surrogate has not been informed of the patient's wishes. One is the "substitute judgment" standard. When using this standard, the surrogate bases a decision on a prior expressed statement of the patient's preferences or on an in-depth knowledge of the personality of the patient and a willingness to do what the surrogate believes the *patient*, not the surrogate, would want in that specific situation. The second standard is that of the "best interest" of the patient. This is obviously a far more nebulous concept and occurs when the surrogate has not had any specific communication with the patient about the specific type of situation and is not cognizant of any particular patient preferences. In this situation, the surrogate is supposed to do what he or she believes is in the best interest of the patient. This is an important distinction to make and emphasizes the difference between doing what the patient would want done in a given situation as opposed to having someone else decide what he or she thinks is best.

A further problem with advance directives that limit full implementation of medical care is the application of such directives in situations for which they were not intended. An example that confronts the acute care surgeon is a healthy patient who has been injured in an automobile crash and has treatable conditions, such as a ruptured spleen or a lung contusion requiring aggressive pulmonary support. Should such a patient not be intubated because of an advanced directive indicating "do not resuscitate"? In such a case, it would be a serious error to respect the advanced directive and not to treat the patient's injuries aggressively. It is clearly probable that the patient would have wanted treatment under these circumstances.

There must also never be confusion when the patient is able to relate his or her preferences to health care providers. Verbal communication takes precedence over any written advance directive. In addition, when there is any confusion about the advance directive, disagreement among family members, or concern that it was not meant for the clinical circumstance at hand, advance directives limiting treatment should be ignored in favor of prudent medical care. In general, it is always wise for acute care providers to err on the side of life and to begin standard medical treatment. Treatment options, such as mechanical ventilation and hemodynamic support, can always be withdrawn at a later time once issues are resolved and the family is present. In such situations, the hospital ethics consultation service can prove very helpful.

Perhaps the major problem, at this point in time, is that there is little evidence that advance directives have made a significant impact on health care delivery in the United States.[21] We, as surgeons rendering acute care, should do all within our power to reverse this situation.

Confidentiality

General Principles

Acute care surgeons are bound by the same rules of confidentiality as other doctors. Especially with the new restrictions imposed by HIPAA, all health care personnel working in the emergency department must be very cognizant of preserving confidentiality. In the hectic morass that is the waiting area of most big hospitals, it is sometimes difficult to take the time to ensure that doctors convey sensitive and private information to patients, families, or surrogates in a full and complete manner, and yet ensure the confidentiality of the information. Certain health information can be very significant in the treatment of a patient, including medication history and psychiatric history. Yet, some patients or families might be reluctant to give such information to the treating physician if the situation is not conducive to confidential communication. Similarly, the families of the patient are most certainly due confidentiality of the information that the physician is going to impart. It is critical for the surgeon to establish a trusting relationship so that the best and most important information relevant to treatment can be given and received. An exception to the confidentiality rule occurs when the law requires disclosure of information to officials, as in the case of certain infectious diseases or when a third party might be injured as a direct result of the physician's failure to report information.

A surgeon's duty to maintain confidentiality regarding information disclosed by the patient has been a long-held medical precept. On occasion, however, the ethical duty to prevent harm to others overrides the duty to keep the confidences of a given patient. Although the law generally prevents the divulgence of confidential information, it also mandates certain exceptions, such as reporting patients with infectious disease and those who are likely to harm others, the latter being elucidated by the famous 1976 Tarasoff case in which nondisclosure of a patient's homicidal thoughts resulted in the death of the threatened person. This case raises the confusing possibility of preventing harm to others becoming a legal not just an ethical duty. It broadens the concept of mandatory reporting to include more than the currently accepted requirements for reporting child, elder, or domestic abuse. Such legal requirements may force us to compromise the ethical norm of respecting our patient's decisions with regard to confidentiality.[2]

Abuse of the Elderly

It is claimed that approximately 2 million elderly Americans are mistreated each year, with a significant number falling into the definition of abandonment. Although mistreatment of elders has occurred for centuries, only recently has society become significantly concerned about it. The problem and concern will increase as the population ages. Those physicians and surgeons who work in the acute care situation are ideally suited to play a significant role in the detection, management, and prevention of elder abuse and neglect. The acute care physician may be the only person, outside the family, who sees the older adult and is qualified to intervene in a preventive way. This means that especially surgeons should be aware of risk factors and their detection. It requires an astute clinician to detect abuse based on history alone. Even in the face of injuries, such as fractures at uncommon sites, the elderly patient may continue to conceal the possibility of abuse for fear of embarrassment or abandonment by the abuser. It may well be the surgeon called to see the patient for injury who picks up clues of old injuries or new injuries in unusual locations, such as on the scalp or behind the ears.

The first priority of the acute care physician is to ensure this victim's safety. The surgeon should never hesitate to ask for social service consultation or to report suspicions to the appropriate adult protective services. Such acts are not breaches of confidentiality; they represent implementation of the most sincere duty of the physician.[22]

Futility and Withholding Treatment

Significant, and perhaps inappropriate, concern continues to exist in medicine with regard to the difference between *withholding* and *withdrawing* medical treatment. This has become more of an issue as the potential for resuscitating critically ill patients has become a reality. Depending on the clinical situation, surgeons and other physicians attribute higher legal risk of one procedure over another.

Apparently because of this fear of legal retribution, or ridicule and condemnation by professional peers, employing full, almost ritualistic, resuscitation has become the default position of those delivering critical care when no advance directive exists. In fact, no physician has ever been successfully prosecuted for withholding or withdrawing of medical care from any dying patient in the legal history of the United States. This leaves one wondering what actually fuels the spheres of legal retribution for making the wrong decision.[23]

The dilemma could of course be alleviated by early meaningful discussion with patients, families, and surrogates with regard to care options at the end of life and honest estimates of prognosis. Studies have shown, however, that many physicians and surgeons fail to take these opportunities. A disturbing example of this inadequacy can be found in the 1995 SUPPORT study. This expensive, multiinstitutional study demonstrated the physicians' failure to meet all outcome markers: failure to include patient and family in pivotal care discussions, failure to provide realistic estimates of outcomes valued by patients, failure to treat pain adequately, and failure to prevent prolonged death in patients with poor prognoses.[23]

Sometimes confusion is created over the venue in which surgical or medical care is delivered. In the usual setting, a decision to withhold further medical treatment is done quietly, often without input from the patient or the surrogate decision maker, whereas withdrawal of ongoing medical treatment can be more obvious and difficult. Some clinicians and ethicists feel that the withholding of acute care medical treatment is more problematic than later withdrawal of unwanted or useless interventions. This discrepancy in the acute care situation probably exists because the physicians involved usually lack the vital information about their patients' identities, medical conditions, and expressed wishes. In addition, perhaps because of frequent, but inaccurate, representations on television, society has come to expect only spectacular results in the delivery of emergency care in the United States. This concept is in marked contrast to the attitude that those clinicians who withdrew treatment (an act leading to death) were more culpable than those who withheld treatment (an omission leading to death); this distinction between acts and omissions is now thought to be more of a difference in psychological preference than an ethical norm.[24] For all of these reasons, despite the fact that the law has clearly spoken, the distinction between withdrawal and withholding of medical treatment will continue to be a challenge.

The surgeon's decision to limit or withhold treatment can be based either on the patient's refusal or on the physician's determination that the treatment would not be of benefit. Although the patient has the ethical and legal right to forego treatment, the physician must be very careful about withholding a treatment that might be beneficial. Such issues are usually intensified by the need for rapid intervention versus the desire to verify the meaning of the patient's current or preexisting desires. The classic example is the patient who is unresponsive, has reversible pulmonary or cardiac disease, needs cardiopulmonary resuscitation, but is said to have a preexisting do not resuscitate order.

Withholding treatment because of a judgment of "futility" is even more of an ethical challenge. A "futile" effort has been defined as "any effort to achieve a result [that is] possible but that reasoning or experience suggests is highly improbable and that cannot be systematically produced." Physicians, as moral agents, should exercise professional judgment in assessing a patient's requests. If the request goes beyond well-established criteria of reasonableness, the surgeon ought not feel obliged to provide it. Some ethicists believe that the appropriate allocation of resources is another important consideration when one is making decisions regarding invasive, costly, or lengthy procedures. John Lantos even stated that, "given limited resources, it is ethically justifiable to limit access to treatments that are expensive and offer minimal benefit. . . . [D]ecisions by doctors to curtail use of those treatments are socially responsible."[25] "Futility" is such a complicated concept that it may be of little use in most situations. The classic challenge is the decision not to start resuscitation when a patient with extensive metastatic cancer and cachexia presents in cardiac arrest. The initial emotional inclination is to treat the patient; however the medical situation, as emphasized by Jonsen et al.,[13] leads to a judgment that such a resuscitation will not be beneficial. This requires the difficult objective determination of ineffectiveness rather than a subjective decision based on the worth of the intervention or on the value of the patient's continued life.[2]

Assertions of futility come about in two contradictory situations. One is when the patient or surrogate wants the doctor to refrain from a further treatment that the doctor thinks is not futile; and the other is when the doctor wishes to refrain from a treatment that he or she believes to be futile. The only measure of what should be done is the standard of care in the given region for similar cases. Dealing with this concept of "futility" or other "end-of-life" concerns is usually only a problem when disagreement arises among the patient, the family, and the health care team.

Many ethicists agree that physicians are under no obligation to render treatments that they deem of little or no benefit to the patient. Many believe that it would be advantageous to abandon the word "futility" and to use instead the construct of "clinically nonbeneficial interventions." We all know that one of the greatest fears of both patients and families is their abandonment by the health care team. It is easy to fall into this trap by declaring that further treatment for a given patient is "futile." When it is decided that certain interventions should be appropriately withheld, special efforts should be made to maintain effective communication, comfort, support, and counseling for the patient, family, and friends. Although we, as surgeons, may not always proceed with potential technologically advanced nonbeneficial interventions, we always must continue to *care* for the patient and the family.[26]

Withdrawal of Treatment

General Principles

Taking into account the preceding discussion, an important line of reasoning for the moral and legal equivalents for the two actions of withholding or withdrawing is that if a medical intervention will not result in the desired or beneficial results intended for the patient, it makes no difference whether the clinician withholds the intervention before beginning it or discontinues its use after it has been started and found to be not effective.[24]

Special moral issues can arise in the care of terminally ill patients. We must be willing to respect a terminally ill patient's wish to forego life-prolonging treatment, as expressed in a living will or through a health care surrogate appointed via a durable power of attorney for health care. Those of us caring for patients in acute care situations, or in general, should also be willing to honor "do not resuscitate" orders appropriately executed on behalf of terminally ill patients. We should also understand the established criteria for the determination of death and should be prepared to assist families in decisions regarding the donation of the patient's organs for transplantation. This involves knowing the specific regulations in our own states and in our own specific institutions, especially the criteria for death and the mechanisms for initiating the conversation relative to organ donation. It is usually not the surgeon, or any member of the treating team, who first raises the issue with family regarding donation of the dying patient's organs.

Applying the Principles

To comply with the principle of autonomy, when a competent patient requests or demands the withdrawal of further treatment, the treating physician is in a situation analogous to that of the patient who initially refuses treatment. Autonomy governs. The acute care surgeon should ensure that the patient is given all the information necessary to allow proper informed consent regarding withdrawal of treatment; but, once this is done, it is the ethical duty of the surgeon to withdraw the specified treatment. This is true no matter what the patient requests, whether it be withdrawal of feeding tubes, ven-

tilators, or nutrition and hydration. As long as the patient is fully aware of the consequences, both short term and long term, his or her stated wishes should be respected and acted on appropriately by the health care team.

The same principle should be invoked when the patient is not able to understand but has indicated in an advance directive a desire with respect to withdrawal of treatment under specified circumstances. It is still the duty of the physician to withdraw the specific treatment because the patient has, in the advance directive, given prior informed consent. The duty of the physician is identical if a designated surrogate requests or demands the withdrawal of treatment. This is the patient speaking through the surrogate, and, once again, autonomy governs.

When the surgeon determines that withdrawal of treatment is appropriate and further treatment would be ineffective, consent of the family or surrogate should be sought. In this situation, it is very important and helpful to know what if any *surrogacy laws* exist. These vary from state to state, and those surgeons faced with potential decision making should know in advance the laws of their state. Where such laws exist, they can be very helpful in delineating the hierarchy of surrogate designation. In the absence of advance directives, surgeons have the responsibility to judge what they believe the patient would want or what is in the best interest of the patient. If no family is available, close friends of the patient may be asked to give their opinions about what the patient would want.

Courts have upheld the principles of autonomy and self-determination, affirming the right to refuse life-sustaining treatment. The classic illustration of this is the 1976 ruling by the New Jersey Supreme Court that Karen Ann Quinlan, a woman in a persistent vegetative state, had the right to decide to be removed from a respirator and that this right could be asserted, on her behalf, by her family. This right was extended to include the withdrawal of nutrition by the 1990 Cruzan case in which the U.S. Supreme Court ruled that a life-sustaining feeding tube could be removed from another young woman in a persistent vegetative state.[20]

Acute care surgeons who have moral or religious beliefs that would preclude them from withdrawing treatment should withdraw from the case. It is important to recognize at the beginning of the clinical encounter the possible need to withdraw treatment so that physicians can extricate themselves at the earliest possible stage. As the clinical course evolves and a surgeon develops a relationship with the family and the patient, it becomes progressively more difficult to leave the treatment team.

Palliative Care

Focusing on making the last months, not minutes, of life meaningful is especially appropriate when death is likely to occur. Chronic progressive diseases such as cancer, congestive heart failure, and chronic obstructive pulmonary disease account for 50% to 70% of deaths compared with the sudden deaths attributed to stroke, heart attack, trauma, and suicide. In the United States, patients' perceptions of human finitude lead them to deny death and to rely on medical achievements that they think will let them live forever. Physicians grapple with their technological power, the imperative to tell the truth about fatal conditions, and despair at denying hope and the promise of cure for their trusting patients. It is probably this mutual self-deception that becomes the central issue in rendering appropriate end-of-life care. It is the management of these intense psychological and spiritual challenges facing terminally ill patients that has come to form the basis of what is called "palliative care."[23]

Palliative care can be briefly defined as the act of total care of patients whose disease is not responsive to curative treatment. Although palliative care has been a major focus in Europe for the past 20 years, interest in the United States only became significant in the late 1990s with an Institute of Medicine report that evaluated end-of-life care. It revealed significant deficiencies in how we manage end-of-life care, including management of pain, nausea and vomiting, dyspnea, depression, and anxiety. McCahill et al.[27] explain that "palliative care is not a concept defined in terms of the amount of time remaining in a patient's life or the terminal nature of his disease. It is defined in terms of the type of need that is being met by the care."

Palliative surgery is surgery for which the major intent is alleviation of symptoms and improving quality-of-life, not necessarily cure. As the ages of the patients increase, surgeons will be progressively involved in performing operations whose desired outcomes are not met. Managing these patients through the entire course of their disease, including death, is an important part of being a good physician and a good surgeon. Surgical emergencies are often the first encounter with older patients, and they often have multiple comorbidities. An example is the 80-year-old person who presents with an acute abdomen. The risk of surgery will be high, the prognosis may be poor, and cure may be impossible. Perhaps offering surgical treatment would even be inappropriate. Thus, acute care surgeons are immediately thrust into contemplating palliative care for the surgical patient, and it becomes clear that surgeons need to be aware of the concepts involved in delivering such care.[27]

Determination of Death

The attending physician has the discretion and the responsibility to determine death. Statutes in different states use different criteria for death. In some cases they have not caught up with the science available. Some states use the "irreversible cessation of cardiopulmonary function" criterion, as do some religions. The complete cessation of respiration and circulation constitutes "death" under this definition. The concept of "intensive care" has advanced dramatically since these statutes were enacted and has superseded this antiquated definition. In most states where this is the statutory definition, the courts have now ruled that "brain death" suffices.

Most states use the brain death criterion. There is debate currently about whether the "whole brain" definition of death is still valid or whether the appropriate ethical standard for definition of death is cessation of "higher brain" function. Higher brain function includes the cognitive functions or the capacity for consciousness. Once there is irreversible cessation of this capability, a judgment usually made in consultation with a neurologist, then death can be declared. Most neurologists are trained to determine whether death has occurred or whether the patient is in a "permanent vegetative state."

In some states the definition of death includes *either* the cessation of cardiopulmonary function *or* irreversible cessation of all brain function, including the brain stem. The health care team should realize that no matter which criterion is being used, it may be appropriate to continue cardiovascular support for the purpose of maintaining perfusion during the eminent birth of a fetus or to sustain viability of transplantable organs.

Organ Donation

Criteria for organ donation are not always clearly understood. Many patients and families are mistakenly concerned about having death declared prematurely just to facilitate the harvesting of organs for transplantation. Here the surgeon's bioethical responsibilities are clear. The medical ethical principle of "patient autonomy" dictates that the desires of the patient and the family be respected.

Federal law requires most hospitals to ask all patients, during their admission for any procedure, whether emergency or elective, about their wishes to be a potential organ donor. Although this can be somewhat of a shock to patients who are coming in for elective surgery, especially a minor procedure, it obviates the need for physicians to make the painful inquiry when a patient is actually facing eminent death. If the admitting personnel ask for this information on a routine basis, the patient is more likely to render a competent decision, and the potential problems of dealing with surrogates, sometimes under difficult circumstances, is alleviated.

However it is obtained, informed consent of the *donor* is required. Most states provide organ donor options on driver's licenses, and many people possess other documents such as donor cards that indicate their desire to become organ donors. In some cases, donors place limits on the organs they want to donate. For example, some donors have indicated that they do not wish to donate their eyes or some other specific organ. Even though patient autonomy should guide the physician, there are times when the family emphatically wants to override the clearly stated intention of the donor. These situations are difficult, and while the surgeon's clear ethical duty is to respect the wishes of the donor, the body of the donor, after death, belongs to the family. The treating physician would be well advised to leave the resolution of this situation up to the transplant coordinator. In fact, it is usually inappropriate for anyone on the treating team to initiate the discussion of organ donation. Most hospitals have in place a procedure whereby the discussion of potential organ donation is initiated by a person specifically trained for this purpose. It is often the transplant coordinator, a social worker, or a hospital chaplain.

Insisting on compliance with the donor's clearly stated wishes, in the face of strong family opposition, does not affect the legal position of the surgeon; it can, however, result in unfortunate lawsuits because of the animosity created with the family. In cases where there are no previously expressed wishes by the potential donor, the family, as custodians of the body, may agree to organ donation. The duty of the physician in this case is to obtain the consent of the family *before* doing anything to preserve the functioning of the organs for potential transplantation.

When there is no surrogate or family or any evidence of previously stated intention to donate, the ethical position of the doctor is less clear. However, absent permission, to do something to the body in a situation that is no longer an emergency, assuming that the organs should be harvested or transplanted, would seriously violate the concept of informed consent. It can be argued that the dead person cannot give informed consent, but the family whose property the body is would have to give their consent to have any procedure done at all to the newly dead person. In cases with no directives at all, the best course of action is to do nothing postmortem.

Ethical and Legal Consultations

Most surgeons rendering emergency care work within an institution, and these institutions usually provide help in sorting out challenging ethical dilemmas in the form of consultations with hospital ethics committee or in-house lawyers. It is critical to realize that utilization of such resources does not commit the surgeon to accepting an arbitrary decision of what is right and what is wrong in a complicated ethical situation. Consultation is meant to provide a process for most expeditiously sorting out the issues that have arisen and for providing rapid access to the potential mechanisms for solving the problem.

Hospital ethics committees are specifically charged to advise physicians, patients, and families who face ethical dilemmas. These situations usually arise when there is disagreement among these groups. Consultation with the ethics committee is usually rapidly facilitated through such agencies such as the hospital nursing service. Consultation should be available, instantly, 24 hours a day. Frequently, it is the hospital chaplain who facilitates the consultation. By bringing in appropriate resources and facilitating meetings with the health care team, patients, and families, the ethics committee should help resolve even the most complicated medical ethical challenges. The hospital ethics committee should be charged with what is the right thing to do for the patient. It should have no vested interest in protecting the institution at the risk of embarking on an action that is ethically unsettled for the good of the patient.

A word of caution, however, is necessary for surgeons rendering emergency care within a given institution. Once "legal counsel" or "risk management" is brought in to deal with a complicated situation, it must be remembered that they work for the institution, their job is to protect the institution, and the advice that they give will be aimed toward that end. This commitment to the institution is important for the physician to realize if there is potential for placing oneself in personal jeopardy. It is also important to realize that legal standards are not always reliable guides to determining what are the best ethical and medical decisions.

Good Samaritan

A Case

The most skilled ear, nose, and throat surgeon in town is out to dinner. At the next table he sees the local crime boss choking to death on a piece of prime beef. What are the ethical and legal ramifications he must consider before performing an acute care tracheotomy? What is he ethically obligated to do? Is the old medical oath binding? Can anyone give consent? Must he identify himself? If he performs the procedure, and there is a bad outcome, is it malpractice? What if he is a medical student instead of a famous surgeon? Is a bad outcome here considered battery? What should the surgeon do when the emergency medical technicians arrive and want to take the dying crime boss to a known inferior local hospital? What are the obligations and risks for the this surgeon?

General Concepts

Good Samaritan acts are deeds in which aid is rendered to a person in need, where no fiduciary or legal obligation exists to provide such aid, and no reward or remuneration for the aid is anticipated. The aid provided can include a survey of this situation, protection of the victim, notification of other care providers, or personal provision of immediate treatment. The Good Samaritan ethic is one that is generally endorsed by our culture, which strongly supports assisting an individual who is in danger or in need of help. Surgeons, especially those trained an emergency care, may be regarded as having a greater responsibility to provide Good Samaritan aid than a lay person by reason of the special training and knowledge and commitment to duty for the benefit of individuals and society that generally drive people to become physicians and surgeons. Clearly, in a situation of sudden medical need, an acute care surgeon will be better able to assess the medical condition of the victim and to render immediate treatment if indicated and feasible. Many believe that the mere status of being a physician entails the duty to use one's skills and knowledge in cases of sudden or acute care need; for some, this duty is an inherent feature of the role and even of the definition of a physician.[28]

Briefly stated, in almost every state, an off-duty surgeon who comes across a person with an acute care medical condition has no legal duty to come to the aid of that person. However, a physician's ethical obligation inspires him to help in such an emergency. All states in the United States have enacted so-called Good Samaritan statutes, which protect the physician from liability incurred for good-faith efforts to help at the scene of an accident or emergency. The ethical duty should far exceed the legal excuse for inaction.[2]

Generally, Good Samaritan acts include the following principles: (1) There is no legal obligation of doctors to answer or treat emergencies. (2) If the doctor chooses to intervene, the expected standard of care is modified by circumstances of the situation. (3) If aid is given, it need be stabilization only and not definitive treatment. (4) Implied consent exists to treat the victim if he or she lacks the capacity to consent. (5) These criteria apply whether or not the physician is paid for his or her services rendered. Despite the establishment of these principles, the extensive coverage in the media of spectacular medical malpractice suits causes many surgeons to develop a strong aversion to the performance of Good Samaritan acts. To alleviate this apprehension, Good Samaritan laws were enacted, the first in California in 1959. Since then every state has enacted such laws. The laws all have the following provisions: there is no legal obligation to provide aid; there is immunity from malpractice suit if aid is provided; there is exception from immunity for gross negligence or lack of "good faith"; acts are restricted to application outside of hospitals; and there is withdrawal of legal immunity if the doctor accepted payment for aid rendered.[28]

Pain Relief and the Doctrine of Double Effect

Confusing Principles

When it comes to adequacy of pain control, especially for patients near the end of life, physicians and surgeons have been caught in a complicated dilemma. On the one hand, most entered medicine to relieve suffering. On the other hand, administration of excessive doses of pain medication can suppress respiration and run the risk of contributing to the death of patients already near the end of life. At the same time that physicians are criticized for not giving enough pain medication to suffering patients, they are also challenged by the law for prescribing medication with the double effect of potentially hastening death. This doctrine of double effect is intended by the courts to recognize the difference between provision of adequate pain treatment that unintentionally cases death and the ordering of medication that intentionally causes a patient's death. This concept of *intent* is confusing not only for the courts but also for the physician who is ordering the pain medication.

Double Effect

The application of the principle of double effect is controversial because it places significant weight on physician intent, which is impossible to prove, and no weight on a patient's right to self-determination. This seems to contradict a paramount principal of American bioethics: patient autonomy. Why, when death is on the line, should concern over the physician's intention take precedent over the patient's informed consent? The physicians fear over misinterpretation of their actions often leads to inappropriate use of pain medication, leaving patients unjustifiably suffering. It is clearly recognized that opioids should be considered early in the care of dying patients and in dosages that often exceed the standard range. These analgesics are effective in not only reducing painful sensation but also in adjusting the sense of well-being, thereby improving the patient's ability to cope with pain. Adjustment of dosage can be aided by using one of the known "pain scales" or by observation of patients' objective signs of distress, especially useful with the non-communicative patient.

Despite the significant effects that opioids have on several components of respiration, respiratory arrest from opioids, in the absence of other central nervous system depressants, is rare. When caring for dying patients, acute care surgeons must acknowledge that they are one part of the often-fragmented medical team. They must accept the goal of providing care when they can, comfort always, consult when necessary, and coordinating the remaining end-of-life issues.[23]

Hastening Death

Because the overwhelming admonition to the physician is "above all, do no harm," society has implored the acute care surgeon, in life-threatening situations, to waive informed consent requirements and to act presumptively to save life or limb in situations where the usual consent is impossible to obtain. This leads to our current default in dealing with the critically ill or moribund unknown patient: resuscitating with a "full code" and asking questions later. This practice is probably acceptable as long as the surgeon realizes that withdrawing life support is just as acceptable as withholding life support initially. The full resuscitation may make it possible to assess the patient's end-of-life desires more fully and carefully. If the initial intervention is unsuccessful or is inconsistent with the patient's preference, it can and should be withdrawn, consistent with the patient's identified goals.

What are ethically frowned upon are such deceitful practices as the "slow code," a charade consisting of a halfhearted resuscitation that seems to allow the acute care surgeon to take the moral middle ground by giving the family a false impression of respecting patient autonomy while knowing full well that the act will not be effective. Experience suggests that this hedge is used fairly commonly. Although no ill is usually intended, the slow code is an indication that the surgeon has not realistically communicated with the patient and family to express the medical opinion that resuscitation, in the face of cardiac or respiratory arrest, would be inappropriate.[23]

The concept of "no code" should be clear and is usually instituted at the request of the patient, his advance directive, or an appropriate surrogate. It is ethically inappropriate for the physician to disrespect the patient's autonomous decision even when faced with despairing surrogates requesting interventions over a clear directive to the contrary. The patient with decision-making capacity is, of course, free to change any prior stipulation, even those written in an advance directive. In the absence of any directive, including a decisional patient, the acute care physician must employ the best interest standard, which requires implementing what a reasonable patient would want done in a similar situation.

To understand these concepts, the surgeon must understand the implications of the three means of accelerating death for patients in the United States: double effect, voluntary euthanasia, and physician-assisted suicide. The rule of double effect, as previously described, involves the dichotomy of treatment versus side effects, where death is the unintended side effect of adequate symptom control. Voluntary euthanasia, that which is requested by the patient, can be either active or passive. Passive euthanasia is the result of withdrawing or withholding life support in situations judged to be medically futile. In the United States, this is both ethically and legally acceptable. On the other hand, active euthanasia occurs when the physician intentionally administers an agent to cause a patient's death. This act is considered unethical and illegal everywhere in the world except in the Netherlands, where it is practiced openly. Physician-assisted suicide

occurs when a physician supplies a death-causing agent to a patient with the knowledge that the patient intends to use this agent to commit suicide. In United States, this practice is legal only in Oregon.[23]

Of great concern to all physicians in the United States is a recent action by the Attorney General of the United States with regard to the Oregon Death with Dignity Act, a law that authorizes doctors to help their terminally ill patients commit suicide. The doctors were allowed to prescribe, but not to administer, such drugs. Attorney General Ashcroft, in 2001, directed that doctors who help their patients commit suicide could be prosecuted under the federal Controlled Substances Act. This was the first example, in United States, of the federal government interceding in the practice of medicine, historically entrusted to state lawmakers. In May 2004, the United States Court of Appeals for the Ninth Circuit, in San Francisco, rebuked the Attorney General and upheld the Oregon law.[29,30]

Know Your Intent

For all physicians, the concept of avoiding killing seems obvious. However, what is a doctor to do when confronted with a situation whereby the administration of sufficient medication to alleviate the pain of a patient might have the secondary effect of diminishing respiration and actually hastening the death of the patient? This is, of course, the crux of the major debate over physician-assisted suicide. There are other situations, such as abortion, where a physician must take avoiding killing into account. Confronting such issues challenges a surgeon not only with the duty to respect the autonomy of the patient but also to be aware of situations that might put the individual doctor in the uncomfortable situation of confronting conflict with his or her own personal beliefs.

In multiple decisions, the courts have emphasized the importance of the distinction between "letting a patient die and making that patient die."[20] This, in our opinion, is the most distressing conflict for the physician who must make such decisions. Physicians know full well that when they give high-dose opioids or withdraw ventilatory support, they may be hastening the patient's death. The callous ones see this as euthanasia and strongly criticize those who claim otherwise. When confronted with this challenge, in a personal communication, Dr. Edmund Pellegrino, one of the most respected medical ethicists, immediately responded with his comforting interpretation of such a situation. In his mind, and in his conscience, he recognizes and acts upon the difference between actively and intentionally hastening a patient's death as opposed to relieving pain and suffering or withdrawing artificial life support, thus "letting nature take its course."

Case Management Scenarios

Case 1: Informed Consent for Trauma

"Friends" drop a 19-year-old male at the front door of the emergency department. He has one gunshot wound to the abdomen with wounds just above the umbilicus and one just lateral to the spine on his back. His blood pressure is 100/50 and heart rate 110. He is awake and alert and denies any drug use. He smells of alcohol, and his speech is somewhat slurred. You inform him that he needs to go to the operating room for an emergent exploratory laparotomy. He says he wants to be left alone and to let him leave the hospital.

Question 1: What are the ethical principles involved in this case?
Autonomy versus beneficence

Question 2: What should you do?
This patient should be taken to the operating room emergently. Obtaining informed consent after a traumatic injury is recognized as a difficult task. Many prominent ethicists believe the pressure and urgency of a traumatic situation make it impossible to have a true informed consent decision, even if the patient has a normal mental status. Shock, drugs, alcohol, head injury, and pain often complicate the trauma patient's cognitive abilities. In these cases, it is commonly considered that the ethical principle of beneficence overrides the patient's autonomy; therefore, the surgeon should do what a "reasonable person" would want done under these circumstances. This does overrule the patient's autonomy, but traumatically injured patients are often unable to make critical decisions in their own best interests. This ethical reasoning is also backed by the legal system, which has consistently ruled that the care provider should treat based on the "reasonable person" scenario.

Question 3: What if he was not drunk?
The patient should, even if in a seemingly perfect mental state, still be taken to the operating room for potentially life-saving surgery. Time is of the essence for these patients, and, even if they are temporarily hemodynamically stable, any delays in treatment may cause unrecoverable injury. Again, the principle of beneficence applies, and the patient should have all required emergent treatments. Many medical centers routinely do *not* obtain any written consents for trauma patients as a matter of practice. Once stabilized, the patients may then be able to make further treatment decisions with the team.

Case 2: Truth Telling and Communication

A 75-year-old Korean man presents to the Emergency Department with symptoms of large bowel obstruction. Eight family members, including four children, accompany him. His wife has died. Your work up includes a Hypaque enema that reveals a constricting colon lesion that is confirmed to be cancer by colonoscopy. The family wishes for you to withhold the cancer operation from their father and to proceed with a decompressive colostomy. They say they have always cared for their father, and there is no reason to worry him about the diagnosis. Especially, they ask you not to use the word "cancer."

Question 1: What are the ethical considerations of this case?
Autonomy and truth telling

Question 2: What do you tell the family?
You should tell the family that you respect their opinion and the care and love that they have for their father but that you are morally and legally obligated to discuss the diagnosis and options with their father because he clearly has decision-making capacity. Then you should discuss the case with their father. The principle of autonomy is very important in this case because the patient has the right for self-determination of his treatment decisions. He might make different decisions than his family would have expected or wanted. The choice must be for what he wants, not for what someone else thinks is "best for him."

Your discussions with the patient and family must also be truthful. If you respect the family's wishes, then you would have to lie to the patient about his potential operation. This is inappropriate in this case. However, there may be cases when the patient has a decreased mental capacity, such as a severely mentally retarded patient; in this case, you must respect the family's decisions for the patient's good, as they are the surrogate decision makers. One should also ensure that family members acting as interpreters for you pass on all information to their loved one. This may require finding an independent interpreter for the patient.

Case 3: Surrogate Decision Makers

A 45-year-old gay man presents to the emergency department after a rollover motor vehicle accident. He is hemodynamically stable but has a decreased mental status and requires intubation. A full-body CT scan reveals a severe brain injury, without other major injury.

The neurosurgeon and you believe this is a devastating injury for which the anticipated outcome is prolonged hospitalization in a chronically bedridden state. His partner of 15 years is given this information and says the patient and he have talked about death and dying many times because of many of their friends' struggles with AIDS. He informs you that his partner, now your patient, told him many times he would not want such aggressive care and should be taken off the ventilator. The patient's mother and sister now arrive, and they wish everything to be done for this patient, whom they have not talked to in over 10 years.

Question 1: What are the ethical principles?
Surrogate decision makers

Question 2: What should you do?
Determination of surrogate decision makers involves both ethical and legal considerations. From a legal standpoint, most states have a specific hierarchy of people who become the surrogate for patients not capable of making medical decisions. The list usually starts with a parent or a spouse. Also, some states have started to recognize same sex partners as the closest surrogate. These factors all need to be taken into consideration when making critical end-of-life decisions.

In this case, it would be wise to keep the patient on the ventilator for the time being until the surrogate problem is worked out. The decision to remove the patient from the ventilator can happen at any time. Discussions between the partner and the family are often useful in working out differences. Time will also let you investigate the situation more fully. Has the patient had recent contact with the family? Are there any issues between the same sex partners? Are there other friends or neighbors who can help confirm or refute issues? Finally, an ethics consult is most helpful for you to work through these problems.

Once a surrogate has been identified, you are ethically responsible to follow his or her wishes as long as they are reasonable and conform with nonmaleficence, or avoiding harm to the patient. For this critically head-injured patient, it is reasonable to remove the ventilator, but it may be more appropriate to discuss with the surrogate that all head injuries are different, and allowing some time to assess for changes would give the medical team a chance to provide a more accurate prognosis.

Case 4: Jehovah's Witness

A 10-year-old girl is brought to the emergency department after being hit by a car while riding her bicycle. She is awake and alert but hypotensive and tachycardic.

A CT scan shows moderate liver and spleen lacerations. You decide she does not need surgery but does need a blood transfusion. Her mother arrives and tells you that they are Jehovah's Witnesses and that she does not want her daughter to "get blood and go to hell." You are very concerned about the patient's hypotension and feel the patient will die without blood.

Question 1: What are the legal and ethical considerations?
Legal surrogacy, beneficence, and autonomy

Question 2: What should you do?
Parents are routinely the decision makers for children under 18 years of age. Consents for surgery are signed by the parent, although older children are usually involved in the decision-making process. In the case of Jehovah's Witnesses, as well as with similar religious restrictions, the legal system has routinely allowed physicians to give life-saving care despite the objections of the parents. The process to circumvent the parents' wishes can usually be accomplished quite expeditiously, because most children's emergency departments have the appropriate legal resources to call for emergency permission to override the parents' objections. One should always be as nonconfrontational as possible with the family, and any therapies that can be initiated to prevent the need for blood products should also be used. However, if the overriding process cannot be completed by the time the child is in extremis, then the principle of beneficence applies, and one should give the child blood products if she is imminent danger of dying without them.

This puts the surgeon in the stressful situation of having to expeditiously make a decision that takes into account the obligation of saving the life of another human being while being respectful of individual religious beliefs and trying to accomplish this all within the constraints of legal liability placed upon the surgeon.

Question 3: What if the child is 16 years old?
This case is slightly different. At this age, the autonomy of the child to assent can be taken into consideration. If the child desires blood products, they can be more freely given. If the child wishes to respect the teachings of her religion, that may also be appropriate. Of course, one should ensure that the minor is making an informed decision and not being pressured into a decision by the family. Most courts also begin to respect children's wishes before they reach the age of 18 years. If the child is mentally capable, a discussion should be held without the parents in the room. In all of these situations, an ethics consultation will help to bring the issues and parties to the best solution possible.

Question 4: What if the 16-year-old has a child?
This case becomes clearer. When a minor has a child, she is considered emancipated and can legally and ethically make her own decisions. Here the decision is based on the discussion with the patient about her wishes, making certain, and documenting, that she understands the gravity of the situation and the implications of her choice.

Case 5: Competency

A 40-year-old poorly compliant diabetic woman presents with wet gangrene of her right foot. You advise urgent amputation but she refuses. You voice your objections but agree to try a course of intravenous antibiotics. The gangrene progresses to the point of sepsis and intubation. There is no family.

Question 1: What are the legal and ethical considerations?
Autonomy and competency

Question 2: What should you do?
Determination of "decision-making capacity" can be a difficult problem and is commonly encountered with the acutely ill patient. The first portion of the problem is determining capacity. Patients must understand the medical problems they have as well as the treatment options and their resulting implications. Many factors can affect decision-making capacity, including mental disease, acute illness (e.g., sepsis), drugs, and underlying medical conditions (e.g., stroke). If you feel that a patient lacks decision-making capacity, a psychiatric consult is not needed, as any physician is able to make this determination.

In this case, the patient appears decisional at first. It was appropriate to initially try a course of intravenous antibiotics. As the patient became more infected and septic, she lost adequate decision-making capacity, especially after she was sedated and intubated. At that point, family surrogates would be helpful, but none is present for this case. Because the patient is not decisional, the principle of beneficence will allow you to perform an amputation to save her life. If the patient recovers from the acute episode, discussions regarding future care can then be held.

This is not the same as legally being declared "incompetent" by a court, with appointment of a legal guardian. In that case, the legal system has determined, after a thorough review, that a person is not able to make decisions for herself. In such cases, the decisions of the legal guardian should be respected.

Case 6: Mass Casualty and Triage

You are working at a small rural hospital and receive word that a commuter plane has gone down nearby. You are informed that four people died at the scene, but nine patients are coming to the Emergency Department (ED) at the same time. Your ED has two nurses, three beds, and one surgeon available in 30 minutes to work in the hospital's one operating room. The patients arrive with the following presentations:

75-year-old man with severe chest injuries, hypotension, and a distended abdomen
74-year-old woman with head laceration that is bleeding, and she complains of leg pain
50-year-old man demanding immediate care with a severely comminuted right arm deformity
42-year-old woman with bruising over the right chest who was stable, but has dyspnea and acute hypotension as the ambulance arrives
35-year-old woman hypotensive, severe head and facial injuries, breathing twice a minute
26-year-old man stumbling around holding a bloody towel over his right eye
19-year-old woman, Olympic athlete (she tells you), with a severe open tibia/fibula and femur fracture; hemodynamically stable
14-year-old girl, obtunded, hypotensive, with severe face, head, and chest trauma
3-year-old boy, crying, with blood in his nose and bruises on his chest

Question 1: What are the ethical considerations governing your choice of who to treat first?
Justice

Question 2: Who do you treat and why?
We will not discuss each individual person, but the basic principles should be followed. You want to provide justice, or fair use of resources for all. Your aim is to save as many people as possible with your limited resources. Considerations of survivability must include degree of injury, age, and ability to quickly resolve a patient's problems. The 75-year-old listed first should probably not be treated first, as his use of resources and poor expected outcome would likely lead to other deaths and morbidities, and there is a high likelihood that he will die anyway. This is not the case when only one patient arrives at a time, and you have the resources to direct all attention to that individual. The 42-year-old is a likely first choice, as a quick needle decompression of the chest may well fix her urgent problems and quickly save her life. The 14-year-old could also be looked at early, as the young survive trauma better, and her major problem may only be provision of an adequate airway.

The objective here is not to give the reader exact answers, but rather guidelines about who to treat and in what order. Ultimately, the decision will depend on who you think can be saved quickly with the least use of resources. You might decide wrongly. Not everyone will be able to be saved, and this is contradictory to what we are always taught as physicians. It would be difficult to watch the elderly man die with his wife next to him, but resources diverted from him may save three or four others. One must also not be distracted by the vocal but only minimally injured patient. In these situations, people like the 50-year-old man only add tension and friction to the situation.

A Final Thought

Perhaps Richard Hayward, who compares a surgeon to the young sea captain in Joseph Conrad's novel *The Shadow-Line*, best describes a successful career in acute care surgery. Hayward explains that there are so many variables in the interaction between patient, surgeon, and disease that it is not surprising that the prediction of results becomes uncertain. Even routine procedures will produce complications that are found to be much more difficult than anticipated. As the surgeon crosses Conrad's Shadow-Line, energy, enthusiasm, ability to make firm decisions and then act upon them, optimism, self-confidence, and resilience in the face of adversity become necessities without which an individual will have difficulty coping with the pressures of a surgical practice, especially when involving the care of critically ill acute care patients. There comes a time when a surgeon must come to terms with the inadequacies and, sometimes, the downright failures of his or her actions that will be the inevitable companions during a surgical life.[31]

References

1. ACEP Ethics Committee. Code of ethics for emergency physicians. Ann Emerg Med 1997; 30:365–372.
2. Derse AR. Law and ethics in emergency medicine. Emerg Med Clin North Am 1999; 17:307–325.
3. Kodner IJ. Ethics curricula in surgery: needs and approaches. World J Surg 2003; 27:952–956.
4. Little M. Invited commentary: is there a distinctively surgical ethics? Surg 2001; 129:668–671.
5. Beauchamp TL, Childress JF. Principles of Biomedical Ethics, 5th ed. Oxford: Oxford University Press, 2001:12–23.
6. Justice Cardoza. *Schloendorff v. New York Hospital* 105 N.E. 92. New York Court of Appeals 1914.
7. Iserson KV. Principles of biomedical ethics. Emerg Med Clin North Am 1999; 17:283–306.
8. Adams J, Larkin G, Iserson K, et al. Virtue in emergency medicine. Acad Emerg Med 1996; 3:961–966.
9. Alexander L. Medical science under dictatorship. N Engl J Med 1949; 241:39–51.
10. Koenig HG. Taking a spiritual history. JAMA 2004; 291:2881.
11. Weber JE. Conflicts of interest in emergency medicine. Emerg Med Clin North Am 1999; 17:475–490.
12. Buckner F. The Emergency Medical Treatment and Labor Act (EMTALA). Medical Pract Manage 2002; Nov/Dec: 142–145.
13. Jonsen AR, Siegler M, Winslade WJ. Clinical Ethics: A Practical Approach to Ethical Decisions in Clinical Medicine, 5th ed. New York: McGraw-Hill, 2002:41–42, 181–182.
14. Burns JP, Reardon FE, Truog, RD. Using newly deceased patients to teach resuscitation procedures. N Engl J Med 1994; 331:1652–1655.
15. Moore GP. Ethics seminars: the practice of medical procedures on newly dead patients—is consent warranted? Acad Emerg Med 2001; 8:389–392.
16. Nee PA, Griffiths RD. Ethical considerations in accident and emergency research. Emerg Med J 2002; 19:423–427.
17. Beecher HK. Ethics and clinical research. N Engl J Med 1966; 274:1354–1360.
18. Rothman DJ. Ethics and human experimentation: Henry Beecher revisited. N Engl J Med 1987; 317:1195–1199.
19. Jacobstein CR, Baren JM. Emergency department treatment of minors. Emerg Med Clin North Am 1999; 17:341–352.
20. Schmidt TA, Zechnich AD. Suicidal patients in the ED: ethical issues. Emerg Med Clin North Am 1999; 17:371–383.
21. Sanders AB. Advance directives. Emerg Med Clin North Am 1999; 17:519–526.
22. Birrer R, Singh U, Kumar DN. Disability and dementia in the emergency department. Emerg Med Clin North Am 1999; 17:505–517.
23. Schears RM. Emergency physicians' role in end-of-life care. Emerg Med Clin North Am 1999; 17:539–559.
24. Iserson, KV. Withholding and withdrawing medical treatment: an emergency medicine perspective. Ann Emerg Med 1996; 28:51–54.
25. Marco CA. Ethical issues of resuscitation. Emerg Med Clin North Am 1999; 17:527–538.
26. Marco CA, Larkin GL. Ethics seminars: case studies in "futility"—challenges for academic emergency medicine. Acad Emerg Med 2000; 7:1147–1151.
27. McCahill LE, Dunn GP, Mosenthal AC, et al. Palliation as a core surgical principle: Part I. J Am Coll Surg 2004; 199:149–159.
28. Daniels S. Good Samaritan acts. Emerg Med Clin North Am 1999; 17:491–504.
29. The rights of the terminally ill. New York Times, May 28, 2004.
30. Liptak A. Ruling upholds Oregon law authorizing assisted suicide. New York Times, May 27, 2004.
31. Hayward R. The shadow-line in surgery. Lancet 1987; Feb: 375–376.

Part IV
System and Curriculum Development

46
Development of a Regional System for Surgical Emergencies (RSSE)

A. Brent Eastman, David B. Hoyt, and J. Wayne Meredith

The Problem—The Solution

In the United States, in the first decade of the twenty-first century, a 60-year-old man run over by a truck may have better access to life-saving care than a man with a perforated viscus or a ruptured abdominal aortic aneurysm. The reason is that many states and counties now have regional systems to coordinate the care of injured patients, but the concept of a geographic plan for *nontraumatic*, but devastating, surgical emergencies is new. The trauma system model is appropriate for these other surgical emergencies and possibly for certain medical emergencies as well, such as stroke and acute myocardial infarction. The concept of trauma system development is based on the principle that the system adds value over and above the efforts of individual practitioners or hospitals.[1–3]

It is historical irony that today there are well-trained and qualified surgeons in most of the country's community hospitals, but there are too few surgeons who are committed to providing emergency department coverage 24 hours a day. Training has improved over the past 30 years to the point that most surgeons who complete an accredited general surgery program are well qualified to perform most acute care operations. Yet surgical coverage in emergency department call panels is a critical health care challenge in the United States. The problem has many compounding causes.

The first is a physician shortage nationwide: some experts estimate that the United States will be short some 200,000 physicians within the next decade, and a large portion of the missing physicians will be specialists in surgery.[4] There is also inadequate reimbursement for providers along with soaring medical malpractice insurance costs. Furthermore, a powerful cultural change has occurred prompting many young surgeons to seek a more balanced life style. The net effect is fewer professional hours devoted to patient care. Finally, the population is aging, with octogenarians representing the most rapidly growing segment, and the resources required for the elderly with acute severe illnesses are greater than for younger patients with the same emergencies (Table 46.1).[5] All of these factors speak to the urgent need for a system designed to coordinate and ensure access to emergency surgical care.

The trauma system model should be strongly considered in addressing the treatment of nontraumatic surgical emergencies (NTSEs). Trauma systems are designed to identify injured patients in the prehospital setting, establish triage guidelines, and institute protocols of care. Furthermore, a trauma system provides for the immediate availability of a coordinated team with the resources necessary to care for critically injured patients. In regions without a trauma system, autopsy records have shown an unacceptable rate of preventable deaths (i.e., deaths of patients who would have survived with appropriate surgical intervention).[6] Lowered rates of preventable deaths reflect the presence of a system that rapidly identifies those at risk and transports them to the appropriate facility.[7,8] An analogous situation may exist for NTSEs.

Figure 46.1 describes the preventable death data derived from the San Diego Trauma Registry. The San Diego Trauma Registry was inaugurated in 1984 with the resultant immediate decline in the number of preventable deaths. This dramatic change is directly attributable to the implementation of all components of a regionalized trauma system plan.

Regionalization: A Concept for Optimal Care

Regionalization, for purposes of this chapter, is defined as creating a system of care, within a defined geographic area, to ensure optimal care for every patient with a life-threatening surgical illness. Regionalization is *not* meant to be synonymous with centralization. Centralization

TABLE 46.1. Aging population and surgery workforce: proportion of work within surgical specialty by age group.

Specialty	<15 Years	15–44 Years	45–64 Years	65+ Years	Total
Cardiothoracic*	0%	0.3%	29.4%	70.3%	100%
General surgery‡	2.6%	12.3%	25.5%	59.6%	100%
Neurosurgery	2.8%	12.9%	39.1%	45.2%	100%
Ophthalmology	0.6%	0.7%	10.8%	88.0%	100%
Orthopedic surgery	0.6%	16.1%	31.8%	51.4%	100%
Otolaryngology	39.6%	22.1%	29.9%	8.4%	100%
Urology	4.0%	6.3%	24.9%	64.8%	100%

*In the 1996 NHDS sample, the incidence rate for specific cardiothoracic procedures in pediatric patients was too small to allow an accurate incidence rate to be reported.
‡Category includes vascular, breast, hernia, abdominal, gastrointestinal, and pediatric procedures.
Source: NHDS and NSAS 1996. Reprinted by permission from Etzioni et al.[5]

would imply that all acutely ill surgical patients be triaged and transported directly to "designated acute care surgery centers." The centralization of most surgical emergencies will not be necessary because most can be appropriately treated at the local community hospital. However, it is essential that any hospital providing acute care be committed to meeting the regionally defined standards. A guiding principle of regionalization of acute care surgery would be to move the patient expeditiously to the level of care commensurate with the severity or complexity of the patient's acute surgical problem.

The architects of a regional plan should

- Conduct a needs assessment
- Document the available resources
- Determine how those resources could be used to guarantee the highest quality and most cost-effective care
- Develop triage guidelines to direct patients to the appropriate facility

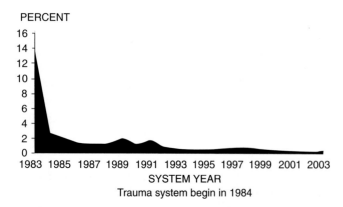

FIGURE 46.1. Preventable-death data derived from the San Diego Trauma Registry. (Reprinted with permission of the County of San Diego Health and Human Services Agency, Emergency Medical Services, Trauma Database, 1983–2003; [UCSD, Palomar Medical Center, Sharp Memorial, Scripps Mercy, Scripps Memorial La Jolla, and Children's' Hospital].)

The following case scenario is an example of what optimal emergency surgical care would look like in a regional system for surgical emergencies (RSSE):

A 60-year-old male, with a history of atherosclerotic cardiovascular disease with hypertension, has sudden onset of back and abdominal pain. The patient lives in a small town with a 50-bed hospital and an emergency department (ED) staffed by contracted acute care physicians. The local ambulance service responds to a 911 call, and the patient is transported to the ED. On initial examination by the acute care physician, the patient is found to have a tender abdomen with tachycardia, hypotension, and a palpable 10cm abdominal aortic aneurysm (AAA). There is one general surgeon on the hospital staff who promptly sees the patient in consultation, makes the correct diagnosis, and immediately contacts a 500-bed tertiary care hospital 150 miles away.

The surgeon in the community hospital speaks directly to the vascular surgeon to whom the patient is being referred. The surgeon-to-surgeon communication expedites the transfer and allows appropriate preparation at the tertiary hospital (i.e., operating room made ready with necessary equipment and staff). Transfer agreements are in place, which further expedites the process of getting this patient to the appropriate level of care. The regional helicopter service is activated and transfers the patient to the tertiary hospital where the previously notified vascular surgeon is awaiting the patient. On arrival, an appropriately staffed and equipped operating room is ready for the acute care repair of a ruptured AAA. The vascular surgeon has the requisite experience, and his practice includes both elective and emergent AAA repairs. The patient has a successful resuscitation and repair of the AAA and is ultimately discharged back to his primary care physician in his home town.

Both the community hospital and the tertiary care hospital contribute appropriate data on this case to the regional acute care surgery registry. These registry data allow quality assessment of the patient's entire continuum of care from the initial 911 call to his discharge from the tertiary care hospital and return to his primary care physician in his home town. The acute care physician and general surgeon at the community hospital are provided a complete summary of the patient's clinical course from transfer to discharge. The surgeon and acute care physician at the community hospital are both invited to participate in the tertiary care hospital's continuing medical education program, including a session on vascular emergencies, which includes ruptured AAA. This educational experience is accomplished with a teleconferencing system, thus allowing the acute care physician and the single general surgeon in the community to participate in the conference while remaining in their own hospitals.

When a trauma system exists, the infrastructure of the system is utilized to expedite care of NTSEs.

The hypothetical scenario describes a patient receiving optimal care in the context of as RSSE. Fundamental to providing such care is the collection and analysis of data, which allows the measurement and monitoring of the quality of care in the system. This scenario certainly occurs in some communities today, but an RSSE would be designed to ensure that it happens consistently for every patient in every community.

Regionalization of any component of the health care system inevitably raises issues of politics, economics, logistics, and quality of care. The political ramifications can be partially mitigated by having practicing surgeons involved in the initial design and implementation of the regionalization process. Political and economic issues can be addressed by ensuring that the regionalization plan includes all qualified and committed surgeons and hospitals in the region and is thus an *inclusive* regional system of care for surgical emergencies. The driving force must be a commitment to a standard of care based on evidence-based best practices with measurable outcome indicators. Ultimately, the success of such a regionalized system of care will rest on the demonstration of improved clinical outcomes and decreased variation in the care of the emergency surgery patient.

Trauma System: A New Paradigm for Emergency Surgical Care

A systems model for regionalization does not have to be reinvented for the critically ill surgical patient. The best working model for effective and efficient regionalization of emergent surgical conditions is the inclusive trauma system (TS) model, which has evolved and been proven effective in the United States over the past 30 years. The most current assessment of TS design and efficacy is provided in the *Trauma System Agenda for the Future*.[9]

The concept of an *inclusive* TS has replaced the prior *exclusive* concept of the traditional individual trauma centers. The Model Trauma Care System Plan[10] describes the basic components. Many of these components, as

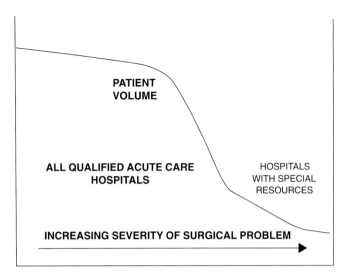

FIGURE 46.2. Regionalized system for surgical emergencies. (Adapted from Eastman et al.[10])

described later, are relevant and applicable to the regionalization of care for NTSEs.

Figure 46.2 shows a conceptual model of an RSSE. The diagram is derived from a similar model for an "inclusive trauma system" that was first described in the Model Trauma Care System Plan of 1992.[10] The triage and distribution of patients in this model should be determined by evidence-based outcome data. As depicted, most acute care surgical problems should be treated in *qualified (meeting established standards of care)* acute care hospitals; however, there may be a subset of particularly critical and complex patients who will require transport/transfer to hospitals with special resources. This model requires strong surgical leadership, cooperation, and direct communications among all health care providers involved, from the onset of acute illness to recovery and/or rehabilitation. The following components were originally described in the Model Trauma Care System Plan[10] and have been modified to reflect application to an RSSE.

Administrative Components

Leadership and System Development

The success of any RSSE will require broad-based commitment and leadership. It has been imperative, in trauma systems, to establish a responsible "lead agency" that is given the necessary authority to develop and implement the system. This is essential when existing patient flow and referral patterns may be altered. Also required are surgical "champions" to lead the development and implementation efforts as well as the participation of all acute care hospitals that receive acute care surgery patients. Any process that will have a major impact on patient care should be communicated to all stakeholders. Appropriate public education about the proposed new system of care will help engender public advocacy, and this will be critical in gaining political support and the necessary funding. It has become increasingly apparent that the public wants and deserves to know the status of health care delivery systems in their community.

A variety of issues must be considered in the development an RSSE, including the following:

- *Needs assessment* studies are essential to any planning process. There must be an accurate understanding of the type and potential volume of acute care surgical patients in the region. The needs assessment then must be correlated with the available resources.
- An *inventory of resources* must antedate any efforts toward developing a system of care. A major factor driving the need for regionalization in the United States is the current shortage of resources, both human and facility. The shortage of physicians, previously alluded to, and the decreasing reimbursement for both physicians and hospitals are contributing to a crisis in the area of emergency department specialty coverage. Without physicians, there is no access to emergency surgical care. Today, many hospital systems are struggling to maintain a positive profit margin even though operating at capacity. This lack of capacity would be critical with the surges in patient volume that would occur in a disaster with mass causalities. The determination of available resources will be essential in designing an RSSE.

Legislation

The field triage guidelines that are commonly utilized in TS to direct transport of the injured patient may not be applicable in the NTSE; therefore, these patients should be transported expeditiously to their local hospital, evaluated, and transferred to a higher level of care if necessary. Such patients would follow the established regional referral patterns, provided that the receiving hospital is committed to meeting the community standards of care given its available resources, and would transfer to a higher level of care as the clinical situation dictates. There will be a cohort of patients transported who clearly require specialized surgical resources (e.g., a patient with a rupturing abdominal aortic aneurysm) for which enabling legislation will be needed to allow direct transport to the appropriate facility. The enabling legislation must address the issues of triage guidelines, and physician coverage of emergency department specialty panels. The designation of such facilities must be based on demonstrated commitment to the standard of care established by the RSSE. The implementation of such a system would require a consensus among the hospitals and the medical and surgical communities. However, *no consideration should supersede the best interest of the patient.*

Finance

Patients with acute surgical emergencies may present a financial challenge to physicians and hospitals. The physicians involved in such emergency surgical care will include not only surgeons but also anesthesiologists, radiologists, neurosurgeons, orthopedic surgeons, and other physicians. As with the trauma patient, patient selection is based on the urgency of the clinical situation, not on ability to pay. Consequently, both physicians and hospitals assume the financial risk for such emergency care. Essential to the planning of a regional system is the establishment of adequate funding sources for those providing this care in an open access environment. The experience derived from attempts at securing funding for trauma systems and trauma patient care may be a good resource in dealing with this economic issue.

The limited access and capacity of our current health care system necessitate planning to ensure that all patients will receive optimal care given the available resources of a given hospital. There may be situations in which there is a well-trained surgeon available, but neither the surgeon nor the hospital is prepared to care for the patient who requires complex surgical procedures and the management of severe critical care problems. These patients will require transfer to a higher level of care. Adequate funding for emergency care, wherever it is provided, is imperative for the sustainability of an RSSE.

Operational and Clinical Components

Public Information and Prevention

Public information and education regarding the establishment of a regional system is crucial and will help to engender public support. Public information should include data documenting the magnitude of the problem and the improved outcomes that can be anticipated with a regional effort. This message should include the available data on the relationship between volume and outcome for the treatment of surgical emergencies. Public support will be essential to gaining funding sources for these high-risk and often under- or uninsured patients.

As with trauma, the patient with an NTSE (as opposed to an elective surgical problem) is dependent on a triage system that ensures the patient is taken to a hospital committed to providing the optimal care. If the initial receiving hospital does not have the resources available, then the patient must be transferred expeditiously to a surgeon and hospital that can provide the appropriate level of care.

Human Resources

The critical shortage of human resources lends a major impetus to the concept of regionalization. Inherent in the design of any regionalized system of care is to provide a structure for a more efficient use of limited resources. As noted, there is already a shortage of surgeons and surgical specialists, but this pattern is also likely to be seen with nurses, technicians, and other ancillary personnel. The system will require the optimal use of these limited resources. Trauma systems with designated trauma centers have facilities with dedicated resources to provide immediate care for injured patients. Included in these resources are trauma surgeons, staffed operating rooms, radiology units, and intensive are units. Currently, many trauma centers also function as a de facto hospital to provide emergency surgical care. Where trauma centers exist this is a desirable situation, because the resources are available and it provides essential operative experience for the trauma surgeons. Yet, because of changing therapeutic options, many injured patients now can be treated nonoperatively. Therefore, the capacity and surgical resources often exist to care for the emergency, nontrauma, and surgical patient.[11] Today, many trauma programs do incorporate the treatment of NTSEs. The benefit of such a program was described at the University of Pennsylvania.[12] As noted earlier, the increased operating experience will be necessary, in the future, to attract general surgeons to pursue a career in trauma surgery. This also helps address the fact that there are a decreasing number of surgical specialists available to provide coverage to many hospital emergency departments in the United States today.

Prehospital Issues

The prehospital component of the system will most often come into play with 911 calls concerning patients with symptoms suggestive of a surgical emergency. Often the specific diagnosis will not be obvious in the field, and the charge of the prehospital provider will be to transport the patient to the nearest hospital that has been predetermined to have the necessary resources and, most importantly, the surgical commitment to care for these emergency surgery patients. Excellent communication systems between prehospital providers and emergency departments will ensure the most appropriate and expeditious care. It should be recognized that some patients with acute surgical conditions will be transported by families in private vehicles, and therefore triage decisions will necessarily be made in the emergency department of the receiving hospital.

Every region has unique challenges with regard to topography, transportation and communication, and they must be addressed in the regionalization plan. For example, a rural region with mountain ranges, severe weather conditions, and limited health care facilities and providers would require much different systems planning than an urban area with a centralized dense population served by multiple acute care hospitals with qualified staff and surgeons.

The emergency medical system linkage will be critical in the event that an emergent surgical patient requires initial transport or interfacility transfer by the emergency medical system prehospital providers. The emergency medical system linkage would vary greatly between a rural and an urban or suburban region and would become a central issue in a natural disaster or act of terrorism with mass casualties. All hospital and physician resources of the regional system would be of vital importance in caring for the victims of such a disaster.

There will be a subset of emergent surgical patients who will require surgeons with special expertise and surgeons who have access to specialty resources. This subset of patients will benefit from expeditious transfer to the appropriate surgeon and facility, as in the case of a ruptured abdominal aortic aneurysm. Conversely, the majority of emergency surgical problems, such as acute appendicitis and acute cholecystitis, will be appropriately treated in the local hospital by surgeons committed to providing the defined, evidence-based standard of care. The essence of an "inclusive" RSSE system is to involve *all* acute care hospitals and providers in the region who are committed to providing the established standard of care. Wherever acute surgical problem is treated, there should be a commitment to collect the data, including prehospital data, necessary to monitor quality and drive continued performance improvement. This monitoring of quality is just as critical for the more common surgical emergencies (i.e., acute appendicitis) as it is for the less common and more complex or resource consumptive conditions (i.e., ruptured abdominal aortic aneurysm).

Definitive Care

Definitive care is defined as the level of surgical expertise and hospital resources required to cope successfully with any life-threatening surgical emergency. Where available and relevant to surgical emergencies, the data on the relationship between volume and outcome should be considered. Definitive care specifically implies the following:

- Prompt availability and commitment of a qualified surgeon and surgical team
- Volume and outcome data demonstrating competence in treating specific surgical emergencies
- Hospital resources such as imaging equipment, operating rooms, intensive care unit beds, and blood bank

Emergent surgical conditions are defined in this chapter as clinical situations that demand the immediate services of a surgeon with access to the necessary resources. A few examples of such surgical emergencies are:

- Acute abdomen secondary to a perforated appendix
- Sepsis from acute gangrenous cholecystitis or perforated diverticulitis
- Acute ischemia to a lower extremity secondary to an arterial embolus
- Ruptured intracranial arterial (berry) aneurysm
- Ruptured abdominal aortic aneurysm

Some of these emergent conditions will be appropriately cared for at the nearest community hospital; however, others may require a higher level of care. It is the profound responsibility of the regional system to ensure that all patients are cared for in a facility with the needed resources and by a surgeon who can provide optimal care.

All hospitals and all surgeons should not be expected to deal with every surgical emergency. The regionalized system would ensure that the acutely ill surgical patient gets to the appropriate level of care in an expeditious manner.

Data on the volume of surgical acute care cases should be available from most emergency department records. However, outcome data will be more difficult to obtain. With the increasing regulatory requirements to publish outcomes of selected surgical procedures, a region would be well served to be proactive in the collection of these data.[13,14] No one is better suited to define the appropriate outcome measures in surgery than is the surgeon providing the care. The failure of surgeons to determine what is relevant will result in abdication of these definitions to regulatory agencies.

Evidence-based clinical outcome studies should establish a quality of care basis for the regionalization of emergency surgical care.[15,16] The more experience that physicians and teams have in treating patients with a particular disease or condition, the more likely they are to create better outcomes and, ultimately, realize lower costs.[17] By performing particular procedures over and over, teams increase their learning opportunities and thereby reduce mortality rates.[15,16] Birkmeyer's data show estimated mortality rates in low-volume compared with high-volume hospitals versus high-risk surgeries (coronary artery bypass graft, coronary angioplasty, elective abdominal aortic aneurysm repair, and esophageal cancer surgery). An RSSE would be designed to direct patients with surgical conditions known to have an established relationship between volume and outcome (i.e., ruptured abdominal aortic aneurysm) to hospitals with the volume and data demonstrating improved outcomes. These data would be necessary to warrant bypassing some hospitals lacking that experience.

The system should be coordinated with the critical care transport system to ensure expeditious transfer of those patients who have complex and emergent surgical conditions requiring a higher level of care. All surgical patients must be ensured access to the appropriate level of care commensurate with their condition in a timely, coordinated, and cost-effective manner.

Evaluation

One of the great lessons learned from the experience of *inclusive* TSs is the power of a system-wide process for evaluating quality of care. A fundamental building block of a regional system must be a data base that facilitates monitoring of the quality of care as measured against evidence-based clinical outcome indicators. Such a data base would require the contribution of at least a minimal data set from every hospital that would receive and treat patients with acute surgical conditions. Trauma registries that have been developed and used extensively could serve as models for data acquisition and the use of these data for performance improvement. The basic elements of a registry should include data that are relevant to assess traditional disease-based outcomes (pneumonia, deep vein thrombosis, pulmonary embolism, and so forth) and provider-based outcomes (e.g., delay in diagnosis and error in diagnosis).[18,19]

Trauma registries have been the basis of the National Trauma Data Bank, which was established by the Committee on Trauma of the American College of Surgeons in 1990. There are currently over 200 trauma centers contributing data on over 750,000 injured patients. Figure 46.3 show some of the data.

A data base similar to the National Trauma Data Bank might be developed for NTSEs. Such a data base would be a powerful tool in the continuous quality improvement process of an RSSE. Any regionalized system must be driven by reliable data (i.e., evidence-based measurements and outcomes).

It is necessary to have defined critical indicators of performance and the ability to measure these indicators and compare them with appropriate standards or benchmarks. A system-wide performance improvement program will help improve care by extending the learning experiences of a single hospital, surgical service, or individual surgeon to the system as a whole. This combined experience will contribute to an improved level of care provided by all of the participants. This is particularly true of low-frequency but high-acuity emergency surgical conditions.

Any system-wide data base and quality performance improvement program must be carefully structured so as to protect its participants under statutes that guarantee the confidentiality of peer review. This protection from discovery has been achieved in the peer review process of many trauma systems.

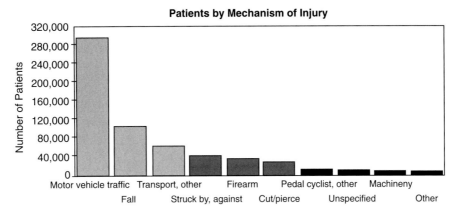

FIGURE 46.3. Example of some of the data from the American College of Surgeons National Trauma Data Bank™ 2004, Version 4.0. Proportional distribution of patients, grouped by mechanism of injury. Total number = 604,266. Bars 1–3 represent blunt mechanisms of injury. Bars 4–6 represent penetrating mechanisms of injury. Bars 7–10 represent unspecified and other mechanisms. (Reprinted with permission of the American College of Surgeons/Committee on Trauma, National Trauma Data Bank. © American College of Surgeons 2004. All rights reserved worldwide.)

Ultimately, it must be quality of care that drives the establishment of a regionalized system for the care of surgical emergencies. Quality must be monitored by a timely peer review process with the development of quality performance improvement plans when an opportunity for "best practice" is identified. An advantage of a regionalized system is the development of a common data base to be utilized in the performance improvement process. A fundamental goal must be to decrease inappropriate variation in the care of patients with surgical emergencies. Achieving a reduction in variation will lead to higher quality and more cost-efficient care. The Veterans Administration's National Surgical Quality Improvement Program (NSQIP) is an excellent example of an outcome-based, risk-adjusted, and peer-controlled program for the measurement and enhancement of the quality of surgical care.[20]

Quality of care is enhanced by establishing measurable, evidence-based, clinical outcome indicators that can be benchmarked, tracked, and reviewed by the regional providers of emergency surgical care. This medical review process is fundamental for achieving success in systemwide quality performance improvement. A cornerstone of successful trauma systems is a "medical audit process" that monitors the quality of care and drives an evidence-based performance improvement program. A medical audit committee (MAC) has been an essential element in the success and sustainability of the San Diego trauma system since 1984.[21] San Diego County contains 43,000 square miles and has a population of approximately 3 million. The demographics range from rural to urban, requiring both air and ground transport systems. The MAC in this trauma system meets once a month, with the confidentiality of the proceedings protected by the Cali-

fornia 1157 Evidence Code. The MAC has representation from the following groups:

• Designated trauma centers (surgeon and nurse)
• Nontrauma community hospitals
• Representatives of key specialty groups (i.e., anesthesia, orthopedics and neurosurgery)
• Medical examiner
• Representatives from San Diego County EMS, which is the lead agency in the trauma system
• Emergency physician representative of the Prehospital Medical Audit Committee (PAC).

At the heart of this process is a common trauma registry data base. Such a data base should be established and protected for confidentiality under statutes protecting the discoverability of peer review documents.

This continued quality improvement (CQI) process, modified for an RSSE, could lead to the development of "best practices," which would in turn positively impact the quality of care provided for emergency surgery patients throughout the region. The composition of a MAC for surgical emergencies might include the following members:

• General surgeon representing each acute care hospital
• Emergency physician representing each acute care hospital
• Representative of the emergency medical system/prehospital providers
• Nurse representing acute care hospitals
• Specialty representatives, for example, anesthesiologist, orthopedic surgeon, and neurosurgeon
• Others appropriate at certain times might be a hospital association representative and insurance and other payer representatives

The number of representatives would depend on the size and population of the region.

Rehabilitation

Rehabilitation is a critical component in the continuum of care of the emergency surgical patient just as it is with the trauma patient. It is imperative that rehabilitation services, either in house or by transfer agreements with a rehabilitation center, be built into the practice of every acute care hospital providing emergent surgical care.

Research

Another distinct advantage of a regionalized system is the opportunity to utilize the system data base to carry out clinical research and outcome studies based on the collective surgical experiences. It is important at the outset of establishing a system-wide data base to define who owns the data and exactly how the data may be accessed and used. The assurance of confidentiality is of paramount importance and will require the use of the hospital institutional review boards for the patient confidentiality component.

Building on a Trauma System

The system components as described are the basis of the current American College of Surgeons Trauma System Consultation program, which is being utilized increasingly by various "regions" (counties, states, groups of states) throughout the United States.[22] Those areas that have instituted a TS would have the basic infrastructure already in place to develop an overarching regionalized system for the care of all surgical emergencies. Utilization of an existing TS may be contemplated only if the surgical leadership, at both trauma and nontrauma centers, of the region concur. Use of the existing TS for the subset of acute care surgery patients who need a higher level of care should be determined to be the best use of available resources and the greatest opportunity for optimal patient care. In those regions where the TS has the capacity and desire to care for these more complex acute care surgery patients, and local emergency departments are unable to provide surgical on-call coverage 24 hours a day, 7 days a week, this arrangement could be a win–win–win situation for the trauma centers, the local emergency departments, and, most importantly, the acute care surgery patient.

Disaster Preparedness

The establishment of an RSSE will provide a valuable resource in the event of a disaster, natural or terrorist, with mass causalities. Current intelligence in the United States indicates that a terrorist act may well utilize explosive or incendiary devices resulting in blast and burn injuries. All disaster preparedness plans should include the integration of existing trauma and RSSE systems when such systems exist.

In summary, in this country today, the patient with an acute NTSE may not have immediate access to life-saving care. Many existing impediments can be mitigated by the establishment of an RSSE. A systems model for regionalization does not have to be reinvented for the critically ill surgical patient. The best working model for efficient regionalization of acute care surgical conditions is the *inclusive* TS model, which has evolved and been proven effective in the United States over the last 30 years. In those regions where trauma systems exist, the planning and resources of the TS will overlap and often be synergistic with those of the RSSE. In some instances the trauma centers with 24/7 immediate availability of surgical resources have already become de facto "acute care surgery centers."

The national shortage of surgeons is another incentive to create regionalized systems of care for the emergency surgical patient. Today, many such patients are taken to emergency departments that lack the needed surgical specialists. A regionalized system would establish triage guidelines to ensure that patients are taken to a hospital with the resources commensurate with their surgical needs. This triage would take place in the field or be based on the judgment of the physician in the first hospital to which the patient is taken.

The design of any RSSE should consider the relationship of volume to outcome. These data will define the subset of patients who would benefit from being directed to a specific hospital and surgeons who have the requisite volume to ensure optimal outcomes.

Wherever RSSEs are developed, they must be designed and implemented based on the regional needs and resources available (i.e., the design of an urban system will be different from that in a rural area). The goal, no matter where the RSSE is located, should be to ensure optimal care to the acutely ill surgical patient given the available resources. Many of the principles that have been developed for the TS will pertain in creating a system of optimal care of the noninjured but devastatingly ill surgical patient.

Acknowledgments. The authors would like to acknowledge the assistance of Samantha Saunders in the preparation of this chapter.

References

1. Nathens AB, Jurkovich GJ, Maier RV, et al. Relationship between trauma center volume and outcomes. JAMA 2001; 285:1164–1171.

2. Eastman AB, Lewis FR, Champion HR, and Mattox KL. Regional trauma system design: critical concepts. Am J Surg 1987; 154:79–87.

3. Eastman AB. Blood in our streets. The status and evolution of trauma care systems. Arch Surg 1992; 127:677–681.

4. Cooper RA, Stoflet SJ, Wartman SA. Perceptions of medical school deans and state medical society executives about physician supply. JAMA 2003; 290(22):2992–2995.

5. Etzioni DA, Liu JH, Maggard MA, Ko CY. The aging population and its impact on the surgery workforce. Ann Surg 2003;238(2):170–177.

6. West JG, Trunkey DD, Lim RC. Systems of trauma care. A study of two counties. Arch Surg 1979;114(4):455–460.

7. Shackford SR, Hollingsworth-Fridlund P, Cooper GF, Eastman AB. The effect of regionalization upon the quality of trauma care as assessed by concurrent audit before and after institution of a trauma system: a preliminary report. J Trauma 1986; 26(9):812–820.

8. Shackford SR, Mackersie RC, Hoyt DB, Baxt WG, Eastman AB, Hamm FN, Knotts FB, Virgilio RW. Impact of a trauma system on outcome of severely injured patients. Arch Surg 1987; 122(5):523–527.

9. Trauma System: Agenda for the Future; American Trauma Society, 2002. http://www.nhtsa.dot.gov/people/injury/ems/emstraumasystem03.

10. Eastman B, et al. The Model Trauma Care System Plan. Washington, DC: Health Resources and Services Administration (HRSA), U.S. Department of Health and Human Services Administration, 1992.

11. Spain DA, Richardson JD, Carrillo EH, Miller FB, Wilson MA, Polk HC Jr. Should trauma surgeons do general surgery? J Trauma 2000; 48:433–437.

12. Kim PK, Dabrowski GP, Reilly PM, Auerbach S, Kauder DR, Schwab CW. Redefining the future of trauma surgery as a comprehensive trauma and emergency general surgery service. J Am Coll Surg 2004; 199(1):96–101.

13. Luft HS, Bunker JP, Enthoven AC. Should operations be regionalized? The empirical relation between surgical volume and mortality. N Engl J Med 1979; 301:1364–1369.

14. Begg CB, Cramer LD, Hoskins WJ, Brennan MF. Impact of hospital volume on operative mortality for major cancer surgery. JAMA 1998; 280:1747–1751.

15. Birkmeyer JD, Siewers AE, Finlayson EVA, et al. Hospital volume and surgical mortality in the United States. N Engl J Med 2002; 346:1137–1144.

16. Birkmeyer JD. High-risk surgery—follow the crowd. JAMA 2000; 283:1191–1193.

17. Dudley RA, Johansen KL, Brand R, Rennie DJ, Milstein A. Selective referral to high-volume hospitals: estimating potentially avoidable deaths. JAMA 2000; 283:1159–1166.

18. Hoyt DB, Hollingsworth-Fridlund P, Fortlage D, Davis JW, Mackersie RC. An evaluation of provider-related and disease-related morbidity in a level I university trauma service: directions for quality improvement. J Trauma 1992; 33:586–601.

19. Hoyt DB, Hollingsworth-Fridlund P, Winchell RJ, et al. Analysis of recurrent process errors leading to provider-related complications on an organized trauma service: directions for care improvement. J Trauma 1994; 36:377–383.

20. Veteraris Administration National Surgical Quality Improvement Program, www.acsnsqip.org/main/about_features.asp.

21. Shackford SR, Hollingsworth-Fridlund P, McArdle M, Eastman AB. Assuring quality in a trauma system—the medical audit committee: composition, cost, and results. J Trauma 1987; 27(8):866–875.

22. ACS Trauma System Consultation Program; http://www.FACS.org/trauma/systems.pdf.

47
Acute Care Surgery: A Proposed Curriculum

L.D. Britt and Michael F. Rotondo

There is no simple origin for this proposed new surgery specialty. On the contrary, the emergence of "acute care surgery" parallels both the development of trauma surgery in the United States over the past three decades and the apparent partitioning or fragmentation of general surgery. In keeping with a Darwinian adaptation process, the birth of acute care surgery should solidify the pivotal role of the broadly trained surgeon. The following is the proposed format and curriculum.

Proposed formats (after 4 years of core general surgery)

Format A (2 Years)	Format B (3 Years)
Year 1:	Year 1:
12 months: Trauma/ emergency surgery/ critical care	12 months: Trauma/emergency surgery
Year 2:	Year 2:
3 months: thoracic	9 months: critical care (SICU/NICU/CCU/burns/PICU)
3 months: transplant/ hepatobiliary	3 months: vascular/ interventional radiology
3 months: vascular/ interventional radiology	
3 months: elective (orthopedics, neurosurgery, plastics)	
	Year 3:
	5 months: orthopedics and Neurosurgery
	3 months: thoracic
	2 months: transplant/hepatobiliary
	2 months: elective (plastics/ pediatric surgery/endosurgery)

I. General
   A. Prehospital/system management
   B. Initial assessment and early resuscitation
   C. Diagnostic imaging
   D. Anesthesia in the emergency setting
   E. Fundamental operative approaches
   F. Nutrition
   G. Critical care

II. Organ systems
   A. Pharyngeal/laryngeal/tracheobronchial
   B. Esophageal
   C. Thoracic
   D. Abdominal wall
   E. Gastroduodenal
   F. Intestinal
   G. Hepatic
   H. Pancreatic
   I. Splenic
   J. Vascular
   K. Urogenital/gynecologic
   L. Orthopedics
   M. Neurosurgical

III. Areas for special emphasis
   A. Acute care surgery in the rural setting
   B. The elderly and acute care surgery
   C. Disaster and mass casualties management
   D. Education: surgical simulation
   E. Prevention: principles and methodology
   F. Advance directives
   G. The nonviable patient and organ procurement

IV. Operative management principles
   A. Management of perforations/injuries
      1. Esophagus
      2. Stomach
      3. Duodenum
      4. Small bowel
      5. Colon/rectum
      6. Bladder
      7. Lung
      8. Cardiac
   B. Management of solid organ injuries
      1. Trachea/bronchus
      2. Spleen (splenectomy/splenorrhaphy)
      3. Liver (hepatic resection/hepatorrhaphy)
      4. Pancreas (major resection/debridements)
      5. Kidney (primary repair, nephrectomy/partial repair)

C. Necrotic tissue: debridements principles
D. Abscess: drainage principles
E. Appendectomy
F. Adhesiolysis
G. Cholecystectomy/cholecystostomy
H. Common bile duct exploration
I. Gastrointestinal resections
J. Colostomy
K. Colostomy reversal
L. Hemorrhoidectomy/rectal prolapse management
M. Gynecologic emergencies
   1. Ectopic pregnancy
   2. Ovarian cyst
   3. Tubo-ovarian abscess
N. Thoracic
   1. Mediasternotomy
   2. Left/right thoracotomy
   3. Wedge and partial lung resection
   4. Cardiac injury repair
   5. Decortication (open and VATS)
   6. Pleurodesis
O. Orthopedic
   1. Intraoperative washouts
   2. Placement of external fixators
   3. Fasciectomies (upper and lower extremities)
   4. Open reduction and internal fixation

P. Neurosurgery
   1. Intracranial pressure monitoring placement (including ventriculostomy)
   2. Burr hole placement
   3. Limited craniotomy
   4. Halo traction
Q. Plastics
   1. Soft tissues, flap construction
   2. Management of hand injury
   3. Management of facial soft tissue injuries

The curriculum for acute care surgery should be competency based as designed by the Accreditation Council for Graduate Medical Education (ACGME). The required competencies are as follows:

- Medical knowledge
- Patient care
- Interpersonal and communication skills
- Professionalism
- Practice-based learning
- System-based learning

This curriculum will also incorporate the "seventh" competency: procedural proficiency.

48
Emergency General Surgery: The Vanderbilt Model

José J. Diaz, Jr., Oscar D. Guillamondegui, and John A. Morris, Jr.

Background

The Concept of Nontrauma Acute Care Surgery

With the evolution of trauma systems in the United States, morbidity and mortality rates from trauma have decreased over the past 30 years.[1-3] Trauma centers are highly organized systems that administer care to the most critically injured patients. This provides a concentrated setting for multispecialty professionals to dedicate themselves to the care of these individuals promptly and efficiently.

During the same 30-year period, general surgery has splintered into various subspecialties and flourished without the burden of care for the complex trauma patient. Yet, general surgeons continued to be responsible for the patient presenting at all hours of the day with an acute surgical problem. For the busy general surgeon, a patient presenting with an acute abdomen is a surgical emergency necessitating an urgent laparotomy. As most surgeons have busy clinics and operative schedules, such a patient would negatively affect clinical productivity.

The patient presenting with an acute abdomen demands immediate surgical attention. The perioperative evaluation and resuscitation must be dictated by the surgeon. Once the patient has been resuscitated, surgery must begin promptly. Commonly, postoperative resuscitation continues in the intensive care unit (ICU), demanding further commitment by the surgeon. In most community practices, this is both an uncommon and an untenable scenario. Within the typical tertiary care center, where the referral pattern and population catchment area is much larger, this can become a routine practice.

Within this framework, the concept of an emergency general surgery (EGS) service (24 hours a day, 7 days a week), dedicated to the care of patients with acute surgical problems and unique characteristics, was developed.

Using a service approach to enhance the available institutional resources, the Department of Surgery can fulfill its mission of providing quality care to both the elective and the acute patient with surgical problems.

The Regional Referral Center

Tertiary care centers have demonstrated to be centers of excellence in multiple fields of surgery.[4-6] This is especially true when time sensitivity, such as with trauma, is a critical factor in good outcomes. This requires a commitment from the institution to gather specialists and create sufficient infrastructure to ensure success. Studies have shown that aggregation of severely injured patients to Level I trauma centers is associated with reductions in mortality and morbidity rates.[7]

The size of the catchment area and the size of the population served help to off-set the significant cost of maintaining such a system. Integration of trauma care services into a regionalized system reduces mortality rates. Studies have demonstrated that tertiary trauma centers and reduced prehospital times are essential components of an efficient trauma care system.[8] Similar results should be attainable in EGS, most notably for the patient presenting with an abdominal catastrophe at a community hospital. Primary care environments may not have the necessary infrastructure to care for such a patient, such as state-of-the-art imaging, around the clock intensivists, large blood banks, and a fully staffed operating room.

The Acute Care Surgery/Trauma Paradigm

Trauma is a disease that occurs regardless of time, and the requisite urgent assessment and management demands life or death decision making. The care of the EGS patient with an acute surgical problem also requires rapid assessment, resuscitation, and timely surgical management. Level I and II trauma centers staffed by critical care–trained general surgeons are readily available to

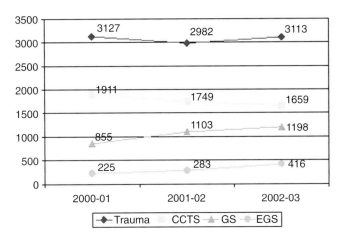

FIGURE 48.1. Admissions per year. CCTS, critical care trauma surgery; EGS, emergency general surgery; GS, general surgery.

handle the admission of the critically injured patient. Hospital trauma centers are regulated by the American College of Surgeons Committee on Trauma (ACS-COT) and/or state agencies for the basic requirements. These centers are more than adequately prepared to manage the patient with an acute surgical problem.

The advent of nonoperative management of blunt abdominal trauma and the results of evidence-based practice have demonstrated improved outcomes for trauma patients. As a result, the operative experience for the trauma surgeon has declined. Significant decreases in injury severity, inner-city violence, and penetrating trauma have occurred over the past 15 years.[9] These changes have had profound effects on the practice of trauma surgeons and on surgical education.[10] Several institutions have incorporated the care of trauma patients and EGS into their practice. Scherer and Battistella[11] studied their experience with combining the care of

trauma patients and general surgical emergencies. The result was a breadth and scope of practice for trauma surgeons that compared favorably with that of nontrauma surgeons. Other groups have traditionally cared for both trauma and EGS patients. Spain et al.[12] demonstrated that a combined program that provides acute care and general surgical care by the trauma service cushioned the impact of variability in trauma volume while maintaining operative skills in an era of increased nonoperative management of many injuries.

Our experience demonstrates that restructuring the Department of Surgery to include an EGS service provides the institution with the opportunity to achieve several goals. Above all, the department can become more productive by increasing elective general surgery *and* EGS hospital volume. As a result of trauma surgeons' participation in EGS, their operative volume has increased despite decreased trauma admissions to the trauma service. There were increases in ICU and operating room utilization of all services. Our initial data suggest that critical care–trained trauma surgeons with broad operative general surgery backgrounds and critical care knowledge are ideal to staff the EGS service (Figures 48.1, 48.2, and 48.3).

Surgical residency programs have suffered at the expense of nonoperative trauma management. The operative requirements established by the Residency Review Committee (RRC) for graduating residents were unattainable in many residency programs because of the high incidence of blunt trauma and the changing patterns of trauma management.[13] This prompted the RRC to decrease the number of operative cases needed to meet the minimum threshold for surgery. Adding acute care surgery cases, with resulting increases in evaluations and resuscitations, on an EGS service will enhance operative experience and enhance graduate medical education.

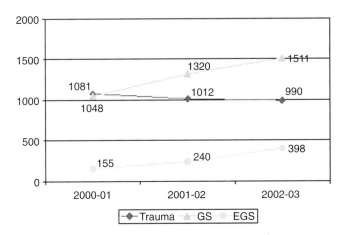

FIGURE 48.2. Operations per year. EGS, emergency general surgery; GS, general surgery.

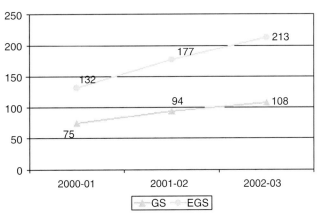

FIGURE 48.3. Intensive care unit admissions per year. EGS, emergency general surgery; GS, general surgery.

System Infrastructure

The Service Concept

Establishment of a service allows for a cohesive group of multidisciplinary providers (attending physicians, residents, medical students, physician extenders, case managers, and social workers) to manage patients and improve communication. Efficient patient care mandates communication between the primary service, other surgical providers, nursing, physical therapy, and case management. Communication is hampered by the number of services involved, the workload of each service, and the institution's training mission. By providing a forum for clear communications among all providers, discharges can be streamlined for complex patients. As health care resources become more constrained, this multidisciplinary model is a viable option for senior physicians to directly impact hospital performance. Daily multidisciplinary rounds shorten length of stay for trauma patients and should demonstrate similar benefits for an EGS service.[14]

The service concept, with the rotation of a fresh surgical team, allows for greater attention to the sickest patients and a rested surgeon for the next surgical patient. As such, management of the patient's disease can occur around the clock. Availability of a residency team for patient evaluation expedites diagnosis and any subsequent operative management.

The Surgical Director

The director of a service oversees the planning and implementation of its mission. Once the mission has been drawn, key elements are put in place for the infrastructure to function efficiently and to deal with problems as they occur. In a "service concept" program where multiple physicians and care givers are involved in a single patient's care, the director plays a key role in ensuring the continuity of the patient's care. This is especially critical for the complex patient with a protracted illness and long hospital stay.

Systems (i.e., practice management protocols) are put in place for process improvement and quality assurance. For example, oversight of multidisciplinary team rounds as a process improvement initiative assists identification of the complex patient. This helps to decrease variability in care and maintain consistency. It also allows for review of outdated policies or protocols and continuous reappraisal of new medical information.

Hospital Support

The Emergency Department

The emergency department (ED) is an important access site for the EGS patient into the system. For the non-trauma surgical patient presenting in shock, the care provided in the ED significantly reduces the progression of organ failure and mortality. Although this period is brief compared with the total length of hospitalization, physiologic determinants of outcome may be established before ICU admission [15].

Creating a collegial relationship with the ED is key to facilitating evaluation, resuscitation, and timely surgical consultation. Development of joint protocols using evidence-based medicine and patient management guidelines for the most common surgical problems allows the ED physician to expedite patient evaluation. The ED is an essential partner with the EGS service, decreasing delays and promoting ED autonomy to function without unnecessary input from the EGS team.

The Operating Room—Urgent/Emergent

Access to a busy operating room is essential for the surgical patient. Most hospitals have criteria for "urgent/emergent" cases. This allows for an equitable system for scheduling acute care cases. Having a universal surgical instrument set for each specialized service also decreases preparation time, costs, and delays during acute care surgical procedures.

Radiology

Twenty-four-hour availability of in-house radiologic services is crucial for the workup of the EGS patient. Although evaluation may well start with plain films of the abdomen, studies demonstrate that the helical computed tomography (CT) scan for the evaluation of abdominal pain has a high sensitivity and specificity.[16–18] Ultrasound continues to be a mainstay for the workup of acute diseases of the biliary tree and must be available 24 hours a day for an EGS service to function at its maximum potential.[19,20]

The era of minimally invasive management is here. The interventional radiologist (IR) is an important consultant for the EGS surgeon when the least invasive, and sometimes the most appropriate, treatment may be angiographic embolization or CT- or ultrasound-guided drainage for immediate control of bleeding or drainage of a closed-space infection. This approach may allow the patient to recover enough physiologic reserve to endure an elective operation.

The Surgical Intensive Care Unit and the Intensive Care Unit Team/Bedside Surgery

The surgical intensive care unit (SICU) team is a critical partner in the care of the EGS patient. Several studies have demonstrated improvement in outcomes and decreased hospital cost by having a dedicated surgical critical care team.[21,22] Coordination of care is essential for complex patients requiring resuscitation, frequent operative interventions, and a subsequent ICU stay.

The "open abdomen" technique is often utilized for the EGS patient with an intraabdominal catastrophe, and bedside surgery is common. Other bedside surgical procedures include percutaneous tracheostomy, bronchoscopy, percutaneous endoscopic gastrostomy, and abdominal washouts. Jointly developed protocols between the EGS and the SICU service utilizing evidence-based medicine should provide a decreased variability and lower the cost of care.

The Hospital Floor

A dedicated hospital floor provides a continuum of care for non-ICU management of the EGS patient. Nursing staff can manage the patient to service protocols and clinical pathways for common problems. Patient care deviating from the protocol can be identified early in hopes of decreasing medical errors, morbidity, and mortality.[23]

Emergency General Surgery Clinic

The EGS clinic has two primary functions: (1) to evaluate posthospital discharges and (2) to manage posthospital care of complex patients. Additionally, it serves as a referral area from the primary care provider's office for minor out-patient surgical problems. A well-staffed clinic allows the surgeon to safely and expeditiously manage simple surgical procedures such as superficial abscesses, perirectal problems, and skin lesions.

Referrals and the Catchment Area

The catchment area for an EGS service includes local or rural hospitals lacking 24-hour surgical expertise or sophisticated ICU care. It also includes primary care physicians and after-hours in-house surgical emergencies. It is critical to have prearranged referral or consult agreements in place. With an EGS team ready and available, transfer times and time to operative intervention decrease, resulting in expeditious treatment of the critical patient.

Intrahospital Communications

Marketing

Once an EGS service is fully functional and referral systems are in place, the service must be marketed as an integrated EGS/critical care product. An outreach program, similar to most regional trauma programs, can be clinically, academically, and financially rewarding. The goal is to demonstrate commitment to serving the clinical and educational needs of the referral base.[23]

Transfer Center

Intrahospital communication is a key aspect of notifying the EGS team of an emergent consult. Establishing one phone number as a single clearinghouse for incoming calls is essential. Access to the EGS service by a referring physician or hospital is facilitated.

Commercial paging systems can be utilized to notify and mobilize several services in times of an emergency. A protocol-driven communication system facilitates appropriate notification of team members for time-sensitive evaluation of the EGS patient. The protocol should also incorporate a tiered EGS response depending on patient acuity.

Transportation

Risks are inherent in the transport of critically ill patients. Protocols are useful in arranging appropriate transportation of such patients. Each institution should have a formalized plan for intra- and interhospital transport that addresses (1) pretransport coordination and communication, (2) transport personnel, (3) transport equipment, (4) monitoring during transport, and (5) documentation. The transport plan should be developed by a multidisciplinary team and should be evaluated and refined regularly using a standard quality improvement process.[24] Lovell et al.[25] evaluated all the factors that can lead to problems during intrahospital transports. Some difficulty or complication occurred in 62% of transports. Of these, 31% were patient related, 45% were related to equipment or the transport environment, and 15% were related to problems in both areas. Many of the difficulties were preventable with adequate pretransport communication and planning. Other problems were directly related to the increased severity of the illnesses of these patients.[25]

Aeromedical Transport

The use of aeromedical transport has significantly improved outcomes for trauma patients. Severity of illness or injury should be the primary justification for aeromedical transport.[26] In one study, major trauma patients transported by aeromedical transport had a better outcome than those transported by ground emergency medical services (EMS). The benefit seen with aeromedical transport was directly related to injury. The state of Maryland has demonstrated a commitment to its citizens and invested heavily in its public safety air medical service. Evaluation of this EMS system suggests that the rapid air transport of victims of traumatic events by specialized personnel has a positive effect on the outcome of severely injured patients.[28]

Critical care expertise during transport to a tertiary care center is essential to the management of the acute care surgery patient. A hospital-based helicopter transport program serves as a logical extension of an institution's emergency care capabilities in an effort to enhance the prehospital and interhospital care of the critically ill.[29] Using conservative patient selection criteria, pretransfer stabilization, and appropriate equipment and medical personnel results in interfacility transfer programs achieving the goal of transferring high-risk patients without adverse impact on clinical outcomes or resource use.[30] When distances are greater than 100 miles, helicopter transport is economically unjustified for interhospital transports where an efficient fixed-wing service exists.[31]

Staffing the Service

The Skill Set

An in-house on-call attending surgeon policy has not been associated with improved outcomes, but a board-eligible or certified surgeon either in-house or immediately available provides improved outcomes in the care of the injured patient. The presence of a trauma and surgical critical care fellowship program, a surrogate for institution commitment to expert subspecialty care, is associated with improved outcomes for critically injured patients. An investment in advanced postgraduate medical education has potential benefits in patient care and outcomes.[32,33] Improved outcomes for the EGS patient would also be expected.

Faculty Coverage

Typically, five to eight surgeons are necessary to provide 24-hour, 7-day-per-week coverage for acute care surgery cases. While on service, their attention should be dedicated to the management of this complex surgical population. Furthermore, graduate medical education should be a secondary goal, as house staff education is an investment in the future of surgical critical care.

Surgical and Medical Subspecialty Consultants

Occasionally, the EGS patient will require input from various surgical and medical subspecialty consultants. A predetermined agreement for priority access to these subspecialists is essential in situations that require such expertise as cardiology, gastroenterology, or obstetrics/gynecology.

The House Staff Team

The EGS service is an exceptional educational environment for graduate surgical education. Opportunities include patient diversity, ability to participate in the evaluation, complex pathophysiology, and unlimited operative experience to challenge all levels of expertise.

The *chief resident* is the captain of the team, responsible to the patient and attending physician for defining and executing the plan of care. The EGS service provides an opportunity for enhancing clinical acumen in time-sensitive situations. Requisite to success is a facile grasp of the pathophysiology of complex surgical diseases from skin and soft tissue infections to intraabdominal catastrophes. The skill set required includes the fortitude to make decisions for surgical versus nonsurgical management of critically ill patients, as well as the operative expertise to execute such operative interventions and the ability to concomitantly mentor junior house staff to the same.

The chief resident also functions as senior consultant to other subspecialty services. Often, surgical pathology occurs in patients admitted to nonsurgical services (i.e., upper gastrointestinal hemorrhage admitted to the medicine service). Diplomatic communication of the patient's surgical needs and need for urgency is important to maintain intraspecialty relationships for future consultation.

The final, and perhaps most important, role of the chief resident is that of educator/mentor. The ability to communicate knowledge into meaningful information for the junior house staff and medical students is essential to personal learning and further strengthens their leadership role.

The *junior resident* on the EGS service is pivotal to the smooth function of the service. This role is designed as a liaison to the hospital. This position is based on the skill to rapidly respond to all consults from the ED and from nonsurgical services across the hospital. To assertively and rapidly identify acute care surgical needs and convey that information in a succinct fashion to the chief resident is essential to the role.

Knowledge of preoperative resuscitation, management of underresuscitated patients, and perioperative antibiotic requirements are crucial to the care of the EGS patient. A successful junior resident also requires the surgical skills for management of lower complexity EGS cases such as uncomplicated appendectomy.

The final requirements of the EGS junior resident are skills to collaborate with the intensivist in the aggressive resuscitation of the unstable patient; at a minimum, these skills include management of mechanical ventilators, manipulation of pulmonary artery catheters, and a broad knowledge of vasoactive cardiac drugs. These skills provide the foundation for quality patient care and smooth operation of the service.

The final member of the house staff team is *the intern*. The nature of the EGS service demands a skill set not typically necessary on a routine general surgical service. This is usually the first time the intern gets to hone the skills of a rapid evaluation and decision-making process. The routine management of the noncritically ill surgical patient is also appropriate to the EGS patient population with one caveat: the complex EGS patient may have long-term needs that may require rehabilitation placement. The multidisciplinary coordination of such a plan is dependent on the intern defining these plans early and collaborating with the appropriate discharge planner.

The EGS service is a powerful forum for the *medical student*. Most medical students will matriculate into a primary care subspecialty. The EGS service is an opportunity for students to learn the pathophysiologic processes that mandate surgical intervention. This exposure is essential to the future development of these students. As for the residents, the EGS service is an introduction to surgical disease, the evaluation process, operative and nonoperative management, as well as intensive and routine care of the complicated surgical patient. This may be the medical student's only opportunity to critically assess a patient from the surgical perspective.

In summary, the EGS service manages a unique subset of patients and disease processes. This complexity allows each level of student, from chief resident to medical student, to have a gratifying educational opportunity.

Physician Extenders

The roles of nurse practitioner and physician assistant were born in the mid-1960s out of a perceived need for nonphysician clinicians (NPCs) in underserved regions of the country.[34] These roles have been more utilized in response to changes in the structure of resident education. The use of NPCs has been shown to reduce physician work load, enhance overall patient care, and improve the morale among the residents.[35,36] In areas where NPCs have the same authority to treat as physicians, comparable patient outcomes have been achieved.[37] Overall, the addition of the NPC enhances the productivity and efficiency of an EGS service.

Responsibility and Credentialing

As the ultimate responsibility for the patient remains in the hands of the physician, delineation of the patient management privileges for the NPC should be a process involving both institution and physician input.[38] The training of physician assistants (PAs) is typically at the baccalaureate level, whereas nurse practitioners (NPs) are required to have a master's level education.[39] The credentials are formulated to identify and promote the skill set unique to the acute care surgery patient. Hospital administration, professional societies, and legal hurdles must be overcome to adequately credential the NPC in order to perform the necessary procedures that are typically handled by the house staff.[40]

The Nonphysician Clinician Skill Set

The skills and activities of the NPC must be defined and then added to the armamentarium of patient care for the EGS team. The traits admired in the prototypical surgical resident could be detrimental for the surgical NPC. Victorino and Organ[36] place a strong emphasis on the patient care and ward responsibilities skills of the NPC, not the manual dexterity and aggressive critical thinking required of the surgical house officer. Unless roles are clearly defined, competition for procedures may breed contempt and resentment between the two resources.[36]

The utilization of the NPC for non-ICU care allows the surgical house staff to concentrate their efforts on the acutely ill patient. By developing a group of NPCs capable of formulating and enacting clinical management guidelines and clinical pathways, there is a marked reduction in the workload of the physician staff. Service coverage, including history and physical examinations, in-patient notes, and daily wound management are all within the scope of practice of the NPC. Routine assessment of the noncomplex clinic patient in the pre- and postoperative setting frees the house staff for complex teaching cases. It has been shown that, in some areas of health care, well-trained NPCs can independently care for 95% of patients without physician input.[41] This approach enhances house staff education without increasing work hours. Ultimately, it also leads to a larger educational tool for the training of future NPCs.[42]

Promoting a Continuum of Care

Case Management

Facilitating patient-focused, cost-effective care throughout the continuum of care is a challenge that requires creativity and resourcefulness. At Vanderbilt University, a case manager or patient care coordinator (PCC) role was developed to improve communication among health care providers, payer organizations, and families by blending the functions of utilization management and discharge planning into a unit-based leadership role. The PCC role is a critical initiative for patients requiring subsequent care at a long-term acute care facility or rehabilitation center.

Social Worker

Because complex illnesses affect the integrity of the patient's support system, a social worker is an effective resource for the family throughout the patient's hospitalization and recovery period. Additionally, social workers are an enormous help when patients travel from great distances to receive care at a tertiary care facility.[43]

Rehabilitation/Extended Care

During the past decade trauma and burn survivors have gone on to specialty rehabilitation. Studies have demonstrated improved patient outcome with a decrease in hospital length of stay and more rapid restoration of function when such resources are available.[44–46] This option is especially important following a protracted ICU stay as the patient may not be ready to be discharged home. Options include rehabilitation, skilled nursing home, or a long-term acute care center (LTAC) to assist with complex needs such as ventilator weaning. In some cases, patients are being transferred directly from the ICU to an LTAC for weaning earlier in their course than previously experienced. Patients are now more severely ill on arrival at the LTAC than in past years, but mortality rates are unchanged; more than half of patients in LTACs continue to be successfully weaned, and survival after respiratory wean protocols is improved.[47]

Similar successes have been demonstrated in medical and cardiac units.[48–50] The ability to maintain ICU bed availability for the critically ill surgical patient depends on established relationships with a variety of extended care facilities. Defining which EGS population may benefit from extended care is essential. Early referral and transfer, once acute surgical needs have been met, is critical to maintaining patient through-put, ensuring that the needs of the community will be met by bed availability.

The Emergency General Surgery Registry

Evidence-based medicine is the conscientious, explicit, and judicious use of current best evidence in making decisions about the care of individual patients.[51] From this laudable goal stems the need for a patient registry in order to fully operationalize the concept of performance improvement. The tools afforded by prospective data collection allow concurrent critical examination of techniques utilized to improve patient care. This process starts with identification of disease-specific and global clinical parameters essential to the analysis of the EGS patient. The greatest hurdle to standardization of care is the clinical handling of a problem that varies among institutions.[52]

The Model

Ideally, the information collected for a database should be easily accessible, clearly defined, and clinically relevant. The data should include patient demographics, physiologic parameters with associated disease processes, and clinical outcomes.[53] The data can then be utilized for institution-specific performance improvement, as well as

an on-going research tool. The process of data collection and assessment should be continually evaluated to define new or on-going issues within the program that need improvement. It must always be remembered: "not all questions of relevance to the care of patients are scientific in their nature and so science cannot ever provide the basis for clinical decision making in any fundamental sense."[54]

Practice Management Guidelines

A recent survey showed that many physicians are wary of practice management guidelines for many reasons: lack of awareness, lack of familiarity, lack of agreement, poor cost-benefit ratio, "cookbook" medicine, and lack of autonomy.[55] The implementation of practice management guidelines should improve quality of care by limiting variability and providing "effective advances" in the daily practice of health care.[56] The foundation for practice management guidelines should be the best clinical data as defined by national organizations and societies or institution-specific algorithms.[53] Examples include stress ulcer prophylaxis, deep vein thrombosis prophylaxis, and ventilator-associated pneumonia protocols. The development team should include physician, NPCs, and pharmacists as well as any institutional-specific member for an appropriate practice management guideline.

The Financial Model

Historical Perspective

Before a dedicated EGS service was developed at Vanderbilt University Medical Center, surgical patients presenting with an emergency were cared for by a mix of general/laparoscopic, oncologic/endocrine, and trauma/critical care surgeons on three separate services within the Department of Surgery. Each maintained a separate budget based on its individual practice goals. With the introduction of an EGS service, the implications of not having a unique budget plan were clear. The needs of the EGS patient and the requirements for a hospital infrastructure (ICU and hospital days, operating room utilization, percent referral to subsequent care facilities) are essential.

The Need for an Emergency General Surgery Service Designation

A fundamental business issue is the inability to track or analyze EGS performance. Unlike trauma, burn, or cardiovascular services, which have descriptive ICD-9 codes, acute care general surgery does not. As this patient population presents with common general surgical problems,

TABLE 48.1. Historical financial and statistical information about the emergency general surgery patient population is collated and summarized by month and by primary payer class.

Financial information

Gross billings	Actual hospital charges from all sources
Collections (pro forma)	Estimated based on prior year actual collections
Expense	Estimated using cost accounting methodologies set forth by the finance department
Net income	Collections less expense

Statistical information

Discharges	Information is captured only after a patient is discharged
Length of stay	Based on that episode of care (readmission is another episode)
Average length of stay	

although at a higher acuity, it is extremely difficult to distinguish them from elective surgical patients.

Designing a system to track a patient population requires changing the culture of the institution. From admission to discharge and across departments a completely separate service-specific category/designation must be created. Such data provide a manometer from which productivity of a new service can be measured. Building the infrastructure and having the ability to plan a service/hospital budget for this high-acuity patient population becomes critical when additional hospital resources are necessary.

The Budget: Basics

Typically, historical financial and statistical information about the EGS patient population is collated and summarized by month and by primary payer class. This information is important in monitoring performance of the product line (Table 48.1).

Analysis

The mainstay of monitoring and improving this business is profitability. Information and methodology can quickly be adapted to analyze change versus past year and performance versus plan (financial and/or statistical). In addition, the above information can yield a great deal of statistics and analysis regarding payer mix changes, payer profitability, cost, and charge per day (per discharge) to name a few variables. The analysis helps for planning for needed hospital resources that a service incurs. This information becomes essential when medical groups and hospitals develop contracts with payers. Being able to accurately define a population one is caring for allows for equitable contracting.

In conclusion, developing a new academic surgical service is complex and requires a significant dedication from the Department of Surgery as well as the institution. A service that cares for surgical emergencies must have access and privileges to multiple different resources of the hospital and physicians. The patient's illness demands it, and any thing less would not be prudent.

References

1. Sosin DM, Sniezek JE, Waxweiler RJ. Trends in death associated with traumatic brain injury, 1979 through 1992. Success and failure. JAMA 1995; 14;273(22):1778–1780.
2. Cornwell EE 3rd, Chang DC, Phillips J, et al. Enhanced trauma program commitment at a level I trauma center: effect on the process and outcome of care. Arch Surg 2003; 138(8):838–843.
3. Mullins RJ, Veum-Stone J, Helfand M, et al. Outcome of hospitalized injured patients after institution of a trauma system in an urban area. JAMA 1994; 271(24):1919–1924.
4. Rathore SS, Epstein AJ, Volpp KG, et al. Hospital coronary artery bypass graft surgery volume and patient mortality, 1998–2000. Ann Surg 2004; 239(1):110–117.
5. Begg CB, Cramer LD, Hoskins WJ, et al. Impact of hospital volume on operative mortality for major cancer surgery. JAMA 1998; 280(20):1747–1751.
6. Birkmeyer JD, Siewers AE, Finlayson EV, et al. Hospital volume and surgical mortality in the United States. N Engl J Med 2002; 346(15):1128–1137.
7. Sampalis JS, Denis R, Frechette P, et al. Direct transport to tertiary trauma centers versus transfer from lower level facilities: impact on mortality and morbidity among patients with major trauma. J Trauma 1997; 43(2):288–296.
8. Sampalis JS, Denis R, Lavoie A, et al. Trauma care regionalization: a process-outcome evaluation. J Trauma 1999; 46(4):565–581.
9. Cherry D, Annest JL, Mercy JA, et al. Trends in nonfatal and fatal firearm-related injury rates in the United States, 1985–1995. Ann Emerg Med 1998; 32(1):51–59.
10. Engelhardt S, Hoyt D, Coimbra R, et al. The 15-year evolution of an urban trauma center: what does the future hold for the trauma surgeon? J Trauma 2001; 51(4):633–638.
11. Scherer LA, Battistella FD. Trauma and emergency surgery: an evolutionary direction for trauma surgeons. J Trauma 2004; 56(1):7–12.
12. Spain DA, Richardson JD, Carrillo EH, et al. Should trauma surgeons do general surgery? J Trauma 2000; 48(3):433–438.
13. Bulinski P, Bachulis B, Naylor DF Jr, et al. The changing face of trauma management and its impact on surgical resident training. J Trauma 2003; 54(1):161–163.
14. Dutton RP, Cooper C, Jones A, et al. Daily multidisciplinary rounds shorten length of stay for trauma patients. J Trauma 2003; 55(5):913–919.
15. Nguyen HB, Rivers EP, Havstad S, et al. Critical care in the emergency department: a physiologic assessment and outcome evaluation. Acad Emerg Med 2000; 7(12):1354–1361.
16. Scaglione M, Grassi R, Pinto A, et al. Positive predictive value and negative predictive value of spiral CT in the

diagnosis of closed loop obstruction complicated by intestinal ischemia. Radiol Med (Torino) 2004; 107(1–2):69–77.

17. Wilson EB, Cole JC, Nipper ML, et al. Computed tomography and ultrasonography in the diagnosis of appendicitis: when are they indicated? Arch Surg 2001; 136(6):670–675.

18. Rosen MP, Sands DZ, Longmaid HE 3rd, et al. Impact of abdominal CT on the management of patients presenting to the emergency department with acute abdominal pain. AJR Am J Roentgenol 2000; 174(5):1391–1396.

19. Patel M, Miedema BW, James MA, et al. Percutaneous cholecystostomy is an effective treatment for high-risk patients with acute cholecystitis. Am Surg 2000; 66(1):33–37.

20. Menu Y, Vuillerme MP. Non-traumatic abdominal emergencies: imaging and intervention in acute biliary conditions. Eur Radiol 2002; 12(10):2397–2406.

21. Pronovost PJ, Angus DC, Dorman T, et al. Physician staffing patterns and clinical outcomes in critically ill patients: a systematic review. JAMA 2002; 288(17):2151–2162.

22. Dimick JB, Pronovost PJ, Heitmiller RF, et al. Intensive care unit physician staffing is associated with decreased length of stay, hospital cost, and complications after esophageal resection. Crit Care Med 2001; 29(4):753–758.

23. Biffl WL, Moore EE, Offner PJ, et al. The Outreach Trauma Program: a model for survival of the academic trauma center. J Trauma 2002; 52(5):840–846.

24. Warren J, Fromm RE Jr, Orr RA, et al. Guidelines for the inter- and intrahospital transport of critically ill patients. Crit Care Med 2004; 32(1):256–262.

25. Lovell MA, Mudaliar MY, Klineberg PL. Intrahospital transport of critically ill patients: complications and difficulties. Anaesth Intensive Care 2001; 29(4):400–405.

26. Rhee KJ, Baxt WG, Mackenzie JR, et al. Differences in air ambulance patient mix demonstrated by physiologic scoring. Ann Emerg Med 1990; 19(5):552–556.

27. Boyd CR, Corse KM, Campbell RC. Emergency interhospital transport of the major trauma patient: air versus ground. J Trauma 1989; 29(6):789–793.

28. Kerr WA, Kerns TJ, Bissell RA. Differences in mortality rates among trauma patients transported by helicopter and ambulance in Maryland. Prehosp Disaster Med 1999; 14(3):159–164.

29. Farnell MB, Sachs JL. Mayo Clinic's hospital-based emergency air medical transport service. Mayo Clin Proc 1989; 64(10):1213–1225.

30. Selevan JS, Fields WW, Chen W, et al. Critical care transport: outcome evaluation after interfacility transfer and hospitalization. Ann Emerg Med 1999; 33(1):33–43.

31. Thomas F, Wisham J, Clemmer TP, et al. Outcome, transport times, and costs of patients evacuated by helicopter versus fixed-wing aircraft. West J Med 1990; 153(1):40–43.

32. Arbabi S, Jurkovich GJ, Rivara FP, et al. Patient outcomes in academic medical centers: influence of fellowship programs and in-house on-call attending surgeon. Arch Surg 2003; 138(1):47–51.

33. Hoyt DB, Shackford SR, McGill T, et al. The impact of in-house surgeons and operating room resuscitation on outcome of traumatic injuries. Arch Surg 1989; 124(8):906–910.

34. DeNicola L, et al. Use of pediatric extenders in pediatric and neonatal intensive care units. Crit Care Med 1994; 22:1856–1964.

35. Spisso J, O'Callaghan C, McKennan M, et al. Improved quality of care and reduction of housestaff workload using trauma nurse practitioners. J Trauma 1990; 30(6):660–663.

36. Victorino G, Organ C. Physician assistant influence on surgery residents. Arch Surg 2003; 138:971–976.

37. Mundinger M, Kane R, Lenz E, et al. Primary care outcomes in patients treated by nurse practitioners or physicians in a randomized trial. JAMA 2000; 283(1):59–68.

38. Schaeffer H, Hardy D, Jewett P, et al. The role of the nurse practitioner and physician assistant in the care of hospitalized children. Pediatrics 1999; 103(5):1050–1052.

39. Cooper R. The growing independence of nonphysician clinicians in clinical practice. JAMA 1997; 277(13):1092–1094.

40. Riportella-Muller R, Libby D, Kindig D. The substitution of physician assistants and nurse practitioners for physician residents in teaching hospitals. Health Affairs 1995; 14:181–191.

41. Polk H. The declining interest in surgical careers, the primary care mirage, and concerns about contemporary undergraduate surgical education. Am J Surg 1999; 178(3):177–179.

42. Abrass C, Ballweg R, Gilshannon M, et al. Process for reducing workload and enhancing residents' education at an academic medical center. Acad Med 2001; 76(8):798–805.

43. Bijttebier P, Vanoost S, Delva D, et al. Needs of relatives of critical care patients: perceptions of relatives, physicians and nurses. Intensive Care Med 2001; 27(1):160–165.

44. DeSanti L, Lincoln L, Egan F, et al. Development of a burn rehabilitation unit: impact on burn center length of stay and functional outcome. J Burn Care Rehabil 1998; 19(5):414–419.

45. Sheridan R, Weber J, Prelack K, et al. Early burn center transfer shortens the length of hospitalization and reduces complications in children with serious burn injuries. J Burn Care Rehabil 1999; 20(5):347–350.

46. Mosenthal AC, Livingston DH, Lavery RF, et al. The effect of age on functional outcome in mild traumatic brain injury: 6-month report of a prospective multicenter trial. J Trauma 2004; 56(5):1042–1048.

47. Scheinhorn DJ, Chao DC, Stearn-Hassenpflug M, et al. Post-ICU mechanical ventilation: treatment of 1,123 patients at a regional weaning center. Chest 1997; 111(6):1654–1659.

48. Scheinhorn DJ, Chao DC, Stearn-Hassenpflug M. Approach to patients with long-term weaning failure. Respir Care Clin North Am 2000; 6(3):437–461, vi.

49. Dennis C, Houston-Miller N, Schwartz RG, et al. Early return to work after uncomplicated myocardial infarction. Results of a randomized trial. JAMA 1988; 260(2):214–220.

50. Stohr IM, Albes JM, Franke U, et al. Outcome of patients after cardiac surgery transferred to other hospitals following prolonged intensive care stay. Thorac Cardiovasc Surg 2002; 50(6):329–332.

51. Hutchinson L, Marks T, Pittilo M. The physician assistant: would the US model meet the needs of the NHS? BMJ 2001; 323:1244–1247.

52. Hampton J. Evidence-based medicine, practice variations and clinical freedom. J Eval Clin Pract 1997; 3(2):123–131.

53. Performance Improvement Subcommittee of the American College of Surgeons Committee on Trauma. Trauma Performance Improvement Reference Manual. Chicago: American College of Surgeons, 2002.

54. Miles A, Bentley P, Polychronis A, Grey J. Evidence-based medicine: why all the fuss? This is why. J Eval Clin Pract 1997; 3(2):83–86.

55. Sox H. Independent primary care practice by nurse practitioners. JAMA 2000; 283(1):106–108.

56. Chassin M. Practice guidelines: best hope for quality improvement in the 1990s. J Occup Med 1990; 32(12):1199–1206.

Part V
The International Communities

49
Acute Care Surgery: United Kingdom

Bernard F. Ribeiro, Simon Paterson-Brown, Murat Akyol, Michael Walsh, Andrew Sim, and Christopher Aylwin

The United Kingdom can, with some justification, claim to be the first country to introduce a modern, comprehensive accident service. Historically, England, Wales, and Northern Ireland were divided into counties, each with a county town, a diocese, a cathedral and bishop, and a hospital. During the reign of Queen Victoria (1837–1901), a large number of hospitals were built; these formed the basis of the United Kingdom's district general hospitals.

In 1888, Robert Jones, a Liverpool surgeon, was given charge of the medical services for the Manchester Ship Canal. Over 20,000 workers were employed to work the 35-mile stretch. Over the 6 years it took to build the canal, Robert Jones built up a network of first-aid posts and hospitals with fully staffed resident doctors and nurses to treat the injured. A railway running the length of the canal united the hospitals. This early example failed to influence future planners, and therefore hospitals and their casualty departments were built in a haphazard manner often to reflect the constituencies of members of Parliament rather than the needs of the population.

When the National Health Service (NHS) was introduced in 1948 for England, Wales, Scotland, and Northern Ireland, the Ministry of Health inherited a casualty service in which there was no discernible plan. The only ray of hope was the Birmingham Accident Hospital. This hospital in the industrial midlands was designed to improve the care of the injured by providing continuous 24-hour coverage from consultant surgeons and anesthetists with good support services.

It achieved world-wide recognition under Professor William Gissane and Mr. Peter London, but the concept of an independent accident hospital manned by trauma surgeons did not find favor, and, as a result, the United Kingdom continues to lag behind in the development of a trauma service.

In 1971, Sir John Bruce of the Joint Consultant's Committee recommended that 32 accident and emergency departments in the United Kingdom be placed under the control of a new type of specialist, namely, a consultant in accident and acute care medicine. There are currently 505 consultants in 240 hospitals in this new specialty providing care across the spectrum of medicine and surgery in England and Wales. The next phase will be to integrate this service with the acute medical and surgical specialties for the benefit of the acutely ill patient.

The introduction of the NHS created a unique system of health care for all, free at the point of need. To sustain a health service through taxation against a background of increased public expectation and choice, new innovations, and rising costs inevitably leads to a rationing of services and the creation of waiting lists.

The increasing trend toward specialization in all branches of surgery has not only developed expertise and improved outcomes but also had a dramatic effect on the provision of acute care services. The role of the generalist is not in doubt in the smaller, remote hospital, but, in the larger urban center, the demand for specialists must be balanced against the need for a comprehensive acute care service. The number of doctors per 1,000 patients in the United Kingdom is among the lowest in the world, and, in order to provide a quality acute care service covering all the surgical subspecialties, there will need to be a massive expansion of surgeons. In 2001, the National Health Service Executive (NHSE) statisticians recorded 1,331 consultants in general surgery—a ratio to population of 1 : 40,000, against a targeted requirement for 1,410 consultants. The projected requirement for 2009 is 2,165, which will produce a shortfall of 246 surgeons.

To make better use of scarce resources and to concentrate services on fewer sites, the Medical Royal Colleges have recommended that the ideal unit for a fully comprehensive medical and surgical service is a hospital serving a population of 500,000.[1] At present, fewer than 10% of hospitals serve a population of 500,000. Some 33% of hospitals cater to less than 250,000. It is envisaged that, for the foreseeable future, hospitals serving populations of between 250,000 and 300,000 will provide the bulk of the acute services for medicine and surgery.

In all the surgical disciplines, there has been a steady rise in acute care activity, reaching 3.5% at the end of the 1990s.[2] This represents over half of all general surgical admissions[3,4] and slightly fewer than half for orthopedics and trauma. Many of the patients are elderly with multiple comorbidities, and it is estimated that in this age group there is a 5% annual increase in the incidence of proximal femoral fractures, with 95% of these patients requiring surgery.[5] A New Deal on Junior Doctor Hours[6] and the European Working Time Directive (EWTD)[7] applicable to all doctors in the European Union will soon make some junior doctors supernumerary in all but name and restrict their hours in hospital. This change will require consultants to assume a greater role in the management of emergencies. The new consultant contract scheduled for implementation in 2004 recognizes this change by including two programmed activities (PAs) per week for acute care work done while on call (4 hours per PA). This is the first time that emergency care has been recognized as work done by consultants. For once, politicians can be forgiven for not appreciating that consultants undertake acute care work, because, historically, funding of the NHS was centered on elective care with no separate provision for emergency care, which was largely provided by junior doctors.

In 1993, the Association of Surgeons of Great Britain and Ireland[8] proposed that surgeons, while on call, should have no other responsibilities likely to delay the treatment of patients. This followed the recommendations of The National Confidential Enquiry into Post-Operative Deaths (NCEPOD)[9] that acute care surgery should not be carried out at night by unsupervised trainees. In orthopedic surgery, trauma teams have achieved this objective, but other specialties have yet to do so. A 24-hour snapshot of acute care general surgery in the United Kingdom[3] showed that most patients seen "on call" arrived between 10 am and 8 pm, a period when most general surgical consultants have other duties. How, then, can we shift the balance of care to meet the growing demand for the emergency admissions?

1. By ring-fencing elective beds, thus separating acute care from elective care, preferably on the same site

2. By encouraging the development of day units and treatment centers with overnight facilities, an initiative the present Labour Government supports

3. By encouraging the concept of "a surgeon of the day" or "surgical team of the week" to manage emergency admissions with dedicated emergency theaters fully staffed with a consultant surgeon and anesthetist available from 9 am to 9 pm—all staff to be freed of their elective duties

4. By improving the care pathway for patients and making greater use of nurse practitioners, physiotherapists, and radiographers to assist in the process

5. By developing an integrated pathway of care for all emergencies—medical and surgical—with a triage for emergencies in accident and emergency (A&E) and links to social services in order to encourage the early discharge of patients.

The reduction in junior doctor hours prompted by health and safety issues both in Europe and the United States has necessitated a review of working practice. It has also called into question how junior doctors are trained. If service delivery is to be provided in the future by consultants, then it is imperative that we separate emergency care from elective care, and, by so doing, create a climate where trainees can receive adequate supervision in both disciplines.

The problem of service provision has been the subject of many reviews by Medical Royal Colleges, specialty associations, and government departments. All recognize the need to provide a comprehensive acute service to a population, but such services are not uniformly distributed or funded. Providing the appropriate workforce to deliver the service in the future will be key to the success of the NHS in the next 50 years.

Emergency General Surgery

Introduction

The care of patients admitted to the hospital with acute care general surgical problems remains one of the most important aspects of general surgical practice,[10] and, with the current trend of increasing emergency admissions throughout the United Kingdom in all medical specialties,[11] this responsibility will undoubtedly increase. Some studies have demonstrated that up to 50% of all general surgical admissions are emergencies,[12] with approximately half involving acute abdominal pain. The workload for the general surgeon is therefore substantial. The NCEPOD has repeatedly demonstrated that the outcome for patients requiring acute care surgery is improved when senior surgical staff is involved not only in the preoperative decision making but also in the surgery and postoperative care.[9] This, of course, has major implications for the staffing structure of the on-call surgical team, the resources required for the care of the emergency patient, and the actual system that needs to be put in place so that optimum care can be delivered.

On-Call Surgical Team

Of all the changes that have occurred in general surgery over the past decade, undoubtedly the reduction in junior doctors' hours,[6] associated with the EWTD,[7] has had the strongest influence, followed closely by the reduced overall period of training as recommended in the Calman report.[13] These two factors together have been estimated to have halved the overall experience available for surgical trainees.[14] Where continuity of care was maintained by the "middle-grade" surgical team in the past, the new schedules currently being put into place are increasingly of a shift pattern where the maximum time worked per week is 48 hours. As a result, the consultant (almost by default) has become the main person ensuring continuity of care for the emergency patients. In itself, this is of course no bad thing and has previously been recommended by the NCEPOD.[9] However, there are two main problems to its implementation. First, the consultant cannot carry out this emergency activity if he or she also has elective commitments. Second, he or she must be supported by junior staff who are not continually changing.

In essence, this means that the consultant and supporting junior staff on call must have no elective commitments, both during the period of on call and for several days afterward, so that the problems can be sorted out. Although there will have to be some change of junior doctors because of the EWTD, these can be kept to a minimum by allocating junior doctors to emergency activities for a defined period of time, perhaps a week, perhaps longer. Their subsequent attachment to elective activities then no longer suffers from the disruption associated with on-call shifts, a state of affairs that enhances both emergency and elective training opportunities. This "emergency team" system, with many adaptations according to local requirements, has now been adopted in many units throughout the United Kingdom since it was first reported in Edinburgh in 1999.[15]

The emergency team (ET), undoubtedly, improves the ability of the consultant general surgeon, as well as the middle-grade team, to provide a safe and effective emergency care, but requires other conditions to be met if it is to be both efficient and cost-effective in terms of lost elective activity for the consultant and training opportunities for the surgical trainees. These include easy access to radiologic imaging, a dedicated acute care operating theatre with full (and senior) anesthetic support available 24 hours each day, enough surgical admissions to make the system worthwhile, and a distinct and dedicated admission area, that is, a surgical assessment unit (SAU) where these patients can be assessed. Many of these patients have equivocal signs and symptoms of acute appendicitis, and the value of "active observation" with reassessment after 2 to 3 hours by the same surgeon, repeated thereafter as necessary, is well established[16] and should be routine in all units. This is only possible if all acute admissions remain in a single identifiable area.

Early Investigation of Patients with Emergency Surgical Problems

For an ET system to work efficiently, the surgical team must have rapid access to diagnostic blood tests and appropriate imaging, which should include plain and contrast radiology, diagnostic and interventional (percutaneous drainage and biopsy) ultrasound, and computed tomography (CT). Furthermore, plain radiographs evaluated by senior radiologists substantially enhances senior surgical assessment of patients with acute abdominal pain resulting in reduced surgical admissions (17).

Many surgical patients admitted as an emergency do not require surgery and, of these, most will require admission for only a day or so, if not less. What has always stood out from all the studies on acute abdominal pain in the past two decades is the high incidence of nonspecific abdominal pain (NSAP), with published figures of 40% or more.[18] However, these patients often require some investigations to help exclude a surgical problem, and one study was able to reduce the overall incidence of NSAP to 27% by selective use of laparoscopy.[19] A randomized trial conducted in 1999 comparing early laparoscopy versus observation for patients admitted to the hospital with suspected nonspecific abdominal pain clearly supports the use of early laparoscopy because of its higher diagnostic accuracy and subsequent improved quality of life assessed 6 weeks after discharge from hospital.[20] Obviously, the sooner these investigations can be carried out the better for all concerned.

Blood Tests

Although blood test results are often useful as baseline information, their influence on the diagnosis of acute abdominal pain remains unclear, with the exception of serum amylase for acute pancreatitis.[21] A quick and reliable dip test has recently been developed[22] to confirm acute pancreatitis by detecting urinary trypsinogen-2 and may compliment serum amylase levels, particularly if they are equivocal. Studies examining the influence of white cell concentration,[23] C-reactive protein,[24] and skin temperature in the right iliac fossa[25] in patients with "query appendicitis" have concluded that serial white cell counts are useful, as compared with a single measurement, and measurement of skin temperature over the right iliac fossa is of little value. Although isolated C-reactive protein levels may also be fairly nondiscriminatory, when they are interpreted with white cell count and both are normal, acute appendicitis is unlikely.[26] Thus, routine measurement of the white cell count in patients with acute abdominal pain can be justified, if simply for achieving baseline data with which to compare subsequent levels depending on clinical progress.

Liver function tests are unlikely to be available during the early assessment of the acute abdomen. They are, however, extremely useful in confirming or refuting the presence of acute biliary disease.[27,28]

TABLE 49.1. Common emergency conditions detectable by abdominal ultrasonography.

Acute appendicitis
Gynecologic disorders (ovarian cysts, ectopic pregnancies)
Acute biliary disease
Small bowel obstruction
Abdominal aortic aneurysm
Free air/fluid/blood
Disruption to solid organs (liver, spleen, and kidney)
Renal tract obstruction

Ultrasonography

Ultrasonography has become increasingly common as a first-line investigative tool for both acute abdominal pain of various causes[29-31] and abdominal trauma,[32] with the ability to detect a wide variety of conditions (Table 49.1). Ultrasound is highly user dependent and, as such, relies on senior radiologic support. Although intensive training courses for surgical trainees can allow them to use ultrasound,[33] because of the time required and the fact that interventional maneuvers are increasingly being adopted, it is best to involve senior radiologic staff at an early stage.

Contrast Radiology

Suspected Upper Gastrointestinal Perforation

Although the erect chest radiograph is recognized as the most appropriate first-line investigative tool for a suspected perforated peptic ulcer, in as many as 50% of patients no free gas may be identified.[34] For many years now, depending on the clinical condition, water-soluble contrast studies have been used to help confirm or refute the presence of perforation,[35] but they will of course not differentiate between the patient without a perforation and one in whom the perforation has sealed. The addition of ultrasound and even CT in this scenario may contribute by revealing free abdominal fluid in the patient whose perforation has sealed spontaneously, and ultrasound has actually been shown to be superior to plain radiographs for the detection of perforations.[31] As has been well understood for quite some time, many patients with perforated peptic ulcers can be managed nonoperatively,[36,37] with which knowledge the assessing surgeon can afford, with most patients, to resuscitate the patient and make efforts to confirm or refute the diagnosis before rushing to acute care surgery. Obviously, only patients in whom there is no leak of contrast should be considered for nonoperative treatment of their perforation.

Small Bowel Obstruction

Surgery for small bowel obstruction is performed for one of two reasons: first, there has been failure of nonoperative management; second, there is a clinical suspicion of impending strangulation. Although plain abdominal radiographs are useful in establishing the diagnosis of small bowel obstruction, they cannot differentiate between strangulated and nonstrangulated gut. The criteria on which strangulated intestine must be suspected are well established: peritonism, fever, tachycardia, and leukocytosis.[38] Even when the diagnosis is suspected, the changes at operation are often irreversible and resection is required. Small bowel contrast studies improve the diagnostic accuracy of small bowel obstruction[39] and can provide useful clinical information for more than three fourths of patients.[40]

The influence on clinical decision making remains to be established. What can probably be agreed on is that failure of contrast to reach the cecum within 4 hours[41,42] and certainly by 12 hours[43] strongly suggests that surgical intervention is likely to be required and therefore better sooner than later.

Large Bowel Obstruction

The management algorithm for large bowel obstruction is now well established, following the more widespread recognition that colonic pseudo-obstruction could not be distinguished from mechanical obstruction on plain x-rays alone.[44,45] Knowing that all patients with suspected large bowel obstruction should now undergo a contrast enema before laparotomy has probably been the most important factor in reducing not only the unnecessary operation rate for pseudo-obstruction but also in the earlier recognition of those patients who require surgery.

Acute Diverticulitis

Most patients who present with symptoms and signs of acute diverticulitis can be managed nonoperatively, with the exception of those patients who have overt peritonitis from perforation. Although ultrasonography in experienced hands might identify a thickened segment of colon, perhaps with an associated paracolic collection of fluid, invariably there is too much gas for adequate assessment, and quite significant collections can go unnoticed. For this reason, clinicians have used other modalities such as water-soluble contrast radiology and CT scanning.[46] The former has the ability to identify a "leak," the latter, a collection. Both of these pieces of information may be of use to the surgeon in reaching a decision to operate, even though the ultimate decision must be based on clinical rather than radiologic criteria. Overall, CT scanning is no more specific than a contrast enema, but it does allow guided percutaneous drainage to be carried out if a collection is identified.[47]

Computed Tomography

The place of CT in the early assessment of the acute abdomen has recently been studied in a randomized controlled trial of 120 patients.[48] Early CT reduced the hospital stay by an estimated 1.1 days (not significant), but significantly improved diagnostic accuracy. It can also be utilized specifically to improve the diagnostic accuracy of suspected acute appendicitis with quite impressive results: 98% accuracy in 100 consecutive patients of whom 53 had acute appendicitis.[49] However, irrespective of the cost and availability issue, care must be taken to ensure that such techniques of investigation are used to compliment rather than to replace the clinical assessment.[50] At present, few if any units would advocate routine use of CT scanning as a first-line diagnostic test for the acute nontraumatic abdomen.

Emergency Theater Availability

It is now well established that most acute care surgical procedures do not need to be carried out overnight, but reducing operations during these inappropriate hours requires that the theater be available during the day. It also goes without saying that there is no point in having an on-call surgical team available and free of elective commitments during the day if they do not have ready access to the theater. Indeed, as could be anticipated, establishment of an acute care theater during the day substantially reduces the amount of out-of-hours operating.[15,51]

Surgical Subspecialization

All general surgeons treating emergency patients must keep up to date in all the subspecialties and be aware of new developments in both diagnosis and early management in order to provide the best care for their patients. However, the increasing trend toward subspecialization in elective general surgery has, not surprisingly, resulted in some consultants becoming increasingly uncomfortable with the broader knowledge and skills they need to maintain for acute care surgery when their elective practice is in an unrelated field, such as breast or endocrine surgery. Although separate on-call schedules for vascular emergencies are now a common feature in the larger hospitals in the United Kingdom, there are an increasing number of hospitals in which subspecialty interunit referrals for complex acute care esophagogastric, hepatobiliary, pancreatic, and colorectal problems are undertaken.[52] This becomes yet another on-call commit-

ment for the increasingly busy consultant. However, there appears to be no doubt that, even within abdominal surgery, acute care subspecialization influences outcome. Patients undergoing acute care colorectal surgery are less likely to have a stoma fashioned if the surgeons operating have a specialist interest in colorectal surgery,[53] and patients with acute biliary disease are more likely to undergo laparoscopic cholecystectomy during their index admission when a subspecialist upper gastrointestinal surgical service is available.[54]

If implemented throughout the United Kingdom, this policy of acute care subspecialization would have widespread and far-reaching effects not only on the surgical schedules within larger hospitals but on the very existence of acute care surgical services in smaller hospitals. Early results from Edinburgh, where upper and lower gastrointestinal surgeries, both elective and emergency, were divided in 2002, have been encouraging,[55,56] although different solutions will need to be tailored to local requirements.

Future Provision of Emergency General Surgical Services in the United Kingdom

With the overwhelming drive to the 48-hour week for both consultants and junior surgical staff, combined with the shortened training program and the further development of surgical subspecialization, the future of emergency general surgical care will almost certainly involve the majority, if not all, of the developments discussed above. Emergency hospitals of the future will have on-call surgical teams, free from all elective activities, to provide state-of-the-art surgical care all the way from initial assessment, through surgery, to postoperative care. This will involve dedicated SAUs, same-day access to appropriate investigations, and 24-hour theater availability. Large hospitals with a high acute care workload at present could probably move to this sort of system fairly rapidly and many have already done so. In those areas where several hospitals currently provide emergency surgical care, a move to a single acute care site and a combined schedule would be advantageous in terms of overall workload and efficiency. These moves would also facilitate the development of subspecialty emergency surgical care. Even though most emergency surgical admissions have either relatively minor or unspecialized problems, most morbidity and mortality is, undoubtedly, associated with the more specialized conditions. With the increasingly litigious nature of the population and the growing evidence in support of emergency subspecialty surgical care, moves toward emergency subspecialization are likely to be irresistible. However, the hospitals in more remote areas will need to work on a different model, as discussed elsewhere in this chapter.

Emergency Surgery and Organ Transplantation

Introduction

Living donor transplantations are the only elective procedures in the field of solid organ transplantation. All other transplantation activity occurs unplanned, in an acute care fashion. Emergencies in the area of organ transplantation can be divided into four types:

1. Organ retrieval from cadaveric donors
2. Cadaveric organ transplantation
3. Super-urgent transplantation
4. Surgical emergencies in organ transplant recipients

Organ Retrieval from Cadaveric Donors

In common with most countries in the developed world, most organ transplants in the United Kingdom are performed using organs from brain stem–dead cadaveric donors. The number of cadaveric organ donors in the United Kingdom over the past decade is shown in Figure 49.1. Table 49.2 compares cadaveric organ donation rates in European countries with those in the United Kingdom[57].

For the provision of organ transplantation and organ retrieval services, the United Kingdom is divided into various regions. At the time of writing, there are 6 cardiothoracic, 7 liver, 8 pancreas, and 21 kidney transplant centers in the United Kingdom. (Kidney transplant centers in London are amalgamated into two alliances, North Thames and South Thames.) Each of these transplant units is responsible for organ retrieval from cadav-

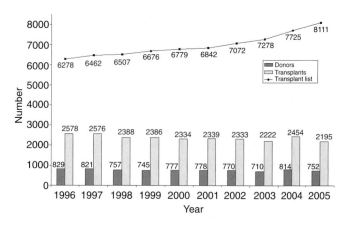

FIGURE 49.1. Number of deceased donors and transplants in the United Kingdom, 1996–2005, and patients on the active and suspended transplant lists at December 31, 2005.

eric donors within their "zone." Potential organ donors are notified to the UK Transplant Service (UKTS) by the regional transplant coordinators.

The UKTS is a government-funded special health authority based in Bristol. It has duties and authority that extend to all four countries of the United Kingdom. The responsibilities of the UKTS include the following:

• Managing the National Transplant Database, which includes details of all donors and patients who are waiting for or who have received a transplant
• Providing a 24-hour service for the matching and allocation of donor organs and making the transport arrangements to get the organs to the patients
• Maintaining the National Organ Donor Register

TABLE 49.2. Organ donation and transplant activity per million population (PMP) in Europe, 2002.[57]

	Euro*	France	Italy	Spain	Scandia[†]	United Kingdom[‡]	ROI[§]
Cadaveric donors (PMP)	1,659	1,198	1,019	1,409	322	766	78
	(13.9)	(20.0)	(18.1)	(33.7)	(13.2)	(13.0)	(20.5)
Cadaveric kidney transplants (PMP)	2,865	2,147	1,464	1,998	610	1,350	140
	(24.1)	(35.8)	(26.0)	(47.7)	(25.1)	(22.9)	(36.8)
Living donor kidney transplants (PMP)	698	108	124	34	254	371	3
	(5.9)	(1.8)	(2.2)	(0.8)	(10.4)	(6.3)	(0.8)
Liver transplants (PMP)	1,257	882	863	1,033	213	712	38
	(10.6)	(14.7)	(15.3)	(24.7)	(8.8)	(12.1)	(10.0)
Heart and heart/lung transplants (PMP)	598	339	312	310	94	175	15
	(5.0)	(5.6)	(5.5)	(7.4)	(3.9)	(3.0)	(3.9)
Lung transplants (PMP)	357	87	60	161	75	112	0
	(3.0)	(1.4)	(1.1)	(3.8)	(3.1)	(1.9)	—

*Euro includes Germany, Austria, Belgium, Luxembourg, the Netherlands, and Slovenia.
[†]Scandia includes Denmark, Norway, Finland, and Sweden.
[‡]Figures taken from National Transplant Database, March 2003. All others are provisional figures from Organizacion Nacional de Trasplantes (ONT).
[§]ROI is the Republic of Ireland.
Note: Definitions of a cadaveric solid organ donor vary among countries.
Source: http://www.uktransplant.org.uk/statistics.

- Improving organ donor rates by funding initiatives in the NHS
- Contributing to the development of performance indicators, standards, and protocols that guide the work of organ donation and transplantation
- Acting as a central point for information on transplant matters
- Auditing and analyzing the results of all organ transplants in the United Kingdom and the Republic of Ireland to improve patient care

Cadaveric donor organs are shared nationally in the United Kingdom. Individual transplant units make their own arrangements for organ retrieval within their "zone." The liver and the thoracic organs are retrieved by respective organ retrieval teams of the region. Kidney retrieval is performed either by the team from the local kidney transplant unit or more commonly by the liver retrieval team.

The present system of organ retrieval from cadaveric donors in the United Kingdom requires each transplant unit to have several on-call staff members available at all times. This is becoming increasingly difficult, especially with the recently introduced regulations with respect to junior doctor training in the United Kingdom and the impending and more restrictive regulations of the EWTD for all staff. The procedure is also logistically complex to organize. It sometimes results in multiple teams, each comprising two or three members of staff from liver, cardiothoracic, pancreas, and kidney transplant units to attend organ retrieval procedures, often in small district general hospitals. Reorganization of cadaveric organ retrieval services for the United Kingdom is presently being considered. One of the options being evaluated is the establishment of four or five multiorgan retrieval teams serving the entire country, each self-sufficient and capable of retrieving all cadaveric donor organs and tissues for transplantation.

Improving road safety and better management of hypertension has resulted in a reduction in the incidence of brain stem death (from trauma and cardiovascular accidents) over the past two decades in the United Kingdom.[58] Changes in neurosurgical practice have also contributed to the decline in the number of cadaveric organ donors.[59] Improvement in cranial imaging methods and clinical experience in predicting outcomes of victims of head injury or cardiovascular accident has led to earlier identification of a group of patients with a poor prognosis. Consequently, such patients are not always considered for ventilation in intensive therapy units; hence they do not develop brain stem death. In severe cranial trauma, procedures such as "craniectomy" (creation of a circumferential bone flap of the skull) prevent brain stem herniation and brain death associated with raised intracranial pressure. The decline in the incidence of cadaveric donation from brain stem–dead donors has not reduced the acute care workload for transplant teams, primarily as a consequence of the expansion in non-heart-beating donations.

Non-Heart-Beating Donations

Brain stem death has been recognized, and the method of diagnosis has been defined by a code in the United Kingdom, since 1979.[60,61] Before this, organs were retrieved from cadaveric donors following the cessation of heartbeat and establishment of death. Non-heart-beating donation (sometimes referred to as asystolic donation) has been revisited recently and is becoming an increasingly important source of organs for transplantation.[62] There are two distinct clinical settings in which non-heart-beating donation takes place, and they have different implications for acute care surgical practice.

Uncontrolled Non-Heart-Beating Donation

Uncontrolled non-heart-beating donation refers to the clinical scenario in accident and emergency departments when individuals are admitted following an out of hospital cardiac arrest and when the resuscitation has been unsuccessful. Provided that the asystolic time does not exceed 30 minutes, organs (usually kidneys; rarely lungs, liver, or pancreas) can be retrieved and successfully transplanted. After the establishment of the diagnosis of death and a period of "stand down" (of between 3 and 5 minutes), two cannulas are inserted, one into the femoral artery and one into the femoral vein through a cut-down in the groin. These cannulas are used to perfuse the organs (the abdominal organs or the whole body) with cold preservation solution. During this period, attempts are made to identify and to contact the next of kin of the deceased in order to seek permission for organ retrieval. If such permission is obtained, the organ retrieval procedure takes place in an operating theater in a similar fashion to that used for brain stem–dead cadaveric donors.

There are obvious logistical difficulties with uncontrolled non-heart-beating donation. It requires round the clock availability and an immediate response from the transplant team. These are compounded further by ethical and legal difficulties. There are only a few transplant centers in the United Kingdom where uncontrolled non-heart-beating donation programs have been successfully established.

Controlled Non-Heart-Beating Donation

Controlled non-heart-beating donation refers to the scenario whereby death of a patient in a hospital is anticipated but is not likely to take the form of brain stem death. If the patient has made an advance directive or the

TABLE 49.3. Activity Summary for the United Kingdom, 2003.

	Kidney	Pancreas	Heart	Heart/Lung	Lung	Liver	Total
Deceased donors	681	88	163	—	149	607	710
Organs donated	1,345	88	163	—	283	607	2,486
Deceased donor transplants	1,297	54	145	15	135	627	2,222*
Living donor transplants	439	0	4	—	0	6	449

*Includes combined transplants: 42 kidney and pancreas, 8 kidney and liver, 1 kidney and heart.
Source: http://www.uktransplant.org.uk/statistics.

wishes and consent of the relatives for organ donation have been ascertained before death, organ retrieval can proceed after a period of "stand down" following asystole and the diagnosis of death. In clinical practice, this type of organ donation is associated with a different set of logistical problems and has different implications for the acute care workload of the transplantation team.

Unlike uncontrolled non-heart-beating donation, the transplantation team does receive some notice of the possibility of organ donation, and an immediate response is not critical. However, even for patients from whom support is withdrawn and death is expected, the time of asystole cannot be reliably predicted. If the time to asystole is prolonged, kidneys may suffer significant ischemic damage. In practice, the transplantation teams arrive in the donor hospital before the support is withdrawn. If asystole does not occur within 3 to 4 hours of withdrawal of support, the organ retrieval is abandoned and the transplantation team leaves.

Cadaveric Organ Transplantation

The urgency of transplant operations depends on the ischemia tolerance of the organs to be transplanted. Heart transplants are the most urgent, and reperfusion of a cardiac allograft needs to be performed no later than 4 to 6 hours after circulatory arrest in the donor. This always requires the presence of two teams working simultaneously. The decision to proceed with heart retrieval is communicated from the donor hospital to the transplantation team in the cardiac transplant center as soon as the organ retrieval team has had a chance to open the chest and confirm the satisfactory condition of the heart. The recipient operation to explant the heart then proceeds simultaneously, and the retrieval team travels back to the cardiac transplant center without delay.

Liver transplantation also requires the availability of a dedicated 24-hour transplant theatre and staff, but organ retrieval and subsequent implantation procedures are done sequentially. The cold ischemia time in liver transplantation is almost always under 12 hours. Pancreas allografts have a slightly greater ischemia tolerance, and a total cold ischemia time of 18 and perhaps up to 24 hours is acceptable.

Kidneys also have a greater cold ischemia tolerance, and kidney transplant operations rarely need to be performed in the middle of the night. Most cadaveric kidney allografts are still implanted with a total ischemic time of less than 24 hours, although successful allograft function after cold ischemia periods of 36 to 48 hours can be achieved.[63] In many kidney transplant units, cadaveric kidney transplantation is performed in general emergency operating theaters and competes with other surgical emergencies for priority. Table 49.3 lists the numbers of cadaveric kidney, liver, pancreas, heart, and lung transplants performed in the United Kingdom in 2003.[57]

Super-Urgent Transplantation

In the area of abdominal organ transplants, the need for a truly urgent life-saving procedure arises only for liver transplantation for patients with fulminant hepatic failure. For patients presenting with fulminant hepatic failure, criteria based on clinical and biochemical parameters reliably allow the selection of those with a poor prognosis.[64] More than 90% of patients who fulfill criteria for poor prognosis die within hours or days. The liver allocation system in the United Kingdom allows transplantation of such patients with the first blood group–compatible liver that becomes available nationally. There is no other provision in the United Kingdom organ allocation system to prioritize patients awaiting organ transplantation on a "may require transplantation sooner than others" because of their clinical condition. With the exception of patients in the United Kingdom requiring "super-urgent" transplantation for fulminant hepatic failure, the individual transplant units have the first choice to use liver allografts that become available within their "zone." Transplant clinicians then have complete discretion to prioritize patients on their own waiting list depending on clinical urgency.

Surgical Emergencies in Organ Transplant Recipients

In common with all surgical procedures, organ transplant operations do have complications, some of which require acute care surgical intervention. Procedures within this category constitute a relatively small proportion of the overall acute care workload of transplantation teams.

A unique situation that falls within this category is primary nonfunction (PNF) or the development of hepatic artery thrombosis (HAT) within the first few days after liver transplantation. Patients whose transplanted liver allograft does not function or those who develop HAT in the early postoperative period require acute care retransplantation to have any chance of long-term survival. The liver allocation system operated in the United Kingdom gives these two conditions the same degree of priority as fulminant hepatic failure. Therefore, patients with one of these three indications (fulminant hepatic failure with poor prognostic criteria, PNF, or early postoperative HAT) for liver transplantation are considered as "super urgent" and receive the first liver allograft that becomes available nationally.

Emergency Vascular Surgery

Introduction

Vascular surgery in the United Kingdom is in the process of emerging as a distinct specialty, separate from general surgery. However, most members of the Vascular Surgical Society of Great Britain and Ireland (VSSGBI) are general surgeons with an interest in vascular surgery as opposed to specialist vascular surgeons. For the year 2001–2002, 398,000 vascular operations were performed in England.[65] An average of 70 arterial operations, 47 interventional radiology procedures, and 81 venous operations are performed per 100,000 head of population per annum, with 30% 40% of arterial conditions presenting as urgent or acute care cases.[66]

To adequately deal with these numbers, a hospital with a vascular service needs a minimum of one vascular surgeon per 150,000 population or one general surgeon with a major vascular interest per 100,000 population. However, a recent survey of 125 hospitals with a vascular unit showed that 45% of hospitals have two vascular consultants, 21% have one consultant, and just 5% have more than four. Interestingly, 43% of these hospitals provided 24-hour-a-day service.[66]

Present Arrangements

In the past, general surgeons dealt with many of the acute care vascular conditions. With increasing subspecialization, however, many surgeons without a specialist vascular interest have become concerned about their ability to treat vascular emergencies adequately. With increasing complexity of treatments, evidence showing superior clinical outcomes with specialist vascular teams,[67,68] and

scrutiny from clinical governance and audit, the argument for specialist treatment for all vascular conditions (including emergencies) is strong. In the same way, with increasing specialization, vascular surgeons become de-skilled in other areas of general surgery. In order to run separate vascular on-call schedules, there is increased pressure on vascular surgeons to withdraw from the general surgical acute care service.[66,69]

There are few hospitals in the United Kingdom with enough vascular surgeons to provide a 24-hour emergency vascular service. In 1998, the VSSGBI recommended a maximum "1 in 4" on-call schedule. Some hospitals have developed strategies to cover this shortfall. The most popular strategy is collaborative clinical networks. Currently, 44% of hospitals participate in such a network, and 23% have firm plans to do so in the future. Within the collaborative network, the on-call surgeon may move between hospitals out of hours to operate on patients, but more commonly the patient is transferred to the on-call hospital. Both methods work well, with no detriment to the patient.[70,71] Another strategy involves a "hub and spoke" network with a centralized service in one major unit supported by several adjacent hospitals. Currently, only 2% of units are committed to this type of arrangement.[66]

Proposals

The report of the VSSGBI working group in 1998 recommended centralization of vascular services from adjacent hospitals onto a single site.[72] However, with the exception of a few large cities, such "hub and spoke" arrangements have proved unworkable. As mentioned earlier, collaborative networks are more popular, but it is likely that in time centralized services will be developed as units realize the advantages of working together more closely.

The EWTD, which applies to all doctors and stipulates a 48-hour working week by 2009, means that trainee surgeons will have much less exposure to acute care general surgery than in the past. In addition, training in elective surgery will also be restricted, and obtaining competence in more than one specialty within general surgery will be difficult. Newly appointed consultant general surgeons will no longer have sufficient experience to deal with vascular emergencies. Therefore, vascular surgeons should manage vascular emergencies. Because of the complexity of the work and the increasing lack of vascular experience among trainees, consultants must now attend for most acute care cases. In 2004, the VSSGBI recommends therefore that the vascular on-call schedule should be at least 1 in 6, and, where networks cover populations in excess of 1 million people, the schedule should be at least 1 in 8. Elective work should be cancelled when on duty.[66]

Trainees

Trainees who apply for consultant posts in vascular surgery should normally have spent the past 2 years of their specialist training in vascular units. These units must have two or more vascular surgeons, and vascular surgery should comprise at least 70% of the unit's in-patient elective workload. By the end of the 6-year training program, trainees should have been involved in at least 200 arterial reconstructions, having been principal operator in a minimum of 20 elective aortic aneurysm repairs, 5 ruptured aneurysms, 20 carotid endarterectomies, and 10 infrapopliteal bypass grafts.[66,73]

Radiology

The continuing emergence of interventional radiology in the diagnosis and treatment of vascular emergencies also requires a 24-hour acute care service to be available. There are few hospitals with enough vascular interventional radiologists to provide such a service. It is recommended that similar collaborative networks be applied, which in the longer term would lead to centralization of adjacent units to include radiologists as well as surgeons working in a single larger unit. To overcome the shortage of vascular interventional radiologists and the increasing role of endovascular surgery in acute care and elective management of patients, the VSSGBI also recommends that future vascular surgeons should develop the skill to undertake interventional radiology procedures and become an essential part of vascular surgical training.[66,74]

Summary

Vascular surgery in the United Kingdom is in the process of changing. With the increasing complexity of treatments, the changes in surgical training, and the expectation of patients to be treated by specialists, the traditional approach to the management of vascular emergencies by general surgeons is no longer appropriate. The continuing emergence of vascular interventional radiology in treatment modalities will act as a catalyst for change. The collaboration or centralization of adjacent, small vascular units in many areas will enable the provision of expert specialist management of vascular conditions 24 hours a day and is essential to promote the best possible care for vascular patients.

Emergency Surgery in Remote and Rural Areas

Introduction

Provision of surgical services to people living in areas distant from major population centers provides challenges to any health care system. The requirement for high-quality surgical care by patients living in isolated areas, where hospital facilities are necessarily limited, are no different from those of patients living close to the fully resourced hospitals of the bigger towns and cities. Although inconvenient, many are willing to travel long distances for nonurgent health care, but they worry about how sudden life-threatening conditions can be safely dealt with away from the centers of excellence. People will continue to live in remote areas, and their surgical needs must be met.

General Principles

Safe systems for managing surgical emergencies in remote communities have been developed over the years and differ from place to place. General principles that apply include the following:

- Operating in the remote community provides the best treatment option for the patient.
- Emergency surgical procedures are only embarked on when there is a genuine clinical need and a realistic chance of a successful outcome.
- The surgeon, anesthetists, and the remainder of the team possess the necessary generic skills to perform procedures that may be necessary in the course of an operation.
- Much surgical work is nonoperative, and the skills, resources, and personnel must be available to provide first class, state-of-the-art treatment.

The kind of acute care surgery performed in a remote community hospital is illustrated by operating data from the Western Isles Hospital, Stornoway, Scotland, between 1996 and 2000 (a project funded by the Remote and Rural Area Resource Initiative [RARARI]). Of the 2,000 procedures carried out in the operating theaters annually, over 300 (including endoscopy) were emergencies. On average, there were 70 upper gastrointestinal endoscopies, 16 appendectomies, 20 exploratory laparotomies (which included 2 perforated peptic ulcers and 4 acute care large bowel procedures), 5 pilonidal or perianal abscesses drained, 25 fractured neck of femurs operated on, and 20 cesarean sections carried out every year. The Western Isles Hospital has two general surgeons, an orthopedic surgeon, and two obstetrician and gynecologists.

Medical and Nursing Staff

Remote and rural hospitals of all sizes must be adequately staffed with properly trained and experienced personnel.[75] It is not possible to employ large numbers of trained medical staff in remote communities, and so increasing involvement of nurse practitioners is helping to ensure that sufficiently skilled personnel are available around the clock. However, because the acute care workload is often low, skill maintenance is an issue, and retraining and refresher courses are required.

Doctors in training do play a role in service provision but are usually at an early stage of training and are present in small numbers. Some are in defined basic surgical training posts, but most are training for general practice.

Each remote and rural hospital serving a population of 20,000 or more will require a core consultant staff of anesthetists, physicians, and surgeons. How many consultants and whether they should be available 24 hours a day, 7 days a week are topics of intense debate.

Surgeons

In the past, surgical services have been provided by dedicated single-handed surgeons. However, working time regulations, quality control, revalidation, (equivalent to recertification in the United States), and changes in lifestyle requirements make these dedicated and selfless individuals something of the past.

Remote and rural surgery is not recognized as a subspecialty of general surgery, and there is no obvious career pathway to lead up to consultant appointments. To think that surgeons trained for specialized district general hospital practice are suitable for posts in remote communities is a failure to recognize the particular surgical needs of hospitals where it is not possible to provide consultants for individual specialties. Remote and rural surgeons must be broad based and multiskilled, and, until they are specifically trained for the work that needs to be carried out in remote communities, problems with recruitment and retention will persist. Notwithstanding the above, the North Scotland Deanery based in Aberdeen funds a fellowship to train a surgeon for a consultant post in a remote community hospital.

The rationale behind having a surgical service in a remote community is twofold: first, to provide an acute care surgical service; and second, to perform as many surgical procedures locally as can be justified by good surgical practice. For a surgeon to maintain the generic skills necessary to manage emergencies, it is important that he or she has an active elective surgical practice. A remote and rural surgeon may carry out 250 operative and 300 endoscopic procedures per year (personal experience, 2001), and, although numbers of individual procedures performed are not great, they are similar to those reported by Ritchie et al.[76] based on the operative logs of general surgeons recertifying in the United States. Unlike larger hospitals, where much of the operative work will be carried out by surgeons in training, in remote community hospitals, consultants perform most of the operations.

Hospitals

Remote and rural hospitals are equipped to deal with those conditions that are likely to occur within its community. Properly equipped accident and emergency departments, wards, operating theaters, and radiologic and laboratory facilities including blood transfusion need to be available.

The remote and rural hospital accident emergency department is unlikely to be busy, but it must be capable of treating emergencies as and when they arise, and it must be able to play a part in any major incident alerts. They are often run by specifically trained emergency nurse practitioners backed up by doctors in training and consultants.

Patient Transport

Fundamental to delivering a remote and rural surgical service is the facility to safely transfer a patient to a larger, better resourced hospital. Deciding who should be transferred depends on the patient's condition and on a determination of the balance between the benefits and drawbacks of travel. On the Scottish islands, emergency transport is by helicopter or fixed wing aircraft, while on the Scottish mainland it can be by air or road. Patient transport is coordinated and organized through the Scottish Ambulance Service. Transportation by sea is well developed in some Scandinavian countries, but not in the United Kingdom, which is surprising as it is an island. Techniques for transportation of seriously ill patients have been well worked out and fall into three main categories.

Patient Transport with Paramedic Escort

Transport with paramedic escort is suitable for the relatively stable patient who does not require major therapeutic maneuvers during transport and is unlikely to present any major medical problems during the flight. Relatives can often travel with the patient in this circumstance.

Patient Transport with Local Medical Support

Transport with local medical support (eg, anesthetist or surgeon) is appropriate for patients who may require ongoing treatment, such as ventilation, during transport. Other patients will be those who may need treatment during the journey, but the ability to do this is often limited. The major drawback of this mode of transport is that it takes a member of the medical staff away from the remote community, and, if that person is the only anesthetist available, the remote community would be without anesthetic coverage for the period of the absence. Because some air ambulances are based at airfields distant from the remote community, returning the attending medical practitioner to his or her base can be difficult.

Patient Transport with a Distantly Based Transport Team

Sometimes the patient is stabilized in the remote community, and a team is dispatched from elsewhere (e.g., the Shock Team in Glasgow, the Pediatric Retrieval Team from the Royal Hospital for Sick Children in Glasgow, or one of the regional neonatal resuscitation teams). Once in the remote community, the team will prepare the patient and effect the transfer as rapidly as possible. In many ways, this is the best way to transport the seriously ill patient from an isolated area, but it does require a team to be sent out, which can add a further delay in commencing definitive treatment. Such delays can be detrimental to patient care and may tie up both local and retrieval team staff for prolonged periods.

One of the attributes of a remote and rural surgeon is the ability to recognize that, despite the fact that he is able to perform a particular procedure, it might, for reasons of patient safety and well being, be better to perform it elsewhere. Frustrating as this can be, the patient's interests come first.

Procedures

Life-Threatening Emergencies Requiring Immediate Surgical Intervention

Facilities must be available for immediate surgical procedures to be carried out in the remote community, and surgeons need to be suitably trained to deal with them:

- Hemorrhage: from vascular injury, intrathoracic and intraabdominal organ damage, and pericardial tamponade resulting from trauma; ruptured ectopic pregnancy; debate surrounds whether acute extradural or subdural hematoma should be surgically evacuated in small isolated hospitals
- Pneumothorax
- Cesarean section for life-threatening maternal problems (obstructed labor, hemorrhage from placenta previa), and fetal distress

Life-Threatening Emergencies Requiring Resuscitation Followed by Expeditious Surgical Intervention

Life-threatening emergencies will fall into one of two categories: those for which skills and resources are available locally and those for which such locally performed surgery is inappropriate. For those patients who can be

operated on locally, it will from time to time be necessary for them to be transferred to an intensive care unit to complete their postoperative recovery. If preexisting disease puts the patient into a high-risk category and management in a remote community will be difficult, transportation of the patient to a center with more extensive facilities may be the best option. Those emergencies for which local surgery can be contemplated include the following:

- Perforated gastrointestinal tract: peptic ulcer, diverticular disease, and following penetrating or blunt trauma
- Intestinal obstruction: with evidence of ischemic bowel
- Intraabdominal sepsis
- Mesenteric infarction
- Major thoracic or pelvic trauma
- Acute upper gastrointestinal hemorrhage (excluding operative treatment of esophageal varices)
- Strangulated external hernias

It is probably unwise to attempt life-saving surgery in a remote community on patients with the following:

- Ruptured aortic aneurysm
- Perforated esophagus
- Ruptured liver (although, if sufficient blood is available, liver packing may have to be attempted)
- Bleeding esophageal varices

Life-Threatening Emergencies That Might Not Require Surgical Intervention

Most remote community hospitals will have a high dependency area that will be capable of moderately sophisticated monitoring but that will have the facility to ventilate patients for only relatively short (up to 12 hours) periods. Some of the patients with the conditions described below may require transfer to a larger center:

- Acute pancreatitis
- Severe head injuries with a surgically remediable problem, severe cerebral contusion and intracerebral hemorrhage
- Burns

Emergencies That Might Become Life Threatening if Not Managed with Expeditious Surgical Intervention

Overall assessment of the patient's condition will determine whether these patients need to be transferred elsewhere:

- Uncomplicated small and large intestinal obstruction
- Irreducible but not strangulated external hernias
- Acute appendicitis
- Infected obstruction to the upper urinary tract

- Major abscesses and empyemas (gallbladder and thorax)
- Evacuation of retained products of conception

Emergencies That Will Lead to Incapacity and Disability if Not Managed by Immediate Surgical Intervention

When specialist expertise or the possible need for additional specialized procedures is required, such patients should be transferred elsewhere. These conditions may require emergency transportation:

- Peripheral vascular occlusion
- Complex fractures, particularly those causing vascular injury (e.g., supracondylar fractures of the humerus)
- Torsion of the testis

Emergencies That Will Lead to Incapacity and Disability if Not Managed by Surgical Intervention

Most emergencies that can lead to incapacity or disability can be managed effectively in remote community hospitals, and to transfer a patient for treatment elsewhere is only necessary when there is severe preexisting medical disease:

- Abscesses: cutaneous, pilonidal, and perianal
- Irreducible but not strangulated hernias
- Fractures and dislocations

Emergency Surgery Outcome

Little information on outcome of the management of patients with conditions requiring emergency surgical care in remote communities exists. Patient satisfaction with the service is obvious by the vociferous objections to any attempt to alter the service by apparent reductions in the locally available clinical service.

Some information gathering has been done in Australia, where the remote and rural surgical service is larger than in the United Kingdom. One particular study of colorectal surgery[77] included data on the management of patients with large bowel obstruction, general peritonitis, and paracolic sepsis, and it demonstrated an 8.3% mortality in 276 patients (15% in those patient >80 years of age). Such figures were considered comparable with those found at many major medical centers.

Although most people will seek the most expert treatment available to manage their own or their relatives' condition, there are times when a patient would "rather take the risk" and stay local than be transferred elsewhere. This can happen particularly with elderly patients, who, if it were a possible outcome, would rather die in their own local hospital than in an unfamiliar place away from their relatives and friends.

Trauma Services in the United Kingdom

Introduction

Severe injury remains a common cause of death and disability in the United Kingdom. Accidents are responsible for 10,000 deaths per year in England and are the most common cause of death in people under the age of 40 years. Approximately 450 children die each year, and 10,000 are permanently disabled. Injuries cost the National Health Service and social services $2.2 billion per annum.[78,79]

A Historical Perspective

In the United Kingdom, acute hospital care is primarily provided by district general hospitals. In addition to the district general hospitals, there are university teaching hospitals that are usually located in large cities and serve as both acute and tertiary-referral hospitals. There are no specialist trauma centers, and there is no trauma system like those found in the United States.[80] Traditionally, ambulances, which may or may not have a trained paramedic on board, are called to the scene of an accident, tend to the injured, and are obliged to take them to the nearest available emergency department, regardless of the facilities within that hospital.

In 1988, Professor D.D. Trunkey, who had reported previously on trauma services in Orange County, in the United States,[81] was invited to review trauma services in the United Kingdom as the British Journal of Surgery Travelling Fellow.[82] Trunkey noted the following: "In general, trauma care is fragmented, disorganized, and has an unacceptably bad outcome. Pre-hospital care of the accident victim is suboptimal.... The patient is usually taken to the nearest hospital without regard to surgical availability."

In 1988, a Royal College of Surgeons of England working party investigated trauma care in England.[82] They concluded that one third of all deaths occurring after major injury were preventable and proposed measures such as enhancing prehospital care, rapid transfer to the best local facility (not necessarily to the nearest), implementing Advanced Trauma Life Support (ATLS) principles, integrating trauma services, and instigating audit and research into injury and systems of care.

In response, the Department of Health supported the development of a regional trauma service in the North West Midlands region based around the North Staffordshire Royal Infirmary and commissioned an in-depth analysis of its performance compared with the orthodox British model of care in two other centers in Lancashire and Humberside. The first analysis of the North Staffordshire Trauma system, between 1990 and 1993, found little evidence of the development of an integrated trauma system and no reliable evidence that such a system improved patients' chances of survival from major trauma in the region.[83] However, after this study period, trauma services in North Staffordshire continued to be developed, and mortality rates fell. A prospective audit of patients with an injury severity score (ISS) of more than 15 has shown a significant decrease in mortality from 26.5% in 1992–1993 to 13% in 1997–1998.[5]

In addition, the UK Major Trauma Outcome Study (MTOS) was established, which collected data from participating hospitals of patients suffering major injury. By the late 1990s, the name had changed to the Trauma Audit and Research Network (TARN) and was receiving data from over 50% of trauma-receiving hospitals in England and Wales.[84]

The Royal College of Surgeons of England's 1988 report stimulated change, and in 1992 Yates et al.[85] analyzed the effectiveness of trauma care in the United Kingdom. Their findings include the following:

• Mortality rates higher in the United Kingdom than in the United States
• Large interhospital variations in performance
• Unacceptable delays before treatment
• Most initial care provided by junior doctors

In 2002, however, an analysis of 129,979 patients from the TARN data base suggested that the fatality rates for major trauma patients reaching hospital alive had not improved in England and Wales since 1994, although a 40% reduction had occurred in the preceding 5 years (1989–1994).[86,87] This lack of change occurred in parallel with a plateau in the level of consultant (attending) involvement in the most severely injured patients. The overall mortality rate for patients with an ISS >9 over the study period (1989–2000) was 6.2%. There is also variation in outcomes among hospitals. The top 10% of hospitals deliver a statistically significant improvement in mortality rate.[87]

Present Arrangements

There is still no nationally coordinated policy for the care of the severely injured. There are 32 ambulance services operating as independent NHS trusts. Individual hospitals are often served by more than one ambulance agency. In all but a few areas, seriously injured patients are still taken to the nearest hospital rather than to a designated hospital with appropriate resources and experienced staff. An exception is the Helicopter Emergency Medical Service, established in 1988 in London and partly funded by the NHS and charitable organizations. Operating during daylight hours, an experienced trauma physician is flown to the scene of accidents within the Greater London area, where life-saving intervention and stabi-

lization may be performed at the scene of the accident. The patient is then transferred to the most appropriate hospital, either by air or by land ambulance, where an awaiting trauma team has been activated.

There are approximately 240 acute care hospitals in England, Wales, and Northern Ireland with emergency departments, but only 22 of these have neurosurgery departments on site. Five hospitals have the full range of surgical services (general surgery [including vascular and paediatric], orthopedics, cardiothoracics, neurosurgery, maxillofacial, and plastics). However, there are well-established systems of referral for head, spine, and burn injuries and an increased willingness to transfer such patients.[85]

Incidence and Costs of Severe Injury

The incidence of severe trauma (ISS >15) in the United Kingdom is estimated to be 4 per 1 million per week. The average acute care hospital is not likely to be called on to treat more than one severely injured patient each week, which suggests that some hospitals may have too little experience to give these patients their best chance of an optimum outcome. It is estimated that on average 1 per 1,000 acute care cases admitted to the hospital are multiply injured patients. Without centralization to larger acute care hospitals, adequate experience in the definitive management of such patients is hard to acquire.[85]

In 1997, a fatal injury was estimated to cost the nation $1.7 million, a major injury $190,000, and a minor injury $15,000. These costs included direct medical expenditures, loss of economic activity, and the human aspects of grief, suffering, and pain. Annual hospital costs for road trauma alone are about $1 billion and ambulance costs are $38 million more.[85]

The Future

The Royal College of Surgeons of England, along with the British Orthopaedic Association, in 2000 published a follow up to their 1988 report titled "Better Care for the Severely Injured." There were several key recommendations in the following areas[85]:

1. A national trauma service: This should be developed based on a "hub and spoke" arrangement among hospitals within a defined geographic area or system. Each system would serve a population of up to 3 million, with a single integrated emergency ambulance service. There would be one major acute care hospital (Level I) in each system with all specialities on site. This would be supported by acute care general hospitals (Level II) acting in partnership with the major acute care hospital and would be able to resuscitate the severely injured and treat most injuries. Some acute care general hospitals would be

designated as Level III, as they may not receive sufficient numbers of major trauma patients to retain the skills of staff or justify the expense required for the reception and resuscitation of major injuries.

2. Prehospital care: Emergency ambulances attending major trauma should have a paramedic trained to the Prehospital Trauma Life Support standard. The paramedic will select the most appropriate receiving hospital and radio ahead to activate the trauma team. Patients with life-threatening trauma or multiple injuries should never be taken to the Level III hospital. The use of helicopter retrieval may be beneficial in isolated locations, especially where distances from the Level I hospital may be great.

3. Interhospital transfer: Protocols for secondary transfers from Level II to Level I hospitals must be in place, with targets for transfer time.

4. Audit and research: A National Trauma Audit Committee should set standards and develop realistic outcome indicators. A National Trauma Audit Research Network should collect data from all hospital trusts receiving severely injured patients, ensuring development, improvement, and monitoring of standards of care.

In addition to these nationwide recommendations, a working party has been set up to develop practical proposals to optimize care, treatment, and transfer of severely injured patients within London. There are approximately 1,400 severely injured patients treated in London per year, with two thirds requiring transfer for specialist care. As in many other parts of the country, current services in the capital are neither well located nor well coordinated. The London Severe Injury Working Group has built on the recommendations of the Royal College of Surgeons of England specifically for the city of London, and suggests the following[88]:

1. Improved patient pathways: faster prehospital response and treatment, optimal prehospital routing (including bypass to specialist centers), and criteria for automatic transfer to specialist care

2. A London-wide trauma system: establishment of networks, clinical governance and auditing, and a system-wide coordination center

3. Pediatric trauma: multispecialist units with a network of approved pediatric trauma admitting hospitals and approved pediatric trauma receiving hospitals around each unit, allowing prompt treatment and transfer of pediatric trauma patients to the most appropriate center

Despite the recommendations, trauma care in the United Kingdom has seen little progress. There is still little prospect of a national trauma service being established, and, to date, only 50% of receiving hospitals provide data to a national trauma audit research network. The nearest the United Kingdom has to a designated trauma center is likely to be the Royal London

Hospital. The Helicopter Emergency Medical Service is based on the helipad on top of the hospital, and, through the efforts of individuals over the last 10 or so years, the hospital has developed toward being a specialist trauma center. There is certainly a degree of a "hub and spoke" model within the local acute care hospitals in terms of secondary transfer, and the Helicopter Emergency Medical Service has the ability to take the severely injured directly to the most appropriate hospital, which is not always the Royal London Hospital.

To improve trauma care in the United Kingdom, a national policy is required with a strong commitment by the government to maintain and increase the current level of consultants involved in major trauma. One hundred percent participation in national auditing is a must to providing quality observational evidence valuable insight into both good and bad practices.[86] Without facing up to such challenges, trauma care in the United Kingdom may continue to plateau.

There is some hope for progress in the near future given the changes in other fields, most notably cancer services. The NHS has embarked on an ambitious plan to improve cancer services nationally with the development of a network of cancer units and cancer centers. Minimum standards of care, multidisciplinary teams, management protocols, and referral patterns have been established for specific malignancies. Cancer units will provide care for most patients with the common malignancies, for example, breast and colorectal. Cancer centers will provide the leadership for the units within their network, monitor standards, and provide treatment for the less common tumors or where data have demonstrated that high volume surgery leads to better outcome, for example, pancreatic, esophageal, and hepatic malignancies.[89,90]

This pattern of care could be adapted to the advantage of injured patients: a trauma system consisting of trauma units providing care for the majority of injured patients and trauma centers providing care for the most seriously injured and leadership within their local network. Trauma systems could then work within a framework of agreed on protocols, referral patterns, and standards of care. The idea of a trauma system for the United Kingdom has been proposed several times to date, but no action has been taken. With the development and acceptance of national standards and programs in other specialities in the NHS, the time for a UK national trauma system may be approaching.

The Emergency Department (Acute Care Facility) of the Future

The emergency department of the future will need more front-line specialists of sufficient seniority to assess new emergency admissions and to make decisions about the

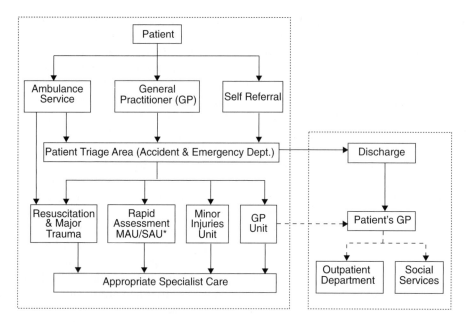

FIGURE 49.2. Proposed integrated pathway for access to emergency care. MAU, medical assessment unit; SAU, surgical assessment unit. (Source: http://uktransplant.org.uk/statistics.)

need for surgery without delay. To achieve this, new integrated pathways of care will be required. The role of nurses, physiotherapists, and radiographers will need to change as they take on a more therapeutic role.[91] To improve patient flow, an effective triage of patients must be established to identify patients who are the most at risk (Figure 49.2).

The Medical Royal Colleges and the Department of Health have agreed to proposals to aid the development of the new emergency departments within the NHS.[92] Only time will tell if this succeeds where others have failed. The implementation of the EWTD in August 2004 has ensured that most trainees do not remain resident on call.[93] New ways of working are requiring separate day and night shifts, and, in order to maximize teaching and training, as much emergency work as possible will be moved from evening and night-time to occur between 9 am and 9 pm.

Several initiatives have been considered. The Out of Hours Medical Team (OoHMT) will provide a mixed team of physicians, anesthetists, surgeons, and nurses to manage the acutely ill patient at night. Consultant surgeons will be available on call, from home, to deal with emergencies requiring urgent surgery at night.

Health care in the United Kingdom is changing rapidly. The reduction in trainee hours, the introduction of independent treatment centers (staffed by overseas doctors), the inclusion of 10 new member states into the European Union, and providing free access for specialists to work in the United Kingdom will all have a significant impact on health care delivery. The NHS has received a substantial boost in funding in the past 2 years, under the current Labour Government. More will be required if services are to be maintained and emergency care given the priority it deserves.

References

1. The British Medical Association, The Royal College of Physicians of London, The Royal College of Surgeons of England. The Provision of Acute General Hospital Service. Consultation Document, July 1998.
2. The Royal College of Surgeons of England. The Surgical Workforce in the New NHS. November 2001.
3. Watkin DFL, Layer GT. A 24-hour snapshot of emergency general surgery in the UK. Ann R Coll Surg Engl 2002; 84:194–199.
4. Chezhian C, Pye J, Jenkinson LR. The next millennium—are we becoming emergency surgeons? A seven year audit of surgical and neurological admissions in a rural district general hospital. Ann R Coll Surg Engl 2001; 83:117–120.
5. The Royal College of Surgeons of England and British Orthopaedic Association. Better Care for the Severely Injured. London, 2000.
6. NHS Management Executive. Junior Doctors, the New Deal. Working Arrangements for Hospital Doctors and Dentists in Training. London: Department of Health, 1991.
7. European Working Time Directive 93/104/EC.
8. Giddings AEB. Organisation of general surgical services in Britain: strategic planning of workload and manpower. Br J Surg 1993; 80:1377–1378.
9. Campling EA, Devlin HB, Hoile RW, Lunne JN. Report of the National Confidential Enquiry into Peri-operative Deaths 1990. London: National Enquiry into Peri-operative Deaths, 1992.
10. Senate of the Royal Surgical Colleges of Great Britain and Ireland. Consultant Practice and Surgical Training in the UK. London, October 1994.
11. Hobbs R. Rising emergency admissions. BMJ 1995; 310: 207–208.
12. Ellis BW, Rivett RC, Dudley HAF. Extending the use of clinical audit data: a resource planning model. BMJ 1990; 301:159–162.

13. Calman K. Hospital Doctors: Training for the Future. The Report of The Working Group on Specialist Medical Training. London: HMSO, 1993.

14. Beecham L. New Scottish CMO criticises training reforms. BMJ 1996; 313:947.

15. Addison PDR, Getgood A, Paterson-Brown S. Separating elective and emergency surgical care (the 50 emergency team). Scot Med J 2001; 46:48.

16. Thomson HJ, Jones PF. Active observation in acute abdominal pain. Am J Surg 1986; 152:522–525.

17. Cochrane RA, Edwards AT, Crosby DL, Roberts CJ, Lewis PA, McGee S, et al. Senior surgeons and radiologists should assess emergency patients on presentation: a prospective randomised controlled trial. J R Coll Surg Edinb 1998; 43:324–327.

18. Gray DWR, Collin J. Non-specific abdominal pain as a cause of acute admission to hospital. Br J Surg 1987; 74:239–242.

19. Paterson-Brown S. The acute abdomen: the role of laparoscopy. In: Williamson RCN, Thompson JN, eds. Bailliere's Clinical Gastroenterology: Gastrointestinal Emergencies, Part 1, London: Bailliere Tindall, 1991:691–703.

20. Decadt B, Sussman L, Lewis MPN, et al. Randomised clinical trial of early laparoscopy in the management of acute non-specific abdominal pain. Br J Surg 1999; 86:1383–1386.

21. Clavien PA, Burgan S, Moossa AR. Serum enzymes and other laboratory tests in acute pancreatitis. Br J Surg 1989; 76:1234–1243.

22. Kylanpaa-Back M-L, Kemppainen E, Puolakkainen P, et al. Reliable screening for acute pancreatitis with rapid urine trypsinogen-2 test strip. Br J Surg 2000; 87:49–52.

23. Thompson MM, Underwood MJ, Dookeran, KA, Lloyd DM, Bell PRF. Role of sequential leucocyte counts and C-reactive protein measurements in acute appendicitis. Br J Surg 1992; 79:822–824.

24. Davies AH, Bernau F, Salisbury A, Souter RG. C-reactive protein in right iliac fossa pain. J R Coll Surg Edinb 1991; 36:242–244.

25. Middleton SB, Whitbread T, Morgans BT, Mason PF. Combination of skin temperature and a single white cell count does not improve diagnostic accuracy in acute appendicitis. Br J Surg 1996; 83:499.

26. Gronroos JM, Gronroos P. Leucocyte and C-reactive protein in the diagnosis of acute appendicitis. Br J Surg 1999; 86:501–504.

27. Dunlop MG, King PM, Gunn AA. Acute abdominal pain: the value of liver function tests in suspected cholelithiasis. J R Coll Surg Edinb 1989; 34:124–127.

28. Stower MJ, Hardcastle JD. Is it acute cholecystitis? Ann R Coll Surg Engl 1986; 68:234.

29. Ogata M, Mateer JR, Condon RE. Prospective evaluation of abdominal sonography for the diagnosis of bowel obstruction. Ann Surg 1996; 223:237–241.

30. Gallego MG, Fadrique B, Nieto MA, et al. Evaluation of ultrasonography and clinical diagnostic scoring in suspected appendicitis. Br J Surg 1998; 85:37–40.

31. Chen S-C, Yen Z-S, Wang H-P, Lin F-Y, Hsu C-Y, Chen W-J. Ultrasonography is superior to plain radiology in the diagnosis of pneumoperitoneum. Br J Surg 2002; 89:351–354.

32. Stengel D, Bauwens K, Sehouli J, et al. Systematic review and meta-analysis of emergency ultrasonography for blunt abdominal trauma. Br J Surg 2001; 88:901–912.

33. Williams RJLI, Windsor ACJ, Rosin RD, Mann DV, Crofton M. Ultrasound scanning of the acute abdomen by surgeons in training. Ann R Coll Surg Engl 1994; 76:228–233.

34. Wellwood JM, Wilson AN, Hopkinson BR. Gastrografin as an aid to the diagnosis of perforated peptic ulcer. Br J Surg 1971; 58:245–249.

35. Fraser GM, Fraser ID. Gastrografin in perforated duodenal ulcer and acute pancreatitis. Clin Radiol 1974; 25:397–402.

36. Donovan AJ, Vinson TL, Maulsby GO, Gewin JR. Selective treatment of duodenal ulcer with perforation. Ann Surg 1979; 189:627–636.

37. Crofts TJ, Park KGM, Steele RJC, Chung SS, Li AKC. A randomized trial of non-operative treatment for perforated peptic ulcer. N Engl J Med 1989; 320:970–973.

38. Stewardson RH, Bombeck CT, Nvhus LM. Critical operative management of small bowel obstruction. Ann Surg 1978; 187:189–193.

39. Dunn JT, Halls JM, Berne TV. Roentgenographic contrast studies in acute small bowel obstruction. Arch Surg 1984; 119:1305–1308.

40. Riveron FA, Obeid FN, Horst HM, Sorensen VJ, Bivins BA. The role of contrast radiography in presumed bowel obstruction. Surgery 1989; 106:496–501.

41. Chung CC, Meng WC, Yu SC, Leung KL, Lau WY, Li AK. A prospective study on the use of water-soluble contrast follow-through radiology in the management of small bowel obstruction. Austr and NZJ Surg 1996; 66:598–601.

42. MJ Brochwocz, S Paterson-Brown, JT Murchison. Small bowel obstruction—the water-soluble follow-through revisited. Clin Radiol 2003; 58:393–397.

43. Chen S-C, Lin F-Y, Lee P-H, YU S-C, Wang S-M, Chang J-J. Water soluble contrast study predicts the need for early surgery in adhesive small bowel obstruction. Br J Surg 1999; 86:1692–1698.

44. Stewart J, Finan BJ, Courtney DF, Brennan TG. Does a water soluble contrast enema assist in the management of acute large bowel obstruction: a prospective study of 117 cases. Br J Surg 1984; 71:799–801.

45. Koruth NM, Koruth A, Matheson NA. The place of contrast enema in the management of large bowel obstruction. J R Coll Surg Edinb 1985; 30(4):258–260.

46. Shrier D, Skucas J, Weiss S. Diverticulitis: an evaluation by computer tomography and contrast enema. Am Coll of Gastroenterol 1991; 86:1466–1471.

47. McKee RF, Deignan RW, Krukowski ZH. Radiological investigation in acute diverticulitis. Br J Surg 1993; 80:560–565.

48. Ng CS, Watson CJE, Palmer CR, et al. Evaluation of early abdominopelvic computer tomography in patients with acute abdominal pain of unknown cause: prospective randomised study. BMJ 2002; 325:1387–1389.

49. Rao PM, Rhea JT, Novelline RA, Mostafavi AA, McCabe CJ. Effect of computed tomography of the appendix on treatment of patients and use of hospital resources. N Engl J Med 1998; 338:141–146.

50. McColl I. More precision in diagnosing appendicitis. N Engl J Med. 1998; 338:190–191.

51. Calder FR, Jadhav V, Hale JE. The effect of a dedicated emergency theatre facility on emergency operating patterns. J R Coll Surg Edinb 1998; 43:17–19.

52. Dawson EJ, Paterson-Brown S. Emergency general surgery and the implications for specialisation. Surgeon. Surg JR Coll Surg Edinb Irel 2004; 165–170.

53. Darby CR, Berry AR, Mortensen N. Management variability in surgery for colorectal emergencies. Br J Surg 1992; 79:206–210.

54. Mercer SJ, Knight JS, Toh SKC, Walters AM, Sadek, Somers SS. Implementation of a specialist-led service for the management of acute gallstone disease. Br J Surg 2004; 91: 504–508.

55. Elson DW, Sa'adedin F, Partridge R, et al. The separation of upper and lower emergency surgery: implications for emergency specialisation. Br J Surg 2004; 91(Suppl 1):62.

56. Anakwe REB, Collie MHS, Bradnock T, Zorcolo L, Bartolo DCCB. A study to assess the impact of a new specialist colorectal unit. Br J Surg 2004; 91(Suppl 1):iv–v.

57. Organ donation and transplant activity per million population (PMP) in Europe 2002. http://www.uktransplant.org.uk/statistics.

58. New W, Solomon M, Dingwall R, McHale J. A Question of Give and Take: Improving the Supply of Donor Organs for Transplantation. Research Report 18. London: King's Fund Institute, 1994.

59. Nicholson M. Kidney Transplantation from Non-Heart Beating Donors. Position paper prepared by the National Kidney Research Fund. Peterborough: NKRF, 2002.

60. Conference of Medical Royal Colleges and Their Faculties in the UK. Diagnosis of brain death. BMJ 1976; 12:1187–1188.

61. Conference of Medical Royal Colleges and Their Faculties in the UK. Diagnosis of death—memorandum issued by the honorary secretary of the Conference of Medical Royal Colleges and their Faculties in the UK. BMJ 1979; i:332.

62. Wijnen RMH, Booster MH, Stubenitsky BM, de Boer J, Heineman E, Kootstra G. Outcome of transplantation of non-heart beating donor kidneys. Lancet 1995; 345:1067–1070.

63. Collins GM, Bravo-Suarman M, Terasaki PI. Kidney preservation for transplantation. Lancet 1969; ii:1219–1222.

64. O'Grady JG, Alexander GJM, Hayllar KM, Williams R. Early indicators of prognosis in fulminant hepatic failure. Gastroenterology 1989; 97:439–445.

65. Department of Health. Hospital Episode Statistics England: Financial Year 2001–02. London: Department of Health, 2002.

66. The Vascular Surgical Society of Great Britain and Ireland. The Provision of Vascular Services 2004. London: The Vascular Surgical Society, 2004.

67. Michaels JA, Browse DJ, McWhinnie DL, Galland RB, Morris PJ. Provision of vascular surgical services in the Oxford Region. Br J Surg 1994; 81:377–381.

68. Samy AK, MacBain G. Abdominal aortic aneurysm: ten year's hospital population study in the city of Glasgow. Eur J Vasc Surg 1993; 7:561–566.

69. The Vascular Surgical Society of Great Britain and Ireland. The Provision of Emergency Vascular Services. London: The Vascular Surgical Society, 2001.

70. Dawson K, McFarland R, Halliday A, Thomas, M. Shared emergency vascular cover between two district general hospitals: implications for a consultant service. Br J Surg 1998; 85:564.

71. Cook SJ, Rocker MD, Jarvis MR, Whiteley MS. Patient outcome alone does not justify the centralisation of vascular services. Ann R Coll Surg Engl 2000; 82:268–271.

72. The Vascular Surgical Society of Great Britain and Ireland. The Provision of Vascular Services. London 1998.

73. The Vascular Surgical Society of Great Britain and Ireland. Training in Vascular Surgery. London: The Vascular Surgical Society, 2001.

74. The Royal College of Radiologists and the Vascular Surgical Society of Great Britain and Ireland. Provision of Vascular Radiology Services. London: The Vascular Surgical Society, 2003.

75. Surgery in Hospitals Serving Isolated Communities. Report by the Working Party of the Royal College of Surgeons of Edinburgh, July 1998.

76. Ritchie WP, Rhodes RS, Biester TW. Workloads and practice patterns of General Surgeons in the United States 1995–1997 Ann Surg 1999; 4:533–543.

77. Birks DM, Gunn IF, Birks RG, Strasser RP. Colorectal surgery in rural Australia: SCARS, a surgeon based audit of workload standards. ANZ J Surg 2001; 71:154–158.

78. Carter YH, Jones PW. Mortality Trends in UK 1979–1997. London: Child Accident Prevention Trust, 2002.

79. Our Healthier Nation—A Contract for Health. London: Department of Health, 1998.

80. Earlam R. Trauma centres: a British perspective. Br J Surg 1999; 86:723–724.

81. Trunkey DD. A time for decisions. Br J Surg 1988; 75:937–939.

82. Commission on the Provision of Surgical Services. The Management of Patients with Major Injuries. London: The Royal College of Surgeons of England, 1988.

83. Nicholl J, Turner J. Effectiveness of a regional trauma system in reducing mortality from major trauma: before and after study. BMJ 1997; 315:1349–1354.

84. Lecky F, Woodfrord M, Yates DW. Trends in trauma care in England and Wales 1989–1997. Lancet 2000; 335:1771–1775.

85. Yates DW, Woodford M, Hollis S. Preliminary analysis of the care of injured patients in 33 British hospitals: first report of the United Kingdom major trauma outcome study. BMJ 1992; 305:737–740.

86. Lecky FE. Trauma care in England and Wales: Is this as good as it gets? Emerg Med J 2002; 19:488–489.

87. Lecky FE, Woodford M, Bouramra O, Yates DW. Lack of change in trauma care in England and Wales since 1994. Emerg Med J 2002; 19:520–523.

88. London Severe Injury Working Group. Modernising Trauma Services in London. Report and recommendations. Unpublished.

89. Begg CB, Cramer LD, Hoskins WJ, Brennan MF. Impact of hospital volume and operative mortality of major cancer surgery. JAMA 1998; 280:1747–1751.

90. Birkmcycr JD, Siewers AE, Finlayson EV, Stukel TA, Lucas FL, Batista I, et al. Hospital volume and surgical

mortality in the United States. N Engl J Med 2002; 346: 1128–1137.

91. The Royal College of Surgeons of England. The Provision of Emergency Surgical Services—An Organisational Framework. London: The Royal College of Surgeons, 1997.

92. Reforming Emergency Care—The Emergency Department. http://www.doh.gov.uk/capacityplanning, 2004.

93. Clarke MD, Anderson ADG, Mackie J. Training the higher surgical trainee within the framework of the European Working Directive (EWTD). Ann R Coll Surg Eng (Suppl) 2004; 86:82–84.

50
Acute Care Surgery: Australia

Thomas Kossmann and Ilan S. Freedman

The ways in which acute care surgical services across the world have developed and are currently delivered vary greatly from one country to another. The evolution of these services is particularly influenced by the interplay of unique geographic and demographic factors in each individual country and is ultimately determined by resources and demand.[1] The mechanisms by which trauma and other emergency surgical care is provided in Australia differ substantially from those in the United States and Europe. This chapter outlines the provision of acute care surgery in Australia as well as Australia's contribution to acute care surgery in the neighboring Pacific Island countries.

Australia is one of the largest countries in the world and has a landmass comparable with the United States or Europe.[2] Much of the land is, however, barren, inhospitable desert (the so-called outback) and is sparsely populated. Australia's population of approximately 20 million people is highly urbanized, with almost 90% of Australians living in several large cities along the coastlines.[1,2] However, despite increasing urbanization, a substantial population continues to live in smaller regional, isolated communities in what is broadly defined as "rural Australia."[3] Many of these people live there permanently, whereas others reside temporarily for purposes of work, holiday, or travel. The towns in these regional areas of Australia generally decrease in size and are further apart as one travels inland. Many of the larger regional towns support well-equipped health care services, but the more remote communities are often situated great distances from medical facilities. Many small rural towns are geographically and socially isolated, but all Australians nevertheless expect equitable access to high-quality health care.

Various management systems have been developed to meet the challenge of providing a sustainable, achievable, and high quality of surgical care to those living in these vast and isolated regions and across the continent of Australia. Optimal care of major trauma injuries entails a multidisciplinary treatment approach and the availability of specialist facilities such as neurosurgery, thoracic surgery, and modern intensive care units that often cannot be provided or are not sustainable in smaller rural hospitals. In Australia, there has consequently been an emphasis in developing mechanisms to rapidly retrieve major trauma patients from rural areas and to deliver them efficiently to the larger metropolitan centers. In contrast, the treatment of nontraumatic general surgical emergencies requires the availability of skillful surgeons and good operative facilities, but transfer of the patient to a major city hospital is seldom necessary. Australia has a proud tradition of training and providing highly skilled and versatile general surgeons who manage the majority of the general surgical emergencies in rural Australia. To enhance the services provided to remote regions, outreach services such as the Royal Flying Doctor Service have been developed.[1] These services have the capability to fly surgical teams to remote rural areas and transfer patients to the larger regional hospitals.

To place Australia's metropolitan and rural acute care surgical services in context, this chapter reviews the geography of the continent of Australia and outlines factors that affect the demographics of the country. The workings of Australia's health care system are explored, and the system of surgical training in Australia is outlined. Important factors that affect the medical workforce and the distribution and provision of surgical services are also considered. Trauma and nontrauma acute care surgery in Australia are considered separately. The supporting role that Australia provides to the health care facilities in its broader region, in particular to the Pacific Island countries, is also described.

Geography and Demography

Australia is the smallest continent and largest island in the world and is situated in the southern hemisphere between the Indian Ocean and the South Pacific. The country is comparable in size to the United States and covers a landmass of approximately 7,682,300 square kilometers.[2] Australia is, however, the world's driest continent and consequently has a much smaller population. The center of the country receives particularly little rainfall and is consequently a vast stretch of sparsely populated desert or semidesert. Australia's population of approximately 20 million people is consequently distributed unevenly across the continent. The majority of the population is highly urbanized, and most Australians live in the capital cities of the states and territories.[1] These cities have developed in close proximity to reliable water supplies or along the coasts around safe harbors, particularly along the fertile southeast coastal strip of Australia. In this region, the cities of Melbourne, Sydney, and Brisbane contain more than half of the entire country's population. A substantial number of people do, however, live in remote regional or rural areas of the country. The larger regional towns serve as industrial centers and provide a wide range of social and medical facilities. Smaller rural towns may, however, contain less than 1,000 people and are frequently surrounded by vast farming or cattle grazing regions. These communities are often geographically isolated from one another and may often be situated hundreds of kilometers from a major city. The further one moves from the coast, the more widespread the rural population centers tend to become.

The population of Australia has increased greatly since the end of World War II and has more than doubled in the past 50 years. This is due in large part to extensive government-supported migration programs and to a lesser extent to an increase in the national birth rate. The majority of the population remains of European extraction, and English is the national language. However, in recent years, migration, particularly from Asia, has increased substantially, and Australia is now a profoundly multiethnic and multicultural society.[1]

The Australian Medical System

Australia operates a universal national health care system that aims to enable all citizens to enjoy an affordable high standard of health care.[1] The system is partially funded by a flat-percentage special income tax levy and is largely supplemented by federal government resources.[4] The major trauma centers, the vast majority of the tertiary teaching hospitals, and most of the small metropolitan and district hospitals are publicly funded. Australia also provides an optional second tier of private hospitals, many of which were originally established by religious or nonprofit organizations. The smaller private hospitals cater predominantly to elective medical and surgical admissions. The major private centers do, however, operate large emergency departments and

provide a full range of specialist acute care surgical services, including cardiothoracic and neurosurgery.

Most Australians requiring either elective or acute care surgery are treated in public hospitals, which involves no direct cost to the patient. Patients with private medical insurance have the option of being treated either in a private hospital or as private patients in public hospitals (semiprivate). This entitles them to minor perks such as choice of individual medical practitioners, but the standard of care provided to private versus nonpaying patients in the public hospitals is equal. The Australian health care system also provides rebates for medical treatment administered outside the hospitals by general practitioners (primary care physicians), specialist physicians, and surgeons who set their own fees.[4] Most choose a fee that relates to the rebate so that patients pay only marginal out-of-pocket fees for services provided outside the hospital. The federal government also operates a Pharmaceutical Benefits Scheme, which makes approved medications available at substantially subsidized cost. A patient's attendance for medical treatment in Australia and compliance with prescribed treatment is thus generally independent of their financial status.[1]

Australia's health care system is by no means flawless in that patients without private medical insurance are sometimes made to endure lengthy waiting periods for elective procedures at the public hospitals. However, patients with conditions requiring urgent treatment generally have no waiting period and enjoy a high standard of service.[1] The Australian health system successfully allows all the country's inhabitants, regardless of financial status, to have fast access to acute care services and any required acute care surgical treatment. The system also ensures that Australians have equitable and affordable access to general practitioners.

Distribution and Provision of Surgical Services

The uneven distribution of Australia's population has led to a markedly skewed distribution of the country's surgeons, with the majority of surgical specialists tending to practice in metropolitan areas of the country. Australia's acute care surgical services were designed with the ramifications of this in mind.[1]

Australia's major cities offer the full range of surgical subspecialties with surgeon-to-patient ratios similar to those in major cities in the United States and the United Kingdom. Modern operating and perioperative facilities, well-equipped intensive care units, and world-class anesthetic services are generally widely available. There is long tradition among Australian doctors for clinical excellence and high standards of technical skills, and the quality of care provided in Australia's major hospitals is comparable to that of most "first world" centers.[1]

In the larger regional towns, with populations of 25,000 to 250,000 people, a wide range of local specialists, such as orthopedic surgeons, urologists, and otolaryngologists, are usually available. Towns with populations between 10,000 and 25,000 people are often situated far from the major cities and are usually too small and too isolated to sustain the services of resident specialist surgeons. These towns instead have several general surgeons who provide a wide range of surgical services. Depending on the size and needs of the local population, specialist surgeons from either the larger regional centers or major cities visit these towns at regular intervals to supplement the services provided by the resident general surgeons. In true rural or remote areas, defined as more than a few hundred kilometers from a major urban area and where the population served is less than 10,000 people, limited surgical services are often provided by general practitioners who have a particular interest in surgery.[5] Some small communities may also enjoy the services of a single resident general surgeon. Local services provide backup and relief when required.

Anesthetic services in regional Australia tend to run in parallel with the general surgical services. General practitioner anesthetists usually service small towns with populations up to 25,000 people, and progressive input from specialist anesthetists is usually provided above that population level.

Acute Care Trauma Surgery in Australia

Australia has a long and successful history of reducing morbidity and mortality from trauma through the aggressive implementation of primary prevention strategies that seek to reduce the environmental and behavioral factors that contribute to major injuries. For example, the state of Victoria led the world in introducing legislation for compulsory wearing of motor vehicle seatbelts and later in the introduction of random breath testing, speed detection, and red-light traffic cameras.[1] These measures had a dramatic effect, and by 1992 the death rate due to road trauma in Victoria was 1.6 per 10,000 vehicles, the lowest for any major developed country in the world.

Despite maximal public prevention measures, some people will inevitably continue to sustain major traumatic injuries. These injuries are often "time critical" in that prompt, appropriate care reduces morbidity and mortality. The literature has increasingly supported the concept that severely injured patients achieve optimal outcomes when treated in major trauma centers that consistently manage large trauma volumes. Most of Australia's states

and territories provide modern, well-equipped tertiary hospitals, but in many states a high percentage of major trauma patients have traditionally been delivered to the nearest emergency department and not necessarily admitted directly to the major trauma centers. To improve the streamlining of major trauma patients to designated trauma centers and to improve the standard of care in the prehospital setting, Australia's states have begun to embrace the concept of integrated trauma systems. To illustrate the development of such a trauma system and the impact of the system on management of major trauma patients, the Victorian State Trauma System is described.

The state of Victoria occupies the southeastern portion of Australia and covers an area of 227,590 square kilometers. It has a population of 4.9 million people, 3.5 million of whom live in Melbourne, the capital city. Several Victorian studies in the 1990s evaluated the management of road traffic fatalities involving people who were alive when the ambulance services arrived and indicated that a significant proportion of deaths may have been potentially preventable.[6-8] Organizational, prehospital, and hospital management and system problems, which included prolonged accident scene times, inadequate prehospital and emergency department life support skills, and the triage of patients to hospitals with inadequate resources were identified.[6-8] The Victorian State Government responded by implementing an advanced and integrated statewide trauma system that aims to provide optimal care from the injury scene through rehabilitation.[9]

Prehospital Care

In remote parts of Australia, injuries are sustained significant distances from a medical facility. Paramedic response times and the standard of prehospital and in-transit care provided can consequently significantly impact a trauma patient's outcome from injury. Integrated, prehospital care is a vital step in the sequence of comprehensive trauma management. In the 1980s, Victoria's metropolitan ambulance services were consolidated into a single prehospital provider for the greater metropolitan area, and in 1992 the state's five rural services were integrated into a single rural ambulance service. All Victorian ambulance services now share common training, dispatch, and clinical practice protocols. A third ambulance division, Air Ambulance Victoria, coordinates a rotary wing service staffed by Mobile Intensive Care Ambulance (MICA) personnel and also operates fixed wing aircraft out of the state capital, Melbourne, to rural centers. The use of transport helicopters facilitates the rapid transfer of seriously injured patients from nearby rural areas to the metropolitan major trauma services. Fixed wing aircraft are utilized for transfers from more distant sites. Transport from remote regions is often coordinated with the Royal Flying Doctor Service.

Designation of Hospitals to Receive Trauma Patients

It is not feasible for every regional hospital to be resourced to the level of a major trauma center. Victorian hospitals have instead been stratified to various trauma care roles, based on resource and geographic considerations.[9] The various tiers provide for different complexities of trauma care, and patients are managed in a service appropriate for their injuries (Figure 50.1).

One major pediatric and two adult hospitals in Melbourne were designated to serve as major trauma services (MTSs).[9] These centers provide 24-hour trauma reception teams and on-site specialist resources. The MTS hospitals deliver definitive care to the majority of the state's major trauma caseload (Figure 50.2) either through primary triage from the accident scene or following secondary transfer. The MTS classification was restricted to ensure that a large caseload of major trauma patients is consistently managed at the MTS institutions. In the metropolitan areas, a second tier of MTSs was designated to receive major trauma patients who, for logistic or safety reasons, are unable to be transported directly to an MTS.[9] These hospitals provide resuscitation and stabilization, establish early consultation with the MTS, and transfer severely injured patients to the MTS at an early opportunity. In some situations, they may provide definitive treatment in consultation with an MTS. A third tier of primary injury services was designated to treat patients with minor injuries. When transporting trauma patients to a hospital, ambulance services generally bypass these hospitals in preference for services of a higher level.[9]

The regional component of the trauma system is also led by the MTSs, but regional hospitals were also strati-

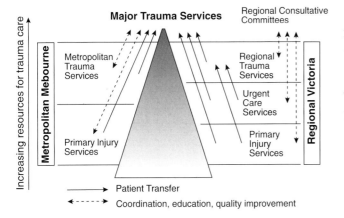

FIGURE 50.1. Structure of the Integrated Victorian State Trauma System. (Courtesy of The Victorian Department of Human Services, Victoria, Australia, with permission.)

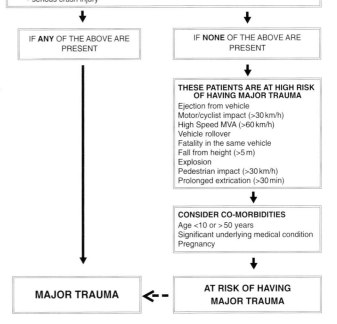

FIGURE 50.2. Prehospital major trauma criteria. (Courtesy of The Victorian Department of Human Services, Victoria, Australia, with permission.)

fied to particular trauma care roles. Regional trauma services (RTSs) located in major regional centers serve as a regional focus for trauma management and receive trauma referrals from the surrounding catchment area. They provide resuscitation and stabilization to trauma patients, establish early communication with the MTS, and transfer major trauma patients to the MTS (Figures 50.1 and 50.3). The RTSs also provide definitive care to a limited number of trauma patients when injuries are assessed as not severe enough to warrant early transfer. Urgent care services in smaller rural communities where higher levels of trauma care are not readily accessible provide resuscitation and stabilization of patients before early transfer to higher level centers, and primary injury services in isolated areas provide initial resuscitation and

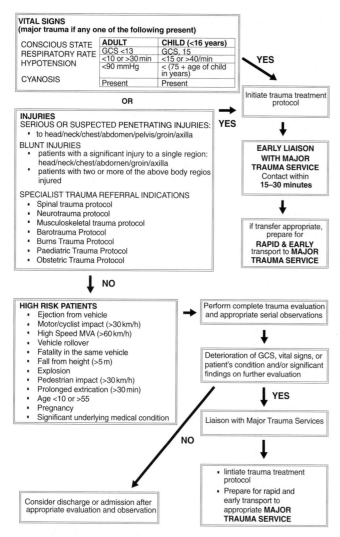

FIGURE 50.3. Major trauma interhospital guidelines. (Courtesy of The Victorian Department of Human Services, Victoria, Australia, with permission.)

and transfer protocols were consequently formulated, and a rapid response retrieval system was designed.[9] Prehospital major trauma criteria were developed using specific physiologic, anatomic, and mechanistic indicators to identify major trauma patients (see Figure 50.2). A 30-minute major trauma bypass protocol was also developed in which patients who fulfill the triage criteria for major trauma and who are within 30 minutes of an MTS are delivered directly to the MTS with the ambulance bypassing nearer non-MTS hospitals (Figure 50.4). This time period was selected so that most patients given average system activation and injury scene times would reach a hospital well within the "golden hour" of trauma care.

Communication processes were also streamlined to provide seamless information transfer, and wider application of mobile systems for early prehospital to hospital communications was instituted. Regional retrieval services coordinate retrieval missions that require treatment at a regional hospital level, but timely liaison with the statewide retrieval system occurs for situations possibly requiring tertiary level care. Simultaneous dispatch of regional and statewide retrieval services is sometimes activated to minimize time transport delays or to provide support to the regional ambulance services or local hospitals. Regular audits of the triage and transfer system's efficacy are performed to verify that the triage and transfer protocols operate as intended. A meticulous trauma registry has been established to record details pertaining to all phases of care for each trauma patient. Regular audits of each component of the system are performed, and system enhancements continue to be made as required.[9]

stabilization before early transfer to the MTS. In less isolated areas, the primary injury services may be designated for bypass so that major trauma patients can be transported from the injury scene directly to the MTS.[9]

Triage, Transfer, and Retrieval Services

The geographic isolation, sparse population, and limited resources in rural Australia were acknowledged in the design of the Victorian State Trauma System. The particular importance of providing a rapid response retrieval system and efficient interhospital transport was also recognized.

The efficacy of patient transfer depends more on the time taken to cover a particular distance and quality of care delivered during interhospital transfer than on the actual distance travelled.[10] Streamlined triage, referral,

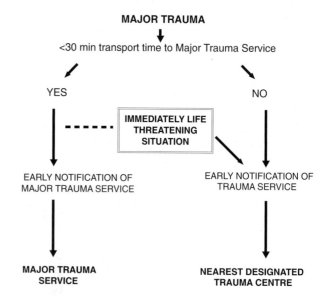

FIGURE 50.4. The 30-minute bypass protocol. (Courtesy of The Victorian Department of Human Services, Victoria, Australia, with permission.)

Trauma Care in the Other States of Australia

The recent implementation of an integrated trauma system in the state of Victoria is likely to spur the development of similar systems in the other states. The way in which these will be designed will be influenced by the demographic and geographic factors particular to each state.[2] For example, the state of Western Australia covers an area of 2.5 million square kilometres but has a population of only 1.8 million people, of whom 1.4 million live in the capital city, Perth. Retrieval distances of 3,000 km between outlying rural towns and Western Australia's Major Trauma Center, located in Perth, are not uncommon, and in such cases lengthy transport times are inevitable.[2] Particular attention to optimizing the standard of care provided in flight is consequently likely to be emphasized in Western Australia.

Nontrauma Acute Care Surgery

The acute care surgical services in Australia's large cities operate in a similar fashion to those in major medical centers in other modern western countries. The system for providing surgical care to Australia's rural population does, however, have several unique features. Acute care surgery in rural Australia is provided by way of several strategies. These include training and providing highly versatile general rural surgeons and development of efficient outreach programs that allow both transport of specialist surgeons to patients in remote regions or retrieval of patients from remote regions and timely transport to larger base hospitals. There has also been an emphasis on development of electronic data transfer mechanisms and interactive audiovisual communication systems to minimize the impact of geographic isolation.

Australia's large regional hospitals generally enjoy the services of a range of resident specialist surgeons, and most also support modern intensive care unit facilities. These hospitals are usually able to provide definitive treatment for most of the surgical emergencies that occur in their local catchment area. In the smaller towns, where resident specialist services may be scarce, the resident general surgeons are often experienced in managing a wide range of conditions. Unlike their city counterparts, many rural surgeons continue to practice as true "general surgeons" and are experienced in definitively managing a wide range of orthopedic, vascular, urologic, and obstetric and gynecologic acute care situations. Major surgery performed by these rural surgeons has subsequently been shown in studies to be of consistently high quality.[11] When definitive care is beyond the means of the general surgeon, the general surgeon is usually able to resuscitate the patient while awaiting either the arrival of a specialist surgeon or the transport of the patient to a larger regional hospital where specialist care can be provided.

In the small towns that have no resident surgeon, the general practitioner is often the first point of call.[5] Many rural general practitioners have sufficient surgical training and experience to treat most minor surgical problems. Many also possess the skills to perform urgent life-saving surgical procedures such as placement of intercostal catheters. More serious surgical problems require either transport of the patient to an appropriate medical facility or utilization of outreach services to deliver appropriate surgical services to the local facility. Prompt and efficient patient transport is facilitated by modern retrieval services. In view of the vast distances from isolated rural towns to larger regional hospitals, efficient air transport services have been developed and are frequently employed.

To facilitate a good understanding of the high level of qualification of Australia's general surgeons as well as specialist surgeons, a brief overview of the surgical training process in Australia is necessary.

Surgical Training in Australia

In view of the uneven population distribution in Australia and the geographically isolated nature of many of the country's rural towns, medical and surgical training in Australia has been designed to ensure that all Australian doctors receive broad exposure to both medical and surgical fields before specializing. Unlike the training model in the United States, where junior doctors enter streamlined residency programs soon after graduation from medical school, in Australia all medical graduates are required to then undertake a 1-year general rotating internship before receiving full registration as a medical practitioner. Rotations in each of medicine, general surgery, and acute care medicine are required, and one rotation usually needs to be completed in a small country hospital.

This concept of mandating broad exposure before allowing more focused training continues for both medical and surgical specialist training.[4] After the internship has been completed, medical school graduates wishing to pursue a career in surgery enroll in the Basic Surgical Training (BST) program, administered by the Royal Australasian College of Surgeons (RACS).[1] The aims of this course are acquisition of the anatomy, physiology, and pathology knowledge prerequisite for a career in surgery as well as attainment of knowledge of the theory and practice of general surgery. The emphasis is not on early specialization. Instead, basic surgical trainees rotate through a wide range of hospital posts, each approximately 3 months in duration, to gain exposure to a wide range of surgical specialties. Rotations in emergency medicine and intensive care are also compulsory requirements of the program. The training posts are generally in public hospitals specifically accredited by the RACS for training purposes. This ensures that appropriate educational facilities and activities are provided.

In addition to the hospital rotations, all basic surgical trainees are also required to complete the Early Management of Severe Trauma course conducted by the RACS. During the BST period, which occupies a minimum of 2 years, trainees also undertake a detailed written examination and practical clinical examinations that test their knowledge base and clinical and technical skills.[4]

After completing basic training and passing the requisite examinations, trainees are eligible to enter advanced training programs, which can be undertaken within the nine recognized specialties of general, orthopedic, pediatric, cardiothoracic, plastic and reconstructive surgery, ophthalmology, neurosurgery, otolaryngology, and urology.[1] These training programs take 4 or 5 years to complete, depending on the specialty. Each specialty has a surgical board that advises with regard to the curriculum, course content, duration of training, selection of trainees, satisfactory completion of training, and maintenance of standards in the specialty. In the final year of advanced training, eligible candidates also complete a second set of examinations that consist of written, clinical, and oral sections and include assessment of knowledge of surgical pathology, operative surgery, and surgical and developmental anatomy. Candidates who pass all sections of these examinations at a high standard are granted the status of provisional fellow until they have completed their full period of training, at which time they become fellows of the college and are entitled to practice independently as specialists.

Rural Surgeon Training

It has been recognized that rural surgeons need broader training than their metropolitan counterparts and also need increased professional support from their colleagues and specialty societies.[12-17] All Australian surgical trainees are required to undertake a portion of their training rotations at a regional country hospital. For surgical trainees who wish to undertake training for rural surgical practice, the RACS has devised a Rural Surgical Training Program (RSTP).[3,12] This program operates as an integral part of the General Surgical Training Program and complements and expands on it to ensure that trainees obtain the skills and experience necessary to provide high standard surgical care to rural centers.[13] The program enables rural general surgery trainees to gain experience in a range of nongeneral surgical disciplines, such as orthopedics and plastic surgery, urology, vascular surgery, pediatric surgery, and thoracic surgery.[14] Experi-

ence in these areas is particularly useful to general surgeons working in a rural center.[12] The program is designed to be flexible and allows rotations to be tailored to an individual trainee's requirements so as to focus on the region in which the trainee intends to practice upon completion of training. For example, with regard to orthopedic surgery, most rural surgeons would be expected to be competent in the management of common closed fractures but would not be expected to undertake joint replacement surgery. The surgical units to which rural trainees are rostered are selected accordingly.

The RACS has also instituted a Rural Continuing Medical Education scheme to better enable rural surgeons to maintain and update their clinical knowledge. Increasing use of tele-conferences, the Internet, and other electronic information services should further decrease the sense of professional isolation previously experienced by rural surgeons.[17]

Surgical Training for General Practitioners

In the more isolated areas of Australia, general practitioners (primary care physicians) are often the only resident medical staff. To ensure that these doctors possess the requisite skills to perform basic first-responder tasks, an Advanced Surgical Skills Training Program for Rural General Practitioners was developed. This is a joint initiative of the RACS, the Royal Australasian College of General Practitioners, and the Australian College of Rural and Remote Medicine. Additional intensive training courses provided by various state rural medical support agencies and that cover various aspects of emergency medicine (including surgery, obstetrics, and ophthalmology) have also been developed to provide supplemental training for general practitioners in rural and remote areas of Australia.

Outreach Services

It is not feasible for the full range of surgical services and facilities to be provided in all of Australia's many sparsely populated rural towns. An array of outreach services, such as the Royal Flying Doctor Service, has consequently been developed.[3,18] Depending on the particular clinical scenario, the facilities, and staff available in each town, these outreach services allow efficient and rapid transport of the patient to a higher level medical center or transport of the appropriate medical and surgical practitioners to the rural site. These outreach services are cognizant of needing to work closely with the on-site medical general practitioner so as to support the local services while simultaneously avoiding de-skilling of local medical staff. Effective outreach services depend on the availability of efficient transport mechanisms. Because of the vast distances that need to be covered in rural Australia, these outreach services tend to operate via air transport.[18]

The world's first aerial medical service was developed in Australia. Still the country's most extensive outreach service, the renowned Royal Flying Doctor and Flying Surgeon Service developed from the vision of a Presbyterian missionary to the outback, the Reverend John Flynn.[2,19] He realized that transporting patients to the hospital by air and enabling doctors to fly to remote areas to provide medical attention would significantly improve the standard of care available in the remote regions of Australia.[1]

The Flying Doctor service was first established in the western part of the state of Queensland in 1928. The original flying teams delivered treatment locally where appropriate or carried patients back to the larger centers for treatment that was beyond local resources. The Flying Surgeon service was established in Queensland in 1959. The initial concept entailed providing a resident general surgeon who would regularly fly out to a number of hospitals in a remote region that extended over more than 500,000 square kilometers. The flying team, consisting of the surgeon, an anesthetist, and the pilot, were able to perform acute care surgery locally with the assistance of local general practitioners or at the larger base hospital after the patient had been transported. The local practitioners managed the patients' preoperative and postoperative care. The inaugural scheme was very successful and led to the establishment of a second Flying Surgeon team in Queensland. This allowed two centers to provide emergency coverage and relief for each other and led to the subsequent development of similar "flying" schemes to provide obstetric and gynecology services to the remote regions of Queensland.

The Flying Doctor and Flying Surgeon service was later expanded to cover the other states of Australia. The service now operates 24 hours a day, 365 days a year and provides comprehensive aeromedical emergency and primary health care services to remote regions of most of the continent. The Royal Flying Doctor Service is also involved in transferring patients between small rural and remote area hospitals and the larger metropolitan medical centers. As vast distances between Australian population centers restrict the use of helicopter transport to near-urban regions, the Royal Flying Doctor Service predominantly utilizes fixed wing aircraft. The service now operates over 40 aircraft from 20 bases and has a staff of over 500 people. The aircraft fleet is constantly being modernized and currently utilizes pressurized aircrafts that are able to fly at high altitude to avoid turbulent weather but can also fly at low altitude when medically indicated.[19] Further improvements to the aircraft facilitate safe landings on short, makeshift dirt landing strips, thereby enabling the Royal Flying Doctor Service to efficiently evacuate patients from remote areas of rough terrain and then transport them rapidly and safely over long distances. Advances in biomedical engineering, such as development of portable invasive pressure monitoring, have further improved in-flight medical treatment.[19] Even in the most remote parts of the Australian continent, no one is currently more than 2 hours away from medical assistance.

The Use of Information Technology in Providing Surgical Services

A number of information technology initiatives have been pursued in Australia to minimize the impact of the geographic isolation experienced in many of the rural areas, to enhance the standard of care delivered to patients, to augment the support provided to local medical staff, and to reduce the strain on Australia's vital but expensive outreach services. For example, many Australian rural and remote hospitals now have access to tele-conferencing, tele-medicine, and satellite communication facilities, which allow real-time interactive audiovisual communication between doctors separated by vast distances.[1] These technologies are used for educational purposes and also have numerous clinical applications. For example, the ability to conduct specialist consultations and referrals over interactive audiovisual communication systems often reduces the need to transfer the patient. A further technological development has been the digitalization of radiology images so that x-ray images can now be transmitted by standard telephone lines to be viewed on a personal computer screen at off-site locations. Specialist surgeons and radiologists located at the larger hospitals are then able to assess the images and assist in surgical decision making.[1]

Prehospital care has also been improved with the advent of new technologies. For example, as an ever increasing number of Australian and foreign tourists are choosing to travel into the rugged interior of the continent or to go sailing along Australia's vast coastline, greater use is being made of global positioning satellite (GPS) devices and emergency position indicating radio beacons (EPIRBS).[2] These transmit a localizing distress signal that is detected by overhead satellite and relayed to rescue stations, enabling injured travellers to be located quickly and retrieved efficiently. The development of new technologies will continue to impact the care delivered to remote regions. It is, for example, conceivable that robotic technologies may one day allow specialist surgeons located in a major city to perform operative procedures in rural areas by remote control.

Challenges to Trauma and Acute Care Surgery in the Developing World

The are significant disparities between mortality rates for injured patients in developed countries, such as Australia, and developing countries in Africa, Asia, and other poorer regions.[20] For example, with the same severity of a major multisystem injury, the probability of survival is six times less in developing nations than in more highly developed countries. This is due to factors such as a lack of triage, transfer, and treatment protocols, deficiencies in education and training, inadequate infrastructure, an absence of necessary resources and personnel, an insufficient supply of consumables, and inadequate coordination between various care providers.[20] In third world countries, emergency surgical care itself is often poorly defined, and clinical decisions are consequently often delayed. The resultant suboptimal care amplifies the tremendous burden of disability experienced in many developing countries and places an overwhelming strain on their underfunded health systems.[20]

Governments, professional organizations, and academic institutions in first world countries such as Australia and the United States have an important role to play in helping to improve the standard of acute care surgery delivered in developing nations. Low-cost interventions, such as efforts aimed at improving the training and education programs in poorer countries, have the capacity to significantly reduce the burden of death and disability experienced there.[20] Australia's involvement in the Pacific Island countries highlights several of these concepts.

Australia is situated in close proximity to a series of small, widely scattered Pacific Island countries in which there is a wide discrepancy between disease incidence and local medical capability.[21,22] Australian surgeons have a proud tradition of volunteering their surgical and teaching skills to assist these communities. Australia has also established several formal outreach programs that aim to improve the quality of medical and surgical care provided to these regions.[21,22]

The Royal Australasian College of Surgeons has established and conducts several of these outreach projects. For example, since 1995 the RACS has operated a Pacific Islands Project (PIP) in which multidisciplinary Australian surgical teams undertake short-term visits (2 weeks) to the 11 Pacific Island countries of Fiji, Samoa, Tonga, Kiribati, Tuvalu, Marshall Islands, Federated States of Micronesia, Cook Islands, Vanuatu, Solomon Islands, and Nauru.[21,22]

The composition of each PIP team varies according the specialty and local clinical, anesthetic, and nursing capability. Most surgical teams consist of two surgeons, an anesthetist, and a theater nurse. All team members provide their services on a voluntary basis, and the project funds travel and accommodation expenses. Arrangements are made for local staff to be attached to the team, and the availability of appropriate staff and facilities is organized and confirmed in advance. Sets of equipment, which include anesthetic equipment, portable operating microscopes, and specialized surgical instruments, were developed for each specialty to allow the respective teams to guarantee a defined service capability in each country.[21] Local practitioners work closely with the PIP teams through all steps of clinical management, and detailed instructions are left with these practitioners with regard to the postoperative care for all patients treated. When necessary, directions for review are passed on to the next visiting team. The delivery of the outreach surgical services is combined with training of local Pacific Island doctors and nurses so that an ultimate goal of self-sufficiency will eventually be attained.[21,22]

Training of local practitioners is an important focus of the PIP. Clinical instruction is delivered to the local practitioners by all team members during the course of their work, and more structured tuition is arranged whenever circumstances permit. Teaching often takes the form of 1-hour lectures, but at its most extensive it also includes all-day seminars. Practitioners from outlying islands travel to and participate in these workshops. In addition to the tuition delivered on the islands, a number of local practitioners who would benefit from further training in Australia are also identified. Through several charitable sources, they are given intensive tuition in Australia for 1 to 3 months or are given the chance to attend major clinical meetings. The improved medical knowledge and skills acquired enables these Pacific Island surgeons to deliver an improved range of primary, secondary, and limited tertiary health services to their peoples.[22]

Ongoing links between Pacific Island health professionals and their Australian counterparts and institutions have also been established. For example, in Fiji the RACS helped formulate a detailed curriculum and the course content for Diploma and Master of Medicine programs in anesthesia, medicine, obstetrics and gynecology, pediatrics, and surgery. The RACS also arranges training attachments in Australia and/or New Zealand for Fijian trainees. In addition, the RACS has recently also extended its outreach program to Papua, New Guinea (PNG). In the PNG project coordinated by the college, specialist medical and surgical teams visit the larger hospitals and some smaller provincial centers to deliver surgical services that would otherwise be unavailable.[21]

The RACS has also extended its assistance program to southeast Asia, where it provides a specialist general surgeon and anesthetist to work full time in Dili, the only surgical hospital in East Timor. The two doctors each work as one of only two such specialists in a country of over 800,000 people. They are required to conduct operations in challenging circumstances, which includes dealing with tropical medicine using very limited resources. In addition to the services provided by the general surgeon, specialist surgical visits are conducted once a month for a week at a time. Support is also provided to train local personnel in surgery and anesthetics and to improve the maintenance of biomedical equipment.

In summary, the design of acute care surgical services across the world is influenced by the interplay of the unique geographic, demographic, resource, and demand factors that affect each particular country. Australia is a vast but scantily populated country, with a population concentrated mainly in several large cities along the coasts, whereas a small proportion of the population lives in smaller, rural towns that are sometimes situated great distances from the major cities. To provide equitable high-quality surgical care to all Australians, various management systems have been designed. The mechanisms for trauma surgery and nontrauma acute care surgery in Australia differ substantially from one another. Optimal trauma care often requires a multidisciplinary approach to treatment. As it is usually not feasible to provide this in the rural setting, mechanisms have instead been devised to efficiently retrieve and rapidly transport these patients to larger medical centers. In contrast, Australia has a long tradition of training highly skilled and versatile general surgeons who are able to manage most nontrauma acute care surgical scenarios in the rural setting. In recent years, the Royal Australasian College of Surgeons has also expanded its role to provide surgical services, clinical support, training, and education to the developing nations of the Pacific Island region. This experience suggests that, across the world, greater logistic support from governments, private organizations, and academic institutions would greatly boost acute care surgical services in the developing world in the short term. Specific attention to training local doctors in acute care surgery and trauma care will increase these countries' capacity to eventually maintain good-quality acute care surgery services of their own.

References

1. Clunie GJ. Surgery in Australia. Arch Surg 1994; 129(1):13–20.
2. Croser JL. Trauma care systems in Australia. Injury 2003; 34(9):649–651.
3. Green A. Maintaining surgical standards beyond the city in Australia. Aust N Z J Surg 2003; 73(4):232–233.
4. Egerton WS. Health care delivery system in Australia and its effect on surgical education and training. World J Surg 1994; 18(5):656–662.
5. Bruening MH, Maddern GJ. The provision of general surgical services in rural South Australia: a new model for rural surgery. Aust N Z J Surg 1998; 68(11):764–768.
6. McDermott FT, Cordner SM, Tremayne AB. Evaluation of the medical management and preventability of death in 137 road traffic fatalities in Victoria, Australia: an overview. Consultative Committee on Road Traffic Fatalities in Victoria. J Trauma 1996; 40(4):520–533.
7. McDermott FT, Cordner SM, Tremayne AB. Management deficiencies and death preventability in 120 Victorian road fatalities (1993–1994). The Consultative Committee on Road Traffic Fatalities in Victoria. Aust N Z J Surg. 1997; 67(9):611–618.
8. Danne P, Brazenor G, Cade R, Crossley P, Fitzgerald M, Gregory P, et al. The major trauma management study: an analysis of the efficacy of current trauma care. Aust N Z J Surg 1998; 68(1):50–57.
9. Review of Trauma and Emergency Services—Victoria 1999. Final Report of the Ministerial Taskforce on Trauma and Emergency Services and the Department Working Party on Emergency and Trauma Services. Melbourne, Victoria: Department of Human Services, 1999.
10. Danne, PD. Trauma management in Australia and the tyranny of distance. World J Surg 2003; 27(4):385–389.
11. Birks DM, Gunn IF, Birks RG, Strasser RP. Colorectal surgery in rural Australia: scars; a surgeon-based audit of workload and standards. ANZ J Surg 2001; 71(3):154–158.
12. Tulloh B, Clifforth S, Miller I. Caseload in rural general surgical practice and implications for training. Aust N Z J Surg 2001; 71(4):215–217.
13. Birks D, Green T. Training, retraining and retaining rural general surgeons: comment. Aust N Z J Surg 1999; 69(12):885–886.
14. Faris I. The making of a rural surgeon. Aust N Z J Surg 1997; 67(4):153–156.
15. Kiroff G. Training, retraining and retaining rural general surgeons. Aust N Z J Surg 1999; 69(6):413–414.
16. Bruening MH, Maddern GJ. A profile of rural surgeons in Australia. Med J Aust 1998; 169(6):324–326.
17. Green A. Ups and downs of rural practice: a surgeon's view. Med J Aust 1999; 171(11–12):625–626.
18. Kierath A, Hamdorf JM, House AK, House J. Developing visiting surgical services for rural and remote Australian communities. Med J Aust 1998; 168(9):454–457.
19. Langford SA. The Royal Flying Doctor Service of Australia. Its foundation and early development. Med J Aust 1994; 161(1):91–94.
20. Joshipura M. Challenges to trauma care in developing countries. Trauma Grapevine 2003; 9:62–63.
21. Theile DE, Bennett RC. The Pacific Islands Project: the first 3 years. Aust N Z J Surg 1998; 68(11):792–798.
22. Theile DE. Improving world health—Australia's focus on the Pacific. Med J Aust 1999; 170(7):295–296.

51
Acute Care Surgery: Japan

Kyoichi Takaori and Nobuhiko Tanigawa

The practice of acute care surgery varies in the international community and depends on many factors, for example, economics, politics, education, hygiene, diet, climate, religion, and social custom. This book is written by authors from those communities where acute care surgery is carried out in well-established forms. In some developing countries, however, acute care surgery cannot be practiced properly because medical resources are not sufficiently supplied, and education for surgeons and medical personnel is not appropriately organized.[1] Acute care surgery is the most common form of surgical practice in developing countries, and one of the purposes of this new textbook is to help bridge the gap between the practice of surgery in developed and in developing countries.

Japan suffered a catastrophe during World War II, and famine and poor hygiene prevailed throughout the country thereafter. The public health in Japan shortly after the war was no better than it is in developing countries today. Nevertheless, by adopting the methodologies of medical education and health care delivery mainly from the United States, outstanding progress has been made in medical care in Japan.[2] Presently, the World Health Organization ranks health attainment of Japan in terms of the average level of population health and health equality as number one among the 191 member countries. The successfully developed medical care system, specific epidemiology, and other factors have characterized acute care surgery in Japan with several unique features. In this chapter, practical highlights of acute care surgery in developing countries and current topics of acute care surgery in Japan are described with an emphasis on nontrauma-related illnesses. Finally, a perspective is offered on the future of acute care surgery in the international communities.

Acute Care Surgery in Developing Countries

Certain infectious diseases occur exclusively in developing countries, the tropics, Africa, or Asia. Therefore, special precautions and therapeutics for these infectious diseases are mandatory in acute care surgery in such communities. Acute care surgery in developing countries can also be complicated by malnutrition resulting from inadequate food supplies. Thermoregulatory disorders also need to be considered, as they affect acute care surgery particularly in tropical countries. Malnutrition, infectious diseases, and thermoregulatory disorders are highlighted here, and managements of these morbidities for acute care surgery in developing countries are described from a practical point of view.

Malnutrition

Poverty and ignorance contribute to malnutrition in developing countries. Prolonged lactation also causes malnutrition in childhood. Typically, there are two forms of malnutrition, marasmus and kwashiorkor.[3] Marasmus, synonymous with "protein-energy malnutrition," is caused by a diet deficient in both calories and proteins. Congenital syphilis and parasitic infection also can cause marasmus. General signs of marasmus include growth failure, weight loss, fatigue, irritability, and lethargy. Kwashiorkor is also known as "malignant malnutrition" or "infantile pellagra" and is caused by inadequate protein intake regardless of the calorie intake. Kwashiorkor is typically characterized by a large protuberant belly, pigment loss in desquamated skin, vitiligo, and reddish hair.

Malnutrition in developing counties usually presents as a combination of marasmus and kwashiorkor. Edema and hypoalbuminemia are prominent features in kwashiorkor patients, and these patients are more susceptible to hypovolemic shock. Because the binding of serum proteins to electrolytes and other molecules may be altered in the presence of hypoproteinemia, particular caution should be exercised to avoid the abrupt development of an electrolyte imbalance during infusion. Kwashiorkor patients are more susceptible to congestive heart failure and lung edema, and their renal, hepatic, exocrine, and pancreatic functions are often hampered. Thus, acute care surgery for patients with malnutrition is inevitably associated with great risks.

Because the function of the immune system is usually suppressed in patients with malnutrition,[4] administration of wide-spectrum antibiotics during and after acute care surgery is desirable. When perioral nutrition becomes feasible, food must be reintroduced slowly: carbohydrates first to supply calories, followed by high-quality protein. Intravenous hyperalimentation, if available, is extremely useful when food intake cannot be tolerated because of ileus, intestinal fistula, or sustained inflammation of the alimentary tract.

Infectious Diseases

Certain infectious diseases are common in developing countries. Representative infectious diseases that necessitate or affect acute care surgery include malaria, schistosomiasis, amebiasis, and ascariasis. Physicians who work in developing countries and those who treat patients traveling to or from endemic countries are encouraged to read the textbooks of medical parasitology, microbiology, and zoology.

Malaria

Malaria remains one of the most life-threatening diseases in tropical countries despite a malaria eradication program by the World Health Organization (WHO) in the 1950s and 1960s and a recently launched campaign to Roll Back Malaria by the WHO.[5] *Plasmodium falciparum* (Figure 51.1) causes malignant tertian malaria, which is the most common form of malaria in the tropics. Malaria parasites are transmitted from one human to another by the bite of infected *Anopheles* mosquitoes (Figure 51.2). In humans, the parasites, in a form of the sporozoites, migrate to the liver, where they mature and release another form, the merozoites. The merozoites enter the

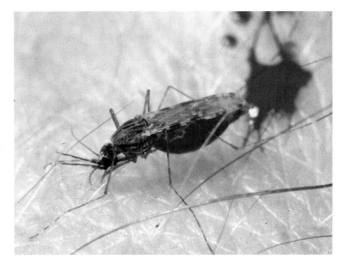

FIGURE 51.2. *Anopheles gambiae*, a carrier mosquito of *Plasmodium falciform*. (Courtesy of Dr. Yukio Yoshida.)

blood stream and infect the red blood cells. Malaria typically causes fever, anemia, and splenomegaly.

It is imperative to treat patients with the prompt administration of antimalarials. Although curative treatment of malaria generally consists of chloroquine or amodiaquine administration, malaria therapy can be complicated by the resistance of certain strains to these drugs, and other regimens may be indicated. When rupture of the spleen with massive hemorrhage occurs, acute care splenectomy is indicated. Malaria occasionally presents with colicky abdominal pain and as an acute abdominal emergency. Major surgery and severe trauma in the presence of malaria may precipitate malaria crises (e.g., cerebral malaria, hyperpyrexia, and hemolytic anemia) and possibly result in death. Transfusion of blood infected with malaria into a patient who has not been previously exposed to the disease may be lethal.

Schistosomiasis

Infections of *Schistosoma* species are common in endemic areas, including *Schistosoma haematobium* and *Schistosoma mansoni* in Africa and *Schistosoma japonica* (Figure 51.3) in Asia. Ova of *S. haematobium* and *S. japonica* are often found in the colon, where they induce a granulomatous response and increase the risk of carcinoma. When schistosomiasis is complicated by intestinal obstruction caused by a granuloma, resection of the lesion is indicated. It must also be noted that a granulomatous nodule of schistosomiasis often contains a carcinoma. *Schistosoma japonica* can parasitize the inferior mesenteric radicles, and the eggs may obstruct microcapillary vessels of the liver, resulting in cirrhosis of the liver (Figure 51.4).

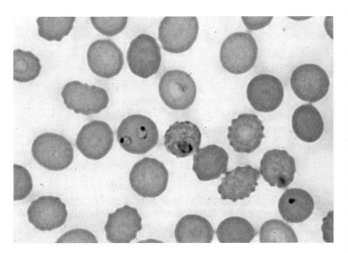

FIGURE 51.1. *Plasmodium falciform*, ring forms, in thin blood films, Giemsa's stain. (Courtesy of Dr. Yukio Yoshida.)

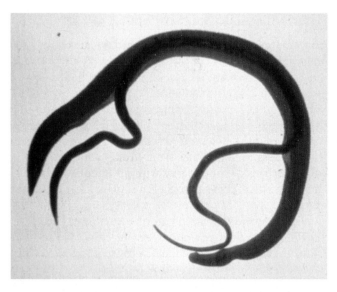

FIGURE 51.3. *Schistosoma japonica*, male and female adults. (Courtesy of Dr. Yukio Yoshida.)

Amebiasis

Tropical and subtropical countries that have poor hygienic conditions are infested with *Entamoeba histolytica*, and at least 40,000 people die of amebiasis annu-

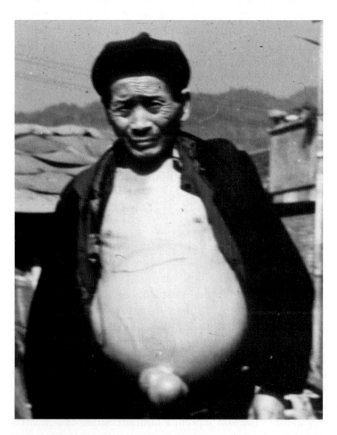

FIGURE 51.4. An Asian patient with liver cirrhosis caused by *Schistosoma japonica*, manifesting massive ascites and umbilical hernia. (Courtesy of Dr. Yukio Yoshida.)

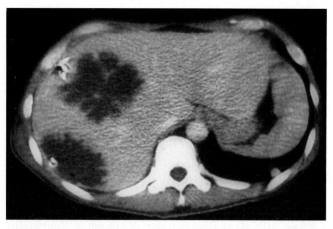

FIGURE 51.5. Abdominal computed tomography scan of a 48-year-old male patient with amebic liver abscesses. Note two low-density areas with foci of calcification. (Courtesy of Dr. Yukio Yoshida.)

ally.[6] Food and drink contaminated with the cysts of *E. histolytica* are the sources of infection. Amoebic colitis is a common presentation and generally responds to treatment with metronidazole, tinidazole, or chloroquine. However, invasive amebiasis of the colon may respond insufficiently to systemic chemotherapy. When invasive amebiasis is complicated by perforation, acute care enterostomy and aggressive peritoneal drainage are indicated in combination with chemotherapy. Unfortunately, the outcome is often fatal. *Entamoeba historica* invading the intestinal wall may metastasize to the liver via portal venous flow and produce a liver abscess, more commonly in the right lobe (Figure 51.5). Percutaneous puncture and drainage of these liver abscesses is indicated when the abscess is large and associated with a septic condition. Administration of metronidazole into the abscess cavity following drainage can also be effective.

Ascariasis

Ascaris lumbricoides is the large intestinal roundworm that causes ascariasis. Although ascariasis is rare in developed countries except in some rural communities, it is far more common in developing countries, and infection rates approach 60% to 100% in some tropical countries. Embryonated eggs of *A. lumbricoides* are passed with the feces, and infective eggs can be swallowed through contaminated foods and dusts. The larvae hatch in the small intestine, undergo an obligatory migration through the liver and lung, grow to reach a length of 1 mm, return to the small intestine, and eventually grow to maturity. Adult male worms reach a length of 20 cm, and females reach 30 cm.

Intestinal ascariasis may produce several symptoms such as intermittent abdominal pain, diarrhea, and

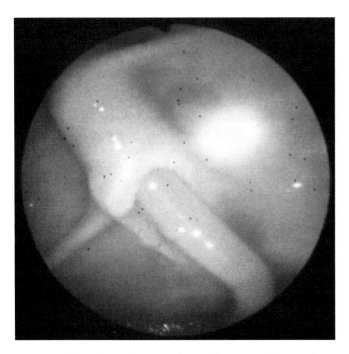

FIGURE 51.6. Endoscopic view of an adult worm of *Ascaris lumbricoides* impacted in the bile duct at the ampulla of Vater. (Courtesy of Dr. Yukio Yoshida.)

anorexia. A mass of packed *A. lumbricoides* may obstruct the bowel and present acute abdominal symptoms of the mechanical ileus, necessitating an acute care laparotomy.[7] The worms tend to force themselves into any aperture that they may encounter. When *A. lumbricoides* migrate upward, they may enter and block the biliary or pancreatic duct, resulting in acute biliary obstruction or acute pancreatitis, respectively (Figure 51.6).[7,8]

Ascaris lumbricoides impacted into the papilla of Vater may be treated either by endoscopic removal of the worm or by surgery (e.g., a choledochotomy or a duodenotomy). When the roundworms migrate into the appendix and cause appendicitis, an appendectomy is indicated. Worms can further migrate into the parenchyma of the liver via the biliary duct and cause liver abscesses or calcifications.

Bacterial Enteritis

Contamination of foods and water with pathogenic microorganisms, for example, *Salmonella* species, *Shigella* species, *Campylobacter jejuni*, and *Yersinia enterocolitica*, is common in poor sanitary conditions. Enteropathogenic bacteria generally cause abdominal pain and diarrhea, and the morbidities are usually treated conservatively. However, bacterial enteritis can be occasionally complicated by perforation, hemorrhage, volvulus, and intussusception, and may result in an acute care laparotomy.[9]

Thermoregulatory Disorders

Extreme climates in tropical countries can cause thermoregulatory disorders. Without the luxury of air conditioning, patients can be susceptible to heat illness or heat exhaustion. Many ambulances, operating theaters, and recovery wards in developing countries do not have air conditioning, even though fever is a usual concomitant of severe trauma, infectious diseases, and major surgery. Heat illness or sometimes heat stroke can occur during and after acute care surgery without adequate environmental control. Hyperpyrexia is a serious life hazard, and rapid reduction of the core temperature by evaporative cooling, immersion into a tub of cold water, and/or ice packing should be exercised. An internal cooling technique is, if available, more ideal because it can avoid shivering. Cold lavage of the pleural or peritoneal cavity may be employed to address hyperpyrexia during acute care thoracotomy or laparotomy, respectively.

In the high inland areas of the tropics, there may be a wide diurnal temperature variation, as much as 30°C, and exposure in mountains can cause accidental hypothermia. A patient with accidental hypothermia should be warmed immediately with insulation, heating blankets, warm bath, or by any available technique until cardiac output is sufficiently restored. Supplementary humidified oxygen and intravenous fluid should be given. Infusion and transfusion should be prewarmed to 40°C. In case of ventricular fibrillation, defibrillation should be attempted. If the repetitive attempts of defibrillation fail, cardiopulmonary resuscitation should be initiated.

It is not uncommon that a patient with profound accidental hypothermia has other illnesses requiring acute care surgery. In such a case, the core temperature should be carefully and continuously monitored and maintained by external warming and/or pleural or peritoneal lavage with warm saline because thoracic or abdominal surgery can further deteriorate accidental hypothermia.

Acute Care Surgery in Japan

In Japan, most general surgeons specialize in gastroenterologic surgery, and most of the general surgeons, thoracic surgeons, cardiovascular surgeons, pediatric surgeons, and some neurosurgeons have joined the Japan Surgical Society (JSS), which has over 40,000 members as of 2004. General surgeons usually undergo 4 or 5 years of postgraduate training in surgery and practice both elective and acute care surgeries under the supervision of senior surgeons, who are authorized by the JSS. If the surgeons pass the subsequent examinations, they are certified by the JSS as a qualified surgeon or a specialized surgeon. General surgeons receive education and training in acute care surgery in the context of these qualifications by the JSS. A number of other societies individually certify qualified specialists who play important roles in acute care surgery in Japan. These other societies include the Japanese Association for Thoracic Surgery, Japanese Society of Pediatric Surgeons, Japan Neurosurgical Society, Japan Society of Anesthesiologists, Japanese Association for Acute Medicine, Japanese Society of Gastroenterological Surgery, Japanese Society for Cardiovascular Surgery, and the Japanese Society for Vascular Surgery.

There are several unique aspects to acute care surgery in Japan. First, the demographics of the patients and diseases are distinctive. Although most of the epidemic diseases, including malaria, schistosomiasis, amebiasis, ascariasis, and tuberculosis, have been effectively eradicated, there are specific epidemic diseases such as anisakiasis in Japan. Infection with *Helicobacter pylori*, a cause of gastritis and a risk factor of gastric cancer, is also prevalent.

Second, the setting of medical centers is unique. There are 170 critical care medical centers throughout Japan.[10] Acute care surgeries are carried out in a number of private hospitals, community hospitals, and university hospitals as well as in the critical care medical centers. Operative theaters are usually equipped with instruments for laparoscopic procedures, even in the rural hospitals. High expectations of the patients have led some Japanese surgeons to perform complex operations such as radical subtotal gastrectomy in the presence of gastric cancer by laparoscopic technique. As a consequence, the skills to perform abdominal acute care surgeries by the laparoscopic approach exist and are employed.

Third, social custom and religious backgrounds are different. Despite the legal approval of transplantations from brain dead donors, there have been few donors so far, presumably because brain death is not readily accepted socially or religiously in Japan. By necessity, living donor transplantation has become common practice and realistically is the sole treatment for fulminant hepatic failure not responding to conventional treatments.

Fourth, health care financing in Japan is independent. Most medical treatments are financed by public medical insurance systems that cover virtually 100% of the Japanese population. The cost for health care is inflating year to year because the population is aging and because further development of medical technologies results in higher expenses. Just as in the United States, medical practice in Japan has become more cost-conscious. Furthermore, evidence-based medicine became a requirement in health care. Recently, several guidelines on the treatment of various diseases have been introduced in Japan. For instance, a guideline for the clinical management of acute pancreatitis was published recently, and medical treatments for acute pancreatitis, including acute

care surgery, are to be carried out following this guideline in Japan. Because most of the evidence that supports the Japanese guideline is from the English literature, recommended managements in the guideline are similar to those in the United States and in European countries. Nevertheless, the guideline also recommends some intensive treatments that are almost exclusively practiced in Japan. Herein, we introduce current topics of acute care surgery in Japan with regard to anisakiasis, gastroduodenal perforation, fulminant liver failure, and acute pancreatitis.

Anisakiasis

Anisakiasis is a disease caused by *Anisakis* larvae, marine nematodes including *Anisakis simplex*, and *Pseudoterranova decipiens* (Figure 51.7). The *Anisakis* larvae are usually found in mackerel, squid, salmon, cod, halibut, rockfish, sardine, and herring. In Japanese society, people enjoy eating raw fish as sushi and sashimi, and it is estimated that anisakiasis develops in over 1,000 Japanese per year. Anisakiasis is also relatively common in the Netherlands, and there are some recent reports from the United States, where sushi restaurants are becoming more popular.[11] The most common symptom of anisakiasis is intermittent cramping abdominal pain of acute onset from 2 hours to 2 days after eating raw or undercooked fish. Anisakiasis involving the intestine may occur as late as 5 days after raw fish ingestion. The diagnosis of anisakiasis is established by endoscopic observation

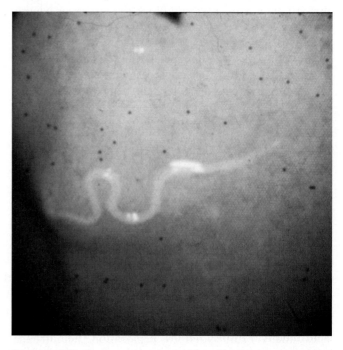

FIGURE 51.7. Endoscopic view of *Anisakis simplex*, larvae, invading the stomach wall. (Courtesy of Dr. Yukio Yoshida.)

of the Anisakis larvae and may be suspected by positive serologic test for immunoglobulin E specific to anisakiasis.

When the Anisakis larvae invade the gastric wall, endoscopic removal of the larvae can cure the disease. On the contrary, when the Anisakis larvae invade the wall of the intestine, a granuloma with circumferential edema is produced and can cause intestinal obstruction.[12] A granulomatous mass with proximal dilatation of the bowel may be detected by computed tomography. A resection of the granuloma is often performed, especially when a neoplastic lesion such as a malignant lymphoma is suspected. However, supportive measures and decompression of the digestive tract with a short tube (nasogastric tube) or long tube (ileus tube) may be all that is needed for intestinal anisakiasis.

Gastroduodenal Perforation

Infection of *H. pylori* induces infiltration of inflammatory cells in the gastric mucosa and may result in the development of digestive diseases such as gastritis, gastroduodenal ulcer, and gastric cancer, although the mechanisms involved in the pathogenicity of *H. pylori*–related illness are not fully elucidated.[13–15] It is also unclear whether or not *H. pylori* infection is epidemiologically related to perforation of gastroduodenal ulcers.[16] Because successful eradication of *H. pylori* cures most gastroduodenal ulcers, surgical interventions such as wide extent distal gastrectomy or vagotomy are no longer frequently practiced. Exceptionally, a distal gastrectomy with or without proximal vagotomy is indicated for patients with gastroduodenal ulcer complicated by pyloric stenosis. When widespread bleeding cannot be controlled completely by endoscopic hemostasis in patients with acute gastric mucosal lesions, a wide extent distal gastrectomy is occasionally indicated. Perforation of a gastroduodenal ulcer is usually an indication for surgery, although a conservative therapy with decompression by a nasogastric tube may be feasible for some patients without deteriorating peritonitis.

The preferred choice of operation for perforated duodenal ulcer is a laparoscopic closure of the perforation by omental patch, as a laparoscopic repair is associated with less postoperative pain, reduced postoperative pneumonia, shorter hospital stay, and earlier return to normal daily activities than a open (laparotomy) procedure (Figure 51.8).[17,18] A laparoscopic omental patch may be performed for perforated gastric ulcer located within 2 cm of the pyloric ring. Open (laparotomy) procedure is indicated when (1) the perforated ulcer is complicated by severe peritonitis; (2) the general condition of the patient is unstable; (3) pyloric stenosis is present; (4) the ulcer is located in the body or cardia of the stomach; (5) the opening of the perforated ulcer is too large (>2 cm); (6)

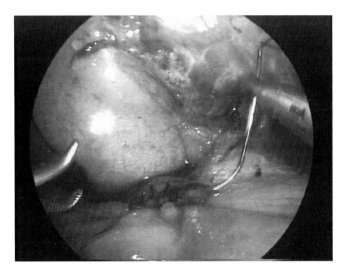

FIGURE 51.8. Laparoscopic closure of a perforated duodenal ulcer.

adhesions caused by the disseminated gastric content are too severe; (7) gastric cancer is suspected; or (8) the surgeon in charge is not used to laparoscopic procedures.

Infection of *H. pylori* and high salt intake are the risk factors of gastric cancer,[19] and gastric cancer is the second leading cause of cancer death in Japan. Patients with early gastric cancer (i.e., carcinoma confined to the mucosa and submucosal layer) are treated with endoscopic mucosal resection (EMR),[20,21] laparoscopy-assisted gastrectomy,[22] or conventional open gastrectomy, depending on the size, depth, degree of histologic differentiation, and other factors. Iatrogenic perforation of the stomach occurs in about 5% of the patients who undergo EMR.[23] In some cases, the perforation can be closed by endoscopic clipping and treated with intubation of a nasogastric tube and systemic administration of antibiotics.[23] However, when there are signs of peritoneal sepsis, acute care surgery is indicated preferably by laparoscopic approach. Closure of the perforation site and intraperitoneal lavage are generally performed. If there is a possibility that carcinoma cells remain at the margin of EMR, a local resection encompassing the possible residual lesion around the site of perforation is indicated. When spontaneous or iatrogenic perforation of advanced gastric cancer necessitates acute care surgery, a laparoscopic procedure is contraindicated because pneumoperitoneum with carbon dioxide may exacerbate peritoneal dissemination of neoplastic cells.

Fulminant Hepatic Failure

One of the most disastrous of the nontrauma emergencies is fulminant hepatic failure (FHF), a severe liver dysfunction caused by sudden loss of hepatocyte function characterized by hepatic encephalopathy and coagulopathy. In Japan, FHF is estimated to affect over 1,000 individuals annually. Whereas drug-induced acute liver failure plays a large role in FHF in the United States, about 90% of FHF cases in Japan are associated with hepatitis A, hepatitis B, non-A, non-B, and non-C hepatitis, and other viral infections.

The treatment for FHF consists of plasmapheresis in combination with continuous hemodialysis and filtration in an intensive care unit. When the conventional medical treatments fail to restore the liver function, a living-donor liver transplantation (LDLT) is the choice of treatment in Japan because cadaver donors are rarely available. Over 400 LDLTs are performed each year for various diseases, such as biliary atresia (Figure 51.9), and about 50 LDLTs are estimated to be carried out for FHF with satisfactory outcome in Japan. A lateral segment or left lobe is usually used for FHF in pediatric recipients, and left plus caudate lobes or the right lobe of the donor liver are used for FHF in adult patients.[24]

Auxiliary partial orthotopic liver transplantation from living donors has been successful in only a limited number of cases.[24,25] Survival rate after LDLT for FHF ranges from 60% to 100%, comparable to the survival rate after cadaver donor transplantation in the United

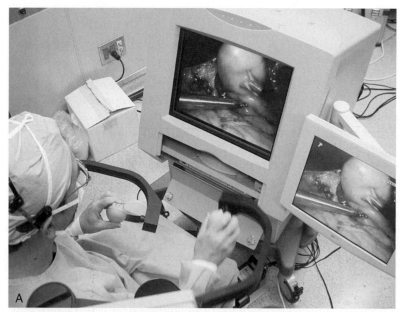

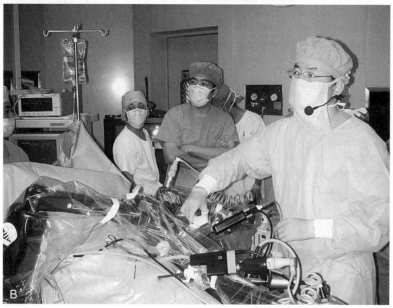

FIGURE 51.9. The ZEUS robotics system. A cholecystectomy was carried out in a teleconference including the European Institute of Telesurgery, University of Strasbourg, France, and the operating theater of Osaka Medical College, Japan. **(A)** The operator and a manipulator (a master robot). **(B)** The patient and robotics arms (a slave robot).

States. A hybrid artificial liver support system utilizing hepatocytes remains an experimental therapy at the present time.[26,27]

Acute Pancreatitis

Approximately 20,000 patients per year suffer from acute pancreatitis in Japan, and 7.2% of the patients died of the disease in 1999. The mortality rate in Japan is comparable to that in the West, at between 7.5% and 17.0%. The etiology of acute pancreatitis includes alcohol abuse (30.1%), gallstones (23.9%), idiopathic (22.7%), exaggeration of chronic pancreatitis (5.6%), endoscopic retrograde cholangiopancreatography (3.9%), surgery (2.6%), endoscopic sphincterotomy (1.7%), drugs (1.2%), and hyperlipidemia (1.2%). The Japanese Society for Abdominal Emergency Medicine and the Japan Pancreas Society, in collaboration with an investigation team sponsored by Ministry of Health, Welfare, and Labor, established a guideline for the clinical management of acute pancreatitis in 2003.[28,29]

Based on reports from both the English and the Japanese literature, the guideline recommends mostly similar practices as those currently used in the United States and other countries.[30–32] However, some intensive treatments such as continuous regional arterial infusion (CRAI) of protease inhibitor and antibiotics are practiced almost exclusively in Japan. According to the original method by Takeda et al.[33], nafamostat mesylate, a potent protease inhibitor, and imipenem, an antibiotic with good penetration into pancreatic tissue, are continuously infused into the celiac artery. They reported that the CRAI treatment significantly reduced the mortality rate compared with systemic infusion of the same drugs[33] and that the CRAI therapy was effective when initiated within 72 hours after the onset of acute necrotizing pancreatitis.[34,35] Their results had been confirmed by other institutions in Japan.[36] In a rat model of necrotizing pancreatitis, it was shown that nafamostat has maximal effects on the pancreas and peritoneal capillary leakage when delivered by way of local intraarterial infusion and that nafamostat shows a greater reduction of lung leukocyte infiltration and capillary leakage when delivered by intravenous route.[37]

In the United States, however, the beneficial effects of the CRAI therapy are not approved clinically. Computed tomography–guided or ultrasound-guided fine-needle aspiration is recommended to confirm pancreatic infection, and a necrosectomy should be indicated in case of infected pancreatic necrosis. Following necrosectomy, continuous closed lavage or open drainage is recommended while conventional drainage with simple drainage tube(s) is not. There is some controversy regarding surgical intervention for noninfected pancreatic necrosis because most of these cases can be treated by the CRAI therapy or conventional treatments.[34]

Acute Care Surgery in the Future

Several practical highlights of acute care surgery in developing countries were mentioned in the first section of this chapter. In reality, however, the demand for acute care surgery is hardly met in the majority of these countries. Even in industrial nations, accessibility to acute care surgery varies from community to community, and the management of acute care surgery is not consistent among centers. It is imperative to obtain harmonization in education, research, and practice in acute care surgery in the future international communities. The following are possibilities for establishing global standards for acute care surgery in the future: the realization of routine tele-surgery in association with education of doctors and medical personnel by telecommunication technologies; international collaboration for application of regenerative medicine to surgical therapeutics; and introduction of a global health care system into the setting of acute care surgery.

Tele-Surgery

Tele-surgery is defined as a surgical procedure carried out from a distance.[38] Advances in telecommunication technologies and application of robotics to surgery have enabled even intercontinental tele-surgery.[38–40] Teleconference, tele-consultation, tele-mentoring, and other tele-medicine systems can be used in combination with tele-surgery (Figure 51.9).[41–43] Tele-surgery provides opportunities to share experiences and expertise of surgery among physicians beyond the barriers of geography, nations, and politics. In the near future, it will become a reality that surgery requiring special techniques and expertise for patients in remote locations or inaccessible circumstances will be tele-manipulated by specialists and that tele-surgery will benefit acute care surgery in the rural areas, remote islands, war zones,[44] and ultimately in space.

Regenerative Medicine

Application of regenerative medicine to acute care surgery is most promising. The initial step has been the topical use of growth factors. It is already well known that growth factors accelerate the healing processes of wounds and burns,[45] and growth factors are now commercially prepared for topical administration. For patients with spinal cord injury, topical administration of neurotrophin 3 may help regenerate the spinal cord.[46] With the development of tissue engineering, cultured

TABLE 51.1. Recommendations of the G8 Global Healthcare Applications Sub-Project (SP)-4.

Standards, Network Reliability, Security, and Application

1. Tele-health applications and networks should adopt as many standards as possible and be harmonized with recommendations of the International Standard Organisation working groups.
2. There is a need to develop a process model for each health care/medical discipline with technical needs defined in terms of quality of service, security, and application interoperability; they should remain understandable to the clinical user.
3. Existing tele-health infrastructures need to be compatible and interoperable with digital dial-up and/or TCP/IP protocols; they should adopt emerging technologies, which have been demonstrated and the least expensive.
4. Tele health systems should receive bandwidth on demand, as appropriate for the application.

Organizational Issues

1. National governments should recognize both health and economic benefits of interoperable tele-health and make health a strategic argument for interoperable tele-health.
2. National governments should create and promote working models toward interoperability and promote industry and health sector partnerships.
3. National governments should implement national and international strategies resolving the issues of licensures, credentialing, and health care provider reimbursement.
4. National governments should recognize the need for national leadership to promulgate consensus building and a vision for a future health care system that fully integrates and benefits from tele-health and tele-medicine.

Human Factors

1. National governments should financially support training and education of health professionals and students in using tele-health instruments.
2. National governments should provide incentives to established health professionals to learn, acquire, and use tele-health and telemedicine-based systems.
3. National governments should provide funding to evaluate key human factors and systems in tele-health.
4. National governments should ensure adequate access to technical expertise among the user community.
5. National governments should support the development of multilingual health information and tele-health systems.

Evaluation of tele-medicine and tele-health

1. Evaluation should be an integral part of all tele-health deployed with the aim to assess whether its application was effective in improving health outcome, appropriate for the needs of the population, reliable, and cost effective compared with other instruments to achieve the same goal.
2. It should assess the systemic aspects and interactions with other instruments, programs, policies, and effects of conditions (e.g., government frameworks).
3. It should measure impacts on the acceptability, workforce distribution, and competence of health personnel.
4. Evaluation should aim at development of evidence-based tele-medicine through good practice documentation, thus improving the key management issues and dissemination.

Medicolegal aspects

1. As infrastructures for the use of PKI evolve, governments must ensure that there is an appropriate legal framework for its use in the health care sector and that dialogue takes place at an international level to ensure interoperability of its use among countries.
2. Patients must give fully informed consent for the use of their personal medical information for health care, evaluation, or research, even if data are anonymous; their use for commercial purposes should be restricted to informed and ethically approved uses. Professional and patient organizations should work together to promote better understanding of privacy and confidentiality.
3. An international group of national representatives must develop ethical and medicolegal guidelines for the practice of tele-medicine; formal work conducted by various groups such as the Einbeck group should be considered as a starting model.
4. The major barrier of health care professional licensing should be resolved by deciding that the tele-medicine activity is occurring at the site of the consultant; the patient should agree that he or she will follow the legal rules at the site of the consultant, as is done currently when the patient travels physically to that site.

Continued work of the G8 SP-4 Working Group

1. The G8 GHAP SP-4 participants wish to pursue their common efforts in international collaboration.
2. Additional forums are required to formulate recommendations on the evaluation and implementation of medical, ethical, legal, and technical aspects of tele-medicine services, including aspects of cross-border services.
3. G8 and other participating countries should provide sufficient funding to their national representatives, experts, and expert centers to pursue their work and disseminate their conclusions and recommendations.
4. The former G8 SP-4 Working Group should collaborate with other international health care organizations, such as the World Health Organization, to facilitate the integration of health tele-matics to health care strategies worldwide.
5. This new international body of experts should report annually on its progress and activities to national health authorities and to citizens through an active Web site.

Source: Reprinted with permission from Nerlich et al.[56]

epithelia became available, and allogenic skin grafts have been employed as scaffolds of epithelial growth after trauma, burn injury, venous ulcers, or bacterial dermatitis.[47,48]

Establishment of embryonic stem cell lines from human blastocytes[49] has led to enthusiasm for therapeutic use of stem cells. Embryonic stem cells are derived from multipotent cells of the early mammalian embryo and characterized by prolonged undifferentiated proliferation and developmental potential to form derivatives of all three embryonic germ layers. However, the investigation of embryonic stem cells is restricted to various extents for ethical reasons in Germany, United States, Japan, and some other nations.

Another cell source for regeneration of tissues and organs has been found in tissue-derived somatic stem cells. It was originally believed that somatic stem cells can differentiate into the tissue or germ layer from which they are derived. However, it has also become apparent that some tissue-derived somatic stem cells can differentiate outside the tissue of their origin.[50,51] Bone-marrow derived stem cells, neural stem cells, umbilical cord cells, and placenta are now considered potential sources of somatic stem cells for regenerative medicine. Expectations are particularly high for bone marrow–derived mesenchymal stem cells because they can differentiate into skin,[52] bone, cartilage, fat (adipocyte), muscle (myocyte), nerve (astrocytes, oligodendrocytes, neurons),[53] blood vessel (endothelium),[54] heart (myocardium), lung (bronchial epithelium, pneumocytes), esophagus (squamous epithelium), stomach (gastric mucosa), intestine (endothelium), liver (hepatocyte, cholangiocytes), and kidney (renal tubules).[55] Furthermore, there is no need to immunosuppress patients treated with autologous bone marrow–derived stem cells. In the future, lost or damaged organs or body parts will be replaced by new tissues regenerated from the stem cells, and acute care surgery will undergo a Copernican revolution.

Global Health Care

The twenty-first century is bringing a borderless world and presenting new challenges in all facets of medical care. Frequent travels abroad and increased migrations of the population require practitioners, including those who engage in acute care surgery, to be more knowledgeable of diseases with specific geographic distributions. The current consensus is that international collaboration is needed to improve the quality and cost efficiency of each field of health care through tele-medicine, tele-health, and health tele-matics. To establish an international concerted collaboration in this regard, national representatives of G7, joined by Russia later on, have organized

the G8 Global Healthcare Applications (GHAP) Sub-Project (SP)-4.[56]

The GHAP SP-4 first focused on the use of tele-medicine tools in acute care medicine. The objective of this first project was to establish a transnational and multilingual acute care system. The study concluded that, from a technological viewpoint, a worldwide telemedicine network is feasible and can be implemented gradually and in steps. Application of global health care to acute care surgery will improve the quality of the practice in not only industrial nations but also in developing countries and may be further enhanced by a series of recommendations by G8 GHAP SP-4 (Table 51.1).

Despite the fluidity of borders between nations, inequalities of economy, of welfare, and of health are further expanding in the world at the present time. It is imperative for a healthier world in the future that global health care systems be applied to all fields of medicine, including acute care surgery beyond the barriers of economics, politics, language, religion, and culture.

References

1. Rennie JA, Janka A. Emergency surgery in Ethiopia. Ann R Coll Surg Engl 1997; 79(6 Suppl):254–256.
2. Inoue K. Surgery in Japan. Arch Surg 1993; 128:1093–1098.
3. Williams CD. Kwashiorkor: a nutritional disease of children associated with a maize diet. Bull World Health Organ 2003; 81:912–913. [Originally published in Lancet 1935; 2:1151–1152.]
4. Field CJ, Johnson IR, Schey PD. Nutrients and their role in host resistance to infection. J Leukoc Biol 2002; 71:16–32.
5. Attaran A, Barnes KI, Curtis C, et al. WHO, the Global Fund, and medical malpractice in malaria treatment. Lancet 2004; 363:237–240.
6. Walsh JA. Problems in recognition and diagnosis of amebiasis: estimation of the global magnitude of morbidity and mortality. Rev Infect Dis 1986; 8:228–238.
7. Ochoa B. Surgical complications of ascariasis. World J Surg 1991; 15:222–227.
8. Hamaloglu E. Biliary ascariasis in fifteen patients. Int Surg 1992; 77:77–79.
9. Cook GC. Gastroenterological emergencies in the tropics. Baillieres Clin Gastroenterol 1991; 5:861–886.
10. Ministry of Health and Welfare Statistics [in Japanese]. Tokyo: Kosei Tokei Kyokai, 2003.
11. Schuster R, Petrini JL, Choi R. Anisakiasis of the colon presenting as bowel obstruction. Am Surg 2003; 69:350–352.
12. Doi R, Inoue K, Gomi T, et al. A case of anisakiasis as a cause of ileum obstruction. Dig Surg 1989; 6:218–220.
13. Matsuhisa TM, Yamada NY, Kato SK, et al. *Helicobacter pylori* infection, mucosal atrophy and intestinal metaplasia in Asian populations: a comparative study in age-, gender- and endoscopic diagnosis-matched subjects. Helicobacter 2003; 8:29–35.
14. Montani A, Sasazuki S, Inoue M, et al. Food/nutrient intake and risk of atrophic gastritis among the *Helicobacter*

pylori–infected population of northeastern Japan. Cancer Sci 2003; 94:372–377.

15. Nishise Y, Fukao A, Takahashi T. Risk factors for *Helicobacter pylori* infection among a rural population in Japan: relation to living environment and medical history. J Epidemiol 2003; 13:266-73.

16. Matsukura N, Onda M, Tokunaga A, et al. Role of *Helicobacter pylori* infection in perforation of peptic ulcer: an age- and gender-matched case–control study. J Clin Gastroenterol 1997; 25(Suppl 1): S235–S239.

17. Matsuda M, Nishiyama M, Hanai T, et al. Laparoscopic omental patch repair for perforated peptic ulcer. Ann Surg 1995; 221:236–240.

18. Siu WT, Leong HT, Law BK, et al. Laparoscopic repair for perforated peptic ulcer: a randomized controlled trial. Ann Surg 2002; 235:313–319.

19. Tsugane S, Sasazuki S, Kobayashi M, et al. Salt and salted food intake and subsequent risk of gastric cancer among middle-aged Japanese men and women. Br J Cancer 2004; 90:128–134.

20. Tada M, Murakami K, Karita H, et al. Endoscopic resection of early gastric cancer. Endoscopy 1993; 25:445–450.

21. Ida K, Nakazawa S, Hiki Y, et al. A prospective study on endoscopic treatment for early gastric cancer in Japan: an interim report. Dig Endosc 2000; 12:19–24.

22. Lee SW, Shinohara H, Matsuki M, et al. Preoperative simulation of vascular anatomy by three-dimensional computed tomography imaging in laparoscopic gastric cancer surgery. J Am Coll Surg 2003; 197:927–936.

23. Ono H, Kondo H, Gotoda H, et al. Endoscopic mucosal resection for treatment of early gastric cancer. Gut 2001; 48:225–229.

24. Uemoto S, Inomata Y, Sakurai T, et al. Living donor liver transplantation for fulminant hepatic failure. Transplantation 2000; 70:152–157.

25. Inomata Y, Kiuchi T, Kim I, Uemoto S, et al. Auxiliary partial orthotopic living donor liver transplantation as an aid for small-for-size grafts in larger recipients. Transplantation 1999; 67:1314–1319.

26. Kawashita Y, Ohtsuru A, Fujioka H, et al. Safe and efficient gene transfer into porcine hepatocytes using Sendai virus–cationic liposomes for bioartificial liver support. Artif Organs 2000; 24:932–938.

27. Fujikawa T, Hirose T, Fujii H, et al. Purification of adult hepatic progenitor cells using green fluorescent protein (GFP)–transgenic mice and fluorescence-activated cell sorting. J Hepatol 2003; 39:162–170.

28. Mayumi T, Ura H, Arata S, et al. Working Group for the Practical Guidelines for Acute Pancreatitis. Japanese Society of Emergency Abdominal Medicine. Evidence-based clinical practice guidelines for acute pancreatitis: proposals. J Hepatobiliary Pancreat Surg 2002; 9:413–422.

29. Hirata K, Mayumi T, Ohtsuki M, et al. [Clinical guideline of acute pancreatitis based on evidences; in Japanese] Nippon Shokakibyo Gakkai Zasshi 2003; 100(8):965–973.

30. Banks PA. Practice guidelines in acute pancreatitis. Am J Gastrocntcrol 1997; 92:377–386.

31. Uhl W, Warshaw A, Imrie C, et al. International Association of Pancreatology. IAP Guidelines for the Surgical Management of Acute Pancreatitis. Pancreatology 2002; 2:565–573.

32. Sarr MG. IAP guidelines in acute pancreatitis. Dig Surg 2003; 20:1–3.

33. Takeda K, Matsuno S, Sunamura M, et al. Continuous regional arterial infusion of protease inhibitor and antibiotics in acute necrotizing pancreatitis. Am J Surg 1996;171: 394–398.

34. Takeda K, Sunamura M, Shibuya K, et al. Role of early continuous regional arterial infusion of protease inhibitor and antibiotic in nonsurgical treatment of acute necrotizing pancreatitis. Digestion 1999; 60(Suppl 1):9–13.

35. Takeda K, Yamauchi J, Shibuya K, et al. Benefit of continuous regional arterial infusion of protease inhibitor and antibiotic in the management of acute necrotizing pancreatitis. Pancreatology 2001; 1:668–673.

36. Nakase H, Itani T, Mimura J, et al. Successful treatment of severe acute pancreatitis by the combination therapy of continuous arterial infusion of a protease inhibitor and continuous hemofiltration. J Gastroenterol Hepatol 2001; 16:944–945.

37. Keck T, Balcom JH, Antoniu BA, et al. Regional effects of nafamostat, a novel potent protease and complement inhibitor, on severe necrotizing pancreatitis. Surgery 2001; 130:175–181.

38. Marescaux J, Leroy J, Gagner M, et al. Transatlantic robot-assisted telesurgery. Nature 2001; 413:379–380.

39. Marescaux J, Leroy J, Rubino F, et al. Transcontinental robot-assisted remote telesurgery: feasibility and potential applications. Ann Surg 2002; 235:487–492.

40. Cheah WK, Lee B, Lenzi JE, et al. Telesurgical laparoscopic cholecystectomy between two countries. Surg Endosc 2000; 14:1085.

41. Malassagne B, Mutter D, Leroy J, et al. Teleeducation in surgery: European Institute for Telesurgery experience. World J Surg 2001; 25:1490–1494.

42. Eadie LH, Seifalian AM, Davidson BR. Telemedicine in surgery. Br J Surg 2003; 90:647–658.

43. Wysocki WM, Moesta KT, Schlag PM. Surgery, surgical education and surgical diagnostic procedures in the digital era. Med Sci Monit 2003; 9:RA69–RA75.

44. Satava RM. Virtual reality and telepresence for military medicine. Ann Acad Med Singapore 1997; 26:118–120.

45. Brown GL, Nanney LB, Griffen J, et al. Enhancement of wound healing by topical treatment with epidermal growth factor. N Engl J Med 1989; 321:76–79.

46. McDonald JW, Sadowsky C. Spinal-cord injury. Lancet 2002; 359:417–425.

47. Green H, Kehinde O, Thomas J. Growth of cultured human epidermal cells into multiple epithelia suitable for grafting. Proc Natl Acad Sci USA 1979; 76:5665–5668.

48. Parenteau N. Skin: the first tissue-engineered products. Sci Am 1999; 280:83–84.

49. Thomson JA, Itskovitz-Eldor J, Shapiro SS, et al. Embryonic stem cell lines derived from human blastocysts. Science 1998; 282:1145–1147.

50. Ferrari G, Cusella-De Angelis G, Coletta M, et al. Muscle regeneration by bone marrow–derived myogenic progenitors. Science 1998; 279:1528–1530.

51. Gussoni E, Soneoka Y, Strickland CD, et al. Dystrophin expression in the mdx mouse restored by stem cell transplantation. Nature 1999; 401:390–394.

52. Alonso L, Fuchs E. Stem cells of the skin epithelium. Proc Natl Acad Sci USA 2003; 100(Suppl 1):11830–11835.

53. McDonald JW, Liu XZ, Qu Y, et al. Transplanted embryonic stem cells survive, differentiate and promote recovery in injured rat spinal cord. Nat Med 1999; 5:1410–1412.

54. Yamashita J, Itoh H, Hirashima M, et al. Flk1-positive cells derived from embryonic stem cells serve as vascular progenitors. Nature 2000; 408:92–96.

55. Krause DS, Theise ND, Collector MI, et al. Multi-organ, multi-lineage engraftment by a single bone marrow–derived stem cell. Cell 2001; 105:369–377.

56. Nerlich M, Balas EA, Schall T, et al. G8 Global Health Applications Subproject 4. Teleconsultation practice guidelines: report from G8 Global Health Applications Subproject 4. Telemed J E Health 2002; 8:411–418.

Index

ISBN 0-387-34470-5

EAN

9 780387 344706 >

Printed in the United States of America.